S0-EKO-301
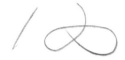

DISORDERS
of the FOOT

Volume 2

MELVIN H. JAHSS, M.D.

Clinical Professor of Orthopaedic Surgery,
Mount Sinai School of Medicine, New York;
Attending Physician and Chief of Orthopaedic Foot
Services, The Hospital for Joint Diseases
Orthopaedic Institute, New York; Attending Physician
and Chief of Orthopaedic Foot Services,
Mount Sinai Hospital, New York, New York

W.B. SAUNDERS COMPANY

Philadelphia   London   Toronto
Mexico City   Rio de Janeiro   Sydney   Tokyo

W. B. Saunders Company: West Washington Square
Philadelphia, PA   19105

1 St. Anne's Road
Eastbourne, East Sussex BN21 3UN, England

1 Goldthorne Avenue
Toronto, Ontario M8Z 5T9, Canada

Apartado 26370 – Cedro 512
Mexico 4, D.F., Mexico

Rua Coronel Cabrita, 8
Sao Cristovao Caixa Postal 21176
Rio de Janeiro, Brazil

9 Waltham Street
Artarmon, N.S.W. 2064, Australia

Ichibancho, Central Bldg., 22-1 Ichibancho
Chiyoda-Ku, Tokyo 102, Japan

Library of Congress Cataloging in Publication Data

Jahss, Melvin, 1921–

Disorders of the foot.

Bibliography: p.

1. Foot – Surgery.   2. Foot – Abnormalities.   3. Foot –
   Diseases.   4. Foot – Wounds and injuries.   I. Title.
   [DNLM: 1. Foot diseases. WE880 D611]

RD563.J33   617'.585   80–50563

ISBN 0–7216–5104–6 (set)

ISBN 0–7216–5106–2 (v. 1)

ISBN 0–7216–5107–0 (v. 2)

Disorders of the Foot

Single Volume   0-7216-5104-6
Volume 1 ‚0-7216-5106-2
Volume 2   0-7216-5107-0

© 1982 by W. B. Saunders Company.   Copyright under the Uniform Copyright Convention.   Simultaneously published in Canada.   All rights reserved.   This book is protected by copyright.   No part of it may be reproduced, stored in a retrieval system, or transmitted in any form or by any means, electronic, mechanical, photocopying, recording, or otherwise, without written permission from the publisher.   Made in the United States of America.   Press of W. B. Saunders Company.   Library of Congress catalog card number 80-50563.

Last digit is the print number: 9   8   7   6   5   4   3   2

CONTRIBUTORS

JAMES A. ARNOLD, M.D.

Assistant Clinical Professor of Orthopaedics, University of Arkansas for Medical Sciences, Little Rock; Attending Physician, Washington Regional Medical Center, Fayetteville, and Springdale Memorial Hospital, Springdale, Arkansas

JAMES E. BATEMAN, M.D., F.R.C.S.(C.)

Surgeon-in-Chief, Orthopaedic and Arthritic Hospital, Toronto, Ontario, Canada

WILLIAM M. BLODGETT, M.D.

Clinical Professor of Orthopaedic Surgery, Wayne State Medical School, Detroit; Senior Staff, Orthopaedic Surgery, Henry Ford Hospital, Detroit, Michigan

MALCOLM A. BRAHMS, D.S.C., M.D.

Associate Visiting Orthopaedic Surgeon, Mount Sinai Hospital, Cleveland; Attending Physician, Mount Sinai Hospital, Suburban Community Hospital, and Shaker Medical Center Hospital, Cleveland, Ohio

PAUL W. BRAND, M.D., F.A.C.S., F.R.C.S.

Clinical Professor of Surgery and Professor of Orthopedic Surgery, Louisiana State University Medical School, New Orleans; Chief, Rehabilitation Branch, U.S. Public Health Service Hospital, Carville, Louisiana

CRAWFORD J. CAMPBELL, M.D.

Lecturer, Harvard Medical School, Boston, Massachusetts; Professor, Albany Medical College, Albany, New York; Visiting Professor of Orthopaedics and Pathology, University of St. Louis School of Medicine, St. Louis, Missouri; Senior Orthopaedic Surgeon, Massachusetts General Hospital, Boston, Massachusetts

TOM P. COKER, M.D.

Assistant Clinical Professor of Orthopaedics, University of Arkansas for Medical Sciences, Little Rock; Attending Staff, Orthopaedic Surgery, Washington Regional Medical Center, Fayetteville, and Springdale Memorial Hospital, Springdale; Consultant, Veterans Administration Hospital, Fayetteville; Team Physician, University of Arkansas, Little Rock, Arkansas

JOSEPH J. CONRAD, M.D., F.A.C.S.

Assistant Clinical Professor of Orthopaedic Surgery, Mount Sinai School of Medicine and Mount Sinai Hospital, New York; Attending Orthopaedic Surgeon, Benedictine and Kingston Hospitals, Kingston; Associate Attending Orthopaedic Surgeon, The Hospital for Joint Diseases Orthopaedic Institute, New York, New York

EDWARD F. DELAGI, M.D.

Professor of Rehabilitation Medicine, Albert Einstein College of Medicine, New York; Clinical Director, Department of Rehabilitation Medicine, Bronx Municipal Hospital, Bronx, New York

JAMES T. DEMOPOULOS, M.D.

Professor of Rehabilitation Medicine, Mount Sinai School of Medicine, New York; Director, Department of Rehabilitation, Beth Israel Medical Center and The Hospital for Joint Diseases Orthopaedic Institute, New York, New York

LIEBE SOKOL DIAMOND, M.D.

Associate Professor, University of Maryland School of Medicine, Baltimore; Director of Clinical Research, Kernan Hospital, Baltimore, Maryland

THOMAS DUCKWORTH, M.D., Ch.B., B.Sc., F.R.C.S.

Professor of Orthopaedic Surgery, University of Sheffield School of Medicine, Sheffield; Consultant Orthopaedic Surgeon, Royal Hallamshire Hospital, Children's Hospital, and Sheffield Area Health Authority, Sheffield, England

MICHAEL G. EHRLICH, M.D.

Associate Professor of Orthopaedics, Harvard Medical School, Boston; Chief, Pediatric Orthopaedics, Massachusetts General Hospital, Boston, Massachusetts

CHARLES H. EPPS, Jr., M.D.

Professor and Chief, Division of Orthopaedic Surgery, Howard University College of Medicine, Washington, D.C.; Chief, Orthopaedic Surgery, Howard University Hospital, Washington, D.C.; Orthopaedic Consultant, Handicapped and Crippled Children's Unit, District of Columbia General Hospital, Veterans Administration Hospital, and Walter Reed Medical Center, Washington, D.C.

PHILLIP M. EVANSKI, M.D.

Associate Professor of Orthopedic Surgery, New York University Medical School, New York; Associate Attending Physician, Bellevue Hospital, New York; Attending Physician, University Hospital, New York; Staff Physician, Manhattan Veterans Administration Hospital, New York, New York

DAVID J. FELDMAN, M.D.

Clinical Assistant, Mount Sinai School of Medicine, New York; Assistant Attending Orthopaedic Surgeon, Mount Sinai Hospital, New York, New York

DOUGLAS E. GARLAND, M.D.

Clinical Instructor in Surgery (Orthopedics), University of Southern California, Los Angeles; Chief, Head Trauma and Problem Fracture Service, Rancho Los Amigos Hospital, Downey, California

RICHARD C. GIBBS, M.D.

Clinical Professor of Dermatology, New York University School of Medicine, New York; Attending Physician, Skin and Cancer Unit of New York University Medical Center, University Hospital, and Bellevue Hospital, New York, New York

MARVIN S. GILBERT, M.D.

Associate Clinical Professor of Orthopedics, Mount Sinai School of Medicine, New York; Associate Attending Physician, Mount Sinai Hospital, New York, New York

J. LEONARD GOLDNER, M.D.

James B. Duke Professor and Chief, Division of Orthopaedic Surgery, Duke University Medical Center, Durham, North Carolina

NATHANIEL GOULD, M.D.

Associate Professor of Orthopaedic Surgery, University of Vermont College of Medicine, Burlington; Attending Orthopaedic Surgeon, Medical Center Hospitals, Burlington, Vermont

ADAM GREENSPAN, M.D.

Associate Professor of Clinical Radiology, Mount Sinai School of Medicine, New York; Associate Attending Physician, Radiology, The Hospital for Joint Diseases Orthopaedic Institute, New York, New York

HAMILTON HALL, M.D., F.R.C.S.(C.)

Assistant Professor of Surgery, University of Toronto, Toronto; Staff Orthopedic Surgeon, Toronto General Hospital and Women's College Hospital, Toronto; Orthopedic Consultant, Ontario Workmen's Compensation Board, Downsview Rehabilitation Center, Toronto, Ontario, Canada

STANLEY HOPPENFELD, M.D.

Associate Clinical Professor, Albert Einstein College of Medicine, New York; Attending Physician, The Hospital for Joint Diseases Orthopaedic Institute, New York, New York

REUBEN HOPPENSTEIN, M.D., F.A.C.S.

Clinical Instructor, Mount Sinai School of Medicine, New York; Attending Neurosurgeon and Co-Chief, Problem Back Service, The Hospital for Joint Diseases Orthopaedic Institute, New York, New York

CHIEN LIANG HSU, M.D., F.R.C.P.(C.)

Radiologist (Retired) and formerly Associate Professor of Radiology, Peiping Union Medical College, Peking, China

JOHN D. HSU, M.D., C.M., F.A.C.S.

Clinical Professor, Department of Orthopedics, University of Southern California School of Medicine, Los Angeles; Attending Orthopaedic Surgeon, Rancho Los Amigos Hospital, Downey, California

CHARLES E. IMBUS, M.D.

Assistant Clinical Professor of Pediatrics and Neurology, University of Southern California School of Medicine, Los Angeles; Attending Pediatrician, Pediatric Neurology Clinic, Rancho Los Amigos Hospital, Downey, California

RICHARD L. JACOBS, M.D.

Professor and Head, Division Orthopedic Surgery, Albany Medical College, Albany; Chief of Orthopedic Surgery, Albany Medical Center, Albany, New York

WILLIAM L. JAFFE, M.D., F.A.C.S.

Associate Clinical Professor of Orthopaedic Surgery, Mount Sinai School of Medicine, New York; Associate Director and Attending Orthopaedic Surgeon, The Hospital for Joint Diseases Orthopaedic Institute, New York; Associate Attending Orthopaedic Surgeon, Mount Sinai Hospital and N.Y. Infirmary Beekman-Downtown Hospital, New York; Consultant Orthopaedic Surgeon, City Hospital at Elmhurst, New York, New York

KENNETH A. JOHNSON, M.D.

Consultant, Orthopedic Surgery, Mayo Clinic, Rochester; Orthopedic Surgeon, Rochester Methodist Hospital, Rochester, Minnesota

ALLASTAIR KARMODY, M.D.

Professor of Surgery, Albany Medical College, Albany; Attending Surgeon, Albany Medical Center Hospital, Albany, New York

HAMPAR KELIKIAN, M.D.

Emeritus Associate Professor of Orthopedic Surgery, Northwestern University Medical School, Chicago; Senior Attending Orthopedic Surgeon, Northwestern Memorial Hospital, Chicago; Assistant Attending Surgeon and Consultant, Augustana Hospital, Chicago; Consulting Orthopedic Surgeon, St. Barnard's Hospital, Henrotin Hospital, and Bethany Methodist Hospital, Chicago, Illinois

BARNARD KLEIGER, M.D.

Clinical Professor of Orthopaedic Surgery, Mount Sinai Medical School, New York; Visiting Professor of Orthopaedic Surgery, Albert Einstein College of Medicine, New York; Consultant, Orthopaedic Surgery, The Hospital for Joint Diseases Orthopaedic Institute, New York; Attending Orthopaedic Surgeon, Albert Einstein College Hospital and Montefiore Hospital and Medical Center, Bronx, New York

JEFFREY T. LAITMAN, Ph.D.

Assistant Professor of Anatomy, Mount Sinai School of Medicine, New York; Member, Graduate Faculty of Biological Sciences of the City University of New York, New York; Fellow, Human Growth and Development Study Unit, Yale-New Haven Medical Center, New Haven, Connecticut

PAUL W. LAPIDUS, M.D.

Professor Emeritus, New York Medical College, New York; Consultant Orthopedic Surgeon and Emeritus Chief of Foot Service, Hospital for Joint Diseases, New York; Consultant Orthopedic Surgeon, Metropolitan Hospital and Polyclinic Medical School, New York, New York

WILLIAM J. LAUNDER, M.S., M.D.

Instructor, Department of Orthopedic Surgery, Johns Hopkins University School of Medicine, Baltimore; Attending Surgeon, The Good Samaritan Hospital, Baltimore, Maryland

JAMES L. LENOIR, M.D.

Clinical Professor of Orthopedic Surgery, Louisiana State University Medical School, New Orleans; Orthopedic Surgeon, New Orleans Charity Hospital and Southern Baptist Hospital, New Orleans, Louisiana

RALPH LUSSKIN, M.D.

Professor of Clinical Orthopedic Surgery, New York University School of Medicine, New York; Attending Orthopedic Surgeon, University Hospital and Bellevue Hospital, New York, New York

JOHN BARRY McCRAW, M.D., F.A.C.S.

Professor of Plastic Surgery, Eastern Virginia Medical School; Active Privileges, Norfolk General, DePaul, Leigh Memorial and Kings Daughters Children's Hospitals; Consultant, USPHS Hospital, Norfolk; U.S. Naval Hospital, Portsmouth; Veterans Administration Hospital, Hampton, Virginia; and U.S. Naval Hospital, Bethesda, Maryland

W. DAVID McINNIS, M.D., F.A.C.S.

Assistant Clinical Professor of Plastic Surgery, University of Texas Health Science Center, San Antonio; Staff, Plastic Surgery, Southwest Texas Methodist Hospital, San Antonio, Texas

ISAAC S. McREYNOLDS, M.D., F.A.C.S.

Associate Clinical Professor of Orthopaedic Surgery, Baylor University College of Medicine, Houston; Consultant Staff, Orthopaedic Surgery, Memorial Baptist Hospital, St. Joseph's Hospital, St. Luke's Hospital, Methodist Hospital, and Medical Arts Hospital, Houston; Attending Staff, Twelve Oaks Hospital, Houston, Texas

ROGER A. MANN, M.D.

Associate Clinical Professor of Orthopaedic Surgery, University of California Medical School, San Francisco; Director, Gait Analysis Laboratory, Shriner's Hospital, San Francisco; Chief of Foot Surgery, Samuel Merrit Hospital, Oakland, California

JAMES W. MILGRAM, M.D.

Associate Professor of Orthopaedic Surgery, Northwestern University Medical School, Chicago; Attending Physician and Chief of Foot Service, Northwestern Memorial Hospital, Chicago; Associate Attending Physician, Children's Memorial Hospital, Chicago; Consultant, Veterans Administration Lakeside Hospital, Chicago, Illinois

JOSEPH E. MILGRAM, M.D., Sc.D.

Professor Emeritus of Clinical Orthopaedic Surgery, Albert Einstein College of Medicine, New York; Director Emeritus, Orthopaedic Surgery, The Hospital for Joint Diseases Orthopaedic Institute, New York, New York

ROBERT F. MURRAY, Jr., M.D., M.S.

Professor of Pediatrics, Medicine, and Oncology and Chief, Division of Genetics and Human Genetics, Department of Pediatrics, Howard University College of Medicine, Washington, D.C.; Attending Physician, Howard University Hospital and D.C. General Hospital, Washington, D.C.

ST. ELMO NEWTON, III, M.D.

Associate Clinical Professor of Orthopedics, University of Washington, Seattle; Chairman, Department of Orthopedics, Swedish Hospital Medical Center, Seattle; Director, Hand Surgery Service, Harborview Medical Center, Seattle, Washington

ALEX NORMAN, M.D.

Professor of Radiology, Mount Sinai School of Medicine, New York; Director of Radiology, The Hospital for Joint Diseases Orthopaedic Institute, New York, New York

JAMES E. C. NORRIS, M.D.

Associate Clinical Professor, College of Physicians and Surgeons of Columbia University, New York; Acting Director, Section of Plastic Surgery, Harlem Hospital Center, New York, New York

J. SERGE PARISIEN, M.D.

Chief of Arthroscopy Service (Diagnostic and Surgical) and Attending Orthopaedic Surgeon, The Hospital for Joint Diseases Orthopaedic Institute, New York, New York

WALTER J. PEDOWITZ, M.D.

Associate Clinical Professor, New Jersey College of Medicine, Newark; Assistant Attending Physician, St. Elizabeth's Hospital and Elizabeth General Hospital, Elizabeth, and Rahway Hospital, Rahway, New Jersey

DONALD M. QUALLS, M.D.

Assistant Clinical Professor, Department of Orthopedics, Jefferson Medical College, Philadelphia; Associate Orthopedist, Lankenau Medical Center, Philadelphia, Pennsylvania

NASIM A. RANA, M.D.

Associate Professor of Clinical Orthopaedic Surgery, Northwestern University Medical School, Chicago; Attending Orthopaedic Surgeon, Northwestern Memorial Hospital and Children's Memorial Hospital, Chicago; Chief, Orthopaedic Service, Veterans Administration Lakeside Medical Center, Chicago, Illinois

MARCEL A. REISCHER, M.D.

Adjunct Assistant Professor, Department of Rehabilitation Medicine, University of Maryland, School of Medicine, Baltimore; Head, Division of Rehabilitation Medicine, Department of Internal Medicine, Franklin Square Hospital, Baltimore, Maryland

HERMAN ROBBINS, M.D., F.A.C.S.

Clinical Professor of Orthopaedic Surgery, Mount Sinai School of Medicine, New York; Director of Orthopaedic Surgery, The Hospital for Joint Diseases Orthopaedic Institute, New York; Chief of Orthopaedic Surgery, St. Clare's Hospital, New York; Attending Orthopaedic Surgeon, Mount Sinai Hospital, New York, New York

GORDON K. ROSE, F.R.C.S., M.B., Ch.B.

Postgraduate Tutor, University of Birmingham, Birmingham; Director of Orthotic Research and Locomotor Assessment Unit and Senior Consultant Orthopaedic Surgeon, Robert Jones and Agnes Hunt Orthopaedic Hospital, Oswestry, and The Royal Shrewsbury Hospital, Shrewsbury, England

G. JAMES SAMMARCO, M.D.

Associate Clinical Professor, University of Cincinnati Medical Center, Department of Orthopaedic Surgery, Cincinnati; Associate Attending Physician, Cincinnati General Hospital, Good Samaritan Hospital, Children's Hospital, Christian R. Holmes Hospital, and Christ Hospital, Cincinnati; Attending Staff, Deaconess Hospital, Cincinnati, Ohio

EARL SCHWARTZ, M.D.

Clinical Instructor in Psychiatry, Mount Sinai School of Medicine, New York; Associate Attending Psychiatrist, Joint Diseases North General Hospital, New York, New York

A. J. SELVAPANDIAN, M.D.

Professor and Head, Department of Orthopedic Surgery, Christian Medical College and Hospital, Vellore, Tamilnadu, South India

MARVIN L. SHELTON, M.D.

Associate Professor of Clinical Orthopaedic Surgery, College of Physicians and Surgeons of Columbia University, New York; Associate Attending Surgeon, Columbia Presbyterian Medical Center, New York; Chief, Orthopaedic Service, Harlem Hospital Center, New York; Attending Surgeon, The Hospital for Joint Diseases Orthopaedic Institute, New York, New York

ROBERT S. SIFFERT, M.D.

Professor and Chairman, Department of Orthopaedics, Mount Sinai School of Medicine, New York; Professor and Chairman, Department of Orthopaedics, Mount Sinai Hospital, New York, New York

SHELDON R. SIMON, M.D.

Assistant Professor of Orthopedic Surgery, Harvard Medical School, Boston; Associate Orthopedic Surgeon, Children's Hospital Medical Center and Brigham and Women's Hospital, Boston; Director, Gait Analysis Laboratory, Children's Hospital Medical Center, Boston; Director of Rehabilitation, Brigham and Women's Hospital, Boston, Massachusetts

FEDERICO SOTELO-ORTIZ, M.D., F.A.C.S., F.I.C.S.

Formerly Professor of Human Anatomy and Instructor of Histology, National School of Medicine, U.N.A.M. Mexico City; Orthopaedic Surgeon, Hospital Sonara, Hermosillo, Mexico

MONROE W. SPERO, M.D.

Clinical Instructor in Psychiatry, Mount Sinai School of Medicine, New York; Attending Psychiatrist,

Joint Diseases North General Hospital, New York, New York

ALFRED J. SPIRO, M.D.

Professor of Neurology and Pediatrics, Albert Einstein College of Medicine, New York; Attending Physician in Neurology and Pediatrics and Director of the Division of Pediatric Neurology, Bronx Municipal Hospital Center, Hospital of the Albert Einstein College of Medicine, and Montefiore Hospital and Medical Center, Bronx, New York

MIHRAN O. TACHDJIAN, M.D., M.S.

Professor of Orthopedic Surgery, Northwestern University Medical School, Chicago; Head, Orthopedics Division, Children's Memorial Hospital, Chicago, Illinois

ALBERT H. TANNIN, M.A., M.D.

Lecturer, Department of Orthopaedic Surgery, Mount Sinai School of Medicine, New York; Assistant Attending Orthopaedic Surgeon, The Hospital for Joint Diseases Orthopaedic Institute, New York; Attending Orthopaedic Surgeon, Benedictine and Kingston Hospitals, Kingston, New York

WILLIAM THOMAS, M.D.

Assistant Clinical Professor of Orthopedic Surgery, Harvard Medical School, Boston; Associate Orthopedic Surgeon, Brigham and Women's Hospital, Barcelona, Spain

ARTHUR W. TROTT, M.D.

Lecturer, Orthopaedic Surgery, Harvard Medical School, Boston; Senior

Associate Orthopaedic Surgeon, Children's Hospital Medical Center, Boston; Associate in Orthopaedic Surgery, Brigham and Women's Hospital, Boston, Massachusetts

ANTONIO VILADOT, M.D.

Professor, Free University of Barcelona; Chief, Surgical Service (del aparato locomotor), San Rafael Hospital, Barcelona, Spain

F. WILLIAM WAGNER, Jr., M.D.

Clinical Professor of Orthopedic Surgery, University of Southern California School of Medicine, Los Angeles; Chief, Foot Service, Los Angeles County–USC Medical Center, Los Angeles; Chief, Ortho-Diabetes Service, Rancho Los Amigos Hospital, Downey, California

R. L. WATERS, M.D.

Associate Clinical Professor, Department of Orthopedics, University of Southern California, Los Angeles; Chief, Surgical Services, Rancho Los Amigos Hospital, Downey, California

THOMAS E. WHITESIDES, Jr., M.D.

Professor of Orthopaedic Surgery, Emory University School of Medicine, Atlanta; Acting Chairman, Department of Orthopaedics, Emory University School of Medicine, Emory University Hospital, Grady Memorial Hospital, Egleston Children's Hospital, and Veterans Administration Hospital, Atlanta, Georgia

CONTENTS

VOLUME I

PART I BASIC FOOT SCIENCE

Chapter 1   The Evolution and Anatomy of the Human Foot.......   1
             William L. Jaffe and Jeffrey T. Laitman

Chapter 2   Biomechanics......................................   37
             Roger A. Mann

Chapter 3   Electrodiagnosis..................................   68
             Marcel A. Reischer and Edward F. Delagi

Chapter 4   Examination.......................................   81
             Melvin H. Jahss

Chapter 5   Physical Examination of the Foot by Complaint........   103
             Stanley Hoppenfeld

Chapter 6   Roentgenographic Examination of the Normal
             Foot and Ankle   116
             Barnard Kleiger, Adam Greenspan, and Alex Norman

Chapter 7   Arthroscopy of the Ankle..........................   139
             J. Serge Parisien

Chapter 8   Surgical Principles and the Plantigrade Foot   144
             Melvin H. Jahss

PART II THE GROWING FOOT

Chapter 9   The Role of the Pediatrician and Pediatric
             Specialties in Identifying Disorders of the Foot........   195
             Robert F. Murray, Jr.

Chapter 10   Developmental Disorders 200
              Arthur W. Trott

Chapter 11   Congenital Deformities 212
              Mihran O. Tachdjian

Chapter 12   Generalized Genetic Disturbances Involving
              the Foot 233
              Charles H. Epps, Jr. and Liebe S. Diamond

Chapter 13   Management of the Foot in Spinal Dysraphism
              and Myelodysplasias 248
              T. Duckworth

Chapter 14   Foot and Ankle Deformities in Cerebral Palsy
              (Static Encephalopathies) 282
              J. Leonard Goldner

Chapter 15   Motor Unit Disease 335
              John D. Hsu and Chien Liang Hsu

Chapter 16   Bone Dysplasias 353
              Alex Norman and Adam Greenspan

Chapter 17   Inverted Talipes and Rotational Deformities
              of the Lower Extremities 374
              James L. LeNoir

Chapter 18   Congenital Vertical Talus and Arthrogryposis 439
              Herman Robbins

Chapter 19   Pes Cavus 463
              John D. Hsu and Charles E. Imbus

Chapter 20   Pes Planus 486
              G. K. Rose

Chapter 21   Tarsal Coalition 521
              Michael G. Ehrlich

PART III THE ADULT FOOT

Chapter 22   The Hallux 539
              Hampar Kelikian

Chapter 23   The Small Toes 622
              Malcolm A. Brahms

Chapter 24   The Metatarsals.. 659
             Antonio Viladot

Chapter 25   Disorders of the Anterior Tarsus and
             Lisfranc's Joint.. 711
             Melvin H. Jahss

             Additional Miscellaneous Conditions....................... 722
             William H. Blodgett

Chapter 26   The Subtalar Complex 727
             Melvin H. Jahss

Chapter 27   The Adult Heel.. 764
             James E. Bateman

Chapter 28   The Ankle 776
             Barnard Kleiger

             Ankle Fusion Versus Total Ankle Replacement:
             An Overview... 811
             Sheldon R. Simon and William Thomas

             Total Ankle Arthroplasty 816
             St. Elmo Newton, III

Chapter 29   Miscellaneous Soft-Tissue Lesions 828
             Melvin H. Jahss

Chapter 30   The Skin 869
             Richard C. Gibbs

Chapter 31   The Toenails... 914
             Paul W. Lapidus

Chapter 32   Plastic Surgery of the Foot and Ankle..................... 939
             John B. McCraw and W. David McInnis

Chapter 33   The Geriatric Foot... 964
             Phillip M. Evanski

PART IV   TUMORS OF THE FOOT

Chapter 34   Tumors of the Foot.. 979
             Crawford J. Campbell

VOLUME II

PART V THE FOOT IN SYSTEMIC DISEASE

Chapter 35   Gout 1014
Nasim A. Rana

Chapter 36   Rheumatoid Arthritis, Other Collagen
Diseases, and Psoriasis of the Foot.......................... 1024
Nasim A. Rana

Chapter 37   Metabolic Disorders and Paget's Disease of Bone 1064
James W. Milgram

Chapter 38   Hemophilia.. 1084
Marvin S. Gilbert and William J. Launder

Chapter 39   The Hemoglobinopathies and the Foot 1095
William J. Launder and Marvin S. Gilbert

Chapter 40   Examination of the Foot with a Neurologic
Disorder... 1107
Alfred J. Spiro

Chapter 41   Disorders of the Lower Extremity in the Stroke
and Head Trauma Patient...................................... 1112
Robert L. Waters and Douglas E. Garland

Chapter 42   Poliomyelitis and the Foot..................................... 1123
Federico Sotelo-Ortiz

Chapter 43   Peripheral Neuropathies Affecting the Foot:
Traumatic, Ischemic, and Compressive Disorders 1169
Ralph Lusskin

Compartment Syndromes 1201
Thomas E. Whitesides, Jr.

Chapter 44   Miscellaneous Peripheral Neuropathies and
Neuropathy-Like Syndromes.................................. 1205
Melvin H. Jahss and Ralph Lusskin

Chapter 45   Charcot Foot.. 1248
Richard L. Jacobs and Allastair Karmody

Chapter 46   The Insensitive Foot (Including Leprosy) 1266
Paul W. Brand

Chapter 47   Reflex Sympathetic Dystrophy Syndrome................. 1287
Kenneth A. Johnson

Chapter 48   Surgical Salvage of the Intractably Painful,
              "Failed" Foot 1295
              Reuben Hoppenstein

Chapter 49   Vascular Diseases of the Foot 1301
              Allastair Karmody and Richard L. Jacobs

Chapter 50   The Diabetic Foot 1377
              Richard L. Jacobs and Allastair Karmody

Chapter 51   Infections of the Foot, Including Leprosy 1398
              Ambrose James Selvapandian

              Yaws 1420
              Donald M. Qualls

Chapter 52   Psychiatric Aspects of Foot Problems 1429
              Monroe W. Spero and Earl Schwartz

PART VI   TRAUMA TO THE FOOT AND ANKLE

Chapter 53   Injuries of the Forefoot and Toes 1449
              William H. Blodgett

Chapter 54   Injuries to the Midfoot and Talus 1463
              Marvin L. Shelton and Walter J. Pedowitz

Chapter 55   Trauma to the Os Calcis and Heel Cord 1497
              Isaac Stephens McReynolds

Chapter 56   Trauma to the Ankle 1543
              Joseph J. Conrad and Albert H. Tannin

Chapter 57   Sports Injuries to the Foot and Ankle 1573
              Tom P. Coker, Jr. and James A. Arnold

Chapter 58   Industrial Injuries to the Foot and Ankle
              and Their Prevention 1607
              Hamilton Hall

Chapter 59   The Foot and Ankle in Classical Ballet and
              Modern Dance 1626
              G. James Sammarco

Chapter 60   Trauma to the Child's Foot and Ankle,
              Including Growth Plate and Epiphyseal Injuries 1660
              Robert S. Siffert and David J. Feldman

Chapter 61   Burns of the Foot 1689
              James E. C. Norris

PART VII   ORTHOTIC FOOT MANAGEMENT

Chapter 62   Padding and Devices to Relieve the
Painful Foot.. 1703
Joseph E. Milgram

Chapter 63   Arch Supports and Miscellaneous Devices 1733
Melvin H. Jahss

Chapter 64   Shoes and Shoe Modifications............................. 1745
Nathaniel Gould

Chapter 65   Orthotic and Prosthetic Management of
Foot Disorders 1783
James T. Demopoulos

Chapter 66   Organization of a Foot Service 1827
F. William Wagner, Jr.

PART VIII   APPENDICES AND INDEX

Appendix 1   Suggested Course Outline for Resident Study
of the Adult Foot and Ankle................................. 1831
F. William Wagner, Jr.

Appendix 2   Suggested Course Outline for Resident Study
of the Child's Foot and Ankle 1835
F. William Wagner, Jr.

Appendix 3   Guide to Basic Literature on the Foot..................... 1837
F. William Wagner, Jr.

Appendix 4   Terminology Utilized in the Field of
Prescription Footwear 1867

Index.. I

DISORDERS
of the FOOT

Part V
THE FOOT IN SYSTEMIC DISEASE

CHAPTER 35

GOUT

Nasim A. Rana, M.D.

Primary gout is a metabolic disease that has its basis in an inborn error in the intermediary metabolism of purines and related compounds. It is characterized by hyperuricemia, recurrent attacks of acute arthritis, deposition of monosodium urate crystals in and around the joints of the extremities, renal disease, and urolithiasis.

The word gout has its derivation from a Latin word "gutta," which means a drop, reflecting the early belief that a poison falling drop by drop into the joint was responsible for the disease. Hippocrates described gout in the foot as "podagra" — "pous" (foot) and "agra" (attack).

Historically, this disease was known to ancient Greeks — Hippocrates (460–370 B.C.), for example, was well acquainted with this entity — and Romans and also has a very prestigious heritage.[20] Renal calculi with uric acid nuclei have been found in a 7000-year-old Egyptian mummy. Alexander the Great, Charles Darwin, Benjamin Franklin, William Harvey, Alexander Hamilton, Henry VIII, John Hunter, Louis XIV, Isaac Newton, Thomas Sydenham, and Cardinal Wolsey are some of the well-known individuals reported to have been afflicted with gout.

Sydenham, who, as just mentioned, suffered from gout himself, gave a classic description of gout in 1683. According to Yü and Katz, Scheele discovered uric acid as a constituent of urine and some renal stones in 1776.[25] A few years later, Wollerton isolated uric acid from gouty tophus and confirmed the relationship between gout and uric acid. In 1876, in his "Treatise on Gout and Rheumatic Gout," Garrod described a test to detect an increased amount of uric acid in gouty patients. Emil Fischer established the relationship between uric acid and purine metabolism. Many others have written about the history of gout.[3, 7, 17]

The hereditary nature of this disease is well known. In at least 50 per cent of the cases, family history of gout can be elicited. Although this disease chiefly affects men, an affected woman from a family in which gout is present may likewise transmit the trait to her offspring. Women carrying the trait usually do not develop hyperuricemia until after menopause, and clinical gout, if it occurs at all, does not appear until some years later.

PATHOGENESIS

Hyperuricemia is the biochemical hallmark of gout. It is not apparent at the time of acute attacks in all patients with gout,

TABLE 35–1. Metabolism of Purine Nucleosides to Uric Acid

ADENOSINE → INOSINE → HYPOXANTHINE
↓ XANTHINE OXIDASE
GUANOSINE → GUANINE → XANTHINE
↓ XANTHINE OXIDASE
URIC ACID

but it is manifested at some time in 98 per cent of patients with this disease.[5] Serum urate levels greater than 7.0 mg/100 ml for men and 6.0 mg/100 ml for women are an indication of hyperuricemia.

Uric acid is the end product of purine metabolism in man (Table 35–1). Because humans are ureotelic, the bulk of nitrogen waste is eliminated by the kidneys as urea, and only about 1.5 per cent of total nitrogen in the urine is in the form of uric acid. In about one third of the patients with gout, a disproportionate amount of dietary nitrogen is excreted as uric acid, and in the remainder the excretion of uric acid is not excessive. In contrast, birds and reptiles are uricotelic and eliminate primarily uric acid, not urea, in the course of nitrogen metabolism. In humans with gout, the uric acid metabolism tends to more or less resemble that of uricotelic species.[9] Holmes has proposed six theoretic bases for hyperuricemia[8]:

I. Increased production of uric acid
    a. Increased biosynethesis of purine de novo
    b. Increased catabolism of nucleic acid
    c. Ingestion of excessive purines in diet
II. Decreased excretion of uric acid
    a. Decreased renal clearance
    b. Decreased gastrointestinal excretion
III. Decreased catabolism of uric acid. The only form of another mechanism has been demonstrated to be operative in patients with hyperuricemia. The decreased catabolism of uric acid is just a theoretic possibility.

Isotopic studies have demonstrated that in a normal individual, the miscible uric acid pool is approximately 1 gram. In an individual with nontophaceous gout, however, this pool is enlarged to 2 to 4 grams, so that in a patient with tophaceous gout, it may be tremendously enlarged.[2] The excess uric acid is largely stored in the tophi. The uric acid in the body fluids is in equilibrium with that in the tophi. This miscible pool can be decreased by the administration of uricosuric drugs, although this change may not be reflected in the serum uric acid levels.

In a normal person not affected by gout, uric acid is excreted mainly in the urine, and some is eliminated by way of tears, sweat, and feces. Uric acid excretion by the kidneys involves three mechanisms, i.e., glomerular filtration, tubular reabsorption, and tubular secretion. Ordinarily, most of the filtrated uric acid is reabsorbed by the renal tubules, and the amount that appears in the urine consists primarily of the portion derived from tubular secretion and, to a lesser extent, from a portion that escaped reabsorption.

PATHOLOGIC FINDINGS AND PATHOGENESIS OF SYNOVITIS INDUCED BY URATE CRYSTAL DEPOSITS

In the evolution of gouty changes in a joint, urate crystals are deposited in the synovial membrane and articular cartilage, and similar deposits are also seen in the subarticular and juxta-articular bones, fibrous capsule, and surrounding soft tissues.[9] The synovial membrane shows proliferation, inflammatory changes, and pannus formation. The articular cartilage usually exhibits deposits of urate crystals and surrounding cell necrosis, which eventually destroys the entire articular surface, resulting in deposition of the crystals in the subchondral bone. Independent tophi are also found in the articular end of bones, giving rise to the typical picture of punched-out lesions in the radiographs (Figs. 35–1 and 35–2). Large deposits of urate crystals are also seen in adjacent bursae, tendons, ligaments, and subcutaneous layers of skin. (Fig. 35–3).

The mechanism of urate deposition is very poorly understood. *In vitro* studies have shown crystallization of urate with changes in pH and sodium concentration, but this has not substantiated by *in vivo* studies. It may be that the proteins of patients with gout cannot bind the urate normally. Katz and Schubert observed that urate deposits occur exclusively in the connective tissues.[10] Proteoglycans selec-

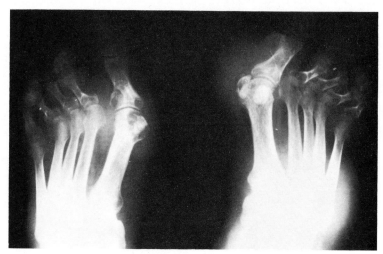

Figure 35–1. *Radiographs of both feet in a patient with chronic tophaceous gout showing a punched-out lesion in the bones around the first metatarsophalangeal joint of the left foot and a large tophus around the right first metatarsophalangeal joint.*

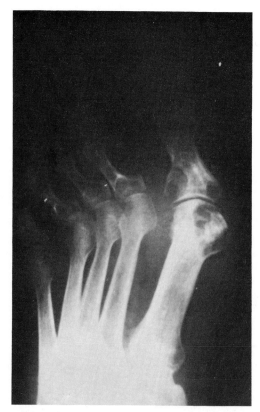

Figure 35–2. *Localized view of the left foot showing a punched-out lesion in the bone due to deposition of urate crystals.*

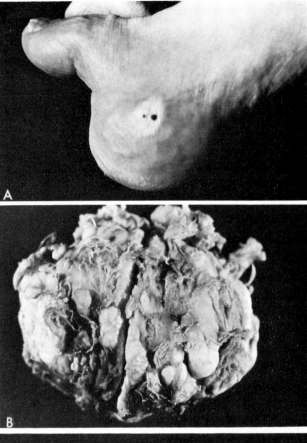

Figure 35–3. (A) Clinical photograph of the right foot of the same patient as in Figure 35–1 showing a large tophus involving the soft tissues of the plantar aspect of right foot that caused problems with footwear. (B) The excised tophus has a lobulated, well-encapsulated appearance. (C) Cross section of the tophus showing septa, pseudocapsule, and urate crystal deposits. (D) A histologic section of the tophus shows crystal deposits (right side of the illustration) surrounded by inflammatory cells and foreign-body giant cells.

Illustration continued on following page

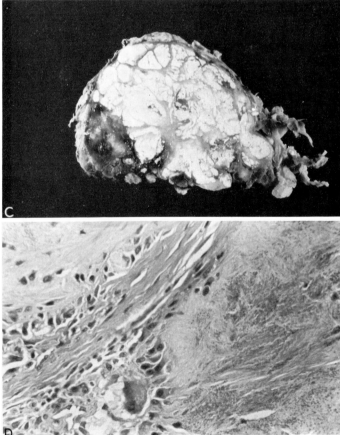

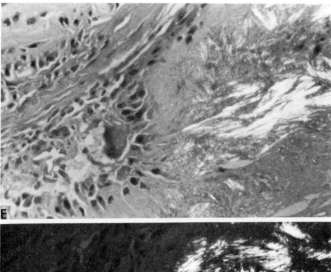

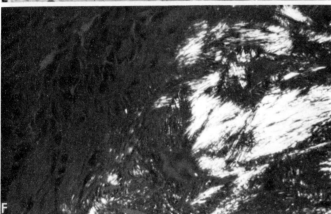

Figure 35–3 Continued. (E) The same section under polarized light shows characteristic urate crystals. (F) The same section stained with De Galantha stain and under polarized light reveals typical urate crystals.

tively augment the solubility of monosodium urate, whereas proteolytic disruption of urate-saturated polysaccharides results in the precipitation of urate deposits *in vitro*; these authors proposed that a similar mechanism might occur *in vivo*. Glycosaminoglycans in protein fractions augment urate solubility, and then there is threefold increase of glycosaminoglycans in patients with gout. For some unknown reason, the connective-tissue metabolism may be accelerated in these patients.[11]

Urate crystals in the joint provoke an inflammatory response. The proposed mechanism for this inflammatory response seems to be that the crystals in the joint activate Hageman factor and kinins, which in turn lead to endothelial permeability. Leukocytes migrate toward the crystals and begin to phagocytose them. This results in the death of the cell and the release of lysosomal enzymes, which induce an intense inflammatory reaction and give rise to a typical acute attack of gout. Schumacher and Phelps studied the changes in the polymorphonuclear leukocyte on ingestion of urate crystals by electron microscopy and found that the urate crystals are phagocytosed by polymorphs and become surrounded by a membrane, with degranulation of the cell.[19] This leads to lysis of the cell membrane and death of the cell.

ACUTE GOUTY ARTHRITIS

Clinical Manifestations

Gout is one of the true intermittent inflammatory types of arthritis. The typical acute attack may appear and then resolve spontaneously after 72 to 96 hours. The initial acute attack is followed by an asymptomatic period that may last from several days to years. Commonly, the initial symptom of an attack of gout is a dull or gnawing sensation in the involved joint. The pain increases in intensity over a period of six to 24 hours, and the joint becomes very warm, erythematous, swol-

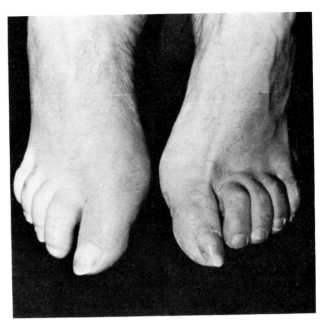

Figure 35–4. *Patient with an acute attack of gout involving the first metatarsophalangeal joint of the right foot.*

len, and exquisitely tender. Sometimes this will be associated with fever. Within 24 to 48 hours, the joint is so painful that the patient refuses to walk. Some cannot even tolerate the pressure of bedclothes.[1] Untreated, the attack of gout usually lasts for a few days and then subsides completely. Acute gouty arthritis usually occurs in men (95 per cent), and the first attack usually takes place in the fourth or fifth decade. Women rarely develop gout before menopause. The patient usually never forgets the acute attack. This typical history helps in making the diagnosis (Figs. 35–4 and 35–5).

Gouty arthritis usually presents as monoarticular arthritis, occurring in the first metatarsophalangeal joint in about 75 per cent of cases. Occasionally, it presents as oligoarthritis or polyarthritis, even during the first attack. About 60 per cent of the patients have the second attack within a year. In general, mental stress, postoperative anxiety, physical trauma, indulgence in food and alcohol, and certain medications can induce an acute attack.

The diagnosis is clinical and is confirmed by the presence of typical monosodium urate monohydrate crystals in the synovial fluid. These crystals are characteristically needle-shaped and exhibit strong negative birefringence.[4] The synovial fluid should be aspirated into a simple tube, without any additive, and a drop of the fluid should be examined under an ordinary light microscope to note the presence or absence of crystals. If crystals are present, this is followed by examination of the fluid under a compensated polarizing light microscope to determine the type of crystal. The biopsy specimens should be collected and fixed in absolute alcohol, for the crystals have a tendency to dissolve in fixatives containing water.

Treatment

The treatment of gout usually involves (1) management of the patient as a whole; (2) treatment of the acute attack; (3) measures directed toward prevention of future acute attacks and development of topha-

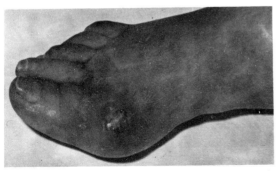

Figure 35–5. *Patient with acute attack of gout of first metatarsophalangeal joint, with a draining tophus and superimposed infection.*

ceous gout and other complications; and (4) management of chronic gouty arthritis and systemic complications, e.g., renal complications.

There seems to be universal agreement about the management of acute attacks of gout. Most physicians will recommend the use of colchicine, which in *in vitro* studies has been noted to inhibit migration of polymorphonuclear leukocytes toward a chemotactic stimulus and to inhibit the increased leukocyte mobility induced by urate crystals. The therapeutic course of colchicine usually consists of oral administration of 1 mg promptly, followed by 0.5 mg every two to three hours until there is relief of joint pain or the patient develops gastrointestinal symptoms, i.e., severe nausea or diarrhea. Diarrhea can be treated with routine antidiarrheal measures, e.g., the administration of paregoric. In the presence of very severe pain, routine analgesics (e.g., codeine) can also be administered. It usually takes 12 hours or more to see the effect of colchicine, and this can also serve as a diagnostic test. Acute gout is the only disorder in which the dramatic response to colchicine occurs consistently.

The colchicine can be administered intravenously in patients who cannot tolerate the gastrointestinal symptoms produced by oral administration. The intravenous route practically eliminates the gastrointestinal toxicity that is produced by the local effect of colchicine on the jejunal and ileal mucosa. Intravenous administration of colchicine is very effective. A single dose of 3 mg will control the acute attack of gout,[21] and response usually starts within six hours of the administration of the drug. Unfortunately, the colchicine solution is extremely irritating to the soft tissues. The veins used for the intravenous administration usually exhibit severe inflammation, and if any drug spills outside the vein, it causes local tissue necrosis. After the acute attack has abated, colchicine in a divided dose of 1.5 mg daily will help to prevent the development of other acute attacks. Phenylbutazone (Butazolidin) or oxyphenbutazone (Tandearil) in doses of 200 mg orally every four hours for two days can be highly effective in controlling an acute attack of gout.

Indomethacin (Indocin) is also very helpful in the management of an acute attack of gout. Twenty-five to 50 mg orally three or four times a day for a few days is very effective, especially when the attack is in the subacute phase.

In fulminating cases, intramuscular or intravenous ACTH (adrenocorticotropic hormone) is very effective. The initial dose varies from 60 to 100 units for the first day, and then it is tapered off slowly. This can be helpful in treating a postoperative acute gout attack when the patient is on intravenous fluids only.

Prevention of Recurrent Gouty Arthritis. Colchicine in small daily doses can be very beneficial in the prevention of recurrent attacks of gouty arthritis. A dose of 0.5 mg of colchicine daily by mouth is sufficient.

CHRONIC GOUTY ARTHRITIS AND TOPHACEOUS GOUT

Clinical Manifestations

The frequency of chronic tophaceous gout as a manifestation of hyperuricemia has been noted to be decreasing. This may be due to early recognition of the problem and good medical management.[16]

If an acute attack of gout is not treated or is treated ineffectively, after an undetermined period a clinical syndrome of tophaceous gout may appear. This is almost directly related to hyperuricemia. If the uric acid levels reach beyond 9 mg/100 ml to 10 or 11 mg/100 ml, the chance of development of tophaceous gout is about 50 per cent.[25]

Tophaceous gout usually presents as symmetric polyarthritis. Tophi can occur anywhere in the body, but are commonly seen at the olecranon, extensor surface of the hand, first metatarsophalangeal joint, Achilles tendon, and the ear. The diagnosis is confirmed by aspiration of the nodule and examination of the aspirate, as discussed previously.

Treatment

Pharmacologic Management

Uricosuric drugs, which increase the elimination of uric acid in the urine, are helpful in the prevention or amelioration of chronic gouty arthritis. The effectiveness of probenecid (Benemid) and sulfinpyrazone (Anturane), a derivative of phenylbutazone, in lowering the high uric acid levels has been well established. Both of these drugs inhibit the renal tubular resorption of uric acid, increase uric acid excretion, and thus reduce serum uric acid levels. Their use can prevent the formation of tophaceous deposits and can also decrease the sizes of tophi that are already present.[24] Probenecid, 0.5 gm twice a day, or sulfinpyrazone, 100 mg three times a day, is very effective and well tolerated. With increasing renal involvement, the uricosuric agents become ineffective, especially if the glomerular filtration rate falls below 20 to 30 ml/minute.

Allopurinol (hydroxypyrazolo-[3,4-d] pyrimidine) is a very potent inhibitor of xanthine oxidase, the enzyme that acts as a catalytic agent in the conversion of hypoxanthine to xanthine and of xanthine to uric acid.[18, 24] By inhibiting uric acid formation, it decreases the serum and urinary uric acid levels. As its action does not depend upon the renal status, this drug is effective even in the presence of poor kidney function. Allopurinol is usually administered in doses of 100 mg two or three times a day in most patients.

By decreasing the uric acid formation with allopurinol and increasing uric acid excretion with uricosuric agents (e.g., probenecid), the rate of disappearance of already existing tophi can be facilitated. The combined use of these drugs can also prohibit or decrease the formation of new tophi.

Surgical Management

Modern drug therapy is of definite value in decreasing and preventing the formation of tophi and chronic tophaceous gouty lesions and arthritis. It is conceivable that some tophaceous material is miscible with general circulation, but some is rather immiscible and avascular and remains despite prolonged drug therapy. There are occasional cases that require removal of tophaceous deposits and reconstructive surgery. Linton and Talbott,[14] Woughton,[22] Larmon and Kurtz,[13] and Kurtz[12] have written extensively on the pathology, indications for surgery, and the various operative procedures beneficial in gout.

Gouty deposits seem to have an affinity for bursae and subcutaneous tissues superficial to the deep fascia, tendons, articular cartilage, and bone. Urate crystals do not invade vessels and nerves, although they often surround or compress them.

According to the authors just mentioned, the various indications for surgery for gout in the foot are:

1. Large tophi interfering with footwear.
2. Painful tophi over the weight-bearing areas.
3. Danger of breakdown and necrosis of skin over a tophus.
4. Draining sinus associated with a tophus.
5. Deformity of toes.
6. Painful destruction of joints.
7. Compression of nerves, vessels, and tendons.
8. Danger of rupture of tendons.

Techniques

Tophi involving soft tissues usually have a definite fibrous capsule, a false capsule. Complete excision of the tophus with its capsule is the treatment of choice, but if for some reason the entire tophus cannot be excised, then as much as possible should be removed, with the rest being curetted out. If it involves the tendon extensively, great care should be taken in removing crystals from the tendon. The integrity of the tendon must be kept to retain its function, which means incomplete removal of the tophus, but this partial removal usually works very well and results in healing of the operative wound.

Chronic draining sinuses over a tophus should be managed by curettage through the sinus or enlargement of the sinus in an anatomic fashion.

If the first metatarsophalangeal joint is grossly deformed and painful, it should be managed either by excision of the first metatarsal head (Mayo procedure) or proximal hemiphalangectomy (Keller operation). This usually provides symptomatic relief. If the toe is grossly deformed, it can be managed by routine standard operations for toe deformities. i.e., arthroplasty or arthrodesis. Amputations are rarely indicated.

Tarsal joint arthritis can again be handled with arthrodesis of the appropriate joint, keeping the general principles in mind.

Surgery is an adjunct to medical treatment, and the patient should be on a regular regimen of antigout drug therapy. With regard to surgical incisions, general surgical principles should again be kept in mind, and one should try to make straight incisions so as not to jeopardize the circulation of the flaps. As much of the tophus as possible should be excised without sacrificing the vital structures. One should just curette the undersurface of the skin as much as possible. Following this, the wound should be thoroughly irrigated and closed over hemovac drains. The foot should be encased in a compression dressing and a plaster of Paris splint. The compression should be continued until the stitches are to be removed. If there is delayed healing of the wound, the wound should be managed with moist saline or Betadine dressings until the wound is healed or well-granulated. Skin grafting is usually unnecessary. The open wound from the sinus and tophus excision can again be managed primarily with moist dressings until complete healing has taken place.

Early diagnosis and proper treatment can save the patient from destructive lesions and large tophi.

SECONDARY GOUT

Secondary gout is present when there is an identifiable and acquired cause for the clinical manifestations of the gout that is not due to the inborn error of the purine metabolism. Instead, the hyperuricemia is attributed to the excessive degradation of the nucleoproteins and nucleic acid in some of the hematologic disorders, such as leukemia and polycythemia rubra vera, and sometimes to a definable renal factor or drugs, e.g., diuretics. Secondary gout is usually controlled effectively with allopurinol.

PSEUDOGOUT (PYROPHOSPHATE ARTHROPATHY, CHONDROCALCINOSIS)

Like gout, pyrophosphate arthropathy is considered a crystal deposition disease. It differs from gout in that calcium pyrophosphate dihydrate (CPPD) crystals are deposited in place of the monosodium urate monohydrate (MSUM) crystals. The CPPD crystals are deposited in the fibrocartilage (menisci), hyaline articular cartilage, ligaments, and tendons. These crystals are radiopaque and show up on radiographs as a diffuse opacity in the soft tissues (like menisci in the knee joint) or as linear calcifications in the hyaline cartilage, quite a distinct line from the subchondral bone.

Crystals are usually rhomboid or acicular in shape (Fig. 35–6). The CPPD crystals have an optical property of bifringence like the MSUM crystals. The CPPD crystals show weak positive bifringence as compared with the strongly negative bifringence of urate crystals. These two

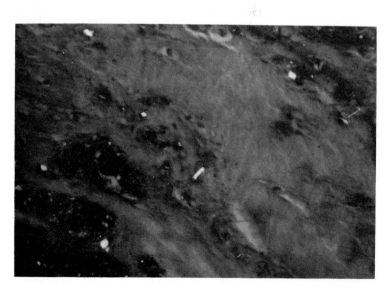

Figure 35–6. *A polarized histologic section showing characteristic CPPD crystals deposited in the soft tissues in a patient with pseudogout.*

types of crystals are distinguished with the help of the compensated polarizing microscope.[4] Bifringence means that after striking the crystal, the incident light is split into two refracted rays vibrating at different angles. The resultant ray with the greater angle of deviation from the optical axis will be slower passing through the crystal, and the ray with the smaller angle will be a fast-moving ray. The crystals are bi-axial. These fast and slow rays bisect the two oblique axes. If a slow ray bisects the optical axis angle, the crystal is optically positive; if the fast ray bisects the optical axis, the crystal is optically negative.

Sometimes, pseudogout is clinically indistinguishable from uric acid gout. McCarty distinguishes five different patterns of CPPD crystal deposition disease, with pseudogout being Type A.[15] This can present as an acute or subacute episode. Like gout, pseudogout can also flare up with the stress of surgery or other medical illnesses. Joint aspiration and crystal identification are necessary to establish the diagnosis. He also mentioned eight confirmed cases of pseudogout involving the first metatarsophalangeal joint ("pseudopodagra").

Pathogenesis

There is no known underlying metabolic abnormality in CPPD-induced arthropathy. Chondrocalcinosis, which is a radiologic finding, also occurs in patients with hemochromatosis, hyperparathyroidism, hypothyroidism, ochronosis, Wilson's disease, diabetes mellitus, and a few other diseases. The initial site of CPPD crystal formation is probably articular cartilage.[15] It is not clear whether the CPPD crystal formation is the primary phenomenon or whether it is a secondary feature. The chondrocyte dies, and subsequently the calcium pyrophosphate crystals are released into the synovial fluid, initiating a synovitis.

Management

The usual nonsteroidal anti-inflammatory drugs (e.g., indomethacin, phenylbutazone) can control the acute attack of pseudogout. Aspiration of the joint and instillation of corticosteroid are sometimes necessary to manage a very severe attack.

REFERENCES

1. Arnold, W. J., and Gröbner, W.: Clinical manifestations of hyperuricaemia. Clin. Rheum. Dis., 3:51, 1977.
2. Benedict, J. B., Forsham, P. H., and Stetten, DeW., Jr.: The metabolism of uric acid in the normal and gouty human studied with the aid of isotopic uric acid. J. Biol. Chem., 181:183, 1949.
3. Bywater, E. G. L.: Gout in the time and person of George IV: a case history. Ann Rheum. Dis., 21:325, 1962.
4. Gatter, R. A.: Use of the compensated polarizing microscope. Clin. Rheum. Dis., 3:91, 1977.
5. Goldthwait, J. C., Butler, C. F., and Stillman, J. S.: The diagnosis of gout: significance of an elevated serum uric acid value. N. Engl. J. Med., 259:1095, 1958.
6. Harper, H. A.: Metabolism of purines and pyrimidines. In Review of Physiological Chemistry. Los Altos, California, Lange Medical Publications, 1967, p. 344.
7. Hartung, E. F.: Symposium on gout: historical considerations. Metabolism, 6:196, 1957.
8. Holmes, E. W.: Pathogenesis of hyperuricaemia in primary gout. Clin. Rheum. Dis., 3:3, 1977.
9. Jaffe, H. L.: Metabolic, Degenerative, and Inflammatory Diseases of Bones and Joints. Philadelphia, Lea and Febiger, 1972, pp. 479–505.
10. Katz, W. A., and Schubert, M.: The solubility of monosodium urate crystals in connective tissue components. J. Clin. Invest., 49:1783, 1970.
11. Katz, W. A.: Deposition of urate crystals in gout. Altered connective tissue metabolism. Arthritis Rheum., 18:751, 1975.
12. Kurtz, J. F.: Surgery of tophaceous gout in the lower extremity. Surg. Clin. North Am., 45:217, 1965.
13. Larmon, W. A., and Kurtz, J. F.: The surgical management of chronic tophaceous gout. J. Bone Joint Surg., 40A:743, 1958.
14. Linton, R. R., and Talbott, J. H.: The surgical treatment of tophaceous gout. Ann. Surg., 117:161, 1943.
15. McCarty, D. J.: Pseudogout — the CPPD Crystal Deposition Disease. Resident and Staff Physician, 71, 1977.
16. O'Duffy, J. D., Hunder, G. G., and Kelly, P. J.: Decreasing prevalence of tophaceous gout. Mayo Clin. Proc., 50:227, 1975.
17. Rodnan, G. P.: A gallery of gout — being a miscellany of prints and caricatures from the 16th century to the present day. Arthritis Rheum., 4:27, 1961.
18. Rundles, R. W., Wyngaaeden, J. B., Hitetchings, G. H., et al.: Effects of a xanthine-oxidase inhibitor on thiopurine metabolism, Hyperuricaemia and gout. Trans. Assoc. Am. Physicians, 76:126, 1963.
19. Schumacher, H. R., and Phelps, P.: Sequential changes in human polymorphonuclear leukocytes after urate crystal phagocytosis. Arthritis Rheum., 14:513, 1971.
20. Talbott, J. H.: Gout, 2nd ed. New York, Grune and Stratton, 1964.
21. Wallace, S. L.: The treatment of the acute attack of gout. Clin. Rheum. Dis., 3:133, 1977.
22. Woughton, H. W.: Surgery of tophaceous gout. J. Bone Joint Surg., 41A:116, 1959.
23. Yü, T. F., and Gutman, A. B.: Effect of allopurinol (4-hydroxypyrazolo-(3,4-d)pyrimidine) on serum and urinary uric acid in primary and secondary gout. Am. J. Med., 37:885, 1964.
24. Yü, T. F., and Gutman, A. B.: Metabolism of gouty tophi by protracted use of uricosuric agents. Am. J. Med., 11:765, 1951.
25. Yü, T. F., and Katz, W. A.: Gout and pseudogout. In Katz, W. A. (ed.): Rheumatic Diseases: Diagnosis and Management. Philadelphia, J. B. Lippincott Co., 1977, pp. 697–730.

CHAPTER 36

RHEUMATOID ARTHRITIS, OTHER COLLAGEN DISEASES, AND PSORIASIS OF THE FOOT

Nasim A. Rana, M.D.

Collagen diseases, especially rheumatoid arthritis, frequently affect the foot and ankle. In many instances, the initial symptoms of the disease may start in the foot. Heel spur pain or hallux valgus may be due to an underlying rheumatoid arthritis rather than to static causes. An unexplained swollen toe may be caused by rheumatoid arthritis or psoriasis. A tenosynovitis may be related to any one of the collagen diseases. A perplexing peripheral neuropathy may be associated with a relatively mild rheumatoid arthritis.

Although psoriasis may be properly classified as a hereditary disorder, it often results in rheumatoid-like changes in the foot and is frequently associated with true rheumatoid changes, with or without associated positive laboratory confirmation.

RHEUMATOID ARTHRITIS OF THE FOOT

Information provided by the Arthritis Foundation states that about five million people suffer from rheumatoid arthritis in the United States.[1] In most of these patients, the foot will be involved. Although

any synovial joint in the foot can be affected first by rheumatoid arthritis, the metatarsophalangeal joints are affected first most frequently.

According to Short and associates, the feet were more commonly the site of initial involvement for rheumatoid arthritis than the hands — 15.7 per cent in the feet as compared with 14.7 per cent in the hands.[40] In 1956, Vainio surveyed 1000 patients with rheumatoid arthritis and found that 85 per cent of 337 men, 91 per cent of 618 women, and 69 per cent of 45 children had foot involvement (Table 36-1).[44]

TABLE 36-1. Foot Involvement in 1000 Rheumatoid Cases*

	NUMBER OF PATIENTS	PER CENT OF FOOT INVOLVEMENT
Men	337	85
Women	618	91
Children	45	69
Total	1000	Average 81.66

*Adapted from Vainio, K.: Ann. Chir. Gynaecol., *45* (Suppl. 1):1, 1956.

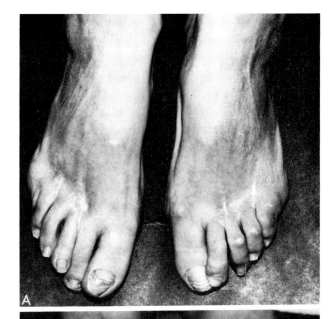

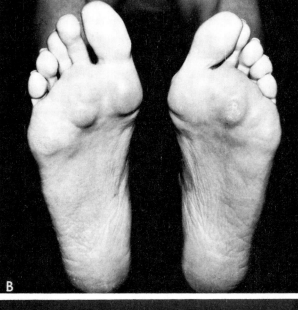

Figure 36–1. (A–C) Clinical photographs and radiograph of the feet of a patient with rheumatoid arthritis who has a tendency to stiffen most of the joints. She had previously undergone bilateral Keller arthroplasty and synovectomy of the metatarsophalangeal joints. Now all the joints are stiff and painful, and bony ankylosis is present.

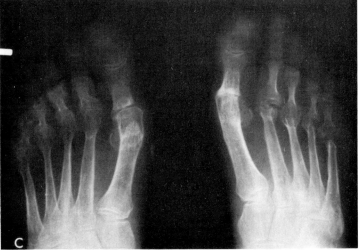

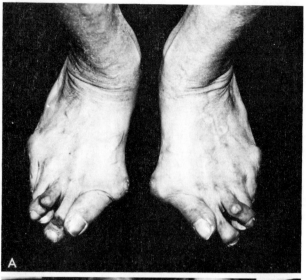

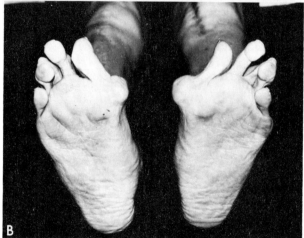

Figure 36–2. (A–C) Patient with marked ligamentous laxity showing marked clinical and radiologic deformities typical of rheumatoid arthritis – splaying, hallux valgus, hammer toes, and pes valgus. The patient is well adjusted to her deformities and, surprisingly, has very little discomfort and has not asked for surgical help.

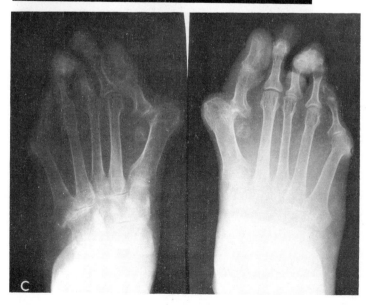

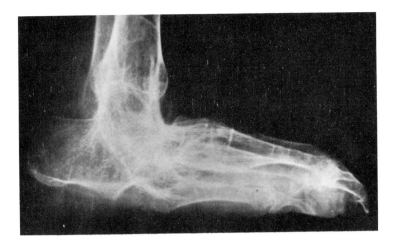

Figure 36–3. *Radiograph of the foot of a patient with rheumatoid arthritis who has bony ankylosis of most of the joints of the extremities. The spine and sacroiliac joints remain free of disease.*

Rheumatoid arthritis is a chronic inflammatory disease belonging to the group of collagen diseases of unknown etiology. There is considerable overlapping of the symptoms of the collagen diseases, but with certain guidelines one can differentiate the various entities. The American Rheumatism Association has provided criteria for the diagnosis of rheumatoid arthritis.[38] A precise diagnosis must be made before proper treatment is recommended. With a good history, physical and radiologic examinations, and appropriate laboratory tests, a specific diagnosis can be made with reasonable certainty.

Clayton has pointed out, and it has been my observation as well, that there are definitely two different clinical types of joint involvement in rheumatoid arthritis.[9] The first is that in which the patients' joints have a tendency to develop progressive stiffening and eventual fibrous or bony ankylosis (stiff type) (Fig. 36–1). The second kind is that type in which there is a tendency toward destruction of bone and laxity of soft tissues, leading to instability (loose type) (Fig. 36–2). Younger patients have a tendency to develop stiffening of the joints compared with patients in whom the disease started later in life. At times, I have noticed that all the tarsal joints are fused and that the foot is essentially one solid piece of bone (Fig. 36–3). In rheumatoid arthritis with the loose type of joint involvement, there is more proliferative and hypertrophic synovitis and bursal enlargement, and the looseness is present in most of the joints in that particular patient.

Clinical Features

Vainio[44] and Calabro[5] presented a clear picture of the clinical and radiographic manifestations of rheumatoid arthritis in the feet (Table 36–2).

Synovitis of the Metatarsophalangeal Joints

As mentioned previously, metatarsophalangeal joints are very commonly involved in rheumatoid arthritis, which usually starts as synovitis. The lateral metatarsophalangeal joints are most frequently the first to be affected, and eventually all five metatarsophalangeal joints are involved. In the early stages, the forefoot is usually tender and puffy. Palpation, move-

TABLE 36–2.   Clinical Study of the Rheumatoid Foot*

AREA OF FOOT INVOLVED	PER CENT OF FOOT INVOLVEMENT
Subtalar and midtarsal joint	66.9
Calcaneal valgus with flatfoot	46.5
Spread foot	33.2
Digitus malleus (hammer toe)	53.2
Hallux valgus	58.8
Hallux rigidus	10.4
Achilles bursitis Tendo periostitis nodules	9.0
Tenosynovitis	6.5

*Adapted from Vainio, K.: Ann. Chir. Gynaecol., *45* (Suppl. 1):1, 1956.

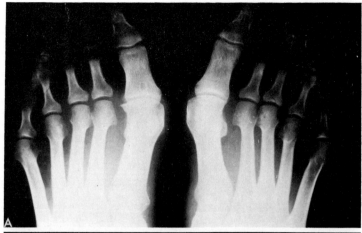

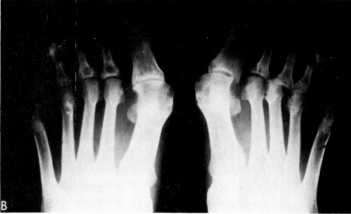

Figure 36–4. (A and B) Progressive rheumatoid changes over a period of four years involving the metatarsophalangeal joints. The radiographs show loss of articular cartilage, bony erosions, and hallux valgus deformities.

ment of the metatarsophalangeal joints, and lateral compression of the forefoot usually cause pain. With increasing synovial and periarticular swelling and joint erosion, forefoot deformities begin to develop (Fig. 36–4).

Splaying of the Forefoot

Because of chronic synovitis and ligamentous laxity, the metatarsals have a tendency to spread, which is more pronounced on weight bearing and eventually results in marked splaying of the forefoot (see Figure 36–2).

Claw Toes

Claw toes occur secondary to metatarsophalangeal joint involvement and may be due to muscle imbalance and involvement of the intrinsic muscles. The proximal phalanges develop progressive dorsal subluxation, causing hyperextension of the

metatarsophalangeal joints. With obvious tension in the toe flexors, the interphalangeal joints develop flexion deformity, which eventually leads to claw-toe or hammer-toe deformity.* Occasionally, I have seen a toe deformity similar to a swan-neck deformity of the finger, in which there is hyperextension of the proximal interphalangeal joint with flexion of the distal interphalangeal joint (Fig. 36–5). Gradually all of the toes drift toward the fibula. With marked splaying, the fifth toe usually drifts toward the tibial side.

With typical clawing, the plantar fat pad shifts distally, exposing the thinner part of the skin to pressure, and with the wearing of shoes and weight bearing, the patient develops painful callosities over the dorsal aspect of the proximal interphalangeal joints and under the plantar aspect of the

---

*Some authors make a distinction between claw toes and hammer toes, but in this chapter the terms will be used synonymously.

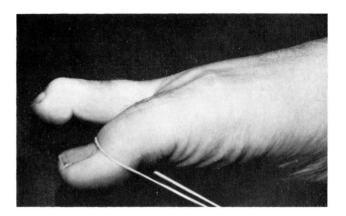

Figure 36–5. Swan-neck deformity of the second toe in a patient with rheumatoid arthritis.

metatarsal heads. In the late stages, these are usually palpable subcutaneously, especially those involving the three central proximal interphalangeal joints and metatarsal heads (see Figures 36–1B and 36–2B).

Hallux Valgus

With progressive splaying of the forefoot and ligamentous and capsular laxity, there is dynamic imbalance and bowstringing of the long extensor of the toe. The big toe typically drifts toward the fibula, resulting in hallux valgus, and at times overrides or underrides the lateral toes. This is usually made worse by the wearing of tight shoes. Hallux rigidus is usually superimposed on this. There is an associated adventitious

bursa over the tibial side of the first metatarsal head, without any significant underlying exostosis; and on rare occasions, there is a hallux varus deformity (Fig. 36–6).

Tarsal Joint Involvement

The subtalar, calcaneocuboid, and talonavicular joints are often involved in rheumatoid arthritis (Fig. 36–7A). In Vainio's study, 71.7 per cent of female patients and 58.2 per cent of male patients with rheumatoid arthritis demonstrated radiologic evidence of involvement of these joints.[44] Involvement of these joints leads to progressive valgus deformity of the hindfoot (Fig. 36–7B) and flattening of the longitudinal arch (Fig. 36–3), especially in pa-

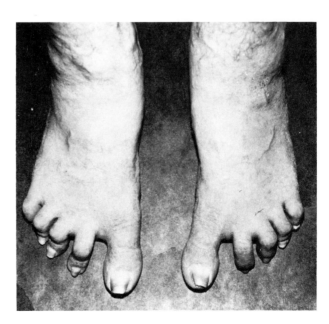

Figure 36–6. Hallux varus deformity.

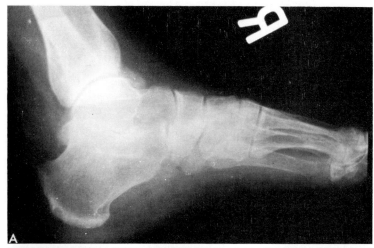

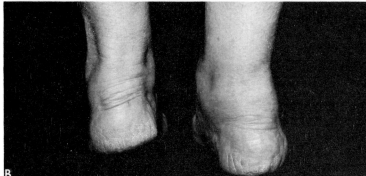

Figure 36–7. Rheumatoid involvement of the subtalar joint (A) leading to valgus deformity of the heel (B).

Figure 36–8. Varus deformity of the heel in a young patient with rheumatoid arthritis – an uncommon deformity.

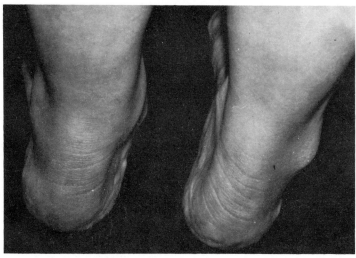

tients with lax ligaments. Sometimes involvement of all the tarsal joints results in total ankylosis (see Figure 36–3).

Varus deformity of the heel and cavovarus or calcaneocavus deformities are rare in rheumatoid arthritis (Fig. 36–8).

Tenosynovitis

As in the hand, tenosynovitis can be found in the foot in rheumatoid arthritis, although the incidence in the foot is relatively lower. Vainio[44] and Kellgren and Ball[25] found tenosynovitis of the foot in 6.5 per cent and 7 per cent of their cases, respectively. Vainio reported that 6.5 per cent of 955 patients had tendon involvement in the foot area.[44] Peroneal and posterior tibial tendons were most commonly involved, with 33 peroneal tendons as compared with 18 posterior tibial tendons

being affected in his study. The tibialis anterior and toe extensors and flexors are less commonly involved.

Tenosynovitis is usually painless and rarely causes a tendon rupture in the foot (Fig. 36–9). It may occasionally cause triggering of the toe.

Bursitis and Nodules

Retrocalcaneal bursitis, tendo-Achillis tenosynovitis, plantar fasciitis, and plantar calcaneal rheumatoid nodules are not infrequent in rheumatoid arthritis. Tendon nodules in the foot can also be found, as in the hand, causing limited range of motion and triggering. Occasionally, a Morton's neuroma is also seen. Bywaters documented 19 cases of heel lesions in rheumatoid arthritis clinically and radiologically.[4] He also presented three pathologic studies of subAchilles bursitis and rheumatoid arthritis nodules on the plantar aspect of the heel.

Special Problems in Rheumatoid Arthritis

Rheumatoid Vasculitis

An increasing number of necrotizing arteritides are being reported in patients with rheumatoid arthritis. These patients usually have a very high titer of rheumatoid factor. Katz has categorized four different types of vasculitis in rheumatoid patients[20]:

1. Vascular congestion of synovial membrane

2. Obliterative endarteritis

3. Subacute inflammation of small-sized vessels

4. Fulminating vasculitis

In the foot, the main concerns are obliterative endarteritis and subacute inflammation of small and medium-sized vessels. The former leads to splinter hemorrhages in the nail and pulp and frank digital gangrene. The subacute inflammation of small vessels usually presents as polyneuropathy, skin ulceration, infarctions, and purpura.

Before undertaking any major surgery, in these patients, a vascular consultation should be obtained, and if there is any doubt about diagnosis, an arteriographic evaluation should be performed. Other-

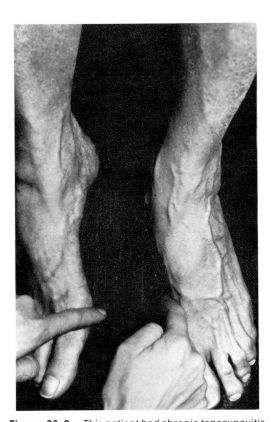

Figure 36–9. *This patient had chronic tenosynovitis of the posterior tibial tendon. After one local steroid injection into the tendon sheath, a valgus deformity of the foot developed owing to rupture of posterior tibial tendon. The lack of inversion of the left foot against minimal resistance is shown.*

wise, major skin flap or even the toes might be lost.

The treatment of rheumatoid vasculitis is not very satisfactory. Nail fold lesions usually do not require any special treatment. Newly developing acute ulcers respond fairly well to corticosteroid therapy. Extensive skin ulceration, visceral lesions, and neuropathy are usually the indications to administer immunosuppressive drugs and penicillamine. Appropriate antibiotics and good local wound care also help to control the infection.

Neuropathies

Rheumatoid neuropathies have also been classified by Katz into the following groups[20]:
1. Peripheral sensory neuropathy
2. Sensory-motor neuropathy
3. Entrapment neuropathies
4. Cervical myelopathy
5. Drug-induced neuropathies

Peripheral sensory neuropathy primarily affects the feet and presents as paresthesias in a stocking-type distribution. This is sometimes manifested in the hands. It is usually associated with other extra-articular manifestations of rheumatoid arthritis, e.g., rheumatoid arthritis nodules.

Sensory-motor neuropathy is usually the result of necrotizing arteritis of the vasa nervorum and causes marked signs of sensory and motor disturbance, e.g., complete footdrop or wristdrop.

Entrapment syndrome in the upper extremities is very common in rheumatoid arthritis, but occasionally tarsal tunnel syndrome can be present in the foot owing to involvement of the posterior tibial nerve around the medial side of the foot, or footdrop can exist owing to involvement of the common peroneal nerve around the fibular neck or in the popliteal area.

Cervical myelopathy is usually secondary to atlantoaxial or subaxial subluxation with compression of the spinal cord, and it is manifested in different ways. Thus, thorough neurologic and radiologic examinations of the cervical spine are essential.

Nonoperative Management of Pain and Foot Deformities in Rheumatoid Arthritis

In the early stages, painful synovitis of the metatarsophalangeal and tarsal joints and tenosynovitis will usually respond to a medical regimen. The patient might require local measures to relieve pressure from these painful areas. The usual physical measures used for management of any painful foot must be kept in mind. Considerable periods of rest to relieve these joints from weight bearing, along with proper footwear, padding, and supports, are helpful. The patient should be advised to wear low-heeled shoes with a wider

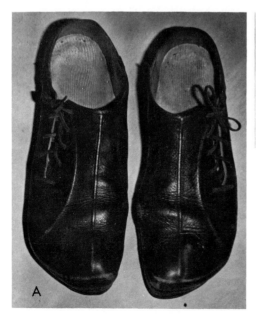

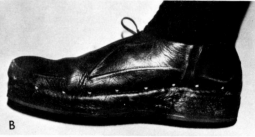

Figure 36–10. (A and B) Space shoes made for a patient with moderate toe deformities and metatarsalgia. So far, the patient has remained pain-free.

toe-box, soft uppers, strong counters, longitudinal arch supports, and appropriate metatarsal weight-relieving pads. The foot inserts can be custom made and can also be made so that they can be used in more than one pair of shoes. If all the metatarsophalangeal joints are painful, I personally recommend a metatarsal bar outside the shoe. I occasionally recommend space shoes, which are custom-made from a plaster-of-Paris mold of the non–weight-bearing foot. The shoe is then made according to the exact shape of the foot, and weight is distributed evenly without distortion (Fig. 36–10).

Mild valgus deformity of the heel can be managed fairly well with proper shoes that have a one-eighth-inch inner heel wedge. Sometimes I prescribe a Thomas heel, although occasionally a UCB shoe insert is needed to control the hindfoot valgus. If there is too much valgus of the hindfoot and it is passively correctable, a short leg orthosis with an outside upright (bar) and an inner T-strap will control the deformity. If the ankle is also involved, a short leg orthosis with two uprights (a double-bar ankle-foot orthosis) would be required. Some patients would object to using these devices, especially one who has poor hand function or in whom there is involvement of other major joints in the lower extremity. If the patient does use an orthosis, however, both the surgeon and the patient can understand and appraise the effect that surgical stabilization would have on the patient's functional capacity and comfort.

Apart from appropriate anti-inflammatory drugs and analgesics, local instillation of corticosteroids into the painful joints, tendon sheaths, bursae, and tender nodules is a good adjunct to conservative nonoperative therapy. I have injected all the metatarsophalangeal joints at the same sitting, with excellent results. This was done in the patients who had painful synovitis of the metatarsophalangeal joints without fixed deformities. One could inject one or two joints in the foot under local anesthetic, but to inject all the metatarsophalangeal joints under local anesthetic is a rather painful procedure, for the needle is not always able to enter the joint on the first attempt. Under mild Pentothal anesthesia, however, it takes barely two minutes to inject all the metatarsophalangeal joints.

Under general anesthesia, the patient has no pain. The joint can be distracted with traction, which makes needle entry into the joint very easy, and a successful injection is always followed by straightening of the toe when the solution distends the joint cavity. The metatarsophalangeal joint is best entered from the dorsal side. In our system, we are not able to bring the patient in as a day case to do multiple injections under general anesthetia. It is not very economical, and all the relevant investigations that are prerequisites to any general anesthesia would have to be performed. The other alternative would be to do these multiple injections under regional ankle block.

Surgery of the Rheumatoid Foot

Surgery is indicated when nonoperative means fail to relieve pain. Sones has said, "From surgery we hope to achieve relief of pain, prevention of destruction of cartilage or tendon, and improvement of overall joint function by increasing or decreasing joint motion, by correction of deformities, by increasing stability, by improving effective muscle forces or by some combination of these measures."[41] Once destruction of cartilage starts, it usually cannot be halted by surgical means. Occasionally, there is an indication for therapeutic tenosynovectomy, but usually the surgery in the foot is performed as a salvage procedure. The main aims are to relieve pain and correct deformities so that the patient can walk comfortably. The extent and type of surgery will depend upon the extent of the painful deformity.

Foot surgery should also be considered in context with the other joints in the lower extremity. If one is planning to do a hip or knee arthroplasty in a patient who has painful forefeet, my advice would be to treat the forefeet first. There are two reasons for this. First, if the foot is painful, the patient is not going to be very comfortable when walking. Second, because the feet are the most dependent part of the extremity, the venous and lymphatic drainage from an area of delayed healing or the unfortunate incidence of infection in the foot can put the prosthetic device in the proximal joints into great jeopardy. I have also noted that patients presenting for forefoot arthroplasty sometimes have low-grade, infected, ingrown toenails. In this case, the infected toenail should be treated first with standard operative procedures, and once that has been achieved, then, and only then, should surgery on the foot be planned. I always look for potential sources of infection in rheumatoid patients prior to any major surgery. Make sure the patient does not have any draining rheumatoid nodules, infected ingrown toenails, drainage from calluses, an infected tooth, or a urinary tract infection.

Surgery on the foot is usually performed under general or spinal anesthesia. Occasionally, a regional block can be utilized for small procedures on the toes. Those patients who are receiving steroid medications or who have received steroids in the past should be managed with supplementary steroids both preoperatively and postoperatively to prevent adrenal gland suppression. I have not used antibiotics routinely for foot surgery.

Preoperatively, flexion-extension lateral radiographic views of the cervical spine should be taken to determine its exact status. In the event of atlantoaxial subluxation, the patient should undergo neurologic examination and should go to the operating room wearing a soft cervical collar to alert the anesthesiologist to the neck problem. Routine and weight-bearing radiographs of both feet should be available prior to surgery. I also recommend the use of a tourniquet, which facilitates surgery and reduces operating time. If surgery is planned on both feet, double teams will cut the surgery time by half.

Procedures

The type of surgical procedures and their indications vary according to the individual's problems and deformities.

Painful Synovitis of Metatarsophalangeal Joints. I have no experience with synovectomy of the small joints of the feet. By the time orthopaedists see the patients with synovitis of the metatarsophalangeal joints, it usually has gone beyond the stage of any therapeutic synovectomy.

Raunio and Laine have reported their experience with synovectomy of the metatarsophalangeal joints of 33 feet (28 patients, five bilateral cases) in rheumatoid arthritis and claimed to have had fairly good results.[36] With regard to relief of pain and radiologic changes, the results were similar; that is, two-thirds were good, one-sixth were satisfactory, and one-sixth were poor, but their longest follow-up was two years, with the average being one and a half years. These results were also influenced by the disease activity; the results improved if the disease remitted and vice versa. The synovectomy of the second to fifth metatarsophalangeal joints was performed through a dorsal transverse incision and then entry to each metatarsophalangeal joint was made longitudinally on one side of the extensor tendon.

Splaying of the Forefoot. Rheumatoid patients usually notice gradual spreading of the forefeet, such that they have to be fitted with wider and wider shoes. Patients usually do not complain of splaying until they develop painful hallux valgus, tailor's bunion, or claw toes with metatarsalgia. Joplin has recommended a sling operation to decrease the splaying.[18] I cannot see the tendon being used as a sling to resist stretching under the weight bearing of the body. Furthermore, this procedure still does not deal with the joint disease, which is the primary problem in rheumatoid arthritis. Joplin also discussed two successful case histories in detail with fairly long follow-ups.[18] In addition to the sling procedure, he also performed proximal interphalangeal arthrodeses with dorsal capsulotomies of the metatarsophalangeal joints and extensor tenotomies to correct the hammer-toe deformities.

I have not recommended correction of painless splaying. In late cases, with excision of metatarsal heads, the forefoot is considerably narrower and can be fitted into relatively normal width shoes.

Morton's Neuroma. If Morton's neuroma is diagnosed and is found to be an isolated problem, it can be excised by any standard approach with predictable good results.

Painful Nodule. A painful nodule over the weight-bearing area in a rheumatoid foot or one interfering with footwear can be excised if the need arises, but they are usually managed nonoperatively.

Isolated Toe Deformity. Table 36–3 outlines some of the standard procedures used for isolated toe deformities in rheumatoid arthritis. Isolated hammer-toe deformity with a painful callus over the dorsum of the proximal interphalangeal joint, without fixed hyperextension contracture of the metatarsophalangeal joint, or with a plantar callus under the metatarsal head is best managed by tenotomy of the long extensor tendon, dorsal capsulotomy of the metatarsophalangeal joint, if necessary, and arthrodesis of the proximal interphalangeal joint. I usually prefer to fuse the proximal interphalangeal joint through a dorsal transverse elliptical incision, excising the callus. The capsule is incised transversely. The joint surface is exposed and removed, and adequate bone is removed

to correct the deformity. The bones are then apposed and fixed with an intramedullary Kirschner wire, which is usually left in for three to six weeks. Even pseudarthrosis in slight flexion is very functional and is usually more desirable then an absolutely straight toe (Fig. 36–11). If there is enough flexion deformity of the distal interphalangeal joint of the toe as well, both interphalangeal joints should be fixed in neutral position. In a hammer-toe deformity without metatarsalgia, I have also obtained good results by performing extension tenotomy, capsulotomy of the metatarsophalangeal joint, and excision of the condyles of the proximal phalanx.

TABLE 36–3. Operations for the Isolated Toe Problems in Rheumatoid Arthritis

YEAR	AUTHOR	ISOLATED HALLUX VALGUS	FLEXIBLE CLAW TOE	FIXED CLAW TOE WITH METATARSO-PHALANGEAL CONTRACTURE	HAMMER TOE WITH PRESSURE OVER THE TIP
1904, 1912	Keller	Proximal hemi-phalangectomy of first toe for hallux valgus bunions			
1937	Thompson	Keller procedure	Proximal interphalangeal arthrodesis	Excision of metatarsal heads	
1950	Key	Modified Keller procedure	Excision of distal half of proximal phalanx, extensor tenotomy, and capsulotomy	Proximal hemiphalangectomy or excision of metatarsal head or both	Distal interphalangeal resection of middle phalanx
1959	DuVries		Plantar condylectomy of metatarsal head for plantar keratosis		
1963	Marmor	Keller procedure	Proximal interphalangeal arthrodesis		
1964	Schwartz-mann		Interphalangeal fusion in flexion		Terminal Syme amputation
1967	Clayton	Keller procedure	Extensor tenotomy	Proximal interphalangeal arthrodesis or partial proximal phalangectomy	Terminal Syme amputation
1969	Thomas		Metatarsal osteotomy for metatarsalgia		
1971	Benson and Johnson	Keller procedure or arthrodesis of metatarsophalangeal joint		Proximal interphalangeal arthrodesis or proximal phalangectomy	
1973	Murray and Inman			Modified DuVries procedure and excision of distal half of proximal phalanx	

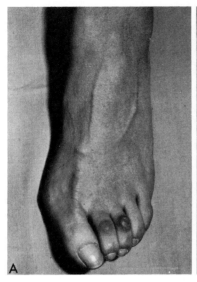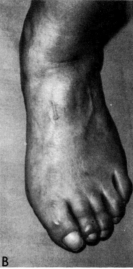

Figure 36–11. *(A) This patient with early rheumatoid arthritis developed painful, isolated hammer toes and callosities. (B) Postoperative appearance following extensor tenotomy and proximal interphalangeal joint fusion. The patient is very pleased with the results.*

An isolated, marked, fixed flexion deformity of the distal interphalangeal joint with a painful callus at the tip can be managed either by a terminal Syme amputation of the toe, removing the distal phalanx and the toenail, or by a dorsal wedge resection of the distal interphalangeal joint, removing as much bone from middle phalanx as is necessary to bring the distal part of the toe into neutral position.

Isolated Hallux Valgus or Hallux Rigidus. This isolated painful deformity of the big toe is best handled by a routine Keller arthroplasty.[24]

Flexible Metatarsalgia. When a patient with rheumatoid arthritis presents with metatarsalgia (pain under the three central metatarsals) and the metatarsophalangeal joint is actively and passively reducible, the patient can be helped by recession-and-dorsal-angulation osteotomy of the metatarsals. Thomas reported that after metatarsal osteotomy, 35 of his 39 patients (90 per cent)[42] had relief of pain. The plantar calluses disappeared, and it was noted that the cocked-up toe deformity was also partially corrected. Joplin recommended peg-and-hole shortening and angulation osteotomy for flexible metatarsalgia.[18] Metatarsal osteotomy should not be performed when the metatarsophalangeal joint is ankylosed or fixed permanently.

Fixed Hallux Valgus and Claw Toes

As discussed previously, many cases of rheumatoid involvement of the foot eventually demonstrate splaying of the forefoot,

hallux valgus, and fixed clawing of the lateral four toes, with painful calluses under the metatarsal heads and over the flexed proximal interphalangeal joints. Pain arises from abnormal weight bearing and mechanical rubbing against shoes, and these patients feel as if they are walking over pebbles or marbles. The toes have lost their normal function in gait. They are not "springy" any more and do not participate in push-off; actually these patients plant their feet as a unit and avoid or, in fact, are unable to have normal heel-toe gait. These feet cannot be fitted into any ordinary shoes.

The role of surgery has been well outlined by Key:

The surgeon is not attempting to return the foot to normal conditions. He is merely attempting to so change its contour that an ordinary shoe which is properly fitted can be worn without causing undue pressure at one or several points, to restore movement to joints where this is desirable and to correct deformities or remove bones which are subjected to undue pressure with weight bearing and cause painful calluses in the skin.[26]

Many surgeons have resected metatarsal heads for various local foot problems at the metatarsophalangeal joints, but as far as surgery of the forefoot in rheumatoid arthritis is concerned, the credit goes to Hoffman, who, in a paper presented to the American Orthopaedic Association in 1911 and later published in 1912,[16] detailed "an operation for severe grades of contracted or clawed toes" and thereby gave us the understanding of forefoot resection arthroplasty and an excellent description of toe deformities. In his discussion, he stated that the operation "is simply to get rid of the metatarsal heads, because they make the patient's life miserable." His operation consists of excision of all the metatarsal heads of the toes and, if necessary, part of the metatarsal necks. He regained the soft-tissue length by resecting bone.

Utilizing the Keller principle of proximal hemiphalangectomy,[24] some surgeons have extended this to the other toes with some trimming of the metatarsal heads.

Key stressed that "deformities are corrected by extensive removal of bone, and movement is restored to joints by wide excision rather than by meticulous arthroplasties."[26]

Over the years, various combinations of resections of metatarsophalangeal joints have been done through various types of incisions. Every surgeon has his own preference. I have summarized the different kinds of bone resections and the incisions in Table 36–4.

Fowler,[14, 15] Kates and associates,[19] and Clayton[6-9] have further strengthened the principle of adequate bone resection. Fowler recommended proximal hemiphalangectomies of the toes and trimming of the metatarsal heads.[14] Clayton established the procedure of excision of all the metatarsal heads and the bases of the proximal phalanges of the first four toes.[6-9] He gives credit to Aufranc[2] for this procedure, except that Aufranc did not remove the first metatarsal head or the base of the proximal phalanx of the fifth toe. Larson[28] and Rhinelander[37] preferred a similar procedure — metatarsophalangeal joint resection of the lateral four toes and Keller's procedure of the first toe. Clayton himself stressed that for severe cases, all metatarsal heads and portions of metatarsal necks should be removed in addition to removal of the proximal halves of the proximal phalanges of the first through fourth toes.[9] Peterson recommended excision of the metatarsophalangeal joints of all five toes in severe fixed deformities of the toes.[34]

Kates and coworkers again followed the principle of Hoffmann and reported good results with excision of all the five metatarsal heads.[19] I have also been very pleased with the results of this procedure.

As shown in Table 36–5, various incisions have been used to achieve this resection arthroplasty. I have become accustomed to doing resection of all the metatarsal heads through a longitudinal incision for the first toe and through transverse dorsal incision for the second through fifth toes.

Forefoot Arthroplasty. I have seen the results of various types of resections and different kinds of incisions. All incisions, whether plantar, dorsal, longitudinal, or transverse, heal equally well. Great care must be taken during retraction to avoid unnecessary pressure on the skin edges from the retractors, and electrocauterization must be used very carefully.

If surgery is planned on one foot, the patient has to be warned that that foot is going to be one size smaller than before the operation. Usually, both feet are involved and require surgery, allowing for conformity of size. I prefer to operate on both feet at the same time, using a two-team approach. This reduces the anesthesia time by half, and it is much more economical. I have not found any increase in morbidity or postoperative discomfort by doing this. These patients are very apprehensive about surgery and think they might not be able to walk for a long time. I allay their fears by taking time to explain the procedure and to assure them that they will be on their feet within a few days of the operation, giving them some statistical results. Always explain the possible complications, especially the occasional need for re-operation, no matter how small the incidence may be.

OPERATIVE PROCEDURE. Under general or spinal anesthesia and tourniquet control, the feet are draped and prepared in a standard fashion. The interphalangeal joints of the toes are manipulated with gentle intermittent pressure to achieve some passive correction of the toe deformities.

A transverse dorsal incision proximal to the web spaces of the second to fifth toes is made through the skin. The deeper dissection is done in a longitudinal fashion to avoid injury to the dorsal veins. Extensor tendons are usually left alone. The second metatarsal shaft is palpated, and the extensor tendons are retracted appropriately on either side. The neck of the metatarsal is exposed subperiosteally, and Davis or

TABLE 36–4. Forefoot Surgery

YEAR	AUTHOR	RESECTION OF BONE	INCISION
1912	Hoffmann	Excision of all metatarsal heads	Plantar transverse
1912	Keller	Proximal hemiphalangectomy of first toe	Longitudinal, inside of foot
1937	Thompson	Tenotomies; proximal phalangectomy; proximal interphalangeal fusion; excision of metatarsal head	Individual toe surgery
1950	Key	Proximal hemiphalangectomy of all five toes, with or without excision of metatarsal heads	Plantar
1951	Larmon	Proximal phalangectomy and plantar condylectomy of second to fifth toes; proximal hemiphalangectomy of first toe	Three dorsal (amputation of little toe, if necessary)
1956	Leavitt	Proximal phalangectomy; plantar condylectomy	Plantar, with excision of wedge of skin
1957, 1960	Fowler	Proximal hemiphalangectomy of all five toes; trimming of all metatarsal heads	Dorsal transverse, cut all extensor tendons and remove plantar wedge of skin
1959, 1960, 1963, 1967	Clayton	Proximal hemiphalangectomy of first to fourth toes; excision of all metatarsal heads	Dorsal transverse
1960	Flint and Sweetnam	Amputation of all toes (authors give credit to other surgeons)	Long plantar flap
1961	Aufranc	Proximal hemiphalangectomy of first to fourth toes; excision of second to fifth metatarsal heads	Dorsal S-shaped for the second to fifth toes; longitudinal for first toe
1963	Marmor	Proximal hemiphalangectomy of all toes; excision of all metatarsal heads	Dorsal transverse
1964	Schwartzmann	Excision all metatarsal heads; occasional proximal phalangectomy	Dorsal transverse or multiple longitudinal
1965	Kelikian	Proximal hemiphalangectomy; excision of metatarsal heads; syndactylization of toes	Dorsal multiple longitudinal
1967	Kates et al.	Excision of all metatarsal heads	Plantar transverse, with excision of wedge of skin
1968	Peterson	Proximal hemiphalangectomy of all toes; excision of all metatarsal heads	Dorsal transverse, with or without extensor tenotomy of the second to fifth toes
1968	Lipscomb	Proximal hemiphalangectomy of all toes; plantar condylectomy of all metatarsal heads	Three dorsal; extensor tenotomy of the second to fifth toes
1969	Joplin	Sling procedure for splayed foot; excision of all metatarsal heads in fixed deformities	Multiple
1971	Benson and Johnson	Proximal hemiphalangectomy of all toes or proximal phalangectomy of second to fifth toes; plantar condylectomy of all metatarsal heads	Three dorsal longitudinal; extensor tendon divided
1971	Jones	Resection of second to fifth metatarsal heads and proximal hemiphalangectomy of first toe, or resection of the metatarsophalangeal joints	Dorsal, plantar
1972	Lipscomb et al.	Proximal hemiphalangectomy of all toes; plantar condylectomy of all metatarsal heads	Three dorsal longitudinal; extensor tenotomy of second to fifth toes; Z-lengthening of extensor hallucis longus
1973	DuVries	Arthrodesis of first metatarsophalangeal joint; excision of bases of proximal phalanges of lesser toes	Two dorsal longitudinal
1978	Kelikian	Fusion of first metatarsophalangeal joint; excision of metatarsal heads of lesser toes; syndactylization of toes	Dorsal multiple longitudinal

TABLE 36–5. Various Incisions for Forefoot Arthroplasty

1. Dorsal transverse incision (single)[6–9, 32, 34, 39]
2. Dorsal longitudinal incisions (multiple)[3, 21, 27, 30, 31, 39]
3. Dorsal transverse incision for the second to fifth toes and longitudinal incision for the first metatarsophalangeal joint[2]*
4. Dorsal transverse incisions with division of all the tendons, along with plantar wedge resection of skin[14, 15]
5. Plantar incision (transverse)[16, 26, 29]
6. Plantar transverse incision with wedge resection of skin[19, 26]

*Incision preferred by author.

small Chandler retractors are inserted subperiosteally on each side of the metatarsal to protect the soft tissues. Then, with sharp dissection, the dorsal capsule of the metatarsophalangeal joint is incised transversely, and the metatarsal head is exposed into the wound by manual flexion of the toe. With the help of a small bone cutter or motor saw, the metatarsal is osteotomized near the neck, and the head is removed by sharp dissection. At times, the head is very adherent to surrounding soft tissues, extremely osteoporotic, and crumbly. It has to be removed piecemeal, making sure no loose piece is left. The cut end of the metatarsal shaft is then smoothed with a small rongeur until no sharp edges can be felt.

The third, fourth, and fifth metatarsal necks are then exposed in a similar fashion. The level of resection is determined by visual alignment with the cut end of the second metatarsal, and all the metatarsals are cut at the same level, one by one, with the cut ends being smoothed as described before.

At the end of this stage, one should make sure that the toes fall into good alignment without any tension and that all metatarsals are cut at the same level. This is the time to do a little more trimming of bone, if necessary.

Attention is then turned to the first metatarsophalangeal joint, which is exposed through a dorsomedial longitudinal incision, deepening the incision through the capsule of the first metatarsophalangeal joint longitudinally. The medial capsule and bursa are then raised as one layer with sharp dissection, and the first metatarsal head and neck are exposed. Soft tissues are protected on each side by Chandler retractors. The first metatarsal head is osteotomized at the same level as the other metatarsals, and the cut end of the metatarsal is smoothed with a rongeur. The adductor hallucis is then released from the proximal phalanx. The big toe is realigned and fixed with an intramedullary Kirschner wire, making sure there is no tension on the soft tissues (Fig. 36–12). Actually, the proximal phalanx is pushed close to the cut end of the metatarsal to avoid any strangulation of the digital vessels by distraction. No soft tissue is interposed. If there is a severe hallux valgus deformity, the extensor hallucis longus tendon might have to be lengthened by Z-plasty. If the first

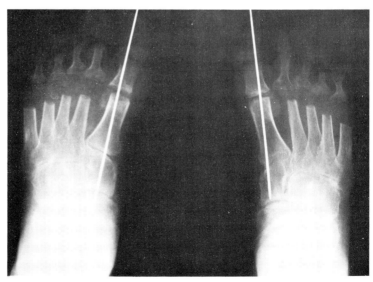

Figure 36–12. Radiograph taken immediately after excision of the metatarsal heads showing that there is no distraction of the first toe after insertion of an intramedullary wire.

metatarsal appears too short in the radiographs, the base of the proximal phalanx of the first toe should be removed (Keller procedure) instead of the head of the first metatarsal.

The wound is irrigated, and a final check is made on the level of resection of the metatarsals to make sure they are all at the same level. The wound is then closed loosely with interrupted sutures.

Postoperative dressings are very important. First dressings are essentially bulky compression dressings. Apart from the tips of the toes, the entire foot and ankle are encased in the dressing. Care should be taken not to put too much fluffed gauze between the toes, for it can cause pressure on the skin or become very hard if soaked with blood. The tourniquet is then removed, and the surgeon should make sure that all the toes have adequate circulation.

Postoperatively, the patient's feet are kept elevated at all times. After two to three days, the patient is allowed to walk a very short distance, for example, to the bathroom. On the fourth or fifth day, the original dressings are changed, and the lateral toes are bandaged and taped downward and toward the first toe. Another compression dressing is applied. The patient is fitted with commercially available postoperative shoes (Fig. 36–13). At this point, the patient stays in bed most of the time, keeping the foot elevated to control postoperative edema but is occasionally allowed to walk short distances with the help of a walker or crutches. By the end of a week or so, the patient is usually walking fairly independently and is discharged from the hospital if there is help available at home. The dressings are changed whenever they feel loose. The stitches and Kirschner wire are removed from the first toe after two weeks.

The patient and his family are taught how to apply dressings and tape to keep the lateral toes in a downward position and toward the big toe, which is itself taped down and in a slightly varus position. The patient can usually soak and clean the feet every third or fourth day and change the dressing. It requires only a 2-inch wide Kling bandage and one 4-inch Ace bandage for each foot and 1-inch and 0.5-inch wide adhesive tape. I usually stress to the

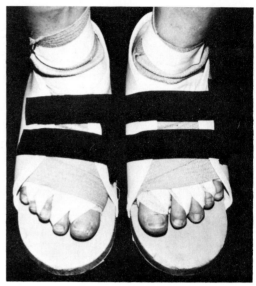

Figure 36–13. *Postoperative dressing and commercially available shoes that are worn after forefoot arthroplasty until the patient is ready to be fitted with regular shoes. These shoes are easy to handle. The black straps are made of Velcro.*

patient that he can gradually increase his activity but that he should still keep the feet elevated as much as possible. I check the patient's progress every two weeks for six weeks, at which time the toes have essentially settled into their final resting position and the patient is fitted with comfortable shoes. I usually recommend shoes with a moderately wide toe-box and low heels. Postoperatively, I have only rarely found it necessary to recommend weight-relieving paddings or metatarsal bars.

RESULTS. Forefoot arthroplasty is the most gratifying operation I know of for a rheumatoid patient. Patients are usually so pleased with the results of this procedure that if further surgery is necessary, they are likely to be very receptive. If indicated at all, I would prefer to operate on the feet of a rheumatoid patient first and thereby gain their confidence. In spite of the tremendous amount of surgery on the forefeet, there is relatively very little postoperative discomfort. The plantar calluses become soft and pain-free and usually disappear over the next two or three months. Patients usually have to readjust and learn a new gait, but they do not need any special instruction. Everyone adjusts readily to his or her own pace. The toes are

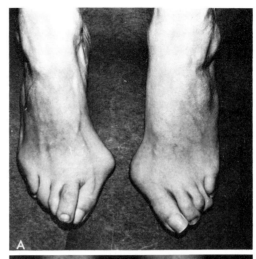

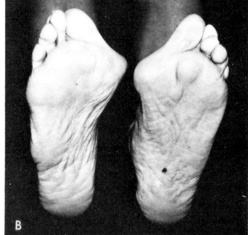

Figure 36–14. *(A–C) Preoperative clinical photographs and radiographs show typical rheumatoid changes – splaying hallux valgus, claw toes, and plantar callosities.*

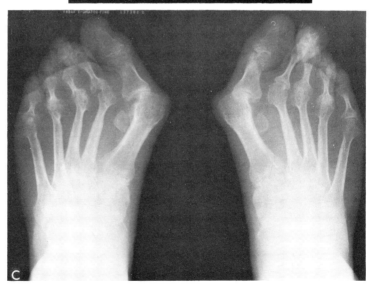

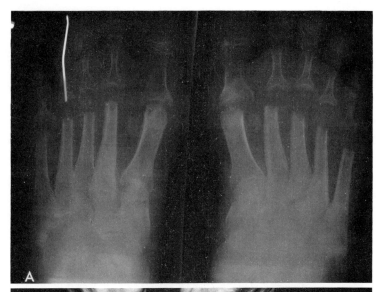

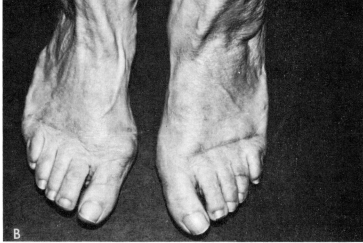

Figure 36–15. See legend on opposite page.

usually well-aligned and have active flexion and extension, but the tips of the toes generally do not touch the floor and do not participate at all in push-off (Figs. 36–14 and 36–15).

COMPLICATIONS. If proper care is taken in handling the soft tissues during surgery, I have not found any problem with wound healing. Healing is not any different in patients receiving steroid therapy from that in patients not receiving steroids. Transverse dorsal, plantar, or multiple longitudinal dorsal incisions all heal well, and one should use the incision or incisions one is familiar with.

If one of the metatarsals is left longer than the others, the patient may develop a recurrence of the painful plantar callus under the end of that long metatarsal

(usually the second or third) (Fig. 36–16). This can be managed by simply trimming the offending metatarsal shaft back to the level of the other metatarsals (Fig. 36–16B, C).

As described previously, a Kirschner wire is placed in the first toe for two weeks (see Figure 36–12). This helps to realign the first toe effectively, but care must be taken not to distract the toe, because that can cause strangulation of the digital vessels. There is no need to insert the wire into the phalanges and metatarsals of the other toes for alignment. That can be achieved by careful dressing and taping of the toes.

Excision of only one or two metatarsal heads should also be avoided, for this invites callus formation under the remain-

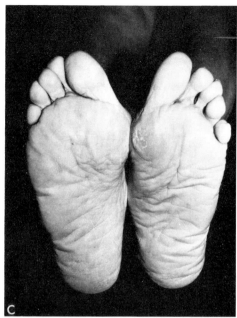

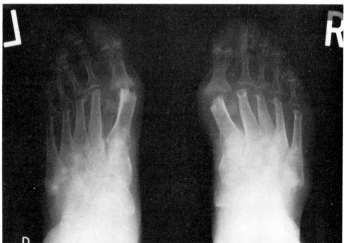

Figure 36–15. *Same patient as in Figure 36–14. (A) The amount of bone resected during forefoot arthroplasty. (B–D) Postoperative appearance of the feet after one year. The toes are well aligned; the plantar callosities have disappeared; and the patient has no pain or functional disability and wears regular shoes.*

ing metatarsal heads (Fig. 36–17). Less radical and more conservative surgery should be considered, such as metatarsal osteotomy with or without proximal hemiphalangectomy and syndactylization. As Clayton has pointed out, if more than three metatarsal heads require surgery, then resection arthroplasty of the entire forefoot provides better weight-bearing alignment.[9]

If the first metatarsal is short, one should not excise the first metatarsal head, but rather perform a regular Keller procedure for the first toe during forefoot arthroplasty.

Resection Arthroplasty. Larmon,[27] Leavitt,[29] Lipscomb,[30] Benson and Johnson,[3] and Lipscomb and associates[31] claimed to have obtained good results with proximal hemiphalangectomy and plantar condylectomy of the metatarsal heads. I have no experience with this procedure, but I have performed surgery on a few patients who had previously undergone this operation. Other authors have claimed good results from proximal hemiphalangectomy and excision of the metatarsal heads with some modifications.[2,6-9,14,15,32,34,43] Finally, Hoffmann,[16] Schwartzmann,[39] Kates and coworkers,[19] Joplin,[18] and Jones[17] report good results following excision of the metatarsal heads.

I prefer to excise all the metatarsal heads, when indicated. Occasionally,

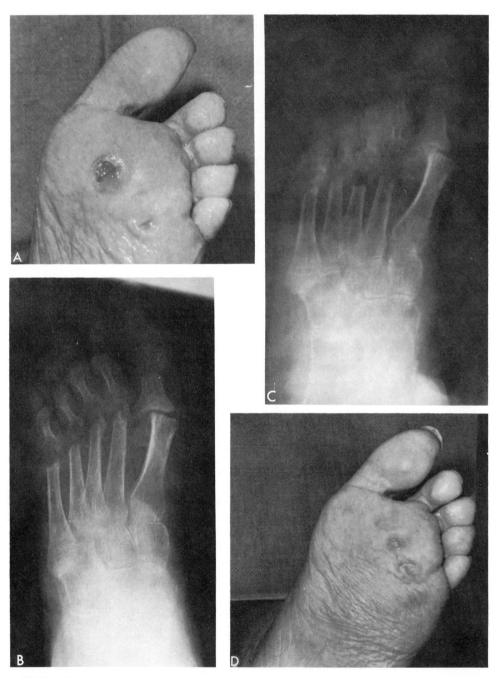

Figure 36–16. *(A) After excision of the metatarsal heads, this patient developed a recurrent callus and ulcer under the resected end of the second metatarsal. (B) A radiograph revealed that the second and third metatarsal shafts were longer than the others, leading to unequal pressure and ulcer formation. (C) Postoperative radiograph after the ends of second and third metatarsal shafts had been trimmed. (D) At the time of the follow-up examination, the pressure calluses and ulcer had disappeared. The callus was not excised at the time of surgery.*

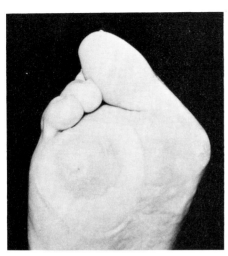

Figure 36–17. *Increasing deformities and pressure keratosis under the fourth and fifth metatarsal heads one year after excision of the second and third metatarsal heads.*

when the first metatarsal is short, I perform a Keller procedure on the first toe. I perform all the resection of bone from the metatarsal side and have found that toes in which all the phalanges have been maintained do not retract and have much better cosmetic appearance. Syndactylization is usually unnecessary.[21] With excision of all the metatarsal heads, especially the first and fifth, the foot is much narrower. I have not found any problem on weight bearing after excising the first metatarsal head in conjunction with the others. Actually, by removing the first metatarsal head, the joint between the sesamoid bones and the metatarsal head—another cause of pain—is also removed. Adequate resection of bone is the key to the success of the operation. Whether the bone is taken from both sides of the metatarsophalangeal joint or just the metatarsal side does not seem to make much difference, as long as there are no prominent down-pitched metatarsal heads and there is a large enough false joint.

Amputation of all the toes, as reported by Flint and Sweetnam,[13] is probably an effective procedure, but I do not think it is any more beneficial than resection arthroplasty of the metatarsal heads. Why sacrifice the toes, which are important cosmetically and esthetically to the patient and the doctor? Having to use toe fillers in the shoes is another drawback of toe amputation.

Midfoot and Hindfoot

As noted previously, Vainio found that 71.7 per cent of 443 female patients and 58.2 per cent of 196 male patients had involvement of the subtalar and midtarsal joints in rheumatoid arthritis.[44] Potter has stressed the importance of recognizing the arthritis in the tarsal joints as a cause of pain around the hindfoot and ankle area, leading to progressive flattening of longitudinal arch and valgus deformity of the hindfoot.[35] (See Figures 36–3, 36–7, and 36–18A). He reported good results in approximately 40 patients who underwent talonavicular fusion for localized talonavicular joint involvement. Clayton[9] and Jones[17] recommend subtalar (Grice-type) fusion or a Gallie-type posterior approach for arthrodesis when the midtarsal joint is mobile and pain-free and when the valgus deformity of the heel is passively correctable.

Painful involvement of the metatarsocuneiform joints is managed fairly well by local arthrodesis.[17]

When there is multiple joint involvement, there is general agreement that the problem is best solved by triple arthrodesis.[3, 9, 17] I also favor a triple arthrodesis for treatment of painful valgus deformity of the hindfoot (Fig. 36–18).

When evaluating hindfoot valgus, particular attention must be paid to the ankle joint to make sure some of the valgus deformity is not secondary to ankle deformity. If that is the case, the patient would also require an operative procedure on the ankle, i.e., pantalar fusion or arthroplasty of the ankle, as a second-stage procedure following triple arthrodesis.

I have also seen very acceptable results from talectomy performed when there is pantalar involvement in rheumatoid arthritis. Murray and Inman also favor talectomy for pantalar arthritis.[33]

All the other joints in the lower extremity should also be elevated before stabilization of the hindfoot or ankle is performed, because hip and knee alignment have marked influence on the foot. Therefore, if the hip and knee require surgical correction, those joints should be operated on first, with the ankle or hindfoot stabilization procedure considered afterward, so as

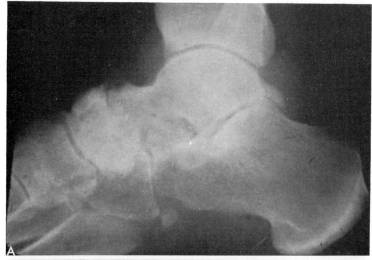

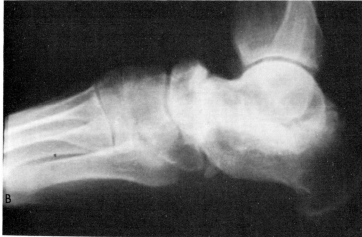

Figure 36–18. *Radiographs of the foot of a patient with painful rheumatoid involvement of the subtalar and talonavicular joints who underwent triple arthrodesis with excellent results. (A) Preoperative radiograph. (B) Postoperative radiograph.*

to have a good final weight-bearing alignment.

In local fusions (stabilization procedures in the foot), additional bone graft material from the tibia or ilium should always be utilized, and this should be explained to the patient beforehand. During a triple arthrodesis in the presence of a mild valgus deformity, a bone graft is usually not required. Be prepared to use a bone graft, if necessary, however. Furthermore, do not hesitate to make an additional incision over the talonavicular joint. Sometimes it is also very difficult to correct severe valgus deformity of the heel because the base of the wedge faces away from the surgeon and the incision. I also favor the use of staples for internal fixation. In addition to clinical alignment with the entire lower extremity, the final align-

ment should also be checked radiographically prior to closure of the wounds.

RHEUMATOID ARTHRITIS OF THE ANKLE

The ankle is not a joint that is commonly affected by the rheumatoid inflammatory process. In Vainio's series of 955 rheumatoid patients, there were 57 females (9.2 per cent) and 27 males (8.0 per cent) who showed clinical involvement of the ankle joint.[58] Tenosynovitis and tendinitis around the ankle were found in 62 of the 955 patients in his series (tibialis anterior — 9; extensor digitorum longus — 8; peroneals — 33; and tibialis posterior —8). Vainio also noticed that the radiographic appearance of 79 out of 716 ankles had

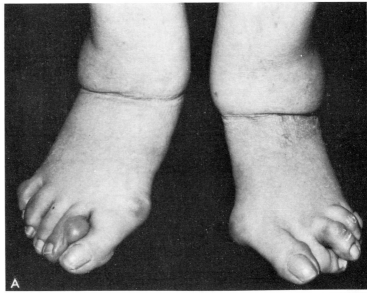

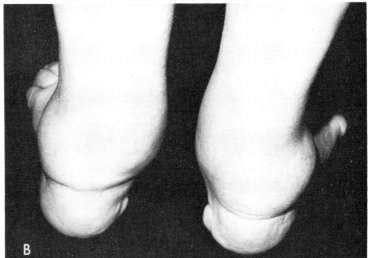

Figure 36–19. Clinical photographs (A and B) and radiograph (C) of a 56-year-old patient with rheumatoid arthritis with ankle involvement of 18 years' duration. The radiograph was taken during a routine joint survey. The anteroposterior radiograph shows involvement of both ankles. Despite the Grade IV changes in the left ankle, the patient had only mild discomfort and did not require any local treatment.

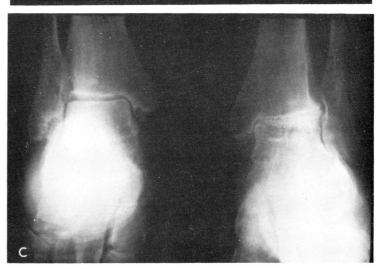

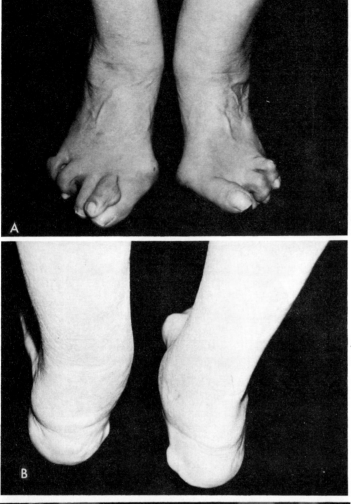

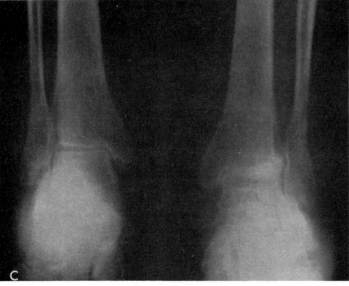

Figure 36–20. Improvement in the appearance of the ankles (A and B) and nearly the same radiologic changes (C) four years later in the same patient as in Figure 36–19. The patient still experienced no functional disability from her ankles.

changed, and in the majority of these patients the duration of the disease was at least seven years; thus radiologic changes in the ankle joint appear relatively late.[58]

Radiologic changes in the ankle usually do not correlate very well with clinical function (Figs. 36–19 and 36–20). There may be loss of articular cartilage in the ankle joint detected on routine radiologic survey of various joints, with either no complaints or minimal discomfort. The ankle joint becomes symptomatic when there is associated loss of subchondral bone and valgus or varus deformity of the ankle joint, the former being the most common. Occasionally, the ankle joint has a tendency toward spontaneous ankylosis. Vainio noticed that five females and two males out of 955 patients had no clinical motion of the ankle joint, and that six females and three males had only 10 degrees of motion.[58] He also commented that the bedridden patients had a tendency to develop plantar flexion contracture owing to the weight of the blankets, and that those patients who walked with two flexed knees had a tendency toward increasing dorsiflexion of the ankle joint.

Treatment

As mentioned before, the ankle joint is one of the less common symptomatic joints. A careful examination of a patient who complains of vague ankle and hindfoot pain will often pinpoint the problem in the other peritalar joints rather than the ankle joint. In a swollen ankle, it is sometimes difficult to differentiate whether the extensor tendons or the ankle joint is the site of synovial swelling.

Ankle joint synovitis responds fairly well to local intra-articular instillation of steroids. Fifty milligrams of hydrocortisone or an equivalent dose of Depo-Medrol or Aristospan is sufficient. This is usually mixed with a few cc of 1 per cent lidocaine (Xylocaine). The joint can be entered very easily through any part of the anterior capsule between the tendons. I prefer the anterolateral site just lateral to the common extensor tendons.

Pain due to hindfoot and ankle deformity can be managed effectively with a corrective below-the-knee orthosis, e.g., double uprights with a fixed ankle and a valgus corrective strap or a polypropylene orthosis. Occasionally, I will immobilize the ankle in a below-the-knee walking cast or orthosis not only to see the effect of immobilization but also to convince the patient of the effect of fusion prior to the actual ankle fusion procedure.

Synovectomy of the Ankle Joint

Jakubowski reported only five cases of synovectomy of the ankle joint performed out of curiosity during tenosynovectomy of the foot, and four of these patients maintained a good clinical result at the end of two years.[53] At the same time, he reported on synovectomies of other major joints in the body (13 hips, 122 knees, 11 elbows, 16 wrists). Vainio also mentions synovectomy of the ankle joint as a useful procedure in the presence of bulky synovitis without erosions on the weight-bearing areas.[59] Peterson stated that "synovectomy of the ankle is rarely considered necessary and normally would be done only in conjunction with additional surgery about the extensor tendons."[34] He further mentioned that synovectomy of the ankle may be indicated occasionally when symptomatic effusion fails to resolve. Clayton, in discussing surgery of the lower extremity in rheumatoid arthritis, mentioned in passing that the "ankle rarely needs fusion. Proper shoe supports and the occasional use of a double upright brace usually will relieve ankle pain. Sometimes later patients may be free of the braces."[48]

My experience has been the same as that of the above-mentioned authors. Therefore, if a patient has persistent chronic synovitis of the ankle joint or associated extensive tenosynovitis, synovectomy alone or combined with tenosynovectomy is indicated. I have found that the classic anterolateral approach is adequate for ankle synovectomy. If the tenosynovectomy is to be performed, then a midline anterior longitudinal incision is more desirable. After the tenosynovectomy is done, the tendons and neurovascular bundle are mobilized and retracted medially and laterally, and the ankle joint is exposed widely by opening the capsule longitudinally. Small rongeurs and pituitary rongeurs are very useful for this. I have also used two separate anterolateral and

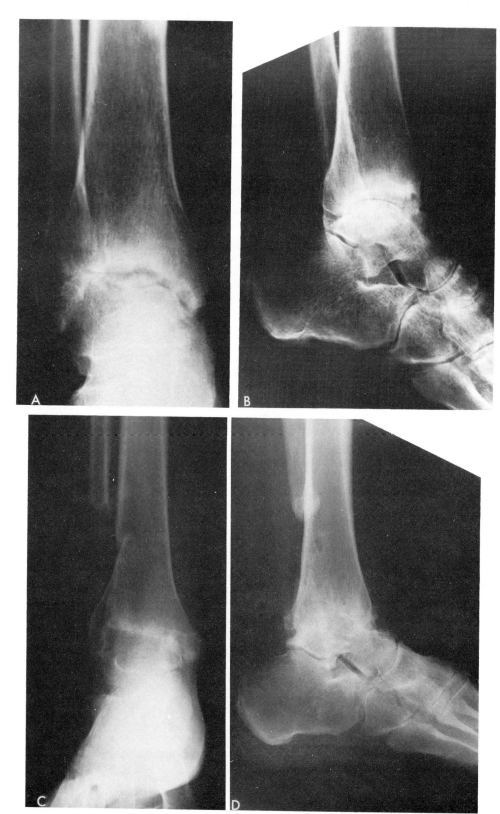

Figure 36–21. *A 54-year-old patient with rheumatoid arthritis had a painful forefoot and ankle joint. His ankle was fused in about five degrees of dorsiflexion. (A and B) Pre-operative rheumatoid changes. (C and D) Solid ankle fusion. Subsequently, the patient underwent forefoot arthroplasty. The patient is very happy with the outcome of both operations and has about 10 degrees of motion in the midtarsal joints, which remain pain-free.*

anteromedial incisions. After the synovectomy, the capsule is repaired, and the ankle is immobilized in compression dressings and a posterior splint. When the initial swelling has subsided, exercises to regain the range of motion are started, but the ankle is protected from weight bearing for about six weeks.

Arthrodesis of the Ankle

When the ankle is extremely painful, the joint is completely devoid of articular cartilage, and the subchondral erosion of the bone is advanced and interferes with the patient's walking, arthrodesis of the ankle is the treatment of choice (Fig. 36–21).[3, 17, 34, 59] Peterson stated, "Arthrodesis of the ankle functions so well that extensive measures to preserve function of the ankle are not warranted."[34] For an irreparable, painful ankle joint, my preference is arthrodesis of the ankle.

The arthrodesis may be achieved fairly easily in rheumatoid patients through any of the standard approaches — anterior, transfibular, and even posterior,[49] with or without compression apparatus. The surgeon should always use the approach with which he is most familiar. Charnley's compression clamps, when used properly, may help to achieve quicker fusion. I prefer to use the transfibular approach with Charnley's compression clamps.[46] The ankle joint is exposed through a lateral incision over the fibula. The fibula is divided approximately 3 inches from its distal tip and is dissected free subperiosteally, except its distal ligamentous attachments below the syndesmosis. The fibula is then turned down and wrapped in a moist sponge. There is a slight overhang of the tibial lip laterally, which is osteotomized. This permits a direct view of the tibiotalar surfaces. Using a motor saw, the joint surfaces are cut transversely to permit accurate contact of the two surfaces. A small additional anteromedial incision is made to make sure that the medial corner of the joint is completely roughened, and one should be able to slide the talus back either by cutting the deltoid ligament or by osteotomy of the medial malleolus. This is very important. Steinmann pins are then passed through the talus and the tibia, and the

compression apparatus is assembled. Sometimes a small Steinmann pin is passed through the heel into the tibia temporarily to maintain the final position. The position is checked radiographically to make sure that there is good contact and position with compression. The final position is very important. One should confirm that the talus is displaced posteriorly and that the ankle joint is fixed in neutral or even in five to 10 degrees of dorsiflexion. I prefer fixation in five to 10 degrees of dorsiflexion; the rheumatoid patient with forefoot involvement walks much better with the ankle joint in this position.

Attention is then directed to the fibula. The fibula is split longitudinally, and the inner half is removed. The lateral surface of the talus is roughened, and the remaining fibula is laid against it. The proximal end of this fibular portion is countersunk into the tibial shaft. The remaining fibula is cut into pieces and packed around the fusion site.

The wound is closed very loosely, and the leg is immobilized in compression dressings and posterior and anterior splints. A few days later, a short leg cast incorporating the compression clamp is applied. The patient does not bear weight on the leg for six to eight weeks, after which the compression apparatus is removed and a new short leg walking cast is applied. This cast has to be changed as needed, but the patient continues to wear it until solid radiologic union is achieved, which may take from three to six months.

If there is a considerable bone loss, the technique of Chuinard and Peterson[47] or that of Campbell and associates[45] may be advisable.

Pantalar Arthrodesis

If a rheumatoid patient has had a previous triple arthrodesis and now has a painful ankle, I would not hesitate to perform ankle fusion. Similarly, if the patient has painful peritalar arthritis (a rare situation), I recommend a primary pantalar fusion, either a one-stage or two-stage procedure, as suggested by Waugh and coworkers.[61] If a patient has multiple joint involvement in the same lower extremity and all of the joints require surgery, the hip and knee should be realigned first, and finally the ankle should be fused into normal weight-bearing alignment for that patient.

Talectomy

As mentioned previously, Murray and Inman prefer talectomy for treatment of pantalar arthritis when it is the dry, stiff type of arthritis.[33] I have observed good results from both pantalar fusion and talectomy in patients with rheumatoid arthritis.

Total Ankle Replacement Arthroplasty

Orthopaedic surgeons overstress the concept that a rheumatoid patient requires motion in every major joint of the lower extremities. The fact is that pain in the ankle, not loss of motion, is the main indication for surgery, and one of the major criteria for good results is relief of pain. That aim can be achieved with arthrodesis of the ankle. Patients who undergo this procedure get along very well, and there is no worry about the problems that pertain to total joint replacement in general, i.e., loosening, implant failure, increasing possibility of infection, and medial and lateral impingement syndrome in the ankle. Greenwald and associates have shown that the ankle joint is subject to forces of considerable magnitude, as much as five times the body's weight during normal walking.[50] There are compressive, medial, lateral shear, and rotational forces across the ankle joint.

Thomas has noted ever increasing numbers of radiolucent lines around total ankle implants,[57] the significance of which is not very clear. In relating this to the presence of radiolucent lines around other total joint replacement arthroplasties in the lower extremity, however, I can project future problems.

The proponents of arthroplasties of the ankle stress bad results of arthrodesis of the ankle, with the major problem being pseudarthrosis, and at the same time, they claim to have no problem at all in fusing an ankle following a failed arthroplasty. It is paradoxic that they have trouble fusing an ankle with good bone stock but have no problem with the fusion when there is bound to be extensive bone loss after removal of both the components of a failed total ankle arthroplasty and the methacrylate.

Morris and Herrick reported on 63 ankle fusions, and only five were performed for rheumatoid arthritis.[54] Heinig and DuPuy reported on 18 ankle fusions, and only one patient had rheumatoid arthritis.[52] With the advent of total ankle arthroplasty, we are suddenly seeing many ankle operations in patients suffering from rheumatoid arthritis. Groth and coworkers reported on 41 Oregon ankle arthroplasties; 13 were done for rheumatoid arthritis, with 100 per cent good results in those 13 cases.[51]

Segal and Stauffer gave their results on 102 Mayo total ankle arthroplasties, 43 of which were performed for rheumatoid arthritis.[56] The postoperative analysis of the rheumatoid patients showed 25 excellent, 13 good, one fair, and four poor results. The patients with good results experienced mild ankle pain. The average follow-up was 23 months the range being six to 44 months). They had to perform 24 re-operations in 20 patients in the entire series of 102 ankles for various reasons — medial and lateral impingement, five with loosening (4.9 per cent), three with deep infection (2.9 per cent), all in rheumatoid patients; four had delayed healing, and malleolar fractures were also noticed. The average postoperative range of motion in the ankle for all the patients in the series was 30 degrees, as compared with 24.5 degrees preoperatively. They also reported on 10 arthrodeses performed after ankle arthroplasty, with nine successful fusions. Their main indication for arthroplasty was to relieve the pain; the motion was only a secondary gain.

Samuelson and Tuke reported on 50 ICLH ankle arthroplasties, 21 of which were performed for rheumatoid arthritis.[55] In the entire series of patients, with follow-up ranging from six months to six years, 21 had mild or no pain, 16 had moderate pain requiring analgesics, and one had severe pain. Six cases were lost to follow-up. Function was increased in 21 cases and remained the same in 16 cases. There were 12 cases of delayed healing, two cases of infection, and two cases of collapsed talus. They also commented on the talomalleolar contact problem and noticed that there was less motion radiologically as compared with clinical measurement of motion and that 10 degrees of dorsiflexion was essential for a good functional arthroplasty.

Waugh compared the results of arthroplasty using his own prosthesis with those of arthrodesis of the ankle[62] and spoke in favor of the arthroplasty, giving the following indications for arthroplasty: (1) motivated older patient, (2) correctable deformity, (3) exercise tolerance less than a block of walking, and (4) willingness to accept arthrodesis as a salvage procedure. Contraindications included: (1) previous infection, (2) marginal circulation, (3) neuropathic joint, (4) weight over 200 lbs,

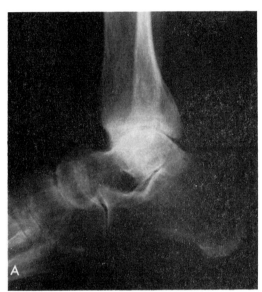

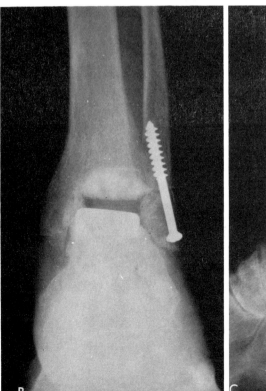

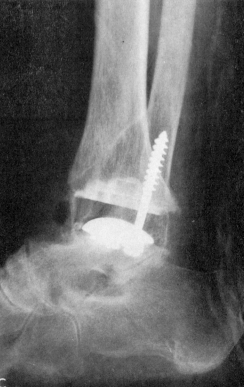

Figure 36–22. *(A) A radiograph of the painful left ankle of a 55-year-old patient with rheumatoid arthritis shows loss of articular cartilage in the ankle and talonavicular joints. (B and C) Total ankle arthroplasty done through a transfibular approach.*

Illustration continued on following page

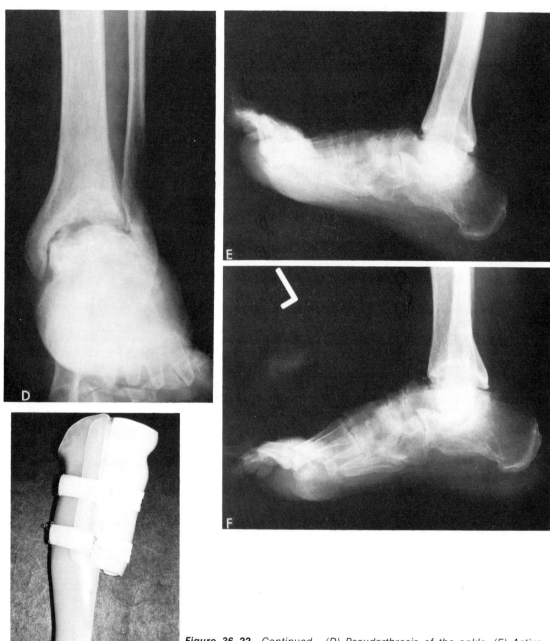

Figure 36–22 *Continued. (D) Pseudarthrosis of the ankle. (E) Active dorsiflexion of the ankle. (F) Active plantar flexion of the ankle. (G) The polypropylene splint used by the patient.*

and (5) inexperienced surgeon. The complications he cited included skin healing problems in rheumatoid patients. The complication rate was 5 per cent, with problems including loosening and poor wound healing. Most of the loosening of the prosthesis occurred on the tibial side. He also commented upon the tibiopedal range of motion in the ankle joint. There were 18 degrees, 45 degrees, and 60 degrees of tibiopedal motion following arthrodesis, arthroplasty of the ankle, and normal ankle, respectively.

It may be that I am biased against arthroplasty of the ankle, and I am inclined to agree with Waring that "arthroplasty of the ankle is never indicated, even when this joint and the tarsal and tarsometatarsal joints are ankylosed."[60] For the time being, fusion of an ankle in proper position is a functionally satisfactory procedure. I have already expressed my feelings about arthrodesis and arthroplasty of the ankle joint. I would like to reiterate that if the ankle joint is the only joint involved, then I would not hesitate to recommend ankle fusion. In a patient who has already undergone triple arthrodesis and then develops a painful ankle, I would still fuse the ankle, but this might be one indication for total ankle arthroplasty. It may be that in the years to come I will change my mind when a solution is found to the biomechanical problem surrounding ankle arthroplasty.

Greenwald and associates have analyzed at least 10 different types of ankle joint implants,[50] and there are many more available on the market. At this time, however, their use should be restricted to their inventors and to centers where the surgeons have access to large patient populations. I agree with Waugh[62] that the inexperience of the surgeon is one of the major contraindications for arthroplasty of the ankle. In my first case of ankle arthroplasty, in 1974, there were the problems of delayed healing and surgical infection, which caused considerable discouragement. The patient did regain a good range of motion and was pain-free but had to be kept on antibiotics, and any attempt at discontinuation of antibiotics would cause a flare-up of infection (*Staphylococcus aureus*, pseudomonas) and pain. Eventually, I had to remove the components and

purposely allowed the ankle to develop a pseudarthrosis. Four years following removal of the components, the patient remained free of any infection and had a very useful, essentially pain-free pseudarthrosis of the ankle joint (Fig. 36–22A–F). He has about 10 degrees of total excursion in the ankle joint. He walks around the house without an orthosis, but for outside activities he feels more confident using a polypropylene appliance (Fig. 36–22G).

JUVENILE RHEUMATOID ARTHRITIS

Juvenile rheumatoid arthritis is a chronic polyarthritis occurring in children and adolescents under 16 years of age. It usually affects the joints, tendon sheaths, and bursae. Because the cartilage covering the epiphyses in the patient of this age is thicker than that in the adult, the bone destruction is long delayed and the disease remains in a reversible stage for a long time.[63] General retardation of growth may be severe if the disease is widespread. Growth usually is not affected if only one joint is involved. Premature appearance of epiphyses in the very young and premature closure of the epiphyseal growth plate in the adult cause some of the major growth disturbances in the bones. Involvement of the metacarpals and metatarsals results in abnormally short rays. Occasionally, overgrowth of the epiphyses or metaphyses also occurs.

The metatarsophalangeal, interphalangeal, tarsometatarsal, and tarsal joints are frequently involved in juvenile rheumatoid arthritis, leading to flexion contractures of the toes, subluxation of metatarsal heads, and hallux valgus deformities; in addition, tarsal joint involvement can lead to varus or valgus deformity of the hindfoot.[64]

During early childhood, treatment consists essentially of medical management and local joint care. Adequate periods of rest and appropriate splinting followed by physical therapy can keep the joints well aligned. Hindfoot deformity, if flexible, is managed by appropriate shoe changes. Once the child stops growing and he or she has a persistent pain and fixed deform-

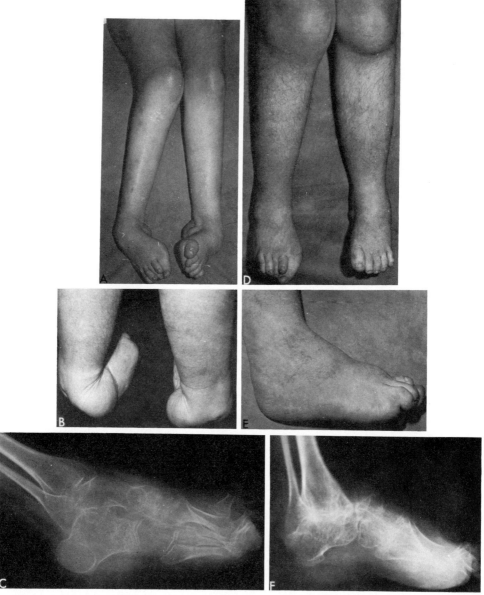

Figure 36–23. *Juvenile rheumatoid arthritis. (A and B) Chronic fixed hip and knee deformities and fixed equinocavovarus deformities of feet. (C) A radiograph of the right foot and ankle shows severe osteoporosis, narrow articular cartilage space, deformities of toes, and severe equinus deformity of the ankle. (D and E) Postoperative clinical results following bilateral astragalectomy and tibiocalcaneal fusion. The patient can now wear oxford shoes with slight raises in the heels. She is able to walk short distances after 20 years of being totally wheelchair dependent and is very happy with the surgical outcome. (F) Postoperative radiograph showing the tibiocalcanceal fusion.*

ity, the problem is handled surgically in the standard fashion, as in adult rheumatoid arthritis. (Fig. 36–23).

REITER'S SYNDROME

Reiter's syndrome classically consists of the triad of conjunctivitis, nonspecific urethritis, and polyarthritis. According to Katz, the triad has been expanded into a hexad or sextad of characteristics, including keratodermia blennorrhagica, balanitis circinata, and mucosal ulceration.[20] Most commonly, it affects males.

The cause of this syndrome is not known. A genetic predisposition has been suspected. Seventy-five per cent of patients have a positive HL-A-B27 histocompatibility antigen.

Jaffe states that pathologically it presents as a synovitis in the joints without any pannus or cortical erosion.[65] The involved synovial tissue is very vascular and edematous and is infiltrated by inflammatory cells, polymorphs, lymphocytes, and plasma cells.

Polyarthritis is usually acute asymmetric in type and sometimes monoarticular. In the foot, the midtarsal joints, metatarsophalangeal joints, and interphalangeal joints of the toes are more commonly in-

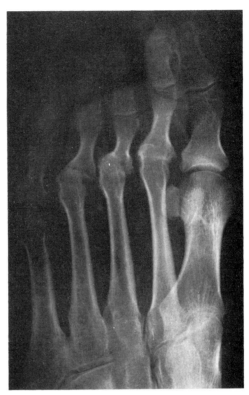

Figure 36–25. *Radiograph of the foot of a patient with Reiter's syndrome showing changes in the second, third, and fourth metatarsophalangeal joints.*

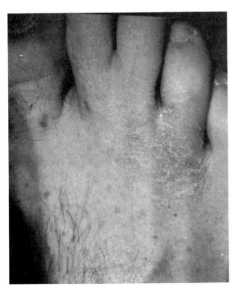

Figure 36–24. *Reiter's syndrome. Scaling of the skin on the dorsum of the right foot. Also note the involvement of the metatarsophalangeal and interphalangeal joints of the toes.*

volved (Figs. 36–24 and 36–25). Tendo-Achillis tendinitis occurs frequently and presents as a painful, tender swelling around the insertion of the heel cord. Plantar fasciitis, periostitis, calcaneal erosions, and calcaneal spurs are also commonly associated with this syndrome. The painful heel is sometimes referred to as "lover's heel." Spontaneous resolution is the rule, but symptoms and signs can linger for months.

Keratodermia blennorrhagica, a pustular lesion, is found on the soles of the feet in about 10 per cent of cases.[20] Later it becomes hyperkeratotic. This is sometimes confused with psoriasis.

In the foot, Reiter's syndrome presents radiographically as para-articular erosions, fluffy periostitis around the Achilles tendon insertion, and calcaneal spurs (Fig. 36–26).

Foot problems associated with Reiter's syndrome are usually managed conservatively by local means, such as a heel lift,

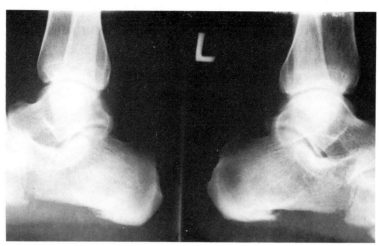

Figure 36–26. *Calcaneal spurs on the plantar aspect of the heels with erosions in Reiter's syndrome.*

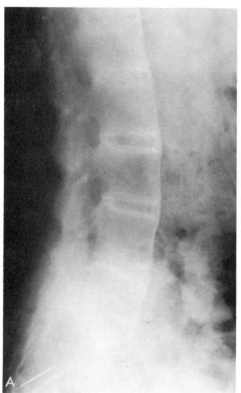

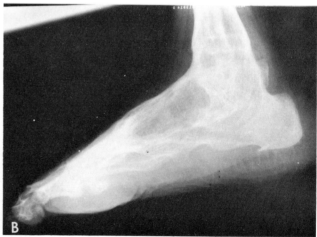

Figure 36–27. *(A) Typical radiographic findings in ankylosing spondylitis include squaring of the vertebral bodies, ossification of the annulus fibrosus, and syndesmophytes. (B) Radiograph of the foot of same patient as in A, showing ankylosis of all the joints of the foot and ankle.*

heel cushion, and local steroid injection therapy.

ANKYLOSING SPONDYLITIS

Ankylosing spondylitis occasionally involves the heel, usually in the form of heel erosions at the tendon insertion site or a calcaneal spur. Owing to the other signs and symptoms of this disease, there is generally no problem in diagnosing this lesion in the heel. Sometimes with marked peripheral joint involvement there can be complete ankylosis of the various joints of the feet (Fig. 36–27).

OTHER CONNECTIVE TISSUE DISEASES

Systemic lupus erythematosus, polyarteritis, polymyositis, and scleroderma can all produce synovitis and effusion in the feet, but joint destruction is rarely seen.[66]

PSORIATIC ARTHRITIS

Seronegative asymmetric polyarthritis associated with psoriasis and typical nail and joint changes causing a sausage-shaped swelling of the digits characterize this type of arthritis. Rheumatoid nodules are also absent. A definite hereditary tendency is suggested by histocompatibility antigen (HL-A).

More often, the psoriasis precedes the arthritis, although the reverse is sometimes true. The arthritis usually starts insidiously. Many joints in the body can be affected by this process, but small joints of the hand and feet are very commonly involved.

In the foot, simultaneous involvement of the distal and proximal interphalangeal joints and the metatarsophalangeal joints gives the toes a sausage-like appearance (Fig. 36–28). Katz described the asymmetric or symmetric types of involvement.[67] The latter produces some of the typical rheumatoid types of deformities. Concomitant psoriatic involvement of the nail and the distal interphalangeal joint is common. Nail changes can suggest a diagnosis of psoriatic arthritis in otherwise undiagnosed cases. The nails are affected twice as often in patients with arthritis as in those with psoriasis alone.

Pathologically, the interphalangeal joints have a very edematous, pale-looking synovial membrane[68] and in the initial stages lack pannus. In chronic involvement, the synovial tissue is more fibrotic and is infiltrated by inflammatory cells,

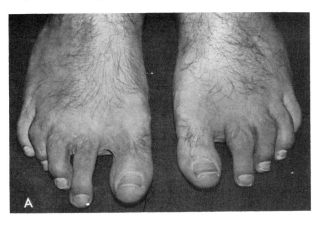

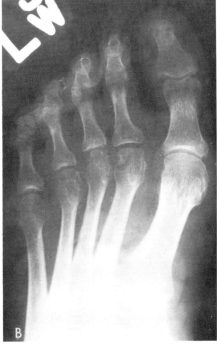

Figure 36–28. *(A) Early psoriatic changes in the forefeet showing typical nail and sausage-type deformities of the toes due to involvement of all three joints of the toes. (B) Early radiographic changes in the same patient, with involvement of the interphalangeal and metatarsophalangeal joints.*

which cause erosions of cortical bone and eventually lead to complete destruction of the joint.

Radiologic features are quite characteristic in the foot. There is predilection for distal interphalangeal joint involvement with erosions of the tufts of terminal phalanges and a pencil-and-cup appearance. Marginal erosions and periostitis are quite common. Eventually, arthritis mu-

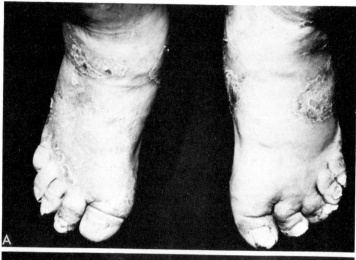

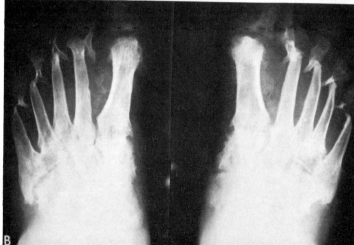

Figure 36–29. (A) Clinical picture of late changes of the feet in psoriatic arthritis showing skin, nail, and arthritis mutilans changes. The patient has no pain or plantar callosities. (B) Radiograph showing arthritis mutilans. (C) Lateral radiograph of foot showing ankylosis of the tarsal joints and involvement of the ankle joint.

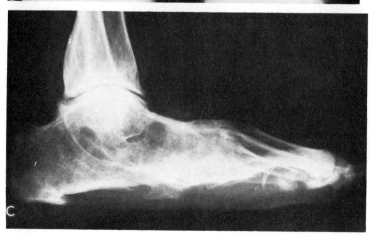

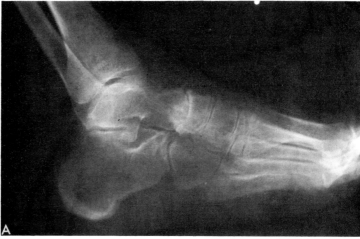

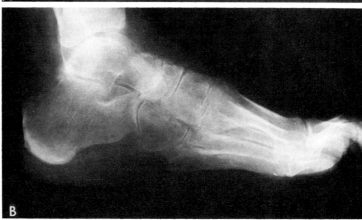

Figure 36–30. (A) Radiograph of the foot of the same patient as in Figure 36–28, showing involvement of the talonavicular joint. Clinically, he had localizing pain in that joint and tenderness and pain on pronation and supination of the foot. (B) The patient responded very well to localized talonavicular fusion. He remains problem free and has no complaint with regard to the subtalar or calcaneocuboid joints.

tilans develops (Fig. 36–29A, B). At times, the tarsal joints are fused into a solid, single block of bone (Fig. 36–29C).

Treatment of psoriatic arthritis of the forefoot is usually nonoperative. Owing to marked resorption of bone, patients generally do not develop any plantar callosities and metatarsophalangeal arthroplasty is not necessary. In the initial painful stages, the interphalangeal joints are usually managed by medical means, i.e., anti-inflammatory drugs and treatment of acute flareups of psoriasis. At times, a local cortisone injection into the joint is necessary. Surgery on the psoriatic foot is uncommon, but the general surgical principles would be the same as in rheumatoid arthritis. In the forefoot, if any joint is to be fused, a bone graft should certainly be utilized to compensate for the lost bone (Fig. 36–30).

I agree with Wright that patients with psoriatic arthritis are not prone to infection following surgery.[69] Owing to the experience obtained from surgery of other psoriatic joints in the body, I have not had any problem making an incision through the psoriatic skin. The scales should be removed from the operative site in preparation for surgery. The wounds usually heal by first intention.

REFERENCES

Rheumatoid Arthritis

1. Arthritis: The Basic Facts. New York, The Arthritis Foundation, 1976.
2. Aufranc, O.: Reconstructive Surgery of the Lower Extremity in Rheumatoid Arthritis. Instructional Course Lectures. Miami, Florida, American Academy of Orthopaedic Surgeons, January 1961.
3. Benson, G. M., and Johnson, E. W.: Management of the foot in rheumatoid arthritis. Orthop. Clin. North Am. 2:733, 1971.
4. Bywaters, E. G. L.: Heel lesions of rheumatoid arthritis. Ann. Rheum. Dis., 13:42, 1954.
5. Calabro, J. J.: A clinical evaluation of the diagnostic features of the feet in rheumatoid arthritis. Arthritis Rheum., 5:19, 1962.

6. Clayton, M. L.: Surgery of the forefoot in rheumatoid arthritis. Arthritis Rheum., 2:84, 1959.

7. Clayton, M. L.: Surgery of the forefoot in rheumatoid arthritis. Clin. Orthop., 16:136, 1960.

8. Clayton, M. L.: Discussion of "Rheumatoid Deformity of the Foot." Paper by L. Marmor. Arthritis Rheum., 6:756, 1963.

9. Clayton, M. L.: Surgical treatment of the rheumatoid foot. In Giannestras, N. J. (ed.): Foot Disorders: Medical and Surgical Management. Philadelphia, Lea and Febiger, 1967, pp. 319–340.

10. Dixon, A. S. J.: The rheumatoid foot. In Hill, A. G. S. (ed.): Modern Trends in Rheumatology 2. New York, Appleton-Century-Crofts, 1971, pp. 158–173.

11. DuVries, H. L.: Intractable keratosis under three metatarsal heads. In Surgery of the Foot. St. Louis, C. V. Mosby Co., 1959, pp. 186–193.

12. DuVries, H. L.: Major surgical procedures for the disorders of the foot. In Inman, V. T. (ed.): DuVries' Surgery of the Foot. St. Louis, C. V. Mosby Co., 1973, pp. 530–533.

13. Flint, M., and Sweetnam, R.: Amputation of all toes. J. Bone Joint Surg., 42B:90, 1960.

14. Fowler, A. W.: The surgery of fixed claw toes. J. Bone Joint Surg., 39B:585, 1957.

15. Fowler, A. W.: A method of forefoot reconstruction. J. Bone Joint Surg., 41B:507, 1959.

16. Hoffmann, P.: An operation for severe grades of contracted or clawed toes. Am. J. Orthop. Surg., 9:441, 1912.

17. Jones, W. N.: Treatment of rheumatoid arthritis of the foot and ankle. In Cruess, R. L., and Mitchell, N. S. (eds.): Surgery of Rheumatoid Arthritis. Philadelphia, J. B. Lippincott Co., 1971, pp. 87–92.

18. Joplin, R. J.. Surgery of the forefoot in the rheumatoid arthritic foot. Surg. Clin. North Am., 49:847, 1969.

19. Kates, A., Kessel, L., and Kay, A.: Arthroplasty of the forefoot. J. Bone Joint Surg., 49B:552, 1967.

20. Katz, W. A. (ed.): Rheumatic Diseases: Diagnosis and Management. Philadelphia, J. B. Lippincott Co., 1977, p. 385.

21. Kelikian, H.: Hallux Valgus, Allied Deformities of the Forefoot and Metatarsalgia. Philadelphia, W. B. Saunders Company, 1965, p. 314.

22. Kelikian, H.: Personal communication, 1978.

23. Keller, W. L.: The Surgical Treatment of Bunions and Hallux Valgus. N.Y. Med. J., 80:741, 1904.

24. Keller, W. L.: Further observations on the surgical treatment of hallux valgus and bunions. N.Y. Med. J., 95:696, 1912.

25. Kellgren, J. H., and Ball, J.: Tendon lesions in rheumatoid arthritis, a clinico-pathological study. Ann. Rheum. Dis., 9:48, 1950.

26. Key, J. A.: Surgical revision of arthritic feet. Am. J. Surg., 79:667, 1950.

27. Larmon, W. A.: Surgical treatment of deformities of rheumatoid arthritis of the forefoot and toes. Quarterly Bulletin of Northwestern University Medical School, 25:39, 1951.

28. Larson, C. B.: Discussion of "Rheumatoid Deformity of the Foot" by L. Marmor. Arthritis Rheum., 6:752, 1963.

29. Leavitt, D. G.: Surgical treatment of arthritic feet. Northwest Medicine, 55:1086, 1956.

30. Lipscomb, P. R.: Surgery for rheumatoid arthritis — timing and techniques: summary. J. Bone Joint Surg., 50A:614, 1968.

31. Lipscomb, P. R., Benson, G. M., and Sones, D. A.: Resection of proximal phalanges and metatarsal condyles for deformities of the forefoot due to rheumatoid arthritis. Clin. Orthop., 82:24, 1972.

32. Marmor, L.: Rheumatoid deformity of the foot. Arthritis Rheum., 6:749, 1963.

33. Murray, W. R., and Inman, V. T.: Vascular and metabolic disorders affecting the foot. In Inman, V. T. (ed.): DuVries' Surgery of the Foot. St. Louis, C. V. Mosby Co., 1973, pp. 282–288.

34. Peterson, L. F. A.: Surgery for rheumatoid arthritis—timing and techniques: the lower extremity. J. Bone Joint Surg., 50A:587, 1968.

35. Potter, T. A.: Talonavicular fusion with bone graft for spastic arthritic flat foot. Surg. Clin. North Am., 49:883, 1969.

36. Raunio, P., and Laine, H.: Synovectomy of the metatarsophalangeal joints in rheumatoid arthritis. Acta Rheumatol. Scand., 16:12, 1970.

37. Rhinelander, F. W.: Discussion of "Rheumatoid Deformity of the Foot" by L. Marmor. Arthritis Rheum., 6:752, 1963.

38. Ropes, M. W., Bennett, E. A., Cobb, W., et al.: 1958 Revision of diagnostic criteria for rheumatoid arthritis. Bull. Rheum. Dis., 9:175, 1958.

39. Schwartzmann, J. R.: The surgical management of foot deformities in rheumatoid arthritis. Clin. Orthop., 36:86, 1964.

40. Short, C. L., Bauer, W., and Reynolds, W. E.: Rheumatoid Arthritis. Cambridge, Harvard University Press, 1957.

41. Sones, D. A.: Surgery for rheumatoid arthritis — timing and techniques: general and medical aspects. J. Bone Joint Surg., 50A:576, 1968.

42. Thomas, W. H.: Metatarsal osteotomy. Surg. Clin. North Am., 49:879, 1969.

43. Thompson, T. C.: The management of the painful foot in arthritis. Med. Clin. North Am., 21:1985, 1937.

44. Vainio, K.: The rheumatoid foot. A clinical study with pathological and roentgenological comments. Ann. Chir. Gynaecol., 45(Supp. 1):1, 1956.

Rheumatoid Arthritis of the Ankle

45. Campbell, C. J., Rinehart, W. T., and Kalenak, A.: Arthrodesis of the ankle. Deep autogenous inlay grafts with maximum cancellous bone apposition. J. Bone Joint Surg., 56A:63, 1974.

46. Charnley, J.: Compression arthrodesis of the ankle and shoulder. J. Bone Joint Surg., 33B:180, 1951.

47. Chuinard, E. G., and Peterson, R. E.: Distraction-compression bone-graft arthrodesis of the ankle. J. Bone Joint Surg., 45A:481, 1963.

48. Clayton, M. L.: Surgery of the lower extremity in rheumatoid arthritis. J. Bone Joint Surg., 45A:1517, 1963.

49. Crenshaw, A. H.: Arthrodesis. In Crenshaw, A. H. (ed.): Campbell's Operative Orthopaedics. St. Louis, C. V. Mosby Co., 1971, p. 1125.

50. Greenwald, A. S., Matejczyk, M. B., and Black, J. D.: Ankle Joint Mechanics and Implant Evaluation. Scientific Exhibit. Meeting of the American Academy of Orthopaedic Surgeons. San Francisco, February 1979.

51. Groth, H. E., Fagan, P. J., and Shen, G.: The Oregon Ankle: A Review of 41 Cases. Paper read before the Meeting of the American Academy of Orthopaedic Surgeons. San Francisco, February 1979.

52. Heinig, C. F., and DuPuy, D. N.: Anterior dowel fusion of the ankle. In Bateman, J. E. (ed.): Foot Science. Philadelphia, W. B. Saunders Company, 1976, pp. 150–155.

53. Jakubowski, S.: Synovectomy in rheumatoid arthritis. In Chapchal, G. (ed.): Synovectomy and Arthroplasty in Rheumatoid Arthritis. New York, Intercontinental Medical Book Corporation, 1967, pp. 4–13.

54. Morris, H. D., and Herrick, R. T.: Ankle arthrodesis. In Bateman, J. E. (ed.): Foot Science. Philadelphia, W. B. Saunders Company, 1976, pp. 136–149.

55. Samuelson, K. M., and Tuke, M. A.: ICLH Ankle Arthroplasty. Paper read before the Meeting of the American Academy of Orthopaedic Surgeons. San Francisco, February 1979.

56. Segal, N. M., and Stauffer, R. N.: Mayo Total Ankle Arthroplasty: Four Years' Experience. Paper read before the Meeting of the American Academy of

Orthopaedic Surgeons. San Francisco, February 1979.

57. Thomas, W.: Personal communication.

58. Vainio, K.: The ankle joint. Ann. Chir. Gynaecol., 45(Suppl. 1):9, 1956.

59. Vainio, K.: Orthopaedic surgery in the treatment of rheumatoid arthritis. Ann. Clin. Res., 7:216, 1975.

60. Waring, T. L.: Arthroplasty. *In* Crenshaw, A. H. (ed.): Campbell's Operative Orthopaedics. St. Louis, C. V. Mosby Co., 1971, p. 1235.

61. Waugh, T. R., Wagner, J., and Stinchfield, F. E.: An evaluation of pantalar arthrodesis. J. Bone Joint Surg., 47A:1315, 1965.

62. Waugh, T. R.: Ankle arthrodesis and ankle arthroplasty: a clinical comparison. Paper presented at the Orthopaedic Society Meeting. Chicago, March, 1979.

Juvenile Rheumatoid Arthritis

63. Ansell, B. M., and Bywaters, E. G. L.: Juvenile chronic polyarthritis. *In* Scoll, J. T. (ed.): Copeman's Textbook of Rheumatic Diseases. Edinburgh, Churchill Livingstone, 1978, pp. 365–388.

64. Vanace, P.: Juvenile rheumatoid arthritis and other rheumatic diseases in children. *In* Katz, W. A. (ed.): Rheumatic Diseases: Diagnosis and Management. Philadelphia, J. B. Lippincott Co., 1977, p. 446.

Reiter's Syndrome

65. Jaffe, H. L.: Metabolic, Degenerative, and Inflammatory Diseases of Bone and Joints. Philadelphia, Lea and Febiger, 1972.

Ankylosing Spondylitis and Other Connective Tissue Diseases

66. Sbarbaro, J. L., and Katz, W. A.: The feet and ankles in the diagnosis of rheumatic disease. *In* Katz, W. A. (ed.): Rheumatic Diseases: Diagnosis and Management. Philadelphia, J. B. Lippincott Co., 1977, p. 189.

Psoriatic Arthritis

67. Katz, W. A.: Psoriatic Arthritis and Reiter's Disease. *In* Rheumatic Diseases: Diagnosis and Management. Philadelphia, J. B. Lippincott Co., 1977.

68. Sherman, M. S.: Psoriatic arthritis: observations on the clinical, roentgenographic and pathologic changes. J. Bone Surg., 34A:831, 1952.

69. Wright, V.: Psoriatic arthritis. *In* Copeman, W. S.: Textbook of Rheumatic Diseases. Edinburgh, Churchill Livingstone, 1978.

CHAPTER 37

METABOLIC DISORDERS AND PAGET'S DISEASE OF BONE

James W. Milgram, M.D.

The diseases that will be discussed in this chapter are often very complex, and any detailed treatment of this subject goes beyond the scope of a textbook on an anatomic region of the body. We have arbitrarily composed a classification of the different conditions that cause changes in bone mineralization and growth (Table 37–1). Paget's disease of bone is discussed separately.

NUTRITIONAL DISEASES OF BONE

Osteoporosis

By definition, osteoporosis is the state of less bone being present than is normal for the patient's age and sex. It is thus a relative condition with age-related parameters. Radiologists estimate that at least 25 per cent of the bone density must be missing for it to be detectable on a clinical roentgenogram. Bone scans do not show abnormalities in most cases. Osteoporosis does occur commonly in the foot and ankle after injury, often to a severe degree. "Disuse" osteoporosis, a transient process that reverses with walking stresses, will not be discussed here. Senile and the related postmenopausal osteoporosis of females are the two forms encountered most often. Osteoporosis, which is a generalized state

of the entire skeleton of the particular patient, is caused by a disparity between the rates of osteoblastic accretion of new bone and osteoclastic removal of old bone. Rather than an increase in osteoclastic activity, there is considerable evidence that osteoblastic activity is less active in some individuals than in others, and over the course of a long time, a normal osteoclastic rate will produce a net amount of less bone in a patient with a lowered, even

TABLE 37–1. Metabolic Disorders That Cause Changes in Bone Mineralization and Growth and Paget's Disease

I. Nutritional Diseases of Bone
  A. Osteoporosis
  B. Hypovitaminosis D
    1. Rickets
    2. Adult osteomalacia
  C. Hypovitaminosis C
  D. Hypervitaminosis A
  E. Heavy-metal poisoning
II. Hormonal Disorders
  A. Growth hormonal disorders
  B. Parathyroid hormone disorders
  C. Thyroid hormone disorders
III. Genetic Forms of Osteomalacia
  A. Hypophosphatasia
  B. Renal resistance to parathyroid hormone
  C. Vitamin D–resistant rickets
  D. Fibrogenesis imperfecta
IV. Renal Osteodystrophy
V. Paget's Disease

slightly lowered, osteoblastic accretional repair rate.

There is a form of osteoporosis that is probably due to increased osteoclasis, but that is usually an iatrogenic disease. Steroid hormones appear to cause the rapid osteoporosis seen in many patients by an elevated activity of body osteoclasts. Cushing's syndrome afflicts the skeleton similarly.

Figure 37–1 illustrates the pathologic section of a first toe with fairly significant osteoporosis. It can be appreciated that the cortex of the bone is paper-thin. Practically no subchondral plate exists under the articular surfaces. Such a state of the skeleton renders it susceptible to deformation with relatively insignificant energies of trauma. Although the spine and proximal femur are the sites of the most significant fractures, the foot and ankle are frequent sites for fractures in an osteoporotic patient. Toe and metatarsal fractures are especially common. Fortunately, a bone with osteoporosis is not deficient in its response to fracture repair, and thus a local, very active osteoblastic response creates an adequate fracture callus in most patients. The problem for the operating surgeon is when the anatomy is disturbed, as with many ankle fractures, and an open reduction is contemplated. The metal screws, plates, and rods do not hold well in the soft, easily crushed bone of an osteoporotic patient. Thus, if possible, osteoporotic fractures should be treated by closed reduction, unless the anatomy of the ankle joint is greatly disturbed. Sometimes Steinmann pins passed through the bones and incorporated into the external cast can maintain adequate position until healing occurs. When screw fixation is inadequate, smooth Kirschner wires can be used temporarily in certain situations. Comminution is frequently present in osteoporotic bone, so that internal fixation may be inappropriate. Transference of weight to an uninjured part of the foot may be useful in the treatment of metatarsal and phalangeal fractures. Therefore, there may be an increased indication for walking casts with heels in these patients.

An osteoporotic patient may present for the first time to a physician for an injury of the lower extremity without a prior diagnosis of osteoporosis having been made. The physician must therefore evaluate the metabolic state of the patient as well as treat the specific presenting disorder. How involved should the work-up be? The most important forms of treatable osteoporosis — osteomalacia, renal disease, and hyperparathyroidism — can be detected by the routine screening SMA-16, which includes values of the serum phosphorus, calcium, and alkaline phosphatase enzyme. Bone marrow dysplasias, such as multiple myeloma, leukemia, and hemoglobinopathies, usually demonstrate abnormalities in peripheral blood counts. Bone marrow cytologic examinations are occasionally necessary. Biopsies are almost never required.

Osteoporosis is most common as a primary disease state, and as such, it is very difficult to treat or alter considerably. The skeleton does not replace the bone tissue that has been resorbed once it is lost. Treatment is aimed at reducing the *rate* of loss by good diet, adequate calcium intake, female hormone replacement, if appropriate, and encouragement of regular physical activity. Usually, however, osteoporosis is a diagnosis of exclusion. Generally, the routine screenings provide the serum calcium and alkaline phosphatase levels, but a test for serum phosphorus has to be ordered separately when appropriate. All three determinations are normal in a patient with idiopathic osteoporosis.

Hypovitaminosis D: Rickets and Osteomalacia

Hypovitaminosis D or rickets in the child is largely an historical disease because it is so rarely encountered today

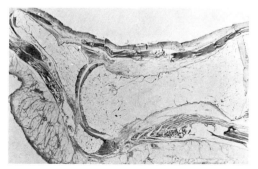

Figure 37–1. *Pathologic section of an osteoporotic first toe.*

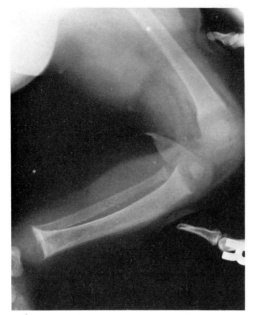

Figure 37–2. Widened and cupped epiphyseal plates in nutritional rickets.

owing to the addition of vitamin D to milk. Florid rickets usually is not seen until after the patient is over one year old. Enlargement of the costochondral junctions (a rosary) and swelling of the ankles and wrists may be early physical findings. Genu

varum and valgum deformities of the legs are seen only in more advanced and neglected cases. There may be a reduction in body weight owing to the generalized nature of the disease and its resultant deformities. Laboratory examinations reveal a depressed serum phosphorus, normal or low serum calcium, and elevated serum alkaline phosphatase levels. Radiographs will show widening of the growth plates with cupping on the metaphyseal side of the plate (where growth is occurring) (Fig. 37–2). As the disease becomes more severe, the epiphysis may not even be discernible, and the cortices of all bones become indistinct (Fig. 37–3). One special form of rickets with marked osteomalacia of the shafts of the bone is seen in cases of biliary atresia (Fig. 37–4). After treatment with vitamin D and an adequate diet, the radiographic changes rapidly revert to normal. Figure 37–5A shows the foot of a six-year-old male with nutritional rickets caused by severe neglect. Figure 37–5B shows the same foot after six weeks of a normal diet with vitamin D supplement (1500 to 5000 IU). The loss of cortical definition and epiphyseal indistinctness have been reversed. The daily requirement of vitamin D is estimated to be 400

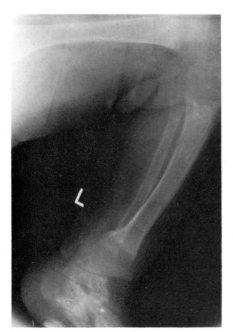

Figure 37–3. Marked osteoporosis and loss of definition in epiphyses in severe case of nutritional rickets.

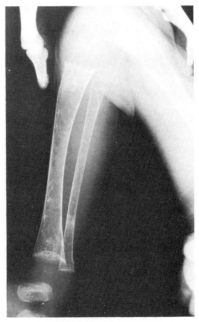

Figure 37–4. Biliary atresia with the osteoporosis of severe osteomalacia.

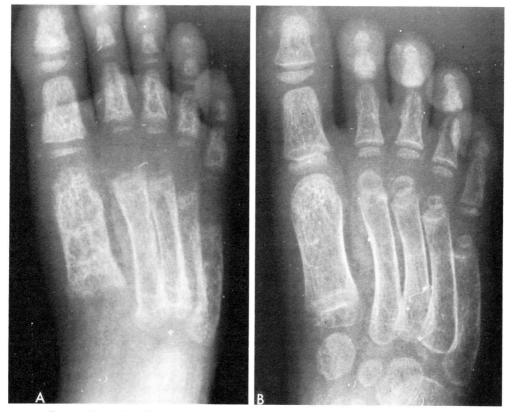

Figure 37–5. *Nutritional rickets. (A) Before treatment. (B) Six weeks after treatment.*

IU. A quart of milk contains this much of the vitamin.

Osteomalacia is a pathologic diagnosis that is made when the trabeculae of bone in histologic sections demonstrate increased and widened osteoid seams, indicating that the bone matrix is not mineralizing properly. Rickets includes osteomalacia of the bone, but in addition, the cartilage cores in the epiphyseal plate do not calcify, so that the hypertrophic zone of the growth plate is greatly widened since the cartilage cells do not die. Concomitant with many cases of osteomalacia is osteoporosis, less bone than normal.

In the growing patient with severe osteomalacia, muscle pull can cause deformation of the softened bone. An anteriorly bowed tibia is encountered occasionally in an adult who had rickets as a child. Genu varum and genu valgum of the knees with secondary varus or valgus ankle deformities may occur. In its severe untreated form the osteomalacic patient presents with grotesque deformities (Fig. 37–6).

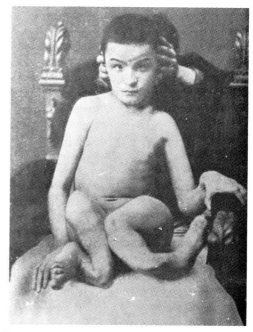

Figure 37–6. *Osteomalacia in a teenager, with grotesque deformities of many bones. (From Looser, E.: Dtsch. Z. Chir., 152:210, 1920.)*

When bowing deformities have occurred, osteotomy of the affected bones may be necessary. Degenerative arthritis of the medial compartment of the knees is seen in middle-aged individuals with significant genu valgum deformity. Osteotomy may avoid the necessity of arthroplasty.

In the adult, significant osteomalacia is only rarely due to dietary deficiency. In our laboratory at Northwestern University, we examined excised bone from many elderly patients, both surgical and post-mortem specimens, and histologic osteomalacia was almost never present unless the patient had a history of significant gastrointestinal disease. Sprue and post-gastrectomy syndromes are the most common forms of adult secondary osteomalacia. They only rarely present with foot complaints. Treatment of the malabsorption syndrome results in an improved intestinal absorption of calcium and vitamin D. The latter is often given as a parenteral supplement.

Hypervitaminosis D leads to excessive calcification in the bone and also in the soft tissues. Excessively dense zones of provisional calcification at the growth plates may be seen at the ankles as well as other sites (Fig. 37–7). Such changes mimic those seen as a result of having

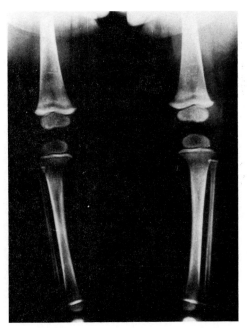

Figure 37-7. *Dense calcification at growth plates in hypervitaminosis D.*

heavy-metal poisoning, which will be discussed subsequently. However, the metastatic calcification of the soft tissues that occurs in vitamin D intoxication is not present in heavy-metal poisoning. Calcinosis universalis must be considered in the differential diagnosis of vitamin D intoxication.

Calcinosis universalis and *calcinosis circumscripta* are syndromes of widespread or localized calcifications occurring in association with collagen vascular diseases, particularly dermatomyositis and scleroderma. The deposits form in injured tissues, but the precise mechanism for deposition is unclear. Patients rarely require surgical procedures to remove the deposits.

Tumoral calcinosis is a condition that is distinct from calcinosis universalis and calcinosis circumscripta. The serum calcium level is normal, although occasionally the serum phosphorus may be slightly elevated. The patient presents with large nodular periarticular deposits of calcium salts. The general health of the patient is unimpaired. Histologically, multicystic spaces are filled with calcium and phosphate crystals separated by fibrous septa containing macrophages, multinucleated giant cells, and chronic inflammatory cells. Treatment consists of surgical removal of the mass, if necessary.

Hypovitaminosis C

Scurvy tends to affect an age group overlapping that of rickets, although scurvy can be manifested in younger patients than rickets. The infant has sufficient vitamin C reserves from its mother. Breast milk contains adequate ascorbic acid, but infants who are bottle fed may require vitamin C supplements. The majority of clinical cases of scurvy in children are seen in the second half of the first year and in the second year of life. Irritability, digestive disturbances, and loss of appetite are frequent clinical symptoms. There may be a general tenderness when the baby is picked up, particularly in the legs when the diaper is changed. The baby may lie without spontaneous movements in a frog-like position at the hips, with the knees also flexed to avoid pain. Edematous swelling along the tibial shafts may be observed. A region of hemorrhage presents as a palpable mass. There are no confirmatory laboratory examinations beyond the radiographs.

The deficiency of vitamin C, or ascorbic acid, affects connective tissue cells of many types. Cells that produce a collagen matrix, fibroblasts and osteoblasts, are unable to manufacture collagen adequately, so that a state of deficiency is produced. Hydroxyproline is not produced for normal collagen. Bone matrix consists of mineralized collagen fibrils. Thus, osteoporosis is a striking feature of scurvy. Osteogenesis imperfecta may be considered in the differential diagnosis. At the growth plates, calcification of cartilage occurs normally, unless there is also concomitant rickets, so that the dense lines of the provisional zone of calcification are present. In the epiphyses, these stand out as rings and are termed Wimberger's rings. Crushing of inadequately supported cartilage cores due to deficient primary bone formation causes even more dense roentgenographic changes relative to the osteoporosis of the rest of the bone.

The periosteum lacks firm attachment, and the *encouche* around the epiphyseal plate is weak owing to deficient bone.

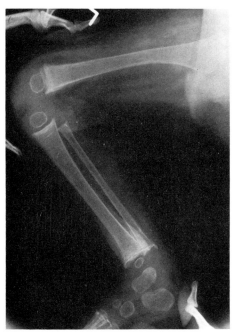

Figure 37–8. *Scurvy in a child's leg, with osteoporosis, Wimberger's rings, and epiphyseal separations.*

Therefore, epiphyseal separation due to minor trauma is frequent in advanced scurvy. Figure 37–8 shows a patient who demonstrates the osteoporosis of scurvy, the ring-like appearance of the epiphyses, and disruption of the epiphyses of the distal femur, distal tibia, and distal fibula. Periosteal new bone is present at all three sites of epiphyseal separation. The bones become normal with ascorbic acid treatment, 100 to 200 mg daily for several months. Infants require 25 to 50 mg of the vitamin daily, children 50 mg, and adults 75 mg.

Hypervitaminosis A

Hypervitaminosis A causes *cortical hyperostosis,* which is frequently first detected in a metatarsal (not the first). The distribution of bones affected differs from that of Caffey's disease (infantile cortical hyperostosis), which is the major problem in the differential diagnosis. The ulna may also be involved. The mandible and other flat bones are spared. There is a history of excessive ingestion of vitamin A, 60,000 units a day, in a typical chronic case. The serum vitamin A level is elevated, and there may occasionally be hypercalcemia. Growth retardation has also been reported.

Infantile cortical hyperostosis is a condition of unknown cause that appears to be inflammatory in origin. The child manifests a low fever, tenderness of the affected bones, and hyperirritability. The skull, mandible, clavicles, scapulas, ribs, and long bones of the extremities (including the metatarsals) may be involved. Radiographs demonstrate soft-tissue swelling and periosteal new bone. There may be an elevated sedimentation rate and serum alkaline phosphatase levels. There is no treatment. Fortunately, the disease usually resolves spontaneously in six to nine months without residual deformities.

Heavy-Metal Poisoning

Heavy-metal poisoning, although much less commonly encountered since an awareness of this problem has led to the introduction of lead-free paints, may be seen in both the long bones of the leg and forefoot and the cancellous bones of the hindfoot. It must be differentiated from osteopetrosis (marble bone disease), which is a genetic disorder of inadequate osteoclast function, and from hypervitaminosis D. Children aged one to six are usually affected. Preventive studies have demonstrated that in areas where leaded paints were used in either rural or urban older neighborhoods, up to 10 per cent of children may have ingested significant amounts of lead. This ingested lead is shared by the skeleton and soft tissues. Whole blood levels above 50 $\mu g/ml$ are considered elevated. When absorbed into the bone, lead atoms may persist in the bone matrix for 25 years. Symptoms of lead colic, acute or chronic encephalopathy, and peripheral neuropathy may be present. Stippled erythrocytes in the peripheral blood and stippled erythroblasts in the bone marrow confirm the diagnosis.

Lead poisoning results in the deposition of lead in the growing centers of bone. Therefore, the metaphyseal side of growth plates will be most affected. The calcified cartilage cores, when containing lead, are apparently capable of thwarting osteoclastic remodeling. Primary trabeculae of bone are also not resorbed. Thus, in a patient with lead poisoning roentgenograms will show dense zones at the growth plates (Fig. 37–9).

Since lead poisoning is seen in the young child who eats flaking paint in his home, recovery may occur with cessation of ingestion. Few patients present with clear symptoms of plumbism. A second period of eating paint will create a second distinct lead line in all of the bones. Parenteral calcium EDTA and BAL (dimercaprol) may be given in the more severe case.

Bismuth is deposited in mineralizing tissues in a way similar to lead. Injectable bismuth compounds may rarely cause poisoning. Figure 37–10 illustrates the leg and foot of a child with two distinct bismuth lines clearly visible in the talus and calcaneus as well as the long bones. Cod liver oil with added phosphorus creates phosphorus lines that are sometimes very striking. In Figure 37–11, the increased dense peripheral zones of the epiphyses

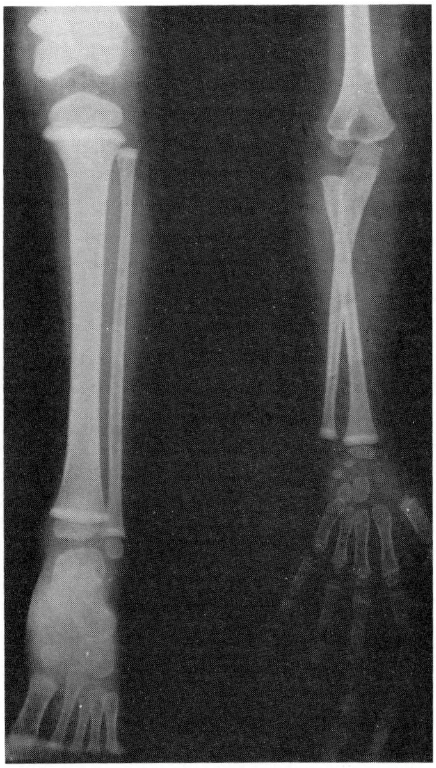

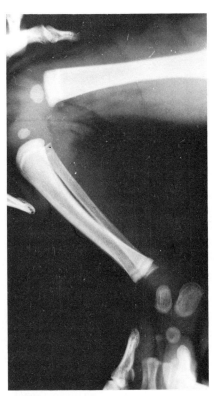

Figure 37–9. Dense, calcified cartilage and increased bone in metaphyseal growing centers in lead poisoning.

Figure 37–10. Increased calcification at epiphyseal growth plates in bismuth poisoning.

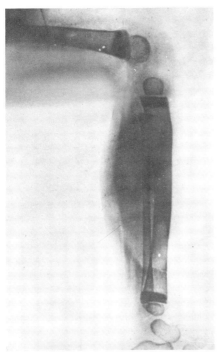

Figure 37–11. *Calcified lines and rings at former growth plate locations that were not remodeled in phosphorus poisoning.*

and cancellous bones of the foot should be noted, as well as the dense bands in the tibia and femur. The radiographic density is due to calcium phosphate crystals. Treatment of all heavy-metal poisoning cases is directed toward discovery and cessation of ingestion of the causative agent.

HORMONAL DISORDERS

Growth Hormone Disorders

Growth hormone deficiency results in retardation of all osseous growth. Bone age is retarded throughout the skeleton, but no specific localized abnormalities are present. Open growth plates may persist into adult life. The child will be a dwarf unless treatment with human growth hormone is given. It is possible to assay growth hormone levels to confirm the diagnosis.

Excess of growth hormone due to adenomas or hyperplasia of the anterior pituitary gland causes gigantism if the onset is during the period when epiphyseal growth is occurring or acromegaly if the onset is in

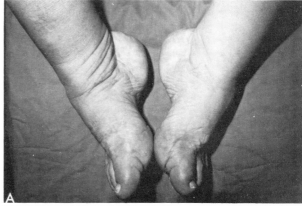

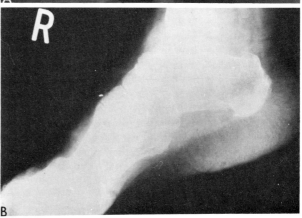

Figure 37–12. *Acromegaly. (A) Thickened heel pads due to hypertrophy of soft tissues. (B) Increased soft tissues in heel pad.*

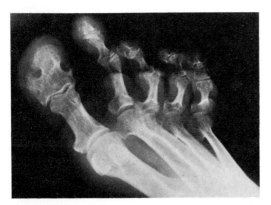

Figure 37–13. *Overgrowth of tufts of distal phalanges and new bone at sites of ligament insertions in acromegaly.*

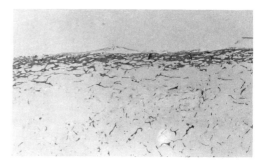

Figure 37–14. *Photomicrograph of primary hyperparathyroidism with resorption cavities permeating the distal tibial cortex.*

adult life. All of the bones are enlarged in the giant owing to epiphyseal cartilage stimulation during the growing period.

Acromegaly causes an overgrowth of soft tissues and also stimulates the formation of periosteal new bone at certain sites. The soft tissues of the feet in an acromegalic patient often thicken (Fig. 37–12A). The lateral radiograph of the foot may demonstrate an enlarged heel pad (Fig. 37–12B). Periosteal new bone at sites of ligament insertion and on the tufts of the distal phalanges creates a characteristic pattern if it is pronounced (Fig. 37–13). The diagnosis is reached by the determination of growth hormone (somatotropin) levels and radiologic study of the pituitary fossa. The arrested acromegalic retains the thickening of the soft tissues that occurred during the active disease process. It does not appear to affect elective surgery of the foot for other problems. Bone healing after fractures and osteotomies occurs normally.

Parathyroid Hormone Disorders

Hyperparathyroidism may present as a form of osteoporosis with a fracture. Rarely, the giant cell tumor seen in association with severe hyperparathyroidism may present in the tibia as a mass. However, today most cases are detected by means of routine blood screening tests before any bone abnormalities have occurred. If the serum calcium is elevated on several successive determinations, a serum parathyroid hormone level can be obtained. Neck explorations for an adenoma of the parathyroids is done if there is a statistical likelihood of a tumor being present.

The radiologic abnormalities of primary hyperparathyroidism are due to bone resorption by osteoclasts. Certain sites are predisposed to recognizable changes. Subperiosteal resorption of the cortices of the phalanges in the feet as well as the hands is an early osseous abnormality. Eventually, a significant degree of intracortical resorption may occur. Figure 37–14 is a photomicrograph of a tibial cortex with severe hyperparathyroidism; many intracortical resorption cavities riddle the entire cortex

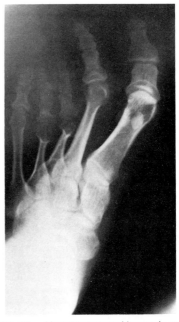

Figure 37–15. *Short metatarsal bones in pseudohypoparathyroidism.*

of the bone. Vessel calcification can be seen in some cases. Reossification may occur with treatment. Rarely, hyperostosis with osteosclerosis is an observed repair phenomenon.

Hypoparathyroidism, a rare disorder most often attributable to iatrogenic causes during thyroid surgery, does not present with foot or ankle abnormalities. A genetic disease termed *pseudohypoparathyroidism* is characterized by short individuals who may have short third and fourth metatarsals and metacarpals (Fig. 37–15). These patients present with a depressed serum calcium level and increased urinary excretion of phosphorus but do not respond to parathyroid hormone, as would a patient with true hypoparathyroidism.

Thyroid Hormone Disorders

Hypothyroid dwarfism is termed *cretinism* in the growing child and *myxedema* when its onset is in adult life. Retardation of growth is the striking morphologic feature of cretinism, but there are other characteristic changes of the soft tissues, as well as severe mental retardation. Therefore, the patient's habitus differs significantly from that of a hypopituitary dwarf. The legs of an adult cretin are disproportionately short in comparison with the measurements of the rest of his body. Treatment with thyroid hormone must be begun early in life to avoid permanent mental retardation.

Hyperthyroidism rarely affects the bones or joints to any significant degree. Osteoporosis is the most common radiological change in hyperthyroidism.

GENETIC FORMS OF OSTEOMALACIA

The diseases discussed under this heading are certain selected hereditary conditions that present with clinical osteomalacia. However, the osteomalacia is the outstanding characteristic of these four disease groups.

Hypophosphatasia is a rare, sometimes fatal disorder, the most prominent feature of which is a profound absence of bone mineralization. Thus, affected infants present with severe rickets at a younger age than patients with either nutritional or renal rickets. Very wide osteoid seams with strikingly deficient mineralization of bone have been reported in those cases examined post mortem. Biopsies from older, less severely affected patients demonstrate rachitic changes at the growth plates. Clinically, the serum alkaline phosphatase level is depressed. Hypercalcemia may also be present. In adult life, pseudofractures or Looser's lines of the long bones may be present.

In contrast to hypophosphatasia is a condition found in a small group of patients who present with elevated alkaline phosphatase levels and varying degrees of osteomalacia and hyperparathyroidism. In the case shown in Figure 37–16, marked osteosclerosis of the skeleton of a 13-year-old boy is demonstrated. Biopsy revealed a true osteosclerosis with more bone per unit volume than normal, but this bone had very wide, abnormal osteoid seams. An increased number of resorption cavities were also present. A *renal resistance to the phosphaturic effects of parathyroid hormone* was demonstrated by metabolic

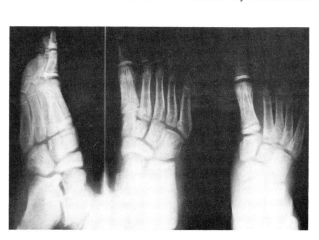

Figure 37–16. *The foot of this 13-year-old patient with renal resistance to parathyroid hormone and osteomalacia demonstrates marked osteosclerosis.*

studies. Thus, the case demonstrates the variation in osteomalacic states from osteoporosis to near normal bone mineralization to osteosclerosis.

The most common form of genetic rickets in children who are otherwise normal is *vitamin D–resistant rickets*, a sex-linked dominant trait. There are several forms of this disease, with certain patients not presenting until the teenage years and others presenting in early adulthood, but the patient with onset in early childhood may present with a deformity of the lower extremities, often genu varum or genu valgum. Hypophosphatemia is present. The child whose knees and ankles are shown in Figure 37–17 required tibial osteotomies on two different occasions to correct severe bow-leg deformities. The deformities may also recur unless the patient is kept under careful metabolic control with high-dose vitamin D therapy. Patients with childhood disease may remit in early adulthood only to have recurrence of clinically significant osteomalacia when older. These patients will present with bone

pain. The synthesized active metabolite of vitamin D, dihydroxycholecalciferol, may prove beneficial in these patients. A seven-year-old female child with widespread fibroxanthomas of many bones in addition to hypophosphatemic rickets is shown in Figure 37–18.

Other patients with neurofibromatosis and unusual giant cell tumors similar to those seen in hyperparathyroidism have been observed. One such case was a 19-year-old female with a giant cell tumor of the distal tibia. Children and adults with this form of hereditary rickets and osteomalacia will frequently present to orthopaedic surgeons for treatment of fractures as well as for lower extremity deformities. Stress fractures may heal with inadequate mineralization, creating radiographic Looser's lines, which may sometimes persist for years. These may be seen in the leg or foot. Dietary phosphate supplements in addition to Vitamin D sometimes improve the more severe cases.

A rare disease of severe osteomalacia has been termed *fibrogenesis imperfecta* (Fig. 37–19). Coarse osteosclerosis with ill-defined fuzzy trabeculae characterizes the roentgenograms of these patients. The

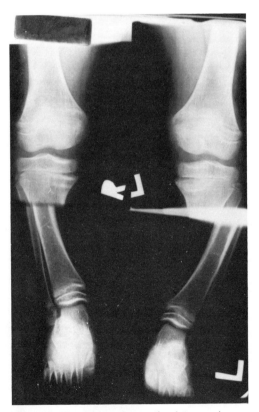

Figure 37–17. *Widened growth plates and severe genu varum in vitamin D–resistant rickets.*

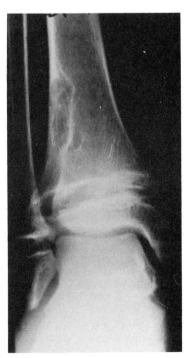

Figure 37–18. *Vitamin D–resistant rickets with unusual fibroxanthoma formation in many bones.*

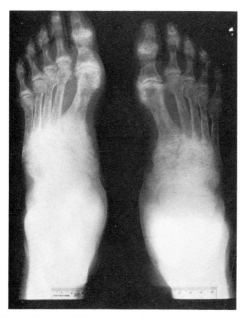

Figure 37–19. *Fibrogenesis imperfecta, a form of severe osteomalacia.*

basic abnormality in this disease is the production of a bone matrix markedly deficient in normal collagen fibers. The fibers are nonrefractile when viewed in a polarizing microscopic field, and it is by means of tissue examination of biopsy material that the diagnosis is made. Treatment with vitamin D analogues is apparently effective.

RENAL OSTEODYSTROPHY

The bone changes that occur secondary to chronic renal disease are osteomalacia caused by the deficiency of active metabolites of vitamin D and secondary hy-

perparathyroidism, which is related to retention of phosphate by the injured kidneys. Phosphate retention and the resultant hypocalcemia stimulate the parathyroid glands to secrete parathyroid hormone, which in turn mobilizes calcium from the bone by osteoclastic resorption. The degree of osteomalacia or secondary hyperparathyroidism varies from case to case and from disease to disease, and in the individual patient whose diet is being varied, who is being treated with various drugs, and who may be dialyzed, the disease varies considerably in response to all of these parameters.

Figure 37–20 is the initial roentgenogram of the feet of a 46-year-old female patient who presented with midfoot pain when walking. No renal disease was known. Stress fractures of metatarsals were discovered as the cause of the patient's rather chronic symptoms. Her blood urea nitrogen was markedly elevated. Eventually, an iliac crest biopsy revealed extensive osteomalacia, despite a rather normal radiographic appearance of the bones. Chronic glomerulonephritis was diagnosed as the underlying disease.

In the child with a renal tubular defect or chronic glomerulonephritis, renal rickets is manifested by widening of the growth plates (Fig. 37–21). As in the other forms of osteomalacia, the total skeletal mass may vary from an osteoporotic state to one of relative osteosclerosis (although that same osteosclerotic bone may be deficient in strength, owing to its poor mineralization).

Secondary hyperparathyroidism varies with the treatment of the patient's hypocalcemia. Long-standing changes can

Figure 37–20. *Radiograph of the feet of a patient with renal osteodystrophy who presented with spontaneous stress fractures due to osteomalacia.*

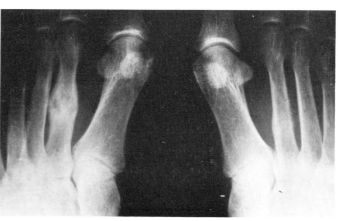

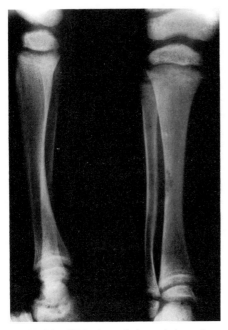

Figure 37–21. *Widening of the epiphyseal growth plates in renal rickets.*

cause true hyperplasia of the parathyroid glands, which then function autonomously, not reacting to the level of ionized calcium in the blood. Subperiosteal resorption and normal weight-bearing stresses can cause epiphyseal fractures that are pathologically similar to Salter-Harris Type I fractures; they do not occur through cartilaginous portions of the growth plates, but in the area of first metaphyseal bone. Figure 37–22 illustrates the feet and ankles of one such very severely affected patient, who succumbed to the disease shortly after these photographs were taken.

Another abnormality seen occasionally in the steroid-treated renal patient, often in association with a renal transplant, is avascular necrosis of the talus. Medullary infarcts of the distal tibia and even of the calcaneus have been reported, but these are not symptomatic, owing to their extra-articular locations. Figure 37–23 shows views of both ankles of a 26-year-old fe-

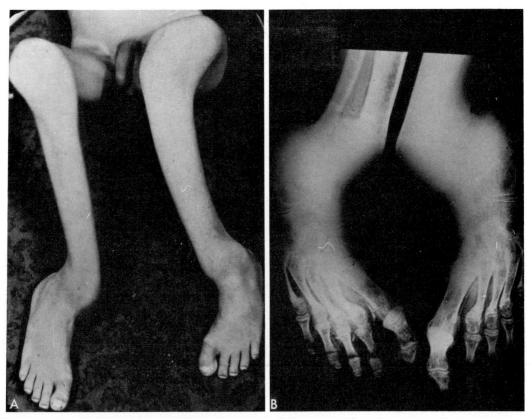

Figure 37–22. *(A) Photograph and (B) roentgenogram of the legs and feet of a patient with severe renal osteodystrophy.*

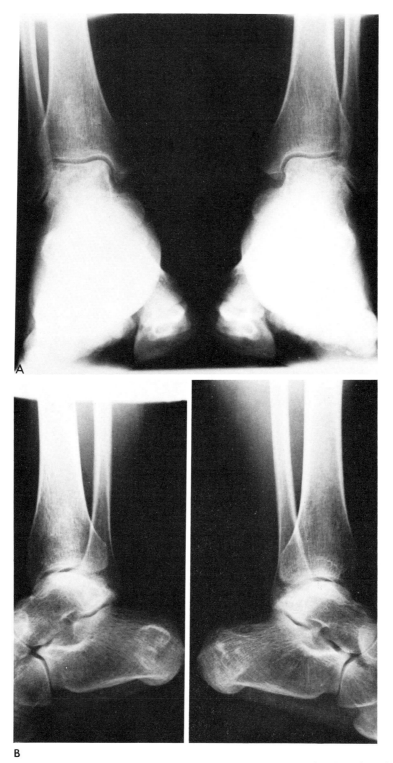

Figure 37–23. (A and B) Steroid-induced avascular necrosis in bilateral tali, calcanei, and distal tibial metaphyses. (From Milgram, J. W., and Riley, L. H., Jr.: Bull. Hosp. Joint Dis., 37:11, 1976.)

male with idiopathic thrombocytopenic purpura who developed infarcts in multiple sites. There are lesions in both talar and calcaneal bones. The femoral and humeral heads and the medial or lateral distal femoral condyles are more common sites for steroid-induced avascular necrosis, but each reported series includes some patients with disease of the ankles. Few of these patients with talar disease have required surgical treatment. A Blair tibiotalar arthrodesis would probably be a preferred method. The etiology of steroid-induced avascular necrosis of bone may be a local hyperplasia of bone marrow fat cells in susceptible patients. The onset of pain and roentgenographic changes are variable in relation to steroid dosage.

PAGET'S DISEASE

Paget's disease of bone is a process that morphologically resembles, at least in part, many of the disorders that have been discussed previously in this chapter. However, unlike all of these conditions, which are generalized, affecting all parts of the patient's skeleton, Paget's disease may be found in certain particular sites that vary from patient to patient. One or a few bones, rarely many different bones, but never all of the bones of any individual patient are involved with the disease. Moreover, in certain cases, the involvement spreads to affect more bones that were not involved previously. Therefore, the pattern of involvement also varies from patient to patient.

As far as can be detected, the bones were normal at the exact site that later in life becomes affected. The patients with true Paget's disease are rarely younger than 35 years of age. Well-developed late sclerotic changes are practically never seen in patients who are in their fourth decade of life. However, active disease is by no means limited to these younger patients. The typical patients are older, perhaps in their sixties or seventies, but

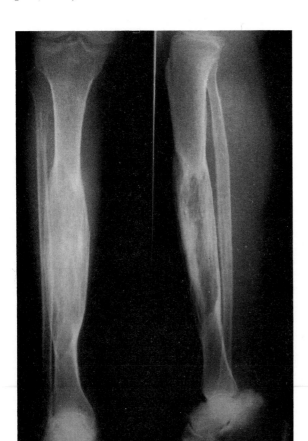

Figure 37–24. *See legend on opposite page.*

often a history of the bowing of a tibia or femur proves that the existence of the disease predated its discovery by several decades. Men and women are equally affected.

The basic etiology of Paget's disease is still unknown. The detection of virus-like particles within a few osteoclasts from certain cases has raised the possibility of a relationship of cause and effect, but the peculiar distribution, progression, temporal course, and ages of affected patients are most unlike other diseases thought to be of viral etiology.

The earliest observable roentgenographic abnormality in a long bone with Paget's disease is resorption of the previously normal cortex. Microscopically, osteoclasts are observed within resorption cavities; however, a purely lytic form of Paget's disease is observed only rarely. In the typical case, increased osteoblastic activity, with the formation of new osseous trabeculae, is juxtaposed to the site of bone resorption. Therefore, the morphology of active Paget's disease is both increased resorption by osteoclasts and increased accretion by osteoblasts. The new bone trabeculae mineralize with a normal width of osteoid seams. Juxtaposition of active bone breakdown and formation of new bone without mineralization defects is the diagnostic histopathology of Paget's disease. Yet despite the marked bone turnover observed histologically in long bones, Paget's disease begins in one area of the bone and then very slowly advances over a period of many years. Figure 37–24 demonstrates progressive involvement of a tibia over two years. Frequently, Paget's disease never progresses to involve more than half of a bone. For instance, the

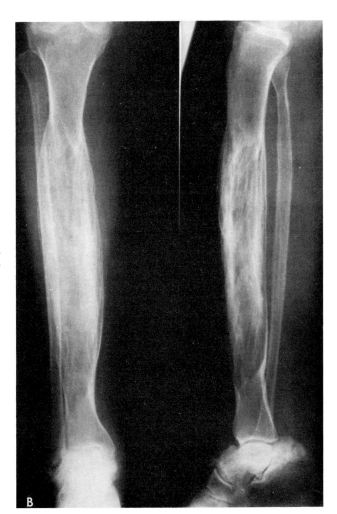

Figure 37–24 Continued. (A and B) Paget's disease of the tibia. Progressive involvement of normal bone over two years.

proximal tibia will show advanced disease, yet the distal half of the same bone will be normal on roentgenograms.

It has been observed by many authors that Paget's disease has a more or less temporal sequence of involvement in any one particular site. The first phase is resorption. Then an active phase, which lasts for years, causes repeated remodeling of an affected bone. The demonstration of a characteristic mosaic pattern of cement lines of the much remodeled bone is cited frequently as a diagnostic histologic finding. Figure 37–25A is a low-power photomicrograph of a distal tibia that demonstrates that there are different types of pathologic alterations in the architecture of the bone. The original cortex is very osteoporotic. In other regions of the specimen, a very fine mesh pattern of the trabeculae can be noted. This change involves the bone near the joint surface and

the original cortex. It also can be observed to form a well-defined zone outside the original confines of the cortex of the bone. This "periosteal" new bone is frequently confusing when interpreted radiologically. Figure 37–25B is a roentgenogram of a slice of this same specimen from a distal tibia. Hazy periosteal radiopacity can be observed, particularly in the more proximal portions of the specimen. Remodeling has caused net loss (osteoporosis) in some regions of the bone and net gain (osteosclerosis) elsewhere. Continued reinforcement of certain trabeculae together with the loss of others creates the coarse trabeculated pattern that is characteristic of this disease. However, eventually Paget's disease enters an inactive third phase when the marrow activity of osteoclasts and osteoblasts fades with reversion back to inactive fat cells. The bone retains its sclerotic radiologic appearance,

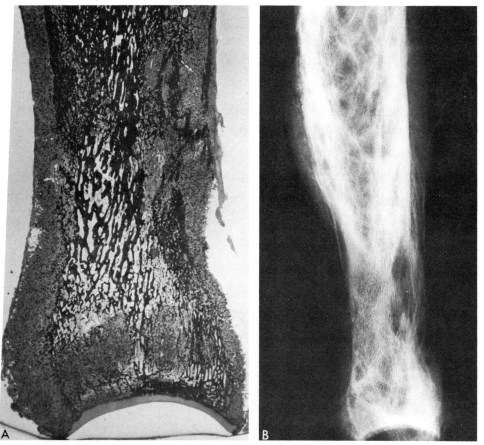

Figure 37–25. Paget's disease involving the distal tibia. (A) Low-power photomicrograph of distal tibia illustrating various types of pathologic alterations in bone architecture. (B) Roentgenogram of a slice of the same specimen from the distal tibia.

and thus roentgenograms are of little use in determining metabolic activity of the disease.

In the distal portion of the lower extremity, the tibia is the bone most frequently involved with this disease. The calcaneus and the talus are affected much more rarely, and the other bones of the feet are practically never observed to have Paget's disease. Ordinarily, either the distal or proximal end of the tibia is the site for the commencement of the disease, although central disease with sparing of the two ends of the bone can occur.

Diagnosis and Evaluation

In the initial evaluation of a new patient, roentgenograms are the means for establishing a diagnosis. It must be remembered that the disease first may be osteolytic in character. In this state, Paget's disease can be confused with neoplastic processes and fibrocystic disease of bone. The oblique, rather sharp demarcation between normal and pagetoid bone is frequently helpful. Figure 37–26 is a lateral radiograph of the ankle of a 69-year-old female that demonstrates all of these features. She had advanced sclerotic disease

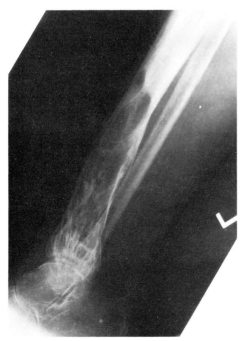

Figure 37–26. *Marked osteolytic changes in the distal tibia of a 69-year-old woman with Paget's disease.*

in the same leg involving the distal femur. This demonstrates that different affected bones may be at different stages of this slowly progressing and insidious disease. Recognition of this ankle lesion as Paget's disease was uncertain, and the patient underwent an open surgical biopsy. Subsequently, she suffered a pathologic fracture through the biopsy site, which healed after a period of external immobilization. I recommend that biopsy be avoided, if possible, since this case is one of three that I observed in which fractures presumably occurred because of biopsies.

If roentgenograms are necessary to establish the diagnosis but frequently do not reflect the degree of activity in a particular case, how is a patient to be evaluated and followed? The bone scan is to be recommended as a screening procedure for a new patient. Silent sites of involvement can be detected, and then appropriate radiographs can document the actual morphologic changes present. To an extent, serial bone scans can be used to follow a treatment program, but scanning is not truly a quantitative examination and is also a fairly expensive and time-consuming procedure.

Serial serum alkaline phosphatase determinations reflect the osteoblastic activity in the particular case and thus provide a simple method of evaluating a patient over the course of time. In fact, detection of Paget's disease may be due to the elevated alkaline phosphatase levels obtained as part of routine screening tests. Some of the highest recorded values from this laboratory test are seen in patients with Paget's disease. Treatment is usually not considered unless the patient's test results show levels over twice normal values.

The urinary excretion of hydroxyproline over a known period of time (usually 24 hours) indicates collagen breakdown. This value is markedly elevated in many patients with Paget's disease, paralleling the degree of elevation of the alkaline phosphatase activity. However, the test is more difficult to perform and thus is too costly for the routine follow-up of the patient with known disease.

In the leg, the presenting symptom of most patients is aching pain in or near the affected portion of the tibia. An increased blood supply is evidenced by the increased warmth of the anterior leg on palpation. In these patients, the vascular activity of the Paget's disease is responsible for the pain, which may occur at rest as well as during weight bearing.

Weight-bearing and gastrocnemius-soleus pulling forces on the tibia when the disease is in its osteolytic and hence weakened phase cause deformity of the bone in many cases. Most typical is a long anteroposterior bowing, sometimes with a so-called saber-shin deformity anteriorly. Varus and valgus deformities of the ankle are less common. I have two patients with significant varus deformities of the ankle that could be improved by corrective osteotomies. It has been reported that osteotomies of a pagetoid bone heal normally.

It will be noted in Figure 37–25 that the articular surface of the ankle is normal. Paget's disease penetrates the subchondral plate of joint surfaces, but it does not affect uncalcified cartilaginous tissue. Patients with Paget's disease that has caused bowing of the femurs and tibias can develop degenerative arthritis of both the ankle and knee joints owing to the abnormal wear on the articular surfaces created by the bone deformity. Therefore, a second possible presenting symptom is weight-bearing pain in osteoarthritic joints that are juxtaposed to bones with the pagetoid process.

A third cause for pain in the leg is a phenomenon that occurs in bowed bones with long-standing and frequently metabolically inactive disease. This phenomenon is known as fatigue or stress fracturing. Propagation of a stress fracture to a full fracture is not uncommon; pathologic fractures in Paget's disease tend to be transverse in configuration. They heal with con-

ventional immobilization. Stress fractures may persist for long periods of time and are definitely the source of weight-bearing pain in some patients.

Two patients with adequately treated early Paget's disease of the tibia had pain despite the absence of stress fractures and arthritis; it was presumed to be related to the weakened nature of the gross osseous architecture. Patellar weight-bearing orthotic devices were prescribed to relieve tibial weight-bearing forces.

The activity of the tibia can be evaluated by means of external measurements of skin temperature over the bone. In a series of serial measurements in patients undergoing metabolic treatment, sequential readings reflected decreased elevations of skin temperature, paralleling lower serum alkaline phosphatase determinations.

Treatment

After an evaluation encompassing the parameters that have been mentioned, a decision to treat a patient with elevated serum alkaline phosphatase levels may be made. There are two currently available drugs that have similar bone-cell–suppressing effects — salmon calcitonin and disodium etidronate, a diphosphonate. They appear to be equally effective, but the diphosphonate has the advantage of being an oral agent. I use a dosage of 10 mg/kg/day. Drug-induced osteomalacia, which could accentuate the stress fracture phenomenon and create more pain as a result, can be controlled by the dosage of the diphosphonate. Obviously, arthritic pain will not respond to metabolic treatment of the active Paget's disease, so that evaluation of pain in each patient is neces-

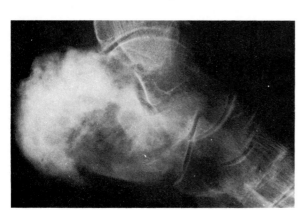

Figure 37–27. *Paget's disease of the calcaneus with secondary osteosarcomatous degeneration.*

sary. Leg pain also occurs as a result of a sciatic nerve compression, which may be associated with spinal stenosis induced by Paget's disease in the spine. Some cases are quite difficult to treat and do not respond to metabolic treatment. Both drugs suppress but do not cure the patient's disease, so periodic evaluations are necessary even after a very gratifying clinical success with drug therapy. A three- or six-month follow-up examination with alkaline phosphatase level determinations is usually sufficient.

Malignant transformation of a bone with Paget's disease is fortunately quite rare, appearing in less than 1 per cent of the patients who manifest clinical disease. Figure 37–27 shows a radiograph of a 68-year-old female who developed osteosarcoma of a calcaneus with Paget's disease. Amputation of the extremity after biopsy confirmation would be appropriate treatment for a malignant tumor arising in Paget's disease. The periosteal active phase of the disease (see Figure 37–25) is sometimes confused radiologically with malignant disease.

REFERENCES

1. Anderton, J. M.: Orthopaedic problems in adult hypophosphatasia. J. Bone Joint Surg., *61B*:82, 1979.
2. Baker, S. L., et al.: Fibrogenesis imperfecta ossium. J. Bone Joint Surg., *48B*:804, 1966.
3. Barry, H. C.: Paget's Disease of Bone. Edinburgh and London, E. and S. Livingstone, Ltd., 1969.
4. Dent, C. E., and Stamp, T. C. B.: Hypophosphataemic osteomalacia presenting in adults. Q. J. Med., *40*:303, 1971.
5. DeRose, J., et al.: Response of Paget's disease to porcine and salmon calcitonins. Am. J. Med., *56*:858, 1974.
6. Frost, H. M.: The Bone Dynamics in Osteoporosis and Osteomalacia. Springfield, Illinois, Charles C Thomas, 1966.
7. Garner, A., and Ball, J.: Quantitative observations on mineralized and unmineralized bone in chronic renal azotaemia and intestinal malabsorption syndrome. J. Pathol. Bacteriol., *91*:545, 1966.
8. Hecht, A., Gershberg, H., and St. Paul, H.: Primary hyperparathyroidism. J.A.M.A., *233*:519, 1975.
9. Jaffe, H. L.: Metabolic, Degenerative, and Inflammatory Diseases of Bones and Joints. Philadelphia, Lea and Febiger, 1972.
10. Katz, A. I., Hampers, C. L., and Merrill, J. P.: Secondary hyperparathyroidism and renal osteodystrophy in chronic renal failure. Medicine, *48*:333, 1969.
11. Khairi, M. R., and Johnson, C. C.: Treatment of Paget's disease of bone (osteitis deformans) with sodium etidronate (EHDP) Clin. Orthop. *127*:94, 1978.
12. Milgram, J. W.: Chronic renal failure, recurrent secondary hyperparathyroidism, multiple metaphyseal infractions, and secondary oxalosis. Bull. Hosp. Joint Dis., *35*:118, 1974.
13. Milgram, J. W.: Radiological and pathological assessment of the activity of Paget's disease of bone. Clin. Orthop., *127*:43. 1977.
14. Milgram, J. W.: Orthopaedic management of Paget's disease of bone. Clin. Orthop., *127*:63, 1977.
15. Milgram, J. W., et al.: Renal resistance to parathyroid hormone with hyperphosphatemic osteomalacia and osteitis fibrosa. J. Bone Joint Surg., *56A*:1493, 1974.
16. Milgram, J. W., and Riley, L. H., Jr.: Steroid induced avascular necrosis of bone in eighteen sites. Bull. Hosp. Joint Dis., *37*:11, 1976.
17. Palmer, P. E. S.: Tumoral calcinosis. Br. J. Radiol., *39*:518, 1966.
18. Pease, C. N.: Focal retardation and arrest of growth of bones due to vitamin A intoxication. J.A.M.A., *182*:980, 1962.
19. Pease, C. N., and Newton, G. G.: Metaphyseal dysplasia due to lead poisoning in children. Radiology, *79*:233, 1962.
20. Rathbun, J. C., et al.: Hypophosphatasia: a genetic study. Arch. Dis. Child., *36*:540, 1961.
21. Reifenstein, E. C., Jr.: The relationship of steroid hormones to the development and the management of osteoporosis in aging people. Clin. Orthop., *10*:206, 1957.
22. Shorbe, H. B.: Infantile scurvy. Clin. Orthop., *1*:49, 1953.
23. Sissons, H. A.: The osteoporosis of Cushing's syndrome. J. Bone Joint Surg., *38B*:418, 1956.
24. Walley, J.: A case of infantile cortical hyperostosis affecting only the clavicle and scapula. J. Bone Joint Surg., *35B*:426, 1953.
25. Wang, G., et al.: Cortisone induced bone changes and its response to lipid clearing agents. Clin. Orthop., *130*:81, 1978.
26. Zadek, R. E., and Milgram, J. W.: Progression of Paget's disease in the tibia. J. Bone Joint Surg., *58A*:876, 1976.

CHAPTER 38

HEMOPHILIA

Marvin S. Gilbert, M.D.,
and William J. Launder, M.D.

HEMATOLOGIC DISORDERS AFFECTING THE FOOT

This is the first of two chapters dealing with hematologic disorders affecting the foot. Musculoskeletal manifestations of hematologic disease are common and are therefore frequently seen in the foot. Many of these changes are generalized or nonspecific for the extremity and are thus beyond the scope of these chapters. However, these signs and symptoms are often the first manifestations of a generalized disorder, and the physician's diagnostic acumen can be taxed. Cutaneous, neurovascular, muscular, and osseous tissues may be affected. Disorders of the erythrocytes, leukocytes, platelets, and plasma proteins must be considered in a general evaluation of the patient.

The hematopoietic system is intimately housed within bone. Increased demands upon this system, as occur in many severe chronic anemias, will force the marrow to expand, eroding the cortex from within, even expanding the normal diameter of growing bone. This process will be discussed in the following chapter on hemoglobinopathies. However, it is rarely seen as a presenting complaint in the foot. Increased red cell production in polycythemia vera may be manifested as a cyanotic appearance of the hands and feet, and although numbness and tingling are common, they occur much more frequently in the hands. Ecchymoses may be noted.

Lymphomas and leukemias frequently have cutaneous manifestations. In addition to nodular infiltration of the skin, pruritus with possible secondary excoriation, hyperpigmentation, and herpes zoster are associated with lymphomas. Cellular hyperplasia, seen in the leukemias, may cause generalized osteoporosis and marrow expansion. A not uncommon complication of this disorder is hyperuricemia. Acute gouty manifestations may occur and are common just after the onset of chemotherapy. The many side effects of these agents are beyond the scope of this chapter.

Multiple myeloma rarely causes symptoms in the foot, but if radiographs are obtained, it is not unusual to see osseous changes in the bones of the feet. Platelet or bleeding disorders are associated with petechiae or ecchymoses but only rarely cause severe disability requiring the care of a foot surgeon. Coagulation disorders, or the hemophilias, do cause severe musculoskeletal disability and will be discussed in detail.

THE HEMOPHILIAS

The hemophilias are a group of congenital disorders of coagulation, transmitted through the female and affecting primarily the male, in which one of several coagulation factors is either nonfunctional or missing. Although the hemophilias are primarily disorders of hemostasis, the most common clinical manifestations are secondary to bleeding into the musculoskeletal system, specifically the joints and muscles. Recent advances in treatment have enabled many patients to avoid deformity and disability and have allowed orthopaedic surgeons to correct established deformities with intensive physiotherapy and surgery.

Hemophilia is a rare disorder affecting approximately one in every 4000 males born live.[1] It appears to have a uniform distribution in all races and countries. It is inherited as a sex-linked recessive trait, with approximately 30 per cent of newly diagnosed cases having no prior family history.[2] This is thought to be due to a high mutation rate.

Factor VIII deficiency (hemophilia A or classic hemophilia) accounts for 80 per cent of all the hemophilias. Factor IX deficiency (hemophilia B or Christmas disease) accounts for most of the rest, with other coagulation factor deficiencies being quite rare.[3] Studies have demonstrated that patients with Factor VIII deficiency produce an immunologically identifiable, but nonfunctioning molecule, as do some patients with Factor IX deficiency.[4] However, some patients with the latter disorder produce no Factor IX molecule at all.

The severity of bleeding correlates well with the procoagulant activity level, and the clinical manifestations of Factor VIII and IX deficiency are indistinguishable. Normal levels vary from 50 to 150 per cent and are slightly increased at periods of stress, exercise, and pregnancy. Patients with levels of less than 1 per cent are defined as having *severe* hemophilia and usually manifest spontaneous, recurrent musculoskeletal hemorrhage. Patients with procoagulant activity levels of 1 to 5 per cent are said to have *moderate* hemophilia and only rarely have spontaneous hemorrhage episodes, but they bleed after mild trauma and have serious bleeding at surgery unless the deficit is corrected. Levels of 5 to 50 per cent are classified as *mild,* and these patients are frequently not diagnosed early. Bleeding after major trauma or surgery is the most common manifestation, and a delay in diagnosis may lead to disastrous results.

Therapeutic Materials for Replacement Therapy

Adequate and immediate replacement of the missing clotting factor is the main-

stay of treatment. All hemarthroses and most muscle hemorrhages require immediate treatment to limit future damage. The motto espoused by Levine is "When in doubt, infuse." Both Factor VIII and Factor IX are very labile, and unless the plasma is frozen fresh, the procoagulant activity is soon lost. Even *in vivo,* Factor VIII has a limited half-life of eight to 12 hours, and Factor IX has a half-life of 12 to 24 hours. By definition, one cubic centimeter of normal plasma contains one "unit" of each factor activity. Therefore, one bag of fresh frozen plasma (250 cc) in a patient having 100 per cent activity of each factor contains 250 units of Factor VIII and Factor IX activity. Several preparations are available for replacement of these factors in the hemophiliac.[5]

Whole Blood. Whole blood is used only to replace blood loss following acute hemorrhage. The low levels of factor activity are insufficient to produce hemostatic levels for most therapeutic purposes.

Fresh Frozen Plasma. Fresh frozen plasma can be effective in the management of most minor bleeding episodes. It contains both Factors VIII and IX. It is universally available, but because of the large volume that must be transfused, levels achieved are limited by circulatory overload. It is useful in children and in patients who require infrequent transfusion. The risks of hepatitis are less than with commercial preparations, which are made from pooled plasma.

Cryoprecipitate. It was not until 1960 that the technique of cryoprecipitation made it possible to concentrate Factor VIII in smaller volumes.[6] Some factor activity is lost in the process, but one bag of cryoprecipitate contains between 50 and 100 units of Factor VIII in 30 cc. This form is also less likely to cause hepatitis than concentrates, but its disadvantages are that it must be kept frozen until use and that the level of factor activity varies from bag to bag.

Lyophilized Concentrates. Freeze-dried concentrates of Factors VIII and IX are commercially available. They come in the form of a powder, which only requires refrigeration and is reconstituted with a small volume of diluent just prior to use. Each lot is assayed, and each vial contains an indication of the number of units therein. Ease of use and predictability of response have made these preparations the most common form used in the United States. The latter makes them especially useful for replacement during surgery.

Analgesic Therapy

Pain following musculoskeletal hemorrhage frequently requires analgesic drugs. Prompt factor replacement will minimize their use. All aspirin and aspirin-containing compounds are contraindicated, because even in small doses, aspirin impairs platelet function and potentiates the bleeding propensity.[7] Similarly, intramuscular injections must be avoided, as they can cause severe hematomas. The use of narcotics must be carefully controlled because of the chronic nature of the disease.

Anti-inflammatory Agents

Anti-inflammatory agents may be useful in the control of the inflammatory responses to a hemarthrosis and of the chronic arthropathy.[8] Short courses of steroids may be used, but nonsteroidal agents predipose to bleeding by a direct effect on the platelets and are irritating to the gastric mucosa. Therefore, they should be used with discretion. Prednisone is used in our clinic if a chronic synovitis persists after hemorrhage. The recommended dosage is 1 mg/kg/day for one week and half that for a second week. For arthritic pain, Motrin, 400 mg three times a day, has been used with moderate success. We are presently doing clinical trials with Tricisate, as it has been shown not to interfere with platelet function. Preliminary results are encouraging.

Methods of Treatment

At the present time, most patients are transfused after the onset of a bleeding episode. This form of treatment is known as *episodic care* and must be started as soon as possible. At most comprehensive care centers, patients are taught to transfuse themselves. *Home care,* or *self-infusion* as it is generally known, has markedly lessened the delay between the onset of symptoms and commencement of treatment. It has significantly decreased the disabling sequelae of hemorrhage.

Prophylactic care is limited to specific indications because of unknown untoward effects and cost. Among these indications are surgery, intensive physical therapy, persistent or recurrent bleeding despite good episodic care, and participation in a high-risk vocation or avocation.

Antibody Formation

Antibodies to either Factor VIII or IX may form in up to 10 per cent of patients with hemophilia and make replacement therapy inadequate owing to the rapid inactivation of the transfused factor.[10] These antibodies (also known as anticoagulants or inhibitors) vary considerably in intensity of inhibition, but continuous replacement of a missing clotting factor may trigger an anamnestic response, rendering treatment useless. This is a devastating complication of the disease, and treatment of these patients should be limited to centers familiar with the special procedures necessary for their care.

Surgical Management

Surgery in the hemophiliac is a major undertaking and, except in emergency situations, should be performed only at centers fully conversant with hemophilia care. These centers must have a diagnostic laboratory capable of performing factor and inhibitor assays. A single lot of concentrated factor is used to maintain predictability of response, and a preoperative infusion study is done to ensure an adequate response and half-life. A factor level of 70 to 100 per cent is achieved just prior to surgery, and a minimal level of 40 per cent is maintained (for most orthopaedic surgical procedures) for 10 days. This is decreased to 25 to 30 per cent for the remaining vulnerable period (i.e., until sutures are removed, healing is completed, and physical therapy programs are completed).[11]

ORTHOPAEDIC CONSIDERATIONS

Hemophilic Arthropathy

Almost every patient with severe hemophilia has some degree of musculoskeletal damage by the time he has achieved skeletal maturity. The joints are the most common sites of hemorrhage in the hemophiliac, accounting for approximately 80 per cent of the bleeding episodes. The commonly affected articulations in order of decreasing frequency are the knees, elbows, ankles, shoulders, and hips.[12] The small joints of the feet and hands are rarely involved, except following trauma. After hemarthrosis, the blood is slowly resorbed, and the joint returns to near normal function. However, recurrence is common, and repeated hemarthroses result in a severe, characteristic arthropathy. The primary site of hemorrhage is the synovium.[13] The severe cartilage destruction that follows may be due to the enzyme liberation associated with the inflammatory response or to a primary effect of iron on the cartilage cells or ground substance (mucopolysaccharides).[14, 15] The joint changes are mirrored in the radiographs, which are frequently characteristic. Early changes include increased soft-tissue density, local osteoporosis, and epiphyseal overgrowth secondary to local hyperemia. These are followed by subchondral irregularity, loss of cartilage space, and early deformity. Subchondral cysts and osteophyte formation are late manifestations.[16]

Treatment of the Acute Hemarthrosis

No joint hemorrhage is so minor that treatment may be deferred or postponed. Hemarthroses associated with mild swelling and pain usually respond to a single infusion, which achieves a factor level of 30 to 40 per cent.[17] If a tense hemarthrosis with secondary muscle spasm has developed, factor levels of 50 per cent are usually required, and infusions may have to be repeated in 12 to 24 hours. Minor hemarthrosis may not require immobilization, but some patients find relief from Ace bandages or splints. For severe pain or deformity, plaster of Paris splints are applied in a position of comfort. Attempts at correction are deferred until bleeding has stopped.

The value of aspiration remains unclear, and it is reserved for very painful, tense hemarthroses and is rarely necessary at the ankle.

Joint rehabilitation must be started as

soon as possible to prevent deformity and atrophy.[18] Isometric exercises may be started immediately, and as soon as the acute symptoms recede, muscle-strengthening and range-of-motion exercises are started. Despite adequate treatment, recurrent hemarthroses are occasionally encountered. This justifies starting a limited period of prophylaxis.

Conservative Rehabilitation

The importance of an ongoing physical therapy program cannot be overstressed.[19] Severe flexion contractures usually require cast correction before this therapy is started. Serial casting or wedging may be tried. Severe joint destruction or the presence of an inhibitor that limits therapeutic possibilities may justify the use of a brace.

Soft-Tissue Hemorrhage

Bleeding into the soft tissues of the extremities is quite common. Superficial hematomas are frequent, but usually resorb without sequelae. Bleeding into deep muscle masses is more significant and, if untreated, may result in adjacent joint contracture, muscle necrosis, and pressure neuropathy. The extent of damage depends on the extent of hemorrhage and the containment provided by fascial compartments. Small hematomas in large muscle masses resorb without complication. Similar hematomas in tight fascial compartments will cause significant ischemic myopathy and neuropathy. On rare occasions, large hematomas may cause vascular compromise and even skin breakdown.

The gastrocnemius-soleus muscle is the most commonly affected muscle. Persistent equinus may be difficult to correct. Bleeding into the iliopsoas fascia is not uncommon, resulting in a femoral neuropathy, and bleeding into the forearm is an orthopaedic emergency.

As with arthropathy, it is of primary importance to stop the bleeding by replacing the missing clotting factor. The limb must be splinted, and motion and weight bearing must be eliminated. Well-padded plaster splints are best for this purpose and should be changed frequently as the contracture decreases. Physiotherapy should be started only after all evidence of acute bleeding has disappeared.

Pseudotumor Formation

Pseudotumor formation is a bizarre manifestation of hemophilia that may be a threat to both life and limb. Its incidence has been estimated at 1 to 2 per cent,[20] but it appears to be on the decline in a well-treated hemophilia population.

There are two clinical patterns to these encapsulated blood cysts.[21, 22] In the adult population, they are most common in the pelvis and femur, areas in which there is proximity of large muscle masses to bone. A history of trauma is common, and these encapsulated hematomas may take up to 20 years to develop. The soft-tissue mass will distort tissues, destroy bone, and interfere with nerve function. Surgical extirpation is required.

In the young hemophiliac, the pseudotumor is most common in the small bones of the foot and hand. Their treatment will be discussed later in the chapter.

Fracture Care

Fractures are not uncommon in the hemophiliac. Osteoporosis and limitation of joint motion predispose to fracture following relatively mild trauma. Fractures about the knee and hip are most common. With adequate treatment, complications are rare and union is usually achieved.

If replacement therapy is started quickly, undue hemorrhage is not a problem.[23] Factor levels of 50 per cent maintained for one week are usually sufficient. Reduction of the fracture and immobilization should be performed, with extra attention being given to prevent neurovascular compromise. Conservative care is preferred, but if open reduction is necessary, the patient should have the presurgical studies mentioned earlier in the chapter. If there is no contraindication, surgery should be performed.

THE FOOT AND ANKLE

Hemophilic Arthropathy

In most reported series, the ankle is the third most common site of joint hemor-

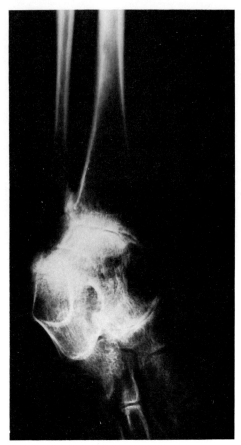

Figure 38–1. Joint-space narrowing, subchondral irregularity, and talar tilt in hemophilic arthropathy.

rhage, following the knee and elbow. However, with the advent of self-infusion, this pattern has begun to change. In the younger patient, the ankle is frequently the first joint in which arthropathy may develop. As the hemophiliac leads a more normal life and participates in sports, the ankle is subjected to continuous strains, which may cause hemorrhage. As arthropathy develops, certain characteristic changes are noted radiographically. Joint-space narrowing and subchondral irregularity are seen most often. Talar tilt is common (Fig. 38–1). Clinically, these changes are first associated with limitation of both dorsiflexion and plantar flexion, but later an equinus contracture develops. Lateral roentgenographs demonstrate flattening of the dome of the talus, with sclerosis and the development of anterior and posterior osteophytes (Fig. 38–2). The role of talar aseptic necrosis as a cause of collapse has not been established.

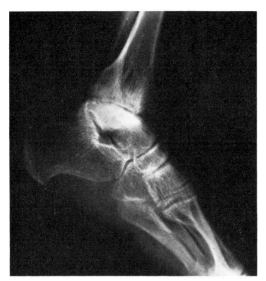

Figure 38–2. *Flattening of the talar dome and sclerosis in hemophilic arthropathy.*

Bleeding into the tarsal joints and other joints of the foot is quite rare. However, it is not uncommon to see degenerative changes at the midfoot and tarsus (Fig. 38–3). The equinus deformity and marked limitation of motion at the ankle put undue pressure stress at these joints, leading to degenerative changes and further stiffness of the foot.

Prevention of deformity by early treatment following hemorrhage cannot be stressed too much. Non–weight-bearing periods should be brief. The wearing of high shoes and boots is useful. With early arthropathy or persistent hemorrhage, posterior plastic splints or leather molded gauntlets may control pain and deformity. On rare occasions, a short leg brace with a Bi-Cal Lock may be necessary. Patellar tendon weight-bearing braces have not proved useful.

If conservative methods fail, surgery can be considered. Synovectomy, with or without joint debridement, has not proved effective at the ankle. An ankle arthrodesis remains the most predictable procedure for control of pain, correction of deformity, and control of hemorrhage. Total ankle replacement remains experimental. The age at which joint replacement is considered in the hemophiliac is much lower than in the general population, and the stresses these patients put on the prosthesis may be considerable. In addition, there may be a problem with loosening secondary to microhemorrhage at the methylmethacrylate-bone junction.

Muscle Hemorrhage

The gastrocnemius-soleus is the most common site of muscle hemorrhage in the hemophiliac. Swelling at the calf and an equinus deformity at the ankle are seen. Factor levels of 50 per cent should be achieved as long as there is evidence of acute hemorrhage. A long leg plaster splint should be applied in a position of comfort, and weight bearing should be eliminated. The splint should be changed every three or four days, and the knee and ankle should be extended as much as comfort allows. It may take over six weeks to achieve a neutral position. Weight bearing

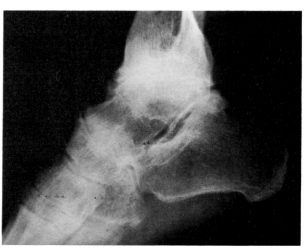

Figure 38–3. *Degenerative changes at the ankle and subtalar joints in hemophilic arthropathy.*

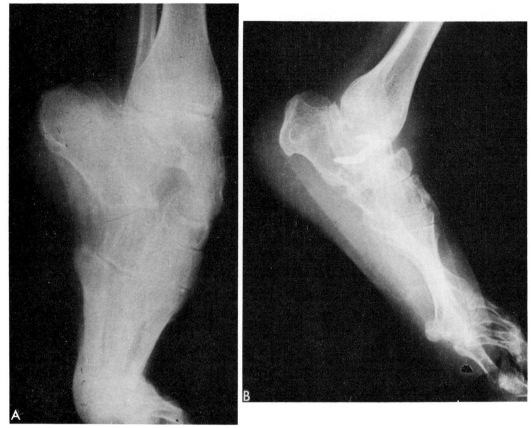

Figure 38–4. *(A) Severe equinus deformity. (B) Correction following Lambrinudi triple arthrodesis.*

should be delayed until the equinus contracture is less than 20 degrees, otherwise stress on the muscle may cause recurrent hemorrhage and place increased strain on the knee.

Once a contracture becomes fixed, it is difficult to correct by nonsurgical methods. Wedge casting may cause damage to the talus and is usually unsuccessful. Passive stretching yields similar results. Tendo-Achillis lengthening should be considered before adaptive changes occur at the ankle.

Frequently, an established Achilles tendon contracture is associated with severe degenerative changes at the ankle and subtalar joints. If the pathology is limited to the ankle, a fusion with wedge resection can be considered. A pantalar fusion may be required. In several patients, in whom there was some painless motion at the ankle, a Lambrinudi triple arthrodesis was found useful in correcting deformity (Fig. 38–4).[24]

Forefoot Problems

Extensive soft-tissue bleeding secondary to trauma at the forefoot has been encountered. Nonsurgical treatment has frequently resulted in rapid return to normal (Fig. 38–5). If neurovascular compromise is feared, presurgical evaluation should be started immediately. The delay required for this may determine whether the surgery is necessary.

Forefoot deformities, either primary or secondary to foot pathology, should be treated as in the nonhemophiliac (Fig. 38–6).

Pseudotumors

Pseudotumors at the foot (and hand) usually occur before skeletal maturity. They differ from the large pseudotumors described in the adult in that a history of trauma is not common and the progression is rapid. Multiple lesions are frequently

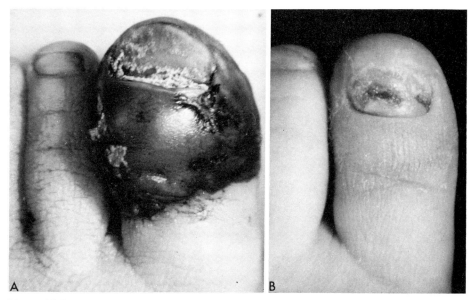

Figure 38–5. (A) Severe hemorrhage following trauma to the great toe. (B) Resolution following replacement therapy.

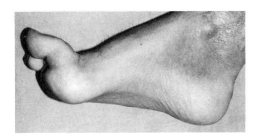

Figure 38–6. Forefoot deformities associated with equinus and cavus deformities.

Figure 38–7. Pseudotumor of the third metatarsal demonstrating cortical expansion and bone destruction.

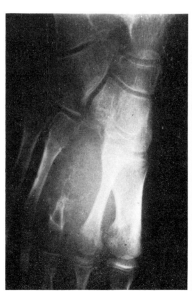
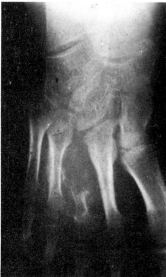

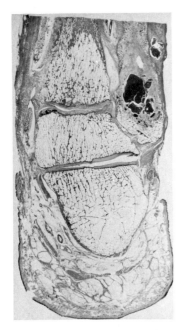

Figure 38–8. *Intraosseous bleeding at the distal fibula.*

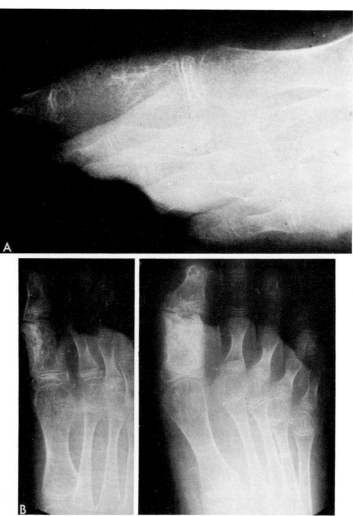

Figure 38–9. *(A) Pseudotumor of the proximal phalanx of the great toe. (B) Resolution following long-term factor replacement and immobilization. (Courtesy of Professor Robert Duthie.)*

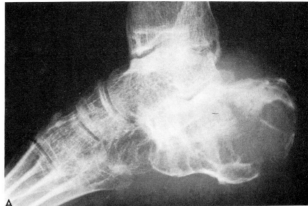

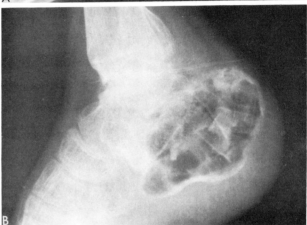

Figure 38-10. *(A) Pseudotumor of the calcaneus. (B) Curettage and grafting of the pseudotumor.*

seen. The radiographs show cortical expansion with bone destruction (Fig. 38–7), and the picture suggests that intraosseous hemorrhage is the cause of the lesion (Fig. 38–8).

These lesions also differ from the large adult lesions in that they frequently respond to nonsurgical treatment.[25, 26] Prophylactic factor replacement and immobilization should be tried first (Fig. 38–9). If this fails, one could try radiation therapy, as it has been reported to be successful in several cases.[27] Curettage and grafting can be limited to those cases in which bone collapse is imminent (Fig. 38–10).

REFERENCES

1. Biggs, R., and Macfarlane, R. G. (eds.): Treatment of Haemophilia and Other Coagulation Disorders. Oxford, Blackwell Scientific Publications, 1966.
2. Graham, J. B.: Mode of inheritance and current research. *In* Brinkhous, K. M., and Hemker, H. C. (eds.): Handbook of Haemophilia. Amsterdam, Excerpta Medica, 1975.
3. National Institutes of Health: National Blood Resource Program. A Pilot Study of Hemophilia in the U.S. Bethesda, Maryland, Department of Health, Education and Welfare, 1972.
4. Rick, M. E., and Hoyer, L. W.: The molecular structures of Factor VIII and Factor IX. Prog. Pediatr. Hematol./Oncol., *1*:1, 1976.
5. Hilgartner, M. W., and Sergis, E.: Current therapy for hemophiliacs: home care and therapeutic complications. Mt. Sinai J. Med., *44*:316, 1977.
6. Pool, J. H.: Cryoprecipitate quality and supply. Transfusion, *15*:305, 1975.
7. Quick, A. J.: Aspirin in hemophilia. *In* Brinkhous, K. M. (ed.): Hemophilia and New Hemorrhagic States. Chapel Hill, North Carolina, University of North Carolina Press, 1970.
8. Kisker, C. T., and Burke, C.: Double-blind studies on the use of steroids in the treatment of acute hemarthrosis in patients with hemophilia. N. Engl. J. Med., *202*:639, 1970.
9. Levine, P.: Efficacy of self therapy in hemophilia. N. Engl. J. Med., *229*:1381, 1974.
10. Shapiro, S. S., and Hultin, M.: Acquired inhibitors to the blood coagulation factors. Semin. Thromb. Hemostasis., *1*:336, 1975.
11. Aledort, L. M.: Hematologic management and surgery in hemophilia. Mt. Sinai J. Med., *44*:371, 1977.
12. Jordan, H.: Hemophilic Arthropathies. Springfield, Illinois, Charles C Thomas, 1958.
13. Swanton, M.: Hemophilic arthropathy in dogs. Lab. Invest., 8:1269, 1959.
14. Sokoloff, L.: Biochemical and physiological aspects of degenerative joint diseases with special reference to hemophilic arthropathy. Ann. N.Y. Acad. Sci., *240*:285, 1975.
15. Hilgartner, M. W.: Degenerative joint disease. Ann. N.Y. Acad. Sci., *340*:285, 1975.

16. Gilbert, M. S., and Cockin, J.: An evaluation of the radiologic changes in hemophilic arthropathy of the knee. *In* Ala, F., and Denson, K. W. (eds.): Haemophilia. Amsterdam, Excerpta Medica, 1973.

17. Kasper, C. K.: Hematologic care. *In* Boone, D.: Comprehensive Management of Hemophilia. Philadelphia, F. A. Davis Co., 1976.

18. Weissman, J.: Rehabilitation medicine and the hemophilic patient. Mt. Sinai J. Med., *44*:359, 1977.

19. Boone, D.: Common musculoskeletal problems and their management. *In* Comprehensive Management of Hemophilia. Philadelphia, F. A. Davis Co., 1976.

20. Gunning, A. J.: The surgery of haemophilic cysts. *In* Biggs, R., and Macfarlane, R. G. (eds.): Treatment of Haemophilia and Other Coagulation Disorders. Oxford, Blackwell Scientific Publications, 1966.

21. Ahlberg, A. K. M.: On the natural history of hemophilic pseudotumor. J. Bone Joint Surg., *57A*:1133, 1975.

22. Gilbert. M. S.: Haemophilic pseudotumor. *In* Brinkhous, K. M., and Hemker, H. C. (eds.): Handbook of Haemophilia. Amsterdam, Excerpta Medica, 1975.

23. Hoskinson, J., and Duthie, R. B.: Management of musculoskeletal problems in the hemophilias. Orthop. Clin. North Am., *9*:455, 1978.

24. Gilbert, M. S.: Reconstructive surgery in the hemophiliac. Mt. Sinai J. Med., *44*:374, 1977.

25. Favre-Gilly, J., Chatain, R., Trillat, A., and Saint-Paul, E.: Pseudo-Tumeur du calcanéum chez un hémophilie. Hémostase, *5*:95, 1965.

26. MacManon, J. S., and Blackburn, C. R. B.: Haemophilia pseudotumor: a report of a case treated conservatively. Aust. N.Z. J. Surg., *29*:129, 1960.

27. Yung Fu Chen: Bilateral hemophilic pseudo tumors of the calcaneus and cuboid treated by irradiation: case report. J. Bone Joint Surg., *47A*:517, 1965.

CHAPTER 39

THE HEMOGLOBINOPATHIES AND THE FOOT

William J. Launder, M.D.
and Marvin S. Gilbert, M.D.

Disorders that alter the structure or production rate of the globin portion of the hemoglobin molecule are termed hemoglobinopathies. Normal adult red blood cells contain a mixture of two basic hemoglobin types, A_1 and A_2. Each of these constituents is derived from two pairs of coiled polypeptide chains and four heme groups (Fig. 39–1). Hemoglobin A_1 contains two alpha polypeptide chains plus two beta polypeptide chains and is represented as $\alpha_2\beta_2$, whereas hemoglobin A_2 is composed of two alpha chains and two delta chains and is represented as $\alpha_2\delta_2$. Healthy adult hemoglobin contains 97 per cent $\alpha_2\beta_2$ plus 3 per cent $\alpha_2\delta_2$ plus a tiny fraction of persistent fetal hemoglobin F or $\alpha_2\gamma_2$. Qualitative and quantitative errors in the composition of this mixture create disorders that may eventually be manifested in the foot.

Sickle cell disease, sickle trait, and hemoglobin SC disease are the most common disorders of structure and are caused by a

NORMAL HEMOGLOBIN A WITH HEMOGLOBIN S VARIANT

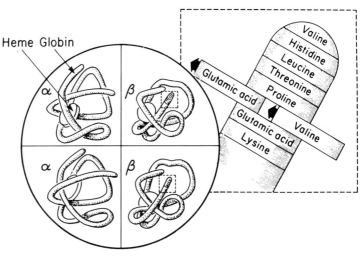

Figure 39–1. *Normal adult hemoglobin is composed of four coiled polypeptide chains plus four heme groups. The substitution of valine for glutamic acid in the sixth position on the beta chain produces hemoglobin S, which is responsible for the symptoms seen in both sickle trait and sickle cell disease.*

single amino acid substitution in the hemoglobin molecule (Fig. 39–1). Each disorder can cause severe leg ulcers, refractory osteomyelitis, and bone infarctions in the foot, as well as systemic changes of variable severity. In sickle cell disease, the majority of hemoglobin is of the abnormal S type, causing the patient to suffer from numerous crises that eventually cause severe disability and shorten the life span. In sickle trait, a smaller amount of the patient's hemoglobin is abnormal, and the symptoms are proportionately less severe. Patients with hemoglobin SC disease have two different, abnormal hemoglobin types, with resultant symptoms that fall somewhere between those of sickle cell disease and sickle trait in severity.

Defects in the rate of hemoglobin biosynthesis also exist and are termed thalassemias. Beta-thalassemias are characterized by underproduction of the beta polypeptide chain and may be seen in the severe major form or the less severe minor form, depending on the number of genes inherited. Characteristic roentgenographic changes are produced in the foot as a result of severe marrow hyperplasia.

Mixed disorders of hemoglobin structure and production, such as sickle cell–beta-thalassemia disease, also exist and are clinically significant. These patients have one normal hemoglobin A gene whose productive capacities are impaired by a thalassemia gene and another gene that produces a structurally imperfect hemoglobin such as hemoglobin S or hemoglobin C. These patients uniformly demonstrate clinical manifestations that are similar to those seen in other sickling disorders.

SICKLE CELL DISEASE

Incidence and Inheritance

Sickle cell disease is clinically manifested in homozygous individuals who carry two of the S-type genes, whereas the less severe sickle trait is seen in heterozygotes or those who have only one S gene. Patients with sickle cell disease received an S-type gene from each parent and will transmit one such gene to each of their children. Those with sickle trait may or may not transmit the gene to their off-

spring. The gene for sickling is equally distributed among males and females and is found most frequently in tropical Africa, Mediterranean countries, the Middle East, and South India. In the United States, 0.25 per cent of blacks are afflicted by the disease, whereas 7.5 per cent carry only one S gene.[1-3,12] The prevalence among other racial groups is low.

Pathophysiology

In sickle cell disease, the globin moiety has been altered by the substitution of valine in place of glutamic acid in the sixth amino acid position (Fig. 39–1). The new hemoglobin S molecule assumes a different tertiary configuration while in the reduced state. This results in the formation of needle-like polymers or tactoids, which induce a change in erythrocyte shape to the familiar sickle or "holly-leaf" form.[4] The sickling phenomenon is directly related to the oxygen concentration. Thus, in patients who are homozygous for HbS, sickling occurs at oxygen tensions that are well within the physiologic range. Increased cellular fragility and eventual hemolysis then result in a chronic hemolytic anemia, erythroid hyperplasia, increased cardiac output, and, occasionally, massive accumulation of hemoglobin degradation products.[5] Microcirculatory stasis will cause tissue hypoxia, which promotes further sickling. A vicious circle is created in which sickling is favored by progressive hypoxia. The final result is tissue necrosis, the replacement of parenchymal cells by fibrous tissue in the viscera, and the proliferation of bony infarcts throughout the skeleton.[6,7]

Diagnosis

Clinical parameters alone are often sufficient to make a diagnosis of sickle cell disease, although laboratory studies are required for its confirmation. The blood smear is typical of a hemolytic anemia, with nucleated red blood cells, target cells, some macrocytes, and occasional sickled cells. Peripheral blood added to sodium metabisulfite (a reducing agent) will initiate gross sickling on microscopic examination. The urinary specific gravity may be low; there is increased bilirubin in the urine and increased urobilinogen in the feces. Hemoglobin electrophoresis demonstrates S-type hemoglobin and fetal hemoglobin F with no A-type hemoglobin present.

Clinical Presentation

Overt manifestations of sickle cell disease are rarely, if ever, seen prior to the age of six months, as immature hemoglobin F must be replaced by the defective hemoglobin S before clinically significant sickling and hemolysis can occur.

The typical child may present at six months of age with jaundice, a chronic anemia, or the first of a lifelong series of "crises." These episodes produce severe abdominal or limb pain or both accompanied by fever, leukocytosis, and occasionally warm, swollen hands and feet.[8] The typical sickle crisis is thought to be precipitated by infection or dehydration and may vary in intensity, typically lasting for a period of several days to weeks.[5, 9, 10]

Recurrent sickle cell crises create visceral and skeletal changes that limit the life span and create many disabilities for the patient. In the kidney, local ischemia and necrosis in the renal papillae, often coupled with pyelonephritis, may lead to microscopic or even gross hematuria. Hyperuricemia secondary to renal failure or from excessive red blood cell turnover may occasionally result in gouty arthritis[11] (Fig. 39–2). Cardiac hypertrophy, pulmo-

nary hypertension, and mitral murmurs are seen in response to the demands of a chronic and severe anemia. Pulmonary vascular congestion and secondary pneumonia are the common responses to vascular stasis due to sickling or direct occlusion by marrow emboli generated in skeletal infarcts. Hepatomegaly and cirrhosis are attributed to the effect of ischemic damage to the liver. The spleen is massively enlarged in early life, owing to sequestration of red blood cells; however, chronic ischemic damage and fibrotic replacement lead to eventual autosplenectomy. Damage in the central nervous system is also secondary to tissue ischemia and manifests with a wide variety of symptoms, including convulsions, headaches, meningeal signs, and vertigo.[5, 9, 10, 12, 13]

The skeletal changes observed in sickle cell disease and its variants can be traced to four pathologic entities commonly seen in this disorder, i.e., marrow hyperplasia, skeletal infarction, osteomyelitis, and growth disturbances.

Marrow Hyperplasia

Marrow hyperplasia is the response of the hematopoietic system to chronic hemolytic anemia and is roentgenographically manifest throughout the skeleton. In the skull, thickening of the calvarium, thinning of the outer table, and a generalized loss of trabecular definition are seen.[4, 5] In the pelvis and ribs, marrow hyperplasia

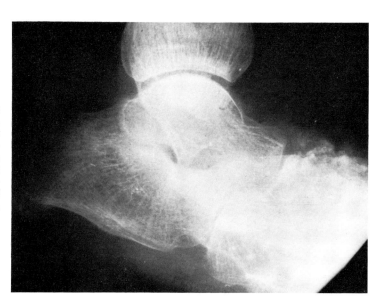

Figure 39–2. *Severe gout in a patient with sickle cell disease. This lateral view of the hindfoot and ankle demonstrates narrowing of the tarsal joint spaces with the deposition of gouty tophi in the dorsal soft tissues. This patient subsequently died in renal failure. (Courtesy of Melvin H. Jahss, M.D.)*

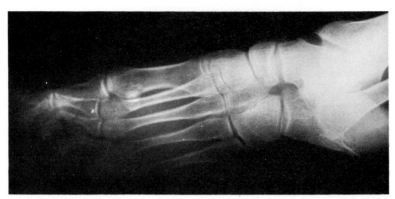

Figure 39–3.   *Bone marrow hyperplasia is expressed as osteoporosis in the foot of this patient with sickle cell disease. The phalangeal and metatarsal cortices are thinned owing to the proliferation of red marrow, while trabecular markings throughout the foot are abnormally well defined. The entire forefoot is elongated, which is typical of the body habitus occasionally seen with this disease.*[37]

results in a subtle loss of fine trabeculations, with cortical thinning. The long bones also respond with cortical thinning and widening of the spaces between diaphyseal trabeculae.[4, 5, 14] In the spine, similar changes are produced as a result of diffuse osteoporosis.

Changes secondary to bone marrow hyperplasia in the foot are due to the fact that children with hemoglobinopathies retain hypertrophic red marrow in the small tubular bones. The result is widening of the medullary canals and intratrabecular spaces by marrow, with thinning of the inner cortical surface. The radiologic appearance is similar to osteoporosis and includes increased translucency of the spongiosa, with sharply defined trabecular markings and thin cortices (Fig. 39–3). These changes are transient, however, and typically regress along with the red marrow by the seventh year.[2, 4, 15]

Skeletal Infarction

Bone infarction is a frequent sequela of the sickling process and is commonly seen in the long bones, the femoral and humeral heads, the vertebral bodies, and the calvarium, and frequently in the hands and feet. In the long bones, small focal infarctions are eventually manifested as purely sclerotic lesions and probably represent an attempt at repair by "creeping substitution"[5, 15, 16] (Fig. 39–4). Larger long-bone lesions are due to infarction of the entire nutrient artery and are occasionally seen in children. Periosteal elevation completely

deprives the cortex of nutrition, resulting in massive cortical necrosis and a "bone-within-a-bone" appearance.[4, 7, 8, 16, 17] Avascular necrosis of the femoral head has been seen in 4 to 10 per cent of older chil-

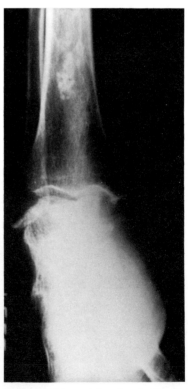

Figure 39–4.   *Old bone infarction in the distal tibia of a patient with sickle cell disease. This mottled, sclerotic lesion probably represents an attempt at repair by "creeping substitution." The surrounding bone appears osteoporotic as a result of marrow hyperplasia.*

dren and adults, and a similar pattern is seen in the humeral head.[1, 7, 8, 16] In the spine, the central three fifths of the vertebrae will appear depressed; the periphery will maintain its original flat surface.[18]

Infarcts in the small bones of the hands and feet produce a characteristic dactylitis, or hand-foot syndrome, which is frequently seen in those with sickle cell disease.[1-6, 8, 14, 17, 19] Episodes occur most commonly between the ages of six months and two years, when the cellular red marrow is most active. During this period, the immature tubular bones of the hands and feet are particularly susceptible to infarction, as they exist in a physiologic milieu that predisposes to hypoxia and sickling. Arterial blood delivered to the metatarsals and metacarpals is depleted of oxygen by the severe metabolic demands of the hyperactive red marrow. The extremities are frequently exposed to relatively low temperature, initiating a vascular response of vasoconstriction and A-V shunting. Furthermore, the metatarsals have few collateral vessels and are dependent on a single blood supply. Oxygen delivery is thus diminished in the face of markedly increased demand, favoring a hypoxic state. Sickling follows with a relative or complete cessation of blood flow, causing infarction and necrosis. Cellular injury results in the stimulation of pain receptors and a localized inflammatory reaction. Intramedullary swelling can then be severe enough to infarct the entire medullary blood supply, with almost complete destruction of the bone.

Bilateral and occasionally symmetric involvement is observed for some unknown reason, although it is distinctly uncommon for both the hands and the feet to be involved at the same time. The patient complains of painful, swollen hands or feet and may have coincident symptoms due to infarcts in the small bones of the wrist and ankle. On examination, the dorsal skin is swollen and painful to the touch, feels warm, and may be voluntarily splinted owing to pain. There is a low-grade fever and neutrophilic leukocytosis.[4] Although symptoms generally subside within 10 to 20 days, recurrence is common.

The early radiologic appearance of small infarctions is usually one of soft-tissue swelling and periosteal elevation (Fig. 39–5). Greater degrees of vascular compromise produce a roentgenographic picture of subperiosteal new bone formation with underlying areas of bony reabsorption about 10 to 14 days after the appearance of clinical symptoms. The diaphysis may appear moth-eaten secondary to bony degeneration and partial absorption.[17] In general, multiple rays are involved, with changes in the proximal phalanges, the metatarsals, and even the tarsal bones being most evident. During the reparative phase, subperiosteal bone formation results in a loss of the diaphyseal waist, parallelism of the cortices, and the production of a fairly characteristic rectangular

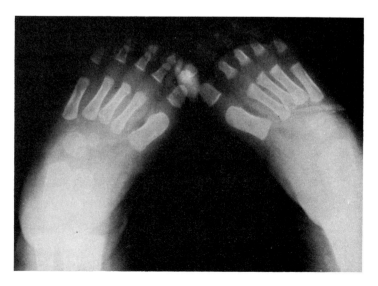

Figure 39–5. *Early changes in sickle cell dactylitis are seen in this anteroposterior roentgenogram of both feet. There is bilateral soft-tissue swelling and early periosteal elevation, which is most evident in the third metatarsal of the left foot.*

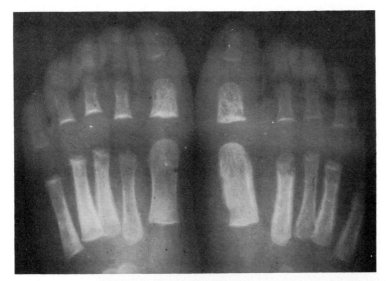

Figure 39–6. This anteroposterior roentgenogram demonstrates the late changes in the feet seen in sickle cell dactylitis. The right metatarsals show destructive metaphyseal changes, which represent absorbed, necrotic bone. Repair is most evident in the remaining metatarsals where subperiosteal new bone formation is under way. The first metatarsal of the right foot has acquired the characteristic "squared-off" appearance.

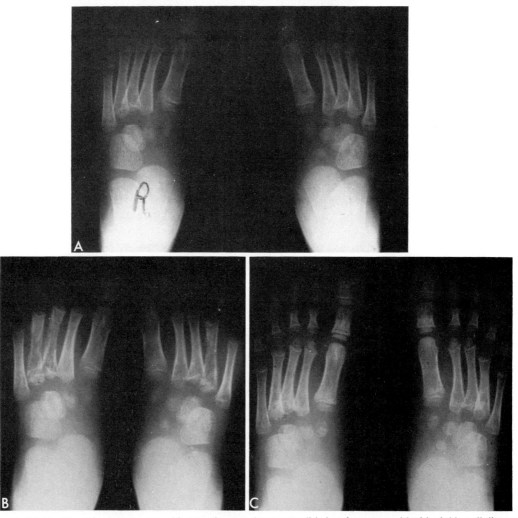

Figure 39–7. Hand-foot syndrome with superimposed osteomyelitis in a four-year-old with sickle cell disease. (A) Four days after admission in crisis this patient had pain, swelling, and periosteal elevation barely seen in the left third and fourth metatarsals and the right fourth metatarsal, indicating an infarction. (B) At two weeks, there was widespread tarsal and metatarsal destruction compatible with the clinical diagnosis of osteomyelitis. (C) At three and a half months bony changes in the foot were almost completely resolved. This child underwent a complete clinical recovery after treatment with IV antibiotics. (Courtesy of Alex Norman, M.D.)

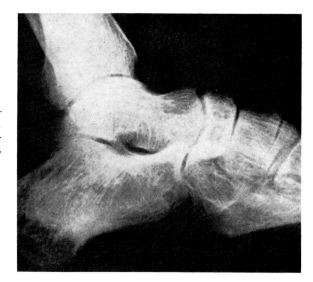

Figure 39–8. *Infarction of the tarsal navicular in a 26-year-old patient with sickle cell disease. There is a central area of radiolucency surrounded by sclerotic bone. (From Legant, O., and Ball, R. P.: Radiology, 51:665, 1948.)*

appearance (Fig. 39–6). Repair of bony damage in the young child, however, is usually rapid and complete and is evident on the roentgenogram within four to eight weeks. Residual deformities are unusual, although shortening of one or more of the tubular bones has been documented.

Treatment is purely symptomatic and consists basically of no weight bearing, analgesics, and reassurance. If osteomyelitis is suspected, care must be taken to avoid the institution of antibiotic therapy until positive cultures are obtained. Such a regimen will avoid masking the symptoms of a fulminant osteomyelitis and will prevent exposure of the noninfected child to potentially harmful drugs (Fig. 39–7).

Bone infarctions are also seen in the tarsal bones in association with dactylitis or as isolated occurrences. Legant and Ball reported a case involving a 26-year-old black male with sickle cell disease who presented with bone infarcts of both the calcaneus and the tarsal navicular. The radiologic appearance was that of central radiolucency surrounded by an area of increased density[16] (Fig. 39–8).

Other Musculoskeletal Manifestations

Chronic anemia, generalized debility, and bony infarcts all take a toll on growth and development. In the foot, individual metatarsals or phalanges may be stunted and develop a short, squat appearance after medullary infarction. Thrombosis of

the nutrient artery can cause infarction of the central portion of the growth plate, while the periphery continues to receive nourishment from the adjacent periosteal vessels. The result is retardation of central growth, with the production of a conical epiphysis and subsequent shortening. Radiologically, this may present as a short, straight, transverse sclerotic line in the diaphysis at the site of growth arrest.[4, 15]

Hyperuricemia is a familiar finding in sickle cell disease, although secondary gout is considered quite unusual.[11] When present, the radiologic and clinical findings are characteristic of the disease (see Figure 39–2).

Osteomyelitis and leg ulcers are two further complications of sickle cell disease that are frequently seen with the other hemoglobinopathies. They are, therefore, considered separately.

Treatment

Analgesics, hydration, and maintenance of electrolyte balance are required during sickle cell crisis and severe infection and for chronic leg ulcers. Patients who require surgery are in a special high-risk category. Care must be taken to correct their low hemoglobin levels prior to anesthesia. Depressant medications should be avoided, while full oxygenation is maintained throughout the procedure. Faulty positioning, tourniquets, spinal anesthesia, and hypovolemia are also relatively contraindicated, as they predispose to localized stasis and subsequent sickling.[20]

SICKLE TRAIT AND HEMOGLOBIN SC DISEASE

Sickle trait is quite common in the United States, occurring with an incidence of 5.5 to 13.4 per cent.[2, 10, 12, 21] Hemoglobin SC disease is seen more commonly in West Africa, the West Indies, and Brazil. The incidence in the United States is only 0.3 to 0.7 per cent in the black population.[21] The severity of each disease is directly related to the concentration of hemoglobin S in the blood. Sickle trait carriers often remain asymptomatic throughout life, whereas an intermediate syndrome is produced in those with hemoglobin SC disease. The sickle cell preparation with sodium metabisulfite and an electrophoretic pattern of only 20 to 40 per cent hemoglobin S establish the diagnosis of sickle trait. There is also a characteristic electrophoretic pattern in hemoglobin SC disease, with less anemia, a greater proportion of target cells, and slowly progressive splenomegaly.

Hand-foot syndrome has been reported in from zero to 28 per cent of those patients with clinically evident SC disease.[2, 22, 23] Reynolds reported a case illustrating a massive old infarction in a 40-year-old patient with hemoglobin SC disease.[15] A dense inner stratum of sclerotic bone had formed within the spongiosa of the distal tibia, calcaneus, and talus to give the classic "bone-within-a-bone" appearance. Changes of this sort were felt to be unusual in the tarsal bones and significant only in that they demonstrated a site of old infarction. Leg ulcers and metatarsal growth disturbances are also seen in this population, with a variable incidence.[22, 24]

THE THALASSEMIA SYNDROMES

The thalassemia genes prevail in Southeast Asia and Mediterranean countries, where the incidence has been reported to be as high as 20 per cent.[12] Thalassemia minor is generally a subclinical disorder due to the inheritance of a single thalassemia gene. The homozygous or double-gene state is termed thalassemia major and is a severe disorder that few survive beyond adolescence. Sickle cell–thalassemia is a mixed disorder that results from inheriting one hemoglobin S gene plus one of the many possible genes that code for thalassemia. The clinical expression of this disease is in great part dependent on the variable severity of the thalassemia syndrome, so that data concerning exact incidence are poor.[25]

The pure thalassemia syndromes may be diagnosed by their characteristic electrophoretic patterns. There is no sickling, but there is an increased resistance to hemolysis in hypotonic saline. The peripheral smear will show thin, pale red blood cells, erythroblastosis, stippling, reticulocytosis, and leukocytosis. The laboratory findings in sickle cell–thalassemia include sickling, hypochromia, microcytosis, target cells, decreased osmotic fragility, and severe hemolytic anemia. The electrophoretic pattern here is 60 to 80 per cent HbS and zero to 29 per cent HbA and may thus be difficult to distinguish from sickle cell disease.

The changes due to marrow hyperplasia are seen to a greater extent with the thalassemia syndromes than with other chronic hemolytic anemias.[25] In the foot, widening of the medullary cavity and cortical thinning may give the metatarsals and phalanges a squared off appearance. Trabecular thinning presents as a prominent reticular pattern, which may actually resemble multiple, small cysts[2, 26] (Fig. 39–9). Extensive hematopoiesis can develop beneath the periosteum in the hands and feet, producing a scalloped cortical edge. As in SC disease, enlarged nutrient foramina in the phalanges are also a frequent finding.[2, 26]

Treatment. Treatment of the thalassemia syndromes is not rewarding, as these patients are generally refractory to any form of therapy. On occasion, however, replacement therapy with iron, vitamins, or transfusion may provide a transient salutary effect.

OSTEOMYELITIS

The incidence of osteomyelitis is increased in sickle cell disease.[14] Gram-neg-

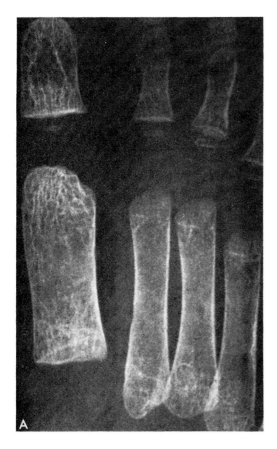

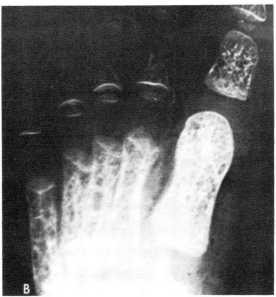

Figure 39–9. *Metatarsal changes due to intense marrow hyperplasia in the thalassemia syndromes. (A) Widening of the medullary cavity has produced thin cortical walls and a rectangular appearance in the first four metatarsals. (B) Alterations in trabecular architecture give the appearance of multiple cystic spaces as a result of compensatory marrow proliferation. (A, from Middlemiss, J. H., and Raper, A. B.: J. Bone Joint Surg., 48B:693, 1966; B, from Baker, D. H.: Ann. N.Y. Acad. Sci., 119, 642, 1964–65.)*

ative organisms, particularly Salmonella, are well known to be responsible for a disproportionate number of these infections.[23, 27]

Several mechanisms may be operating to predispose the sickler to Salmonella osteomyelitis. Normal individuals occasionally experience silent gram-negative bacteremias. In the sickler, however, serious bacteremias can arise as a result of bowel infarction or the relative deficiency of the reticuloendothelial system in filtering the portal circulation. Infection may then follow in areas of bone infarction in which host defenses are minimal.

The affected patient usually presents with local signs of inflammation, fever, leukocytosis, an increased erythrocyte sedimentation rate, and increased serum bilirubin. The initial lesion typically occurs in the diaphysis of a long bone, unlike that in the nonsickler in whom metaphyseal involvement is most common.[14, 27] Less common sites have been reported in the ribs, spine, sternum, hands, and tarsal bones.[15, 28] Golding and coworkers reported a case in which the entire calcaneus collapsed after such an episode.[8] Furthermore, Salmonella infections of the metatarsals and phalanges have been seen secondary to clinically evident dactylitis and leg ulcers. The majority of cases have multiple sites of involvement. The roentgenographic features include massive cortical destruction with periosteal elevation and occasionally overabundant involucrum formation. Multiple foci distributed bilaterally and often symmetrically are fairly characteristic. In addition, "cortical fissuring," a translucent line parallel with the shaft, may appear to split the cortex and currently serves as an almost pathognomonic sign of sickle cell hemoglobinopathy[4, 5, 29] (Fig. 39–10).

Treatment. Ampicillin is generally effective in the treatment of gram-negative organisms and is indicated when infection is suspected. If an infection is clinically obvious, however, chloramphenicol is the drug of choice, as the frequency of resis-

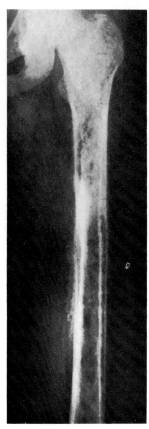

Figure 39–10. *Cortical fissuring in the femoral shaft of a sickler with Salmonella osteomyelitis. The translucent line parallel to the diaphysis is an almost pathognomonic sign of sickle cell hemoglobinopathy. (From Reynolds, J., et al.: Am. J. Roentgenol. 118:378, 1973.)*

tance by Salmonella strains is far less.[27] Care must be taken to closely monitor hematopoietic function with its use. Intravenous antibiotics are generally continued for a period of three to six weeks, depending on the clinical response.

The role of surgical decompression is altered in this disease, as previous diaphyseal infarction invalidates heroic attempts to prevent cortical sequestration. The indications for surgical drainage should be limited to gaining tissue for bacteriologic cultures or for the drainage of an obvious subperiosteal abscess. The results of appropriate treatment are gratifying, with complete radiologic resolution usually seen within a year. Chronic osteomyelitis or pyarthroses are decidedly rare.

LEG ULCERS

Chronic leg ulcers are a frequent finding in sickle cell disease, with reported incidences ranging from 25 to 100 per cent.[13, 30, 31] Skin breakdown is less common in hemoglobin SC disease and sickle cell–beta-thalassemia.[23] The average age of occurrence has been reported as 15 years,[32] it being an uncommon occurrence in young children and seen with less prevalence in those who survive into the fourth decade.[33] The overall incidence appears reduced in well-developed countries, where proper footwear protects the lower leg from accidental trauma. Currently, there are several theories that might account for the development and persistence of leg ulcers, although none have been proved. One theory holds that minor lesions, such as an insect bite, become infected and fail to heal owing to deficient circulation. Another theory notes the existence of lesions that appear spontaneously with the development of a shallow crater and heal rapidly if proper hygiene prevents supervening infection. These lesions are thought to be due to primary vascular thrombosis and tissue infarction. A poor blood supply prevents active healing of these ulcers or the delivery of antibiotics to the site of infection.[31]

Leg ulcers in sicklers classically present on the medial or lateral aspect of the distal tibia, although any area on the leg may be affected, including the sole and dorsum of the foot. Song reported that one third of the patients in his study had bilateral lesions, which were occasionally multiple and were most frequently present on the medial aspect of the distal tibia.[30] These lesions present as sharply marginated, "punched-out" craters with a roughly oval or circular shape (Fig. 39–11). The base usually consists of greyish granulation tissue, although it may be filled with dried serum and fibrinous slough, giving a yellow appearance. The borders of the lesions are generally irregular and elevated, with some undermining. Healing, which is prolonged and plagued by recurrence, takes place with the production of rough, irregular scars, which are usually surrounded by a pigmented border or areola. Recurrence can occur at any time, resulting in a lesion as big as or bigger than the initial ulcer.

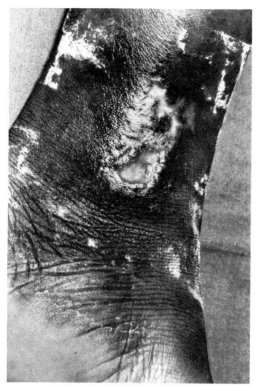

Figure 39–11. *Healing leg ulcer on the medial aspect of the ankle of a patient with sickle cell disease. The crater base is filled with greyish granulation tissue. (Courtesy of Melvin H. Jahss, M.D.)*

Radiologic changes were reported by Ennis in 75 per cent of ulcers in his study.[34] Acutely, periosteal reaction may be seen under the ulcer or even extending the entire length of the fibula or tibia. Occasionally, this subperiosteal new bone formation may have an "onion-skin" appearance or the "sunburst" appearance characteristic of osteogenic sarcoma. Sequestrum formation has also been reported in this group.[35] All of these radiologic abnormalities in the acute and semi-acute stages have, however, been reported to resolve in the course of ulcer healing. Chronic changes include the elaboration of cancellous or sclerotic ivory-like osteomas underlying the ulcer, seen in 19 per cent of Ennis' cases.[34] Periosteal reaction may present as irregular widening of the bone, with the occasional elaboration of bony spicules.

Treatment. Classically, treatment consists of frequent wet-to-dry dressing changes with a mild antiseptic coupled with bed rest for several weeks or even months. Elastic stockings are applied to prevent additional trauma and to decrease resting venous pressure. Antibiotics are employed in the face of obvious infection. Healing may be rapid in small- to moderate-sized ulcers with this regimen, but the recurrence rate is devastatingly high. Wolfort and Krizek reported that only four of 205 conservatively treated ulcers (2 per cent) remained healed for two years.[31]

Surgical intervention has also had uniformly poor results. Debridement of an obviously unhealthy crater base generally results in recurrence within several weeks and further delay in healing. Pinch grafts, split-thickness grafts, and cross-leg flaps have all been discouraging, with a 96 per cent two-year recurrence rate reported.[31]

More recently, intensive transfusion, oral zinc therapy, and disloughing creams have come into favor. Transfusions can achieve a transient rise in hemoglobin levels, which may lead to ulcer healing over a period of weeks. Zinc sulfate or zinc acetate administered as 25 mg of elemental zinc orally every four hours has been demonstrated to increase hemoglobin levels by 10 per cent and to accelerate ulcer resolution.[36] Disloughing creams such as Debrisan have also promoted rapid healing. Recurrence, however, appears inevitable. Conservative methods have, therefore, remained the method of choice, with surgery being reserved for exceptionally large ulcers or those in which primary healing is delayed. Prevention is encouraged by the use of elastic stockings and aggressive treatment of early lesions to prevent infection.

REFERENCES

1. Sennara, H., and Gorry, F.: Orthopedic aspects of sickle cell anemia and allied hemoglobinopathies. Clin. Orthop., *130*:154, 1978.
2. Middlemiss, J. H., and Raper, A. B.: Skeletal changes in the hemoglobinopathies. J. Bone Joint Surg., *48B*:693, 1966.
3. Carroll, D. S., and Evans, J. W.: Roentgen findings in sickle cell anemia. Radiology, *53*:834, 1949.
4. Diggs, L. W.: Bone and joint lesions in sickle cell disease. Clin. Orthop., *52*:119, 1967.
5. Reynolds, J.: Radiologic manifestations of sickle cell hemoglobinopathy. J.A.M.A., *238*:247, 1977.
6. Rowe, C. W., and Haggard, M. E.: Bone infarcts in sickle cell anemia. Radiology, *68*:661, 1957.
7. Chung, M. K., Alavi, A., and Russell, M. D.: Management of osteonecrosis in sickle cell anemia and its genetic variants. Clin. Orthop., *130*:158, 1978.

8. Golding, J. S. R., MacIver, J. E., and Went, L. N.: The bone changes in sickle cell anemia and its genetic variants. J. Bone Joint Surg., *41B*:711, 1959.

9. Harrison, T. R., et al.: Principles of Internal Medicine, 6th ed. New York, McGraw-Hill, 1970, p. 1621.

10. Harvey, A. M., et al.: The Principles and Practice of Medicine, 18th ed. New York, Appleton-Century-Crofts, 1972, p. 562.

11. Ryckewaert, A., and Kuntz, D.: Etiologic varieties of hyperuricemia and gout. Adv. Nephrol., *3*:29, 1974.

12. Wintrobe, M. M.: Clinical Hematology, 6th ed. Philadelphia, Lea and Febiger, 1967.

13. Serjeant, G. R.: The Clinical Features of Sickle Cell Disease. New York, North Holland Publishing Co., 1974.

14. Burko, H., Watson, J., and Robinson, M.: Unusual bone changes in sickle-cell disease in childhood. Radiology, *80*:957, 1963.

15. Reynolds, J.: The Roentgenological Features of Sickle Cell Disease and Related Hemoglobinopathies. Springfield, Illinois, Charles C Thomas, 1965.

16. Legant, O., and Ball, R. P.: Sickle cell anemia in adults: roentgenographic findings. Radiology, *51*:665, 1948.

17. Diggs, L. W.: Anatomic lesions in sickle cell diseases. *In* Abramson, H., Bertles, J. F., and Wethers, D. L. (eds.): Sickle Cell Disease. St. Louis, C. V. Mosby Co., 1973.

18. Reynolds, J.: A re-evaluation of the "fish-vertebrae" sign in sickle cell hemoglobinopathy. Am. J. Roentgenol. Radium Ther. Nucl. Med., *97*:693, 1966.

19. Pearson, H. A.: Sickle cell anemia: clinical management during the early years of life. *In* Abramson, H., Bertles, J. F., and Wethers, D. L. (eds.): Sickle Cell Disease. St. Louis, C. V. Mosby Co., 1973.

20. Shapiro, V. D., and Poe, M. F.: Sickle cell disease: an anaesthesiological problem. Anesthesiology, *16*:771, 1955.

21. Becker, J. A.: Hemoglobin SC disease. Radiology, 88:503, 1962.

22. Barton, J. C., and Cockshott, W. P.: Bone changes in hemoglobin SC disease. Radiology, 88:523, 1962.

23. Robinson, M. G.: Clinical aspects of sickle cell disease. *In* Levere, R. D. (ed.): Sickle Cell Anemia and Other Hemoglobinopathies. New York, Academic Press, 1975, p. 96.

24. Reynolds, J.: Roentgenographic and clinical appraisal of sickle cell–hemoglobin C disease. Am. J. Roentgenol. Radium Ther. Nucl. Med., 88:512, 1962.

25. Reynolds, J., Pritchard, J. A., Ludders, D., and Mason, R. A.: Roentgenographic and clinical appraisal of sickle cell beta-thalassemia disease. Am. J. Roentgenol. Radium Ther. Nucl. Med., *118*:378, 1973.

26. Baker, D. H.: Roentgen manifestations of Cooley's anemia. Ann. N. Y. Acad. Sci., *119*:641, 1964–1965.

27. Engh, C. A., Hughes, J. L., et al.: Osteomyelitis in the patient with sickle cell disease. J. Bone Joint Surg., *53A*:1, 1971.

28. Barrett-Connor, E.: Bacterial infection and sickle cell anemia. Medicine, *50*:97, 1971.

29. Wigh, R., and Thompson, H. J.: Cortical fissuring in osteomyelitis complicating sickle-cell anemia. Radiology, *55*:553, 1950.

30. Song, J.: Pathology of Sickle Cell Disease, 1st ed. Springfield, Illinois, Charles C Thomas, 1971.

31. Wolfort, F. G., and Krizek, T. J.: Skin ulceration in sickle cell anemia. J. Plast. Reconstr. Surg., *43*:71, 1969.

32. Diggs, L. W., and Ching, R. E.: Pathology of sickle cell anemia. South. Med. J., *27*:839, 1934.

33. Gueri, M., and Serjeant, G. R.: Leg ulcers in sickle-cell anemia. Trop. Georgr. Med., *22*:155, 1970.

34. Ennis, J. T., Gueri, M. C., and Serjeant, G. R.: Radiologic changes associated with leg ulcers in the tropics. Br. J. Radiol., *45*:8, 1972.

35. Brown, J. S., and Middlemiss, J. H.: Bone changes in tropical ulcer. Br. J. Radiol., *29*:213, 1956.

36. Brewer, G. J.: A view of the current status of antisickling therapy. Am. J. Hematol., *1*:121, 1976.

37. Whitten, C. F.: Growth status of children with sickle-cell anemia. Am. J. Dis. Child., *102*:101, 1961.

CHAPTER 40

EXAMINATION OF THE FOOT WITH A NEUROLOGIC DISORDER

Alfred J. Spiro, M.D.

The cardinal rule in evaluating the patient with a neurologic problem involving the foot should be not to ignore the rest of the body. Obviously, although the patient's primary complaint may stress the neurologic aspects of the problems of the foot, these complaints may merely represent a peripheral segment of a more generalized disorder. The section that follows will stress the examination and testing of the foot, but it is emphasized that a *standard* neurologic assessment is to be performed in addition to the general examination in every instance. Special attention should be given to the examination of the skin, head, back, and *all* extremities. The neurologic examination includes evaluation of the mental status, cranial nerves, motor system (tone, strength, gait and station, abnormal movements, and coordination), sensory perception, reflexes, and autonomic nervous system. It is beyond the scope and intention of this chapter to detail the entire examination, but certain features relevant to the neurologic foot will be listed.

PRIMARY ASPECTS OF THE NEUROLOGIC EXAMINATION

The Skin

The patient should be questioned concerning the presence of cold feelings in the extremities, which may suggest trophic changes. Changes in the skin and nails that may be indicative of trophic effects should be looked for in *all* extremities. These include drying or tightening of the skin and ulcerations. If ulcerations are present, it should be ascertained if they are painful or painless.

The patient should also be asked about the presence of "birthmarks" on himself or members of his family. Examination for evidence of a neurocutaneous disorder, such as café au lait spots, subcutaneous lumps, or port-wine stains, should then be carried out. Of the neurocutaneous disorders, neurofibromatosis may have profound effects on the central and peripheral nervous system and, therefore, on the foot. Hairy moles over the spine, sometimes associated with diastematomyelia, and dermal sinuses, especially over the cranial and caudal portions of the spine, should be looked for.

The Head

Comparison of measurements of the patient's largest fronto-occipital circumference with percentile tables of normal values will enable the examiner to detect deviations from the normal circumference. Abnormally large or small heads, not necessarily obvious to casual observation, may reflect comparable abnormalities in brain size and may thus have profound effects on the feet.

Observations of the face for the presence of characteristic changes suggesting chromosomal disorders such as Down's syndrome should not be neglected, since these syndromes are often associated with abnormalities of the foot. The so-called "myopathic face," which signifies weakness of some of the mimetic musculature, or inability to close the eyelids against resistance may offer a clue to the correct diagnosis of a more generalized muscular disorder — for example, one of the many types of muscular dystrophy — even though the presenting problem is one referable to the foot.

The Back

Winging of the scapula, which is enhanced if the patient is asked to push against a wall with his elbows flexed, and forward sloping of the shoulders may be associated with a more generalized disorder, facioscapulohumeral muscular dystrophy, which might present with problems related to weakness of the feet. Scoliosis, examined for in the prescribed manner, may be associated with several neurologic and neuromuscular disorders that involve the feet, e.g., Friedreich's ataxia, progressive spinal muscular atrophy, and muscular dystrophy of several types.

Examination for back pain, especially low back pain, is obviously an integral part of the examination of every patient in whom lower extremity radicular pain, weakness, or sensory disturbances are present.

The Extremities

In addition to the evaluation of bones and joints, muscle wasting should be looked for. Characteristic patterns, such as the "stork legs" seen in Charcot-Marie-Tooth disease or Friedreich's foot, may be very revealing; when a problem with the feet is encountered, the clinician should examine the patient's hands carefully to detect an analagous problem, such as weakness or wasting of the intrinsic muscles. In some instances, especially when the diagnosis is not completely clear-cut, it is advisable to evaluate members of the patient's family to document the presence of a genetic disorder, such as Charcot-Marie-Tooth disease.

The Cranial Nerves

A disorder of mobility of the eyes (e.g., partial or total external ophthalmoplegia), when found in conjunction with neurologic disorders of the foot, such as weakness, may indicate the presence of a more generalized disorder. Weakness of the facial, pharyngeal, and tongue musculature also has a great deal of significance in pointing to a more generalized disorder when coupled with weakness of the distal extremities. Fasciculations, atrophy, and myotonia of the tongue should also be looked for. Fasciculations of the tongue together with atrophy document the presence of denervation. Tongue myotonia, examined for by sharply tapping over the surface of the tongue with the narrow edge of a tongue depressor, can assist the clinician in confirming the diagnosis of myotonic dystrophy. The sternocleidomastoid muscle, when small and strand-like, provides a clue that the patient may have myotonic dystrophy. The presenting complaint of patients with this disease may center around their walking problems, because of selective weakness of the anterior tibial muscles.

The Motor System

If ambulatory, the patient's gait should be evaluated, and, if possible, he should be observed walking up and down stairs and running to detect subtleties of pelvic girdle weakness. For further signs of pelvic girdle weakness, the patient should also be watched while getting up from a chair without using his arms for support, getting up from a table from the prone position, attempting to pick up an object from the floor, and doing deep knee bends. The patient should be asked to walk on his heels and on his toes, hop on either foot, and walk on the lateral and medial borders of the foot so that weakness of the anterior and posterior compartments of the lower leg can be detected. If these maneuvers are all performed normally, it is unlikely that significant muscle weakness is present. Tandem gait forward and backward, abnormalities of which may indicate ataxia, should also be observed.

If there is any abnormality in the afore-mentioned tests or any question of weak-ness, manual muscle testing should be performed. The reader is referred to stand-ard manuals for the proper techniques.

As stressed previously, if the patient complains of weakness of the feet, or if weakness is detected by functional or manual muscle testing, the upper extremi-ties, especially the hands, should then be tested manually for weakness.

Station is tested by asking the patient to stand with his feet together, initially with the eyes open and then with the eyes closed. He should not waiver from the original position. Significant waivering may indicate a posterior column disorder.

Abnormalities of tone, the resistance to passive stretching, should also be looked for. The flail hypotonic foot and the spastic plantar flexed extremity can be readily recognized, but minor alterations of tone may be more difficult to detect.

While the patient is being observed, fasciculations of the muscles should be noted. Sometimes they can be accentuated after a light tap with a reflex hammer over the muscle. Myotonia will not be detected in the feet; the thenar eminence should be tapped briskly with a reflex hammer to observe the slowed relaxation of the thumb (percussion myotonia), or the pa-tient should grasp the examiner's hand and attempt to let go quickly in order to elicit reflex myotonia. Tremors of the fingers at rest or on volitional movement should also be looked for. Athetosis, chorea, and dys-tonia, abnormal movements that may be associated with a neurologic disorder of the foot, should also be noted. It should be stressed that in dystonia musculorum de-formans, the complaints may be entirely referable to the foot, and the neurologic examination may be entirely normal. The patient should be requested to perform the finger-to-nose and heel-to-shin tests for dysmetria for detection of a cerebellar component.

Reflexes

The ankle jerks (S1, S2) can be readily elicited by having the sitting patient dan-gle his legs and position his feet so that they are slightly dorsiflexed. The Achilles tendon is then briskly tapped with a reflex hammer. If the reflex is not readily elicit-ed, it can be reinforced by asking the patient to couple his flexed fingers togeth-er and attempt to pull them apart. The patient can also be instructed to kneel on the seat of a chair with the ankles extend-ing unsupported over the edge. In the bedridden patient, the hip can be partially flexed and externally rotated and the knee partially flexed so that the ankle is posi-tioned over the opposite shin. After slight dorsiflexion, the tendon can be tapped with a reflex hammer. The reflex can be graded by a numerical system from zero to four (zero —no response; one — hypoac-tive; two and three — normal; and four — hyperactive). The right and left ankle jerks are also compared for difference in re-sponse.

Other deep tendon reflexes are tested for in the prescribed manner. Clonus at the ankle may be tested for in a relaxed patient by sharply dorsiflexing the foot; pressure is then maintained in the same direction.

Neurologists use many methods to elicit the Babinski reflex, and caution must be used in its interpretation. In general, the reflex may be tested for by running the end of the handle of a reflex hammer, a key, or the examiner's thumbnail along the lateral side of the heel toward the fifth toe, and then across the ball of the foot to the great toe. The response in the great toe, flexor or extensor, should be noted, but it may not always be easily distinguished from a withdrawal from the stimulus. An extensor plantar response (positive Babinski reflex) is indicative of corticospinal tract dysfunc-tion and is a very important sign.

Sensory Perception

Several types of sensory perception are tested in an attempt to document abnor-malities and to help distinguish root from peripheral nerve abnormalities. For this purpose, the examiner must have a basic knowledge of dermatomal and peripheral nerve distribution (see standard texts).

The examiner can test for diminished touch perception by using a piece of cotton or his fingers (lightly) as a stimulus and asking the patient if he experiences any differences when touched in different areas. In using a pin to search for an area of hypesthesia (diminished pain perception), the examiner should proceed from an area of anesthesia or hypesthesia to a normal area. The stimuli should be presented slowly to avoid temporal summation. Symmetric regions of both extremities should be tested and compared for alterations of touch and pain perception. The sensory perception of distal and more proximal regions of the same extremity should also be compared for evidence of "stocking" hypesthesia or hypalgesia, indicative of a peripheral neuropathy. "Glove" sensory disturbances should also be looked for in the upper extremities.

If a lesion involving the lower spinal cord or roots is being considered, or if urinary symptoms accompany the neurologic complaints, the presence or absence of perianal sensation should be ascertained.

Vibratory perception, tested with a 128 Herz tuning fork, should not be neglected. The examiner can use his own limbs as a control to provide a semiquantitative test. Subtle abnormalities of the peripheral nerves or posterior columns can sometimes be identified with this test. For example, in peripheral neuropathies, while position sense is usually maintained, *peripheral* vibratory testing is invariably positive. Vibratory sense must be tested over the first metatarsal (and metacarpal) heads, since in peripheral neuropathy the more distal areas of the arms and legs are involved.

Joint position sense is tested for in the lower extremities by holding the great toe on its side (which eliminates the sense of touch) and moving it up or down slightly and asking the patient, without his observing the action, which way the movement was performed. Irregularities can help identify posterior column abnormalities.

Autonomic Nervous System

If a history of urinary incontinence, frequency, or urgency is obtained or if sacral sensory disturbances are noted, a cystometrogram may be included as part of the patient's neurologic evaluation.

ANCILLARY STUDIES

Blood, Urine, and Radiographic Studies

It is beyond the scope of this chapter to describe the individual situations in which complete blood counts, glucose tolerance tests, urine analyses, spinal fluid examinations, myelography, radiographs of the spine, computerized axial tomography of the lower spine, and tests for pernicious anemia, are needed in the evaluation in the patient with a neurologic foot disorder, since these are described under individual entities.

Serum creatine phosphokinase (CPK) determinations can be very useful in the diagnosis of muscular dystrophy and other disorders of muscle that may involve the feet. In addition, CPK can be useful in identifying certain clinically uninvolved carriers.

Electrodiagnostic Studies

These studies include electromyography (EMG) and sensory and motor nerve conduction velocity determinations. The EMG, which is done with needle electrodes (which are somewhat painful to the patient), enables the examiner to detect abnormalities in clinically uninvolved muscles and to document or detect myotonia and helps to distinguish neuropathic from myopathic processes, with certain limitations. It must be remembered that electromyography is a somewhat subjective procedure, and the results must be interpreted by someone well versed in the technique. Despite these problems, the EMG can be rather characteristic of certain disorders, e.g., inflammatory myopathies (polymyositis) and myotonia. Another important feature is that several muscles can be tested.

Denervation can be identified in a resting muscle by the presence of fibrillations and positive sharp waves. Normally, resting muscles are electrically silent. On minimal volitional activity, it can be seen that the single motor unit potentials are of longer duration than normal and of higher amplitude. They may also be polyphasic.

In "primary" muscular disorders, the EMG reveals electrical silence at rest, similar to normal. The single motor unit potentials recorded on minimal volition are of low amplitude and brief duration.

Nerve conduction velocity determinations, both motor and sensory, are more objective tests, and they are less uncomfortable for the patient since surface electrodes can generally be used. These tests can be extremely useful in diagnosing root and peripheral nerve disorders and entrapment syndrome. Further details about electromyography and electrodiagnostic testing are found in Chapters 2 and 3, respectively.

Muscle and Peripheral Nerve Biopsies

Biopsies of skeletal muscle or peripheral nerve can be performed *if needed* in the study of motor unit disorders; however, in either case, the procedure should be performed in a manner that will provide tissue for maximal usefulness with respect to clinical diagnosis. To accomplish this, the biopsy must provide well-oriented and virtually artifact-free tissue.

Muscle Biopsy. Muscle biopsies are generally performed when diseases such as spinal muscular atrophy, muscular dystrophy, inflammatory myopathy, or congenital myopathy are suspected. The muscle biopsied should be one affected by the disorder but not severely wasted. Recent electromyography or acupuncture should not have been performed in the muscle because of the artifacts associated with these procedures. The patient can be sedated prior to the procedure, which can be somewhat painful, and the tissue overlying the muscle, but not the muscle itself, can be infiltrated with a local anesthetic.

An incision approximately 3 cm long is made over the muscle belly parallel to the muscle bundles; it is then carried down to the superficial fascia, and the wound is spread with a self-retaining retractor. The fascia is incised in the same direction as the bundles, and the retractor is replaced under the fascia. Specimens can be taken, always parallel to the bundles. A section approximately 2 cm by 5 mm by 5 mm can

then be removed carefully, either by using a clamp made for that purpose or by suturing the section to an applicator stick to maintain orientation. Orientation is critical to enable the pathologist subsequently to cut cross sections, which are best suited for diagnostic purposes. The tissue can be used for preparing formalin-fixed sections and for quick freezing (without fixation) in liquid nitrogen for histochemical studies, an essential part of the evaluation. Smaller sections can be taken for glutaraldehyde fixation for electron microscopy.

With this method, the muscle biopsy, when indicated, can be a very useful addition to other diagnostic procedures.

Peripheral Nerve Biopsy. Nerve biopsies, which should not be performed unless facilities for the proper evaluation of the tissue are available, can be useful in the diagnosis of certain degenerative disorders of the nervous system, periarteritis nodosa, and diseases in which the peripheral nerves are enlarged. Less clinically useful information is obtained in chronically evolving distal symmetric polyneuropathies of metabolic or toxic origin.

Biopsy of the sural nerve can be performed under local anesthesia in the area lateral to the Achilles tendon.

Care should be taken to identify the nerve, since the appearance of the vein is rather similar. For most studies a 3- to 4-cm section is adequate. The specimen should be fixed *slightly* stretched.

REFERENCES

1. Asbury, A. K., and Connelly, E. S.: Sural nerve biopsy: technical note. J. Neurosurg., 38:391, 1973.
2. Mayo Clinic: Clinical Examinations in Neurology, 4th ed. Philadelphia, W. B. Saunders Company, 1976.
3. Medical Research Council: Aids to the Investigation of Peripheral Nerve Injuries. London, Her Majesty's Stationary Office, 1975.

CHAPTER 41

DISORDERS OF THE LOWER EXTREMITY IN THE STROKE AND HEAD TRAUMA PATIENT

Robert L. Waters, M.D.,

and Douglas E. Garland, M.D.

STROKE

Hemiplegia is the most common neurologic deficit following a cerebrovascular accident (CVA) and occurs in almost 50 per cent of all strokes.[2] The majority of the spontaneous neurologic recoveries occur within the first six months. Spasticity or flaccidity of the lower extremity often requires bracing at the ankle joint to enable ambulation. In the following months, gait usually improves as neurologic function returns and as the patient learns to cope with his disability. If spasticity or flaccidity persists, bracing may be a continued requirement. Surgery for spasticity or tendon transfers may be performed after six to nine months have elapsed, as there will be little neurologic change after this period.

The correct surgical procedure depends on visual gait analysis and not an examination at the bedside or with the patient in a chair. Spasticity changes with verticality, and which muscles to release or transfer can only be determined after observing the patient ambulate.[3] Kinesiologic electromyography is an important aid and gives a more precise insight into the actions of muscles during ambulation. If available, it confirms and adds to the visual analysis of the abnormal gait.

Stroke patients generally have a mature bony skeleton in contradistinction to the child with neurologic disturbances of the lower extremity. It is generally not necessary to perform bone or joint procedures to balance the foot and toes. Correction of deformities during gait is obtained by proper orthotic management and appropriate tendon releases and transfers.

Equinus, varus, and toe curling alone or in various combinations are the most common disabilities in the lower extremity and most frequently require bracing or surgery or both. Commonly, all the deformities may occur in the same patient.

Equinus

Initially, excessive plantar flexion is secondary to spasticity (it is rarely secondary to flaccid dorsiflexors). Later, it may be due to spasticity or myostatic contractures, especially in the neglected patient or in a patient who has not been ambulatory. In normal gait, the heel strikes the floor first. Spasticity in the gastrocnemius-soleus group causes the patient to bear weight initially on the forefoot and secondarily on the heel. If the spasticity is severe, the heel may not contact the floor. In order for the heel to contact the floor, the tibia must extend backwards, thus causing hyperextension of the knee. The ability to place the heel on the ground should not lead to the belief that there is no spasticity of the gastrocnemius and soleus muscles. Hyperextension of the knee will allow a plantigrade position of the ankle and gives an erroneous impression of a normal gastrocnemius-soleus, when, in fact, it is spastic. Inspection of the knee at midstance and observation of the forefoot in early stance will aid in the diagnosis of a spastic calf in difficult situations.

Equinus due to mild spasticity commonly responds to a rigid ankle-foot orthosis (AFO) to restrict plantar flexion. Heel height may be increased to compensate for mild persistent equinus. Most hemiplegics, however, have difficulty ambulating with an elevation of more than 2.5 cm on their heel.

Surgical correction of equinus is indicated when satisfactory orthotic response cannot be obtained or if spasticity is significant enough to require bracing and an attempt is being made to make the patient a brace-free ambulator. The patient's heel should firmly contact the sole of the shoe, and the patient should walk without a hyperextension thrust of the knee. Commonly, equinus may not be initially detected when the patient stands quietly. After he takes a few steps, however, the spasticity will increase, and the heel will begin to "piston" out of the shoe. This piston-like motion can be detected in the following manner: A mark is placed on the patient's sock at the top of the heel counter when the heel is in firm contact with the sole of the shoe. As the patient ambulates, the mark will be observed to rise out of the shoe.

An anesthetic block of the posterior tibial nerve at the knee is usually indicated at this time. This is accomplished by injecting 10 ml of 1 per cent lidocaine into the proximal aspect of the popliteal fossa. (See Figure 14–5B.) The nerve lies in the midline, deep to the heads of the gastrocnemius and superficial to the artery and vein. In the absence of a fixed contracture, the triceps surae will be paralyzed, and the heel will not "piston" out of the orthosis. This allows the patient, as well as the physician, to foresee the results of surgery. It is of further benefit in that the gastrocnemius-soleus group may mask the strength of the anterior muscles. By blocking the gastrocnemius and soleus muscles, activity of the tibialis anterior and toe extensors will be more readily visualized. It can then be determined if sufficient dorsiflexion strength is present to allow brace-free ambulation. If varus of the forefoot is still present, a split anterior tibial tendon transfer (SPLATT) should be considered at the time of the tendo-Achillis lengthening (TAL) in order to maintain a balanced foot (see "Varus").

Lengthening of the Achilles tendon may be an open or a percutaneous procedure. We prefer modification of the Hoke triple hemisection tenotomy performed percutaneously. At surgery, the knee is extended and the ankle is dorsiflexed, which places tension on the Achilles tendon. It further draws the tendon posteriorly away from the neurovascular structures. The tendon itself is palpated or even visualized from the musculotendinous junction to its insertion on the os calcis. The first hemisection is made on the medial aspect of the tendo Achillis above the os calcis. The second hemisection is on the lateral aspect of the heel cord midway between the os calcis and the musculotendinous junction, and the final hemisection is again on the medial aspect just distal to the musculotendinous junction. The ankle is then dorsiflexed to neutral but not beyond. A short leg cast is applied with the ankle in approximately five degrees of plantar flexion. The plaster should not be applied with the ankle in dorsiflexion since excessive lengthening may occur and plantar flexion weakness could result. The cast is worn for six weeks, and the patient is allowed to ambulate. The ankle is then protected for an additional six weeks with an AFO during the day and a posterior splint at night.

If active toe flexion or slight spasticity of the toe flexors is present prior to surgery, long toe flexor release is performed at the time of Achilles tendon lengthening, even if toe flexion was not painful. This is easily accomplished at the arch of the foot (see "Toe Deformities"). Correction of the equinus causes a relative shortening of the long toe flexors. Consequently, patients with asymptomatic toe curling prior to surgery may have toe curling and pain after surgery.

Plantar Flexion Weakness

Plantar flexion weakness is a common residuum of strokes and is frequently overlooked by the physician. Overlengthening of the Achilles tendon more commonly results in plantar flexion weakness demonstrable during gait than in a pes calcaneus deformity. This pattern is difficult to detect at first for the unsuspecting physician. A patient with plantar flexion weakness will employ one of two abnormal gait patterns. In the first pattern, the ankle is excessively dorsiflexed in stance with some compensatory knee flexion; the patient stabilizes the knee and, consequently, the ankle with his quadriceps. This gait pattern is usually detected early after the CVA. Most patients eventually assume the second gait pattern, since the first pattern places an excessive demand on the quadriceps. In the second pattern, the patient hyperextends his knee at heel-strike, locking it in extension with the tibia extended backwards from the vertical. This allows his body to remain in front of the axis of rotation of the knee during stance and keeps his knee locked in extension. Also, through hyperextension of the knee and backward extension of the tibia, the patient can now keep the center of gravity of the body behind the ankle joint, thus avoiding excessive ankle dorsiflexion and preventing knee flexion. Thus, the patient stabilizes the limb by keeping his body weight in front of the knee joint while at the same time behind the ankle joint. This latter pattern closely resembles the knee hyperextension thrust caused by excessive plantar flexion (equinus). One means of differentiating the two is that patients with plantar flexion weakness bear weight primarily on the heel during the initial phase of stance, while those with equinus deformity generally strike the floor with their forefoot in the initial stance phase. As in equinus, the hyperextension due to plantar flexion weakness can also be corrected by an orthosis that restricts excessive plantar flexion.

Inadequate Dorsiflexion

Inadequate dorsiflexion in the swing phase of gait is due to flaccidity or paresis of the tibialis anterior. As previously mentioned, spasticity of the gastrocnemius-soleus may mask activity of a weakened tibialis anterior and give the impression of relative inadequate dorsiflexion. Anesthetic posterior tibial nerve block will allow one to predict if the activity of the tibialis anterior is sufficient to dorsiflex the ankle. Gait electromyography performed on these patients generally fails to demonstrate suitable muscles for tendon transfer to restore dorsiflexion because they are inactive during the swing phase.[4] Transfer of tendons such as the tibialis posterior for tenodesis is not a reliable procedure. If spasticity of the gastrocnemius-soleus prevails, the tenodesis will stretch out. If a weak calf persists, tenodesis may actually cause persistent dorsiflexion of the foot, and an unstable ankle may result. Isolated footdrop secondary to a cerebrolvascular accident is rare and should be corrected with an AFO.

Varus

It is not uncommon for a patient to be ambulatory without devices and to have a varus deformity of the foot during stance, causing weight bearing on the lateral edge of the foot. Often, callosities will be present over the lateral border of the foot. Such a patient may do well when walking on a flat surface in the office; however, it will be more difficult for him to ambulate on uneven terrain or to walk down steps. Surgical correction of the varus is indicated at this time and also when, despite application of a well-fitted orthosis, the foot twists into varus in the shoe (Fig. 41–1).

Five muscles may contribute to this varus deformity. These muscles are the tibialis anterior, the soleus, the flexor hallucis longus, the flexor digitorum longus, and the tibialis posterior. When the soleus significantly contributes to the varus deformity, equinus is also present. The contribution of the soleus to varus will then be diminished by heel cord lengthening. Similarly, when the long toe flexors contribute to varus, toe curling is also present

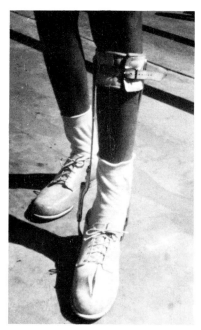

Figure 41-1. *Varus persists despite a well-fitted shoe and brace. The lateral malleolus is abutting the lateral upright. (From Waters, R. L., Perry, J., and Garland, D.: Clin. Orthop., 131:54, 1978.)*

and its contribution to varus will also be eliminated by long toe flexor release.

It is uncommon for the posterior tibial tendon to be active after a cerebrovascular accident.[4] A block of the posterior tibial nerve in the popliteal fossa will demonstrate if the posterior compartment muscles and soleus were causing some hindfoot varus. If the posterior tibial tendon is released or transferred anteriorly in combination with a SPLATT and TAL, there is a possibility that a planovalgus foot will occur, with excessive eversion of the forefoot. This is not an uncommon deformity and usually occurs if there has been preexisting pes planus. These patients may experience collapse of the medial arch and complain of pain.

Palpation and observation of the anterior tibial tendon reveal that this muscle is the main deforming force responsible for forefoot varus. If forefoot varus is corrected, hindfoot varus is usually not a problem. A split anterior tibial tendon transfer (SPLATT) is a procedure that reliably corrects varus deformity of the forefoot. The principle behind the SPLATT is to transfer the lateral or distal portion of the anterior tibial tendon to the cuboid and

third cuneiform, thus creating an eversion force of the forefoot, which neutralizes the varus pull of the remaining anterior tibial muscle (Fig. 41-2).

The SPLATT procedure is performed as follows: Through a medial longitudinal incision in the arch of the foot, the distal one half to two thirds of the anterior tibial tendon is freed from its insertion, and a suture is placed around the free end. This is easily identifiable, since the tendon inserts on the first cuneiform and first metatarsal, and it is in this natural plane that the initial split is made. The second incision is made just lateral to the tibial crest at the musculotendinous junction of the tibialis anterior. The pre-tibial fascia and the retinacular ligaments are then divided by passing scissors between the two incisions from proximal to distal. The tendon suture is then delivered into the proximal incision. By merely applying traction on the suture, the anterior tibial tendon will divide in a natural plane. This division should be continued into the musculotendinous junction. A third incision is made over the cuneiform and cuboid bones. By palpating the base of the fifth metatarsal

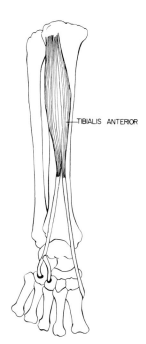

Figure 41-2. *The SPLATT procedure. The anterior tibialis muscle is split and transferred to the lateral side of the foot and inserted into the cuboid and third cuneiform. (From Waters, R. L., Perry, J., and Garland, D.: Clin. Orthop., 131:54, 1978.)*

bone, these two bones can be reliably located. The incision is nearly parallel to the Langer's line of the foot. The incision begins at the extensor tendons and continues to the peroneus brevis tendon. In the mid aspect of the wound, the peroneus tertius tendon and the short toe extensors are commonly identified. Drill holes are placed perpendicularly in the bone at the ends of these incisions. The holes are widened with a curette. The tibialis anterior muscle is then passed subcutaneously on top of the retinacular ligaments to this third incision. The tendon is passed from the lateral to the medial drill hole. It is frequently passed under the short extensor tendon, which allows the bulk of the tendon to remain free from the underlying skin, and is sutured to itself. Passage of the transferred tendon subcutaneously allows it to bowstring anteriorly and increases its mechanical advantage over the ankle.

Following surgery, a short leg walking cast is applied. After six weeks, the cast is removed, and an AFO is worn during the day and a posterior splint at night. This treatment is then continued for four and a half months to insure satisfactory tendon healing.

Equinovarus

In most patients equinus, varus, and toe curling occur together (Fig. 41–3). The SPLATT procedure, Achilles tendon lengthening, and toe flexor release are performed simultaneously. After the transferred tendon has been protected for six months, some patients are able to ambulate without an orthosis. Even though some patients may still be required to wear an orthosis, they are now more braceable. They may be stable enough to ambulate short distances in the house without donning a brace. With time, footdrop may recur owing to stretching of the tibialis anterior caused by anterior tibial weakness or overactivity of the gastrocnemius-soleus in relation to the tibialis anterior muscle. Varus does not generally recur. If necessary, an AFO more than adequately controls the patient's foot at this time.

In an effort to prevent recurring equinus without excessively lengthening the Achilles tendon, the flexor hallucis longus or flexor digitorum longus or both can be

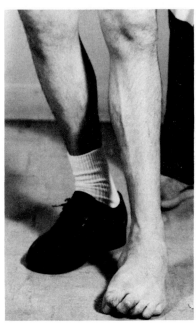

Figure 41–3. A head trauma patient demonstrating the common triad of toe curling, equinus, and varus.

transferred through the interosseous membrane to the dorsum of the foot. This procedure is performed mainly in the young, active patient whose toe flexors were demonstrated to be active in the swing phase of gait either by electromyography or by inspection. This procedure is not performed on the elderly, since it requires more surgical time and dissection, and their life span is greatly decreased by the CVA. If both the flexor hallucis longus and flexor digitorum longus are active, only the flexor hallucis longus is transferred. Transfer of the toe flexor tendons is performed by releasing the tendons in the foot, and the same incision as for the SPLATT procedure is employed. The tendons are then tagged. A second incision is made along the medial aspect of the shank of the leg. The tendons are delivered into this proximal wound by applying tension on the tendons. The flexor hallucis longus muscle is stripped from its distal origin on the tibia, fibula, and interosseous membrane. The distal muscle fibers are then removed from the tendon by sharp dissection. A third incision is made anteriorly over the interval between the extensor hallucis longus and extensor digitorum longus, and a window is created in the interosseous membrane. The window should be sufficiently proximal on the shank (8 to 10 cm above the ankle mortise) so that there is sufficient distance between the tibia and fibula for the tendon and its attached fibers to pass freely. The tendon is then passed posteriorly to anteriorly. The great toe flexor is delivered to the lateral aspect of the neurovascular bundle. The flexor hallucis longus tendon is then transferred to the lateral aspect of the foot, as previously described in the SPLATT procedure, either with a SPLATT or by itself.

Toe Deformities

Excessive toe flexion (toe curling) is usually characterized by inactive toe extensors and frequently causes pain. Correction of the deformity is achieved by releasing the flexor hallucis longus or flexor digitorum longus or both tendons. If only one or two toes are involved or are painful, tenotomy may be performed at each individual toe. If all of the toes are involved, the tenotomy is more easily performed by sectioning the flexor hallucis longus and the tendon of the flexor digitorum longus in the sole of the foot distal to the insertion of the quadratus plantae muscle.

An incision is made along the medial aspect of the foot along the upper border of the abductor hallucis (Fig. 41–4). The incision is the same as that employed for initiation of the SPLATT procedure. The abductor is reflected plantarward. The second layer of the foot can be entered by releasing the origin of the medial short flexor to the great toe. Fat is encountered, and the common toe flexors can then be identified within it and released. At this time, also, if one wishes to transfer the toe

flexors anteriorly, they may be tagged and the appropriate operation continued.

After release of the long toe flexors, there may be some persistent flexion of the proximal interphalangeal joints, which is secondary to spasticity of the short toe flexors. This rarely causes discomfort, and treatment frequently is not indicated. If the patient does experience continued toe pain, the flexors of the individual toes are released at the metatarsophalangeal joint.

Orthosis-Free Walking

Surgery is most commonly performed to make the foot more correctable in a brace or to allow the patient to be a brace-free ambulator. If there is clinical evidence of impaired proprioception, surgery for brace-free ambulation is not indicated. Even though the foot may be corrected by the orthosis, the weight of the brace and anterior-posterior pressure applied by the shank cuff are necessary for sensory input during ambulation. When varus is the only significant gait impairment for which an AFO is worn, a SPLATT procedure has proven so reliable that most of these patients will ambulate without an orthosis after surgery. When treating equinus or equinovarus, the tibialis anterior may not be sufficiently strong to prevent recurrent footdrop in the swing phase of gait. In the young, the toe flexors should be transferred anteriorly to prevent this problem.

HEAD TRAUMA

Neurologic recovery in the head-injured patient differs from that in the stroke patient. Recovery can be divided into three

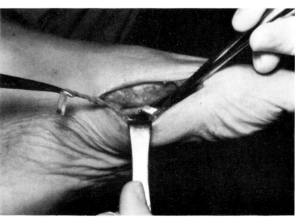

Figure 41–4. *The incision made on medial arch of the foot. One of the long toe flexor tendons has been delivered into the wound. (From Waters, R. L., Perry, J., and Garland, D.: Clin. Orthop., 131:54, 1978.)*

phases: acute, subacute, and stable.[1] Definitive surgical procedures should be delayed until at least 18 months have elapsed, after which there will be little neurologic recovery.

Surgery may be indicated in the subacute phase of recovery when spasticity is preventing rehabilitation or in some patients who have not had rehabilitation and have acquired fixed deformities.

As a general rule, the same surgical procedures as previously described for the stroke patient may be utilized in the head trauma patient for management of the foot and ankle during the stable phase of recovery. Patterns of spasticity are more predictable in stroke patients and do not vary as much as in head trauma patients. Also, during the subacute phase, spasticity is frequently more significant in head-injured patients than in stroke patients, and a more aggressive form of therapy and surgical program are often indicated.

Equinus and Extensor Rigidity

Following acute head trauma, spasticity and extensor rigidity are frequently present, especially if there is brain stem involvement. Proper positioning of the limbs, passive range of motion exercises, and splints are the basic methods of contracture prevention. Rigidity may be quite severe at this time, and a circular plaster cast is often indicated to prevent or correct equinus.

When spasticity and rigidity are severe and passive range of motion cannot be achieved, a padded cast applied after the joint is held in the maximum position of correction is the best method of treatment. The casts are changed every 7 to 10 days until the deformity is corrected or until no further correction can be obtained. A lidocaine nerve block at the posterior tibial nerve is indicated at this time. This will decrease spasticity and allow a better positioning of the ankle prior to application of the cast (Fig. 41–5).

At times, equinus cannot be corrected by the aforementioned measure. This interferes with standing, transferring of weight, and ambulation (Fig. 41–6). A phenol injection to the motor branches of the posterior tibial nerve will interrupt nervous flow to the gastrocnemius-soleus.

As neurologic recovery occurs, so does recovery of the injected nerve. Achilles tendon lengthening should not be performed, since neurologic recovery may take place and pes calcaneus or plantar flexion weakness could result.

Phenol injection to the posterior tibial nerve is an open procedure, and only the motor branches are selected, since the loss of sensation is bothersome and can potentially precipitate causalgia. The posterior tibial nerve is exposed through a midline longitudinal incision. It begins at the popliteal crease and extends distally approximately 8 to 10 cm. The posterior tibial nerve is identified between the heads of the gastrocnemius muscle. The motor branches to the gastrocnemius and the soleus are identified with the aid of a nerve stimulator. It is not uncommon to find several motor branches innervating each head. Once identified, these motor branches are injected with 3 per cent phenol in glycerine. Care should be taken to isolate the nerve from the surrounding musculature with a moist sponge. After these branches have been identified and injected, the soleus should be retracted distally. At this time, motor branches to the tibialis posterior, flexor hallucis longus, and common toe flexors can be identified. They are usually separate from the main nerve, which continues distally as a combination sensory and motor nerve to the foot. These motor branches should also be injected. Failure to inject the motor branches to the toe flexors may cause considerable toe curling postoperatively. This may prevent patients from ambulating, because they are frequently very sensitive to pain. Postoperatively, a short leg cast is applied. Any residual deformity can then be corrected by serial casting.

Toe Deformities

Toe deformities in the head-injured patient are more difficult to treat than those in the stroke patient. They also cause pain more frequently. Different types of deformities occur owing to differing patterns of muscle imbalance. Surgical procedures must be individualized, and no one surgical procedure can be applied to all deformities.

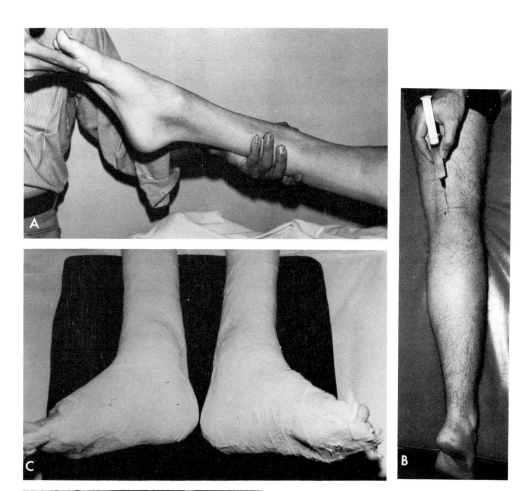

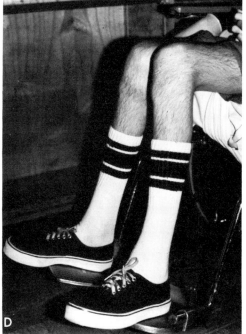

Figure 41–5. *A head-injured patient who demonstrated brainstem involvement and extensor rigidity. (A) Severe equinus that was in a relatively fixed position. (B) Administration of a lidocaine block to the posterior nerve in the popliteal fossa. (C) Position of ankles after repeated lidocaine blocks and serial casting. (D) Patient's legs after severe rigidity had subsided.*

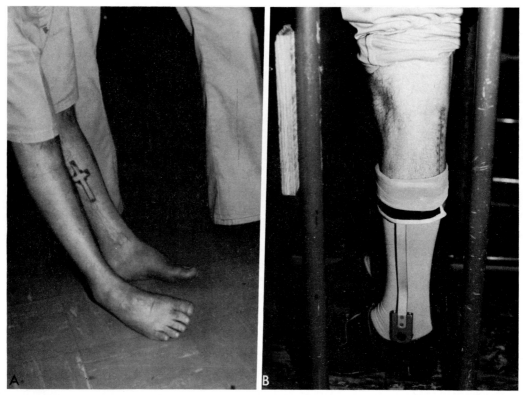

Figure 41-6. *A head-injured patient who developed severe equinus when attempting to stand. He could not be braced. (A) Extreme equinus and backward extension of the tibia. (B) An open phenol nerve block to the motor branches of the posterior tibial nerves aided in bracing and standing.*

Unless a fixed deformity is present, bony resection or phalangectomy is contraindicated. Ligamentous and bony structures provide inherent stability. Without this support, deviation of the toes may occur dorsally, plantarly, or laterally. The exception to this rule is when dorsal callosities are present in association with fixed contractures of the proximal interphalangeal joints. Proximal interphalangeal joint resection and arthrodesis are performed to maintain stability. Appropriate tendon releases must also be undertaken at this time.

As in surgery performed in stroke patients, the objective is to release overactive muscles responsible for painful deformities. This is most frequently accomplished by release of the long toe flexors. Short toe flexor activity will frequently be unmasked once this is accomplished. Inspection of the toes preoperatively will often aid in determining which group of muscles is overactive. If toe curl-ing, as seen in stroke patients, is not present but there is more flexion at the proximal interphalangeal joints, the short toe flexors are presumed to be overactive. This point can be further proved by blocking the posterior tibial nerve at the ankle, which will anesthetize the short flexors (and intrinsic muscles). If the deformity is diminished, tenotomy of both the long and short flexors is then performed through transverse incisions on the volar aspect of each toe. If the anesthetic block at the ankle has no effect on the toes, release of the common flexors through the arch of the foot is indicated. Loss of active toe flexion is not a significant problem. Rarely, the lateral four toes may assume an intrinsic-plus posture of flexion of the metatarsophalangeal joints, with extension of the interphalangeal joint of the great toe (Fig. 41–7). This may be presumed to be due to hyperactivity of the intrinsic muscles. It may also be demonstrated in conjunction with a hyperextended great toe. This de-

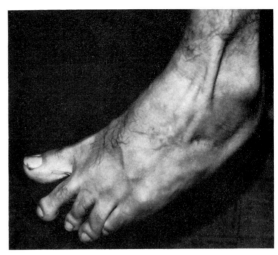

Figure 41–7. *The same head-injured patient as in Figure 41–3 after TAL, toe flexor release with reinforcement anteriorly, and SPLATT. Note the prominent SPLATT and toe flexor transfer. Note also that the toes now demonstrate intrinsic spasticity and extension of the great toe.*

formity may be caused by positive tonic grasp or Babinski's response. It is triggered each time the sole of the foot contacts the ground. Once again, a block of the posterior tibial nerve at the ankle joint should diminish all activity of the short flexors and intrinsic muscles. If this occurs, surgical correction may be obtained by release of the intrinsics and the short toe flexors, which is accomplished by dorsal longitudinal incisions in the second, third, and fourth web spaces. The intrinsics and flexors are identified and transected.

Transfer of the long toe flexors to the extensors (Girdlestone-Taylor procedure) is not recommended in the spastic patient. Electromyographic studies reveal that the long toe flexors often remain active during the terminal stance and early swing phases. Toe flexor transfer to the extensor hood then acts to flex the metatarsophalangeal joints and extend the interphalangeal joints. Consequently, passive dorsiflexion of the metatarsophalangeal joints will be prevented during the terminal stance and pre-swing phases of gait. This will impede roll-off and may cause pain.

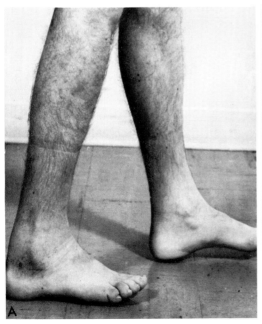

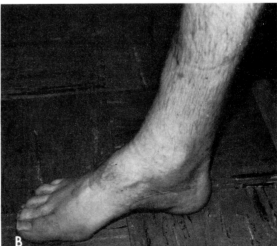

Figure 41–8. *This head-injured patient underwent an early TAL. (A) The patient now has a calcaneus foot and a weak gastrocnemius-soleus muscle. (B) The anterior muscles have been lengthened.*

Excessive Dorsiflexion at the Ankle

Although not seen in the stroke patient, excessive dorsiflexion of the ankle during the stance and swing phases may be detected occasionally in the head trauma patient. This may also be iatrogenically induced if a TAL is undertaken prior to the stable phase for spasticity or early contracture release with normal return of neurologic recovery. Both deformities are treated in a similar manner. An incision is made over the distal tibia and the common toe extensors and tibialis anterior are lengthened. Postoperatively, the extremity is held in a short leg walking cast for six weeks and an AFO for four and a half months, with a posterior splint being worn at night. Although rarely indicated, this is a reliable operation (Fig. 41–8).

Equinovarus

For the most part, equinovarus in the head trauma patient is handled the same way as in the stroke patient. The timing is different, however, since definitive surgery in the head trauma patient should not be undertaken until one and a half years after injury. The other difference is that the toe flexors are more commonly transferred to the dorsum of the foot for added dorsiflexor strength and for prevention of recurrent footdrop. These patients are generally younger than the stroke patients, with a longer time left to live and better sensation, and we usually attempt to make them brace-free. The tibialis posterior is more likely to remain active in these patients than in stroke patients. If significant hindfoot varus is present, a Z-plasty lengthening of its tendon at the ankle is indicated.

REFERENCES

1. Garland, D. E., and Rhodes, M. E.: Orthopedic management of brain-injured adults. Clin. Orthop., *131*:111, 1978.
2. Garland, D. E., and Waters, R. L.: Orthopedic evaluation of the hemiplegic stroke. Orthop. Clin. North Am., 9:291, 1978.
3. Perry, J.: Orthopedic Evaluation and Treatment of the Stroke Patient. Part II: Examination: A Neurologic Basis for Treatment. AAOS Instructional Course Lectures, Vol. 24. St. Louis, C. V. Mosby Co., 1975, p. 26.
4. Perry, J., Waters, R. L., and Perrin, T.: Electromyographic analysis of equinovarus following stroke. Clin. Orthop., *131*:47, 1978.

CHAPTER 42

POLIOMYELITIS AND THE FOOT

Federico Sotelo-Ortiz, M.D.

Poliomyelitis is an acute infectious disease produced by virus Type I, II, or III. The first symptoms are usually respiratory or gastrointestinal, and sometimes even those may not be apparent. The virus reaches the central nervous system by the blood stream, with special affinity for the anterior horn cells of the spinal cord and some motor nuclei of the brain stem. Poliomyelitis used to be endemic in all countries, with a higher incidence in summer and autumn. Flies have been blamed as carriers of the virus, and the condition was and is particularly apparent in slums and in undernourished people and those families living in poor, filthy conditions. Feces seem to be the reservoir of the virus. The flies, the vectors, pick the virus up there, transporting and depositing the infection in food and on dishes, hands, and so on. Lack of elementary knowledge of hygiene and cleanliness opens the door for this contagious disease.

Since the advent of prophylactic vaccines, the incidence of poliomyelitis has greatly diminished. In highly developed countries, a case occurs only occasionally; therefore, in these countries orthopaedic surgeons are no longer trained in the management of and surgery for polio. This is not so in underdeveloped countries[1] or "countries under development," where poverty, lack of education, filthy living conditions, poorly organized Health Departments, and lack of federal funds to eradicate this malady unfortunately main-tain records of low (or even high) endemic poliomyelitis. In our private practice, mainly in summer and autumn, we still see more than a dozen "fresh" cases, and for years we have performed surgery two or three times a week for cases of residual paralysis following poliomyelitis. It is known that the disease primarily attacks children under one year of age, but it may attack older children and, once in a while, adults. The eradication of poliomyelitis in highly developed countries resulted in neglect of facilities once available for acute, subacute, and residual cases. Physiotherapy and rehabilitation departments and diagnostic and therapeutic facilities disappeared or were converted for other uses, as no more cases of polio were seen. Mechanical lungs or respirators were dismantled. As a result, when a sporadic case of poliomyelitis presents, diagnosis is difficult, treatment in the acute phase is not properly carried out, and residual paralysis is incorrectly managed, jeopardizing the life of the patient by improper surgery or fitting of the wrong braces.

Advances in orthopaedic surgery should not be limited to orthopaedic surgeons in highly developed countries but should be available to orthopaedic surgeons all over the world. Because there are so many underdeveloped countries and "countries under development" where poliomyelitis is still prevalent, we must endeavor to bring the elementary knowledge and technology of the management of poliomyelitis in the foot to the surgeons in those areas, who need this knowledge to treat the people affected with polio who come to them for help.

PATHOLOGY AND CLASSIFICATION OF STAGES

For detailed accounts of the pathology and management of the acute contagious phase of poliomyelitis, the reader is referred to textbooks and the voluminous literature on this subject. Only a few elementary notes will be presented here. It must be remembered that mild cases of polio, with paresis of one or more muscles, may become evident in a child after a practically symptomless onset or just a slight "cold" or gastrointestinal distress. For practical purposes, the course of poliomyelitis may be divided into three classic phases. The first is the *acute phase*, which is subdivided into a febrile infectious subphase that lasts for about 15 days after the onset and a noncontagious subphase that lasts for about 15 days more. The other subdivisions of the acute phase are the preparalytic and paralytic subphases. In general, the acute infectious subphase may be considered to end two days after the return of normal temperature.

The second phase of poliomyelitis, the *convalescent phase*, may be defined as the period of varying degree of recovery that may take from one to one and a half years. At the end of the acute phase and the beginning of this phase, there is usually a lapse when the muscles are painful, tender, and "spasmodic." The final phase is the *residual phase*, when no more recovery is to be expected.

DIAGNOSIS

The acute stage of poliomyelitis is very often misdiagnosed, as 20 per cent of patients or more do not show signs of paralysis or muscular tenderness (spasm manifested in the erectors of the spine and those of the nucha by positive Kernig sign). Therefore, many of the so-called abortive cases may pass as an acute gastrointestinal condition, a febrile sore throat, or a cold. The real acute stage is usually manifested by malaise, fever, cephalalgia, vomiting or nausea, diarrhea, and loss of appetite.

These symptoms may vary in intensity and duration and may disappear within a few days. The condition may end just like that, with no diagnosis of abortive poliomyelitis being made, if the possibility of polio was not considered by the physician. The only harm at this point is the spreading of the disease to other children, adolescents, or adults. However, if tenderness or weakness of the muscles appears and the patient experiences difficulty in walking or in using the upper extremities even in the slightest degree, the physician should suspect the presence of poliomyelitis, and a more thorough examination should be performed.

The test for Kernig's sign is usually positive; muscle tenderness (spasm) is present, as is weakness of the asymmetric muscles; and general symptoms are more noticeable. Laboratory tests are mainly useful for differential diagnosis; there is slight leukocytosis, with an increase in polymorphonuclear leukocytes, and the sedimentation rate is moderately elevated. Examination of the spinal fluid may provide some information if it is done during the first two weeks; the number of cells is moderately increased (to 250 or 300 per mm^3, mainly by lymphocytes), and the protein level goes up slowly, sometimes to 300 or 350 mg per 100 ml. Where there is painful spasm of the muscles at this stage, these muscles should not be tested for strength, and not even galvanic or faradic currents should be used for diagnostic purposes. Once the acute stage is over (disappearance of all general symptoms, no muscular spasm, and good general condition of the patient), usually about one month after the onset, muscle testing and galvanofaradic testing may be performed without affecting the comfort of the patient or the evolution of the condition.

Differential Diagnosis

Nonabortive poliomyelitis is easily diagnosed. In addition to the general condition of the patient, muscle spasm, Kernig's sign, onset of even the slightest asymmetric paralysis, and laboratory tests will lead to the correct diagnosis and prompt and proper treatment. As already stated, the acute febrile stage of polio may be misdiagnosed as a cold, a gastrointestinal infection, rheumatic fever, scurvy, or even the pseudoparalysis of congenital lues, meningitis, a tumor of the nervous system, Erb's palsy, Guillain-Barré syndrome, or an hysteric condition. The physician must perform a thorough examination of the patient. A complete blood count, examination of the spinal fluid, and radiographic studies, if necessary (e.g., for scurvy, syphilis, or osteomyelitis) may be helpful.

Once the acute stage is over (four weeks after onset), muscle tests and electrodiagnosis can be used. In any child who is able and willing to cooperate, we use clinical examination of the muscles, but in infants and children who are unable or unwilling to cooperate, we utilize electrodiagnosis, that is, muscle testing by galvanofaradic currents.

The foot per se has very small muscles that are rarely affected by polio. All the important muscles of the foot have their origins on the tibia and fibula and are inserted on the foot; therefore, their involvement in poliomyelitis is reflected in the foot and not in the leg. Involvement of some thigh muscles may be reflected in the foot, as will be discussed later.

In our experience, the muscles affected by paralysis following poliomyelitis, in descending order, are: (1) quadriceps, in the thigh, (2) tibialis anterior, (3) peronei, (4) gastrocnemius, (5) tibialis posterior, (6) hamstrings, (7) intrinsic muscles of the foot, and finally in fewer cases, (8) extensors and flexors of the small toes and extensor and flexor hallucis longus.

EXAMINATION

When the acute contagious stage with muscle spasm is over, the patient can be examined without harm or discomfort. The two methods we use are (1) clinical examination and (2) electrical stimulation of the muscles with galvanofaradic currents. The clinical examination is the most important. As mentioned previously, galvanofaradic diagnosis is only used for small children or for uncooperative children or adults to perform a clinical examination or to complete it. Sometimes, galvanofaradic examination is done as an adjunct to the clinical examination to provide information about prognosis and possible recuperation of the involved muscles.

We use the Weiss galvanofaradic machine. When a muscle does not respond to a normal faradic stimulation (up to 7 on the scale of intensity of the Weiss machine), we use galvanic currents. Twenty milliamperes is the maximum power we use to try to obtain a response. Patients cannot tolerate higher power. If the muscle responds to faradic stimulation below 7, it is felt that there is a possibility of recuperation, and adequate treatment is instituted. If there is no response with an intensity of 7, the prognosis is poor. The prognosis is also poor if response is not obtained with 8 to 10 ma of galvanic stimulation, and if higher power is required or no response is obtained, there is no hope of recovery, and final decisions may be made about treatment, according to the guidelines that will be presented subsequently. We use special charts to record the results of the electromuscular tests.

Clinical Examination

If the patient has not started to walk and is being seen for the first time, the mother usually gives the history of the infant, mentioning whether or not he had a febrile period or gastrointestinal distress or if he received an "injection" that left him with a limp leg or foot or both. Involvement of other parts of the body will not be discussed in this chapter; only the foot and parts of the lower extremity that have influence on the foot (i.e., the thigh muscles, leg muscles, and muscles of the foot itself) will be dealt with, as our interest here is only in those muscles that affect the foot if they are damaged by poliomyelitis.

After the history is taken, the clinical examination is performed and, as in any other condition involving the feet and lower extremities, must include:

1. General inspection.
2. Observation of gait, if any.
3. Observation of standing, if possible.
4. Observation of aids used for walking.
5. Observation of gross visible deformities.

A more detailed clinical examination is then performed, which consists of:

1. Electromuscular diagnosis, if necessary.
2. Clinical muscle testing.
3. Detailed examination of deformities.

4. Notation of the degree of manual correction of deformities.
5. Radiographic studies.
6. Laboratory tests, if necessary.
7. Photographs or movies of the patient showing deformities, gait, and standing, which will be used for comparison with post-treatment results.

General Inspection

When the patient enters the office, it is noticed whether he walks by himself (if old enough to do so), is brought in a wheelchair, or is carried in the mother's arms. If the patient walks, immediate note is taken of his gait, whether there is a limp or a hanging extremity, and the position of the body and the extremities while the patient moves around or stands. The quality of the clothing worn by the patient and parents and the degree of cleanliness are also noted to estimate their approximate social and economic level. This inspection provides a general idea of the patient's gait, standing, aids for walking, and gross visible deformities, but these aspects should be scrutinized on physical examination of the patient.

Physical examination comprises the points mentioned after general inspection and those of the detailed clinical examination.

Gait

The patient may move around with or without any appreciable limp. If present, the limp may be unilateral or bilateral. The patient may move by quadruped ambulation or by squatting or sitting on his buttocks, or he may walk with aids. The abnormal gait may be the result of deformities. The gait should be observed with the patient fully dressed and then without clothes and shoes; if the patient wears braces or uses aids, those should be removed, too, in order to assess his potential to walk without them. When the patient is examined without clothing or aids, the gait can be fully appreciated. For example, a patient with quadriceps palsy either hyperextends the knee or supports it with the fingers, pressing above the knee each time the foot is on the floor and placing the knee in extension. After his normal gait has

been observed, such a patient is then instructed to walk on his tiptoes and on his heels. If he has difficulty or is unable to do the former, the plantar flexors of the foot (the triceps surae) are weak or have no power; if he cannot do the latter, the dorsiflexors of the foot (the tibialis anterior, extensor digitorum longus, and, to some extent, the extensor hallucis longus) are involved.

Standing

While standing, the patient is examined from the front, back, and both sides. From the side, deformities such as genu recurvatum, limitation of extension of the knee, cavus, flatfoot, calcaneus, equinus, atrophy of the leg, flexion contracture of the hip, lordosis, and flexion contractures of the toes can be noted. From the back, inversion or eversion of the heel and foot and genu valgum or varum can be observed. The same deformities seen from the back — inversion or eversion of the foot, deformities of the toes, and other disorders — are observed from the front, but more accurately.

Aids

By this time, the type of aids, if any, used by the patient has been noted. If the patient is being seen for the first time, the aids may be the result of the parents' or the patient's ingenuity. If the patient is old enough to walk and is able to do so, he may use a cane or crutches; he may wear shoes with or without modifications and deformities; or he may move around in a wheelchair or in a cart pulled by someone else. If the patient is not a "new case," he may wear different types of braces and shoes, with or without modifications, and may use proper crutches and canes.

After the patient walks and stands utilizing his aids, they are removed, and the patient is observed walking and standing without them. All changes in both situations are written on the patient's chart.

Gross Visible Deformities

Gross visible deformities are noted during the general inspection and examination of the patient's gait. The patient may have a completely limp extremity or extremities that make him unable to walk or stand owing to complete involvement of all the muscles (thigh, leg, hips, knees, or ankle [equinus]); inversion or eversion of the foot; cavus, valgus, or calcaneus deformities or a combination of these; hyperextension of one or both knees (genu recurvatum) — most cases of which are due to quadriceps palsy; valgus or varus deformities of the knees; internal or external rotation of the legs (tibial rotation); apparent shortening of the lower extremity due to contractures or real shortening or both; or atrophy of the extremity.

From the general inspection and observation of gait, standing, aids, and gross visible deformities, an important advanced clinical impression can be gained before the final one is reached through the detailed clinical examination. For example, a patient walking with genu recurvatum due to quadriceps palsy almost surely has developed a compensatory equinus deformity of the foot so that the foot can be placed flat on the floor when the knee is hyperextended. Steppage gait usually results from a paralyzed tibialis anterior. Eversion of the foot or flatfoot is due to palsy of the tibialis posterior, which, in most cases, is associated with palsy of the tibialis anterior and good or normal peronei. An inversion deformity may be associated a priori with loss of power in the peronei and good tibial muscles. This inversion deformity may also be associated with a cavus or calcaneus deformity, the latter caused by lack of power in the triceps surae. Uncomplicated cavus is usually attributed to involvement of the small muscles of the foot, which secondarily causes toe deformities (e.g., claw toes, hammer toes, and painful calluses on the sole over the anterior metatarsal arch). A weak quadriceps may result in a flexion contracture of the knee, which occurs when the patient spends most of his time in a wheelchair or sitting with the knees flexed, or a flexion contracture of the hip. Total absence of power in the tibialis anterior may result in a flatfoot.

A good, powerful gluteus maximus, which inserts into the gluteal line of the femur and the leg (through the iliopectineal band or Maissiat's band), along with a good tensor fascia lata, may cause development of a valgus deformity of the knee, usually associated with external rotation of the tibia and foot. Deformities located as high as the hip may result in secondary deformities of the foot. Most primary deformities of the foot in poliomyelitis, as noted, are secondary to poliomyelitis affecting the leg muscles.

Following the observation of the gross visible deformities, detailed clinical examination of the lower extremity is performed.

Electromuscular Diagnosis

Our use of this method has been described previously.

Clinical Muscle Testing[5, 6]

This is the most important part of the examination, because the decision about which muscle or muscles will be used to replace the power of the paralyzed muscles will be based on the results of this testing.

Testing of the muscles of the leg and foot and those of the thigh that have an indirect influence on the foot is usually done with the patient sitting on the edge of an examining table with the knees flexed and the feet hanging down and with the examiner sitting in front of the patient. If the patient is unable to sit up, the testing should be performed with the patient lying on the table. The patient must be able to understand what he is asked to do and do it or try to do it. When a child is uncooperative or scared, we usually try to perform muscle testing several times on consecutive days until the patient becomes confident and is not afraid.

Our clinical rating for muscle power ranges from 0 to 5.

0 = Absent — no evidence of contractility.

1 = Trace — evidence of slight contractility; no joint motion.

2 = Poor — complete range of motion with gravity eliminated.

3 = Fair — complete range of motion against gravity.

4 = Good — complete range of motion against gravity with some resistance.

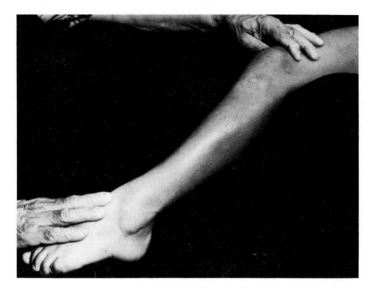

Figure 42–1. *Testing of the quadriceps.*

5 = Normal — complete range of motion against gravity with full resistance.

From the practical surgical point of view, we consider those muscles with a power rating of 3 or more as usable. When there is hope for recuperation (recovery or convalescent stage), we consider using those muscles with ratings of 1 or more, because we try our best to attain the highest level of recuperation. When there is no hope for recuperation (residual phase), muscles with power ratings of 3 or more are considered for use. When this residual phase is reached and no more recovery is expected, we determine if any type of surgery is indicated. The power ratings of the muscles of both sides should always be

written on the patient's chart so that the progress of muscle recuperation can be followed or attainment of the residual phase can be determined.

Quadriceps. To test the quadriceps, the patient is instructed to extend the knee. If he can do this, the power rating of the quadriceps is at least 3. The same test is then tried against resistance, with the examiner's right hand placed in front of the ankle for resistance on the left extremity and the left hand placed in front of the ankle for resistance on the right extremity. The palm of the hand not being used to provide resistance feels the degree of contracture of the quadriceps (Fig. 42–1). From personal experience, if the patient is

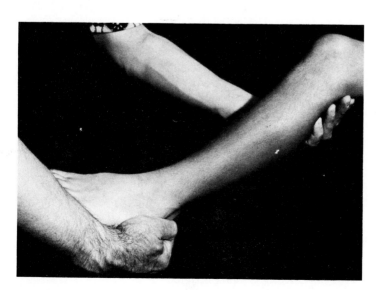

Figure 42–2. *Testing of the hamstrings.*

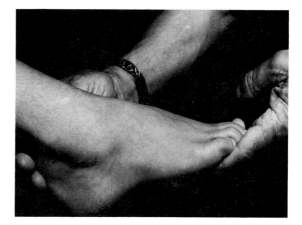

Figure 42–3. *Testing of the triceps surae.*

still able to extend the knee, the power rating of the muscle is 4 or 5.

Hamstrings. To test the hamstrings, the patient is instructed to bend the knee without resistance. The thumb and second and third fingers of the examiner's hand (the left hand is used for the left side and the right hand for the right side) are placed on the popliteal space, with the thumb over the medial hamstrings (gracilis, semi-tendinosus, and semimembranosus) and the other two fingers over the biceps (Fig. 42–2). The strength of contracture is felt and rated. Different ratings may be found for the medial and lateral hamstrings.

For testing against resistance, the palm of the examiner's right hand is used for the left extremity and that of the left hand for the right extremity and is placed in a cupped position over the heel. The patient is instructed to bend the knee against this resistance, and the lateral and medial hamstrings are rated (the rating is 4 or 5 if the

patient can do this). The patient may try to trick the examiner by swinging the leg with the thigh in external rotation, using the sartorius when there is no power in the hamstrings.

Triceps Surae. To test the triceps surae on the left side, the patient is instructed to plantar flex the foot, and the palm of the examiner's right hand is placed over the triceps surae and Achilles tendon to feel any muscular contraction if no motion can be detected on the ankle and to determine the degree of tension of the tendon. The fingers of the examiner's left hand are placed under the metatarsal heads of the left foot to test against resistance. (See Fig. 42–3.) To test the triceps surae on the right side, the opposite hands are used.

Tibialis Posterior. To test the tibialis posterior, if the patient has plantar flexion power, he is instructed to plantar flex the foot and bring the forefoot into adduction while the right hand of the examiner

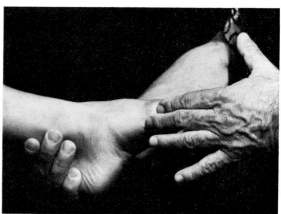

Figure 42–4. *Testing of the tibialis posterior.*

clasps the left heel and the fingers feel the contracture, if any, of the tendon, distal and posterior to the medial malleolus. With the left hand, resistance is then exerted over the medial side of the head of the first metatarsal to rate the power of the muscle. (See Figure 42–4.)

If the patient is a child, he is told to try to touch the finger of the examiner with his big toe with the foot in equinus, while adducting the forefoot.

If there is no power in the gastrocnemius, the foot is brought into equinus with the left hand and the same hand is used to test the power against resistance.

To test the right tibialis posterior, the opposite hands are used.

Tibialis Anterior. To test the tibialis anterior on the left side, the patient is instructed to invert the left foot and then dorsiflex it, while the examiner's right fingers palpate the tendon in front of the ankle. Care must be taken to avoid dorsiflexion of the great toe, as a powerful extensor hallucis longus may be confused with the tibialis anterior, and the tibialis anterior could be rated as a working muscle when the extensor hallucis longus is really doing the work (Fig. 42–5). Resistance may be added by placing the left hand over the forefoot and the medial side of the first metatarsal. If the patient is a child, he is told to try to push or touch the examiner's fingers by bringing the foot up and twisting it into inversion. (See Figure 42–6.)

The right tibialis anterior is examined using the opposite hands.

Peronei. It is practically impossible both clinically and by electromuscular

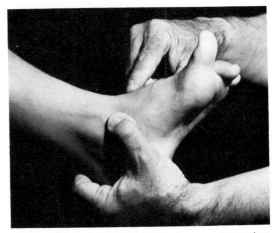

Figure 42–5. *Extensor hallucis longus attempting to do the work of an absent tibialis anterior.*

testing to differentiate the separate power of each peroneal muscle. Therefore, when examined, they are taken as a group, the peronei. To test the peronei on the left side, the patient is instructed, if able, to plantar flex the foot and then bring the forefoot into abduction (without any eversion). While the patient is doing this, the examiner clasps the heel with his left hand and with the fingers feels the peroneal tendons distal and posterior to the lateral malleolus. The right hand can then be used to add resistance at the fifth metatarsal (Fig. 42–7). If the patient is a child, he is told to try to push or touch the examiner's hand with the outer edge of his foot in equinus.

To test the right peronei, the opposite hands are used.

Theoretically, the function of the peron-

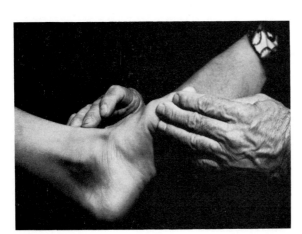

Figure 42–6. *Testing of the tibialis anterior. The extensor hallucis longus is relaxed.*

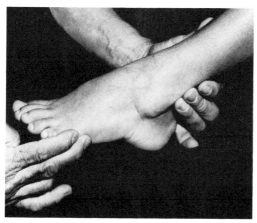

Figure 42–7. *Testing of the peronei.*

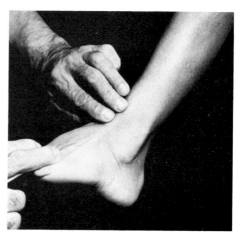

Figure 42–8. *Testing of the peroneus tertius.*

eus longus, which is distinct from that of the peroneus brevis, could probably be determined by its plantar flexion effect on the first metatarsal. When the patient everts his foot against resistance, the head of the first metatarsal should depress.

Peroneus Tertius. To test the left peroneus tertius, the patient is instructed to evert and dorsiflex the foot. The tendon can be felt with the examiner's left finger, while the right hand may apply resistance over the forefoot (Fig. 42–8). The opposite hands are used to test the right peroneus tertius.

Extensor Hallucis Longus and Flexor Hallucis Longus. To test the extensor hallucis longus and flexor hallucis longus of the left foot, the examiner's right hand holds the heel with the foot at a right angle. The patient is instructed to dorsiflex and plantar flex the hallux. Resistance is then applied with the left forefinger for both flexion and extension. A partially powerful extensor is unable to hold the distal phalanx in extension against pressure on the nail (distal phalanx) of the big toe. (See Figures 42–9 and 42–10.) For the right foot, the hands are placed the other way around.

Extensor Digitorum Longus and Flexor Digitorum Longus. These two muscles are tested in a way similar to the extensor hallucis longus and flexor hallucis longus, but instead of applying resistance with the forefinger, the examiner's fourth and fifth fingers are placed across the dorsal aspect of the toes to test for dorsiflexion, and the second and third fingers are placed across the plantar aspect of the toes to test for plantar flexion (Figs. 42–11 and 42–12).

Figure 42–9. *Testing of the extensor hallucis longus.*

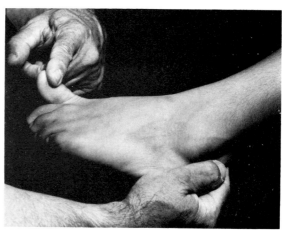

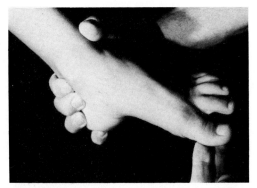

Figure 42–10. *Testing of the flexor hallucis longus.*

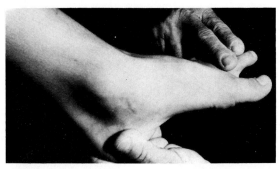

Figure 42–11. *Testing of the extensor digitorum longus.*

The hands are switched to test the muscles of the right foot.

Deformities of the Foot Following Poliomyelitis

A system can be established to classify deformities of the foot following polio. This is the end result of a complete, organized examination of the patient, as outlined previously, and full knowledge of the anatomy and its functions. Anatomy should be well known — the relationships of different structures, the nerve supply, and the action of muscles responsible for involvement of the foot in polio, as well as the knowledge of the muscles, bones, and joints in the areas that will undergo treatment.

In general, many deformities in the child can be prevented, but the majority of patients that we see are those neglected children, adolescents, or adults with established deformities.

Established Deformities

1. Primary equinus due to lack of power in the dorsiflexors of the foot or equinus secondary to other deformities of the extremity, such as genu recurvatum due to lack of power in the quadriceps.
2. Equinus due to lack of power in the dorsiflexors, but with good or normal peronei and tibialis posterior.
3. Eversion of the foot that may develop into paralytic pes planus owing to lack of power in the tibialis posterior and that is very often associated with palsy of the tibialis anterior. The peronei are in good or normal condition.
4. Flatfoot without any other deformity due to lack of power in both the tibialis anterior and tibialis posterior and good or normal peronei and gastrocnemius.
5. Flatfoot without any other deformity due to total absence of power in the tibialis anterior.
6. Inversion of the foot from lack of power in the peronei and persistence of a

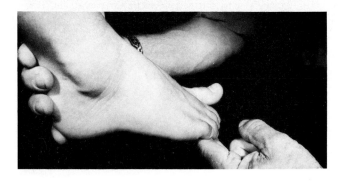

Figure 42–12. *Testing of the flexor digitorum longus.*

good or normal tibialis anterior and tibialis posterior or lack of power in one of the tibial muscles (posterior).

7. No deformity but lack of dorsiflexion power due to a very weak or powerless tibialis anterior. The extensor digitorum longus or the extensor hallucis longus or both may be involved to a greater or lesser degree, aggravating the lack of power to dorsiflex the foot. Good or normal peronei, tibialis posterior, and triceps surae are present.

8. Calcaneus, which is the result of a poor or powerless triceps surae and may be associated with a cavus deformity.

9. Calcaneus and cavus from lack of power in the dorsiflexors and triceps surae.

10. Adduction of the forefoot without inversion may be present when there is an imbalance between the peronei and the tibialis posterior, with predominance of the latter. There is a lack of power in the tibialis anterior.

11. Cavus of the foot alone has been attributed to involvement of the small muscles or the predominance of the plantar muscles, among other causes.

12. Claw toes may be the result of predominance of the extensors of the toes and imbalance of the interosseous and lumbrical muscles. More often, they are a consequence of cavus deformity.

13. Shortness of the foot.

Degree of Manual Correction of Deformities

In children and sometimes in adults, many deformities can be manually corrected while the patient is being examined. This implies that muscular, ligamentous, or capsular contractures have not become fixed or that the structures involved can still be stretched by hand. Some examples of deformities that may be corrected manually are equinus, inversion, or eversion of the foot, pes planovalgus, adduction or abduction of the forefoot and toe deformities. If a deformity can be manually corrected in a child and the deformity is not amenable to definitive correction by surgery, braces or other aids can be used to maintain the correction until the proper age for surgery is reached.

Radiographic Studies

Radiographs are useful for differential diagnosis of other conditions, e.g., scurvy, osteomyelitis, syphilis, and fractures. Later, radiographs are helpful in determining the bone age of the foot, whether the epiphyses are continuing to grow or not, the degree of atrophy of bones and shortness, and the amount of bone deformity.

Laboratory Tests

As indicated previously, laboratory tests are useful for differential diagnosis in the initial stages.

Photographs and Movies

Photographs and movies are part of the file of the patient and are used for comparison of the post-treatment results with the original condition of the patient.

TREATMENT

Initial Stage[2]

In the acute febrile stage of poliomyelitis, the patient is usually confined to the infectious ward of the hospital and is under the care of pediatricians and internists or specialists in infectious diseases, although the orthopaedic surgeon must be called in to initiate measures to prevent early deformities. The orthopaedic surgeon must be aware of the onset of the "spasmodic" phase, which begins 48 hours after the acute febrile phase is over; the first phase is considered the contagious phase of poliomyelitis. The patient is put under the orthopaedic surgeon's care after this phase. I must comment that we have very rarely seen another case of polio among children of the same family when an acute case of polio has not been promptly diagnosed. The ill child may remain among his siblings for all or part of the contagious phase, and none of the others develop even a larvate or abortive case of the disease.

During the painful spasmodic stage, treatment is restricted to the application of hot, moist packs, rest, sedatives, analgesics, and protection of the involved extremities.

In the specific condition of poliomyelitis related to the foot, it must be remembered that practically all the calf muscles originate in the leg, but by their sites of insertion, they act on the foot. The foot itself contains only the "small muscles of the foot." The importance of paying utmost attention to the muscles of the leg involved by polio is reflected in their effect on the function of the foot. Therefore, in general, attention here will be limited to muscles that may directly or indirectly affect the foot. For example, deformities of the knee may affect the foot, such as a hyperextension deformity of the knee that may cause equinus of the foot. During the acute painful stage of poliomyelitis, the lower extremity must be placed in neutral position with regard to internal and external rotation and abduction and adduction with the aid of sandbags. The knee must be kept in slight flexion (about 10 degrees) by placing a soft roll made of a towel or a sandbag under the most proximal posterior aspect of the calf. The foot should be kept at a right angle by placing a padded wooden board or box under it, supporting the sole. The mattress must be positioned so that enough space is left between it and the foot board of the bed to allow the feet to hang down between the mattress and the foot board when the patient is lying face down. While the patient lies face down, a rolled soft towel must be placed over the mattress so that the fronts of the distal ends of the legs (just above the ankles) rest on the folded towel and the knees are kept at about 10 degrees of flexion. The patient should be turned at least every hour on his sides and face down, keeping the extremities in the correct position. During the acute, painful, spasmodic period, manipulation of joints and massaging of muscles should be avoided as long as these procedures are uncomfortable and involved muscles hurt.

During the painful spasmodic phase, the application of hot, moist packs helps to relieve the patient's pain and discomfort. As a rule, we advise that application of the packs be started when the patient awakens in the morning. We leave the packs on for a period of an hour, and after removing them, allow the patient a two-hour rest. If the patient is asleep, he should not be disturbed either to apply or to remove

packs. The last packs are applied just before the patient goes to sleep at night, but they should not be left on overnight. Packs are made to the size of the patient. They wrap completely about the thigh and buttock and the calf and foot. Those for the thighs and buttocks are triangular, and those for calves and feet are rectangular. They are made of a rather thick, woolen fabric. The triangular pack for the thigh is made large enough so that its base will be just above the knee when wrapped around the thigh, covering the anterior and posterior muscles, and its apex will cover the buttock. The two rectangular packs should cover the calf and the foot. The knee, ankle joint, and toes must not be covered by the wet, hot packs. The packs are held in place with safety pins. After the packs are removed, they should be washed with soap and water and dried; otherwise they may develop fungi or mold.

The routine is to make the triangles and rectangles of a double layer of fabric. A layer of plastic of the same size and shape is cut. Both layers of fabric and plastic are sewn together. A third set of triangles and rectangles of the woolen fabric is then cut. A pot of boiling water must be ready to begin the application of the moist, hot packs. The pack to be applied is immersed in the hot water and is then withdrawn and swiftly wrung, maintaining the plastic layer inside. (When polio was endemic in the United States, special electric pots and wringers were available for this purpose.) The moistened and hot pack is then tested over the dorsum of the hand, and when the temperature is not too hot to burn the patient, the pack is placed over the dry fabric triangle or rectangle and wrapped securely around the thigh, calf, and foot, respectively, with the moistened, hot layer in contact with the skin. The packs are fixed with safety pins and left in situ, as previously described. This treatment is usually continued until the painful spasm subsides, which is usually about four weeks. A warm tub bath can be used, too, when available. A month after onset of the disease, application of moist, hot packs is discontinued and the residual paralysis is evaluated.

Small, uncooperative, or hysterical children may not help the examiner in the clinical evaluation of the residual stage of poliomyelitis. In these cases, we use electrical (galvanofaradic) tests. The machine we have been using for years is that designed by the late Dr. Weiss from the Hospital for Joint Diseases in New York. In all other cases, we rely on clinical testing of the power of the involved muscles.

As stated before, involvement of the thigh muscles may affect the foot, and testing of muscles may have to be done by synergic groups in many cases.

Recovery Stage and Prevention of Deformities

In children, if there is a tendency for development of a deformity, the following measures may be taken until the proper age for surgery, if required, is reached.

If equinus is present, the foot should be fitted with a drop-foot brace. This can be the classic metal brace with two uprights either with a caliper with incorporated shoe or, as we prefer, with a metal footplate and ankle cuff. With the latter type of brace, the child can wear any low-heel shoe. Plantar flexion of the brace should be limited to 5 degrees, with free dorsiflexion. Another brace that may be prescribed is the drop-foot brace made of polypropylene. We have started to use this polypropylene brace to the satisfaction of both patients and parents. It should have a strap at its upper end, a strap at the ankle to hold the heel well down in the brace, and another strap at the metatarsal heads.

If there is a tendency toward eversion or paralytic pes planus, a good orthopaedic shoe with a steel shank, Thomas heel, and insole metal arch will give good support to the foot. If a tendency toward equinus exists with the eversion, any of the braces for equinus will support the arch and prevent eversion.

Inversion of the foot may be prevented by the use of a lateral wedge oversole and heel, provided the shoe is a good one. Any of the braces for equinus will also help considerably.

If the tendency toward eversion or inversion is too great, however, we advise the short leg brace with two uprights, and, as noted before, we prefer the one with a footplate and ankle cuff. If the tendency is toward eversion, an ankle T-strap is added, which is fastened laterally to the lateral upright and pulls the ankle outwardly. The T-strap is attached the other way around if there is a tendency toward inversion.

If there is no tendency toward equinus but the dorsiflexors are weak or powerless, in order to avoid steppage gait, any of the braces mentioned for equinus may be prescribed.

Calcaneus may be prevented by the use of braces similar to those indicated for drop foot, but the limitation of ankle motion should be to dorsiflexion, permitting only 5 degrees of foot extension and free plantar flexion.

If a tendency toward adduction of the forefoot is noticed, abductor shoes may be prescribed.

Pure cavus of the foot is very difficult to prevent with braces or shoes. Even metatarsal bars and other devices usually do not help.

Claw toes are usually associated with cavus deformity and may be prevented by the use of metatarsal bars and avoidance of shoes that are too small and crowd the toes, promoting development of the deformity.

SURGERY IN ESTABLISHED DEFORMITIES

Equinus. If the deformity is established in a child less than seven years old, we try first to correct the equinus by a plaster cast that slowly brings the foot dorsally while stretching the triceps surae. The plaster is applied with the knee flexed, so that if the contracture is from the gastrocnemius, this muscle is relaxed while the plaster is applied to correct the equinus. This plaster cast is changed every one or two weeks, increasing the dorsiflexion of the foot with every new cast applied.

If no correction can be obtained with casts or if the patient is a child over seven years of age or an adult, we do an open Achilles-tendon lengthening through a medial longitudinal incision. Sometimes the posterior capsule of the ankle and the corresponding ligaments must be sectioned. The correction must not go beyond a right angle. A plaster boot is applied with the foot in the corrected position (at a right angle) and is removed one month after surgery, when stitches, if nonabsorbable, are removed.

In long-standing cases, it is sometimes impossible to obtain full correction of the equinus because as the talus has become incongruous in equinus, the anterior part of its tibial articular surface has grown broader than normal and does not fit into the tibiofibular mortise.

Equinus secondary to genu recurvatum requires correction of the knee deformity prior to correction of the equinus condition. If hyperextension of the knee is present with lack of power in the quadriceps and hamstrings, correction of this deformity should be performed, although a brace to control hyperextension of the knee will have to be fitted to prevent recurrence. If there is lack of power in the quadriceps with poor, good, or normal hamstrings, the genu recurvatum should be surgically corrected, followed by transfer of the bilateral hamstring tendons to the patella (Mayer's technique). Surgical lengthening of the Achilles tendon should not be attempted until the hyperextension of the knee is corrected. If the equinus is not fixed and if there is a normal or good tibialis anterior, the correction of the genu recurvatum alone will allow the foot to rest at a right angle on the floor, and no other procedures will be needed. If stabilization of the foot cannot be performed because the patient is too young for bone surgery (less than 8 to 10 years of age), the child should be fitted with a drop-foot brace until the tarsal bones have matured enough, as demonstrated radiographically, for bone and tendon surgery.

Equinus from Lack of Power in the Dorsiflexors, Peronei, and Tibialis Posterior with Good or Normal Triceps Surae. Achilles-tendon lengthening may be done, followed by one month of immobilization in plaster. This is followed by the fitting of a drop-foot short leg brace if no deformity of the foot is present. If any osseous deformity exists, it must be corrected in the same surgical session after tendon lengthening if the patient's bones are mature enough, and the drop-foot brace is fitted after three months of immobilization in a plaster boot.

If there are no muscles that can be transferred anteriorly and a strong gastroc-nemius-soleus exists, the medial half of the gastrocnemius-soleus, or less frequently, the lateral half, may be used for dorsiflexion power.[28] A preliminary triple arthrodesis is done. Through a long vertical incision, the medial half of the gastrocnemius-soleus and the medial half of the Achilles tendon are isolated and tubed with the aponeurosis and then transferred subcutaneously anteriorly into the middle cuneiform (see Figure 42–34). If the lateral half of the gastrocnemius-soleus is to be used, it is transferred anteriorly to the middle cuneiform through the interosseous space. The leg is immobilized in a long leg cast for six weeks, and ambulation is initiated eight weeks postoperatively.

Eversion of the Foot and Paralytic Pes Planus. This deformity is the result of tibialis posterior or, often, tibialis anterior involvement. An imbalance, created by good or normal peronei, leads to this situation. Routinely, if eversion of the heel and forefoot is present in addition to the flattening of the longitudinal arch, we first stabilize the foot (triple arthrodesis) through a slightly oblique incision on the dorsolateral aspect of the tarsus, correcting eversion of the heel and forefoot and modeling a normal longitudinal arch. A plaster cast is applied. Two months later, the plaster cast is removed and a peroneal transfer is performed using Mayer's technique. These two procedures, triple arthrodesis and peroneal tendon transfer, will be described subsequently.

When the pes planus is due to lack of power in the tibialis posterior with a good tibialis anterior and peronei, we perform our procedure of stabilization of the talonavicular joint, provided there is hypermobility of the first metatarsal segment. This procedure will be described later. This situation does not require any tendon transfer. If equinus is present with this condition, the tendo Achillis is lengthened through a medial longitudinal incision, as a second step, but not during surgery for flatfoot.

Paralysis of the Tibialis Anterior and Posterior with Good or Normal Peronei and a Good or Normal Gastrocnemius Resulting in Flatfoot Deformity Only. In this situation, we have found that stabilization of the first metatarsal segment, which must be hypermobile, to restore the longitudinal arch of the foot is the only osseous surgery required. After plaster immobilization for two months, a peroneus longus transfer to replace the power of the tibialis anterior will achieve a perfect result.

Inversion of the Foot (Usually the Result of Peroneal Palsy). In this condition, the tibialis anterior and posterior are usually in good or normal condition, but sometimes the tibialis posterior may have no power. In this situation, besides inversion of the foot, there may be adduction of the forefoot and even equinus. If the latter is present, the Achilles tendon should be lengthened as the first step in the corrective stabilization of the foot, and a plaster cast is applied. After two months, the plaster cast will be removed and a tibialis anterior transfer performed (Mayer's technique, which will be described later). The lack of power in the tibialis posterior is disregarded.

No Deformity, with a Lack of Dorsiflexion Power from Weakness or Absence of Tibialis Anterior Power. Involvement of the extensors of the toes and hallux will aggravate the lack of dorsiflexion power. In any case, stabilization of the foot followed by peroneal transfer (Mayer's technique) will correct the problem.

Calcaneus. This deformity is the result of weakness or lack of power in the triceps surae. Correction of the bone deformity is performed as part of a triple arthrodesis, as will be described subsequently. Transfer of the peroneus longus (or brevis, if the peroneus longus is not suitable or if it had to be transferred to replace the lack of power in the tibialis anterior) to the Achilles tendon is then performed (our technique is described later).

Calcaneus and Cavus from Lack of Power in the Dorsiflexors and Triceps Surae. Correction of the deformity by stabilization, which consists of a dorsal cuneiform resection of the midtarsus, correction of the calcaneus, and probably sectioning of the plantar fascia, is followed by three months of immobilization in plaster. A short leg brace must be provided to limit extension and flexion of the foot if there is no power in the peronei. If both peronei are good or normal, two months after corrective surgery of the deformity we transfer the peroneus longus to the

Achilles tendon, close to its insertion on the os calcis (see the description of the technique that follows). This is followed by one month of plaster immobilization with the foot in equinus. After the plaster is removed, the foot is left free, and when the patient loosens his ankle and is able to reach a right angle with his foot (passive motion), the peroneus brevis is transferred forward to the dorsum of the base of the second metatarsal to replace the lack of power of the foot dorsiflexors (tibialis anterior). If one of the peroneal muscles is poor and if there is a good or normal tibialis posterior, we utilize the good peroneal muscle to replace the power of the triceps surae and transfer the tendon of the tibialis posterior forward to the dorsum of the foot.

Adduction of the Forefoot without Inversion. This may be present if an imbalance exists between the peronei (poor or powerless) and the tibialis posterior, with predominance of the latter, and if there is lack of power in the tibialis anterior and a good or normal triceps surae.

The bone deformity must be corrected by wedge osteotomy (with the base of the wedge positioned laterally). Two months later, the tendon of the tibialis posterior is transferred forward to the dorsum of the foot in an attempt to replace the power of the tibialis anterior. Otherwise, a dropfoot brace can be fitted or a posterior bone block operation performed.

Cavus of the Foot with Normal Long Muscles. This deformity has been attributed to imbalance of the small muscles of the foot with predominance of the plantar muscles. In such a situation, we perform a cuneiform resection of the midtarsus with a dorsal or dorsolateral base. The apex of the bone resection is in a plantar position, and we do not remove any bone at the plantar apex in order to avoid shortening of the foot and to increase the length of the foot. If all the muscles are normal, no other procedures are required. As soon as the cavus is corrected, the tibialis anterior begins to function normally.

Claw Toes. In most cases, claw toes are the result of a cavus deformity. Many times, with correction of the cavus and raising of the metatarsal arch, the deformity of the toes is automatically corrected. However, if there are contractures of the plantar or dorsal skin and capsules, surgical correction is necessary. For a description of the different surgical techniques the reader is referred to Chapter 23.

Shortness of the Foot. We have lengthened the foot, depending on its shortness, from 1 to 2 cm, performing a transtarsal osteotomy and inserting bone blocks in between. This technique will be described later.

GENERAL RULES FOR SURGERY OF RESIDUAL POLIO OF THE FOOT

There are several general rules that should be kept in mind when performing surgery to improve the condition of a patient with residual polio of the foot.

1. While the patient is in the acute stage or the recovery stage, no surgery for rehabilitation should be performed. Not until definitive and permanent lesions are established should the surgeon formulate a plan for surgical rehabilitation.

2. When the patient has reached such a stage, which, as noted previously, is usually a year after onset, his condition must be evaluated, and after evaluation a step-by-step plan is formulated.

3. With regard to the patient's age, there are a few operations that can be performed as soon as the patient is able to stand or has reached the age to stand and walk:

a. Flexion contracture of the hip should be corrected as soon as possible.

b. Flexion contracture of the knee should be corrected as soon as possible.

c. Weakness or complete palsy of the quadriceps should be corrected at any age by hamstring transfers, if these muscles are strong enough.

4. Stabilization of the hip, knee, and ankle should not be done for polio at any age. There is always something more functional than a stiff joint.

5. Lengthening of the tendo Achillis should be done as early as possible to avoid narrowing of the mortise or widening of the talus, which then will not fit into the tibiofibular space.

6. Transfer of the tendons of the leg to replace the power of muscles of opposite action should not be done prior to stabilization of the foot; otherwise, a reverse deformity may develop.

7. Therefore, stabilization and correction of foot deformities should be performed prior to tendon transfers, and arthrodeses must not be performed until the bones of the midtarsus have reached maturity, as confirmed radiographically and by age (eight to ten years of age). Annual radiographs are taken until such maturity is noted.

8. Except for the aforementioned transfers that can be performed at any age, those tendon transfers that should not be performed until bone maturity has been established, as just described, are peroneal transfers, transfers of the tibialis posterior and anterior, and medial gastrocnemius transfers.

9. Following stabilization of the foot for peroneal transfer, the application of a well-molded, below-the-knee plaster boot is required. A long leg cast is not necessary. The plaster boot should be skintight and split as soon as it has set, as will be explained later. If the surgeon has no experience with skintight plaster, minimal padding should be used so that the plaster boot is snug, well-molded, and well fitting.

10. As soon as the patient is in the recovery room or his own room, the leg must be elevated at least 40 to 50 cm above his chest to prevent swelling of the foot as much as is possible. As soon as the plaster is split in the operating room, whether it is skintight or not, it should be separated from the skin at least from the base of the toes up to the mid-leg and then molded again over the foot and leg.

11. When bone surgery of the foot is performed, mainly for stabilization, there is a greater tendency for the foot to swell. Ice bags applied to the dorsum of the foot for 48 hours may help to prevent this.

12. A plaster boot should never be applied without plantar support for the toes; otherwise, after three months in plaster, a flexion contracture of the toes may develop. By the same token, the dorsal aspect of the toes must be left free, so that the patient can exercise them daily by routine extension. If such exercising is not done, the toes may become stiff.

13. Dorsal cuneiform resections of the tarsus for cavus or varus or both do not shorten the foot. On the contrary, if performed properly, they lengthen it, as will

be shown subsequently when the resection is described.

14. Claw toes can be corrected at any age, provided there is no arthrodesis to be performed between immature joints.

15. When performing a tendon transfer, one should always try to use the tendon sheath of the paralyzed tendon to insure a good gliding mechanism.

16. Transfer of tendons of opposite action (e.g., flexor to extensor) tends to give results that are not as good as those with transfer of tendons having similar or the same action.

17. Transfer of tendons should be done in such a way that the transferred tendon lies in the straightest line from its muscle origin to the new site of implantation. The more angled this line, the poorer the results.

18. Anchorage of transferred tendons to bone should be strong enough that after a month of plaster immobilization, there is no danger of detachment of the anchored tendon.

19. When a tendon is transferred, no weight bearing should be permitted for one month, for the tendon, by contraction of the parent muscle, may detach from its insertion.

20. Normally weak tendons cannot replace the power of strong tendons in function, e.g., the tensor hallucis longus cannot replace the tibialis anterior and if transferred, will result in a plantar-flexed big toe. Sometimes weak tendons can be used for tenodesis, to limit some arc of motion.

21. Poorly conceived surgery for polio, inventing surgical procedures, and improvising techniques, which are all results of lack of proper knowledge of and training in surgery for polio, may do irreparable harm to a foot that was amenable to surgical rehabilitation before such improper surgery was performed.

22. The anatomy of the leg and foot, the action of the muscles, the mechanics of anatomic structures, and the pathology and anatomy of deformed structures must be understood perfectly by the surgeon.

SURGICAL TECHNIQUES

Routine techniques will be described first, followed by alternative procedures.

Stabilization of the Foot

For stabilization of the foot (triple arthrodesis — talonavicular and calcaneocuboid — and tarsal resections), we prefer to use a slightly modified Ollier incision. This incision, on the dorsolateral aspect of the tarsus, starts at the lower limit of the calcaneocuboid joint and extends upward and forward to the lowest part of the talonavicular joint. Its length depends on the size of the foot, but it normally measures from 4 to 6 cm. We routinely use a cotton stocking or a narrow stockinette, so that the shape of the foot can be appreciated if a deformity is being corrected or, if there is no deformity to be corrected, to avoid producing one. The skin edges of the incision can be protected with the stockinette or stocking by placing three Mitchell skin clips on each lip of the incision.

The peroneus brevis is easily identified and is protected. The skin is undermined to expose the soft tissues of the sinus tarsi. The extensor digitorum brevis muscle fibers are then detached from the cuboid and calcaneus all the way to the sinus tarsi. All fatty tissue is removed from the sinus tarsi. The dorsal calcaneocuboid ligament and capsule, bifurcate ligament, dorsal calcaneonavicular ligament, dorsal cuboideonavicular ligament, and talonavicular capsule are detached from the talus, navicular, os calcis, and cuboid, lifting with them all the tendons and vessels that run along the dorsum of the foot. This detachment is performed systematically from the lateral border of the extensor digitorum brevis upward and medially until the talonavicular and calcaneocuboid joints are exposed. Most of the dorsal surface of the navicular and the neck and head of the talus, as well as the cuboid and the floor of the sinus tarsi, are left bare of ligaments and capsules. The sinus tarsi is denuded of all ligaments and capsules, including the origin of the extensor digitorum brevis. Then, with a thin osteotome about 2 cm wide, the first part of the bone surgery is started. If there is no tarsal deformity, a thin layer of cortex and the cartilage are resected from the articular surfaces of the calcaneocuboid and talonavicular joints. If there is tarsal deformity, such as cavus or adduction or abduction of the forefoot, a corresponding wedge is resected. Care should be taken that the apex of the wedge to be resected is really an apex or the point at which the two planes of the angle of the wedge join; otherwise the foot will be shortened. To insure proper wedge resection, the surgeon can make an outline on paper of the radiograph of the foot, cutting the proper wedge on the outline of the radiograph to obtain an approximate idea of the bone wedge to be resected. He may also start by resecting a small wedge of bone and, by progessive removal of slices of bone, attain the proper resection.

The osteotomized foot should be placed in the corrected position, with attention to proper apposition of the osteotomized surfaces. No soft tissues should interpose between the bones to be in contact, so that union will take place. Any inversion or eversion of the foot may be corrected by rotating the forefoot in relation to the hind part of the osteotomy. If satisfactory correction has been achieved and perfect apposition obtained, the second step of the triple arthrodesis is initiated. When the sinus tarsi has been completely denuded of all soft tissue, the three facets of the subtalar joint — posterior, middle, and anterior — are exposed. A lamina spreader is used to separate the talus and the os calcis. With a narrow osteotome, the cartilage and a thin layer of bone cortex are removed from both the middle and anterior facets of the subtalar joint. Then, after the posterior facet of the joint is opened as much as possible with the lamina spreader, a thin, narrow osteotome (about 1 cm wide) is used to remove the cartilage and a thin layer of cortex from the articular surfaces of the joint. If there is varus or valgus deformity of the heel, resection of the talus is done so that the remaining surface does not have the contour of the normal articular surface (concave from behind forward) but has a flat, horizontal surface. Valgus or varus deformities of the heel are corrected by resecting the articular surface of the os calcis in a wedge fashion, with the base of the wedge being lateral for inversion of the heel or medial for eversion. Following this resection, both flat surfaces should fit well, so that a good union will be obtained. Any small defect in the resected surfaces should be packed with bone that has been resected from the tarsus. While the foot is held in the corrected position, the apo-

neurosis and extensor hallucis brevis are sutured with interrupted, plain catgut stitches so that all the bone surfaces and the sinus tarsi are covered. The skin is sutured in the usual manner. When a great deal of padding is to be used with the plaster cast, so that a poor grip of the foot is expected and displacement of the forefoot may occur, staples may be used to fix the forefoot to the hindfoot. A below-the-knee plaster boot is applied either unpadded (skintight) or with the least possible padding. The back of the heel should always be well padded with cotton to avoid a painful heel and pressure sores. The plaster is split down to the skin from the toes to the upper middle third of the leg, following the midline of the foot and leg, as noted under the general rules for surgery.

To avoid postoperative swelling, the leg is elevated at least about 40 to 50 cm above the chest of patient as soon as surgery has been completed. When there is no more impending swelling, the patient can get out of bed into a wheelchair and then can begin to use crutches. Two weeks after surgery, the stitches of the stabilization are removed (if nonabsorbable suture material has been used) without changing the plaster boot. This incision sometimes heals by second intention. If tendo-Achillis lengthening has been performed, the stitches are left untouched until final removal of the plaster boot. If the wound is healed, or after healing by second intention, the plaster boot is closed with a plaster of Paris bandage and a walking iron or heel is incorporated into it. Unnecessary changing of casts may result in loss of the correction obtained. No weight bearing is permitted until the end of the sixth postoperative week. If no tendon surgery is expected to be performed, the plaster boot is left in place for another six weeks, after which it is removed and full weight bearing started. If the foot and leg swell after removal of the plaster, elevation of the foot at night is advised, and the application of an elastic bandage in the morning and whirlpool massage may also be helpful. If tendon surgery is planned, the plaster is removed two months after stabilization and the tendon transfer is then performed.

Cuneiform Resections. The approach

is the same as described above for stabilization of the foot. The soft tissues (extensor digitorum brevis and extensor digitorum longus tendons and tarsal dorsal ligaments and capsules) are detached and separated from the dorsum of the tarsus, as described for stabilization of the foot. The sinus tarsi is left untouched. Once the dorsolateral aspect of the tarsus (head of the talus, anterior part of the calcaneus, dorsal aspect of cuboid and navicular) is exposed and bared of soft tissues with a broad osteotome (about 2 to 3 cm wide), the wedge resection of the tarsus is performed in accordance with the principles established in the last section of this chapter (Osteotomies for Cavus Deformities).

Care should be taken that the apex of the wedge resected is placed at the lower plantar limit of the talonavicular joint. The plaster boot with the least padding is left on for two months if tendon transfers have been planned, and then they are performed. Otherwise, the plaster is left on for three months, and weight bearing is started six weeks after bone surgery has been performed.

Stabilization of the First Metatarsal Segment. We do this stabilization for flatfoot (our own unpublished technique) when hypermobility of the first metatarsal segment (navicular, first cuneiform, and first metatarsal) is present, as well as for paralytic flatfoot due to lack of power in the tibialis posterior. The talonavicular joint is fused through a 5- or 6-cm incision over the medial border of the foot at the level of the joint. It is fixed with a staple,

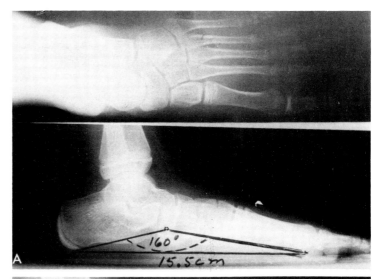

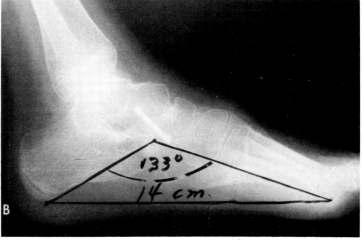

Figure 42–13. (A) Pes planus with a 160-degree arch and a length of 15.5 cm. (B) After stabilization of the first metatarsal segment at the talonavicular joint, the arch is 133 degrees and the length is 14 cm.

and the space left after denuding the anteroinferior surface of the talar head and the navicular articular surface of cartilage is packed with bone chips from the bone bank or from the patient's iliac crest. The first ray is left in maximum plantar flexion, and the plaster boot remains in place for six weeks, with the foot in equinus position. It is usually unnecessary to split the plaster. It must be skintight or have the least possible padding and must be well molded over the longitudinal arch of the foot. At the end of six weeks, the plaster boot is changed for a new one, with the foot positioned at a right angle but keeping the arch of the foot well molded. A walking device is incorporated into the boot, and weight bearing is allowed. Three months postoperatively, the plaster is removed, and normal shoes are recommended, as no more support will be necessary for the corrected flatfoot. If paralytic flatfoot follows weakness or total paralysis of the tibialis anterior, one of the peroneal tendons should be transferred to replace the power of the tibialis anterior eight weeks after stabilization of the first metatarsal segment. Figure 42–13A shows a flatfoot with an arch of 160 degrees with a length of 15.5 cm. After surgical correction by stabilization of the hypermobile first metatarsal segment (talonavicular joint fused in correct position), the arch was reduced to 133 degrees with a length of 14 cm (Fig. 42–13B).

Eversion or Inversion of the Os Calcis. This is corrected by a subtalar fusion. If this deformity is present when stabilization is performed, the surgical correction is as was described previously (i.e., stabilization of the foot or triple arthrodesis). If the only deformity to be corrected is valgus or varus of the os calcis, a subtalar fusion is performed through the same incision as is used for triple arthrodesis and through the sinus tarsi in the same way it is done as a final step in triple arthrodesis, by correcting the os calcis varus or valgus by resection of the corresponding wedge from the os calcis. Three months of plaster immobilization are required, and weight bearing is permitted at the end of the sixth postoperative week. Wedge osteotomy of the os calcis may also be performed following Dwyer's technique.

Bone Blocks. Bone blocks may be used when no muscle is available to correct loss of power in the gastrocnemius or the extensors of the foot (e.g., the tibialis anterior). The *posterior bone block* is performed through a posteromedial incision over the edge of the Achilles tendon. If a fixed equinus deformity is present, the tendon is lengthened. The technique used most frequently is that of Campbell.[3] The *anterior bone block* limits dorsiflexion. It may be used when there is an imbalance between the dorsiflexors and the plantar flexors with peronei that lack power and are therefore unsuitable for transfer to help the gastrocnemius. The anterior bone block is inserted into the neck of the talus through an anteromedial, medial, or anterolateral incision. After any bone block implant, a plaster boot must be worn for three months with the foot at a right angle. Weight bearing may be permitted six weeks after surgery.

Calcaneus. If this deformity is present with a cavus deformity, it should be corrected during triple arthrodesis with wedge resection of the tarsus. While performing the subtalar arthrodesis, the subtalar articulation is resected in a manner similar to that described previously for correction of varus or valgus deformity of the heel. However, instead of resecting a wedge with a lateral or medial base from the calcaneus, the base of the wedge resected should be located posteriorly. It will then be seen that the heel is "too long" posteriorly. To obtain a normal appearance of the heel, it is pushed forward, slipping the os calcis under the talus. A space then appears between the talus and the navicular and should be well packed with the bone wedge removed from the os calcis and from the tarsus if cuneiform resection has been performed for a concomitant cavus deformity. The foot increases in length from 1 to 2 cm. A well-molded plaster boot holds the foot in the corrected position, and the post-treatment care is the same as that after triple arthrodesis. If a tendon transfer is necessary and possible to help replace the power of the gastrocnemius, it is performed two months after stabilization.

Transfer of Muscles of the Leg

Mayer has described the general principles of tendon transfer, and the reader is referred to his classic monograph.[7]

Peroneal Tendon Transfer

For transfer of the peroneal tendons, we use Mayer's technique with a little modification. The operation is performed with a tourniquet applied above the knee.

A long, curved incision with its convexity forwardly placed, extending over the middle three fifths of the lateral aspect of the leg, exposes the sural fascia (Fig. 42–14). The skin and subcutaneous tissue are separated from the fascia from the crest of the tibia to beyond the lateral intermuscular septum, with care being taken not to cut the fascia. The emergence of the musculocutaneous nerve is identified if it is in the exposed area. Sometimes the emergence of the musculocutaneous (superficial peroneal) nerve is farther distal and

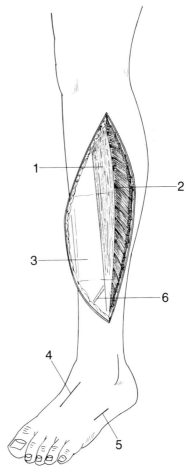

Figure 42–15. *(1) Peroneus longus. (2) Soleus. (3) Sural fascia covering the peronei, extensor digitorum longus, and tibialis anterior. Outline of fascial flap cuts. (4) Incision for anchorage of the peroneus longus tendon over the dorsum of the foot. (5) Incision for section of the peroneus longus over the cuboid. (6) Musculocutaneous nerve.*

cannot be found in the exposed area as a reference point. The distance from the tibial crest to the lateral intermuscular septem is divided into four parts. The fascia is incised with a knife for one fourth of that mentioned distance from the crest of the tibia backwards and perpendicular to the axis of the leg, then from the lateral intermuscular septum forward for another fourth of the distance. The level of the emergence of the musculocutaneous nerve is taken as the distal limit of the aponeurotic flaps in the process of being cut. About 6 to 10 cm above this, depending on the length of the leg, the fascia is incised in a similar manner (Fig. 42–15). With a

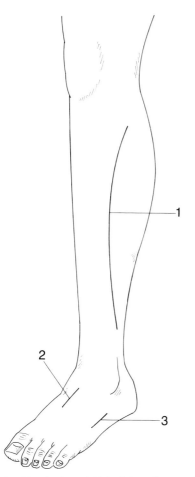

Figure 42–14. *(1, 2, and 3) Incisions for transfer of the peroneal tendons to compensate for lack of power in the tibialis anterior.*

pair of small tendon scissors, an anterior incision is made following the crest of the tibia, joining the first two cuts of the fascia, and another incision following the lateral edge of the intermuscular septum joins the second two incisions. Two flaps of fascia are formed; the posterior flap is folded forward and the anterior one is folded backward. With very fine silk (4–0), which is anchored first at the fascia 0.5 cm proximal to the flaps, the free edges of the everted flaps are sutured, using a continuous Cushing-Lembert type of intestinal suture, so that the edges will be invaginated and the silk buried. After the last stitch has been made, the suture is anchored about 0.5 cm distal to the flaps, into the fascia. The two everted flaps of fascia joined in this way will form a gliding surface for the peroneal tendon being used (Fig. 42–16).

With a pair of small scissors, the fascia is incised over the tendons of the peronei from the distal incision for the flaps to the distal end of the skin incision. A small 1.5- to 2-cm incision following the direction of the peroneal tendons is made to expose these tendons at the level of the cuneiform bone (Fig. 42–14). If the peroneus longus is good or normal, this muscle will be the one to be transferred. The tendon is easily identified over the cuneiform, as it is the most posterior or plantarward one. With a button hook at the tendon over the cuneiform and another one, or an Allis or tendon clamp, at the lower end of the leg incision, the tendon of the peroneus longus can be identified by pulling it distally, making sure that the peroneus brevis is not the tendon grasped. Once it is certain that the tendon is that of the peroneus longus, it is cut transversely with a sharp knife at the cuboid level. Using a Desmarres retractor, an Allis clamp, or even the little finger, the tendon is pulled out proximally. Mayer extends the incision

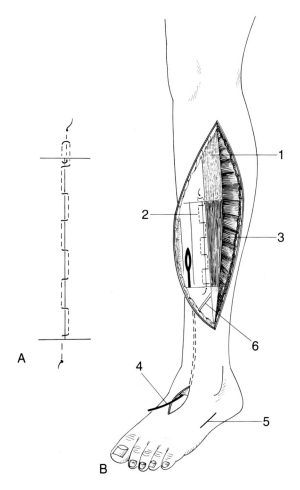

Figure 42–16. *(A) Schematic drawing of closure of the turned-out flaps of the sural fascia, showing in detail the Cushing-Lembert suture. (B) [1] Peroneus longus. [2] Fascial flaps turned out and sutured for muscle gliding. [3] Soleus muscle. [4] Eyed probe introduced through the tibialis anterior sheath and coming out at the anchorage incision. [5] Incision for tendon section. [6] Musculocutaneous nerve.*

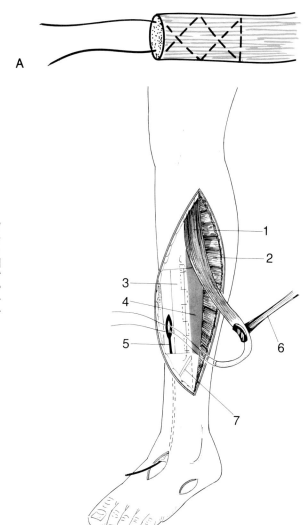

Figure 42-17. *(A) Detail of the Mayer-Bunnell suture of the tendon. (B) [1] Peroneus longus freed all the way up. [2] Soleus. [3] Sural fascia sutured to make a gliding bed for the muscle. [4] Peroneus brevis. [5] Eyed probe with catgut threaded through it for its passage through the tunnel of the tibialis anterior. [6] Desmarres retractor holding the tendon and muscle. [7] Musculocutaneous nerve.*

down around the back of the lateral malleolus to the cuboid bone to expose the tendon completely. With No. 2 chromic catgut, a Mayer-Bunnell type of suture is attached to the distal end of the cut tendon (Fig. 42–17). This will serve for anchorage.

An eyed probe, curved to the anterior curvature of the ankle, is introduced between the fascia and the paralyzed tibialis anterior, through the opening of the fascia and all the way through the tunnel of the tibialis anterior until the round tip of the probe is felt over the dorsum of the foot, the navicular, and the first or second cuneiform bone. The ends of the catgut are introduced through the eye of the probe

for a length of about 10 cm. A longitudinal incision about 3 or 4 cm long is made on the dorsum of the foot over the distal end of the probe to expose it (Figs. 42–14 to 42–16). The probe is pulled out, and the catgut is grasped out of the anchorage incision. With an Allis clamp, the stump of the peroneal tendon must be led to the entrance of the tibialis anterior tunnel, avoiding twisting or buckling of the tendon and muscle, while the tendon is pulled out of the incision on the dorsum of the foot by the attached catgut (Fig. 42–18). If necessary, to avoid constriction, a longitudinal incision of the fascia is made proximal to the flaps, over the muscle. Throughout the surgical procedure, the

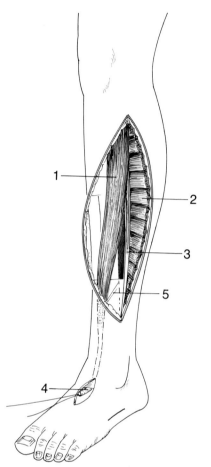

Figure 42–18. *The peroneus longus tendon (1) has been passed through the tibialis anterior tunnel, gliding over the turned-out fascial bed. It emerges at the anchorage incision (4), under the anterior transverse tarsal ligament. (2) Soleus. (3) Peroneus brevis. (5) Musculocutaneous nerve.*

tendon and soft tissues must be kept moist with saline solution. The tendon must not be touched with the hands or sponges; it should be handled with Desmarres retractors, avoiding contact with the stockinette. The fascia distal to the flap incisions is then closed with size 0 plain catgut, followed by closure of the subcutaneous tissue and skin.

The distal stump of the peroneal tendon is fixed with chromic catgut to the surrounding tissues of the cuboid to prevent dorsiflexion of the first metatarsal and formation of a dorsal bunion. The technique for anchoring the tendon is as follows: The navicular bone is freed by separating the dorsiflexors, but it is not denuded of soft tissue. With a thin osteotome, a T-shaped trap door is opened at the site of fixation.

We do not fix the transferred tendon to the medial side of the navicular, but to its dorsal aspect at the level of the second cuneiform, unless a flatfoot due to lack of power in both tibial muscles or in the tibialis anterior alone is being corrected (see previous discussion). In the latter situation, we fix the transferred tendon more medially to the navicular. As dorsiflexion is desired more than inversion, the tendon should be fixed more laterally than Mayer advised. The trap door in the bone is 2 to 3 cm long, with the horizontal arm of the T about 1 cm in length and proximally situated. The cancellous bone is pressed with an instrument to compact it, if it is soft enough, or it is curetted off to make a trough to accommodate the tendon. With a sharp, heavy needle, the ends of the catgut are passed about 0.5 to 1 cm apart, just distal to the T-shaped trap door, and are tied with the tendon under palpable tension as a cord at the anterior aspect of the ankle and with the foot of a right angle with the leg. Then, by crossing the catgut to close the trap door, a suture is made with a blunt needle strong enough to pass the bone cortex and the tendon under it. The catgut suture over the trap door looks like a tied shoelace. The tying knot is made proximally (Fig. 42–19). The skin is closed. An unpadded plaster boot or one with the least possible padding is applied, with the foot at a right angle without inversion or eversion. The plaster is split from the base of the toes to the middle of the calf or more, and the foot is elevated as usual. When there is no danger of swelling, the patient starts walking on crutches for four weeks, after which the plaster and stitches are removed. Rehabilitation is started as soon as the plaster boot is removed.

When the peroneus longus is weak and the peroneus brevis is good or normal, the latter is transferred, with the same good results. Mayer used to perform tendo-Achillis lengthening, triple arthrodesis, and peroneal transfer in one surgical session, in less than the allowable tourniquet time of one hour and 30 minutes.

Tibialis Anterior Transfer

With a tourniquet in place above the knee joint, the tibialis anterior is exposed

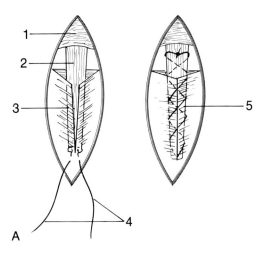

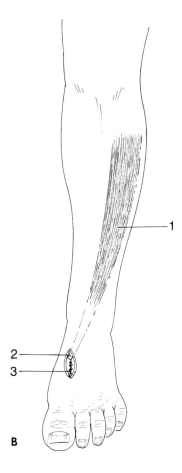

Figure 42–19. *(A) Anchorage of the tendon in detail.*
[1] Anterior transverse tarsal ligament. [2] Peroneus
longus tendon. [3] T-shaped trap door. [4] Emerging
tendon threads. [5] Trap door closed with a shoelace
suture, anchoring the tendon. (B) Anterior view of the
leg showing the transposed peroneal tendon. There is
no angulation whatsoever. [1] Peroneus longus mus-
cle. [2] Transverse tarsal ligament. [3] T-shaped trap
door closed and tendon anchored.

by means of a longitudinal incision of the skin and subcutaneous tissue extending from the junction of the lower and middle thirds of the leg to the navicular (Fig. 42–20). The fascia and retinaculum are slit with a pair of small scissors (such as those used for hand or eye surgery). The tendon is sectioned at the navicular level and is detached from its mesotendon with the small scissors. The freed tendon is threaded with No. 2 chromic catgut in the same manner as advised for the peroneal tendon (Mayer-Bunnell suture). A long and curved eyed probe is introduced through the extensor digitorum longus tunnel, with its tip emerging around the base of the fourth metatarsal. The tip of the probe is felt under the skin, and a 2- to 3-cm longitudinal incision is made. The extensor tendons are retracted, and the tip of the probe can be grasped (Fig. 42–21). The two ends of the catgut are threaded through the eye of the probe, leaving

about 10 cm of the end of the catgut free off the eye. The probe is pulled down and out until the catgut emerges from the wound. The tibialis anterior tendon is then directed with an Allis clamp so that it will not buckle or twist while being pulled out from the distal wound. The fascia and retinaculum are closed with a continuous suture of size 0 plain catgut, followed by closure of the subcutaneous tissue and skin in the usual manner.

A bed is prepared for anchorage of the tibialis anterior tendon in exactly the same manner as described for the insertion of the peroneal tendon. A bed or trap door is made over the proximal part of the fourth metatarsal and part of the cuboid. The remainder of the anchorage procedure is the same as that for the peroneal tendon (Fig. 42–22). The tendon must have the same tension at the ankle as that noted for the peroneal transfer, with the foot at a right angle. A plaster boot is applied as

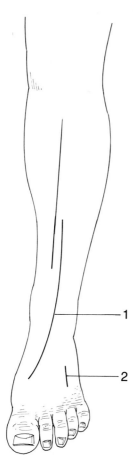

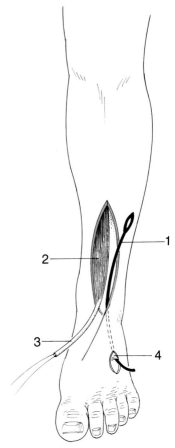

Figure 42–20. *Incisions for transfer of the tibialis anterior tendon to replace the lack of power in the peroneus longus. (1) Incision to free the tibialis anterior. (2) Anchorage incision on the lateral side of the dorsum of the foot.*

Figure 42–21. *Eyed probe (1) introduced through the extensor digitorum longus tendon sheath tunnel, emerging at 4, under the anterior transverse tarsal ligament. (2) Tibialis anterior muscle. (3) Threaded tendon.*

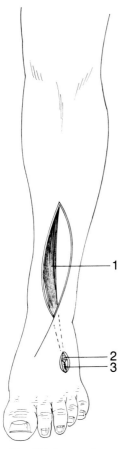

Figure 42–22. *The tibialis anterior tendon has been transferred and anchored. (1) Tibialis anterior. (2) Anterior transverse tarsal ligament. (3) T-shaped trap door closed and tendon anchored.*

most medialward, but further up (proximally), the tendon and then the muscle will be in front of and higher up laterally than the flexor digitorum longus. The flexor hallucis longus is retracted laterally, protecting and avoiding the posterior tibial vessels and nerve. The tendon, which is rather long, and part of the origin of the tibialis posterior are freed up to the proximal level of the skin incision. The tendon is sectioned at its insertion and threaded with No. 2 chromic catgut as described previously.

A small hole is opened in the interosseous membrane about 5 to 8 cm above the

after peroneal transfer and is removed after one month, when the stitches may be removed and rehabilitation started.

Tibialis Posterior Transfer

We use the Putti-Mayer technique for this tendon transfer. An incision is made from in front of and below the medial malleolus, following the back of the malleolus and then the front of the medial border of the Achilles tendon up to the junction of middle and lower thirds of the leg (Fig. 42–23). The tibialis posterior tendon is easily identified in the medial side of the foot, running medially and downward toward the medial malleolus. It is in direct contact with the malleolus and inserts into the tubercle of the navicular. In the posterior aspect of the ankle, it is the

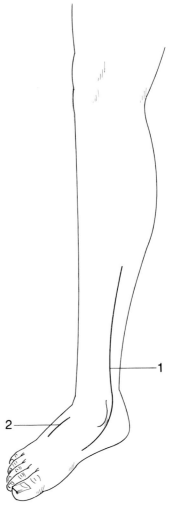

Figure 42–23. *Incisions for forward transfer of the tibialis posterior tendon. (1) Incision for exposure of the muscle and tendon. The tendon will be sectioned at the navicular level. (2) Anchorage incision.*

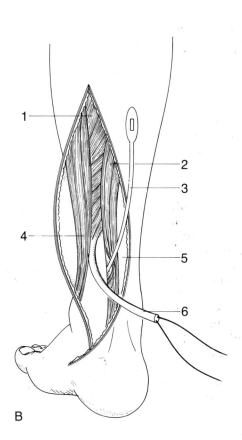

Figure 42–24. *(A) [1] Eyed probe introduced from behind forward through a very low slit in the interosseous membrane, emerging over the dorsum of the foot under the anterior transverse tarsal ligament. (B) Posterior view of the ankle and lower leg. [1] Tibialis posterior. [2] Flexor hallucis longus. [3] Eyed probe introduced through a slit in the lowest part of the interosseous membrane to emerge over the dorsum of the foot. [4] Flexor digitorum longus. [5] Achilles tendon. [6] Threaded tibialis posterior tendon. (C) Anterior view of the ankle and lower leg. [1] Interosseous membrane. [2] Slit in the membrane and emerging tendon of the tibialis posterior. [3] Anchorage incision and threaded tendon emerging under the anterior transverse tarsal ligament.*

A

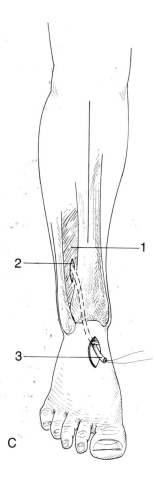

B

C

lower end. The hole, which is for the tendon and not for the muscle, is about 1 cm in diameter. The eyed probe is introduced through that hole, close to the tibia and following the tibialis anterior tendon, emerging distal to the ankle joint (Fig. 42–24A,B). The tip of the probe is felt under the skin, and a longitudinal incision of approximately 3 cm is made over the middle of the tarsus, following the third metatarsal line. The catgut is threaded into the eye of the probe and pulled out of the dorsum of the foot with the probe (Fig. 42–24C). The tendon, as usual, is guided to the hole in the interosseous membrane with an Allis clamp to avoid twisting or buckling. The wound for the exposure of the tendon and muscle is closed, the fascia and flexor retinaculum with size 0 plain catgut and the subcutaneous tissue and skin in the usual manner. The tendon is anchored in the same way as described previously for the peroneal tendon. Tension is also the same as noted earlier, as is the application of the plaster boot with foot at 90 degrees. The plaster and stitches are removed at the end of four weeks, and rehabilitation and full weight bearing are started. This transfer of the tibialis posterior tendon never works as well as the peroneal and tibialis anterior transfers, but it may at least serve as a tenodesis, preventing or correcting a drop foot.

Peroneal Transfer for Paralysis of the Triceps Surae

Transfer of the Peroneus Longus Tendon to the Achilles Tendon. If there is lack of power in the triceps surae and a subsequent calcaneus deformity, with or without cavus or cavovarus and with or without a good tibialis anterior, but with good or normal peronei, the procedure we follow is stabilization with correction of the calcaneus and, if cavus or cavovarus is present, midtarsal wedge resection to correct it. Two months after bone surgery, a lateral incision is made from the junction of the middle and distal thirds of the leg to the insertion of the Achilles tendon, and the peroneal muscles and Achilles tendon are exposed down to the insertion of the latter (Fig. 42–25). The peroneus longus is identified over the cuboid through a small incision, as described in the technique for

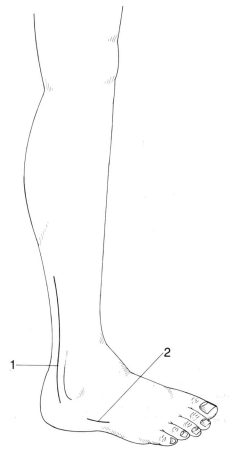

Figure 42–25. *Incision for (1) exposure and (2) section of the peroneus longus muscle and tendon, which will compensate for the lack of power in the triceps surae.*

peroneal transfers. The tendon of the peroneus longus is sectioned; the distal stump of the tendon is fixed to the tissues around the cuboid; and the small incision is closed. The Achilles tendon is then slit transversely with a sharp knife at its insertion on the os calcis, making a buttonhole 1 cm long (Fig. 42–26A). The peroneus longus tendon is pulled out of its paramalleolar tunnel and is threaded with No. 2 chromic catgut. A clamp is introduced lateromedially through the slit in the Achilles tendon and is used to grasp the catgut threaded in the peroneus longus tendon and to pull it out along with the tendon. Thus, the tendon emerges through the slit in the Achilles tendon. The peroneus longus tendon is pulled cephalically, while the foot is held in equinus. When the peroneus longus tendon is tight, the

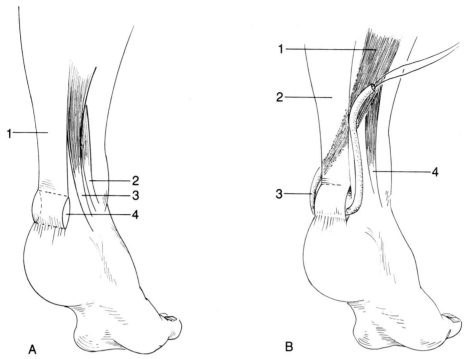

Figure 42–26. *(A) [1] Achilles tendon. [2] Peroneus brevis. [3] Peroneus longus. [4] Buttonhole or slit made on the Achilles tendon just above its insertion. (B) [1] Peroneus longus. The tendon of the peroneus longus is passed in front of the Achilles tendon [2] and from medially outward through the slit in the tendo Achillis [3] and is brought proximally to form a loop. The peroneus longus tendon will be anchored under tension to itself [4] and to the tendo Achillis with the foot in plantar flexion.*

recurrent part of it is fixed to the Achilles tendon from above downward, using the chromic catgut that is threaded to it (Fig. 42–26B). The sural fascia is closed with size 0 plain catgut, and the subcutaneous tissue and skin are closed in the usual manner. A plaster boot is applied with the foot in equinus and is worn for one month. At the end of one month, the plaster and stitches are removed, and rehabilitation and walking are started. If there is lack of power in the dorsiflexors of the foot (primarily the tibialis anterior), the next step in the procedure is the transfer of the peroneus brevis anteriorly to the dorsum of the foot, as described previously. This transfer can be performed only after the patient is able to achieve passive dorsiflexion of the foot to a right angle. If one of the peroneal muscles is weak, the strong one is used for the triceps surae, but if the tibialis posterior is good, that may be transferred forward, as described earlier, to balance the foot. If there is no power in the

tibialis posterior, a posterior bone block may be done to avoid drop foot.

For a good gait, transfer of either the peroneus longus or the peroneus brevis is sufficient for triceps surae function, provided the muscle power is normal. If both muscles are weak, both may be transferred. If there is associated lack of power in the dorsiflexors of the foot, however, one of the peroneal muscles must be left for anterior transfer.

Treatment of Claw Toes and Hammer Toes

For a description of the treatment of claw toes and hammer toes, the reader is referred to Chapter 23.

Correction of Knee Deformities Affecting the Foot

As stated previously, some deformities of the knee may secondarily affect the foot and give rise to a transitory or permanent deformity. Therefore, a brief description of the techniques used for the management of such conditions will be presented.

Hyperextension of the Knee (Genu Recurvatum, Back Knee)

To correct this condition, we perform a posterior capsulorrhaphy of the knee (our own unpublished technique). It is done by means of two lateral incisions long enough to expose the femoral shaft just above the femoral condyles and the lateral and medial aspects of the knee. A transverse drill hole is made in the femoral shaft just above the condyles, exposing a small surface of the bone by separation of the fibers of the vasti. By blunt dissection, all the soft tissues and structures are separated from the back of the capsule to avoid any perforation during subsequent maneuvers that could accidentally damage vessels or nerves. Bilateral slits of about 1 cm are made just behind the collateral ligaments and at the level of the joint space. A curved clamp is introduced from the medial to the lateral side through those slits, moving behind the cruciate ligaments and in front of the posterior capsule. The clamp is used to grasp the tip of an 18-gauge stainless steel wire, which is pulled out medially. This wire is passed under the tendon of the adductor magnus and then from inside outward through the transverse drill hole in the femoral shaft. The wire is cut, so that both ends can be twisted with either a surgical wire twister or a pair of pliers, as we use. The wire circle is made smaller and smaller, while the knee goes into flexion from folding of the overstretched posterior capsule. When the knee cannot go beyond 20 degrees of flexion, twisting of the wire is discontinued; the wire is then cut, and the twisted stump is buried into the soft tissues.

The capsule slits are closed with X stitches of No. 1 or 2 chromic catgut. The aponeurosis, subcutaneous tissue, and skin are closed in the usual manner. A posterior plaster of Paris splint is applied from below the gluteofemoral fold to the toes, with the knee in about 30 degrees of flexion. After 10 to 15 days, the stitches are removed. The splint is removed six weeks postoperatively.

Active and passive motion of the knee is started, and when full extension is possible, anterior transfer of the hamstrings should be performed to replace the power of the paralyzed quadriceps, which is the cause of the genu recurvatum.* Otherwise, the deformity will recur. During the transfer of the hamstrings, the wire used for the capsulorrhaphy is removed. In a growing child, if the wire is not removed in due time, the growing force of the femur will break the wire; however, there is no harm from the wire if it is broken and not removed (Fig. 42–27). If there are no hamstrings strong enough to be transferred, the patient should be fitted with a brace to prevent recurrence of the deformity.

We have never practiced any of the osteotomies recommended for hyperextension of the knee, as the deformity is the result of overstretching of the posterior capsule of the knee as the patient tries to stabilize the joint on walking because of lack of power in the quadriceps or in both the quadriceps and hamstrings.

Flexion Contracture of the Knee

This deformity may be the result of (1) powerful hamstrings with lack of power in the quadriceps and no measures taken to prevent the contracture or (2) lack of power in both the quadriceps and hamstrings or lack of power in the former with good hamstrings, with the patient sitting most of the time with the involved knee flexed, neglecting to prevent the flexion contracture deformity. If there are good or normal hamstrings, they should be transferred as soon as the flexion contracture is corrected. If a flail knee is present, a brace should be provided to prevent recurrence.

We use a conservative method to correct flexion contracture of the knee. A cotton stocking or stockinette is applied to permit sliding of the skin under the plaster. The heel and thigh below the gluteofemoral fold are protected by heavy piano felt, which may be split in a purse-like manner

---

*Editor's Note: A second type of back knee may occur secondary to weak calf and hamstring muscles. This may be accentuated by fusing the ipsilateral ankle in equinus, which increases the backward thrust of the knee.

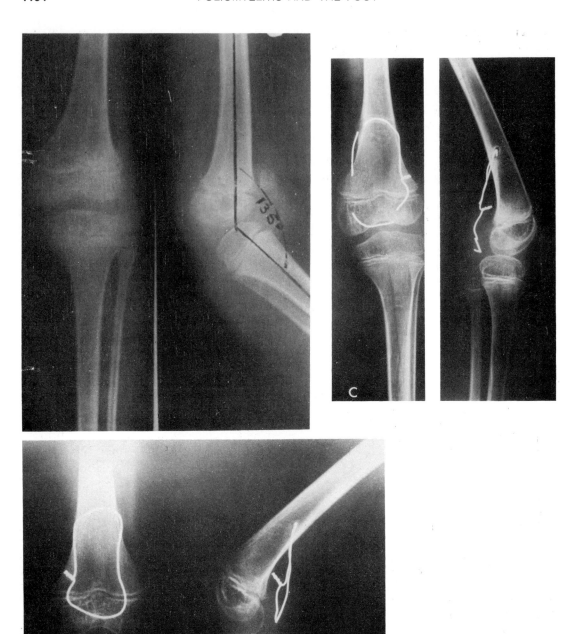

Figure 42–27. *(A) Genu recurvatum of 135 degrees from lack of power in the quadriceps with normal hamstrings. (B) Genu recurvatum corrected. Wire complete. (C) Wire broken by growth. Deformity corrected.*

and filled with cotton. The padding for the heel is molded into a cup shape to accommodate the heel. A similar piece of cupped padding is made to protect the anterior aspect of the knee from pressure. The knee padding is covered with paper to prevent the plaster from adhering to the padding. A long leg plaster cast is then applied from below the groin to the tips of the toes. While the plaster is setting, the maximum "comfortable" correction is initiated by manual pressure over the knee and counterpressure on the heel. On the next day, when the plaster is dry, a pair of hinges are incorporated into the sides of the cast at the knee joint, and a walking iron is incorporated into the foot of the cast. One week later, the plaster is cut transversely on the back of the knee and a wedge is removed from the front of the cast at the knee joint, so that two separate sections are formed, joined by the hinges. With the patient positioned face down on a table, the knee is extended a few more degrees, and a wooden block is inserted into the opening of the plaster slit on the back of the knee and held in place with adhesive tape. Every week or two, the knee is extended a few more degrees, and the wooden block in the back of the cast is changed for a larger one. This procedure requires patience, and the patient must not feel continuous discomfort after every session of stretching. Otherwise, a sore may develop over the heel or patella. Full extension can be obtained with this method from flexion contractures of more than 90 degrees.

Surgical extension has been advocated (i.e., section of the flexors of the knee and capsulotomy), but a sudden surgical extension is dangerous to vessels and nerves. In a few cases, mainly with pronounced flexion contracture of the hip, the extension of both joints can be obtained by skeletal traction above the ankle joint, adding weight to the traction every four or five days until the correction is obtained. We have added up to 20 to 30 kg.

Transfer of the Hamstrings

As stated previously, after correction of a flexion deformity of the knee, one of two conditions could be present: (1) A flail knee (no power in the hamstrings and quadriceps). In this situation, we provide the patient with a long leg brace to prevent recurrence of the deformity. The brace must have a knee lock and a knee cap, so that the patient will be able to sit down and the cap in front of the patella will keep the knee straight. (2) If there is no power in the quadriceps, but good or normal hamstrings, soon after the corrective plaster has been removed and before the knee starts going back into flexion, we perform a hamstrings transfer to replace the quadriceps power. The technique is essentially that of Mayer.

General Rules for Transfer of the Hamstrings. The lateral muscle to be transferred will always be the biceps femoris. On the medial side, the first choice is the sartorius, but sometimes the sartorius is not strong enough and the gracilis, semitendinosus, or semimembranosus may have to be utilized instead. The best muscle should always be used. If the biceps is usable but none of the medial hamstrings are in good condition, use any of them, for if only one acting muscle is transferred (e.g., the biceps), a lateral dislocation of the patella will occur from the pull of the transferred muscle. Therefore, it is imperative to use two muscles, one from each side. No matter how weak the muscle of the opposite side is, it should be transferred so that it will act mechanically to prevent the patella from being dislocated by the pull of the strong side. The medial hamstrings are usually found to be weak or to lack power more often than the biceps.

Always anchor the muscles to be transferred to the patella. When there has been flexion contracture of the knee, even after it has been corrected, it may be found that the hamstrings to be transferred — most often the biceps — do not reach the patella. They will have to be anchored to the quadriceps tendon as close to the patella as possible. The hamstrings to be transferred must be freed as high as possible, so that they will run down in an almost straight line, without any angulation. The transfer must be made under the femoral fascia, over the paralyzed quadriceps, and the undermining must be done well, so that the transferred muscle is not strangled between the fascia and the quadriceps. After correction of the flexion contracture, the Maissiat band is very tense and may have to be split transversely, so that the

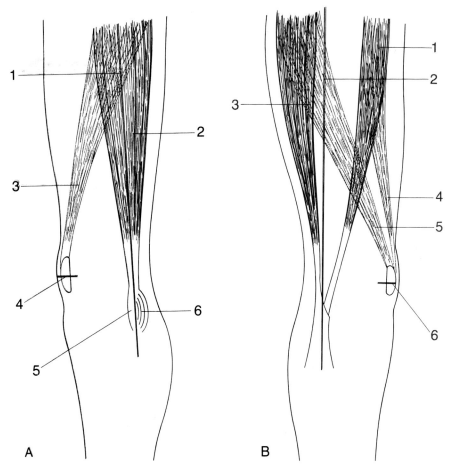

Figure 42-28. *(A) Biceps transfer to replace the lack of power in the quadriceps. [1] Lateral incision for the biceps transfer. [2] Crural biceps muscle. [3] New site of transferred biceps anchored in the patella. [4] Transverse incision over the patella for anchorage of the hamstring. [5] Fibular head. [6] Lateral popliteal (common peroneal) nerve. (B) Medial aspect of the thigh and knee showing the transfer of the medial hamstrings. [1] Sartorius. [2] Line of incision. [3] The medial hamstrings. [4] New position of sartorius, if transferred. [5] New position of any of the medial hamstrings, if transferred. There is no angulation of the transferred muscles. [6] Transverse incision over the patella for anchorage of the hamstrings.*

Illustration continued on opposite page

biceps is not constricted between the fascia and the quadriceps.

Technique. A tourniquet is placed at the base of the thigh. A longitudinal incision is made on the lateral side of the thigh from just distal to the tourniquet to the fibular head and over the biceps, which is easily felt (Fig. 42–28). The skin is protected in the routine manner. The femoral fascia is incised along the skin incision, and the biceps is exposed. The tendon is freed from front to back on its medial

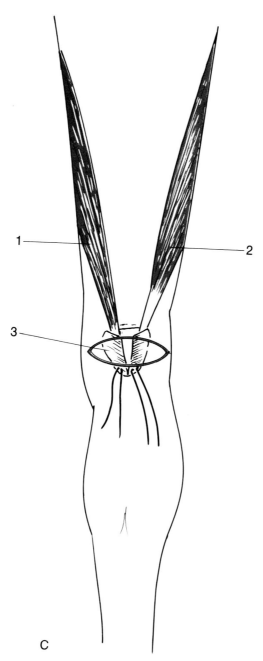

Figure 42–28. *Continued. (C) Anterior view of the thigh and knee showing the transferred hamstrings. There is no angulation of muscles or tendons. [1] Sartorius. [2] Biceps. [3] Patella and T-shaped trap door.*

Illustration continued on following page

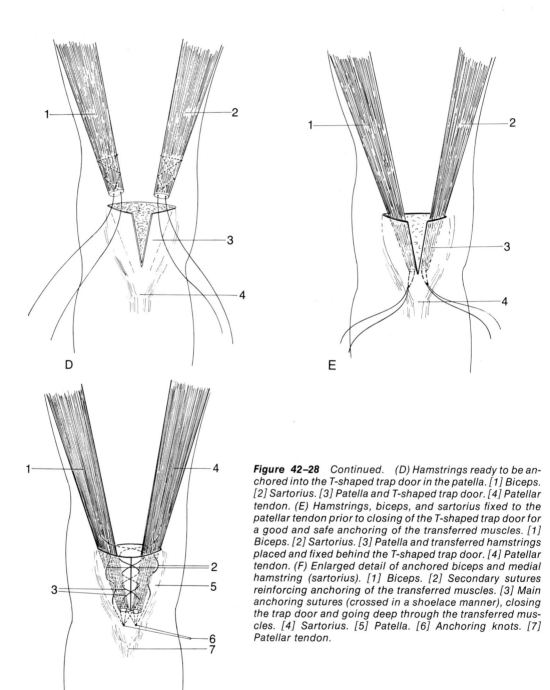

Figure 42-28 *Continued. (D) Hamstrings ready to be anchored into the T-shaped trap door in the patella. [1] Biceps. [2] Sartorius. [3] Patella and T-shaped trap door. [4] Patellar tendon. (E) Hamstrings, biceps, and sartorius fixed to the patellar tendon prior to closing of the T-shaped trap door for a good and safe anchoring of the transferred muscles. [1] Biceps. [2] Sartorius. [3] Patella and transferred hamstrings placed and fixed behind the T-shaped trap door. [4] Patellar tendon. (F) Enlarged detail of anchored biceps and medial hamstring (sartorius). [1] Biceps. [2] Secondary sutures reinforcing anchoring of the transferred muscles. [3] Main anchoring sutures (crossed in a shoelace manner), closing the trap door and going deep through the transferred muscles. [4] Sartorius. [5] Patella. [6] Anchoring knots. [7] Patellar tendon.*

aspect, leaving the lateral popliteal nerve under the soft tissues. A hemostatic clamp is introduced anteroposteriorly and close to the inner surface of the tendon, and the tip is made to emerge on the posterior border of the tendon. With a pair of scissors, the back of the muscle is then freed as high as possible from the femoral fascia. The same is done on the anterior border of the muscle. The tendon is freed distally with care down to its fibular insertion. This is a dangerous step, for two structures must be identified and avoided. The first is the lateral peroneal nerve, which passes medial to the tendon and then in back of it, to surround the fibular head. If care is not taken, this nerve may be injured. The second structure is the lateral collateral ligament of the knee, which is a narrow, very white band that blends with the biceps tendon on inserting into the fibular head. Dissection should be used to separate these two structures.

Once the biceps tendon has been isolated, it is detached from its fibular insertion with a knife. Chromic catgut No. 2 is used to thread the tendon, which is grasped with a wide Allis clamp. With the fingers or a periosteal elevator, the short head is detached as high as possible from its origin on the linea aspera femoris. A transverse incision of the skin is made over the patella. This incision is made somewhat longer than the width of the patella to avoid undue skin retraction. The incision is made all the way down to expose the suprapatellar expansion of the quadriceps tendon. The crural fascia is undermined from the quadriceps on the dorsal and lateral aspects of the lower thigh, using first a curved clamp and then a pair of curved scissors. When the tip of the clamp or scissors emerges on the medial side of the posterior edge of the Maissiat band, the scissors or clamp is opened to separate the femoral fascia from the underlying quadriceps. The scissors are used to separate that border of the iliofemoral band from the lateral intermuscular septum, all the way up and down, so that the transferred biceps tendon will not be constricted under the fascia. If the iliofemoral fascia is too tight, a transverse incision, as extensive as is necessary, is made on it to eradicate the tightness. The fingers may be used to undermine the fascia. A curved

clamp is introduced through the incision over the patella, deep to the undermined fascia, and is made to emerge on the posterior border of the Maissiat band. The catgut threaded in the biceps tendon is grasped with this clamp and is pulled out of the patellar incision. Care must be taken to avoid twisting the muscle or the tendon. The crural fascia is closed by a continuous suture with No. 1 chromic catgut. The subcutaneous tissue and skin are closed in the usual manner.

A similar longitudinal incision is made on the medial side of the thigh, down to the proximal part of the medial tibial condyle (Fig. 42–28B). The first muscle to identify is the sartorius; if it is in good condition, the crural fascia is slit, and the muscle is uncovered from the proximal end of the incision to the tibial condyle. The muscle is isolated from the saphenous nerve (a branch of the femoral nerve), which runs attached to the deep surface of the muscle before becoming superficial, and from the areolar tissue. When the muscle has been denuded down to its slender tendon, the tendon is cut and threaded in the usual manner with No. 2 chromic catgut and is freed with the fingers and/or scissors as high as possible. The medial crural fascia is undermined and handled just as for the biceps femoris, and the muscle is passed between the fascia and the paralyzed quadriceps to emerge out of the patellar incision. The fascia, subcutaneous tissue, and skin are closed. If the sartorius is not suitable for transfer, the best hamstring should be transferred.

The final step is anchoring of the tendons to the patella. First, a T-shaped trap door is made on the dorsum of the patella. The horizontal part of the T corresponds to the base of the patella, cutting the most superficial layer of the quadriceps tendon as it reaches the patella. In children, in whom the patella is still soft, a knife may be used to lift the trap door, but in older children or adults, an osteotome may have to be used. Then, as far distally as possible, the lateral threads are passed from the inside out of the trap door, using a heavy needle. The tendon of the biceps is usually the first to be anchored. The tendon is pulled distally after the ends of the catgut have been made to emerge. The tendon is introduced under the lateral side of the trap door with an Allis clamp, and the catgut is tied. The medial tendon is then anchored on the medial side of the trap door in a similar manner (Fig. 42–28C). Using a noncutting needle, the trap door is closed with the ends of the catgut. During closure of the trap door, the catgut is passed through the tendons to provide good anchorage. The suturing and closure of the trap door are performed distally to proximally (Fig. 42–28D). The prepatellar bursa and fascia are closed with size 0 plain catgut. The skin is closed in the usual manner. When the tendons to be transferred cannot reach the patella, they should be anchored to the quadriceps tendon, as close as possible to the patella. For that purpose, a 2- to 3-cm longitudinal slit is made on each side, and the tendons are buried and anchored under the cover of the quadriceps tendon fibers. A posterior plaster of Paris splint applied from the gluteofemoral fold to the tips of the toes keeps the knee in extension for six weeks, at which time it is removed. The stitches are removed at the end of two weeks. After the plaster splint has been removed, flexion and extension motion, rehabilitation, and walking are started. When 90-degree

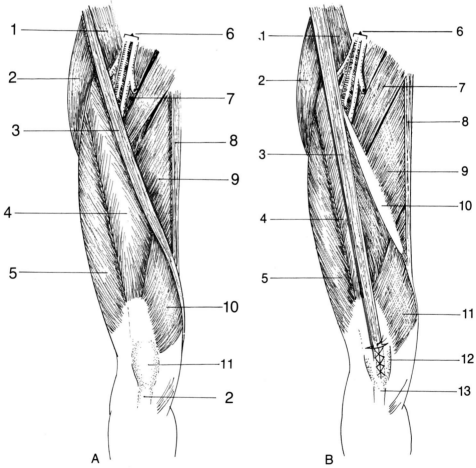

Figure 42–29. (A) Muscles of the front of the thigh. [1] Iliopsoas. [2] Tensor fasciae latae. [3] Sartorius. [4] Rectus femoris. [5] Vastus lateralis. [6] Femoral vessels and nerve. [7] Adductor longus. [8] Gracilis. [9] Adductor magnus. [10] Vastus medialis. [11] Patella. [12] Patellar tendon. (B) Sartorius has been transferred laterally to replace the lack of power in the biceps femoris. [1] Iliopsoas. [2] Tensor fasciae latae. [3] Sartorius transferred laterally and anchored to the middle of the patella. [4] Rectus femoris. [5] Vastus lateralis. [6] Femoral vessels and nerve. [7] Adductor longus. [8] Gracilis. [9] Adductor magnus. [10] Hunter's canal. [11] Vastus medialis. [12] Patella. [13] Patellar tendon.

Illustration continued on opposite page

flexion of the knee is obtained, any subsequent surgery of the foot may be performed.

Although in most instances the medial hamstrings may be the poor muscles and the biceps may be in good or fair condition, the reverse may occur.

If the biceps is very weak or has no power, it can be replaced by laterally transferring the sartorius, which originates on the anterosuperior iliac spine. Care should be taken to avoid damage to its nerve supply, which is rather proximal (Fig. 42–29). If the sartorius is used alone, the anchorage in the patella should be done exactly in the middle of it. Thus, an unbalanced pull of the muscle that could result in a medial or lateral subluxation of the patella will be avoided.

Genu Valgum and Genu Varum

Genu valgum and genu varum deformities are corrected by deangulation osteotomies. The fibula should be osteotomized first through a 2- to 3-cm incision, usually at or below the junction of the proximal and middle thirds of the leg. The osteotomy of the fibula should be oblique. The fascia and skin are closed. An incision is made extending down medial to the tibial tubercle and following the anterior tibial border and long enough for the tibial osteotomy. The tibia is freed of muscular origins all around the proximal part of the shaft and the distal surface of the tibial condyles. The osteotomy may be performed just above or just below the insertion of the patellar tendon. The osteotomy that we prefer is arch-shaped, with the convexity positioned proximally.

The osteotomy is outlined with multiple anteroposterior drill holes, passing through both cortices of the tibia, and is carefully completed with a thin osteotome or a wide, curved gouge, avoiding fracture of the tibia. Once the osteotomy is performed, the deformity (simple valgus or varus) is corrected. We use different methods to hold the osteotomy, depending on the age of the patient. In rather young children, after correction of the deformity and avoidance of a hyperextension or flexion deformity, the correction can be maintained with a plaster cast applied from below the groin to the tips of the toes, with the knee in semiflexion. In adults, special staples may have to be used; we use an inverted Neufeld nail, which holds the proximal fragment and is introduced from the anterolateral aspect of the lateral tibial condyle to the posteromedial aspect of the medial tibial condyle. The plate of the nail has to be shaped to the proximal end of the tibia. The nail is bent at the angle formed by the nail and the plate to a right angle or less, depending on the shape to be given to the plate. The plate is fixed on the lateral aspect of the tibia with the corresponding screws. Suturing is done in layers, leaving suction or a drain to avoid

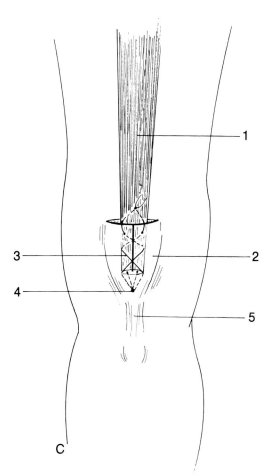

Figure 42–29 *Continued. (C) Detail of anchoring of the sartorius to the middle of the patella. [1] Sartorius. [2] Patella. [3] Anchoring suture crossed in a shoelace manner, closing the trap door and going deep to the sartorius. Transfer should be made at the middle axis of the patella to avoid any late secondary lateral subluxation of that bone. [4] Anchoring knot. [5] Patellar tendon.*

hematoma after release of the tourniquet. No plaster immobilization is required, and motion of the knee is initiated early.

If a derotation osteotomy is to be performed (which is usually associated with genu valgum), the same steps are followed, except that the osteotomy is transverse to allow derotation of the distal fragment of the tibia and correction of the angulation at the same time. Sometimes a gap is left at the site of the osteotomy, opening toward the side of the concavity of the valgus or varus. In this instance, filling the gap with bone chips from the bone bank or from the patient's iliac crest may be necessary. The fragments are held in place as mentioned previously.

Flexion Contracture of the Hip

If unilateral, flexion contracture of the hip is corrected through a small 2- to 3-cm incision extending down from the anterosuperior iliac spine. Through that approach, all contracted structures are sectioned down to the capsule, if necessary; these include the sartorius, tensor fascia lata, anterior crural fascia, rectus femoris, capsule and if necessary, the psoas-iliacus. These sections are done while an assistant holds the opposite lower extremity at full flexion at the knee and hip and another assistant tries to extend the contracted hip. When all the contractures have been released, the affected limb will rest on the operating table while the opposite one is held in full flexion at the knee and hip. Only the skin is sutured. Buck's extension is applied after surgery with 2 or 3 kg of weight. The opposite limb is placed over a stool, chair, or wooden box that is covered by a pillow, with the hip and knee in 90 degrees of flexion.

The patient is kept in traction for six weeks to avoid recurrence of the contracture. He may be allowed to be face down in bed, provided the traction is maintained and the opposite limb hangs out of the bed with the hip in 90 degrees of flexion and the knee flexed and resting over a pillow-covered stool or chair.

If the other hip also has a flexion contracture, it can be corrected in the same way, but not less than three months after the first one has been operated on.

If there are flexion contractures of the knee or other deformities, these must be corrected before correction of the flexion contracture of the hip. Whether it is associated with flexion contracture or not, abduction contracture of the hip may be corrected by extending the incision a few centimeters over the iliac crest to release the abductors (i.e., the tensor fascia lata and the gluteus medius and minimus) from their origins.

As noted previously, we have corrected flexion contracture of the hip and knee by skeletal traction applied to the tibia above the ankle. However, patient follow-up is mandatory to avoid recurrence.

Contracture of the Plantar Fascia

If the plantar fascia is contracted, we release it through a longitudinal incision about 1 cm over the middle of the dome of the plantar surface of the foot.

Other Surgical Alternatives

Other surgical techniques that may be used as possible alternatives to our routine procedures will now be presented. For triple arthrodesis, we have used the Dunn-Brittain technique,[8] but we feel that with this technique, excessive bone is removed and too much shortening of the foot may result. The technique of Siffert and associates[9] is similar to the one used by us, but it is made more complicated by the beak left at the head of the talus to hold it under the navicular and by plantar displacement of the foot.

Triple arthrodesis performed in a foot with a calcaneocavus deformity without pushing the foot forward, as described by us, leaves a long heel projecting backward, and the foot does not increase in length.

Astragalectomy was in vogue after it was described by Whitman[10] and later by Thompson,[22] but it became less popular with improved alternative surgical techniques.

The Lambrinudi-Hart operation for talipes equinus[11] is more complicated than triple arthrodesis combined with tarsal wedge resection, and the correction obtained is not as satisfactory.

The extra-articular subtalar arthrodesis of Grice[12] is a rather easy procedure (Fig.

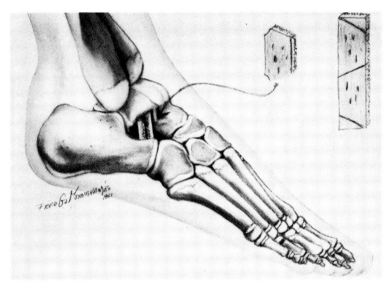

Figure 42–30. *Grice extra-articular subtalar arthrodesis of the foot. (From Grice, D. B.: J. Bone Joint Surg., 34A:927, 1952.)*

42–30). However, it does not prevent secondary forefoot deformities if tendon transfers are performed. This procedure is to be applied to children under 10 years of age, before tarsal bone maturity is reached. However, as stated previously, pes planovalgus, equinus, and other deformities can be prevented and controlled by proper shoes and braces, among which is the popular polypropylene drop-foot brace. The surgeon must not become impatient and perform surgery that may later require further procedures to correct deformities resulting from the premature surgery.

Osteotomies for Cavus Deformity

A cavus deformity may be geometrically conceptualized by measuring it as a triangle, which we will call the *cavus triangle* or the triangle of the arch of the foot. This triangle is placed in the sine of the cavus deformity, and its apex corresponds to the plantar point below the apex of the cavus,

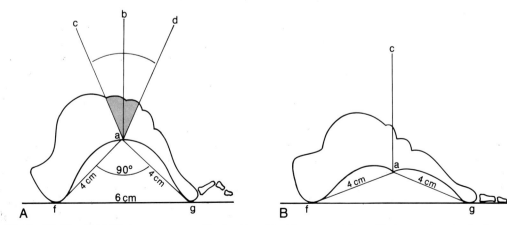

Figure 42–31. *(A) A 90-degree cavus with a foot length of 6 cm, requiring a 45-degree dorsal osteotomy on the apex of the cavus deformity. (B) After the 45-degree osteotomy at the apex of the cavus deformity, the foot length increased from 6 cm to 8 cm. The dorsal lump over the apex of the cavus has disappeared.*

which is normally located between the head of the os calcis and the tarsal navicular. The two sides of this cavus triangle correspond to the lines from the apex *a* to the point of the os calcis and head of first metatarsal where they touch the floor (lines *a-g* and *a-f*) (Fig. 42–31A). The base of the triangle (*f-g*) is the length of the foot from the heel to the head of the first metatarsal (the length of the longitudinal arch of the foot). The normal line to *f-g* passing through the apex *a* of the triangle is the *apex line (b-a)*. Lines *d-a* and *c-a* bisected by *b-a* form the *angle of osteotomy*, which is 45 degrees in this particular case, with a cavus of 90 degrees.

If there is a theoretical cavus that measures as an isosceles triangle with an apex angle of 90 degrees, sides (*a-f* and *a-g*) measuring 4 cm each, and a base (*f-g*) measuring 6 cm, there will be an osteotomy angle *c-a-d* of 45 degrees (Fig. 42–31A).

If an osteotomy is performed with a dorsal base, with its apex exactly at *a*, the apex of the deformity, and if this osteotomy measures 45 degrees (*c-a-d* angle), a bone wedge of 45 degrees will be removed, and on bringing the forefoot up in front of line *c-a*, closing the 45-degree gap of the osteotomy, line *c-a* will overlap with line *d-a*. The cavus deformity will be very nicely corrected, and the foot will have a more normal shape. The length of the arch will increase from 6 cm to 8 cm (Fig. 42–31B).

If the same cavus deformity of 90 degrees is present (Fig. 42–32A), but the same dorsal osteotomy of 45 degrees (in our example 1 cm forward to point *a* over line *a-g*) is performed, it will fall over the base of the metatarsals or over the cuneiforms. On closing the gap of the osteotomy by bringing up the forefoot until lines *j-e* and *k-e* overlap, the foot will acquire an odd shape and will increase only 1.5 cm in length (from 6 cm to 7.5 cm). Line *a-g* will be broken into two lines, *a-e* and *e-g*, forming an obtuse angle whose apex points toward the floor. That is why the foot (Fig. 42–32B) acquires an odd shape and less length when tarsal osteotomies are done beyond the apex angle of osteotomy (*c-a-d* in Figure 42–31A).

Figure 42–33A shows a cavus deformity of 85 degrees with a foot length of 11 cm

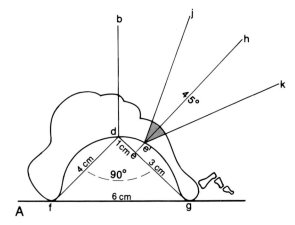

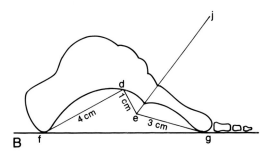

Figure 42–32. *(A) Same cavus deformity as in Figure 42–31. A 45-degree osteotomy is to be performed in front of the apex of the cavus. (B) After the osteotomy, the lump on the apex of the cavus remains, giving the foot an odd shape. Foot length increased to only 7.5 cm.*

and claw toes. Wedge osteotomy at the apex of the cavus deformity resulted in a normal foot shape (105-degree arch angle), anatomic correction of the claw-toe deformity, and lengthening of the arch from 11 cm to 14 cm.

Cole's anterior tarsal wedge[21] with a dorsally based osteotomy is done in front of the apex of the arch of the cavus. The bone cuts are made, the posterior one through the navicular and the cuboid and the anterior one as far as the base of the metatarsals, if necessary, depending on the severity of the deformity.

The apex of the cavus curvature should always be at Chopart's articulation, well behind Cole's site of osteotomy. That is why Cole's osteotomy leaves a lump behind the osteotomy site. However, just as in the osteotomy performed at the apex of the cavus curvature (namely at the head of talus and navicular and cuboid), Cole's osteotomy does not shorten the foot but

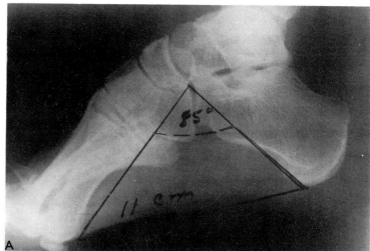

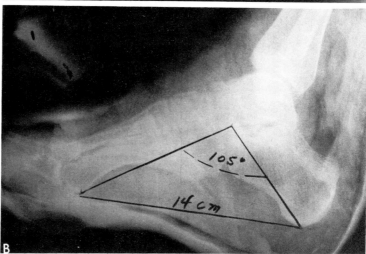

Figure 42–33. (A) An 85-degree cavus deformity. Foot length is 11 cm. (B) After wedge osteotomy at the apex of the cavus, the arch of the foot measured 105 degrees and the length of the foot was 14 cm.

makes it longer (Fig. 42–32B) — but not as long as the osteotomy we use.

Japas' osteotomy[13] is a more complicated procedure. It is an osteotomy performed in front of the apex of the cavus curvature. It must be stressed that the purpose of distal tarsal wedges, such as those of Cole and Japas, is to preserve subtalar function, especially in patients with nonparalytic "idiopathic" cavus. Such feet are stable and require no hindfoot wedges.

McElvenny and Caldwell's technique for correction of cavus deformity consists of a first metatarsal-medial cuneiform arthrodesis or, in more severe cases, inclusion of the navicular in the arthrodesis.[14] It may be applied to a very select group of cases in which no tendon transfer will be performed or in cavus deformity involving

only the first metatarsal segment (if the whole tarsus and metatarsus are involved, the cavus deformity must be flexible). Fixed cavus deformity involves the tarsal and metatarsal segments.

Most dorsal bunions due to elevation of the first metatarsal are the result of lack of fixation of the proximal stump of the distal part of the peroneus longus sectioned over the cuneiform for transfer, since the peroneus longus is a plantar flexor of the first metatarsal. This suture acts as a tenodesis. If the peroneus longus is transferred in the presence of a relatively strong tibialis anterior, which is its antagonist, the first ray will elevate, causing formation of a dorsal bunion. Another cause of dorsal bunion formation is the use of the extensor hallucis longus to replace the tibialis anterior.

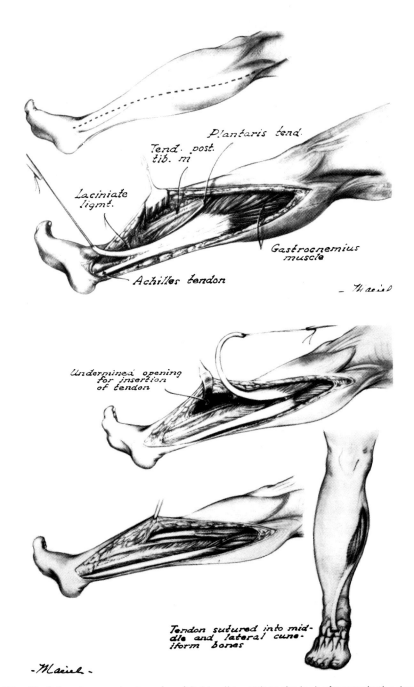

Figure 42–34. *Medial gastrocnemius transfer of Caldwell to replace the lack of power in the dorsiflexors of the foot. (From Caldwell, G. D.: Clin. Orthop., 11:81, 1958.)*

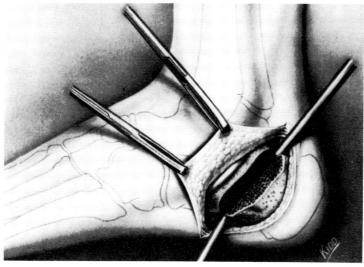

Figure 42–35. *Dwyer's osteotomy of the calcaneus. (From Dwyer, F. C.: Osteotomy of the calcaneum for pes cavus. J. Bone Joint Surg., 41B:80, 1959.)*

This replacement usually has disappointing results. Two main techniques have been advocated, that of Lapidus[15] and that described by Hammond.[16] We think that the latter technique, which consists of a dorsal opening wedge fusion of the first metatarsal-medial cuneiform joint, is easier.

Arthrodesis of the ankle has been advocated as a solution for flail foot. There are several techniques, such as those of Steindler,[17] Liebolt,[18] Barr and Record,[19] the classic anterior fusion with a sliding graft from the tibia, the compression technique of Charnley,[20] the distraction compression bone graft of Chuinard and Peterson,[24] the transfibular fusion of Horwitz[25] and Adams,[26] posterior arthrodesis, such as that of Campbell,[3] posterior intra-articular arthrodesis, and other variants of the technique, such as of White.[27]

Medial gastrocnemius transfer, as described by Caldwell,[28] to supply extensors of the foot when no peronei are available seems to be a rational procedure (Fig. 42–34), but we have no experience with this method. Dwyer's technique of osteotomy by removing a wedge from the os calcis[29] is a rather simple procedure to correct varus deformities of the heel and may be used to correct valgus deformity by inserting a wedge graft at the osteotomy gap (Fig. 42–35).

REFERENCES

1. Huchstep, R. L.: Poliomyelitis. *In* Woodruff, A. H. (ed.): Medicine in the Tropics. Edinburgh, Churchill Livingstone, 1975.
2. Tachdjian, M. O.: Pediatric Orthopedics. Philadelphia, W. B. Saunders Company, 1972, Vol 2, pp. 944–1010.
3. Crenshaw, A. H. (ed.): Campbell's Operative Orthopaedics, 5th ed. St. Louis, C. V. Mosby Co., 1971, Vol. 2, pp. 1517–1581.
4. Giannestras, N. J.: Foot Disorders: Medical and Surgical Management, 2nd ed. Philadelphia, Lea and Febiger, 1973, pp. 302–330.
5. Kendall, H. O., Kendall, F. P., and Wadsworth, G.: Muscles: Testing and Function, 2nd ed. Baltimore, Williams and Wilkins, 1971, pp. 146–173.
6. Daniels, L., and Worthingham, C.: Muscle Testing, 3rd ed. Philadelphia, W. B. Saunders Company, 1972, pp. 60–75.
7. Mayer, L.: Tendons, ganglia, muscles, fascia. *In* Lewis' Practice of Surgery. Hagerstown, Maryland, W. F. Prior Co., 1942, Vol. 3, Chapter 5.
8. Dunn, N.: Suggestions based on ten years experience of arthrodesis of the tarsus in the treatment of deformities of the foot. *In* The Robert Jones Birthday Volume. London, Oxford University Press, 1928, pp. 395–407.
9. Siffert, R. S., Forster, R. I., and Nachamie, B.: Beak triple arthrodesis for correction of severe cavus deformity. Clin. Orthop. *45*:101, 1966.
10. Whitman, R.: The operative treatment of paralytic talipes of the calcaneus type. Am. J. Med. Sci., *122*:593, 1901.
11. Lambrinudi, C.: New operation on drop foot. Br. J. Surg., *15*:193, 1927.
12. Grice, D. B.: An extra-articular arthrodesis of the sub-

astragalar joint for correction of paralytic flat feet in children. J. Bone Joint Surg., *34A*:927, 955, 1952.

13. Japas, L. M.: Surgical treatment of pes cavus by tarsal V-osteotomy. Preliminary report. J. Bone Joint Surg., *50A*:927, 1968.

14. McElvenny, R. T., and Caldwell, G. D.: A new operation for correction of cavus foot; fusion of the first metatarso-cuneiform-navicular joints. Clin. Orthop., *11*:85, 1958.

15. Lapidus, P. W.: Dorsal bunion: its mechanics and operative correction. J. Bone Joint Surg., *22*:627, 1940.

16. Hammond, G.: Elevation of the first metatarsal bone with hallux equinus. Surgery, *13*:240, 1943.

17. Steindler, A.: The treatment of flail ankle: panastragaloid arthrodesis. J. Bone Joint Surg., *5*:284, 1923.

18. Liebolt, F. L.: Pantalar arthrodesis in poliomyelitis. Surgery, *6*:31, 1939.

19. Barr, J. S., and Record, E. E.: Arthrodesis of the ankle for correction of foot deformity. Surg. Clin. North Am., *27*:1281, 1947.

20. Charnley, J.: Compression arthrodesis of the ankle and shoulder. J. Bone Joint Surg., *33B*:180, 1951.

21. Cole, W. H.: The treatment of claw foot. J. Bone Joint Surg., *22*:895, 1940.

22. Thompson, T. C.: Astragalectomy and the treatment of calcaneovalgus. J. Bone Joint Surg., *21*:627, 1939.

23. Brittain, H. A.: Architectural Principles of Arthrodesis, 2nd ed. Edinburgh, E. and S. Livingstone, Ltd., 1952.

24. Chuinard, E. G., and Peterson, R. E.: Distraction-compression bone-graft arthrodesis of the ankle. A method specially applicable in children. J. Bone Joint Surg., *45A*:481, 1963.

25. Horwitz, T.: The use of the transfibular approach in arthrodesis of the ankle joint. Am. J. Surg., *55*:550, 1942.

26. Adams, J. C.: Arthrodesis of the ankle joint. Experiences with the transfibular approach. J. Bone Joint Surg., *30B*:506, 1948.

27. White, A. A., III: Yet another ankle fusion. Exhibit at A.A.O.S. Meeting, Las Vegas, Nevada, 1973.

28. Caldwell, G. D.: Correction of paralytic foot drop by hemigastrosoleus transplant. Clin. Orthop., *11*:81, 1958.

29. Dwyer, F. C.: Osteotomy of the calcaneum for pes cavus. J. Bone Joint Surg., *41B*:80, 1959.

CHAPTER 43

PERIPHERAL NEUROPATHIES AFFECTING THE FOOT: TRAUMATIC, ISCHEMIC, AND COMPRESSIVE DISORDERS*

Ralph Lusskin, M.D.

Compartment Syndromes

Thomas E. Whitesides, Jr., M.D.

Disorders of peripheral nerves affect the foot in several ways, producing paresis or paralysis of intrinsic and extrinsic muscles, sensory defects, pain phenomena, and contractures. These, in turn, have the potential for inducing secondary changes in the foot, which increase disability and which may put the foot at risk from pressure ulcers, sepsis, and neuropathic arthropathy.

The effects of motor nerve disease on the foot were studied intensively when poliomyelitis was prevalent. The studies of Duchenne[7] laid the basis for understanding the results of specific motor deficits on both the adult's and the child's foot. Attention was directed toward the structural and functional results of pure motor neuron disease. Surgical therapy consisted

of joint resections and stabilization by arthrodesis and tendon transfers. Orthoses that could protect, stabilize, and motorize the paralyzed foot were developed and were used extensively. Prosthetic techniques have now been applied to these orthoses, resulting in even better fit and function.

In recent years, the more complex problems associated with mixed peripheral and central nerve trunk disorders have been given more attention, and many syndromes produced by chronic nerve compression and irritation have been identified. The late sequelae of peripheral neuropathies have proved to be a major challenge and are often the most disabling clinical manifestations of systemic diseases such as diabetes and alcoholism.

With improved vascular surgical techniques and resultant limb salvage, the problem of the late sequelae of neural ischemia has become evident. Neurovascular syndromes are associated with arteri-

*The clinical cases presented in this section and the neurologic procedures described were performed in conjunction with A. Battista, M.D., at New York University Medical Center, New York, New York.

al injury, Volkmann's contracture, and compartment syndromes. As the attention of neurologists, orthopaedists, and neurosurgeons has been directed toward the treatment of these disorders, technical advances have led to improved diagnosis and therapy. Electromyography and nerve conduction studies have permitted better identification of the type and level of nerve lesion and improved monitoring of recovery from disease or surgery. Magnification by loupe and operating microscope has permitted much more accurate surgery and has improved the results of nerve suture, grafting, and neurolysis. Newer orthotic techniques have been developed to allow a more normal life for those with irrevocable neural disorders or joints destroyed after sensory denervation and have resulted in reduced risk of sepsis and amputation.

This chapter will review the anatomy of the nerves of the foot and leg, present a system of examination as an aid to diagnosis and discuss the diseases of nerve that affect the foot and their treatment.

NERVE STRUCTURE

The structure of the peripheral nerve fiber, funiculus, and trunk (Fig. 43–1) is reviewed in detail by Sunderland.[55] Myelinated and unmyelinated fibers are surrounded, protected, and supported by Schwann cells. The additional shielding provided by myelinated fibers is interrupted at 0.1- to 1.8-mm intervals by the nodes of Ranvier. Conduction along unmyelinated fibers is by continuous depolarization. The myelinated fibers conduct by skip depolarization from node to node, i.e., *saltatory conduction,*[14] which explains the higher conduction rates in the large myelinated fibers. The complex organization of these two cell systems is vulnerable to trauma and has limited reordering capacity once distorted.

Nerve fibers and their Schwann cells are gathered into funiculi that are also contained by *endoneurial* connective tissue cells and collagen fibers. The endoneurium packs between the nerve fibers, gathers fibers into small bundles, and contains capillaries fed by arterioles and drained by venules in the perineurium. The nerve fibers within each funiculus take an undulating course, which creates a visual phenomenon — the *spiral bands of Fontana.* When the nerve is stretched, the nerve fibers straighten until their elastic limit is reached before rupturing.

The funiculi are surrounded and bound by the *perineurium,* which is a rather dense fibrous structure ranging in thickness from 1.3 to 100 μ. The perineurium protects the nerve fibers and *maintains intrafunicular pressure. Breaking the perineurium* leads to *immediate herniation* of intrafunicular tissue. When axon fibers degenerate, the funiculus shrinks and the perineurium contracts.

The perineurium plays a major role in maintaining the integrity of the nerve trunk under tension,[58] and also acts both as a diffusion barrier and as a pathway for

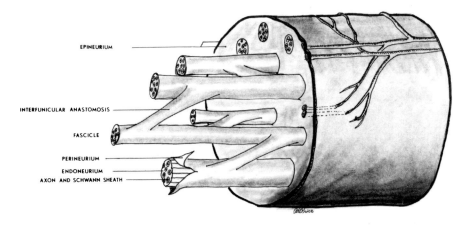

EPINEURIUM

INTERFUNICULAR ANASTOMOSIS

FASCICLE

PERINEURIUM
ENDONEURIUM
AXON AND SCHWANN SHEATH

NERVE TRUNK

Figure 43–1. *Diagram of the nerve trunk (mixed peripheral nerve) showing the important structural units.*

nutrition. It is an excellent barrier to infection. When it is penetrated, the conduction within a funiculus is seriously impaired, whereas removing the epineurium, as in neurolysis, is without harmful effects. Nerve roots lack perineurium and, as a result, the nerve fibers in the roots are more exposed than those in the peripheral nerves.

The funiculi with their perineurial sheaths constantly divide, branch, and anastomose within the nerve trunk. Small nerve bundles pass between the funiculi, forming a plexus along the course of a nerve. This makes accurate repair of nerve defects difficult and presents an obstacle to intraneural neurolysis, necessitating magnification for such procedures.

The localization within the nerve trunk of fibers innervating a particular region tends to become less defined centrally, whereas near the region of nerve branching, continuity of bundles may be rather good for a considerable distance within the nerve.

The funiculi and their perineurial sheaths are surrounded by a rather loose areolar tissue that is concentrated at the surface of the nerve. This investing sheath is the *epineurium*. The epineurium fixes the nerve either loosely or somewhat firmly to surrounding tissues and permits undulations in the nerve. It is thinnest (22 per cent of the nerve diameter) at certain points of fixation (i.e., the ulnar nerve at the medial epicondyle) and thickest at sites where nerves cross joints. The sciatic nerve epineurium is unusually thick and constitutes from 70 to 80 per cent of the nerve cross section.[56]

BLOOD SUPPLY OF NERVES

The nerves are supplied by arteriae nervorum, which have many arrangements. These vessels may approach nerves from different directions at different sites. There is probably no true mesoneurium.[35]

The intraneural blood supply consists of longitudinally directed macroscopic arterioles that are supplied at varying intervals by the arteriae nervorum. These arterioles anastomose with proximal and distal vessels. Occasionally, a dense vascular plexus may form on the surface of a nerve (e.g., ulnar nerve in the upper arm), but usually this does not occur. A network of arterioles, precapillaries, and capillaries leads from the surface vessels. The arterioles pursue an irregular course within the nerve, branching repeatedly to longitudinally arranged fine vessels. Four systems of vessels may be distinguished: surface, interfunicular, perineural, and intrafunicular. These vessels become progressively finer from without inward. Only capillaries are found within the nerve bundles. These vary in density from 36 to 64 per mm^2, averaging 50 capillaries per mm^2. The density is highest in the newborn and lowest in the elderly.[29]

Because of the anastomoses within the nerve trunk, the nerve can function despite interruption of one or several nerve arteries. Although the axon receives much of its metabolic drive from the distant cell body, it is still dependent on some local vascularity to maintain its function. Since intra-axonal flow velocities are probably 40 to 70 mm/day maximum,[34] local ischemia can have a major effect on axon function. There are limits to the effectiveness of the intraneural vascular system when multiple regional arteries have been divided. Physical deformation of a nerve, especially compression, can also obstruct its vascular supply.[45] This interference with the blood supply of nerves can result in failure of conduction without physical change or demonstrable damage, or may lead to severe destruction of nerve tissues, depending on the duration and intensity of the ischemia. There is a venous drainage system that parallels the arterial supply and is vulnerable to compression as well. Nerve edema follows differential blockage to venous outflow.

There appear to be two tissue spaces in the nerve, one *endoneurial* and confined by the funicular perineurium and the other *a lymphatic capillary network in the epineurium*. The endoneurial space has some connection with the subarachnoid space, and both central and distal flow may occur within this system.

NEUROANATOMY OF THE FOOT AND LEG

The long muscles that power the foot are innervated, for the most part, by the peroneal and posterior tibial nerves in the proximal third of the leg. The posterior tibial nerve enters the leg in the middle of the popliteal region, where it lies quite superficially just beneath the deep fascia. Injury or disease that produces denervation of the posterior tibial nerve is quite serious, as the resulting sensory deficit of the sole of the foot may lead to loss of the foot. Ulceration with sepsis followed by osteomyelitis is the common sequence.

Common Peroneal Nerve

The common peroneal nerve is a satellite of the biceps femoris tendon in the thigh and crosses the lateral aspect of the popliteal space. Before it passes beneath the deep peroneal fascia on the lateral aspect of the fibula, it lies unprotected against the back of the head of the fibula. At this point, the nerve is extremely vulnerable to pressure (Fig. 43–2). It may be damaged during surgical approaches to the lateral aspect of the knee, as it is tethered distally. Thus, any surgical approach in this region in which the common peroneal nerve is not identified places the nerve at risk.

In the popliteal region, before crossing the neck of the fibula, the peroneal nerve gives rise to the *lateral cutaneous nerve of the leg* and sends the *sural communicating nerve* to join the *sural branch of the posterior tibial nerve*. The *sural nerve* runs deep to the deep fascia of the calf to the lower third of the leg. It then becomes superficial and runs just behind the fibula and lateral malleolus to innervate the lateral aspect of the sole of the foot. When this nerve is removed cleanly for autografting and the patient has been told to expect the resultant sensory deficit, there is usually a minimal deficit and rarely any pain. When the nerve is traumatized or transected inadvertently by incision a bit too far posteriorly or below the fibula, the resultant anesthesia or hypesthesia seems profound, and any discomfort or pain is most annoying.

Saphenous Nerve

The saphenous nerve sends its terminal branch along the medial aspect of the calf behind the tibia. It ends anterior to the medial malleolus to innervate the anterior medial aspect of the foot and must there-

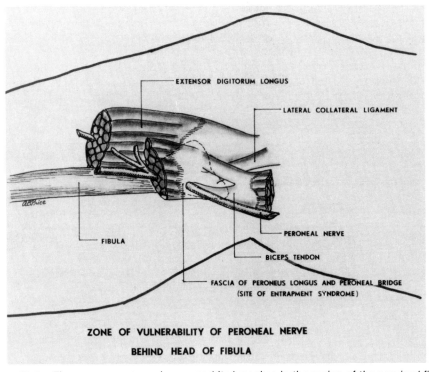

Figure 43–2. *The common peroneal nerve and its branches in the region of the proximal fibula.*

fore cross the distal medial face of the tibia 5.0 to 7.5 cm above the tip of the medial malleolus. The nerve should be avoided during approaches to the medial malleolus.

Posterior Tibial Nerve

The posterior tibial nerve in the lower third of the leg runs beneath the deep fascia behind the flexor digitorum longus tendon. It lies in a somewhat loose but definable sheath along with the posterior tibial artery and its two veins. The veins cross the nerve proximally and distally while the artery (which lies in front of the nerve) sends its lateral plantar branch across the nerve to accompany the *lateral plantar nerve* arising from the division of the posterior tibial nerve. Behind and below the medial malleolus the neurovascular bundle is covered by the flexor retinaculum. This dense band runs to the posterior calcaneal tubercle and contains the sheaths of tibialis posterior, flexor digitorum longus, and flexor hallucis longus. Beneath these structures lies the deltoid ligament.

Any extensive dissection of the medial or posterior ankle ligaments should be preceded by exposure and displacement of the neurovascular bundle.

The *medial calcaneal nerve* is a branch of the posterior tibial nerve. It pierces the flexor retinaculum along with a small artery and innervates the skin of the heel pad. This nerve runs directly under the posterior calcaneal tubercle and may be involved in the painful heel syndrome.

The posterior tibial nerve divides beneath the flexor retinaculum. Its branches, the medial and lateral plantar nerves, pass beneath the abductor hallucis, the most superficial muscle originating from the medial aspect of the calcaneus. Here the nerves may be entrapped by bands or anomalies of the abductor hallucis. Release of this muscle from its attachment to the navicular bone will expose the nerves in the foot.[19] The medial plantar nerve is analogous to the median nerve, and the lateral plantar nerve is analogous to the ulnar nerve. The medial plantar nerve innervates the 3½ medial digits, the lateral plantar nerve the 1½ lateral digits. In the foot both nerves lie beneath the plantar

fascia. The lateral nerve crosses the foot beneath the flexor digitorum brevis, giving off its superficial sensory branch before passing deep and medial on a skeletal plane to supply the small muscles of the lateral aspect of the foot, the interosseous muscles, and the adductor hallucis.

The medial plantar nerve innervates the four medial muscles: the abductor hallucis, flexor digitorum brevis, flexor hallucis brevis, and lumbricalis.

The terminal sensory branches of the medial and lateral plantar nerves penetrate the superficial fascia of the foot and pass to the toes on the plantar surface of the transverse metatarsal (deep transverse) ligament. In this region or just distal to it, the interdigital branches may become involved in an irritative or compressive/irritative lesion, e.g., an interdigital neuroma. It appears that structural abnormalities or gait patterns that increase stress to the lateral metatarsal regions contribute to this disorder.

Peroneal Nerve

The dorsum of the foot is innervated by the two branches of the peroneal nerve — superficial and deep (Fig. 43–3). It is their relationship to the deep fascia of the foot and ankle that gives them their names, for the superficial division penetrates the deep fascia of the leg at the junction of mid and lower thirds and lies just beneath the skin. At times it is visible in the foot. The deep branch runs with the anterior tibial artery and vein beneath the extensor retinaculum between the extensor hallucis longus and extensor digitorum longus. It sends its motor branch beneath extensor digitorum longus tendons to innervate the extensor brevis and then continues on a skeletal plane to the dorsum of the first web space — sending terminal branches to the opposing dorsal surfaces of the first and second toes.

The greater portion of the dorsum of the foot receives sensory innervation from the branches of the superficial peroneal nerve. These nerves are quite superficial and may be easily injured. Transverse incisions often create small, painful neuromas. Compression of the foot by tight bandages or casts can create a pattern of persistent dysesthesias and pain. Long-distance run-

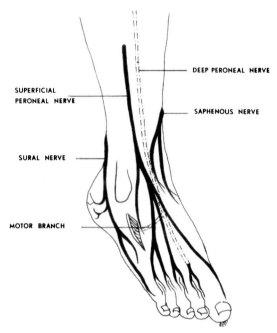

Figure 43–3. *The nerve supply to the dorsum of the foot — peroneal divisions, saphenous nerve, sural nerve. There is considerable variation in the arrangement of the superficial nerves. All are vulnerable to trauma.*

ners may develop a neuritis of a sensory branch of the superficial peroneal nerve. This is relieved by not lacing the eyelet in the running sneaker, which is causing the friction. The point at which the superficial peroneal nerve penetrates the deep fascia of the leg is occasionally a site of neuropathy. Tapping the region may produce distal paresthesias when this compressive neuropathy is present, and pressure on this point may reproduce the pain.

The terminal branch of the superficial peroneal nerve lies on the dorsomedial aspect of the first metatarsophalangeal joint and first toe. Incisions for bunion surgery pass over this nerve, which must be protected. At times the nerve lies on top of a first metatarsal head exostosis and is compresssed against the shoe.

PERIPHERAL NEUROPATHIES

Symptomatology

Peripheral nerve disorders may be roughly classified into interruptive and irritative lesions, with mixed patterns often

being present. The interruptive lesions lead to diminished function — sensory, motor, and sympathetic. When these lesions develop quickly, the patient will usually notice and report a change in function; however, when the lesion develops slowly, the patient may ignore or not appreciate the reduced sensation or motor power. Complaints may then focus on the late sequelae of a functional deficit, e.g., tripping, turning an ankle, or stubbing a toe. Corns, calluses, ulcerations, and deformities produced by dislocating joints or cryptic fractures may appear without warning. Infections from ignored foreign bodies, paronychia, or deep calluses may also develop. Normal adjustment of pressure on the forepart of the foot is controlled in part by differential action of the flexors of the toes.[9] Thus, when paralysis of the intrinsic musculature is present, the dynamics of pressure transfers change and interface overload produces calluses.

The irritative lesions that are seen in partial nerve damage will often produce early complaints. Pain is the most common cause for medical contact, but paresthesias and dysesthesias, such as burning sensations (if present), can cause the patient to seek help.

Since exact localization of symptoms is important in determining the source of the disease, each sympton should be characterized by its exact spatial and temporal parameters. Physical irritation of a single nerve produces pain in the distribution of that nerve with some regional spread, and the pain is most often increased by use of the part. Diffuse neuropathies, in contrast, involve multiple nerves or spinal segment regions, and symptoms are often accentuated by rest and relieved by activity.

One must be aware that spinal cord disease may first appear as localized weakness and atrophy. Posterior column or pyramidal tract disease should be considered whenever a peripheral pattern emerges, but these disorders are rarely accompanied by pain.

Neurologic Examination of the Foot

Successful diagnosis requires an inquiring mind and a trained eye. Whereas complaints of paralysis and anesthesia would make the need for a careful neurologic examination obvious, the necessity for such an examination in the presence of callosities or ulceration over a deformity may not be as apparent. A careful assessment of *sensory, motor,* and *sympathetic* neural function is most important whenever the foot is examined.

The neurologic examination is performed, in part, concomitantly with the orthopaedic examination. Evaluation of the dynamics of the foot implies a study of both form and function. The gait pattern is evaluated first. This is studied with the patient disrobed, a simple but often neglected dictum. Movements of the back, hip, knee, and ankle should be observed. The patient then is asked to heel walk and toe walk. Trendelenburg and Rhomberg tests should be performed.

The examination should reveal the presence of many disorders. Is there an antalgic gait and, if so, does the pain derive from a back, hip, knee, heel, or metatarsal disorder? Is there stiffness or contracture of any joint? Is there paralysis of calf or anterior tibial muscles? Spasticity is often missed in the initial evaluation. Is there ataxia or other signs of posterior column disease? Do the normal rotations of the subtalar joints take place during stance phase?

The foot and leg are then inspected for atrophy and deformity. The pattern of atrophy must be noted and documented. The stork leg of Charcot-Marie-Tooth disease, the anterior compartment atrophy of peroneal palsy, and the intrinsic foot atrophy of many peripheral neuropathies can all give an immediate clue to the type and localization of disease. When there is atrophy of the feet and legs, inspect the hands and arms. Look for abductor hallucis atrophy — an important clue to peripheral neuropathy. Next, study the foot for deformity. Is there a fixed or a functional deformity? A fixed deformity cannot be corrected by the examiner's hands, whereas a functional deformity can be. The range of motion and attitude of ankle, subtalar, and tarsometatarsal joints should be identified. The position of the toes and metatarsal heads should be studied during standing and walking and when non–weight-bearing. Foot contractures are first studied with the knees flexed; the knees should then be straightened to demon-

strate the effect of gastrocnemius tightening on the deformity.

Cavus, calcaneus, varus, valgus, and equinus deformities of the entire foot and of the forepart of the foot; claw toes; hammer toes; and rigidity and flexibility are assessed. Luxation of the metatarsophalangeal joints is often a late result of muscle imbalance caused by peripheral nerve disease. This luxation intensifies the down thrust on the metatarsal heads during the later part of stance phase and accentuates callosities under the metatarsal heads. When there is a sensory deficit, as in diabetic neuropathy or posterior tibial nerve injury, sepsis can develop beneath these calluses.

The skin should be checked for moisture. Peripheral nerve disease is often accompanied by sympathetic denervation with dry, thin skin resulting. This skin is more vulnerable to abrasion and sepsis.

The nerves of the foot and leg should be examined, using their exact anatomy as a guide. When nerve damage or disease is present, each nerve should be palpated and tapped gently over its course. The presence, intensity, and localization of the Tinel sign should be identified and recorded.

Documentation is important. Although descriptive reports are useful, a drawing or photograph may be valuable in recording data, especially when multiple system (skin, skeletal, joint, and nerve) data are to be preserved. A simple drawing outlining motor, sensory, and vascular deficits makes an important record of the extent of disease. Photography, using an instant camera such as the Polaroid SX-70, is most useful in recording deformity and disease. It is a valuable tool for the surgeon as a pre- and postoperative document and can quickly bring complex data to mind when a review of the case is undertaken.

When the nerves of the foot are examined, proximal nerve function should also be evaluated. Reflex, sensory, and motor testing of the entire leg, thigh, and gluteal region often reveals diffuse or proximal localization of disorders that manifest themselves as foot problems. The following nerves should be tested: superior and inferior gluteal, obturator, femoral, lateral femoral cutaneous, sensory branches of T12 and L1 crossing the pelvis, and sciatic (tibial and peroneal components). These should be evaluated for motor and sensory deficits as well as palpated for tenderness.

The sensory examination of the legs should include testing for position sense, deep pain, vibration, and temperature. Dorsal column diseases and other spinal cord disorders, such as extrinsic tumor or syrinx, may manifest themselves by protopathic and other long-tract sensory deficits.

Pain

Pain is produced by irritative neuropathy. A pain pattern can be most devastating and will often demand great patience and a multidisciplinary approach if control is to be achieved. In these instances, careful evaluation of the personality is often required. The exact circumstances of the injury and the inner meaning of the injury to the patient must be sought. The solution may involve combined regional surgery and judicious psychologic treatment. Cutaneous electrical stimulation, regional nerve blockade, and hypnotic techniques may be indicated, but psychologic factors must be evaluated.

A 23-year-old former Israeli soldier complained of severe burning pain following multiple surgical procedures for missile wounds of the right shoulder joint. Reconstruction had included a hemiprosthesis. Rest pain predominated but extreme hypersensitivity of the traumatic and surgical scars was present. Psychiatric evaluation revealed a profound sense of guilt over his survival when a peer group of seven friends had been killed in the same half-track. Local blockade with lidocaine and corticosteroids helped reduce his pain and hypersensitivity, and his coming to understand the deeper meaning of his continued symptoms permitted acceptance of residual hyperesthesia and pain, with rather quick subsidence of the neural hyperirritability. Many similar post-traumatic foot and leg disorders have such a double etiology and should be appropriately evaluated.

The sympathetic nervous system should be studied. Sympathetic denervation leads to absence of sweating, poor response to heat and cold, and perhaps to reduced resistance to physical stress. In irritative lesions of the sympathetic nerve fibers, a true causalgia may develop. This is a disorder of overactivity of the sympathetic nervous system characterized by burning pain and hot, dry skin. Sympathetic nerve blockade often improves symptoms.

Associated Manifestations of Peripheral Neuropathies

Deformities have been mentioned in the preceding section. Paralysis of the posterior tibial nerve will lead to various degrees of calf weakness, depending on the level of the lesion. The deformity produced involves the calcaneus with an excess range of dorsiflexion of the ankle. Some clawing of the toes (hyperextension of metatarsophalangeal joints and flexion of interphalangeal joints) may develop owing to intrinsic paralysis. When the deformity is flexible (functional), the lack of ground reaction forces, especially at push-off, may protect the foot skin from overload. When a contracture of the leg is present, as in combined vascular-neural lesions, this effect may be lost, and pressure ulcers may develop under the forepart of the foot.

Peroneal nerve paralysis leads to foot-drop and an equinus deformity. Overactivity of the partially innervated extensor digitorum or hallucis longus when the main weakness is anterior tibial (a frequently encountered situation) will produce rather severe clawing of the forepart of the foot. Sudden deformations of the foot may be produced by neuropathic arthropathies; often these deformities result from a painless fracture into a joint. At other times the deformity develops slowly, as tarsometatarsal or intertarsal joint destruction progresses.

Most bone changes following peripheral nerve disease can be ascribed to immobilization and disuse. Many of the so-called trophic factors in nerve injuries, i.e., contractures and ulceration, are associated with insensitivity and vascular compromise due either to direct vessel injury or disease or to tight bandaging and swelling. Radiographic changes are nonspecific, but give a clue as to the degree and type of injury.

Charcot (Neuropathic) Deformity

This disorder was originally described as a manifestation of involvement of the spinal cord. It is now understood to develop in the presence of any neuropathy that leads to a sensory deficit in a joint when mobility and function, especially gravitational loading, are preserved. Charcot deformity is seen in syringomyelia, spina bifida, diabetic neuropathy, and occasionally after peripheral traumatic neuropathy. It is also seen in the various congenital indifference-to-pain syndromes.

Neuropathic arthropathy or deformity presents, for the most part, as a more or less rapid deformation and swelling of the foot, ankle, and knee and as a displacement or disintegration of the hip or shoulder. The more central joints often are not involved in the absence of spinal cord disease.

The acute episodes of joint dislocation and fragmentation seem to be initiated by fractures that involve the metaphyses of the metatarsals and enter the metatarsocuboid joints, as well as fractures of the tarsal bones and of the articular ends of the tibia, femur, and other long bones. In addition, fractures of the shafts of metatarsals and long bones are seen.

If treated with prolonged immobilization and weight transfer orthoses, these fractures will heal and the deformed joints will stabilize, but if left unprotected, rather grotesque deformities will develop. Surgical stabilization procedures are followed by a rather high rate of sepsis and nonunion.

The pathogenesis of these lesions has not been clearly defined, as in many instances the disorder develops quickly without evidence of trauma or unusual stress.

DISORDERS OF THE NERVES

Table 43–1 classifies traumatic and ischemic nerve disorders by etiology. The response of the axon to disease or injury is limited, and many noxious agents may produce a similar result in the nerve. Since treatment and progress are often determined by the cause of the pathologic change, this etiologic classification has been useful.

The effects on the foot of such injuries are determined by the degree of injury, the nerves involved, and the presence or absence of irritative lesions. Nerve lesions may follow or accompany treatment and may be produced by factors such as direct injury and compression/ischemic lesions from unchanged limb position or tight dressings. Injuries produce mixed nerve lesions with combinations of contusion, stretch, and ischemia. Closed and open fractures can be accompanied by nerve laceration, contusion, crush between skeletal fragments, stretch, intra- and extraneural hematoma, and late compression by callus. Vascular injury may accompany or follow a fracture, with resultant neuropa-

TABLE 43–1. Nerve Injuries, Traumatic and Ischemic Neuropathies*

DIRECT INJURY

1. Laceration—complete and partial
   (a) External wounding
   (b) Internal wounding—fracture fragment, contusion
   (c) Direct laceration of surgically exposed nerve
2. Crush and contusion
3. Stretch or traction injury
4. Thermal injury
   (a) Cooling and freezing
   (b) Heat
   (c) Electrical burn
5. High velocity and other missile wounds—mixed lesions with excess scarring
6. Radiation injuries
7. Injection of noxious substances within the nerve

COMPRESSION PHENOMENA

1. Tourniquet palsy
2. External compression
3. Internal compression

ISCHEMIC NEUROPATHIES

1. Nontraumatic in origin
   (a) Arterial embolism
   (b) Occlusion of arteriae nervorum
      (1) Polycythemia vera
      (2) Sickle cell disease
      (3) Bacterial endocarditis
   (c) Vascular spasm secondary to injection of harmful substance
2. Traumatic in origin
   (a) Ischemia due to compression and stretch
   (b) Ischemia due to damage to arteriae nervorum
   (c) Ischemia due to damage to main arterial supply to limb, ischemic paralysis
   (d) Ischemic factor in combined neurovascular injury

ENTRAPMENT MONONEUROPATHIES

*Adapted from Sunderland, S.: Nerves and Nerve Injuries. Edinburgh, Churchill Livingstone, 1978.

thy. Compression against a cast can compromise a nerve trunk, and swelling of the limb within a cast produces an ischemic myopathy and neuropathy, i.e., Volkmann's contracture.

Nerve Injuries and Traumatic Neuropathies

Interruptive Lesions

Nerve injuries are usually classified by the degree of injury to the axon. Seddon[48, 49] graded the lesions as (1) *neuropraxia*, a conduction deficit without axonal destruction; (2) *axonotmesis*, axonal disruption without destruction of endoneurial (Schwann cell) tubes; and (3) *neurotmesis*, gross nerve disruption. The grade 3 lesions may occur from either contusion or stretch without destruction of the epineurium with a dense intraneural neuroma.

With the advent of more aggressive surgical approaches to injury, Sunderland's classification[54] is perhaps a more accurate one. Sunderland classifies nerve injuries into five degrees plus irritative lesions (Fig. 43–4). These are:

First degree injury: Conduction deficit without axonal interruption.

Second degree injury: Axon severed without breaching of the endoneurium. There is breakdown of myelin and wallerian degeneration. Electromyographic changes of denervation occur, and regeneration follows the pattern of axonal regrowth.

Third degree injury: Disintegration of axons with disorganization of the internal structure of funiculi. Minor changes take place in the perineurium. Regeneration is irregular and residual deficits are expected.

Fourth degree injury: Axonal rupture with funicular and perineurial disruption. The nerve bundles become disorganized and are no longer sharply demarcated from the epineurium. Continuity of the nerve trunk remains intact, but the trunk through the involved segment becomes a tangled mass of connective tissue, Schwann cells, and neural elements. Injury of this degree rarely exhibits spontaneous functional recovery.

Fifth degree injury: Loss of continuity of the nerve trunk.

Many injuries will result in partial or mixed lesions. The course of recovery and end result will depend on the exact pathologic findings. Mixed lesions may combine all types of injury from first to fourth degree.

Clinical Significance of the Degree of Injury.   The degree of injury determines the pattern of recovery and the requirements for successful surgery, when performed.

First degree injury (neuropraxia) is followed by rapid recovery, often within hours. Nevertheless, in some instances, the pattern of recovery takes several weeks to evolve, and an irritative phase with pain, paresthesia, and hyperesthesia may

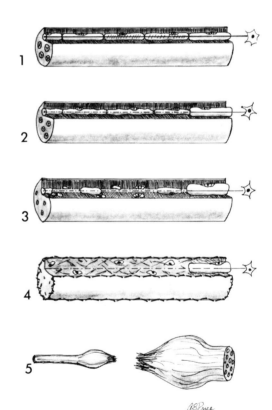

Figure 43–4.   *Five degrees of nerve injury. The nerve funiculus, axon, and Schwann sheath are represented in 1 to 4. The entire trunk is seen in 5. First degree injury corresponds to neuropraxia; second and third degree with axonotmesis; fourth degree injury involves perineurial as well as endoneurial disorganization and results in a degree of damage equivalent to fifth degree injury — neurotmesis. (Adapted from Sunderland, S.: Nerves and Nerve Injuries. Edinburgh, Churchill Livingstone, 1978.)*

predominate. Predictive factors include the nature, intensity, and duration of the injury. When neuropathy is associated with undisplaced fractures, tourniquet use, tight boots, or brief, nondestructive blunt trauma, rapid recovery is to be expected. When ischemia from tight bandaging or casts is a complicating factor, a more prolonged recovery pattern, lasting some weeks, is to be expected. When comminuted fractures indicate dissipation of much energy in the region or if severe contusion is present, the more severe degrees of nerve injury may be present.

Second degree injury will usually recover at a pace determined by axon regeneration (1 to 2 mm/day). The rate of sensory recovery can be monitored by observing the distal migration of the point of sensitivity of the nerve to gentle tapping (Tinel's sign). During the period of recovery, which may be quite prolonged when a popliteal, high thigh, or lumbar plexus lesion is present, contractures and ulcerations may develop as a result of motor imbalance and sensory deficit. The foot must be protected with appropriate insoles, braces, and stretching exercises. The patient must be taught careful inspection of the foot twice daily. Soft, clean stockings should be worn. Burns from hot baths are to be avoided. The toenails should be trimmed carefully and the nail grooves cleaned by using an orangewood stick.

In *third degree injury*, regeneration will be blocked by inter- and intrafunicular fibrosis as well as by disorganization of Schwann cell tubes. Pain may become persistent. As soon as it is evident that the recovery from nerve injury is slowed or absent, careful nerve exploration should be considered. The type of trauma will often indicate the need for early surgery, but if irreversible fibrosis of the denervated muscle is to be avoided, early nerve surgery is also required. By six months the pattern of recovery should be evident, and a decision as to intervention should be made.

Fourth and *fifth degree injuries* may not be distinguishable unless an open injury has revealed the state of continuity of the nerve. Both lesions require careful nerve reconstruction. When the repair of nerve laceration is immediate, it is possible to avoid resection of neuromas and autografting. Once neuroma and fibrosis are present, the lesion must be cut back to intact fascicles and the nerve repaired without tension.

Axon Regeneration and Reinnervation of Motor End Plates. Reinnervation of muscle after axon disruption involves the reinnervation of existing motor end plates rather than the *de novo* production of new end plates.[47] Three weeks after section of the sciatic nerve and repair, tiny axon sprouts (0.5 to 0.8 μ) appear. These contain axoplasm with a few mitochondria. When these axons reach the region of the end plate (a specialized Schwann cell that partially covers the terminal axon and overrides a specially modified region in the underlying muscle surface membrane), neurofilaments and vesicles containing axoplasm can be seen entering the end plates. Increasing numbers of vesicles then develop in the end plate.

De novo formation of end plates can occur when a nerve end is directly implanted into denervated muscle. This has not been demonstrated to have clinical significance, however, as only a few muscle fibers can be so innervated.

Irritative Lesions

Of great interest to orthopaedists and neurosurgeons are irritative lesions. These may result in phenomena such as muscle twitching, fasciculations and spasms, abnormal sweating and vasomotor disturbances, paresthesias, spontaneous pain, and abnormal response to heat and cold. They may be present alone, with progressive nerve disease, or during the recovery phases of many lesions. These irritative phenomena are seen in association with many traumatic and ischemic lesions and with other neuropathies. They can be most disabling and in their most severe form produce true causalgia.

In certain instances, perineural and intraneural (interfascicular) cicatrix can be demonstrated as one factor in interruptive and irritative lesions. Careful neurolysis, both extra- and intraneural, with preservation of fasciculi, has resulted in improved motor and sensory function and marked reduction in irritative symptoms in both mixed and pure irritative lesions.

Ischemic Neuropathy

Ischemia plays an important role in many traumatic neuropathies and can produce a severe neuropathy independently. The pure ischemic neuropathies are seen following arterial embolism[2] and accompanying small vessel embolism in diseases such as polycythemia vera, sickle cell dis-

ease, and bacterial endocarditis. These neuropathies are usually of abrupt onset. When major arterial occlusion has occurred, there will be muscle ischemia in addition to the nerve ischemia, and the resultant paralysis and contracture will be caused by the combined lesions. Nevertheless, the neural lesion is at times a major factor in the disorder and may be partially reversible — especially if irritative symptoms such as pain and dysesthesias are present (Fig. 43–5A to D).

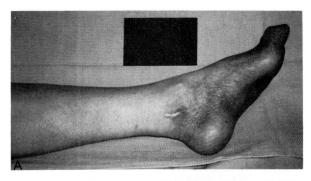

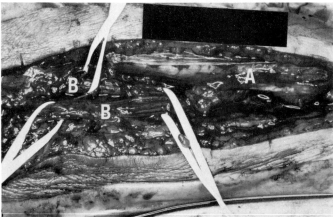

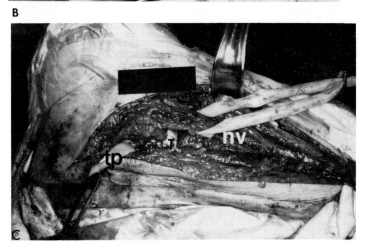

Figure 43–5. (A) Ischemic neuropathy secondary to an arterial embolus in a 70-year-old male. There was severe pain on the plantar surface of the foot and a fixed equinus deformity with claw toes. (B) Operative photograph showing release of the posterior tibial neurovascular bundle, neurolysis of the posterior tibial nerve, and division of the Achilles tendon (A — Achilles tendon; B — neurovascular bundle). (C) Operative photograph showing the neurovascular bundle held by a Penrose drain (n.v.), the posterior tibial tendon turned down (t.p.), and the dome of the talus exposed (T). Complete capsulotomy of the ankle joint with release of all medial and lateral tendon sheaths and lengthening of the tibialis posterior, flexor digitorum longus, and flexor hallucis longus have been performed.

Illustration continued on opposite page

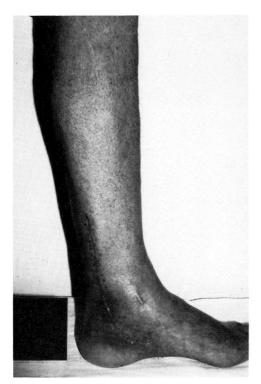

Figure 43-5 Continued. (D) Status one month following surgery. The foot is plantigrade. Pain and dysesthesias in the posterior tibial nerve distribution have been eliminated for the most part. The patient walks with a simple plastic orthosis and wears a standard shoe.

Ischemic nerve lesions accompany Volkmann's contracture when thickening of endoneural collagen can be found.[20] These changes are similar to those found after arterial occlusion or injury. In severe cases, complete nerve scarring is found (fourth degree injury) with axon destruction and degeneration.

The combination of nerve ischemia and nerve compression produces a more intense lesion than either factor alone.[55] Rather prolonged ischemia can be tolerated by the nerve trunks under controlled conditions; however, when compression is added to ischemia, the nerve is much less tolerant to injury, and nerve function can degrade several days later with associated late axon damage. Endoneural edema plays a role in this situation.[35, 36] Thus, continuous compression of a nerve can produce lesions from first through fourth degree, with ischemia playing a role.

In the leg, ischemic lesions are seen after direct injury to the femoral and pop-liteal arteries, after prolonged compression of the peroneal nerve behind the head of the fibula, and after closed injuries of the leg such as fractures of the tibia and fibula. In addition, swelling or hemorrhage into a tight fascial compartment may be associated with neural as well as muscle ischemia.[53] The foot is commonly involved in ischemic paralysis (in which sensory deficits and irritative phenomena, such as pain, may be severe), especially if direct nerve injury is also present. Causalgia-like pain and dysesthesias may develop, but true causalgia requires direct nerve injury.

Compression Injuries and Neuropathies

Compression injuries comprise a group of interesting lesions, many of which are amenable to effective therapy. If injuries caused by direct nerve crush and contusions resulting from short-acting forces are excluded, a group of subacute and chronic lesions remain that are classified in Table 43-2.

Compression neuropathies may vary in severity from first through fourth degree injuries. Physical pressure itself leads to degrees of conduction block and eventually to axonal disruption. Vascular compression may also play a role in the development of compression neuritis, as venous congestion and capillary stasis occur at low levels of compression and block of the vasa

TABLE 43-2. Compression Lesions of Nerves*

EXTERNAL COMPRESSION
1. Unrelieved compression against a firm object — table, bed, or cast — commonly a peroneal palsy
2. Tourniquet palsy
3. Habitual postures — occupational

INTERNAL COMPRESSION
1. Fractured callus causing progressive paralysis
2. Constricting band of fibrous tissue
3. Enlarging aneurysm with and without nerve fixation by scar
4. Enlarging tumor or ganglion
5. Compression within a confined space due to swelling of tissues and/or fibrosis
6. Pressure from hematoma within confined space; trauma and hemorrhagic diathesis due to disease or anticoagulation

*Adapted from Sunderland, S.: Nerves and Nerve Injuries. Edinburgh, Churchill Livingstone, 1978.

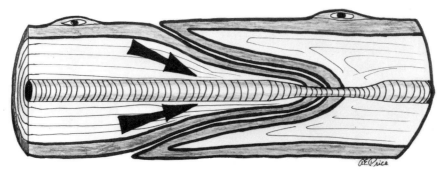

Figure 43–6. *Invagination of Schwann sheaths from compressed into noncompressed segments (Adapted from Sunderland, S.: Nerves and Nerve Injuries. Edinburgh, Churchill Livingstone, 1978.)*

nervorum results at higher pressure. Friction (thought to constitute a separate category of lesion by Sunderland) may lead to increasing intra- and extraneural fibrosis and so to interference with nerve function. In *tourniquet palsy*, invagination of Schwann sheaths from the compressed into the noncompressed nerve segment has been demonstrated, and pressure necrosis of the nerve trunk may be produced with enough pressure[52] (Fig. 43–6).

Recovery from compression neuropathy depends on the degree of injury and the duration of force application, as fibrosis seems to correlate with prolonged compression as well as with the intensity of compression. Although first degree lesions should recover immediately if only the gross axon structure is considered, they often take several days to recover because of disorganization or physiologic damage to internal axon structure (microtubules and filaments) or to Schwann cells, vascular channels, or endoneural cells.

Second degree lesions recover according to the rate of axon regeneration, varying from 1 to 4 mm/day and averaging 2 mm/day. Regeneration is slower in the leg, especially distally, with rates of 1 to 2 mm/day in the lower leg and 1 mm/day in the foot.[57]

Hoffmann-Tinel Sign. Distal tingling on percussion over a nerve marks the most distal point of regenerating sensory axons. This sign is quite useful in mapping nerve regeneration. Scarring due to local lesions and nerve repairs will slow the rate of regeneration.

In some compression neuropathies, especially those involving the peroneal nerve behind the head of the fibula, the rate and degree of recovery do not correspond to the anticipated severity and mechanism of injury. Instead of the first or second degree lesions that should have been produced, third degree lesions characterized by fibrosis within and between the fascicles have developed. A vascular component may also be present to explain the severity of the lesions.

Although motor nerve fibers are usually more susceptible to compression, are the first to fail, and the last to recover, this is not always true. Most compression neuropathies recover by the sixth month; when they do not, intraneural fibrosis and disorganization have occurred. Neurolysis, both external and internal, offers some hope for improvement. When severe third and fourth degree lesions are present with no further chance of recovery, resection of the lesions with autografting can improve the outlook in selected cases.

Treatment of Nerve Trauma and Neuropathies Due to Trauma

An attempt must be made to assess the level of the lesion and the degree of injury. The mechanism of injury can give a clue to the severity of the nerve pathology and the course of recovery to be expected.

Laceration of nerves in the thigh, leg, or foot must be suspected and searched for in any external wound and whenever a fracture has been displaced. The extent of nerve injury is often concealed by the state of consciousness of the patient immediately after injury. Circular casts applied after acute injury or surgery can also conceal the extent of nerve injury as well as contribute to vascular neuropathies.

The first step in management of the lesion is *prevention*. After acute trauma or skeletal surgery, medial and lateral plaster splints applied over adequate padding will serve to protect the limb while permitting inspection and testing for neural and vascular function. Misguided attempts at perfect reduction and immobilization in severe fresh fractures often create more problems than they solve.

When an immediate complete or partial nerve deficit follows wounding or surgery, a fifth degree lesion (neurotmesis) must be suspected. Circumstances may dictate a delay in repair, e.g., multiple injuries or coma. The metabolic activity of the nerve cell is greatest three weeks after injury. Nevertheless, when nerve transection is suspected, it is best to explore the lesion as soon as practicable (especially if the lesion follows surgery) because fibrosis of the wound following healing makes the identification and mobilization of the injured nerve more difficult. This problem is minimal soon after the injury. The surgery must be performed with due understanding of the anatomy and physiology of the individual nerve involved, with an adequate plan for repair or reconstruction, with preparation of the other limb for possible autografting, and with adequate magnification available to effect a good repair.

Specific syndromes of nerve injury are treated as follows:

Since a sensory deficit of the plantar surface of the foot creates great risks, laceration or disruption of the *sciatic nerve* (Fig. 43–7A to D) warrants early repair or reconstruction. Sciatic nerve injuries accompanying dislocation of the hip should be given an opportunity to recover spontaneously following closed reduction. Open reductions of acetabular fractures associated with hip dislocation should include exposure of the sciatic nerve to seek the causes of palsy, if present, and to protect the nerve in the absence of injury. Wounds to the sciatic nerve that accompany fracture may be rather severe and include laceration, contusion, and traction injuries. The sciatic nerve is not routinely observed during surgery for femoral fractures, so that once the skeletal and any vascular problems have been managed, the nerve should be explored if its recovery does not follow the course expected for first or second degree lesions.

The posterior tibial and peroneal nerves may be injured in the popliteal-knee region by direct or indirect violence. The extent of the functional deficit will be apparent from clinical examination and electrodiagnostic studies. Wounds associated with laceration, severe crush injuries, and knee dislocations will lead to nerve lesions that cannot be expected to recover spontaneously. Exploration of the nerve is therefore indicated.

The *peroneal nerve* is vulnerable behind the head of the fibula. Neuropathies may be produced by direct contusion or by compression against unyielding objects. Many instances of neuropathy develop when the unconscious or debilitated patient lies with the leg somewhat externally rotated and does not move it. The point of vulnerability is behind the fibular head, where the nerve lies against bone. The nerve then penetrates the dense deep fascia of the peroneus longus and is protected by that muscle as it winds around the fibula to trifurcate (see Figure 43–2).

Neuropathies in this region (Figs. 43–7E to G, 43–8) may be produced by direct trauma during open surgery when the proximity of the nerve to bone is not appreciated and by compression due to an extrinsic or intrinsic mass such as ganglion. Some lesions develop without apparent cause. Recovery from compression tends to be less satisfactory than would be anticipated by the nature of the injury. It is in this instance that neurolysis has been recommended. Removal of the head of the fibula to decompress the nerve is often useful. In most instances, exploration will reveal intraneural fibrosis. Often the lesion is left untreated except for orthotic support of the paralyzed muscles until fibrosis of the anterior tibial and peroneal muscles has occurred. The lesion usually affects the anterior tibial muscle most and the peroneal muscles least.

Neurolysis

Neurolysis was advocated by Babcock[1] in his review of experiences during World War I. He noted improvement in nerve function and the relief of pain after external neurolysis. *Hersage*, the internal decompression of a nerve by multiple longitudinal incisions, was advocated for

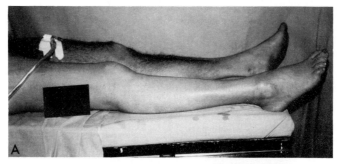

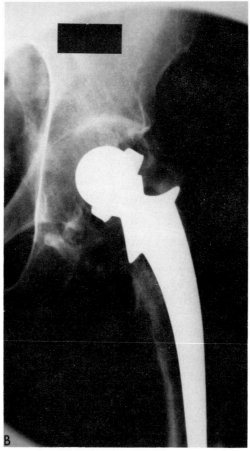

Figure 43–7. *(A) Sciatic neuropathy following fracture of the acetabulum and femoral head and total hip replacement. There is fixed equinus deformity and complete peroneal palsy. (B) Radiograph of hip showing total hip replacement.*

Illustration continued on opposite page

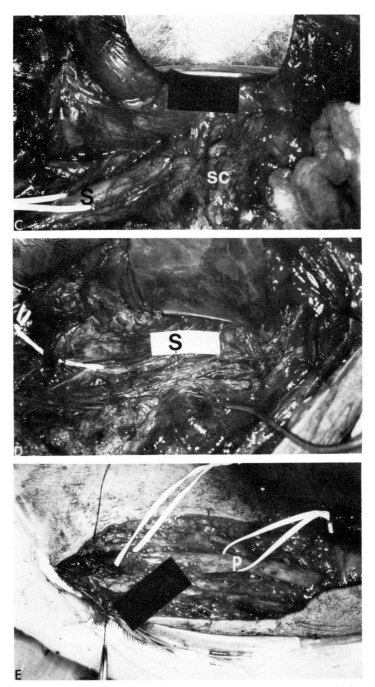

Figure 43–7 Continued. (C) The sciatic nerve is exposed posterior to the hip joint (S). Vessiloop around the nerve and extensive scarring (SC) are noted. (D) Decompression and neurolysis of the sciatic nerve (S). (E) Exploration of the common peroneal nerve at the head of the fibula; localization of the lesion by positive Tinel's sign; scarring found behind fibula (P — peroneal nerve).

Illustration continued on following page

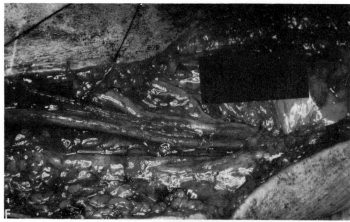

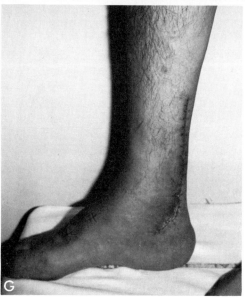

Figure 43–7 *Continued. (F) Appearance following neurolysis of the branches of the common peroneal nerve. (G) Status following second operation, which consisted of exploration of the posterior tibial nerve and vessels, capsulotomy of the ankle joint with release of the medial retinaculum and tendon sheaths, and tendo-Achillis lengthening. There was partial recovery of sensation on the dorsum of the foot, but no motor recovery.*

lesions-in-continuity when internal fibrosis was present. Magnification was not used. Curtis and Eversmann[6] reported improved results after carpal tunnel decompression when an internal neurolysis of the median nerve was performed under magnification.

Neurolysis has been applied successfully in a group of elderly patients when post-traumatic and compressive neuropathies of axillary, median, and ulnar nerve lesions were decompressed.[33] Relief of prolonged extraneural compression has been followed by immediate return of sensation.[32]

Sunderland[55] recommends neurolysis under some circumstances and believes that immediate return of function can be demonstrated in some patients following

this surgery. In addition, when previously arrested progressive axon regeneration appears to have resumed following neurolysis, success can be ascribed to the procedure. Such findings have been reported by Lusskin and associates.[38]

According to Sunderland[55] neurolysis offers some reasonable chance of success if performed in appropriate instances. It may be undertaken under several circumstances:

1. To relieve pain due either to adhesions that fix the nerve or to constricting bands that deform the nerve and obstruct its blood supply.

2. To assist regeneration by freeing adhesions that block axon regrowth.

3. When progress of regeneration is suddenly arrested.

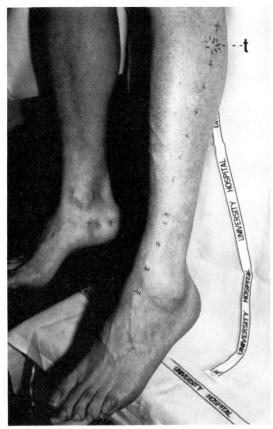

Figure 43–8. *Patient with "radicular" pain on the left leg of nine months duration accompanied by footdrop. A herniated nucleus pulposus was suspected. Electrodiagnostic studies showed a conduction deficit at the head of the fibula. The photograph demonstrates footdrop, positive Tinel's sign along the course of the peroneal nerve, and the zone of tenderness behind the head of the fibula (t). There was no history of trauma. Peroneal nerve exploration revealed cicatrix behind the head of the fibula. Release of the peroneal nerve resulted in full recovery.*

4. When premature exploration has demonstrated the nerve to be intact but bound in scar.

5. Following unsatisfactory recovery after nerve suture.

6. In the surgical treatment of painful leprous neuritis in which intrafunicular lesions may be managed by internal neurolysis. This is the only instance in which the perineural tubes themselves should be opened.

In the lower half of the leg, traumatic, ischemic lesions may be seen after contusion or crush injuries, fractures, and skeletal surgery. Ischemic neuropathy may be present alone or in conjunction with these

injuries. Not only is the sensory deficit serious and the motor loss disabling, but deformities compound the situation and may preclude the wearing of a shoe. Pain, paresthesias, and dysesthesias are frequently encountered. Ischemic neuropathies accompanying Volkmann's paralysis were not considered amenable to therapy,[20] but recent experience using magnification for internal neurolysis has shown improvement of some lesions (see Figures 43–7 and 43–11A to E).

Operative Techniques in Neurolysis. The limb is prepared and draped from the tips of the toes (or fingers) to the hip (or shoulder). Another limb should be prepared for possible removal of donor nerve, should autografting prove desirable and feasible. Since surgery may be prolonged, an indwelling bladder catheter is introduced under sterile conditions. Epidural anesthesia is quite useful in many of the lower limb procedures. The shoulder is protected with a chest pad if the lateral position is used. This position is quite useful for combined common peroneal–peroneal division explorations and when a proximal sciatic nerve exploration is required at the time of peroneal nerve surgery.

The incision should be generous and must allow for complete exposure of the nerve in the zone of injury. Dissection will have to include uninvolved nerve proximally and distally. The incision should curve across joint creases. Z-incisions are very useful around joints, as they will produce the least scar contraction. The incision should be marked with a skin pen and short crosshatches cut just through the epidermis to permit accurate reapproximation at the closure. Previous scars are usually excised. If extensive scar is present and flaps are required to close the wound, preliminary plastic surgical reconstruction or the assistance of a plastic surgeon in planning and performing the closure may be appropriate.

Often an arterial trunk will be involved in scar. Therefore, plan for exposure and control of the artery proximal to the region of injury. When the artery is exposed, a strand of vessiloop should be passed around it twice. A clamp holding the vessiloop will permit compression of the artery without damage if vascular repair is required. 6–0 Tevdek and an atraumatic needle should be available to repair an arterial tear or incision. Veins should be preserved whenever possible and major tears repaired with Tevdek sutures.

A tourniquet is not necessary or desirable when operating upon the post-traumatic or ischemic nerve. Bleeding should be reduced by elevation of the limb (Trendelenburg position for foot and leg surgery) and the use of bipolar cautery tip.

Magnification aids accurate hemostasis as well as the dissection of the nerve from surrounding scar. Loupes (2.5×) should be used as soon as the nerve or neurovascular bundle is located proximal to the lesion. Dissection then proceeds into the scar, with removal of external scar. The nerve must be approached distally as well in order to work backward to the zone of injury. When dissection is difficult, the nerve trunk can be better differentiated from scar following the injection of normal saline, without preservatives, into the nerve, using a No. 30 needle.

Once the nerve is exposed and its branches identified and released, an intraneural neurolysis can be performed. For this procedure an operating microscope with magnification up to 30× is essential. Electrical nerve stimulation during the procedure is quite useful. This permits identification of functioning motor branches in the scar and may reveal improved motor conduction as the neurolysis proceeds. Paralytic agents must be stopped 20 minutes prior to the use of nerve stimulators. When selective epidural anesthesia has been administered, some information about sensory function may be available from electrical stimulation. Disposable single pole electrode stimulators are not as useful as larger devices with variable outputs and double electrodes. The fascicles are teased apart using microscissors, with care being taken to preserve the anastomosing interfascicular axon bundles.

Joint/skeletal procedures such as capsulotomy, tenotomy, and osteotomy can be performed with relative ease and safety once the neurolysis is completed; since the nerve and accompanying vessels will have been mobilized, they can be protected.

The deep fascia is not closed over the lysed or repaired nerve. When immobilization is required after surgery, a bulky soft bandage made of sheet wadding of narrow width, 2 to 3 inches, should be applied first. Plaster splints that do not circle the limb may be used to reinforce this dressing. The foot pulses can be monitored through holes in the dressing. A final cast may be applied when the wounds have healed.

When the posterior tibial nerve is involved in the leg or behind the medial malleolus, exploration for decompression and neurolysis can be useful for two reasons. First, the neurolysis may have a beneficial effect on the pain phenomena and sensory deficit despite existing advanced muscle fibrosis. Second, the mobilization of the nerve and posterior tibial artery permits extensive capsulotomy of ankle and subtalar joints, even in the elderly patient.

Within the foot, the posterior tibial nerve and its branches, the medial and lateral plantar nerves, are subject to injury from lacerations and fractures. Nerve repair and/or neurolysis may be undertaken under magnification to relieve the motor and sensory deficits that may result.

Injuries to the peroneal nerves in the lower half of the leg and in the foot result in relatively minor motor deficits, but the sensory loss may be quite annoying (Fig. 43–9A to C). Irritative phenomena are important in peroneal nerve injuries, with and without ischemic neuropathy. Pain on the dorsum of the foot and toes may be severe. In this instance the first step is to utilize local nerve blocks to localize the lesion, reduce pain for varied lengths of time, and distend the perineural cicatrix. Repeated nerve blocks may reduce the dysesthesias and pain. Localization of the lesion and transient response to nerve blocks may guide successful neurolysis or proximal nerve section when a traumatic neuroma is present (Fig. 43–10A to F).

Physical Modalities

Physical therapy modalities have been used in an attempt to improve nerve regeneration. After denervation, massage, electrical stimulation, heat, and ultrasound have not been demonstrated to improve the outlook for either nerve regeneration or joint flexibility.

Although gentle manipulation of affected joints can maintain flexibility in the absence of ischemic injury, there is no evidence that forceful passive stretching will be successful. The patient must perform the therapy if it is to be useful. The therapist should guide, not perform, treatment.

Orthotic Management

Once a fixed contracture has developed, it should be accommodated by the shoe or orthosis or else surgically corrected. A

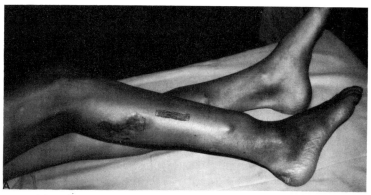

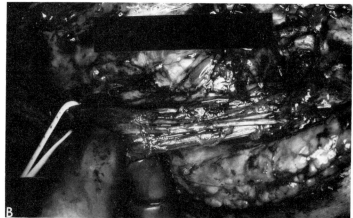

Figure 43–9. (A) Posterior tibial and peroneal palsy following severe fractures of the tibia and fibula. Ischemia may have played a role in the etiology. There was severe pain in the foot, and the patient requested amputation. (B) Operative photograph showing peroneal nerve after external and internal neurolysis. Fascicles can be seen. (C) Photograph of patient standing without pain one and a half years after surgery. He has returned to work.

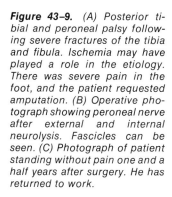

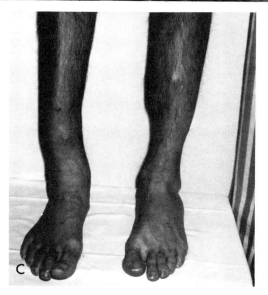

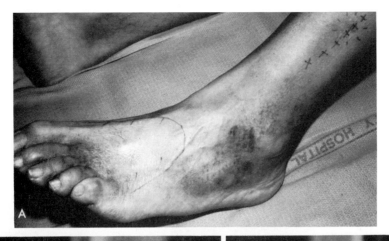

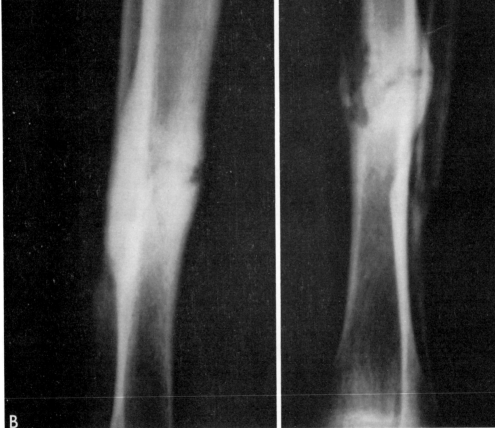

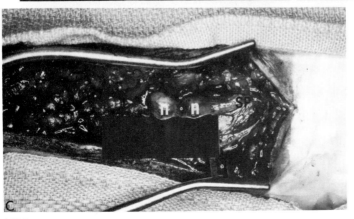

Figure 43-10. *(A) Superficial and deep peroneal palsy and posterior tibial neuropathy following fracture of the tibia. There is a superficial scar and a positive Tinel's sign over the point of penetration of the superficial peroneal nerve through the deep fascia. (B) Radiographs of the leg. (C) Operative photograph shows double neuromas of the superficial peroneal nerve at the level of the deep fascia of the leg (SP — superficial peroneal nerve; n — neuromas). Dysesthesias were relieved by proximal fascicular ligation under an operative microscope. (Technique of A. Battista, M.D.)*

Illustration continued on opposite page

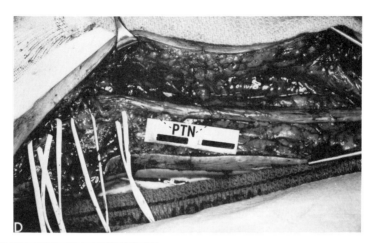

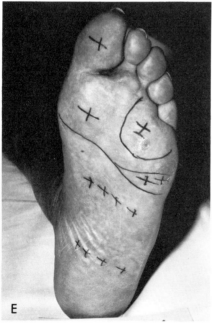

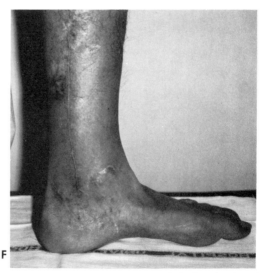

Figure 43–10 *Continued.   (D) Operative photograph showing posterior tibial neurolysis in the distal portion of the leg and branches of the posterior tibial vessels exposed and protected under the medial retinaculum of the foot (PTN — posterior tibial nerve). (E) Plantar surface of the foot six months after posterior tibial neurolysis (+ — normal sensation; + + + + — hyperesthesia). (F) The patient standing 20 months after posterior tibial neurolysis and six months after superficial peroneal nerve ligation proximal to the neuromas. The patient experienced minimal discomfort and is working.*

fixed equinus should be treated by heel elevations and varus of the foot by medial support. Only that element of the deformity that is increased under gravitational loading can be corrected by bracing.

Custom-molded inner soles, especially those using newer foamed plastics such as Plastazote, can better distribute ground reaction forces in order to prevent or minimize callosities and pressure ulcers.

Support of the denervated muscle is important to prevent overstretch. This improves the gait pattern and protects destabilized joints from luxation. Custom-designed plastic orthoses or metal bar orthoses attached to the shoe or to plastic foot pieces have proved useful. When the gastrocnemius and/or soleus is to be protected, one must use a rigid foot piece, a strong ankle joint with dorsiflexion stop or a fixed ankle joint, and a calf band that is wide and high to distribute the forces that are generated at the anterior shank.

Once there has been breakdown on the plantar surface of the denervated foot, salvage requires the use of an orthosis that transfers weight from the shank to the foot. The patellar tendon-bearing (PTB) brace has been effective in managing the Charcot foot and peripheral neuropathy associated with diabetes.[16]

Orthopaedic Reconstruction and Releases for Peripheral Nerve Injury in the Foot and Leg (Figs. 43–11A to E and 43–12)

The management of fixed contractures by capsulotomy has been mentioned. Protection of nerve and vascular supply is essential during this procedure. Stabilization procedures (arthrodeses) have also been used successfully. These are most helpful in treating deformities of the toes and subtalar joints. Footdrop (functional equinus) after peroneal nerve injuries is not managed well by ankle arthrodesis, as stresses are transferred to the midtarsal, intertarsal, and tarsometatarsal joints, and late degenerative arthropathies may develop. If there is a sensory deficit on the plantar surface of the foot, ankle fusion that produces excess pressures on the forepart of the foot may lead to ulceration.

Tendon transfers to control footdrop and varus can be quite useful. The posterior tendon transfer through the interosseous space to the dorsum of the foot works well. The foot must be protected by an orthosis with a plantar flexion stop for many months.

Timing of Orthopaedic Procedures. The timing of tendon transfers deserves comment. It has been customary to wait until the end results of nerve surgery are fully realized before undertaking such procedures. Since the best of nerve repairs will result in partial recovery only and since tendon transfers cannot function at normal strength, there is little to be gained by prolonged delay in completing orthopaedic procedures after the neural surgery is performed. The age of the patient will often determine the course of treatment. When peroneal palsy is present in the elderly person, the disorder is usually managed by an orthosis even if nerve repair or neurolysis is undertaken. In the young patient, the full orthopaedic reconstructive program can be undertaken in the presence of pronounced paralytic instability. Neural repair should be followed by subtalar arthrodesis and then by posterior tibial tendon transfer. In many instances subtalar (triple) arthrodesis will not be required once growth has ceased, but in children the skeleton will deform under the influence of unbalanced forces and surgical stabilization is often required.

Stabilization of Charcot joints has been attempted in the past, often unsuccessfully. This was true even when the arthropathy was produced by tabes dorsalis. Arthrodesis is accompanied by risk of sepsis, by high rates of nonunion, and also by problems associated with stress transfer to adjacent bones and joints. Orthotic management of these lesions using rigid custom-designed plastic orthoses and weight-transferring orthoses is acceptable and often quite successful.

Claw toes are amenable to proximal interphalangeal joint arthrodesis and capsulotomy of the metatarsophalangeal joints when subluxation has developed. Diaphysectomy of the proximal phalanges may also be effective.[21] In advanced cases, the joint resection procedures such as the Hoffman metatarsal head resection may be required to correct deformity. When plantar ulcers are present, conservative surgery

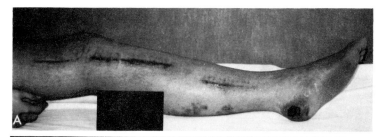

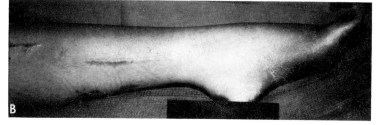

Figure 43–11. Combined neurolysis and joint release. (A) Fourteen-year-old male five months after dislocation of the knee with popliteal and posterior tibial artery injury. Reconstruction of circulation by arterial bypass has been performed. Fasciotomies were required. Severe pain and fixed contractures followed. (B) Eight months after surgery. Heel ulcer has been treated by debridement and a skin graft. Angiography showed that the posterior tibial artery was the only arterial supply to foot. Equinus has increased despite exercise regimen. (C) Operative photograph showing neurolysis of the posterior tibial nerve, exploration and displacement of the posterior tibial artery, and exposure of the tendo Achillis and medial tendons (AT — Achilles tendon; nv — neurovascular bundle; TP — tibialis posterior).

Illustration continued on following page

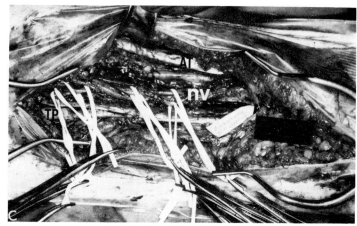

will often salvage the foot. Deep ulcers are treated by excision of infected bone, the use of protective padding or casts, and appropriate bactericidal antibiotic therapy.

Entrapment Neuropathies

Entrapment neuropathies constitute a subgroup of compression neuropathies that are due to (1) the gradual constriction of anatomic structures about a nerve or (2) the chronic compression of a nerve against an adjacent unyielding fibrous or skeletal structure. They are quite interesting in that these lesions have been recognized rather late (within the past 20 years) and the site of compression is often removed from the site of symptoms or signs. In addition, the insidious and mild nature of the compression phenomenon is out of proportion to the annoying and often disabling symptoms.

The entrapment neuropathies produce sensory and motor changes and are usually painful. The pain is referred to the distribution of the involved nerve. Since a small sensory nerve can be affected, the distribution of pain to this nerve may not appear typical of a nerve lesion, and local or more distal causes may be considered or treated before the true nature of the lesion is appreciated.

The sensory deficits of entrapment neuropathies are often rather subtle and appear somewhat later than the pain. Since superficial nerves are usually involved, it is superficial sensation that is most affected.

The relationship between fiber size, nerve function, and vulnerability to compression has been shown to be incon-

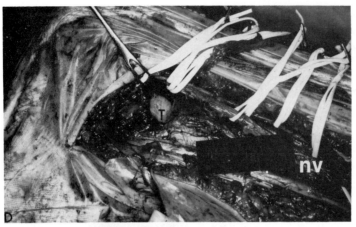

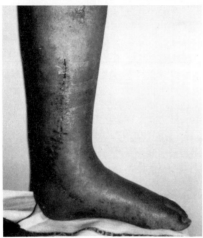

Figure 43–11 Continued. (D) Operative photograph showing complete capsulotomy of the ankle, tendo-Achillis lengthening, and lengthening of the tibialis posterior, flexor hallucis longus, and flexor digitorum longus. Neurovascular structures are displaced (nv — neurovascular bundle; T — talus). (E) Patient standing on plantigrade foot six weeks following surgery. Pain has subsided. Sensory recovery in posterior tibial distribution followed. The patient has returned to school with adequate protection of the foot.

stant.[12, 13] In addition, it has been shown that individual fibers vary in size and myelin thickness along their length.[59]

The time of appearance of motor deficits in relation to sensory deficits in the development of the disorder is also inconstant. Certainly, there is varied evidence as to which fibers are more vulnerable to compression. Many authors feel that sensory fibers are more resistant to compression than are motor fibers. Sunderland[55] feels that although motor and sensory fibers react differently to pressure and ischemia, the pattern is not predictable. In entrapment neuropathies involving a mixed motor-sensory nerve, it is often difficult to quantitate motor deficits until rather late in the evolution of the disorder.

When a mixed trunk nerve or motor nerve is involved in this type of disorder, electromyography and nerve conduction studies can be useful in identifying and localizing the lesion.[14]

An important clinical finding in entrapment neuropathies involving sensory or mixed nerves is the presence of tenderness over the point of entrapment. Often, pain will be referred to the distal region of primary symptomatology. When compression has produced axonal interruption, a Tinel sign may be elicited at the point of compression.

Stretch of a nerve may also reproduce symptoms. Inversion plantar flexion of the foot–ankle complex applies longitudinal tension to the peroneal nerve. This maneuver can serve as a mechanism of injury to the nerve at its point of fixation at the neck of the fibula and can reproduce pain resulting from such a lesion — much as performing the Lasègue test stretches the roots of the lumbar plexus over a herniated intervertebral disc. Similarly, the superficial peroneal nerve may be put under tension by plantar flexion of the ankle and produce pain from entrapment at its point

Figure 43–12. This patient had a depressed fracture of the lateral tibial plateau with genu varum and peroneal nerve palsy secondary to direct trauma. Surgery consisted of peroneal neurolysis, osteotomy of the tibia, and release of the proximal tibiofibular joint. Operative photograph illustrates the area of injury to common peroneal nerve at the head of the fibula (P — common peroneal nerve). The branches traced well into the upper third of the leg. White pointer shows cicatrix (SC). Magnification permits dissection in the anterior compartment with protection of the branches of the anterior tibial artery and vein.

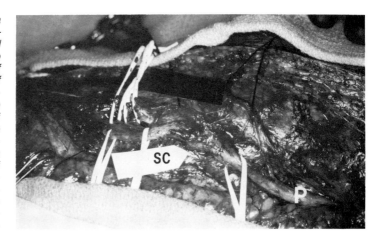

of penetration through the deep fascia in the lower third of the leg. The plantar interdigital nerve can be stretched, and so reproduce metatarsalgia, by dorsiflexion of the toes when the foot is also dorsiflexed.

Proximal reference of pain and associated hypersensitivity of the nerve trunk, the Valleix phenomenon, can also be seen in entrapment phenomena[5, 23, 27] and may obscure the diagnosis. When proximal symptoms are relieved by distal nerve block, the distal lesion usually has caused the proximal nerve hyperirritability.

The treatment of entrapment phenomena is surgical decompression of the involved nerve if local blockade and extraneural nonirritating corticosteroid injections do not suffice. Often, external decompression is satisfactory; however, when prolonged disease has led to intraneural fibrosis, residual motor deficits and sensory disturbance may persist. Intraneural fibrosis is often present once motor denervation has occurred. The latter is evidenced by atrophy and fibrillation potentials and/or sharp spikes on electromyography. Intraneural neurolysis using magnification has proved helpful in the treatment of the carpal tunnel syndrome[6] and has been successful in the management of lower extremity lesions when intraneural fibrosis was present.[37] However, intraneural neurolysis is not without dangers because of both the interfascicular plexus structure of the nerves and the axonal changes that can result from such surgery. Studies have demonstrated no significant vascular injury following intraneural neurolysis, but some endoneural scarring and axonal damage are produced

by the procedure.[46] Nevertheless, remarkably little return of fibrosis follows. After careful intraneural neurolysis, immediate improvement of sensation tends to persist and is often followed by some motor recovery.

The nerves of the foot and ankle that have been reported to be involved in entrapment neuropathies and the clinical pattern and findings in these disorders will next be reviewed.

Peroneal Nerve

The common peroneal nerve may be affected by any lesion at the head and neck of the fibula. Ganglia of the nerve in this location can produce a gradually developing peroneal neuropathy.[3, 10, 61] These ganglion cysts may or may not communicate with the proximal tibio-fibular joint and may be intra- or extraneural. The common peroneal nerve is composed of openly arranged funiculi in this area,[55] and degenerative cysts can thus intrude into or develop within it. Osteomas or osteochondromas of the neck of the fibula can produce a similar lesion, as can an enlarged fabella.[39]

The important anatomic arrangement of the neck of the fibula is the bridge of dense fascia overlying the two heads of the peroneus longus muscle. The superficial head attaches to the head of the fibula and adjacent tibia, whereas the deep head attaches to the neck of the fibula below the nerve. The nerve moves under this bridge during subtalar joint motion. Entrapment is produced by fibrosis that fixes the nerve or by an expanding lesion beneath the nerve. Entrapment under the peroneus longus fascial bridge (the fibular tunnel) has also been reported.[11, 25]

Peripheral entrapment neuropathy is characterized by a state of altered transmission due to mechanical irritation from adjacent anatomic structures.[50] Episodes follow direct trauma or injuries to the foot and ankle but may occur without obvious cause. Lateral leg and/or ankle pain and "weak ankle" are often the presenting findings. Footdrop may be present. Relief by external decompression is usual, but some patients do not improve following extraneural surgery. Idiopathic lesions occur and should be treated before complete fibrosis of the musculature has developed.

Electrical studies show localized conduction slowing in the region of compression in many cases.[14, 44] The site was confirmed by the electrical studies of Brown and associates.[4] Slowing of sensory conduction velocities across the fibular head and neck region, compared with distal velocities, is often diagnostic. Nevertheless, electrodiagnostic tests may fail to distinguish between localized peroneal nerve entrapment and lumbar disc lesions.[51]

The symptoms of common peroneal nerve entrapment include paresthesias and pain along the outer aspect of the foot and leg. Findings include hypesthesia in the peroneal distribution; weakness of the anterior tibial and peroneal muscles, leading to footdrop and repeated ankle injuries; and tenderness at the site of entrapment.

Although eversion weakness is appreciated by most surgeons examining the foot, weakness of plantar flexion of the first metatarsal may not be noted unless searched for. The peroneus longus muscle is the plantar flexor of the first ray. It maintains the longitudinal arch of the foot and is important as an invertor of the subtalar joint by its action on the first metatarsal in the last part of stance phase. Weakness of the peroneus longus muscle leads to increased pressure under the second and third metatarsal heads. Painful metatarsalgia and/or calluses then develop at the points of increased pressure.

Treatment is by decompression and neurolysis. Not all lesions are cured by external decompression because of intraneural fibrosis.[55] Therefore, the peroneal nerve should be exposed under magnification and intraneural neurolysis performed when fibrosis is present within the nerve.

Compression neuropathies of the peroneal nerve can develop as a result of lesions that occur somewhat proximally in the popliteal region. These neuropathies have developed following aneurysm, ganglion of lateral meniscus, and enlarged fabella.

The *lateral cutaneous nerve of the calf* and the *sural communicating nerve* have been involved by entrapment as they pierce the deep fascia in the upper third of the leg.[17] These branches of the peroneal nerve emerge in the popliteal region from the medial aspect of the nerve. When they are involved in compressive states, pain is referred to the lateral aspect of the leg and/or dorsolateral foot. Local anesthetic blocks at the point of tenderness usually relieve the pain.

Superficial Peroneal Nerve

This nerve pierces the fascia of the leg at the junction of the middle and lower thirds and is subject to entrapment at this site. The entrapment may follow fracture of the leg when additional factors such as contusion and vascular compromise may have occurred. Many cases are idiopathic; others follow plantar flexion-inversion injuries of the foot and ankle.

The nerve is purely sensory in this region so that the symptoms from entrapment consist of pain and hypesthesia on the dorsal and lateral surface of the foot and ankle. The pain may be reproduced by inversion of the plantar flexed foot and by pressure over the point of penetration of the nerve through the deep fascia.

There is considerable variation in the anatomy of the superficial peroneal nerve.[26, 60] It pierces the deep fascia as one nerve in 75 per cent of the population and as two nerves in 25 per cent, with the medial branch penetrating higher than the lateral. The sural nerve may innervate greater or lesser zones on the dorsum of the foot and toes.

Local anesthetic blocks at the point of tenderness in the leg are of diagnostic and therapeutic value. The injection of 3 to 5 ml of anesthetic at the level of the deep fascia should relieve symptoms. The injection can be supplemented by noncrystalline corticosteroids. Occasionally, surgical decompression is required.

Dorsal Cutaneous Nerves of the Foot

There are three sensory nerves on the dorsum of the foot. The *medial* and *intermediate dorsal cutaneous nerves* of the foot derive from the superficial peroneal nerve. The *sural nerve* sends its terminal branch to the lateral portion of the foot (but it may reach the medial border). When the sural nerve is absent in the foot, the most lateral branch of the superficial peroneal nerve is called the *lateral dorsal cutaneous nerve.*

The intermediate dorsal cutaneous nerve can be seen and palpated in most individuals by plantar flexing and inverting the foot. It mimics an extensor tendon or vein.

These nerves are vulnerable to direct trauma to the foot. Compressive phenomena can develop from cicatrix, tight shoes, and tight boots, especially ski boots. Painful dysesthesias may develop after plantar flexion-inversion sprains of the ankle. A dorsal osteophyte at the tarsal or tarsometatarsal joints may lead to pressure irritation of these nerves.

Localization of the lesion is aided by injection of local anesthetic into the point of tenderness. Often, permanent improvement can follow anesthetic/steroid instillations. External compression from a boot or shoe is treated by appropriate change in footwear and protective pads that redistribute pressure.

Deep Peroneal Nerve

The deep peroneal nerve emerges from the leg along with the anterior tibial artery (dorsalis pedis) at the midanterior aspect of the tibia in front of the ankle joint. It runs lateral to the anterior tibial and extensor hallucis longus tendons and sends a motor branch beneath the long toe extensor to the point where it innervates the extensor brevis muscle. That innervation may be replaced by an *accessory deep peroneal nerve* that derives from the superficial peroneal nerve and enters the foot behind the lateral malleolus.[14] This variant may lead to diagnostic error when lesions of the deep peroneal nerve are studies clinically and by electromyography.

The deep peroneal nerve runs beneath the fascia in the foot to its distal third. It may be entrapped between a skeletal lesion on the dorsum of the foot and the deep fascia, with accentuation of symptoms by any pressure on the dorsum of the foot over the lesion. Common lesions include osteoarthritic hypertrophic bone ridges at the naviculo-cuneiform and first metatarso-cuneiform joints and bone prominence (osteoma or bossing) of the medial cuneiform. Local tenderness will be present, and hypesthesia on the dorsum of the first web space may be found. Occasionally a Tinel sign is present. When there is a skeletal prominence beneath the nerve, surgical decompression is usually required if a closed shoe is to be worn. The deep fascia is divided and the nerve protected while the skeletal lesion is removed.

Posterior Tibial Nerve

The posterior tibial nerve is not often affected by entrapment disorders of the calf or leg, as it is well protected by muscle. Nevertheless, it is vulnerable during its passage under the soleus arch as it leaves the popliteal region.

In the ankle region, this nerve passes beneath the deep flexor retinaculum along with the posterior tibial artery. Here it divides into its terminal branches, the medial and lateral plantar nerves, and is subject to compression similar to that seen in the carpal tunnel syndrome. This compression produces the *tarsal tunnel syndrome.*[15, 24, 25]

The symptoms of this disorder consist of hypesthesia, pain, and paresthesias of the sole of the foot. The pain often has a burning character and may be accentuated by ambulation or recumbency. Night pain is similar to that seen in the carpal tunnel syndrome. Sensory symptoms precede motor changes, which take the form of paresis and then paralysis of the intrinsic muscles of the foot.[55] Tarsal tunnel syndrome has been associated with leg cramps, numbness, burning, and paresthesias of the feet in pregnancy, and objective conduction deficits in the posterior tibial nerve have been documented in these instances.[18]

This syndrome often develops insidiously but may be related to excess walking or injuries to the ankle region. An association with direct trauma, compression, and vascular insufficiency is often present.

Findings of numbness in the sole of the foot, direct tenderness behind and below the medial malleolus, a positive Tinel sign, conduction deficits, and denervation of the abductor hallucis may be present in any combination. Proximal spread of symptoms and signs is often observed. Electrodiagnostic studies should document the lesion, when present. Given a maximum normal latency of 6.1 msec for the medial plantar nerve and 6.7 msec for the lateral nerve, any excess is considered abnormal.[22] Several authors have found latencies between 6.1 msec and 9 msec in this disorder.[8, 14, 22]

The tarsal tunnel itself is composed of the medial malleolus superiorly, the flexor retinaculum superficially, and the medial aspect of talus and calcaneus on its deep surface. The abductor hallucis muscle arises from the flexor retinaculum. Beneath this muscle the posterior tibial vessels and medial and lateral plantar nerves pass into the foot. The veins that accompany the tibial vessels also participate in the compression process. Inflation of a tourniquet to compress venous outflow increases symptoms of the tarsal tunnel syndrome.[28]

Treatment is surgical, once the diagnosis has been established. The flexor retinaculum is divided, and a neurolysis is performed proximally and distally. Internal neurolysis should be performed if the nerve itself is fibrotic or if there has been major trauma or vascular insufficiency in the region.

Medial and Lateral Plantar Nerves

These nerves have been involved in entrapment syndromes, usually as they pass under the abductor hallucis muscle. Medial plantar neurapraxia (jogger's foot)[43] has been described as a syndrome of burning heel pain, aching in the arch, and reduced sensation on the sole of the foot

behind the great toe. It is postulated that running with the foot in valgus position produces the disorder. Lidocaine injections into the point of tenderness where the abductor hallucis crosses the tubercle of the navicular bone should relieve the pain. Nonirritating steroid infiltration of the region, rest, and a change in the position of the foot at ground contact should relieve the disorder.

Plantar Interdigital Nerves

The *plantar interdigital nerves* are the terminal sensory branches of the medial and lateral plantar nerves. A disorder of these nerves (usually in the third interspace between the third and fourth metatarsal heads) is known as *interdigital neuroma*, or *Morton's metatarsalgia*.[40] Symptoms consist of severe pain in the metatarsal region. The pain is often poorly localized but at times clearly radiates into the toes. Usually the third and fourth toes are involved, but all or any can be. The pain usually develops during ambulation and necessitates rest and often removal of the shoe.

The lesion is well known, but has not been regularly included in the entrapment neuropathies. It is considered to be a disorder of the intraneural connective tissue and is characterized by formation of a thickening of the nerve at its point of bifurcation into the proper digital nerves. Vascular phenomena have been implicated in interdigital neuroma,[41] but these have not been demonstrated in recent studies.[30] The anatomic determinant of the lesion appears to be the relation of the plantar digital nerve to the deep transverse metatarsal ligament between the heads of the metatarsals. The nerve, with the vascular bundle running to the toes, passes below the ligament and emerges between the slips of the plantar fascia that run to the toes. With dorsiflexion of the toes and the metatarsophalangeal joints, the nerve and vessels are angulated over the leading edge of the transverse ligaments.[24, 25] The third nerve is formed from a conjunction of the medial and lateral plantar nerves and is relatively more fixed than the other digital nerves and is more vulnerable.

Several factors can accentuate stress on this nerve during walking. These include a high arch (cavus) configuration, weakness of the intrinsic toe flexors and the peroneus longus muscle, and high-heeled shoes. The intrinsic muscles restrain dorsiflexion of the toes, and the posterior tibial and peroneus longus muscles produce a varus rotation of the foot during the last part of stance phase, all reducing pressure on the metatarsal head region. A dynamic gait pattern reduces stress, whereas a passive pattern leads to higher loading. Repeated trauma at the edge of the ligament or under it can produce nerve irritation and fibrosis, as well as irritation and fibrosis of the digital vessels.

A study of 105 cases of Morton's metatarsalgia by light and electron microscopy demonstrated neural lesions in 75.[30] Findings included thickening and hyalinization of the walls of the endoneural vessels, endoneural edema, hypertrophy of the neural connective tissue, and demyelinization of nerve fibers without wallerian degeneration. In late cases there was diffuse intermingling of perineural cells with epineural tissue, the nerves being transformed into cords of connective tissue. Under the electron microscope, connective tissue cell processes were similar to those of other compression neuropathies and were not due to primary vascular disease or local inflammation. There were no neoplastic changes.

Treatment of interdigital neuroma has included stress-transfer shoe correction, exercise programs that strengthen the foot musculature and modify the gait pattern, and surgical excision of the irritated nerve. Each of these programs deserves some consideration.

Since the digital nerve is compressed over the leading edge of the transverse metatarsal ligament, a shoe correction that lessens pressure on the metatarsal heads and reduces dorsiflexion of the metatarsophalangeal joints will reduce pain and, in many instances, lead to gradual resolution of the lesion. Required shoe modifications include a well-fitted oxford-type shoe, a metatarsal bar and pad, and a low heel. To avoid excess pressure on the forepart of the foot, there must be adequate space in the shoes. Lateral compression on the foot creates excess loading in the middle of the metatarsal head row and does not allow for varus rotation of the subtalar joint and

plantar flexion of the first metatarsal at the end of stance phase. Longitudinal support and containment of the mid- and hindfoot control the shape of the foot and permit normal intertarsal rotations during gait. The metatarsal bar acts in two ways, to concentrate ground reaction forces posterior to the point of nerve sensitivity and to reduce metatarsophalangeal dorsiflexion at toe-off. To accomplish these, the bar must be placed posterior to the metatarsal heads, not under them. In addition, the bar should be contoured, similar to a rocker bar.

To ensure adequate position of the bar in the shoe, the distance from the posterior edge of the metatarsal heads to the back of the heel must be measured and specific instructions given as to placement. The bar is often placed erroneously under, not behind, the metatarsal heads. The bar is best positioned between the two soles of a support shoe, not on the undersurface of the outer sole. A contoured-soled clog will have a similar effect and blocks metatarsophalangeal motion. It can be prescribed as an alternate shoe for indoor wear.

A metatarsal pad set behind the point of tenderness is also useful. Placement is determined by measuring the distance from the back of the heel to the region to be protected.

Foot exercises can be useful if performed properly and if they serve as a guide for a more dynamic gait pattern. The goal is to strengthen the peroneus longus, tibialis posterior, and intrinsic foot musculature. The patient toes in and rolls to the outer side of the foot (inversion of subtalar joint), curling the toes at the same time. This accentuates cavus (pronation at the first metatarso-tarsal joint). Ambulation for one to two minutes with the heel of the leading foot just touching the toe of the following foot is performed two to three times daily. The patient should be encouraged to do the exercises during the day while wearing shoes and standing. This strengthens the musculature and reduces pressure on the affected nerve. Picking up marbles with the toes serves as a useful drill for the ambulation exercise.

Surgical excision of the "neuroma" is advocated as an acceptable and effective procedure and is often curative. Once the irritative lesion is excised, a true neuroma develops at the cut nerve end. If this neuroma is exposed to pressure or if it becomes bound to scar between the metatarsal heads, severe pain may develop. Disability can then be greater than prior to excision. Pain may require extensive secondary surgical procedures to divide the nerve farther back in the foot. To avoid this situation, certain precautions should be taken. If the standard dorsal approach is used, the transverse metatarsal ligament must be divided to ensure excision of the proper digital nerve behind the metatarsal heads and transverse ligament. Magnification is useful to distinguish nerve from vessels and to avoid excess scarring when a block excision is performed.

The plantar approach to the lesion by a transverse incision near the plantar metatarsophalangeal joint crease is quite useful. This permits adequate demonstration of all structures in the region. The nerve can be resected behind the ligament with ease, and scarring is minimal following this approach. Magnification is helpful in this procedure.

Following surgery the forepart of the foot must be protected. A sneaker is useful as a postoperative shoe for two weeks. Protective oxford shoes and/or clogs should be worn for several months to avoid the occasional problem with excess pain. The patient should be prepared for these steps to obtain a successful result.

Sural Nerve

The sural nerve arises from the tibial nerve 3 cm above the knee joint. It lies deep beneath the deep fascia in the popliteal region and proximal leg. The nerve runs between the heads of the gastrocnemius in 38 per cent of specimens and on the soleus in 40 per cent.[26] It then pierces the deep fascia of the leg two thirds of the distance from the knee to the heel and gives off cutaneous branches to the distal quarter of the leg, lateral cutaneous branches to the heel, and branches to the dorsum of the foot. In 40 per cent of specimens the sural nerve receives an anastomotic branch from the peroneal nerve, i.e., the sural communicating or lateral sural nerve. When the medial and lateral sural nerves unite, a true sural nerve is formed. In the other instances the nerves pass separately to the distal leg and foot.

The medial sural nerve can be trapped as it passes through the deep fascia of the leg, but in most cases it is post-traumatic scarring behind the lateral malleolus that produces a compressive phenomenon. Pringle and associates[42] reported on four cases of sural nerve entrapment relieved by neurolysis. Localized tenderness with pain and paresthesias referred to the lateral aspect of the foot were present in three cases.

Painful Heel Syndrome

This is a disorder, usually of unknown etiology, that produces intense pressure-related pain in the heel. About 10 per cent of cases can be ascribed to a rheumatoid or systemic inflammatory disorder. Although many physicians believe that the ossification in the origin of the plantar fascia, called a "heel spur," is causative, there is no statistical correlation between this ossification and the disorder. In any event, the ledge of bone lies horizontally rather than vertically and would not be expected to cause pain.

Of interest is the relation of the calcaneal branches of the medial plantar nerve and sural nerve to the deep fascia and inferior surface of the posterior calcaneal tubercle. The character of the pain is quite similar to that in other entrapment neuropathies. Weight transfer modification of the shoe usually relieves the disorder although anti-inflammatory drugs such as indomethacin (Indocin) may be required as well. When the pain is intense and tenderness is localized, injections of local anesthetic and nondepository and noncrystalline corticosteroids may be useful, but the injections are quite painful.

COMPARTMENT SYNDROMES

Thomas E. Whitesides, Jr., M.D.

Compartment syndromes of the extremities were initially described in the forearm, the classic description being that of Volkmann. The necessity for early fasciotomy has been recognized for decades. The pathologic findings of the infarct in the forearm have been well established by Seddon, and the surgical principles of infarct release, tendon neurolysis, and tendon transfers to improve sensation and function in the hand and to avoid the severe contractures have been long and well established.

Compartment syndromes of the lower extremity are probably more common than those in the upper extremity. In the upper extremity the hand is the involved terminal organ; in the lower extremity the involved organ is the foot. There are four well-defined fascial compartments in the leg. The anterior and peroneal compartments are fascially bound enclosures in which muscles are present and nerves pass. The posterior musculature of the leg is contained in two other compartments that are quite different. The gastrocnemius and soleus are in a superficial compartment containing no neurovascular bundles passing to the foot. This compartment is not rigidly bound by fascia and rarely is involved in a compartment syndrome. The deep posterior compartment contains extrinsic musculature to the foot and, more importantly, contains the tibial nerve and vessels to the foot. Infarction of this compartment causes pathologic changes in the foot that correspond to those seen in the usual compartment syndrome in the volar aspect of the forearm — plantar flexion deformity at the ankle, loss of sensation due to neural involvement, and clawing of the toes secondary to intrinsic imbalance and contracture.

Compartment syndromes occur when there is swelling of the muscular contents of the compartment beyond the elastic limits of the surrounding fascia, thus resulting in an increased pressure in the compartment. When this pressure rises to a level sufficient to impede circulation to the structures in the compartment for a long enough period of time, functional damage occurs to the nerve and muscle.

Scarring then can also occur in the muscle and secondarily involves the nerve. The causes of swelling in the compartments are many — trauma to the leg with or without fracture, temporary ischemia due to arterial occlusion, bleeding and swelling secondary to operative procedures, burns, overuse, inappropriate intra-arterial drug injection, chronic external pressure occurring secondary to positioning in patients comatose from drug abuse or central nervous system problems, and others.

Recent studies have suggested that the tissues of the leg can tolerate four hours of ischemia with little, if any, residual permanent damage. Eight hours of total ischemia yields complete infarction and involvement of both neural and muscular structures. Ischemia of six hours is crucial in that swelling occurs that may prolong the ischemia. With fasciotomy, quite dramatic recovery may take place; without fasciotomy, progression to a totally scarred muscle with secondary nerve involvement may occur. Measurement of tissue pressure is not available as a clinical tool. Considerable argument still goes on as to what level of pressure is tolerable over what period of time before ischemia occurs. I am of the conviction that capillary perfusion to tissues inside compartments ceases completely at diastolic pressure. Peripheral pulses are generally present with no evidence of distal ischemia at that point. However, the patient may exhibit severe pain and neural loss. Circulation begins diminishing rapidly as the tissue pressure rises to within 20 mm Hg of diastolic pressure. If this situation occurs, fasciotomy is urgent (certainly if distal neural deficits and paralysis are present).

Isolated compartment syndromes of the foot and hand have been reported to me verbally from a number of sources and have generally been secondary to burns and direct trauma (e.g., crush injuries). Markedly elevated tissue pressures have been observed, and fasciotomy has been felt to be effective in providing relief. Those procedures done in the foot have been via the medial approach of Arnold Henry, taking down the "master knot" and thus opening the entire plantar aspect of deep foot anatomy. Wound closure has usually been by secondary intent and occasionally by delayed closure.

Contractures involving the superficial posterior compartment are less common, as the gastrocnemius-soleus muscles are not in a tight fascial compartment. Such contracture generally causes a pure equinus deformity without neural embarrassment, as no neural or vascular structures pass through this compartment en route to the foot. Thus, this compartment syndrome is very rare.

Isolated peroneal compartment syndromes are unusual. Owing to the involvement of the superficial peroneal nerves, slightly more sensory loss occurs and loss of strength of the peroneal musculature is present in these disorders. Neurolysis would be difficult but severance of the peroneal tendons in the presence of severe contracture would seem appropriate. This is a rare syndrome and generally requires little treatment other than a stable shoe.

Anterior compartment syndrome, which results in infarction of all musculature with loss of the deep branch of the peroneal nerve, causes one of two situations as regards the foot. In either instance there is a mild loss of sensation and loss of function of the short toe extensors (this is of little consequence). There is either a "drop-foot" gait or the compartment forms a contracture in a shortened position — thus creating a tenodesis that holds the foot up. This latter situation would seem more favorable, as an orthosis is not needed. In the presence of an isolated anterior compartment syndrome with a "drop-foot" gait, appropriate tendon transfers or the use of orthotic devices to compensate for the dropfoot situation could be used when clinically appropriate. The presence of an iatrogenic but fortuitous tenodesis should likely be left unchanged.

Isolated infarction of the deep posterior compartment is most common following tibial fractures. It is devastating in that an equinus contracture, more severely involving the flexor hallucis longus than the other muscles, is generally present as a result of muscle infarction. Frequently, the great toe will forcefully plantarflex when the foot is dorsiflexed, owing to the severity of this contracture. More important, there is loss of sensation in the sole of the foot and a loss of innervation to the intrinsic musculature. A clawfoot results, with claw deformities of the toes and inability to dorsiflex the forefoot effectively as a result of the unopposed extrinsic extensors. In addition, alterations of the sole of the foot are often present secondary to the loss of sensation. In the acute phase, the same principles established by Seddon for treatment of the volar musculature to the hand and median nerve are applicable to this lower extremity compartment. Resection of the infarct to release contractures in the deep posterior compartment is indicated, along with neurolysis of the tibial nerve. This procedure is done with the patient prone. A long posteromedial incision is made, carrying out a Z-lengthening procedure of the Achilles tendon. The soleus muscle is then detached from its tibial origin up proximal to the soleus bridge, exposing the deep posterior compartment throughout its length. The tibial nerve is neurolysed throughout the length of the muscular scarring and either the contracted muscles are excised or the tendons are severed or lengthened. Reconstruction of the foot in the latter situation would require correction of the fixed hammer toe deformity, plantar fasciotomy (if appropriate), and an intrinsic muscular reconstruction either by transfer of a flexor tendon to the extensor mechanism (if the flexor musculature still works) or by transfer of the extrinsic long toe extensors to the metatarsal necks to provide forefoot dorsiflexion. Other tendon transfers are generally neither effective nor available and orthoses are not helpful unless provision is made for a "dropfoot" or ankle instability. If contracture and lack of sensation cause a severe deformity and if persistence or recurrence of ulceration is a problem, an amputation through a more proximal sensible area may become necessary.

Involvement of all four compartments is rather common. The problem that then predominates in the leg is generally the equinus contracture and the loss of function of the tibial nerve. As the foot is otherwise flaccid, a dynamic clawing contracture is not likely. In this situation, neurolysis of the tibial nerve may be indicated even some months following injury in the hope of obtaining protective sensation. Release of contractures to allow orthotic devices to position the foot for a plantigrade gait is indicated. If satisfactory foot posture cannot be so obtained, a reconstructive procedure of the bony architecture may be in order (triple arthrodesis, os calcis osteotomy, and so forth). However, if the lack of sensation persists and recurrent ulceration cannot be managed, an amputation at a level with appropriate sensation (preferably below the knee) is in order and yields a more continually functional lower extremity for an active patient.

The above descriptions apply to the adult patient. If the compartment syndrome and its secondary problems occur in the face of future bony growth, secondary deformities and shortening can occur and more complex situations are likely to arise. Combinations of treatment may then be in order.

REFERENCES

1. Babcock, W. W.: A standard technique for operations on peripheral nerves with special reference to the closure of large gaps. Surg. Gynecol. Obstet., 45:364, 1927.
2. Benjamin, H. A., and Nagler, W.: Peripheral nerve damage resulting from local hemorrhage and ischemia. Arch. Phys. Med. Rehab., 54:263, 1973.
3. Brooks, D. M.: Nerve compression by simple ganglia: A review of thirteen collected cases. J. Bone Joint Surg., 34-B:391, 1952.
4. Brown, W. F., et al.: The location of conduction abnormalities in human entrapment neuropathies. J. Can. Sci. Neurol., 3:111, 1976. Cited in Sunderland, S.: Nerves and Nerve Injuries. Edinburgh, Churchill Livingstone, 1978.
5. Carrel, J., and Davidson, D.: Nerve compression syndromes of the foot and ankle. J. Am. Pod. Assn., 65:322, 1975.
6. Curtis, R. M., and Eversmann, W. M., Jr.: Internal neurolysis as an adjunct to the treatment of the carpal tunnel syndrome. J. Bone Joint Surg., 55-A:733, 1973.
7. Duchenne, G. B.: The Physiology of Motion (1867). Philadelphia, J. B. Lippincott, 1949 (Kaplan, E. B., translator and editor).
8. Edvards, W. G., Lincoln, C. R., Bassett, F. H., III, and Goldner, J. L.: The tarsal tunnel syndrome, J.A.M.A., 207:716, 1969.
9. Elftman, H.: Dynamic structure of the human foot. Artif. Limbs, 13:49, 1969.
10. Ellis, V. H.: Two cases of ganglia in the sheath of the peroneal nerve. Br. J. Surg., 24:141, 1936.
11. Fettweis, E.: A cause of sciatic pain: Nontraumatic peroneal nerve compression. German Med. Month, 13:535, 1968. Cited in Sunderland, S.: Nerves and Nerve Injuries. Edinburgh, Churchill Livingstone, 1978.
12. Gasser, H. S.: Conduction in nerves in relation to fiber types. Ass. Res. Nerv. Ment. Dis., 15:35, 1935.
13. Gasser, H. S.: Pain producing impulses in peripheral nerves. Ass. Res. Nerv. Ment. Dis., 23:44, 1943.
14. Goodgold, J., and Eberstein, S.: Electrodiagnosis of Neuromuscular Diseases. 2nd Ed., Baltimore, Williams and Wilkins, 1977
15. Goodgold, J., Koppell, H. P., and Spielholtz, N. J.: The tarsal tunnel syndrome: Objective diagnostic criteria. N. Engl. J. Med., 273:742, 1965.
16. Gristina, A. G., Thompson, W. A. L., Kester, N., Walsh, W., and Gristina, J. A.: Treatment of neuropathic conditions of the foot and ankle with a patella-tendon bearing brace. Arch. Phys. Med. Rehab., 54:562, 1973.
17. Haimovici, H.: Peroneal sensory neuropathy entrapment syndrome. Arch. Surg., 105:586, 1972.
18. Helm, D. A., Nepomuceno, C., and Crane, C. R.: Tibial nerve dysfunction during pregnancy. South. Med. J., 64:1493, 1971.
19. Henry, A. K.: Extensile Exposure Applied to Limb Surgery. 1st Ed. Baltimore, Williams and Wilkins, 1945.
20. Holmes, W., Highet, W. B., and Seddon, H. J.: Ischemic nerve lesions occurring in Volkmann's contracture. Br. J. Surg., 32:259, 1944.
21. Jahss, M.: Diaphysectomy for severe acquired overlapping fifth toe and advance fixed hammering of the small toes. In Bateman, J. E., (ed.): Foot Science. Philadelphia, W. B. Saunders, 1976, pp. 211–221.
22. Johnson, E. W., and Ortiz, P. R.: Electrodiagnosis of tarsal tunnel syndrome. Arch. Phys. Med., 47:776, 1966.
23. Keck, C.: The tarsal tunnel syndrome. J. Bone Joint Surg., 44-A:180, 1962.
24. Kopell, H. P., and Thompson, W. A. L.: Peripheral entrapment neuropathies of the lower extremity. N. Engl. J. Med., 56:262, 1960.
25. Kopell, H. P., and Thompson, W. A. L.: Peripheral Entrapment Neuropathies. Baltimore, Williams and Wilkins, 1963.
26. Kosinski, C.: The course, mutual relations and distribution of the cutaneous nerves in the metazonal region of the leg and foot. J. Anat., 60:274, 1926.
27. Kummel, B. M., and Zazanis, G. A.: Shoulder pain as the presenting complaint in carpal tunnel syndrome. Clin. Orthop. Rel. Res., 92:227, 1973.
28. Lam, S. J. S.: Tarsal tunnel syndrome. J. Bone Joint Surg., 49-B:87, 1967.
29. Lang, J.: Uber das Bindegewebe und Die Gefasse der Nerven. Z. Anat. Entw-Gesch., 123:61, 1962.
30. Lassman, G., Lassman H., and Stockinger, L.: Morton's metatarsalgia. Virchow's Arch. Pathol. Anat., 370:307, 1976.
31. Lemont, H.: The branches of the superficial peroneal nerve and their clinical significance. J. Am. Pod. Assn., 65:310, 1975.
32. Leonard, M.: Immediate improvements of sensation on relief of extraneural compression. J. Bone Joint Surg., 51-A:1282, 1967.
33. Levine, J., and Spinner, M.: Neurolysis in elderly patients. Clin. Orthop. Rel. Res., 80:13, 1971.
34. Lubinska, L.: Axoplasmic streaming in regenerating and in normal nerve fibers. In Mechanism of Neural Regeneration. Progress in Brain Research. Vol. 13, Amsterdam, Singer and Schade, 1964. Cited in Sunderland, S.: Nerves and Nerve Injuries. Edinburgh, Churchill Livingstone, 1978.
35. Lundborg, G.: Ischemic nerve injury: Experimental studies on intraneural microvascular pathophysiology and nerve function in a limb subjected to temporary circulatory arrest. Scand. J. Plast. Reconstr. Surg., Suppl. 6, 1970.
36. Lundborg, G.: Limb ischemia and nerve injury. Arch. Surg., 104:631, 1972.
37. Lusskin, R., and Battista, A.: Internal neurolysis after post-traumatic and post-ischemic neuropathies. (Unpublished data).
38. Lusskin, R., Campbell, J. B., and Thompson, W. A. L.: Post-traumatic lesions of the brachial plexus. Treatment by transclavicular exploration and neurolysis or autograft reconstruction. J. Bone Joint Surg., 55-A:1159, 1973.
39. Mangieri, J. V.: Peroneal nerve injury from an enlarged fabella. J. Bone Joint Surg, 55-A:395, 1973.
40. Morton, T. G.: A peculiar and painful affection of the

fourth metatarsophalangeal articulation. Am. J. Med. Sci., 71:37, 1876,

41. Nisson, K. I.: Plantar digital neuritis — Morton's meta-tarsalgia. J. Bone Joint Surg., 30-B:84, 1948.

42. Pringle, R. M., Protherve, K., and Mukherjee, S. K.: Entrapment neuropathy of the sural nerve. J. Bone Joint Surg., 56-B:465, 1974.

43. Rask, M.: Medial plantar neurapraxia (jogger's foot). Clin. Orthop. Rel. Res., 134:193, 1978.

44. Redford, J. B.: Nerve conduction in motor fibers to the anterior tibial muscle in peroneal palsy. Arch. Phys. Med., 45:500, 1964.

45. Roberts, J. T.: The effect of occlusive arterial diseases of the extremities on the blood supply of nerves. Experimental and clinical studies on the role of the vasa nervorum. Am. Heart. J., 35:369, 1948.

46. Rydvik, B., Lundborg, G., and Nordbord, C.: Intraneural tissue reactions induced by internal neurolysis. Scand. J. Plast. Reconstr. Surg., 10:3, 1976.

47. Saito, A., and Zacks, S. I.: Fine structure observations of denervation and reinnervation of neuromuscular junctions in mouse foot muscle. J. Bone Joint Surg., 51-A:1163, 1969.

48. Seddon, H. J.: Clarification of nerve injuries. Br. Med. J., 2:237, 1942.

49. Seddon, H. J.: Three types of nerve injuries. Brain, 66:237, 1943.

50. Sidney, J. D.: Weak ankles: A study of common peroneal entrapment neuropathy. Br. Med. J., 3:623, 1969.

51. Singh, N., Behse, F., and Buchthal, F.: Electrophysiological study of peroneal nerve palsy. J. Neurol. Neurosurg. Psychiatr., 37:1202, 1974.

52. Speigal, I. J., and Lewin, P.: Tourniquet paralysis: Analysis of three cases of surgically proved peripheral nerve damage following use of rubber tourniquet. J.A.M.A., 129:432, 1945. Cited in Sunderland, S.: Nerves and Nerve Injuries. Edinburgh, Churchill Livingstone, 1978.

53. Subotnick, S.: Compartment syndromes in lower extremities. J. Am. Pod. Assn., 65:342, 1975.

54. Sunderland, S.: A classification of peripheral nerve injuries producing loss of function. Brain, 74:491, 1951.

55. Sunderland, S.: Nerves and Nerve Injuries. Edinburgh, Churchill Livingstone, 1978.

56. Sunderland, S., and Bradley, K. C.: The cross-sectional area of peripheral nerve trunks devoted to nerve fibers. Brain, 72:428, 1949.

57. Sunderland, S., and Bradley, K. C.: Rate of advance of Hoffmann-Tinel sign in regenerating nerves. Arch. Neurol. Psychiatr., 67:650, 1952.

58. Sunderland, S., and Bradley, K. C.: Stress-strain phenomena in human peripheral nerve trunks. Brain, 84:102, 1961.

59. Sunderland, S., and Roche, A. F.: Axon-myelin relationships in peripheral nerve fibers. Acta Anat., 33:1, 1958.

60. Variations in the distribution of the cutaneous nerves on the dorsum of the foot. Report of Committee of Collective Investigation of the Anatomical Society of Great Britain and Ireland. J. Anat. Physiol., 26:1891.

61. Wadstein, T.: Two cases of ganglia in the sheath of the peroneal nerve. Acta Orthop. Scand., 2:221, 1931.

Compartment Syndromes

62. Ashton, H.: Critical closure in human limbs. Br. Med. Bull., 19:149, 1963.

63. Bradley, E. L., III: The anterior tibial compartment syndrome. Surg. Gynecol. Obstet., 136:289, 1973.

64. Burton, A. C.: On the physical equilibrium of small blood vessels. Am. J. Physiol., 164:319, 1951.

65. Burton, A. C.: Physical principles of circulatory phenomena. In Hamilton, W. F., (ed.): Handbook of Physiology. Vol. 1, Washington, D.C., American Physiological Society, 1962.

66. Cooper, R. R.: Alterations during immobilization and regeneration of skeletal muscle in cats. J. Bone Joint Surg., 54-A:919, 1972.

67. Dahlback, L. O.: Effects of temporary tourniquet ischemia on striated muscle fibers and motor end-plates. Scand. J. Plast. Reconstr. Surg., Suppl. 7, 1970.

68. Dahn, I., Lassen, N. A., and Westling, H.: Blood flow in human muscles during external pressure or venous stasis. Clin. Sci., 32:467, 1967.

69. French, E. Z., and Price, W. H.: Anterior tibial pain. Br. Med. J., 2:1290, 1962.

70. Harman, J. W., and Guinn, R. P.: The recovery of skeletal muscle fibers from acute ischemia as determined by histologic and chemical methods. Am. J. Pathol., 25:741, 1948.

71. Henderson, Y., Oughterson, A. W., Greenberg, L. A., and Searle, C. P.: Muscle tonus, intramuscular pressure and the venopressor mechanism. Am. J. Physiol., 114:261, 1936.

72. Henry, A.: Extensile Exposure. 2nd Ed. Baltimore, Williams and Wilkins, 1970.

73. Jennings, A. M. C.: Some observations of critical closing pressures in the peripheral circulation of anesthetized patients. Br. J. Anaesth., 36:683, 1964.

74. Kelly, R. P., and Whitesides, T. E., Jr.: Transfibular route for fasciotomy of the leg. In Proceedings of the American Association of Orthopaedic Surgeons, J. Bone Joint Surg. 49-A:1022, 1967.

75. Leach, R. E., Hammond, G., and Stryker, W. S.: Anterior tibial compartment syndrome. Acute and chronic. J. Bone Joint Surg., 49-A:451, 1967.

76. Lewis, T.: Vascular Disorders of the Limbs. London, Macmillan, Inc., 1935.

77. Matsen, F. A., III, and Clawson, D. K.: The deep posterior compartment syndrome of the leg. J. Bone Joint Surg., 57-A:34, 1975.

78. Paton, D. F.: The pathogenesis of anterior tibial syndrome. An illustrative case, J. Bone Joint Surg., 50-B:383, 1968.

79. Pellegrino, C., and Tranpini, C.: An EM study of degeneration atrophy in red and white muscle fiber. J. Cell Biol., 17:327, 1963.

80. Rorabeck, C. H., Macnab, I., and Waddell, J. P.: Anterior tibial compartment syndrome: a clinical and experimental review. Can. J. Surg., 15:249, 1972.

81. Scully, R. E., Shannon, J. M., and Dickerson, J. R.: Factors involved in recovery from experimental skeletal ischemia in dogs. Am. J. Pathol., 39:721, 1961.

82. Seddon, H. J.: Volkmann's ischemia in the lower limb. J. Bone Joint Surg., 48-B:627, 1966.

83. Vogt. Quoted by Horn, C. E.: Acute ischaemia of the anterior tibial muscle and long extensor muscles of the toes. J. Bone Joint Surg., 27:615, 1945.

84. von Volkmann. R.: Verletzungen und Krankheiten der Bewegungsorgane. Handbuch der allgemeinen und speciellen Chirurgie, 1872.

85. Walker, J. W., Paletta, F. X., and Cooper, T.: The relationship of post-ischemic histopathological changes to muscle and subcuticular temperature patterns in the canine extremity. Surg. Forum, 10:836, 1959.

86. Whitesides, T. E., Jr., Harada, H., and Morimoto, K.: The response of skeletal muscle to temporary ischemia: an experimental study. In Proceedings of the American Association of Orthopaedic Surgeons. J. Bone Joint Surg., 53-A:1027, 1971.

87. Whitesides, T. E., Jr., Haney, T. C., Morimoto, K., and Harada, H.: Tissue pressure measurements as a determinant for the need of fasciotomy. Clin.Orthop., 113:43, 1975.

88. Whitesides, T. E., Jr., Harada, H., and Morimoto, K.: Compartment syndromes and the role of fasciotomy, its parameters and techniques. AAOS Instructional Course Lectures, 26:179, 1977.

89. Wiederhielm, C. A., and Weston, B. V.: Microvascular, lymphatic, and tissue pressures in the unanesthetized mammal. Am. J. Physiol., 225:992, 1973.

90. Willhoite, D. R., and Moll, J. H.: Early recognition and treatment of impending Volkmann's ischemia in the lower extremity. Arch. Surg., 100:11, 1970.

CHAPTER 44

MISCELLANEOUS PERIPHERAL NEUROPATHIES AND NEUROPATHY-LIKE SYNDROMES

*Melvin H. Jahss, M.D.,
and Ralph Lusskin, M.D.*

Peripheral neuropathy is a general classification indicating degeneration of a sensory and/or a motor nerve or nerves anywhere from the root to the most terminal endings, including the ganglion, nerve trunk, or more distal segments. Specific neurologic disorders, toxins, metabolic disorders, and systemic diseases may affect one or more portions of the peripheral sensory or motor systems. The classification of peripheral neuropathies is based upon these specific disorders and diseases. When the etiology is unknown, the initial diagnosis is often made by determining which of the specific nerve elements are damaged. Peripheral nerve function may be damaged or interfered with by direct trauma, compression, oxygen deprivation, direct toxic action, scar tissue, local infiltration, tumors, loss of blood supply, genetic defects, neurologic degenerative disorders, and infection; as well as by interference with electrical, metabolic, or chemical modes of nerve transmission; congenital lack of development of the means of transmission; more central damage or cerebral interference with or indif-ference to nerve transmission; and even by allergic and immune responses. Peripheral neuropathy may be a discrete localized entity but, more often, is part of a more generalized neurologic or systemic disorder.

Peripheral neuritis may be primarily a sensory neuritis, a motor neuritis, or a sensorimotor neuritis. When more than one nerve is involved, the term polyneuritis is used; however, if only one nerve is involved, the disorder is called a mononeuritis. A neurologic disorder may be essentially a multiple motor neuritis, as in the Guillain-Barré syndrome, although most forms of polyneuritis are sensorimotor in type. The majority of cases of polyneuritis tend to be symmetric and involve essentially distal nerve elements. However, the level of involvement may occur much more proximally, and sensory and motor damage may even be asymmetric and spotty, as in the nerve root involvement of lues or in multiple sclerosis.

Patients with peripheral neuropathy or a neuropathy-like condition, even if it is only a minor part of a more generalized neurologic or systemic disorder, are usually not only unaware of their neuropathy but of the underlying disorder as well. More often than not, the symptoms are minimal, often quite vague, and seemingly nonanatomic, such as leg cramps. Patients are unaware of the diagnostic significance of their symptoms. Thus, they may not voluntarily describe an important symptom such as numbness of their feet and only do so when specifically asked. Superficial examination may give little more information, except possibly to reveal a small ulcer or just an old scar on a foot or end of a toe. Such persons often remain undiagnosed for many years without receiving proper care. They may lose one or both legs from secondary chronic or fulminating infection before a diagnosis is established, usually by a more comprehensive workup incidental to a hospital admission.

Early diagnosis, however, is usually possible if the examiner is made aware of the significance of the seemingly unimportant subjective complaints along with certain apparently innocuous objective findings. These diagnostic "leads" can be amplified by the astute clinician with careful history-taking combined with neurologic, orthopaedic, and systemic examination to pinpoint the pathology as well as the underlying etiology. Additional laboratory and specialized diagnostic tests or biopsy specimens (nerve, muscle) may be necessary to fully establish the diagnosis.

SENSORY AND PROPRIOCEPTIVE SYSTEMS

In order to comprehend any patient's neurologic findings, it is necessary to know how to test for the various neurologic elements and to understand the anatomic basis of any abnormal findings. Although orthopaedists are well versed in respect to the motor system, they may be at a loss in regard to the various pathologic subtleties of the sensory and proprioceptive systems, which are usually the diagnostic cues in detecting the various peripheral neuropathies.

What are the various elements of sensation and how do afferent impulses affect the reflex arc?[20] Sensation consists of pain,

temperature, touch, and pressure discrimination, which are initiated distally from specialized nerve endings and mediated by chemical transmission. All sensory fibers, exclusive of those of the autonomic nervous system, are of the large myelinated A type. Pain and temperature fibers have the smallest diameter (2 to 5 μ) and slowest conduction velocity (12 to 20 m/sec).[21] The autonomic C-type pain fibers are of the smallest and slowest variety and are nonmyelinated.

Pain consists of skin pain, determined by pinprick, as well as deep and periosteal pain. Deep pain includes visceral pain as felt with abdominal cramps, gallbladder pain, pain of vascular occlusion, headache pain, and birth pain. Deep pain objectively is determined most commonly by supraorbital pressure and squeezing the heel cord. Periosteal pain may be readily determined with a needle. Root pain, as in lues and in some forms of sensory neuropathies, is described as knifelike or as girdle pain. Incomplete peripheral nerve lesions may cause paresthesias or in larger nerve trunks may result in major causalgia. Paresthesias of the tips of the toes are characteristic of early changes in subacute combined degeneration caused by pernicious anemia. Sympathetic nerve pain is often accompanied by vasomotor changes such as excess sweating and increased warmth and redness, as seen in minor causalgia associated with Sudeck's atrophy. The response of this pain to steroids and sympathetic nerve block is well documented. One should also be aware of the phantom pain of amputated limbs and the thalamic pain of stroke patients, as well as the severe thalamic pain associated with long-standing causalgias. Pain fibers enter the dorsal roots and then relay to the contralateral lateral spinothalamic tract to the thalamus. Pain has cerebral connections. There is a pain center in the supramarginal gyrus of the parietal lobe (pain asymbolia)[114] as well as the awareness or nonawareness of pain as a noxious stimulus, as seen in congenital indifference to pain. In such patients, pain of all types may be felt as tickling. Finally, there are different thresholds of pain in different individuals, as well as pain mitigated by strong emotional response, such as fear. Anatomically, there is an overlap in regard to pain peripherally and, therefore, evaluation of touch is more clinically accurate peripherally. However, in dorsal root lesions loss of pain is more accurate than touch owing to overlap to touch by adjacent roots.[20] One must also keep in mind that peripheral sensory nerves also overlap and may vary anatomically. Thus, resection of a plantar interdigital neuroma results in minimal or, more often, no sensory loss. Transection of a small sensory nerve, nevertheless, should be avoided, as it may result in annoying tender neuroma formation.

Temperature discrimination is mediated by the same type of nerve fibers as pain and runs up the same tracts. In congenital indifference to pain, the patient is able to discriminate temperature differences, but cannot feel the pain of burns.

Sensation also includes *touch* and *pressure,* which are mediated by medium-sized A-type myelinated nerve fibers of 5 to 12 μ diameter with conduction velocities of 30 to 70 m/sec.[21] Touch sensation includes two groups. The first is light touch and light pressure. Fibers of this group enter the posterior roots, decussate to the ventral spinothalamic tracts, and then travel to the thalamus and parietal lobe. Some fibers probably also run up the posterior column, as damage to this column may lead to some decrease of touch. The second component of touch is known as tactile discrimination and includes deep pressure, two-point discrimination, and vibratory sense. These fibers also enter the dorsal roots, as do all afferent nerves, but then travel up the posterior column to the ipsilateral gracilis and cuneus and then to the thalamus and parietal lobe. Their course is the same as proprioceptive fibers. Vibratory sense is an excellent means of determining peripheral nerve, dorsal root, or posterior column damage, as it tends to diminish markedly or disappear early in the course of neurologic disease. Touch, on the other hand, due to sensory overlap peripherally and the usual incomplete involvement in peripheral neuropathy, frequently appears relatively normal and is difficult to evaluate. Deep sensibility is a term used to include vibratory sense associated with proprioception, i.e., position sense and movement. In peripheral neuropathy, position sense (e.g., in

the hallux) tends to be maintained long after vibratory sense is lost.

The last of the sensory-afferent components is proprioception. Proprioceptive fibers are the largest of the A type, fibers measuring 12 to 20 μ in diameter, and have the fastest conduction velocity of 70 to 120 m/sec.[21] Proprioception involves position sense and the stretch reflex arc, such as the deep tendon reflexes. Proprioceptive fibers also enter the dorsal roots and posterior column. They then travel up the spinocerebellar tracts, whereas other fibers go to the gracilis and cuneus on their way to the thalamus and parietal lobe. Specific proprioceptive distal nerve endings are present in the joint capsules, aponeuroses, tendon sheaths, and musculotendinous junctions, which are sensitive to pressure.[100] The nerve endings at the foot and toes are much more sensitive to minor degrees of motion than are those higher up at the musculotendinous junctions.

Proprioceptive fibers from the muscle spindles make up the afferent arm of the deep tendon reflexes. Loss of these fibers causes loss of tendon reflexes, such as the knee jerk or ankle jerk. The proprioceptive fibers synapse with the anterior horn cells along with pyramidal tract fibers, some of which are inhibitory. Therefore, pyramidal tract damage via damage to the lateral cord or brain stem (e.g., stroke) causes *release* of the proprioceptive system with *increase* of the deep tendon reflexes. Thus, in posterolateral sclerosis (associated with pernicious anemia) if the major damage is to the posterior column (proprioceptive fibers), there will be decrease in the deep tendon reflexes. If, as occasionally happens, the major damage is to the lateral (pyramidal) column, the deep tendon reflexes may be increased. Confirmatory evidence of pyramidal tract damage would be a positive Babinski sign. To further complicate matters, posterolateral sclerosis is associated with a sensorimotor polyneuritis. If either the distal afferent proprioceptive fibers or the efferent motor fibers are sufficiently damaged, the reflex arc will be broken, with absent reflexes. Confirmatory evidence of the peripheral nature of the disorder would be "glove and stocking" sensory loss, vibratory loss in the toes, and atrophy of the foot intrinsics.

The reflex arc also contains an efferent

or motor component, which, if interrupted at any level, will also cause abolition of deep tendon reflexes. This may occur distally (as in peripheral motor or sensorimotor neuropathies), higher up in the motor or ventral root (as in a herniated disc), or in the anterior horn cells (as in amyotrophic lateral sclerosis or poliomyelitis). An L5–S1 herniated disc may involve the S1 motor root, which is the main motor root responsible for the ankle jerk. Isolated root involvement, whether sensory or motor, has classic peripheral distribution. In general, deep tendon reflexes are frequently not of diagnostic value, as they are often markedly decreased in many normal individuals. Older patients often normally have depressed ankle jerks. Of greater significance are differences of deep tendon reflexes between the left and right sides or differences in activity between ankle jerks and knee jerks compared with the deep tendon reflexes of the upper extremities.

In summary, all sensory and proprioceptive afferent fibers enter the dorsal ganglia and dorsal nerve roots. Therefore, complete damage to these areas results in loss of all these modalities, including the associated deep tendon reflexes, without muscle atrophy if there is no concomitant motor nerve damage. This is the anatomic basis of hereditary sensory neuropathy. Similarly, if a neuropathy causes a peripheral polyneuritis of a sensory or sensorimotor type, all the afferent fibers may also be destroyed. This causes a similar clinical picture, but is associated with "glove and stocking" sensory nerve loss plus loss of distal proprioception, sensory discrimination, and reflexes (e.g., loss of position sense, vibratory sense, and ankle jerks, respectively).

Although the clinical examination will determine the anatomic sites of nerve damage in neurologic entities involving the foot, electrodiagnostic testing will elucidate more specific neuropathologic changes. Such testing will differentiate the axonal neuropathies seen in alcoholics from the demyelinating neuropathies seen in diabetics. Similarly, testing will also confirm interstitial neuropathies as seen in Charcot-Marie-Tooth disease and vasculitis neuropathy superimposed upon a diabetic neuropathy (see Chapter 3).

CLASSIFICATION OF PERIPHERAL NEUROPATHIES

An abbreviated classification of the causes of various peripheral nerve lesions and neuropathies is shown in Table 44–1, along with a few syndromes that may be confused with peripheral nerve pathology. Many of the diseases are rare and in others the peripheral nerve pathology represents only a minor facet of a more widespread neurologic or non-neurologic systemic disease. In many cases, the classifications merge or overlap, since spinal degenerative diseases and metabolic disorders are more often than not hereditary, whereas neurotoxins, metabolic diseases, and vitamin deficiencies all relate to their metabolic effect on the nervous system. In general, the classification is useful in assisting the examiner to obtain an appropriate history and to evaluate the patient not only neurologically but systemically in relation to the specific classifications and possible disease entities. Since treatment and prognosis are often determined by the source of the pathologic change, this classification is pragmatic. Traumatic, ischemic, and compressive neuropathies were classified separately in Chapter 43.

GENERAL EXAMINATION AND DIFFERENTIAL DIAGNOSIS OF THE NEUROPATHIC FOOT

As previously noted, most patients with neuropathic feet present a minimum of complaints. Such patients are usually adults. Pain is not a frequent symptom, since there is often associated sensory involvement. Thus a relatively painless ulcer on the foot or toes should immediately arouse suspicion. Many patients have no active ulcer, but rather healed, scarred areas from prior ulceration. These too are usually asymptomatic, whereas in a normal individual such areas would cause considerable distress. A trophic ulcer may precede any clinical evidence of a slowly developing neuropathy. Normal feet do not develop ulcers. In adults, foot ulcers are due to sensory nerve or vascular impairment, or both (as in diabetic polyneuropathy). Normal pedal pulses do not exclude vascular impairment, as the dis-

TABLE 44–1. Classification of Neuropathy and Neuropathy-like Syndromes Associated with Hereditary-Congenital, Metabolic, and Systemic Diseases°

1. Hereditary and Congenital Sensory Neuropathies
   a. Congenital indifference to pain including Riley-Day syndrome (familial dysautonomia)
   b. Hereditary sensory neuropathy—congenital and hereditary (familial) types
   c. Overlap syndromes—familial sensory neuropathy with anhidrosis
2. Spinal Lesions
   a. Benign cauda equina tumors
   b. Dysraphism and thecal tethering
   c. Spinal cerebellar diseases including Friedreich's ataxia
   d. Horn and root diseases including Charcot-Marie-Tooth disease and Roussy-Lévy syndrome
   e. Overlap syndromes—sensory neuropathy with spinal cord involvement
   f. Syringomyelia
3. Toxic Neuropathies
   a. Alcoholic peripheral neuropathy
   b. Heavy metals (lead, phosphorus, thallium, arsenic, mercury), methyl alcohol, Jamaica ginger paralysis, organic insecticides, and industrial products
   c. Drug-induced
4. Vascular Disorders
   a. Vasculitis
   b. Diabetic mononeuropathy multiplex
   c. Posterior tibial artery syndrome
   d. Hemoglobinopathies
   e. Leukemia (?)
5. Infections
   a. Leprosy
   b. Syphilis, yaws
   c. Diphtheria
   d. Herpes zoster
6. Metabolic and Endocrine Disorders
   a. Diabetes (plus vascular causes?)
   b. Porphyria
   c. Refsum's disease
   d. Uremic neuritis
   e. Hyperpituitarism
   f. Myxedema
   g. Acanthocytosis
   h. Tangier disease
   i. Gestational, with toxemia (?)
   j. Malignancy (?)
7. Vitamin Deficiencies
   a. Beriberi—thiamine (vitamin B_1)
   b. Pellagra—B complex vitamins
   c. Pernicious anemia—vitamin B_{12}
   d. Alcoholic
8. Direct Infiltration and Interstitial Neuropathies
   a. Primary amyloidosis
   b. Leukemia
   c. Progressive hypertrophic neuritis (Dejerine-Sottas syndrome)
9. Inflammatory Autoimmune Vasculitis
   a. Rheumatoid arthritis
   b. Periarteritis nodosa
   c. Systemic lupus erythematosus
   d. Scleroderma
10. Allergy (?)
    a. Guillain-Barré syndrome
    b. Multiple sclerosis
    c. Serum sickness

°Adapted from Merritt, H. H.: a Textbook of Neurology, 5th Ed., Philadelphia, Lea & Febiger, 1973; and Walton, J. N.: Brain's Diseases of the Nervous System, Oxford, Oxford University Press, 1977.

ease may be in the smaller arteries of the foot. Diabetic neuropathy may be associated with normal or high normal blood sugar levels. A glucose tolerance test should be performed in all patients with suspected neuropathy, even those with normal blood sugar concentrations.

Foot ulcers occur at sites of undue weight bearing, such as under the metatarsal heads and interphalangeal joint of the hallux; at areas of shoe pressure, as the end of a toe; or in areas of shear, as over the plantar lateral aspect of the forefoot. Significantly, a subungual ulcer may develop from pressure of the hallux against its nail bed caused by the toe box of a shoe. The ulcer is not obvious under the intact nail, but may be suspected by noticing a drop of pus oozing out from the free nail edge (Fig. 44–1). On careful inspection, the nail will be seen to be lifted from its bed, and some subungual purulent-sanguineous material will be noted. Removal of the nail will reveal the ulcer, which may penetrate the underlying tuft. There may be some neuropathy but vascular impairment is usually found.

Many patients with neuropathy of some duration will develop secondary infection under their toe ulcers associated with bone destruction and absorption. Surgical ablation of such toes without ever establishing a diagnosis is quite common. Occasionally, such toes remain viable, with some distortion or even gigantism (infectious gigantism).

Any child who develops a foot ulcer has a neuropathy unless proved otherwise. The possibility of congenital indifference to pain should be considered in the young child, and hereditary sensory neuropathy should be sought in teenagers and young adults, in which age group this disorder usually first becomes manifest. Rarely, a benign cord tumor or thecal tethering may occur, which is often suggested by a dimple, excess hair, sinus, or localized subcutaneous fat over the sacral area.

Patients with neuropathy may occasionally complain of vague leg cramps. Fasciculations, often not noted by the patient, may be brought out by sharply flicking the muscle with one's finger. Such fasciculations are more diagnostic of muscle degeneration, as seen in amyotrophic lateral sclerosis, than of peripheral neuropathy.

Most patients with peripheral neuropathy will have considerable atrophy of the subcutaneous tissues and intrinsic muscles of the foot. The skin over the sides of the foot appears loose (Fig. 44–2). The muscle atrophy is due to peripheral motor involvement. Since the motor neuritis usually does not extend significantly proximal to the ankle, muscle power about the

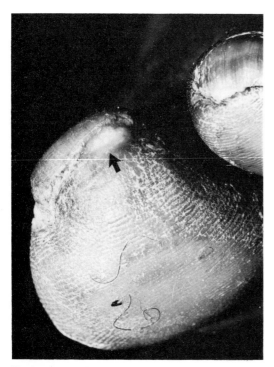

Figure 44–1. *Subungual drop of pus (arrow). It usually occurs under the nail of the hallux.*

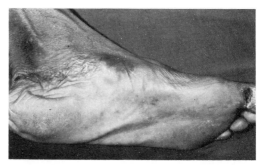

Figure 44–2. *Soft-tissue atrophy of the sides and the sole of the foot of a patient with alcoholic peripheral neuropathy. Note the old skin graft covering a previous ulcer over the medial side of the base of the hallux.*

foot and ankle is normal, and there are no secondary deformities.

Small muscle atrophy alone does not cause pes cavus or hammer-toe deformities. However, the presence of pes cavus, with or without hammer toes, is often of neurologic significance. Spinocerebellar diseases, such as Friedreich's ataxia, and hereditary neurologic disorders, such as Charcot-Marie-Tooth disease, are frequent causes of pes cavus. Charcot-Marie-Tooth disease is a fairly common disorder. It is one of the few neurologic disorders with a sex predilection, males being affected about three times more often than females, and may occur in a mendelian dominant pattern or sporadically. Charcot-Marie-Tooth disease is usually associated with a motor neuropathy involving especially the peroneal nerves and will be discussed separately. Suffice it to say, all patients with pes cavus require careful neurologic workup. Pes cavus may antedate the clinical appearance of an underlying neurologic disorder by years. Conduction velocity studies, however, may be positive at this time. Positive family history will further corroborate the diagnosis.

Many patients, when asked, will admit to some numbness of their feet and, occasionally, of their hands as well. Careful neurologic workup, especially sensory, is necessary. This includes touch, superficial and deep pain discrimination, temperature discrimination, position sense, and, above all, vibratory sense using a 128-v.p.s. tuning fork. These sensory and proprioceptive modalities should first be determined about the foot and then compared with higher levels at and above the knee, as well as in the upper extremities. Loss of vibratory sense distally over the first metatarsal head is frequently the only early clinical sign of a peripheral neuropathy as well as an early sign of Friedreich's ataxia.

The presence of vibratory sense over the first metatarsal head does not necessarily indicate normal vibration sense. More subtle quantitative loss is determined by leaving the tuning fork over the metatarsal head until the patient no longer feels vibration. The fork is then rapidly placed over a more proximal bony site. If vibration is felt here, one may conclude that there is loss of vibratory sense peripheral-

ly, since vibratory sense is normally about equal proximally and distally.

Such testing is especially important in the hereditary sensory neuropathies in which clinical neurologic findings may be minimal. One must remember that in peripheral polyneuritis, including the polyneuritis of diabetes and alcoholism (which are by far the most frequent causes), the sensory and motor findings are mainly distal — of the "glove and stocking" type. Therefore, testing only proximal to the ankles will often prove negative. As previously noted, loss of afferent proprioceptive fibers will result in loss of deep tendon reflexes, especially the more distal ankle jerks. Different neuropathies vary in their involvement of the motor and various sensory elements and will be discussed separately under "Peripheral Polyneuritis."

Miscellaneous neurologic findings may be present, such as pyramidal tract and cerebellar signs, especially in more generalized neurologic disorders involving the spinal cord and nerve roots.

Charcot joints are frequently overlooked while examining neuropathic feet. They may present as relatively nonpainful bony thickenings about Lisfranc's joint and may be mistaken for osteoarthritis. Charcot joints are not particularly tender and may be found in the ankle, talus, or metatarsophalangeal joints. They may initally present as a slightly warm, moderately tender, reddish, indurated area over a joint. X-ray studies, at this stage, are usually negative. However, acute joint destruction and dislocation may occur in four to six weeks. Treatment of Charcot joints basically consists of allowing healing while maintaining a plantigrade foot (Fig. 44–3) and is discussed in Chapters 45 and 46. One should not confuse bone absorption and joint destruction occurring under a chronic trophic neuropathic ulcer with a true Charcot joint (Fig. 44–4). Finally, the presence of multiple metatarsal fatigue fractures associated with extensive periostitis and tendency toward nonunion is typical of the Charcot foot. These fractures are usually associated with Charcot metatarsophalangeal joints (Fig. 44–5). Charcot joints are by far the most common in diabetic neuropathies, the incidence having been reported as 2.4 per cent in 500 dia-

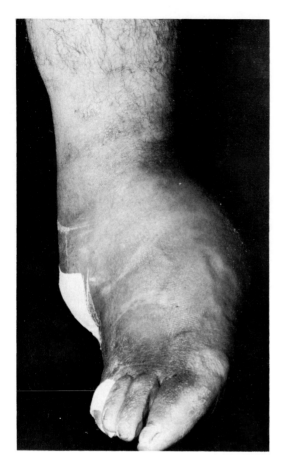

Figure 44–3. *Untreated diabetic Charcot ankle that spontaneously dislocated medially, with the lateral malleolus sloughing through the skin. Secondary infection necessitated amputation.*

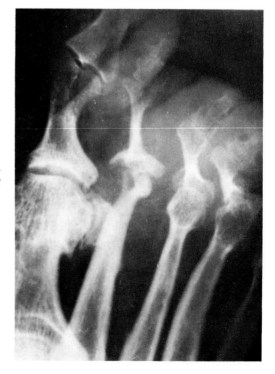

Figure 44–4. *Chronic ulcer under the second metatarsal head causing secondary pseudo-Charcot joint changes.*

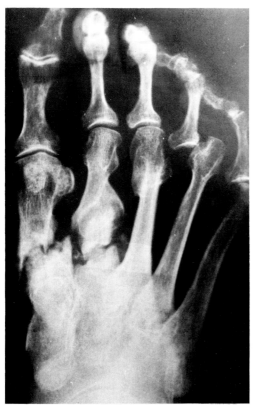

Figure 44–5. *Charcot (diabetic) metatarsals with metatarsophalangeal joint involvement. Note the dislocations of the fourth and fifth metatarsophalangeal joints before evidence of any bone changes.*

betic feet.[65] However, approximately 50 per cent of diabetic patients treated at the orthopaedic foot clinic of the Hospital for Joint Diseases have clinical evidence of neuropathy, since they are the ones who invariably develop skin breakdown and require orthopaedic management. It is most likely that in a group of diabetic patients an increasing percentage of them will ultimately develop peripheral neuropathy over time.

A Charcot joint in young children is relatively rare and is usually due to some form of congenital indifference to pain. In older children and in young adults, it may occur in hereditary sensory neuropathy, but is less frequent. It rarely occurs in association with Charcot-Marie-Tooth disease or secondary to peripheral nerve injuries. True Charcot joints are rarely seen in alcoholic neuropathies but appear rather as pseudo-Charcot joints secondary to joint destruction from overlying chronic trophic

ulcers. Finally, Charcot joints may rarely be due to or coincidental with other systemic diseases[88] (Figs. 44–6 and 44–7).

The mechanism of the development of Charcot joints has been attributed to continued weight bearing in a relatively insensitive, partially damaged joint with limited proprioceptive sense. Yet this hardly explains the often acute onset of Charcot joints, from an initially normal-appearing joint on x-ray examination to complete disorganization within four to six weeks.[77] Nor does it explain Charcot changes with normal proprioception in congenital (cerebral) indifference to pain, in which all nerve endings are anatomically intact, except for the cerebral unawareness of pain. Finally, if just lack of pain plus continued weight bearing are the instigating factors, how does one explain the development of Charcot changes in non–weight-bearing joints, such as the rapid dissolution of a shoulder joint in multiple sclerosis or syringomyelia?[77] Other unexplained changes include the peculiar formation of bone detritus and fragmentation; the often rapid resorption of bone, as in the talus; and finally the slow, spontaneous healing that occurs in spite of continued ambulation. Also of interest is that Charcot joints may develop in treated luetics, despite complete reversal of their serologic findings.[77]

Other anatomic defects are occasionally associated with more widespread neurologic disorders, such as mental retardation, scoliosis, and nerve deafness. Finally, family history is frequently of diagnostic significance. Many hereditary neurologic disorders are mendelian dominant, recessive, or sporadic. Thus, Charcot-Marie-Tooth disease may be either dominant or sporadic. Hereditary sensory neuropathy may be either congenital or familial (dominant) with clinical differences in each. The sensory loss in congenital forms is more widespread and may be associated with dull intelligence, whereas the familial form mainly involves sensory loss in the feet and legs with normal intelligence. In general, the hereditary neurologic disorders, whether transmitted or sporadic, tend to develop and appear clinically in patients in their second and third decades. In comparison, congenital neurologic disorders, such as congenital indifference to pain,

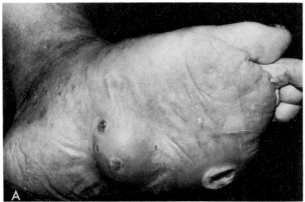

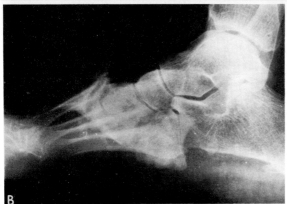

Figure 44–6. *(A) Charcot neuropathy secondary to arteritis from hemoglobinopathy (Bronx-Riverdale disease). Note the plantolateral prominence due to dislocation of the cuboid. (B) Lateral radiograph showing Charcot involvement of Lisfranc's joint with plantar dislocation of the cuboid. (C) Anteroposterior radiograph revealing the Charcot changes of Lisfranc's joint. The changes in the first metatarsophalangeal joint are pseudo-Charcot changes secondary to an overlying chronic trophic ulcer.*

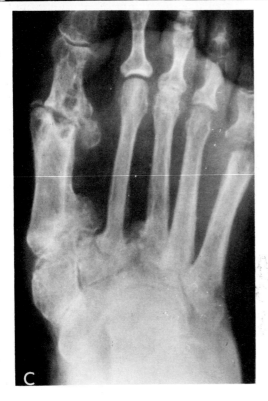

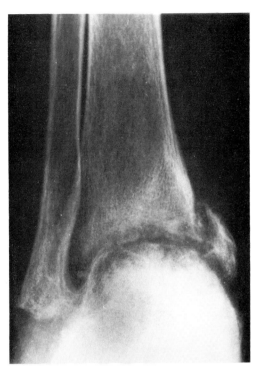

Figure 44–7. *Diabetic Charcot ankle associated with rheumatoid arthritis.*

In general, although orthopaedists are not expected to be aware of or diagnose each rare neurologic disorder, they should be able to suspect neurologic defects or a neuropathy and confirm it clinically. Although electromyographic studies may differentiate neurologic from muscular disorders, the use of conduction velocity studies should not be overlooked. The latter should include sensory conduction studies, since routine motor studies will be negative in the purely sensory neuropathies. Furthermore, the kinship of patients with suspected hereditary neurologic disorders should be investigated, remembering that positive findings in delayed velocity studies may precede the clinical appearance of the disease by years[75] and that members of a family may have abortive forms (formes frustes) of the disease. Genetic counseling in such cases is in order.

may appear clinically at birth, although they may not be diagnosed for several years.

Ethnic distribution has been documented. Congenital indifference to pain is found exclusively in Ashkenazi Jews. Charcot-Marie-Tooth disease and pes cavus in general are relatively rare in blacks.

Special testing is of importance when a peripheral neurologic disease is suspected, not only to establish the etiology but to diagnosis specific neurologic subgroups or overlap syndromes. For example, a sensory neuropathy may be diagnosed clinically and confirmed by *sensory* conduction velocity testing. Nerve biopsy specimens will then differentiate congenital indifference to pain from congenital sensory neuropathy and hereditary sensory radicular neuropathy, since such specimens are normal only in congenital indifference to pain. Genetic studies will further differentiate congenital indifference to pain, as some studies reveal D-trisomy mosaicism.

PERIPHERAL POLYNEURITIS

As noted, peripheral polyneuritis may be defined as a generalized degeneration of the distal elements of the peripheral nerves. It therefore involves the distal portions of the extremities, usually the foot. When the neuropathy is more severe, involvement may occur up to the knee; occasionally, the hands may be affected as well, but to a lesser degree. Peripheral polyneuritis is usually bilaterally symmetric and most frequently affects both motor and sensory components. Other types of peripheral neuritis also exist that may be either multiple or mononeuritis and may affect either sensory or motor or both sensory and motor elements. When the motor involvement extends proximal to the ankle, muscle weakness and imbalance will occur. Thus, in Charcot-Marie-Tooth disease, in which there may be considerable involvement of the peroneal nerves, equinovarus deformities may develop.

Although peripheral polyneuritis usually affects both motor and sensory components, it varies in degree and is usually incomplete. Thus, casual neurologic examination of a patient with relatively advanced polyneuritis may confirm the presence of touch, pinprick, and gross temperature discrimination. There will be a quantitative difference, however, if one also tests more proximally at or above the knee. As a rule, no specific nerve or nerve root distribution is found, the sensory findings roughly being of "glove and sock" or "glove and stocking" distribution. Since the motor involvement is also distal, there is no apparent motor weakness. Careful motor examination, nevertheless, will reveal atrophy of the intrinsic muscles of the foot, often with inability to spread the toes or abduct the hallux.

Frequently, the neuropathy is part of a more extensive involvement of the central nervous system, as in Charcot-Marie-Tooth disease or multiple sclerosis. When reviewing the old records of a patient with long-standing multiple sclerosis, it is not unusual to find an initial diagnosis of a sciatica attributable to a herniated disc, which in reality was a neuropathy of the sciatic nerve caused by the multiple sclerosis.

Neuropathies may also present individual characteristics. Thus, neuritis caused by diabetes, beriberi, and arsenic affects both motor and sensory components. Lead poisoning, Jamaica ginger (triorthocresyl phosphate contaminant) poisoning, and pellagra primarily affect the motor components, whereas hereditary sensory neuropathy affects only the sensory nerves. Amyloidosis and leprosy typically affect the smaller, myelinated, slower-conducting A nerve fibers, resulting in a dissociated sensory loss of pain and temperature, while preserving vibratory and position sense with intact deep tendon reflexes.[95] The patchy distribution of nerve involvement in leprosy is due to the fact that the bacillus thrives better in the exposed cooler parts of the skin, such as the face and tips of the ears.[95] Direct infiltration of a nerve (interstitial neuritis) may cause palpable nerve trunk thickening, as in leprosy and progressive hypertrophic neuritis. Periarteritis nodosa may cause multiple interstitial neuritis with nerve trunk tenderness. Individual neuropathic characteristics include pronounced tremors in mercury poisoning and paresthesias of the tips of the toes in pernicious anemia. Porphyrinuric polyneuritis may simulate Landry's ascending paralysis, and the polyneuritis of terminal cancer may occasionally simulate amyotrophic lateral

sclerosis. The pathologic and physiologic findings of the neuritis vary with the underlying etiology. Thus, a hemoglobinopathy may lead to arteritis, which, in turn, causes peripheral neuritis[88] (see Figure 44–6A to C). The peripheral neuritis, in turn, may result in Charcot joints. Whether the small vessel disease of diabetes plays a part in the development of diabetic neuropathy is as yet open to debate.

Electrodiagnostic Studies in Peripheral Neuropathy

Peripheral neuropathies are manifest by dysfunction or absent function in the nerve trunks. They tend to be grouped into those disorders that result in axon degeneration and those that produce demyelinization. These pathologic states can be identified by differences in electromyographic and nerve conduction studies.

Axon loss leads to denervation of muscles, which produces fibrillations and positive sharp waves. During the regeneration phase, polyphasic potentials appear. These changes are not characteristic of demyelinating neuropathies.

Nerve conduction studies also demonstrate changes due to varied degrees of axon loss. The total number of functioning units, motor or sensory, will determine the intensity of the sensory or motor action potential produced by electrical stimulation of the nerve trunk or skin.

The measurement of conduction velocity reflects the state of axon myelinization and the organization of the Schwann cells. Normally, myelinated nerve fibers conduct impulses not by continuous depolarization but by the discontinuous depolarization of the axon zones that are free of myelin at the nodes of Ranvier. This leads to the high-speed conduction seen in normal nerves. With demyelinization, this normal skip (saltatory) conduction between the nodes of Ranvier is lost, resulting in slower continuous transmission of nerve impulses.

Among the disorders demonstrating demyelinization are Guillain-Barré syndrome, diabetic polyneuropathy (as opposed to diabetic mononeuropathy), and Charcot-Marie-Tooth disease. Segmental or localized nerve conduction defects are seen in entrapment neuropathies, such as tarsal tunnel syndrome, but here the conduction velocity along the nerve trunk is normal. These electrodiagnostic changes will be briefly summarized under the appropriate sections for the different neuropathies. For further detail on electrodiagnostic testing see Chapter 3.

DIABETIC NEUROPATHY

The classification of diabetic neuropathy is outlined in Table 44–2.

Diabetic peripheral neuropathy, its sequelae and treatment, is discussed in Chapters 45 and 50. This section consists of an overview of the diabetic neurologic syndromes and their pathologic findings.

Diabetic Polyneuropathy

Diabetic peripheral neuropathy is by far the most common form of neuropathy. It is symmetric and sensorimotor in type and is the prime cause of Charcot joints and perforating ulcers, both of which have been previously discussed.

Diabetic polyneuropathy was often considered to be of vascular origin as a result of disease in the vasa nervorum. However, it has been shown that most patients with this disorder will have few vascular lesions in the nerve trunks.[29] The primary lesion appears to be segmental axon demyelination, which tends to be peripheral and concentrated at the nodes of Ranvier.[103] There is Schwann cell proliferation and some increase in endoneural tissue.

Axon degeneration is present in severe cases. Degenerative changes in dorsal root ganglia or anterior horn cells are neither primary nor significant. Since the pattern of recovery varies from rapid to slow, de-

pending on the presence or absence of axon degeneration, it is apparent that demyelinization is the primary lesion in most instances. Even in severe lesions in which the intra- and extramedullary portions of the dorsal roots are demyelinated, the dorsal ganglion cells are little affected.[29] Wallerian degeneration will take place when a severe focus of demyelinization develops. Following this, axon regeneration may be slow and incomplete. The neuropathic nerve exhibits increased susceptibility to external pressure, which can further complicate the disorder.

Diabetic Mononeuropathy and Mononeuropathy Multiplex

Diabetic mononeuropathy and asymmetric mononeuropathy multiplex have been ascribed to multiple infarcts in peripheral nerves. These disorders are asymmetric, predominantly motor neuropathies involving one or several nerves. They are often accompanied by pain. The few cases studied histologically have not shown significant obliteration of the blood supply of nerves, despite infarcted lesions associated with the nerves.[86, 87] In contrast to diabetic polyneuropathy, diabetic mononeuropathies are of rapid onset and tend to recover in 3 to 18 months. Pain in the back or leg has led to unnecessary laminectomy when myelography demonstrated some spinal abnormality. Although some authors have suggested that spinal surgery might be appropriate if myelographic changes were present, most authors caution against this.[86, 87]

These diseases may be related to *diabetic amyotrophy*, which has been thought to involve the motor end-plate. Sensory losses have been described in diabetic amyotrophy and conduction deficits have been demonstrated.[40] The symptom pattern of amyotrophy, "asymmetrical pain, weakness, muscle wasting, areflexia in the legs without objective sensory disturbance, occurring in middle aged patients with diabetes of short duration,"[38a] is well within the pattern described in asymmetric diabetic mononeuropathy.

Diabetic Neuropathic Cachexia

Diabetic neuropathic cachexia affects males in the sixth decade. Symptoms in-

---

TABLE 44–2. Classification of Diabetic Neuropathy*

I. Somatic (peripheral) neuropathy
   A. Diabetic polyneuropathy
   B. Asymmetric neuropathy
      1. Mononeuropathy
      2. Mononeuropathy multiplex
      3. Diabetic amyotrophy
   C. Diabetic neuropathic cachexia
II. Visceral neuropathies
III. Secondary manifestations in the foot
   A. Neuropathic ulcer
   B. Neuropathic arthropathy (Charcot)
   C. Diabetic septic foot

*Adapted from Ellenberg, M.: Metabolism, 25: 1627, 1976.

clude profound weight loss, up to 60 per cent of body weight, and an extremely painful symmetric peripheral neuropathy, anorexia, depression, and impotence. The diabetes may be mild. The neuropathy is not associated with evidence of micro-angiopathy.[34]

Diabetic neuropathies are accompanied by elevated cerebrospinal fluid levels in 80 per cent of cases. Recovery in one year is the rule.

Whereas the acute mononeuritic diabetic neuropathies are ascribed to local vascular lesions, the segmental demyelinization of polyneuropathy appears to be a function of metabolic deficits in the Schwann cells, which produce myelin in the course of spiral investiture of the axon.[34] There is often a marked discrepancy between the severity of pathologic findings and the relative paucity of clinical findings.

Another pathologic finding in peripheral neuropathy is at the motor end-plate, where abnormalities are found in juvenile diabetes. Thus, these abnormalities appear to be a pathologic basis for the variable course and unpredictable outcome in the neuropathies of diabetes.

Neuropathic Ulcer

The neuropathic ulcer is painless and develops in a warm foot, often one with good pulses. This disorder is related to diabetic neuropathy more than to vascular disease in the foot.[10, 35, 65] Circulatory changes may be present, but are not obvious. Often the small metatarsal and plantar arch arteries are affected. Abnormal differentials between the ankle/brachial pressures and the toe/ankle pressures have been found.[35]

The sensory deficit does not always follow a predictable pattern. Although plantar sensory denervation has been noted,[36, 101] in many instances the plantar sensory deficit has been restricted to the region immediately surrounding the ulcer.[10]

Sympathetic Denervation in Diabetic Polyneuropathy

Vasoconstrictive/vasodilative responses are abnormal in diabetic neuropathy.[73] Digital vessels show cold hypersensitivity and lack of vasodilation following central body warming. This pattern is a manifestation of the sympathetic denervation that accompanies polyneuropathy[79] and that was first described by Pavy in 1885. The sympathetic denervation appears to play a significant role in the poor foot tissue stamina present in these patients.

The hands and feet receive their sympathetic nerve supply via the peripheral nerves. When galvanic skin resistance is used as an indicator of sympathetic nerve activity, both hyper- and hyporeactivity can be demonstrated. Once the peripheral vasoconstrictive musculature has been denervated, there is an increased response to circulating adrenergic chemical mediators. There is also an enhanced local vasospastic reaction to cooling, which persists despite body heating. This denervation hypersensitivity leads to cold hypersensitivity.[73] Lack of sweating may lead to poor resistance to shear forces because of reduced surface lubrication. In addition, the skin resistance to microtrauma and microbial infection may be reduced.

The diagnosis of diabetic neuropathies is based on the findings of chemical or clinical diabetes and electrodiagnostic changes. Before the clinical manifestations of the disease are apparent, the sensory neuropathy is heralded by an abnormal sensory nerve action potential. Delay in conduction and attenuation of the evoked potential in the sural nerve yield early diagnostic information and correlate well with the presence of demyelinization.[43] There is also an early effect on motor conduction.

When the clinical disease appears profound, conduction velocity deficits can be demonstrated. Fibrillation potentials are present only with axon degeneration and may be absent in polyneuropathy. They are, however, seen in the mononeuropathies, which have been shown to derive from nerve infarcts. The findings in diabetic amyotrophy are those of mixed lesions with abnormal spontaneous activity and conduction deficits. The disease affects proximal muscles more than distal.

Hyperinsulin neuropathy has been described,[22, 62, 74] but whether this disorder and diabetic polyneuropathy are two distinct entities has not been clarified.

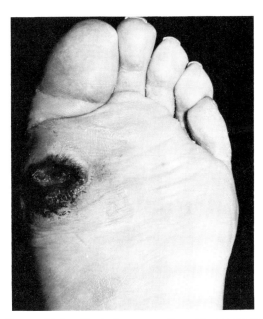

Figure 44–8. *Alcoholic neuropathy with skin ulceration under the first metatarsal head.*

Charcot changes in the forepart of the foot in diabetic neuropathy should be distinguished from pseudo-Charcot-like changes seen in alcoholic neuropathy. In the diabetic, true Charcot changes of the metatarsophalangeal joints may occur with, but usually without, associated local infection and are most frequently multiple (Fig. 44–12A to C). Changes often occur rapidly and are associated with absorption, fragmentation, subluxations, and dislocations. Typically, the dislocations may occur before any bone changes are seen on x-ray films (see Figure 44–5). There are usually associated fatigue fractures of the metatarsal shafts, frequently multiple. These fractures are atypical, as they involve any metatarsal shaft, even in its mid-diaphysis, and are usually associated with excessive periostitis. All these changes are more typical of the diabetic Charcot forefoot and do not occur with alcoholic peripheral neuropathy.

ALCOHOLIC PERIPHERAL NEUROPATHY[29]

By far the two most common peripheral polyneuropathies are diabetic and alcoholic, the former being relatively more common and more serious because of the asso-ciated vascular impairment and the frequent occurrence of Charcot joints. Alcoholic peripheral neuropathy is invariably seen in males, usually in the late third or fourth decade. The patients typically have numbness of their feet, soft tissue foot atrophy, decreased vibratory sense over the first metatarsal head, and increased conduction velocity times. Touch, temperature discrimination, and skin pain are usually felt in the feet, and position sense in the toes is invariably maintained.

The patient's complaints are usually related to plantar ulcerations that are relatively painless. Personal hygiene and nutrition are usually poor. The plantar ulceration occurs most frequently under the first metatarsal head (Fig. 44–8) or under the interphalangeal joint of the hallux. Joint involvement ultimately develops under the ulcer and, in more acute cases, may result in infection, with or without sequestration of a sesamoid (Fig. 44–9A and B) or even of the entire metatarsal head (Fig. 44–10). A less severe but more chronic type of infection is much more common and leads to underlying bone absorption, periostitis, and even pencil sharpening of a metatarsal head (see Fig. 44–4). Chronic infection of a toe may lead to gigantism, especially of the hallux (Fig. 44–11). These soft tissue and bone findings are due to the chronic infection and are not Charcot changes. Why Charcot changes are relatively rare in alcoholic neuropathy is another enigma of the etiology of Charcot joints.

The bone changes seen under an alcoholic trophic ulcer should not be treated like an osteomyelitis, i.e., with open surgery, drainage, saucerization, or excision of a metatarsal head. Such radical surgery leads only to a true osteomyelitis, and excision of a metatarsal head results in thrusting excess weight bearing on the adjacent metatarsal heads, thereby compounding the problems. If treatment is directed essentially toward healing the soft tissue infection and evenly distributing the weight-bearing tread, the ulcer will not only close but the underlying bone will heal and sclerose without sequestration, flare-up, or further bone problems. The simplest treatment is bed rest, appropriate antibiotics, antiseptic soaks,

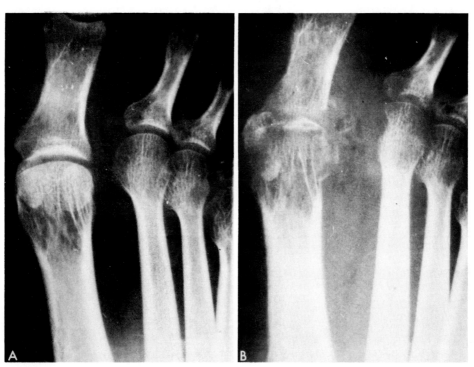

Figure 44–9. *(A) Acute first metatarsophalangeal infection from a deep underlying ulcer. (B) In this radiograph taken two and a half weeks later, note the joint narrowing and the dissolution and fragmentation of the sesamoids.*

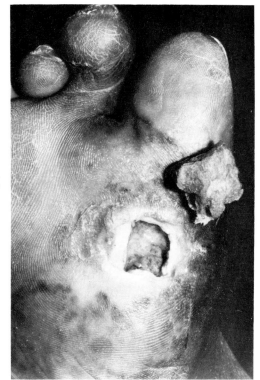

Figure 44-10. Deep ulcer leading to acute first metatarsophalangeal infection with spontaneous sequestration of the first metatarsal head.

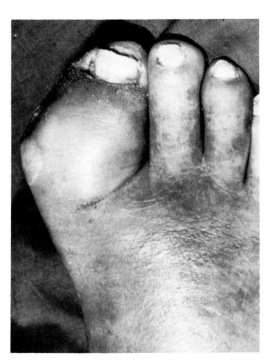

Figure 44-11. Gigantism of the hallux secondary to chronic infection.

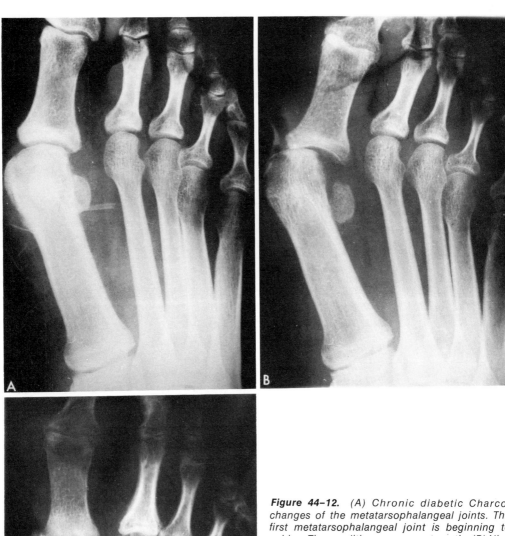

Figure 44–12. (A) Chronic diabetic Charcot changes of the metatarsophalangeal joints. The first metatarsophalangeal joint is beginning to sublux. The condition was asymptomatic. (B) Nine months later. There is further dislocation of first metatarsophalangeal joint and mild subluxation of the second metatarsophalangeal joint. (C) Fifteen months later. There is complete dislocation of the first metatarsophalangeal joint with partial absorption of the first metatarsal head, as well as Charcot changes of the second, third, and fourth metatarsophalangeal joints with extensive periostitis. The condition was still asymptomatic.

and antiseptic whirlpool therapy, followed by custom-made shoes with custom 1-inch-thick cork rubber adjustable Levy molds. The outer soles should consist of thick rubber wedgies or occasionally 3/16-inch tapered rubber heels with rubber metatarsal rocker bars. Wells are made in the inner soles under any bony prominences. Patients with neuropathy do not always take kindly to total-contact casts, which are an alternative method of treatment. In general, patients with alcoholic neuropathy do not usually develop the widespread infections, abscesses, or sloughs seen in those with diabetic neuropathy. In the latter disorder, these findings are due to the associated vascular impairment. Patients with alcoholic neuropathy rarely develop true Charcot joints, but rather the pseudo-Charcot joints described earlier. Because of their foot problems, these patients frequently can be convinced to participate in an alcohol rehabilitation program. The neuropathy, however, persists in spite of subsequent abstinence from alcohol. This is probably due to axon degeneration and fibrosis.

Although alcoholic peripheral neuropathy may be classified in the vitamin deficiency group of neuropathies, there are enough significant clinical and pathologic differences to warrant separate discussion. Along with nutritional deficiency there is probably a direct toxic effect of alcohol on the nervous system. The complete reversal of neuropathy by replacement therapy does not occur in alcoholic neuropathy. Furthermore, ethanol and its breakdown product acetaldehyde interfere with many cellular functions involving the transport and binding of calcium. This may lead to cardiac muscle damage as well as to skeletal myopathies, both reversible acute and irreversible chronic.

A combined sensorimotor neuropathy with bone changes in the forepart of the foot has been described in alcoholic neuropathy. The authors consider the hallmarks of this neuropathy to be distal muscle wasting, muscle weakness, absent ankle jerks, and diminished cutaneous vibration and position sense.[105]

In alcoholic neuropathy, demyelinization has been demonstrated with segmental axon thinning.[26] Conduction slowing is the early electrodiagnostic change. Later in the course of the disease, degeneration of dorsal root ganglia, anterior horn cells, and peripheral axons takes place. Fibrillations may accompany such changes. Thiamine replacement alone may be insufficient to treat the clinical disorder; pyridoxine and folic acid may be needed.[41]

Associated foot problems in alcoholics include poor foot hygiene with infections and ulcerations above the foot and in the lower leg, soft tissue changes secondary to chronic venous and lymphatic stasis, and occasionally frostbite. The recurrent infection and lymphatic stasis may lead to a pseudoelephantiasis.

PERIPHERAL NEUROPATHY IN RHEUMATOID ARTHRITIS AND OTHER COLLAGEN DISEASES

The connective tissue disorders or other collagen diseases associated with autoimmune reactions are accompanied by several forms of central nervous system and peripheral nerve disease. In some instances, the first manifestation of the disorder may be in the foot, with peripheral neuropathies and neuritis leading to paralysis or pain. In certain cases, the neuropathy may be related to changes in steroid therapy — usually to abrupt withdrawal of the steroids.

In addition to the neuropathy of rheumatic diseases, neuropathies may be found in proliferative neoplastic disorders and metabolic disorders manifested by increased circulating globulin, such as amyloid diseases and myeloma.[52, 109]

Table 44–3 lists the collagen diseases and summarizes those in which peripheral neuropathies that affect the feet and legs have been noted, as well as the central nervous system disorders seen in these conditions. These diseases overlap. Angiitis and deposition of immune complexes within the nerves (fibrinoid) have been documented in various proportions in many rheumatoid disorders.

Raynaud's phenomenon is often associated with collagen disease causing sensory deficits (i.e., numbness) in addition to vascular insufficiency, cold intolerance, peripheral vasospasm, and pain. This is more apt to occur in the hands than in the feet.

When angiitis leads to skin breakdown in the feet, any associated neuropathy will intensify the clinical disorder. The resultant problem requires careful management because of possible secondary infection and malum perforans pedis leading to osteomyelitis.

Arteritis in rheumatoid arthritis may be indistinguishable from polyarteritis nodosa and is often accompanied by progressive neuropathy. This neuropathy develops slowly, is sensorimotor in type, and is accompanied by pain and paresthesias.

Diffuse and localized forms may be encountered.

The neuropathy of rheumatoid arthritis may consist of a mild, symmetric sensory neuropathy (group I) or a severe fulminating sensorimotor mononeuropathy (group II).[16] The mild form of sensory neuropathy is usually symmetric, and there is an associated autonomic neuropathy with reduced sweating. The symmetric polyneuropathy is not due to compression or vasculitis. The severe (group II) disorder is considered to be vascular-induced mononeuropathy or mononeuropathy multiplex and is an ominous finding (Fig. 44–13A and B). Vasculitis in the peripheral

TABLE 44–3. Central Nervous System (CNS) Diseases and Peripheral Neuropathies Associated with Collagen Disorders†

COLLAGEN DISORDER	CNS DISEASE	PERIPHERAL NEUROPATHY	
		DPN*	MN and MNM**
Rheumatoid arthritis (RA)	Spinal cord compression	Entrapment syndrome	
Necrotizing arteritis of RA		+	+
Ankylosing spondylitis			
Systemic lupus erythematosus	Convulsions Psychosis Guillian-Barré polyradiculitis	+	+
Polyarteritis nodosa	Transverse myelitis Cerebral syndrome Anterior spine artery thrombosis Usually cranial- headache seizures, hemiparesis, optic atrophy	+	+
Giant cell arteritis		+	+
Thrombotic thrombocytopenic purpura	Coma, convulsions, bleeding		+
Dermatomyositis Polymyositis Polymyositis associated with carcinoma		+	
Scleroderma	Spinal cord compression	+	
Allergic vasculitis and serum sickness	Convulsions Coma	+ (mononeuropathic radiculitis, usually upper extremity)	
Granulomatous arteritis		+	
Rheumatic fever	Hemiplegia Embolism Diffuse arteritis Chorea	Myoclonus	

Key: * = Diffuse polyneuropathy, ** = mononeuropathy and mononeuropathy multiplex, + = present.
† Adapted from Aita, J. A.: Neurologic Manifestations of General Diseases. Springfield, Illinois, Charles C Thomas, 1964.

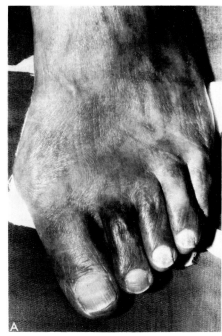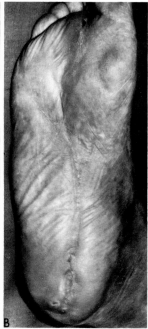

Figure 44–13. *A 52-year-old male with rheumatoid arthritis and Felty's syndrome complicated by vasculitis. The vasculitis resulted in bilateral footdrop from a peripheral sensorimotor polyneuritis as well as superficial gangrene of the toes. The response to Cytoxan was excellent, with resolution of the footdrop and gangrene. Atrophy of the subcutaneous tissues and small muscles, along with the sensory loss, resulted in plantar ulceration and infection, requiring open drainage. When the wound healed, the patient was fitted with custom-made shoes, SACH heels, and metatarsal rocker bars. The shoes incorporated one-inch-thick cork rubber, custom-made, adjustable Levy molds. (A) Resolving gangrene with residual discoloration of the second toe. (B) Healed plantar incision. There is slight drainage proximally.*

nerves with occlusive changes in the vasa nervorum leads to axon degeneration.[82] Immunofluorescent techniques show immune globulin deposition in some nerves.[16] Nevertheless, there is not always a good correlation between vasculitis and thrombosis and the demyelinization and/or axon degeneration. In addition, there may be vascular changes in the diffuse polyneuropathy group I lesions.[113]

In the mild sensory neuropathies, the sural nerves (group I) show varying degrees of axon degeneration and demyelinization, whereas in the severe cases (group II), there is advanced degeneration of myelinated fibers.[113]

Demyelinization may appear without vasculitis, but the more severe changes are seen when vasculitis leads to infarction of nerves.

Mononeuritis multiplex is also seen in cases of polyarteritis nodosa, both associated with rheumatoid arthritis (RA) and without RA.[14] The lateral popliteal (peroneal) nerve is most frequently involved. Foot and leg pain and footdrop appear. The patients are at great risk for generalized arteritis. Some cases occur while high-dose steroids are being used, whereas others appear when steroids are abruptly discontinued. Still other cases appear in the absence of steroid therapy.[49]

The pathologic findings of peripheral neuropathy include demyelinization, loss of axons, degeneration of axon sheaths, and increased perineuronal and intrafascicular fibrous tissue. Small vessel disease in the foot may accompany the neuropathy. Lesions in the vasa nervorum have been reported associated with polyarteritis.[14, 38] As with other neuropathies involving the peroneal nerve, footdrop and plantar ulceration may develop and should be managed by appropriate surgical and orthopaedic programs.

Results of electromyographic and nerve conduction studies are related to the nerve pathology present[43] and include slowed motor conduction due to demyelinization and fibrillation due to axon degeneration. The two processes are independent, and electrodiagnostic studies may show mixed patterns.

Accompanying RA are compressive nerve phenomena related to tenosynovitis in enclosed spaces, e.g., the carpal and tarsal tunnels. In this instance clinical and electrodiagnostic findings would be localized to the single nerve involved unless there was a concomitant diffuse neuropathy.

Other collagen-vascular diseases with neuropathic manifestations include systemic lupus erythematosus (SLE), scleroderma, polyarteritis, Sjögren's syndrome, and dermatomyositis.[56] These neuropathies may be compressive or primary. Vasculitis and immune globulin deposition have been reported in different cases.

Systemic lupus erythematosus is characterized by widespread fibrinoid changes and leukocytic infiltration, especially in the walls of small vessels. Its manifestations include joint disease, cutaneous eruptions, urticaria, purpura, multiple system disease, and hematologic disorders including anemia, leukopenia, and elevated sedimentation rate, and hypergammaglobulinemia. Many neurologic manifestations have been reported. Central nervous system manifestations include convulsive disorders and psychosis. Polyradiculitis and neuropathy — both diffuse polyneuropathy (group I) and multiple mononeuropathy (group II) — occur. Polymyositis may be present. In children, more fulminating psychosis and spinal cord disease leading to quadriplegia are seen.

Polyarteritis (periarteritis nodosa) is seen in many rheumatoid diseases. It may appear acutely or insidiously. Multiple system involvement is the rule, and peripheral neuropathy occurs in 30 to 50 per cent of patients. The neuropathy may be the initial presentation and can be poly- or mononeuritic.[14] The disorder may be accompanied by polymyositis, radiculitis (single or multiple), and transverse myelitis. The neuropathy is usually persistent and progressive with pain, paresthesias, and weakness. Motor loss predominates. Cerebral symptoms are common.[38]

Dermatomyositis and *polymyositis* are poorly defined entities that overlap with other collagen disorders. Fifteen per cent of cases are related to distant neoplastic disease. Raynaud's phenomenon, dysphagia, arthritic manifestations, and electromyographic changes are seen. Other connective tissue diseases are often present.

Scleroderma may be accompanied by peripheral neuropathies. Polymyositis, cerebral involvement secondary to renal disease, and reduced gastrointestinal motility may appear. The neuropathy may precede the appearance of skin changes.

Sjögren's syndrome is a connective tissue disorder that may have manifestations of all the other diseases of this type, including peripheral neuropathies and arteritis. Keratoconjunctivitis and salivary gland enlargement are the hallmarks of this disorder.

As a result of the association of peripheral neuropathies with collagen diseases, all patients presenting with neuropathies should be studied for autoimmune disorders. Hemogram, sedimentation rate, differential blood counts, and latex fixation and other rheumatoid factor tests are indicated. If the sedimentation rate is elevated, tests for SLE and abnormal globulins should be ordered. The search for distant neoplasm should include a general physical examination, rectal examination, chest x-ray study, and test for gastrointestinal bleeding.

Treatment for peripheral neuropathies of rheumatic origin should be conservative. First, protect the sole of the foot with molded shoes or custom insoles. A plastic orthosis will support the paralyzed anterior tibial and peroneal muscles. When chronic neuropathy leads to clawing of the toes, metatarsal callosities will often appear. Hammer-toe surgery can be performed under local or regional anesthesia with considerable benefit. The patellar tendon–bearing brace can be used when a severe sensory deficit has developed. If a fixed equinus has developed as a result of Achilles tendon (gastrocnemius-soleus) contracture, Achilles tenotomy is useful. An orthosis with a locked ankle joint may be used to stabilize the foot and ankle after surgery, reducing the need for postoperative casting.

HEREDITARY SENSORY NEUROPATHY

Hereditary sensory neuropathy, although relatively rare, is frequently undiagnosed for years and may be more common than presumed. It is classified according to congenital and hereditary (familial) types.[78] The congenital form is mostly sporadic (nonhereditary), has some islands of normal sensation, is nonprogressive, and may actually improve to a degree. Intelligence may be defective. The familial variety is dominantly inherited with onset in late childhood, affects primarily the distal legs, and is progressive. Intelligence is normal. In both types, there is loss of myelinated nerve fibers and of dermal nerve endings, as demonstrated by sural nerve and skin punch biopsy specimens. Since only sensory nerves are involved, only sensory conduction velocity is delayed and must be tested for specifically. There is loss of superficial and deep pain, touch, and temperature perception. The motor system is intact. Variations of hereditary sensory neuropathy have been described along with overlap syndromes. Thus, a form of sensory neuropathy with anhidrosis has been described in mentally defective persons.[84] It is inherited in a recessive pattern, occurs at birth, and involves the small dorsal root axons and not the distal myelinated nerves. Touch perception is present, but there is loss of temperature and pain perception. The autonomic dysfunction and self-mutilation are similar to that seen in familial dysautonomia. In his case reports of hereditary sensory neuropathy, Denny-Brown noted lightening pains suggestive of dorsal root involvement; decrease of all sensory modalities including touch, temperature, and vibratory sense; decreased deep tendon reflexes, and mendelian dominance with onset at 20 to 30 years of age.[24] He also noted degeneration of the peripheral nerves, as well as the S1 and T1 dorsal root ganglia. Patients also had progressive bilateral nerve deafness with atrophy of the cochlear and vestibular ganglia. In Hicks' cases of hereditary sensory neuropathy, touch and vibratory sense were about normal, there was no lightening pain, and there was late involvement of the upper extremities.[51a] However, there was degeneration of the dorsal root ganglia.

Overlap Syndromes: Sensory Neuropathy with Spinal Cord Involvement

Three overlap syndromes are Refsum's disease, lumbosacral syringomyelia, and Charcot-Marie-Tooth disease with hereditary sensory neuropathy.

Refsum's disease[89], which is a familial recessive disorder, is a lipid storage disease associated with increased excretion of phytanic acid. Pain and temperature senses are lost, vibratory sense is decreased, and there is minimal loss of touch. Also present are cerebellar phenomena (ataxia), peripheral paresis, increased albumin and globu-

lin in the cerebrospinal fluid, concentric limitation of visual fields with atypical retinitis pigmentosa, and, usually, respiratory paralysis within four to five years.

Familial lumbosacral "syringomyelia"[57] is an autosomal dominant disorder starting at about 10 years of age with upper motor and pyramidal tract involvement accompanied by a spastic paraparesis. Sensory neuropathy occurs later, causing secondary trophic ulcers of the feet and legs.

Hereditary sensory neuropathy with Charcot-Marie-Tooth disease is a mendelian dominant disorder.[30] Pes cavus and hammer toes may occur as early as five years of age, followed by trophic foot ulcers in the third decade. Other findings include peroneal muscular atrophy with weak anterior tibial and peroneal muscles and decreased tough, pain, vibratory, and position sense in the lower extremities, as well as depressed ankle jerks. Occasionally, there is some atrophy of the hand intrinsics and a history of lancinating leg pain. Meissner's corpuscles are absent on skin biopsy specimens. The patient's main problems are related to the sensory neuropathy, namely the trophic foot ulcers, secondary infection, absorption of underlying bone, and, ultimately, almost complete loss of the feet.

Congenital Indifference to Pain

Congenital indifference to pain is a birth defect characterized by cerebral indifference to pain in the presence of an anatomically intact nervous system.[12] It is subdivided into congenital indifference and familial dysautonomia, or Riley-Day syndrome, and overlaps with familial sensory neuropathy with anhidrosis.[69, 84]

The disorder may occur sporadically or be associated with D-trisomy mosaicism. Intelligence is normal. There is a complete loss of all forms of pain sensation (superficial and deep); however, the patients can normally feel touch, tickle, temperature, vibratory, and position sense and have normal nerve conduction, nerve biopsy specimens, and autonomic function. Deep tendon reflexes are normal. The corneal and gag reflexes may be reduced. Although temperature is perceived, extremes of temperature in the form of pain are not felt, so that severe burns or frostbite may readily occur. Deep pain secondary to fractures, pleuritic pain, headache, toothache, and visceral pain are not felt. Trophic ulcers and Charcot joints in the lower extremities are frequent and lead to serious orthopaedic sequelae. Fractures usually heal, but nonunion may occur.[72] Minor sprains and fractures, if left untreated (because patients are asymptomatic), may lead to Charcot changes.[69] A slightly warm joint with effusion should be treated with caution in spite of minimal x-ray changes, since Charcot joints may develop. Anatomic restitution of joint fractures or of Charcot joints is not only impossible but unnecessary, as these patients manage very well without discomfort on deformed and/or arthritic joints. The feet, however, should be kept plantigrade to distribute weight bearing evenly in order to avoid secondary plantar ulceration.

Delayed sensory conduction studies have been noted in cases of congenital indifference to pain with or without anhidrosis.[69]

Familial dysautonomia,[90] which is present at birth, is inherited as an autosomal recessive trait in Ashkenazi Jews. Mentality is dull to normal and is associated with typical facies, emotional lability, temper tantrums, and self-mutilation, the last with biting and partial destruction of the tongue, lips, and fingers. To date, no definite anatomic pathologic findings have been noted. Early signs include feeding and swallowing problems. There is a lack of tearing, poor temperature control, increased vasovagal sensitivity, increased tracheal secretion, excessive sweating, and postural hypotension, all attributed to dysfunction of the autonomic nervous system. These findings, along with the poor swallowing reflexes, cause major anesthesia problems during surgery, including severe hypotension occasionally associated with cardiac arrest and postoperative bronchopneumonia, atelectasis, cyclic vomiting, and spiking temperatures.[59]

Other consistent findings are incomplete distribution of indifference to all forms of pain, scoliosis,[63] absent or hypoactive deep tendon reflexes, absent corneal reflexes, absence of fungiform papillae on the tongue, abnormal esophageal motility, no axon flares on histamine skin testing, and excess homovanillic acid (HVA).[84] Homovanillic acid is derived from epinephrine and norepinephrine, the excess of which is probably related to the exaggerated sympathetic responses found in these patients. Finally, "trophic" foot ulcers and corneal ulcers are found, as a result of the pain insensitivity. Although Charcot joints are allegedly rare in familial dysautonomia, one series[115] reported a 7.7 per cent incidence of osteochondritis, including osteochondritis of the talus. Since epiphyseal fragmentation is typical of Charcot changes in the developing skeleton,[27] cases of "osteochondritis" should be considered as Charcot pathology.

Treatment

Treatment of indifference to pain and the hereditary sensory neuropathies is quite difficult and frustrating in regard to the foot and ankle problems.[104] Loss of pain in the lower extremities and especially in the feet occurs in all the sensory neuropathies and includes the lack of pain

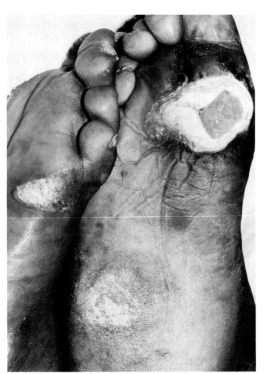

Figure 44–14. Previously undiagnosed hereditary sensory neuropathy in a 37-year-old black male. Note the ulcer under the pressure area of the first metatarsal head and the old healed ulcer over the shear area of the lateral fifth metatarsal head on the opposite foot.

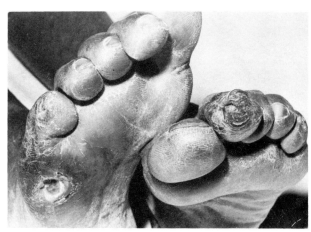

Figure 44–15. *Hereditary sensory neuropathy in a 19-year-old black male. His brother has the same disease. Note the keratotic scar at the end of the second toe of the left foot and the fresh ulcer over the lateral fifth metatarsal head of the right foot.*

related to extremes of temperature. Shoes have to be checked for pebbles and nails, and irritation from sock lining creases must be prevented. Thin rubber sneaker soles may be penetrated by sharp objects, and barefoot walking is to be avoided. Despite good foot care, "trophic" ulcers develop under areas of excessive weight bearing, as under the metatarsal heads (Fig. 44–14); over areas of shoe contact, as the tips of the toes (Fig. 44–15); over the dorsum of the toes, if they are hammered (deformed from secondary infections); or over areas of shear. Since the ulcers are pain-free, they are invariably neglected by the child or adolescent. Secondary infection occurs with underlying bone destruction, absorption, and occasionally draining sinuses with sequestration. Loss of grossly infected deformed toes is relatively common. Wounds will ultimately heal, but are followed by painless scar formation with a tendency to repeated breakdown. The usual custom-made shoe with 1-inch-thick adjustable Levy molds, as previously described, is indicated. Excess calluses are trimmed, and overhanging callous edges of trophic ulcers are also trimmed to provide better drainage. Antibiotic whirlpool baths, foot soaks, systemic antibiotics, and so forth are the standard treatment. In the presense of draining ulcers, polyethylene closed celled, medium-soft arch supports, which are washable, may be used.

Most children, however, are uncooperative both in following conservative treatment programs and in limiting their activities. In younger children, physical discipline is impossible, as spanking causes no discomfort. Older children and

teen-agers resent their physical limitations and lack insight in regard to the dangers of their trophic ulcers or Charcot joints, since they feel no pain. They almost perversely indulge in all sports.

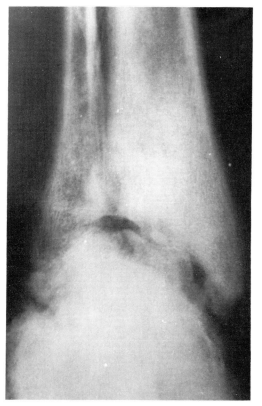

Figure 44–16. *Virulent secondary infection of foot and ankle in a 16-year-old white male with hereditary sensory neuropathy. Note the acute extensive cortical absorption and periostitis. Acute toxicity and sepsis made emergency amputation mandatory.*

Acute fulminating uncontrolled infection may lead to emergency limb ablation (Fig. 44–16). Chronic recurrent ulcers result in piecemeal spontaneous or surgical loss of toes or rays of both feet. In the end stage, amputation is necessary because of the presence of a useless, indurated, distorted, fetid mass of infected bone and soft tissue. Such patients have almost unrecognizable feet with multiple, draining sinuses; ulcerations; massive, dirty, granulating areas; and tissue loss along with areas of gigantism caused by chronic infection. These feet are essentially pain-free. In other instances in which patients have been more cooperative and have received careful orthopaedic and orthotic supervision, the feet are in much better condition. Nevertheless, there may ultimately be almost complete absorption of the forefeet secondary to local chronic and recurrent

infections and Charcot destruction. Such patients may walk surprisingly well on distorted hindfoot stumps without discomfort (Fig. 44–17A to D).

Other relatively common problems related to the foot include pressure heel ulcers from bedrest, splints, braces, or traction used for fractures of the legs.[27] Pin traction infections also occur. Problems may occur from casts, as well as from foreign objects placed inside the cast. Arterial or venous occlusion inside a cast may be relatively asymptomatic or may cause moderate discomfort.[91]

Epiphyseal damage occurs either as an osteomyelitis overlying an ulcer or from Charcot changes. Charcot changes are more frequent in congenital indifference to pain than in the hereditary sensory neuropathies or familial dysautonomia. Outstanding findings of Charcot changes in

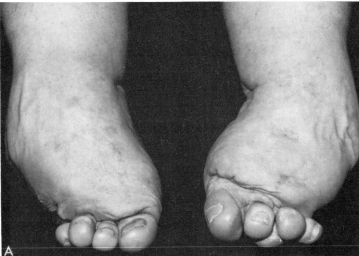

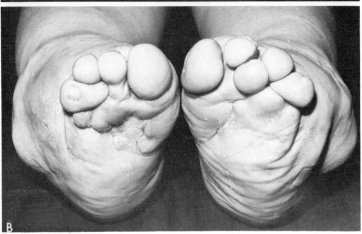

Figure 44–17. *A 44-year-old woman with hereditary sensory neuropathy. The family history was strongly positive, including her mother, brother, and son. All sensory modalities are present in the feet but quantitatively decreased. The upper extremities are clinically normal. The patient had had recurrent plantar infections since she was 16 years of age, but had no recent skin breakdown. She walks unassisted without discomfort in custom-made shoes. (A) Note nubbins of toes and foreshortened forefeet. (B) The plantar view reveals old healed ulcers. There is considerable soft-tissue and small muscle atrophy.*

Illustration continued on opposite page

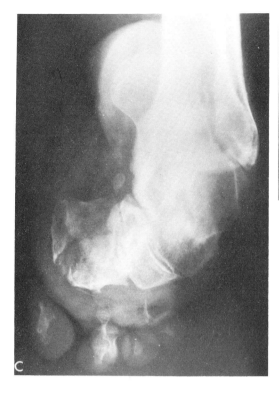

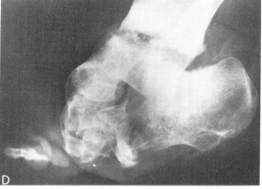

Figure 44–17 *Continued. (C) Anteroposterior radiograph of the left foot. The metatarsals have been completely absorbed, and only a few remnants of the phalanges remain. The calcaneus lies obliquely and the talar head is displaced laterally. The remnants of midtarsus lie transversely, with the toes pointed forward. (D) A lateral radiograph reveals that the lower tibia has been absorbed along with the body of the talus. The midtarsal bones point plantarward as well as medially, while the toes remain in a normal plane.*

children consist of asymptomatic joint dislocations and epiphyseal fragmentation and absorption.[51, 91] In the tarsus, exclusive of the talus, there is relatively mild bony thickening and distortion, which may be readily overlooked (Fig. 44–18A and B). In the ankle, however, there is obvious swelling (Fig. 44–18A) and minimal warmth, but no redness, pain, or tenderness. Minor epiphyseal plate injury is revealed occasionally by the production of a bony spur extending from the metaphysis just above the epiphyseal plate in the ankle (Fig. 44–18C). The spurs are asymptomatic and occur as incidental findings on routine x-ray examinations. Charcot ankles in children involve essentially the body of the talus, which rapidly absorbs (Fig. 44–18D). Partial reconstitution occurs (Fig. 44–18E) with moderately severe but painless residual deformity. In the adult, Charcot ankle changes are frequently revealed by fragmentation of the malleoli with subluxation of the mortise. These changes may occur acutely (Fig. 44–19A and B). In general, Charcot joints are treated conservatively over a prolonged period of time until the slow healing stage results in bone reconstitution and stability. Meanwhile, the foot may be kept plantigrade, remembering that throughout this time casts and braces may cause ulceration of these asymptomatic feet. Epiphyseal damage may lead to asymmetric growth.

SPINAL CORD DISORDERS WITH ASSOCIATED NEUROPATHY

Degenerative Cord Lesions with Neuropathy

Generally, in degenerative neurologic diseases the longest axons are affected first, and therefore findings occur relatively early in the feet.

Charcot-Marie-Tooth disease (peroneal muscular atrophy),[106] the most common of the spinal degenerative disorders, is managed mainly by the orthopaedist. It may occur as a mendelian dominant trait, sporadically, or even as an X-linked recessive trait. Classically, most patients have bilateral symmetric pes cavus or equinovarus deformities associated ultimately with hammer toes. The high arches are usually

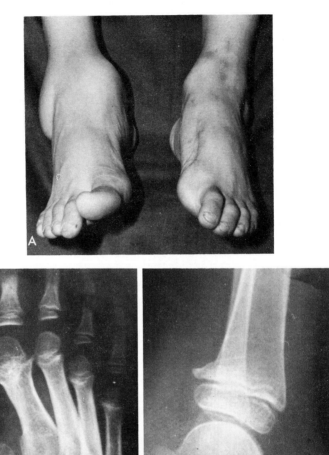

Figure 44–18. *(A) Asymptomatic, clinically subtle Charcot Lisfranc's joint on the left side and obvious Charcot ankle on the right side in a seven-year-old boy with congenital indifference to pain. Note that the left hallux has been amputated owing to prior infection. (B) Radiograph of the left foot. Note the dislocation of Lisfranc's joint without associated bone changes. (C) As noted, the boy had congenital indifference to pain. Note the posterior tibial metaphyseal spur.*

Illustration continued on opposite page

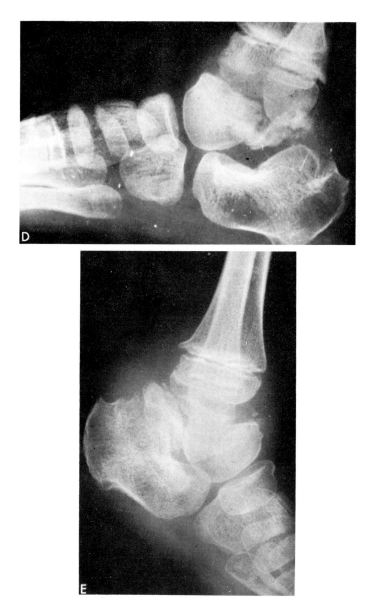

Figure 44–18 *Continued.* *(D) Radiograph of the Charcot right ankle. Note the collapse of the body of the talus. (E) Seventeen months later, the body of the talus is starting to reconstitute.*

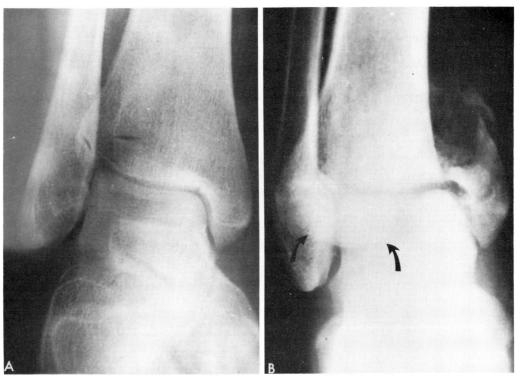

Figure 44–19. *(A) Swollen, asymptomatic ankle in a 26-year-old male with hereditary sensory neuropathy. The initial radiographs were normal. (B) Six weeks later, trimalleolar fragmentation was present. Arrows point to a posterior malleolar fragment.*

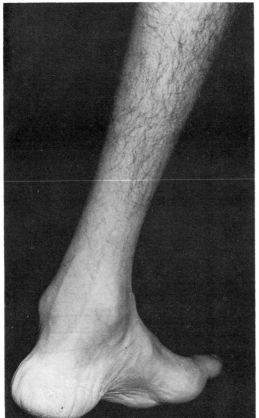

Figure 44–20. *Charcot-Marie-Tooth disease in a 26-year-old white male with bilateral calcaneus deformity. Note the atrophy of the calf muscles.*

noticed early in childhood. Rarely, the feet are normal or even flat. Calcaneus is extremely rare. The one patient seen (Fig. 44–20) walks comfortably without any support. Males are affected slightly more frequently than females. The disease is relatively rare in blacks, as are all forms of pes cavus. Differences in the severity of motor involvement vary dramatically from the more severe cases (in which almost all the lower leg muscles may be considerably paralyzed by the end of the second decade), to moderate cases (in which mild peroneal nerve involvement is revealed by the middle of the third decade), to the mildest cases (in which minimal objective neurologic findings without muscle weakness are detected in the fourth decade).

In the more severe and probably least common form, which appears early in life, there is decided weakness of the lower leg muscles with atrophy, a relatively unsteady gait, and various degrees of bilateral footdrop. The last is due to weakness of the extensor hallucis longus, extensor digitorum longus, and tibialis anterior muscles. Usually there is considerable weakness of the foot extensors and evertors, which are supplied by the common peroneal nerve. Within a few years intrinsic atrophy of the hand muscles appears. Treatment consists of triple arthrodesis and anterior transfer of the tibialis posterior muscle if there is an associated footdrop (Fig. 44–21).

The slightly later appearing, more classic form reveals equinovarus with relatively normal gait and good muscle power. Leg atrophy is relatively mild, and there is mild to moderate weakness of the peroneal muscles. Knee jerks and especially ankle jerks are lost. Intrinsic hand atrophy tends to be mild and usually occurs about 10 to 15 years later than the leg findings. Triple arthrodesis is usually advised to correct the cavus. Hammer-toe surgery may also be required. Supplementary tendon transfer in these cases is usually not necessary.

There are also the "formes frustes,"[102] which are usually overlooked and which may possibly be the most common form. Such patients also have pes cavus and ultimately develop hammer toes. One form reveals associated generalized absence of deep tendon reflexes, including those of the upper extremities. Some of these patients may have other mild classic stigmata of intrinsic hand atrophy and peroneal muscular weakness. All sensory modalities are normal, including vibratory and position sense. Another described kinship (Roussy-Lévy)[92, 93] included pes cavus, hammer toes, late onset of walking, generalized absence of deep tendon reflexes, normal sensory examination, absent abdominal reflexes, slight hand tremors, positive Romberg sign, and equivocal Babinski sign.

Finally, in the mildest of cases, the neurologic examination may be entirely negative except for intrinsic foot atrophy and pes cavus. However, conduction velocity studies may be positive. Mild neurologic findings suggestive of Charcot-Marie-Tooth disease may then appear years later.[75]

In the mild cases with pes cavus and normal muscle power, tarsometatarsal wedge resection gives satisfactory results.

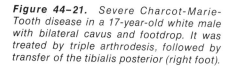

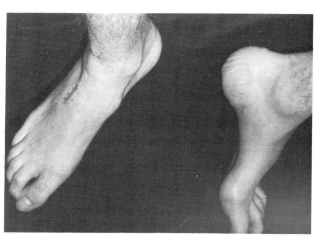

Figure 44–21. Severe Charcot-Marie-Tooth disease in a 17-year-old white male with bilateral cavus and footdrop. It was treated by triple arthrodesis, followed by transfer of the tibialis posterior (right foot).

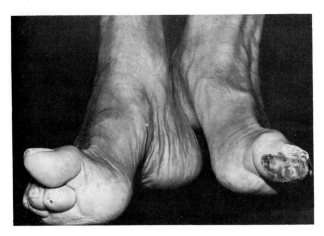

Figure 44–22. *Charcot-Marie-Tooth disease in a 54-year-old white male. There was a positive family history. The patient had severe cavus, hammer toes, atrophy of the intrinsic muscles, and extensive sensorimotor neuropathy of the lower legs. However, the ulcerations were relatively minor, not deep nor indolent. Note the beginning of superficial necrosis of the skin over the pulp of the left hallux.*

In the moderate and severe cases, peripheral sensory neuropathy and posterior column signs may occur, but are usually relatively mild. These include loss or decrease primarily in vibratory and position sense and, less constantly, in touch, pain, and temperature perception. Approximately 3 per cent of patients develop pressure ulcers (Fig. 44–22). Optic atrophy occasionally occurs. There may be peripheral nerve thickening, not unlike progressive hypertrophic polyneuritis, and muscle fasciculations and cramping occasionally develop. The pathologic changes correlate with the clinical findings and include degeneration, especially of the ventral horn cells and dorsal root ganglia, and, to a lesser extent, of the dorsal roots and the peripheral nerves, especially the peroneal nerve. The peripheral nerves reveal an interstitial neuritis.

Electrodiagnostic studies demonstrate pronounced slowing of conduction velocity, to 2 mm/sec.[43]

Although motor conduction is affected at first, sensory action potentials are eventually involved, with delayed conduction, reduced amplitude, and absence of response. Electromyography reveals neuropathic changes in the denervated muscles, which ultimately become fibrosed and electrically silent. There may be impairment of the autonomic nervous system with postganglionic sympathetic denervation. This leads to impaired sweating, low tear production, and skin temperature regulation independent of body temperature.[55]

Treatment of Charcot-Marie-Tooth disease is discussed in Chapter 19 (Pes Cavus). Even in the more severe forms of the disease, life span is normal.

Cerebellar Ataxias

The cerebellar ataxias occur much less frequently than the Charcot-Marie-Tooth group of disorders. The most common form is Friedreich's ataxia, which is also discussed in Chapter 19. Like the Charcot-Marie-Tooth group, Friedreich's ataxia is also hereditary or sporadic, but the onset is earlier in life, usually at five to ten years of age, although ataxia may be seen as early as two to three years of age. It involves the dorsal half of the spinal cord. Degeneration of the posterior column results in early loss of vibratory sense and, to a lesser degree, of position sense. Ankle jerks and knee jerks are also lost early. Pyramidal tract involvement causes a positive Babinski sign, and cerebellar involvement results in ataxia and nystagmus (70 per cent of cases) and, at a later stage, in dysarthria. Orthopaedic manifestations include frequent scoliosis and pes cavus. Occasionally, optic atrophy and deafness occur. Some loss of pain, temperature, and touch sensation occurs late. Cardiac fibrosis is a common finding. Many of the patients have an infantile physique and young-looking facies. Most patients die about 20 years after onset of the ataxia. Abortive forms occur, so that a sibling may have only pes cavus. Patients with other forms may have cavus plus nystagmus. Finally, Friedreich's ataxia may overlap with the other degenerative cerebellar diseases or with the Charcot-Marie-Tooth group of disorders.

Intra- and Extradural Lesions

Occasionally, plantar ulceration and Charcot-like changes in the feet may be noted with spinal dysraphism and with benign cauda equina tumors, usually associated with thecal tethering (Fig. 44–23A).[18, 42] Suspicion should be aroused by stigmata over the lower spine, including dimpling, a sinus tract, an abnormal hairy patch, or localized subcutaneous thickening (e.g., lipoma). The earliest finding is usually a small unexplained pressure ulcer appearing on the foot or toe in adolescence. Ultimately, but very slowly, chronic recurrent ulceration, bone absorption, and Charcot-like changes occur. Even at this time, abnormal neurologic findings may be lacking. There is no muscle weakness, nor are there any sensory changes. Conduction velocity studies may show slight delay. Myelography is diagnostic (Fig. 44–23B).

Treatment consists of excision of the tumor, thecal release, and continued conservative treatment of the damaged feet. Skin grafting may be successful. Of interest is the reported release of thecal tethering done in a patient with idiopathic pes cavus followed by definite clinical improvement.[58]

INTERSTITIAL NEUROPATHY

Multiple interstitial neuritis may occur secondary to periarteritis nodosa with associated nerve trunk tenderness. The neuritis may occur by direct invasion, as in leukemia, or from primary amyloidosis. In addition, vincristine sulfate, a drug used for childhood leukemia, is neurotoxic and may cause a sensorimotor peripheral neuropathy by demyelination. Motor function may return four to six months after withdrawal of the drug.

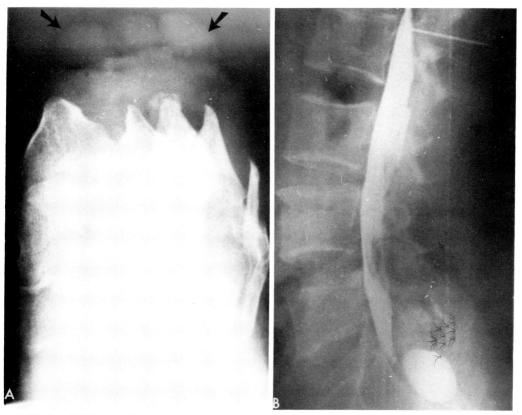

Figure 44–23. *(A) Pseudo-Charcot foot of a 37-year-old male. The first and fifth toes were amputated for ulcerations and for specimen examination. Soft-tissue outlines (between arrows) of the nubbins of the three middle toes are visualized on this radiograph. The bones of these toes and of the distal portions of the metatarsals have slowly and completely spontaneously been absorbed. (B) Myelogram revealing the outlines of an intra- and extradural lesion, which on exploration was found to be a lipoma.*

Another rare disease is progressive hypertrophic polyneuritis (Dejerine-Sottas syndrome), which may be allied to the Charcot-Marie-Tooth group.[30] It is usually familial. The onset is most frequently in infancy, with poor walking and inability to run. This is followed by numbness of the hands and feet that is associated with shooting pains. All sensory modalities are affected. There are often coarse muscle fibrillations, as seen occasionally in Charcot-Marie-Tooth disease. Ultimately, equinovarus deformities, claw hands, areflexia, slowly progressive muscle weakness, ataxia, and increased cerebrospinal fluid protein levels develop, and, occasionally, a positive Romberg sign occurs. Classically, one finds nontender, firm, palpable thickening of the peripheral nerves and their branches, including the posterior auricular nerve. Occasionally, the muscle wasting may be more proximal, and kyphoscoliosis and nystagmus may be found. Ulcerations are rare. The ultimate prognosis is wheelchair confinement at about 20 years of age, paraplegia, and decreased life expectancy.

In general, there is an overlap, not only within the disorders of the Charcot-Marie-Tooth group and the various spinocerebellar diseases,[93] but between these two major groups as well. In the same family, one may find relatives with Charcot-Marie-Tooth disease, Friedreich's ataxia, and Dejerine-Sottas disease, as well as formes frustes of pes cavus.

METABOLIC NEUROPATHIES

Metabolic neuropathies may be primary, as a result of metabolic disorders that may either interfere with neuromuscular function or infiltrate peripheral nerves (as in primary amyloidosis), or secondary to the effects of another systemic disease. They may also be produced by toxins that interfere with or damage neuromuscular function.

The primary metabolic disorders include the previously mentioned Refsum's disease (lipid storage disease), porphyria, and diabetes. In porphyria, the attacks may be precipitated by drugs, especially barbiturates, and also alcohol. Symptoms are those of a polyneuropathy, especially motor, along with cerebral signs, including epilepsy. Urinary porphyrin excretion is increased.

Peripheral Neuropathy Associated with Renal Failure

Although the dysfunction of the central nervous system associated with uremia had been noted for many generations, the polyneuropathy of peripheral nerves was identified and quantitated only relatively recently.[7]

A physiologic peripheral nerve dysfunction that is associated with the azotemic state and is often subclinical has now been recognized. This state of altered function develops into a clinical peripheral polyneuropathy that is more pronounced distally, is greatest in the legs, and especially involves the peroneal nerve. The polyneuropathy is reversible at first if the azotemia is corrected, but becomes profound and irreversible if long-standing renal failure persists.

With the use of renal dialysis, more cases of clinical neuropathy were noted, as survival times increased. Sensory deficits tended to recover, but when clinical renal failure persisted, profound irreversible neuropathy was noted. Recovery is rare when severe motor and sensory losses have occurred during dialysis, but is improved following renal transplantation.[108]

The neuropathy of renal failure is not related to the underlying cause of the kidney disease. Chronic glomerulonephritis, diabetic renal disease, and other nephropathies produce the same disorder, although diabetic neuropathy can be further complicated by renal failure, when present.

Four clinical types of peripheral neuropathy associated with renal failure have been identified:[7]

1. Mononeuropathy of a pressure palsy type involving peroneal or ulnar nerves. This develops in the debilitated patient who remains too long in one position.

2. A mild distal sensory neuritis associated with absent ankle jerks.

3. Dysesthesias — the burning feet or tender sole syndrome with no objective sensory, reflex, or motor findings.

4. A severe sensorimotor polyneuritis, most often affecting the feet and legs below the knee.

Many of the subclinical and clinical manifestations of the disorder have been quantitated by electrodiagnostic studies, and the late anatomic changes in the peripheral nerves have been documented. The majority of patients with azotemia demonstrate slowed conduction velocities in one or more segments, irrespective of clinical signs. This is an integral part of the uremic syndrome and is related to the degree of azotemia that develops when renal function, as measured by creatinine clearance, falls to 10 per cent of normal.[76] Distal latency is not affected. Reduced sensory action potentials are mainly due to increased temporal dispersion of the signals.

This often reversible finding is not explained by axon demyelinization and degeneration but favors the theory that toxic factors inhibit the transmembrane sodium pump, resulting in the reduction of current density at the nodes of Ranvier. Urea and creatinine, per se, do not produce this effect, but azotemic serum does.

When the more profound sensorimotor polyneuropathy develops in a chronically diseased, usually dialyzed, uremic patient, segmental demyelinization can be demonstrated.[28] It is in these more seriously ill patients that this defect in Schwann cell function appears. This is presumed to be due to metabolic effects and can be identified in teased specimens.

In patients dying of renal failure, neuropathic changes beyond demyelinization include severe axonal damage with wallerian degeneration, foam-type phagocytes containing free fat, and a paucity of inflammatory cells.[108]

The "restless leg" syndrome has been related to decreased motor conduction velocity, but since sensory and motor conduction velocities tend to be affected concomitantly,[76] this may be a spurious correlation. Painful, burning paresthesias of the feet may be related to dietary deprivation, as symptoms can disappear within days of initiating a normal, balanced diet. This disorder is not corrected by vitamin therapy alone.[108]

The differential diagnosis of the symmetric, severe polyneuropathy of azotemia includes amyloid-myeloma neuropathy, diabetic neuropathy, and the neuropathy of inflammatory autoimmune diseases, such as polyarteritis nodosa and systemic lupus erythematosus.[19] Pernicious anemia must also be considered, as ataxia may be present in uremic patients.

Treatment. Obviously, the presence of azotemia should be sought for in any peripheral neuropathy. Once the diagnosis has been suggested by findings of renal failure, the efforts of the orthopaedist should be correlated with those of the internist/nephrologist and neurologist.

Orthopaedic management is usually conservative and includes ankle orthoses for footdrop and fixed equinus and appropriate shoes with soft custom-made inner soles in cases of sensory deficit.

Surgical correction of deformities should rarely be undertaken because of the impaired capacity of azotemic patients to handle the stress of surgery. Since most equinus deformities can be accommodated by heel elevation, Achilles tendon lengthening procedures will seldom be necessary. When performed, the deformity is corrected by a simple tenotomy under local anesthesia. A long-acting anesthetic, such as bupivacaine without epinephrine, should be used. The patient should be returned to an ambulatory status almost immediately, using small doses of analgesics to control whatever pain is not tolerated.

ENDOCRINE NEUROPATHIES

Acromegaly may cause nerve entrapment syndromes and, less commonly, peripheral neuropathy secondary to hypertrophic nerve changes. More frequent and severe changes may occur in pituitary gigantism, probably because of the earlier onset of the pituitary disease. Charcot changes have been described in the feet and ankles of such patients.[23]

NUTRITIONAL NEUROPATHIES

Although the classic descriptions of the nutritional diseases were those of single factor deficiencies (e.g., thiamine in beriberi), multiple deficiencies usually exist when such clinical disorders are now encountered. This is probably also true in many instances of alcoholic neuropathy.

Nutritional neuropathies are usually mixed motor and sensory polyneuropathies with "glove and stocking" sensory changes and distal muscle weakness. They include beriberi (vitamin B_1 deficiency), pellagra (B complex vitamin deficiency), subacute combined degeneration (vitamin B_{12} deficiency), and, possibly, to some degree, alcoholic polyneuritis.

Denny-Brown[25] reported on the neuropathies following dietary restriction. Beriberi produced fixed contraction of the calf muscles with symmetric foot drop and wasting below the knee. There was stocking hypesthesia and loss of ankle jerks. The neuritis developed rapidly in one to three days.

In pellagra, glossitis and angular stomatitis are common, but neuropathy is rare and clinically severe polyneuritis is not seen. The neuropathy of pellagra is thought to be produced by associated thiamine deficiency rather than a nicotinamide deficit.[41, 64] Some patients respond very slowly after replacement therapy, presumably because of axon degeneration.

A syndrome of "burning feet" is associated with a diet restricted to cereals. Retrobulbar neuritis may be present, and there are associated motor disorders, including an ataxic and a spastic form. Combined disorders also occur.[25]

Subacute combined degeneration (posterolateral sclerosis)[71, 110] is seen in pernicious anemia or related diseases in which there is either decrease in gastric intrinsic factor (sporadic, familial, or following gastrectomy) or decreased absorption of vitamin B_{12} (sprue). In pernicious anemia, the onset occurs at about 15 years of age. There is degeneration of the posterior lateral cord (posterior column and pyramidal tract), peripheral nerves, and cerebellar tracts. Early findings include typical paresthesias of the tips of the toes and occasional stabbing pain. There is "glove and stocking" sensory loss, in which upper extremity involvement follows that of the lower extremities. Posterior column involvement results in decreased vibratory and pain sensation. Later there is muscle weakness and ataxia with a positive Romberg sign and ultimately a positive Babinski sign. In about 50 per cent of patients, ankle jerks are absent, but these are occasionally increased secondary to pyramidal tract involvement. Glossitis is of diagnos-

tic significance and is probably caused by the anemia. There may be mental changes, including confusion and paranoia, and later bowel problems. Some patients will not reveal any anemia and the sternal marrow may also be normal. In such cases, diagnosis may be made by finding decreased vitamin B_{12} in the serum or by a positive Shilling test, which determines urinary output following oral administration of radioactive vitamin B_{12}. Previously, pernicious anemia was a fatal disease. Currently, however, administration of vitamin B_{12} will not only prevent progression of the disorder but will clear up the polyneuropathy, although the spastic element tends to remain.

MISCELLANEOUS VASCULAR AND HEMATOLOLOGICALLY RELATED NEUROPATHIES

Acute neuropathy may occur in association with hemorrhagic diseases such as thrombocytopenic purpura and hemophilia or from toxic thrombocytopenic purpura secondary to medication such as penicillin.[13] It may also occur iatrogenically from anticoagulants. The neuropathy may be caused by bleeding into the nerve sheath or by ischemia from arterial occlusion. Rarely, a hemoglobinopathy may result in a vasculitis that causes a peripheral neuropathy (see Figure 44–6A to C). Neuropathy is not seen in sickle cell disease.[44] Leukemia may cause nerve involvement by local infiltration.

The neuropathy caused by the vasculitis of collagen disease and diabetic mononeuropathy multiplex have already been discussed.

Pseudo-neuralgic pain caused by arterial occlusion or narrowing is well known. The posterior tibial artery syndrome consists of vascular compromise of this artery, which produces symptoms similar to those in the tarsal tunnel syndrome.

The nerve damage associated with various compartment syndromes is discussed elsewhere (see Chapter 43).

PERIPHERAL NEUROPATHY IN LEPROSY

Leprosy often presents as a slowly developing neuropathy involving the hands and/or feet. More fulminating secondary infection may follow sensory deprivation of the feet. Local infection with *Mycobacterium leprae* may involve the soft tissues and bones of the foot, further complicating the disease. Loss of terminal phalanges or entire toes is quite frequent as sensory loss, trauma, and infection progress.

The key to therapy is early diagnosis, before the more serious sequelae develop. The disease is endemic in many parts of South and Central America and is seen sporadically in the United States. In addition to antibiotic therapy to control the *M. leprae* bacillus and secondary bacterial invaders, surgical therapy of the involved nerves sometimes improves the neuropathies when localized lesions can be identified. Naturally, appropriate surgical therapy for localized sepsis should be used along with antibiotic treatment.

Only a brief overview of lepromatous neuropathy will be presented, as leprosy is covered in more detail in Chapter 46.

The neuropathy of leprosy usually presents insidiously with gradual, progressive loss of sensation in the hands and feet. Weakness and atrophy then appear. The clinical picture includes symmetric hand and foot weakness, reduced sensation, and electrodiagnostic changes revealing both denervation (fibrillations and positive sharp waves) and nerve conduction deficits with increased distal latencies, decreased amplitudes, prolongation of compound muscle action potentials, reduced motor conduction velocities, and low or absent sensory potentials in the arms or legs. Of interest and diagnostic importance is the preservation of deep tendon reflexes. The neuropathy develops as a mixed disease characterized by axon changes (leading to degeneration) and demyelinization with loss of saltatory conduction and resultant conduction velocity deficits.[95]

Two types of leprous nerve lesions can develop — lepromatous and tuberculoid. Both may be present in the same patient. In lepromatous lesions, *M. leprae* organisms are numerous, there is intense fibrosis of the nerve, and granulomas are not present. Tuberculoid lesions show granulomatous zones and few bacilli.

The neuropathy that develops involves sensory, motor, and sympathetic fibers. Anesthesia, poor skin nutrition, and calluses secondary to dynamic imbalances

and contractures occur. This leads to secondary infection of soft tissue and bone. The pattern that may develop includes granulomas in the skin and deeper soft tissues that are produced directly by the leprosy bacillus. Leprous osteomyelitis may also be present.

In leprosy, neuritis occurs selectively in the tibial nerve above the ankle and the common peroneal nerve at the knee, causing anesthesia of the foot with relatively normal plantar power. The involvement of the tibial nerve is below its section supplying the ankle but above its section supplying the subtalar joint, resulting in the frequent occurrence of Charcot changes in the subtalar joint compared with that in the ankle.[47] In one series of 400 patients,[112] 23.5 per cent revealed evidence of Charcot changes, which may also occur following insufficient immobilization after arthrodesing procedures. Peroneal muscle weakness results in fixed varus deformity with ulceration and absorption of the lateral column of the foot. This may lead to unstable medial subluxation of the foot. These changes are not of the Charcot type.[47] Similarly, the forefoot absorption seen in leprosy is also due to chronic plantar ulcerations with secondary underlying bone dissolution.[47]

Leprous neuropathies can be arrested and at times reversed by appropriate chemotherapy, if treatment is begun before irrevocable internal disorganization of the nerve trunk fibers has developed.

Constriction of the neurovascular bundle in the tarsal tunnel has been demonstrated in leprosy.[81] Surgical decompression of the posterior tibial neurovascular bundle by epineural neurolysis has been followed by relief of pain and healing of many ulcers in lepromatous feet.[81] Positive findings in the tarsal tunnel are reported in all patients with tuberculoid, lepromatous, and mixed neuritis. Lesions include thickening of the flexor retinaculum and the perineurovascular connective tissue, fibrous thickening of the tibial nerve, arterial thrombosis and narrowing, and local congestion.

The differential diagnosis of lepromatous neuropathy includes the neuritis of amyloidosis and, in the presence of renal disease, uremic neuropathy. Both these disorders may be present in the leprous patient. In addition, tuberculosis is a known complication, with involvement of the kidneys. Interstitial nephritis produced by immune complexes may also develop. The neuritis of amyloidosis is usually familial. This disease presents as a dissociated sensory loss with loss of pain and temperature sensation and preservation of position and vibration sense, not unlike early leprosy neuropathy. There is, however, a profound autonomic neuropathy with episodic diarrhea, impotence, reduced sweating, and postural hypotension in amyloid neuropathy. Electrodiagnostic findings are those of normal nerve conduction velocities with severe reduction of sensory and motor action potentials. The neuropathy of renal failure develops in the presence of rather pronounced azotemia. It is a diffuse sensorimotor disease, and deep tendon reflexes are abolished. The diagnosis is usually obvious because of the advanced renal disease and the absence of the patchy neuropathy of leprosy, as well as the absence of visible peripheral tissue changes.

TOXIC, ALLERGIC, AND MISCELLANEOUS NEUROPATHIES

Toxic polyneuritis and neuritis occur from drugs,[79] organic substances, and heavy metals, including ethyl alcohol, methyl alcohol (optic atrophy), and Jamaica ginger poisoning. In Jamaica ginger poisoning, the toxic action is caused by the contaminant triorthocresyl phosphate, which mainly results in a motor paralysis with bilateral wrist drop and footdrop. Other causes include lead poisoning, which leads to motor paralysis, and arsenic (rat poison) poisoning, which results in pain, sensory "glove and stocking" anesthesia with flaccid paralysis, rash, and herpes zoster.[45] Thallium (depilatory creams) causes sensorimotor involvement, sometimes associated with retrobulbar neuritis. Mercury poisoning may also cause neuropathy.

Toxic neuropathy may be associated with toxemia of pregnancy and with malignancy.[111]

The allergic group of neuropathies includes serum sickness, Guillain-Barré syndrome, and multiple sclerosis. Serum sickness may cause C5 (deltoid) paralysis or

involvement of the entire brachial plexus. Guillain-Barré syndrome is a progressive ascending motor paralysis with some associated sensory changes. Multiple sclerosis may involve any part of the central or peripheral nervous system and, as previously noted, may cause Charcot joints.

NEUROPATHY ASSOCIATED WITH CARCINOMA

Approximately 6.6 per cent of cancers result in neuromuscular damage, especially carcinomas of the ovary and lung. Since carcinoma of the lung is more frequent and 14 per cent of lung cancers cause neuromuscular damage, this lesion is responsible for 50 per cent of all cases of neuropathy due to malignancy. Different forms exist, including encephalitic neuropathy, mixed polyneuropathy, and myelopathy, and may occasionally simulate amyotrophic lateral sclerosis. Electromyographic studies will show muscle and nerve degeneration, but patients may have relatively normal conduction velocity studies. In myelopathy, there is generalized muscle weakness, especially proximally, but relatively sparse pathologic findings. The muscle weakness may antedate the symptoms of the malignancy by years. One should also note that elderly patients with carcinomatosis often have concomitant heart disease and are on diuretics. Diuretic therapy may result in low serum potassium levels, which may also cause some muscle weakness. However, such patients do not have much weakness in spite of very low potassium levels, since there is minimal change in the potassium concentration ratio (e.g. low extra- and intracellular potassium). Occasionally, a sensory neuropathy may occur in association with bronchogenic carcinoma as a result of involvement of the dorsal root ganglia. It involves both upper and lower extremities, causes considerable paresthesias, and may occur with or without motor involvement.

MOTOR NEURITIS

Multiple motor neuritis, as seen in Landry's ascending paralysis (Guillain-

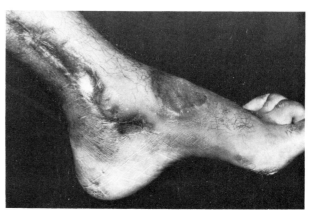

Figure 44-24. *War injury to the common plantar nerve and the posterior tibial artery. There was surprisingly little disability, except for the mild fixed ankle equinus and hammer toes.*

Barré syndrome) or heavy metal poisoning, may cause permanent paralysis, such as flail feet requiring surgical stabilization. Aside from trauma (Fig. 44–24), diabetes is the most frequent cause of mononeuritis, usually motor, of the lower extremities, such as neuritis of the femoral or obturator nerve. Spinal pathology (Fig. 44–25) such as a herniated disc, osteophytes, spinal stenosis, or a localized metastatic lesion may primarily affect a nerve root, simulating a peripheral motor neuropathy. However, there is a root distribution of findings rather than a peripheral nerve distribution. Neuritis of the peroneal nerve over the fibular neck causes local tenderness and Tinel's sign, footdrop, and hypesthesia, especially over the dorsum of the foot between the first and second metatarsals (deep peroneal nerve). It may be caused locally by trauma, scar formation, compression, tumors such as a ganglion or neurilemoma, or may occasionally be idiopathic. Motor involvement is also found in com-

partment syndromes and may be obscured by the secondary contractures and joint stiffness, which, in turn, are due to the edema and massive muscle necrosis. This form of motor involvement is discussed in Chapter 43. Unsuspected vascular damage may occur in association with peripheral nerve damage and may require arteriography. The vascular status will then determine not only any vascular surgery indicated but the extent of foot surgery permissible for the deformities caused by the ischemia, edema, and nerve damage. Rarely, peripheral nerve injuries cause Charcot-like changes in the foot (Fig. 44–26).

Motor paralysis is usually treated by bracing; orthoses; tendon transfers, with or without joint stabilization; and, of course, nerve exploration when indicated. It must be stressed that when there is an accompanying sensory component (including proprioceptive), joint stabilization rather than maintaining a more flexible plantigrade

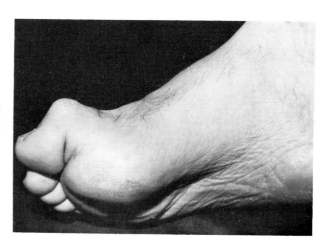

Figure 44-25. *Multiple unilateral fixed hammer-toe deformities in a patient with a fracture of spine with spinal cord injury after laminectomy.*

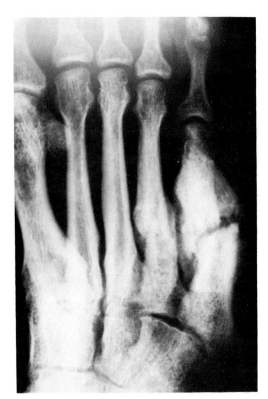

Figure 44–26. *Injury to the posterior tibial nerve and the popliteal artery. The Charcot-like changes in the fourth and fifth metatarsals are probably related to a slight fixed varus deformity of the forefoot (march fractures plus periostitis from an underlying trophic ulcer).*

foot may lead to increased tendency for plantar skin ulceration or breakdown and Charcot-like joints, as seen following subtalar and ankle fusion in myelodysplasia.

PERIPHERAL MONOSENSORY NEURITIS AND NEUROMAS

Sensory neuritis refers to an inflammatory or invasive process involving a sensory nerve. A localized neuritis may be produced by local nerve thickening simulating a neuroma, such as a plantar interdigital neuroma. A neuroma is a reactive process that is due to local nerve injury. One always occurs when a nerve, normal or otherwise, is resected. Thus, the removal of a plantar interdigital "neuroma" (interstitial neuritis) results in true neuroma formation of varying degrees, approximately 10 per cent of the lesions being symptomatic. In general, sensory neuritis and neuromas cause pain, paresthesias, local tenderness, and usually a positive Tinel sign.

Aside from plantar interdigital neuromas, sensory neuritis may occasionally be seen from local shoe pressure over the dorsolateral aspect of a hammered fifth toe. Neuritis of the proper digital nerve is seen secondary to bunions from abnormal weight-bearing pressure as a result of associated medial rotation of the hallux. It should be differentiated from bunion pain. On surgical exploration, the nerve reveals an elongated thickening.

Sensory neuromas are often iatrogenic and occur most frequently secondary to foot surgery. The most common lesions are sural neuromas from lateral foot incisions and, to a lesser extent, from anterior ankle incisions involving a branch of the superficial peroneal nerve. As noted, sensory neuromas occur following resection of a plantar interdigital neuroma or resection of nerve tumors in the foot. They are rarely symptomatic following interruption of a fine branch of the superficial peroneal nerve over the dorsum of the foot and, for some reason, are extremely rare following surgical interruption of a digital nerve related to the hallux or small toe. However, there may be slight numbness of the hallux, especially when the dorsal medial digital branch is cut when making a curved dorsal medial surgical approach. A straight midline medial approach is therefore preferable. When symptomatic, sensory neuromas should be treated appropriately (see Chapter 43).

Iatrogenic neuromas can usually be prevented by avoiding cutting fine sensory nerve branches (as discussed in Chapter 8). Once they occur, resection is most likely to result in recurrence, especially in hypersensitive individuals. Local anesthetic agents, with or without injectable steroids (0.25 ml of each), may be tried, but such treatment is usually unsuccessful.

Exploration may reveal bulbous neuroma formation at the proximal end of a previously resected or severed nerve. At other times the cut end appears normal, but may be adherent to skin or adjacent scar tissue. Prevention of painful neuroma includes avoiding pressure and traction on the nerve end.

In the cases in which a painful neuroma may have to be explored, the operating microscope is useful in identifying the branch embedded in grossly similar-appearing scar tissue. Nerve bundles may be identified using 20 to 25× magnification. Fascicular ligation has been useful (see Chapter 43).

SUMMARY AND CONCLUSIONS

The neuropathies form an extremely diversified etiologic group of entities, some relatively common and others quite rare. Many are primarily related to other medical disciplines, especially neurology, but frequently to pediatrics, internal medicine, and even hematology. In some cases, the presenting primary complaints and findings are mainly localized to the feet and ankles, whereas in others occult foot symptoms play only a minor role in a much more widespread neurologic or systemic disease. In either case, early and accurate diagnosis is necessary, not only to initiate appropriate treatment but to avoid secondary complications and irreversible damage, to evaluate the prognosis, and even to provide genetic counseling.[90]

REFERENCES

1. Adams, R. D., and Sidman, R. L.: Introduction to Neuropathology. New York, McGraw-Hill, 1968, pp. 55–83.
2. Afifi, A. H., and Sabra, F. A.: Treatment of toxic and drug-induced neuropathies. Mod. Treat., 5:1236, 1968.
3. Andersson, R., and Bjerle, P.: Peripheral circulation, particularly heat regulation reactions, in patients with amyloidosis and polyneuropathy. Acta Med. Scand., 199:191, 1976.
4. Andersson, R., and Hofer, P. A.: Primary amyloidosis with polyneuropathy. Acta Med. Scand., 196:115, 1974.
5. Antes, E. H.: Charcot joint in diabetes mellitus. J.A.M.A., 156:602, 1954.
6. Appenzeller, O., and Kornfeld, M.: A chronic peripheral neuropathy with mosaic Schwann cells. Arch. Neurol., 27:322, 1972.
7. Asbury, A. K., Victor, M., and Adams, R. D.: Uremic polyneuropathy. Trans. Am. Neurol. Assn., 87:100, 1962.
8. Babcock, W. W.: Nerve association: A new method for the surgical relief of painful or paralytic affections of nerve trunks. Ann. Surg., 46:686, 1907.
9. Barley, C. C., and Root, H. F.: Neuropathic foot lesions in diabetes mellitus. N. Engl. J. Med., 236:397, 1947.
10. Barrett, J. P., and Mooney, V.: Neuropathy and diabetic pressure lesion. Orthop. Clin. North Am., 4:43, 1973.
11. Bauman, J. H., Girling, J. P., and Brand, P. W.: Plantar pressures and trophic ulceration — An evaluation of footwear. J. Bone Joint Surg., 45-B:652, 1963.
12. Baxter, D. W., and Olszewski, J.: Congenital universal insensitivity to pain. Brain, 83:381, 1960.
13. Bigelow, N., and Graves, R.: Peripheral nerve lesions in hemorrhage diseases. Arch. Neurol. Psychiatr., 68:819, 1952.
14. Blechen, S. S., Lovelace, R. E., and Cotton, R. E.: Mononeuritis multiplex in polyarteritis nodosa. Quart. J. Med., 32:193, 1963.
15. Boehm, H. J.: Diabetic Charcot joint. N. Engl. J. Med., 267:185, 1962.
16. Buchanan, W. W.: Peripheral neuropathy in rheumatoid arthritis. In Scott, J. T. (ed.): Copeman's Textbook of Rheumatic Diseases. Edinburgh, Churchill Livingstone, 1978, pp. 340–341.
17. Butler, J. D., and Block, L. D.: Posterior column diseases as they affect the foot. J. Am. Podiatry Assn., 65:357, 1975.
18. Camera, P.: Lesioni trofoneurotiche in stato disraficio. Minerva Ortop., 6:400, 1955.
19. Case Records, Massachusetts General Hospital: Case no. 42–1962. N. Engl. J. Med., 266:1378, 1962.
20. Chusid, J. G.: Correlative Neuroanatomy and Functional Neurology. 16th Ed. Los Altos, Cal., Lange Medical Publications, 1976, pp. 190–195.
21. Chusid, J. G.: Correlative Neuroanatomy and Functional Neurology. 16th Ed. Los Altos, Cal., Lange Medical Publications, 1976, p. 70.
22. Danta, G.: Hypoglycemia peripheral neuropathy. Arch. Neurol. (Chicago), 21:121, 1969.
23. Daughady, W. H.: Extreme gigantism: Analysis of growth velocity and occurrence of severe peripheral neuropathy and neuropathic arthropathy (Charcot joints). N. Engl. J. Med., 27:1267, 1977.
24. Denny-Brown, D.: Hereditary sensory radicular neuropathy. J. Neurol. Neurosurg. Psychiatr., 14:237, 1951.
25. Denny-Brown, D.: Neurological conditions resulting from prolonged and severe dietary restriction. Medicine, 26:41, 1947.
26. Denny-Brown, D.: Special problems concerning beriberi: The neurological aspects of thiamine deficiency. Fed. Proc., 17(Suppl. 2):35, 1958.
27. Dimon, J. H., III, Funk, J. F., and Wells, R. E.: Congenital indifference to pain with associated orthopedic abnormalities. South Med. J., 58:524, 1965.
28. Dinn, J. J., and Crane, D. L.: Schwann cell function in uraemia. J. Neurol. Neurosurg. Psychiatr., 33:605, 1970.
29. Dolman, C. L.: The morbid anatomy of diabetic neuropathy. Neurology, 13:135, 1963.
30. Dyck, P. J., Kennel, A. J., Magal, I. V., and Kraybill, E. N.: A Virginia kinship with hereditary sensory neuropathy: Peroneal muscular atrophy and pes cavus. Mayo Clin. Proc., 40: 695, 1965.
31. Dyck, P. J., and Lambert, E. H.: Lower motor and primary sensory neuron disease with peroneal muscular atrophy. I. Neurologic, genetic and electrophysiologic findings in hereditary polyneuropathies. Arch. Neurol., 18:603, 1968.
32. Dyck, P. J.: Peripheral neuropathy. Med. Clin. North Am., 52:895, 1968.
33. Eisen, A. A.: Electromyography and nerve conduction as a diagnostic aid. Orthop. Clin. North Am., 4:885, 1973.
34. Ellenberg, M.: Diabetic neuropathy: Clinical aspects. Metabolism, 25:1627, 1976.
35. Faris, I.: Foot lesions in diabetic patients. Med. J. Austral. 1:628, 1977.
36. Faris, I.: Small and large vessel disease in the development of foot lesions in diabetes. Diabetologia, 11:249, 1975.
37. Feldman, R., Hayes, M. K., Youries, R., and Aldrich, F. D.: Lead neuropathy in adults and children. Arch. Neurol., 34:481, 1977.
38. Ford, R. G., and Siekert, R. G.: Central nervous system manifestations of periarteris nodosa. Neurology, 15:114, 1965.
38a. Garland, H. T., and Taverner, D.: Diabetic myelopathy. Br. Med. J., 1:1405, 1953.

39. Geist, F. D.: Chromatolysis of efferent neurosis. Arch. Neurol. Psychiatr. (Chicago), 29:88, 1933.

40. Gilliat, R. W.: Nerve conduction in human and experimental neuropathies. Proc. Roy. Soc. Med., 59:989, 1966.

41. Goldblatt, D.: Treatment of deficiency and alcoholic neuropathies. Mod. Treat., 5:1249, 1968.

42. Golding, C.: Museum Pages III. Spina bifida and epiphyseal displacement. J. Bone Joint Surg., 42-B:389, 1960.

43. Goodgold, J., and Eberstein, S.: Electrodiagnosis of Neuromuscular Diseases. 2nd Ed. Baltimore, Williams and Wilkins, 1977.

44. Greer, M., and Schotland, D.: Abnormal hemoglobin as a cause of neurologic disease. Neurology, 12:114, 1962.

45. Gupta, S. K., Helal, B. H., and Kiely, P.: The prognosis in zoster paralysis. J. Bone Joint Surg., 51-B:593, 1969.

46. Hakstian, R. W.: Perineural neuropathy. Orthop. Clin. North Am., 4:945, 1973.

47. Harris, J. R., and Brand, P. W.: Patterns of disintegration of the tarsus in the anaesthetic foot. J. Bone Joint Surg., 48-B:4, 1966.

48. Harrison, M. J. G., and Faris, I.: The neuropathic factor in the aetiology of diabetic foot ulcers. J. Neurol. Sci., 28:217, 1976.

49. Hart, F. D., Golding, J. R., and Mackenzie, D. H.: Neuropathy in rheumatoid disease. Ann. Rheum. Dis., 16:471, 1957.

50. Harty, M.: Metatarsalgia. Surg. Gynecol. Obstet., 136:105, 1973.

51. Heller, L. H., and Robb, P.: Hereditary sensory neuropathy. Neurology, 5:15, 1955.

51a. Hicks, E. P.: Hereditary perforating ulcer of the foot. Lancet, 1:319, 1922.

52. Hofer, P. A., and Andersson, R.: Postmorteus findings in primary familial amyloidosis with polyneuropathy. Acta Pathol. Microbiol. Scand., 83(Sect. A):309, 1975.

53. Horwitz, M. T.: Normal anatomy and variations of peripheral nerves of leg and foot. Arch. Surg., 36:626, 1938.

54. Jacobs, J. G.: Observations of neuropathic (Charcot) joints occurring in diabetes mellitus. J. Bone Joint Surg., 40-A:1043, 1958.

55. Jammis, J. L.: The autonomic nervous system in peroneal muscular atrophy. Arch. Neurol., 27:213, 1972.

56. Joynt, R. J., and Goldstein, M. N.: Treatment of neuropathies accompanying inflammatory, vascular and neoplastic conditions. Mod. Treat., 5:1263, 1968.

57. Khalifeh, R. R., and Zellweger, H.: Hereditary sensory neuropathy with spinal cord disease. Neurology, 13:405, 1963.

58. Kochs, J.: Spontanheilung einer Fussdeformität bei Spina Bifida Occulta nach Laminektomie. Münch. Med. Wochenschr., 74:1877, 1927.

59. Kritchman, M. M., Schwartz, H., and Papper, E. M.: Experiences with general anesthesia in patients with familial dysautonomia. J.A.M.A., 170:529, 1959.

60. Krittner, A. E.: A technique for salvage of the infected diabetic gangrenous foot. Orthop. Clin. North Am., 4:21, 1973.

61. Lam, S. J.: A tarsal tunnel syndrome. Lancet, 2:1354, 1962.

62. Lambert, E. H., Mulder, D. W., and Bastron, J. A.: Regeneration of peripheral nerves with hyperinsulin neuropathy. Neurology (Minneapolis), 10:851, 1960.

63. Levine, D. B.: Orthopaedic aspects of familial dysautonomia. In Hardy, J. H. (ed.): Spinal Deformity in Neurological and Muscular Disorders. St. Louis, C. V. Mosby Co., 1974.

64. Levy, F. H., Spies, T. D., and Aring, C. D.: Incidence of neuropathy in pellegra. Am. J. Med. Sci., 6:840, 1940.

65. Lippman, H., Perotto, A., and Farrar, R.: The neuropathic foot of the diabetic. Bull. N.Y. Acad. Med., 52:1159, 1976.

66. Lithner, F.: Cutaneous erythema with or without necrosis, localized to the legs and feet — a lesion in elderly diabetics. Acta Med. Scand., 196:333, 1974.

67. Lithner, F.: Cutaneous reactions of the extremities of diabetes to local thermal trauma. Acta Med. Scand., 198:319, 1975.

68. Lithner, F.: Skin lesions of the legs and feet and skeletal lesions of the feet in familial amyloidosis with polyneuropathy. Acta Med. Scand., 199:197, 1976.

69. MacEwen, G. D., and Floyd, G. C.: Congenital insensitivity to pain and its orthopaedic implications. Clin. Orthop. Rel. Res. 68:100, 1970.

70. Mann, R., and Inman, V.: Phasic activity of intrinsic muscles of the foot. J. Bone Joint Surg., 46-A:469, 1964.

71. Merritt, H. H.: A Textbook of Neurology. 5th Ed. Philadelphia, Lea & Febiger, 1973, pp. 624–651.

72. Mooney, V., and Mankin, H. J.: A case of congenital insensitivity to pain with neuropathic arthropathy. Arthrit. Rheum., 9:820, 1966.

73. Moorehouse, J. A., Carter, S. A., and Doupe, J.: Vascular responses in diabetic peripheral neuropathy. Br. Med. J., 1:883, 1966.

74. Mulder, D. W., Bastron, J. A., and Lambert, E. H.: Hyperinsulin neuropathy. Neurology (Minneapolis), 6:627, 1956.

75. Munsat, T. L.: Neurological evaluation. In Hardy, J. H. (ed.): Spinal Deformity in Neurological and Muscular Disorders. St. Louis, C. V. Mosby Co., 1974, p. 35.

76. Nielson, J. K.: The peripheral nerve function in chronic renal failure. VI. The relationship between sensory and motor nerve conduction and kidney function, azotemia, age, sex and clinical neuropathy. Acta Med. Scand., 194:455, 1973.

77. Norman, A., Robbins, H., and Milgram, J. E.: The acute neuropathic arthropathy — A rapid, severely disorganizing form of arthritis. Radiology, 90:1159, 1968.

78. Ogden, T. E., Robert, F., and Carmichael, E. A.: Some sensory syndromes in children: Indifference to pain and sensory neuropathy. J. Neurol. Neurosurg. Psychiatr., 22:267, 1959.

79. O'Sullivan, D.: Drug-induced neuropathies. Bull. Postgrad. Comm. Med. Univ. Sidney, 26:180, 1971.

80. Ozeran, R. S., Wagner, G. R., Reemer, T. R., and Hill, R. A.: Neuropathy of the sympathetic nervous system associated with diabetes mellitus. Surgery, 68:953, 1970.

81. Palande, D. D., and Azhayuraj, M.: Surgical decompression of posterior tibial neurovascular complex in treatment of certain chronic plantar ulcers and posterior tibial neuritis in leprosy. Int. J. Leprosy, 43:36, 1975.

82. Pallis, C. A., and Scott, J. T.: Peripheral neuropathy in rheumatoid arthritis. Br. Med. J., 1:1141, 1965.

83. Petrie, J. G.: A case of progressive disorders caused by insensitivity to pain. J. Bone Joint Surg., 35-B:399, 1956.

84. Pinsky, L., and DiGeorge, A. M.: Congenital familial sensory neuropathy with anhidrosis. J. Pediatr., 68:1, 1966.

85. Pogonowska, M. J., Collins, L. C., and Dobson, H. L.: Diabetic osteopathy. Radiology, 89:265, 1967.

86. Raff, M. C., and Asbury, A. K.: Ischemic mononeuropathy and mononeuropathy multiplex in diabetes mellitus. N. Engl. J. Med., 279:17, 1968.

87. Raff, M. C., Sangalang, V., and Asbury, A. K.: Ischemic mononeuropathy multiplex associated with diabetes mellitus. Arch. Neurol., 18:487, 1968.
88. Ranney, H. M., Jacobs, A. S., Udem, L., and Zalusky, R.: Hemoglobin Riverdale-Bronx and unstable hemoglobin resulting from the substitution of arginine for glycine at helical residue $\beta 6$ of the B polypeptide chain. Biochem. Biophys. Res. Commun. 33:1004, 1968.
89. Refsum, S.: Heredo-pathia atactica polyneuritiformis: A familial syndrome not hitherto described. Acta Psychiatr. Neurol. 38(Suppl.):1, 1946.
90. Riley, C. M., and Moore, R. H.: Familial dysautonomia differentiated from related disorders. Pediatrics, 37:435, 1966.
91. Rose, G. K.: Arthropathy of the ankle in congenital indifference to pain. J. Bone Joint Surg., 35-B:408, 1953.
92. Roussy, G., and Lévy, G.: Sept cas d'une maladie familiale particuliére: Troubles de la marche, pied bots et aréfléxie tendineuse généralisée, avec, accessoirement, légère maladresse des mains. Rev. Neurol. (Paris), 33:427, 1926.
93. Roussy, G., and Lévy, G.: A propos de la dystasie aréflexique héréditaire. Rev. Neurol. (Paris), 62:763, 1934.
94. Rydick, B., Lundborg, G., and Nordborg, V.: Intraneural tissue reactions induced by internal neurolysis. Scand. J. Plast. Reconst. Surg., 10:3, 1976.
95. Scully, R. E. (ed.): Case Records of the Massachusetts General Hospital. Peripheral neuropathy and renal failure in a young Mexican woman. N. Engl. J. Med., 300:546, 1979.
96. Shumacker, H. B., Jr.: Causalgia. III-A. General discussion. Surgery, 24:485, 1948.
97. Siegler, M., and Refetoff, S.: Pretibial myxedema — A reversible cause of drop foot due to entrapment of the peroneal nerve. N. Engl. J. Med., 294:1383, 1976.
98. Sinha, S., Munictroodappa, C. S., and Kozak, G. P.: Neuroarthropathy (Charcot joint) in diabetes mellitus. Medicine, 51:191, 1972.
99. Staal, A.: The entrapment neuropathies *In* Vinkin, P. J., and Bruyn, G. W. (eds.): Handbook of Clinical Neurology. New York, American Elsevier, 1970, pp. 285–325.
100. Stilwell, D. L., Jr.: The innervation of deep structures of the foot. Am. J. Anat., 101:59, 1957.
101. Stokes, I., Faris, I. B., and Hotton, W. C.: The neuropathic ulcer and loads on the foot in diabetic patients. Acta Orthop. Scand., 46:839, 1975.
102. Symonds, C. P., and Shaw, M. E.: Familial claw-foot with absent tendon-jerks: A "forme fruste" of Charcot-Marie-Tooth disease. Brain, 49:387, 1926.
103. Thomas, P. K., and Lascelles, R. G.: Pathology of diabetic neuropathy. Quart. J. Med., 35:489, 1966.
104. Thorne, R. P., Levine, D. B., and Axelrod, F. B.: Management of familial dysautonomia. Orthop. Nurses Assoc. J., 5:37, 1978.
105. Thornhill, H. L., Richter, R. W., Shelton, M. L., and Johnson, C. A.: Neuropathic arthropathy (Charcot forefeet) in alcoholics. Orthop. Clin. North Am., 4:7, 1973.
106. Tooth, H. H.: The peroneal type of progressive muscular atrophy. A Thesis for the Degree of M.D. in the University of Cambridge, London, H. K. Lewis, 1886.
107. Trotter, J. L., Engle, K., and Ignacyak, T. F.: Amyloidosis with plasma cell dyscrasia — an overlooked cause of adult onset sensorimotor neuropathy. Arch. Neurol., 34:209, 1977.
108. Tyler, H. R.: Neurology disorders in renal failure. Am. J. Med., 44:734, 1968.
109. Waldenström, J. G.: Amyloid. Acta Med. Scand., 199: 145, 1976.
110. Walton, J. N.: Brain's Diseases of the Nervous System. Oxford, Oxford University Press, 1977, pp. 940–987.
111. Walton, J. N.: Brain's Diseases of the Nervous System. Oxford, Oxford University Press, 1977, pp. 867–874.
112. Warren, G.: Tarsal bone disintegration in leprosy. J. Bone Joint Surg., 53-B:688, 1971.
113. Weller, R. O., Bruckner, F. E., and Chamberlain, M. A.: Rheumatoid neuropathy: A histological and electrophysiological study. J. Neurol. Neurosurg. Psychiatr., 33:592, 1970.
114. Winkelmann, R. K., Lambert, E. H., and Hayles, A. B.: Congenital absence of pain. Arch. Dermatol., 85:325, 1962.
115. Yoslow, W., Becker, M. H., Bartels, J., and Thompson, W. A. L.: Orthopaedic defects in familial dysautonomia. J. Bone Joint Surg., 53-A:1541, 1971.
116. Zimmerman, E. A., and Lovelace, R. E.: The etiology of the neropathy in acute intermittent porphyria. Trans Am. Neurol. Assn., 93:294, 1968.

CHAPTER 45

CHARCOT FOOT

Richard L. Jacobs, M.D.,
and Allastair Karmody, M.D.

At least 24 different causes of neuropathic arthropathy have been described (Table 45–1). Changes in the foot and ankle have been reported in many, but not all, of these disorders. Diabetes mellitus, by far the most common cause of neuropathic arthropathy in our experience, has a predilection for changes in the lower extremities, although any other area of the body can be involved. Syringomyelia is a much less frequent cause and involves the upper extremities much more often than the lower.

The common feature in these various problems is that motor function is not as severely affected as are sensory modalities in patients who develop Charcot joints. Protective pain sensation is lost in varying degrees. Early on, there may be appreciable pain, although more often the pain is not commensurate with the degree of destruction seen on physical examination and roentgenography. The common misunderstanding is that a painful joint cannot, by definition, be a Charcot joint. This is not so.

Near-normal mobility is thus maintained in an extremity with a loss of normal protective pain sensation. Trauma that would usually elicit pain and awareness of injury (such as sprained ankle, metatarsal fracture) is ignored, and normal use is continued. If the patient is fortunate, the injury may heal without sequelae. If further injury is superimposed before healing can occur, the entire cycle of recurrent trauma with injury and repair reaction can be initiated. Some observers characterize Charcot joints as "the worst degenerative arthritis you will ever see." An everyday analogy that most will have experienced is the patient receiving a regional nerve block for dental work. If he eats before sensation returns, part of his intake may include buccal mucosa. Could this be called a transient Charcot mouth?

Charcot originally attributed bone and

TABLE 45–1. Etiologic Factors in Neuropathic Arthropathy

Diabetes mellitus°
Lues°
Syringomyelia°

Alcoholism
Amyloidosis
Amyotrophic lateral sclerosis
Arachnoiditis
Cerebral palsy
Cerebral vascular accident
Congenital insensitivity to pain
Cord trauma
Cord tumor
Elephantiasis
Hereditary insensitivity to pain
Hereditary sensory radicular neuropathy
Lead poisoning
Leprosy
Peripheral nerve injury
Pernicious anemia
Poliomyelitis
Root trauma
Spina bifida with meningomyelocele
Steroids – intra-articular or systemic
Yaws

°Three most common causes.

joint changes to a loss of central "neurotropic influence" on the peripheral nervous system. Virchow and von Volkmann, in often acerbic exchanges of views, disputed this with Charcot. Their theory of continuing trauma to an insensitive structure is still held. To Charcot, however, goes priority for the first comprehensive description of bone and joint changes in patients with neurologic disease (syphilis).

CLINICAL PRESENTATIONS OF CHARCOT FOOT AND ANKLE PROBLEMS

When first detected, these changes may be described according to any of several different clinical or anatomic patterns.

Acute vs. Chronic. The following classic description of acute neuropathic joint disease was provided by Charcot: A soldier had been in apparent good health, but suffered from previously undetected lues. At the end of a 30-mile march with field pack, he had a marked disturbance of gait, and both hip joints were found to have disintegrated!

The usual clinical pres ntation of acute neuropathy of the foot and ankle is sudden, unexplained swelling, which may or may not be painful (Fig. 45–1). The patient may recall specific trauma, but, just as commonly, does not. As with any injury, the affected area may be painful to palpation, and local temperature is increased. If the injury and repair reaction is sufficient, there may be erythema of the overlying skin. If the examiner is not cognizant of the neurologic changes, the diagnosis may be missed, and many cases are often initially treated as gout, rheumatoid arthritis, or infection. The diagnosis usually becomes more apparent as laboratory results are received (negative tests for rheumatoid arthritis, normal uric acid level, and normal white count and differential in an afebrile patient; smears and cultures of aspirated fluid are negative for microorganisms).

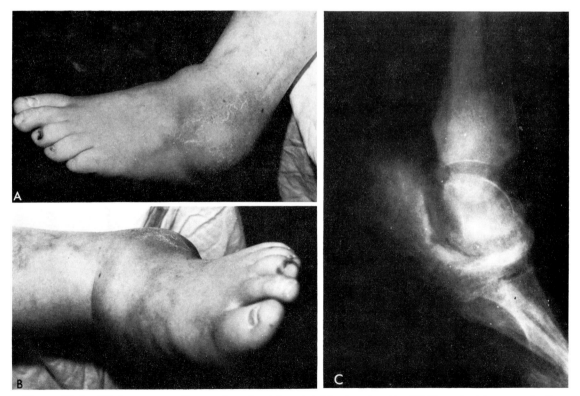

Figure 45–1. *(A) A warm, swollen, and moderately painful foot and ankle. (B) There had been gradually increasing deformity with recent acute onset of the other findings. An acute injury was probably superimposed. (C) Major subtalar destruction is shown roentgenographically. There was injury and repair reaction with no infection; widespread debridement could lead to loss of the foot. The patient is diabetic.*

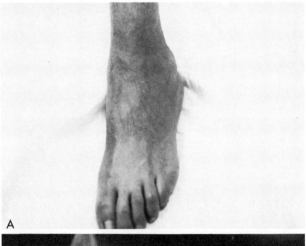

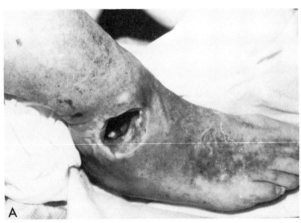

Figure 45–2. *(A) Minimal soft-tissue swelling with increasing valgus deformity and (B) chronic subtalar destruction in a luetic.*

Figure 45–3. *(A and B) Primary destruction of the ankle joint in tertiary lues. With increasing instability, there was ulceration into the ankle joint.*

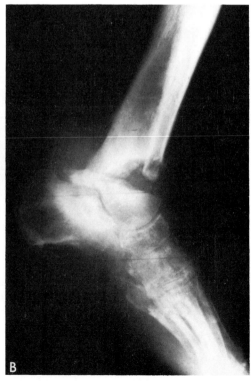

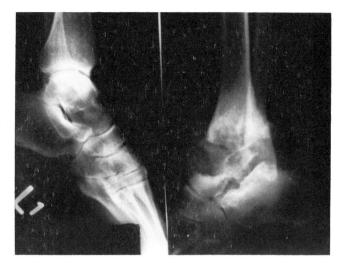

Figure 45–4. *Distintegration of the talus and subtalar joint in a luetic.*

The chronic form of Charcot foot changes (Fig. 45–2) probably represents the cumulative effect of repeated injuries; in this situation, more time elapses between each of the episodes of repeated trauma. Some slight distortion results from each successive injury, and this contributes to the picture of increasing deformity. There may be little soft-tissue swelling; what is commonly called "swelling" is actually structural deformity. There is no erythema in the chronic form. What swelling is seen is the result of traumatic synovitis secondary to joint destruction, and this is usually obvious clinically. Neuropathic joint disease must be considered in any foot with increasing structural deformity of whatever type.

By Anatomic Location. Milgram,[13] a former associate of Steindler at the University of Iowa, once gave a classic description of the neuropathic changes he had encountered in feet (predominantly of luetic patients):

1. Primary destruction of the ankle joint (Fig. 45–3).

2. Primary destruction of the subtalar joint, or "melting away" of the head of the talus (Fig. 45–4; see also Figure 45–1C).

3. Midtarsal destruction (the most common pattern) (Fig. 45–5).

4. Destruction of the joints between the metatarsals and cuboid and cuneiforms (Lisfranc's joint[s]) (Fig. 45–6).

To these, we perhaps can take the liberty of adding destruction of the metatarsophalangeal joints (Fig. 45–7). Any foot may show a mixture of these patterns, and spontaneous fractures of the metatarsal shafts are also fairly common.

Hypertrophic vs. Atrophic. This adds still another dimension to the description of neuropathic joints. Steindler[18] called attention to the difference between atrophic and hypertrophic changes. In the former, neuropathic joints simply seem to

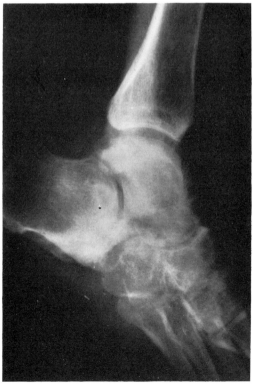

Figure 45–5. *Neuropathic changes in Chopart's joint in a diabetic.*

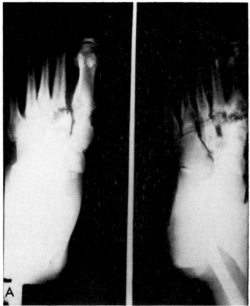

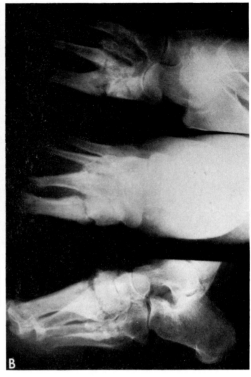

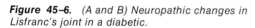

Figure 45–6. *(A and B) Neuropathic changes in Lisfranc's joint in a diabetic.*

"melt away." With increasing neuropathic change, the joint surfaces are progressively effaced, and there is relatively little evidence of fragmentation. The predominant picture is absorptive.

Hypertrophic changes are characterized by massive destruction of joints, much fragmentation, and a great deal of new bone formation. The predominant picture is proliferative.

MICROSCOPIC FINDINGS

Changes in the central and peripheral nervous systems have been exhaustively reported in the literature for the various etiologic fractures, but these changes do not lie within the scope of the present discussion.

As mentioned earlier, the overall changes in neuropathic arthropathy have sometimes been referred to as "the worst case of degenerative arthritis" to be seen. Curtiss[6] describes a synovial fluid effusion similar to that of traumatic arthritis. The fluid is usually clear, but may be bloody from recent trauma. The total nucleated cell count is not elevated, and the glucose concentration in the synovial fluid is only

slightly lower than that in the peripheral blood. The mucin precipitate is at least fair, and, in the case of syphilis, positive serologic findings are often obtained on joint fluid examination.

Synovial changes have been described. Because of the destruction of the joint surfaces, small fragments of bone and cartilage debris are often found embedded in the synovium. Horowitz[9] reports a series of 24 patients with such changes. His control series of 30 patients showed only two persons (both with advanced degenerative arthritis) with similar changes. This article has frequently been cited to demonstrate "a pathognomonic change in Charcot joints," a claim never made by Horowitz. Neither did he claim priority to the description; Barth,[1] Potts,[15] and King[11] made similar observations in earlier years.

We have also seen similar joint changes in patients with ochronosis. In all, these synovial changes are highly suggestive, but not diagnostic, of Charcot joints.

COMPLICATIONS

Spontaneous Fractures. The term implies that these fractures, especially in

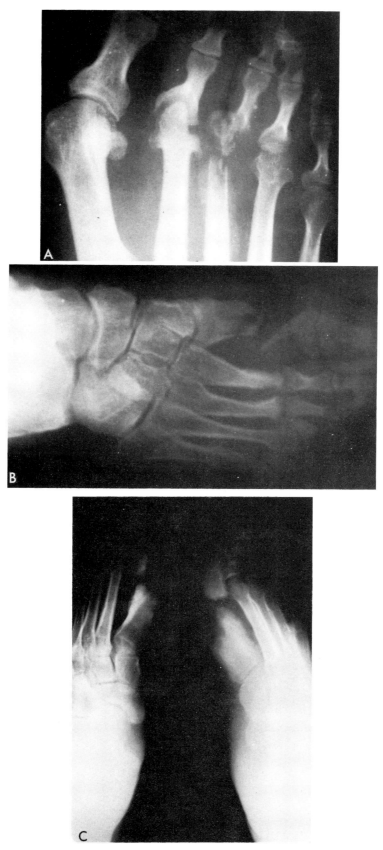

Figure 45-7. (A–C) Metatarsophalangeal joint changes, all in diabetics.

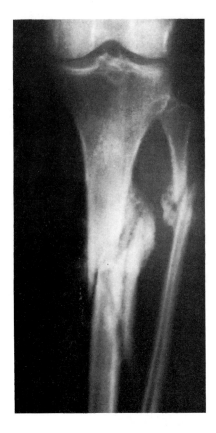

Figure 45–8. Painless spontaneous fracture of the shaft of the tibia in a luetic. Eventual healing occurred with prolonged immobilization.

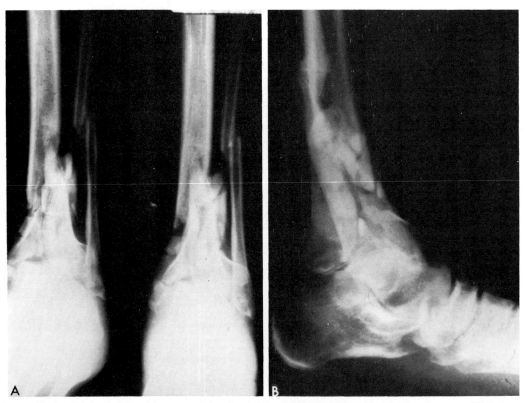

Figure 45–9. (A) Comminuted fracture of the distal tibia and fibula with ankle joint involvement. (B) Pain was very minimal at any time. This luetic patient regained stability after prolonged immobilization.

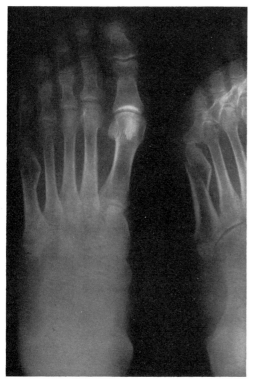

Figure 45–10. *Spontaneous fractures of both the neck and the base of the fifth metatarsal in a diabetic.*

long bones, occur spontaneously with no associated trauma. Indeed, we recall one of our patients, a middle-aged man with tertiary lues, who sustained a helical fracture through the isthmus of his femur simply by crossing his legs! He felt a painless "pop" as he did so, and then had painless instability. This is more the exception than the rule. If closely and repeatedly questioned, most patients will recall some initiating episode such as a misstep on a flight of stairs, direct trauma to the foot, stubbing the toes, or walking long distances (fatigue fracture). This will be followed by varying degrees of discomfort or pain, swelling, and local increase in temperature. The symptoms are usually not commensurate with the clinical findings and are often overlooked or ignored. This is the more common cause of the "spontaneous" fracture (Figs. 45–8 to 45–10).

In our experience, spontaneous fractures are more common in luetics with Charcot joints than in diabetics with this disorder. This is similar to the experiences of Kredel and of Steindler,[19] each of whom

noted about a 25 per cent incidence of spontaneous fractures in luetic patients with Charcot joints. It should be emphasized that we are here considering fractures of bone *not* involving joints. If all fractures involving joints were to be included, almost all patients with Charcot joints would have spontaneous fractures as well.

There is abundant mention of spontaneous fractures of bones of the feet in both the recent and older literature. Charcot mentioned this finding frequently in his writings.

Deformity. Spontaneous fractures by themselves may lead to deformity. A fracture through the tuber of the os calcis may cause apparent valgus or varus of the hindfoot, just as is seen following the various types of corrective calcaneal osteotomies done for pre-existing deformity (Figs. 45–11 and 45–12). Combined fractures through the metatarsals can cause lateral deviation of the forefoot or even rocker-bottom deformity.

More frequently, deformity is secondary to progressive destructive joint changes. Extreme valgus or varus deformity may occur with destructive changes in the subtalar or ankle joints, or both. Extreme lateral deviation of the forefoot can occur as Lisfranc's or Chopart's joints disintegrate (Figs. 45–13 to 45–16).

The rate of these changes can vary tremendously, according to the cause of the deformity. In our experience, progression is the most relentless in syringomyelia, does not seem to be as rapid in the average case of syphilis, and is the least rapid in diabetes.

Again, the classic textbook description of such deformity is that it is "painless." This is not strictly so. A few patients may have appreciable pain, and many at least moderate discomfort. In the usual case, however, the severity of the symptoms is far less than would be expected in a person with normal pain sensation and the same bone changes. The diagnosis does *not* hinge upon the complete absence of pain, and the early descriptions emphasize this point as much as current accounts do.

Soft-Tissue Injury. Mal perforans ulcers developing over normally occurring bone prominences will be discussed elsewhere in this book, and several examples

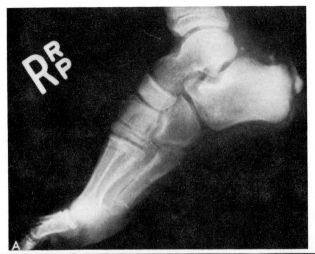

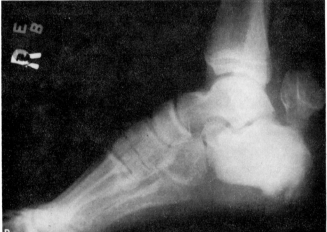

Figure 45–11. *(A) Initial symptoms of painless swelling of heel with the changes shown in this roentgenogram. (B) The correct diagnosis was not considered, and this degree of deformity was seen 32 months later. (C) Seven years later came the finding of sensory deficit and the realization that this was a neuropathic foot. There is fixed deformity, loss of plantar flexion, and difficulty in shoeing.*

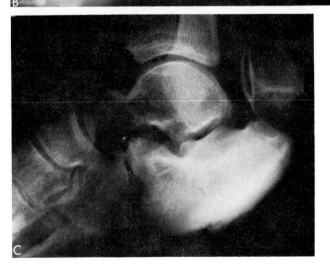

Figure 45–12. *Changes similar to those shown in Figure 45–11 that occurred in a young male after sensory loss secondary to excision of a spinal cord tumor.*

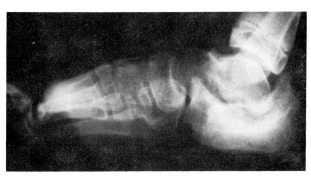

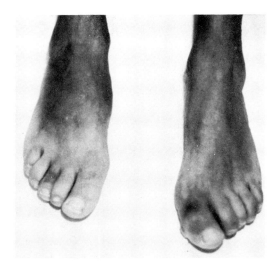

Figure 45–13. *Note the subtle thickening of the left forefoot. This is due to neuropathic involvement of Lisfranc's joint in a diabetic.*

Figure 45–14. *A further degree of the same type of change as that shown in Figure 45–13 in another diabetic; there is now a mal perforans ulcer over a newly weight-bearing bony prominence as the forefoot begins to deviate and the longitudinal arch is effaced.*

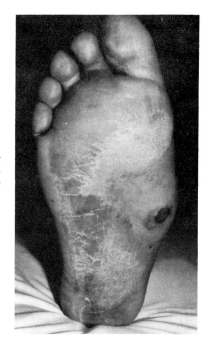

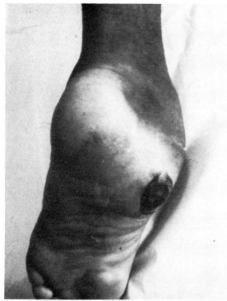

Figure 45–15. Subtalar neuroarthropathy in a diabetic with even more extreme deformity and ulceration. Prolonged immobilization followed by a protective orthosis is indicated.

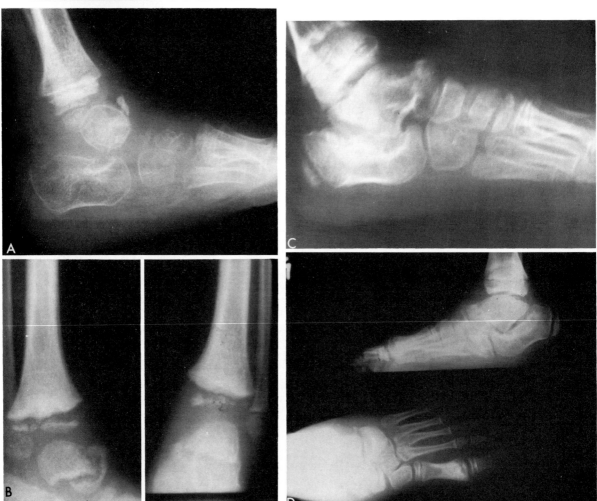

Figure 45–16. (A) Early deformity of the talus and calcaneus in a young patient with Riley-Day syndrome. There was established calcaneal deformity and a recent talar fracture. (B) The same talar changes seen six months later. (C) Changes after another forty months. (D) The final result five years after the first roentgenograms were taken. Many other problems precluded the usual treatment of prolonged immobilization, which would have been useful in lessening the degree of deformity.

have been given in this chapter as well. A somewhat similar lesion can occur over new areas of pressure that occur as a consequence of deformity.

A common sequence is the development of neuropathic changes in Chopart's joint. There is increasing lateral deviation and pronation of the forefoot. The longitudinal arch is, in effect, flattened, and the head of the talus becomes weight bearing. In addition to the swelling of the forefoot caused by deformity and by injury and repair reaction, ulceration may now occur beneath the head of the talus, and the entire complex is often mistaken for widespread infection or "gangrene" (a term too often used, in our experience) (Figs. 45–14 and 45–15).

A more devastating change occurs as the subtalar and/or ankle joint becomes involved. As this occurs, the foot goes into increasing valgus or varus deformity. Progression seems most rapid when the deformity is varus. In this instance, the malleoli may eventually become weight bearing, and the overlying soft tissue can ulcerate as a result of continued lack of protection. Major ulceration can occur into the ankle and subtalar joints. Salvage of such a foot can be one of the most difficult and time-consuming endeavors in orthopaedic surgery (see Figure 45–3).

MANAGEMENT

Control of Neuropathy. Correlation between the degree of the neuropathy and the degree of arthropathy is not absolute. Generally, however, there *is* a correlation. Scattered reports cite clinical improvement in patients (mainly diabetics) with arthropathy after their neuropathy has improved. Certainly, antibiotic treatment of the patient with tertiary lues or strict dietary and chemical control of the diabetic have more than passing merit.

Local Debridement. When there is ulceration and superimposed infection, the usual surgical principles hold. Any collection of pus and necrotic material should be debrided and drained. This is discussed more completely in Chapter 50 on the diabetic foot. Appropriate antibiotics should be started, usually parenterally (intravenous route preferred). A careful evaluation of the situation is required. Charcot joint changes of deformity and fragmentation should *not* be mistaken for "osteomyelitis" and then widely debrided simply because there may be an overlying ulcer. The foot in Figure 45–1 would *not* benefit from debridement, and the feet in Figures 45–14 and 45–15 will require, at most, local debridement *only*.

If ill-advised, overambitious debridement destroys whatever stability may be left in the foot, the results can be catastrophic. With the further loss of stability, the foot may well distintegrate rapidly; the surgeon has contributed additional trauma and destabilized an already decompensated foot and ankle. Only experience can tell what the magnitude of such efforts should be, but in the average case one always has the opportunity of repeating the debridement, if necessary.

Immobilization. A simple and often neglected remedy is available to even the most inexperienced. This has been mentioned time and again, even in the earlier literature on the subject, and Johnson[10] has reiterated the time-proven principles. Charcot joints demonstrate, after all, a combination of injury and repair reactions; therefore, the *usual* treatment of injury and repair reactions should prove of some value.

Consider a few instances of injury and repair reactions in normal patients without neuropathy. We may treat a sprained ankle by cast immobilization or use of crutches; the extremity is put at rest. Swelling, local increase in temperature, and pain gradually diminish with healing. The same sequence can hold with a fracture of the base of the fifth metatarsal, an ankle fracture, or any other traumatic event. The common factor is that the extremity is put at rest while nature heals the injury.

This same sequence can, and usually will, follow in the adequately protected neuropathic foot (Fig. 45–17). Immobilization, usually by a total-contact short-leg plaster cast, is probably the best protection, and the patient is given crutches with touch–weight bearing on the affected extremity. The major difference between healing in the neuropathic and normal foot is the length of time required for immobilization. With timely changes of plaster (every four weeks or so), continuous immobilization is maintained until soft tissue swelling has been reduced and until the local increase in temperature (which reflects the activity of the injury and repair reaction) has subsided. This can be determined either by the sense of touch (accurate to within about 2° C) or by direct measurement with a thermistor. We usually continue immobilization even beyond this point for another month or so. Five to six months in plaster is not at all uncommon.

Roentgenograms of the foot may be of minor value in further determining the *length* of immobilization, if they show increasing callus formation and filling in of defect areas. Needless to say, they will *not* show evidence of reconstitution of bone contour or destroyed joint surfaces. Their

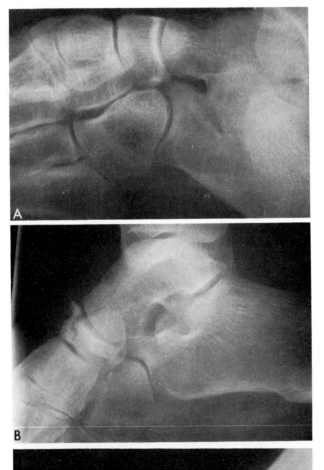

Figure 45–17. *(A) There was no roentgenographic evidence of injury in this diabetic woman with painless swelling in the region of the talonavicular joint. In retrospect, she recalled "numbness" of feet even before this episode. (B) The painless swelling continued and new roentgenograms taken 18 months from the time of the first showed compression and fracture of the navicular. A temporary restriction on weight bearing was recommended. (C) Two years from the time of the first roentgenogram, the navicular is completely destroyed. There was increasing deformity and now almost complete anesthesia of the foot. The diagnosis of neuroarthropathy was established, and plaster immobilization was continued for almost four months. The foot was then cool and there was no roentgenographic evidence of progression. A polypropylene splint has been worn almost habitually for the last four years, and there has been no further change.*

greatest value is to provide pictorial evidence that the lesions are not progressing (i.e., that therapy has halted the sequence). We place much more emphasis on the physical examination of the foot and ankle than on roentgenographic changes to determine the length of immobilization.

After the plaster has been removed for the final time, we find it important to continue with protection of the extremity. Our experience with double upright braces with or without various strap arrangements has not been good. A more effective and esthetic appliance is the Texas Rehabilitation Institute type of polypropylene splint, usually worn in conjunction with extra-depth shoes (Fig. 45–18). For the first few months, the patient is instructed to wear the orthosis continually whenever up and about. With caution, he can then go without it for increasingly longer periods of time, although it must still be worn for prolonged walking and in situations in which reinjury is likely, such

as heavy physical activity. If the patient objects to continuing total use of the brace and wishes to lessen his dependence on it in the manner just described, it is imperative that he check his feet for unexplained warmth or swelling at frequent intervals. Even one injury is potentially serious. We discuss the physiology and care of neuropathic feet at great length with all our patients and find that such preventive medicine can forestall months of treatment.

Role of Surgery. Most experienced orthopaedic surgeons are aware of the disastrous consequences that can follow poorly conceived surgery on Charcot joints (Figs. 45–19 to 45–22). No less an authority than Ridlon once cautioned that *any* such surgery was folly, and in many cases this is still so. If an already unstable joint is further attacked, the progression of the disease may be accelerated. A casual attempt at fusion may lead to a truly catastrophic, wildly unstable pseudarthrosis.

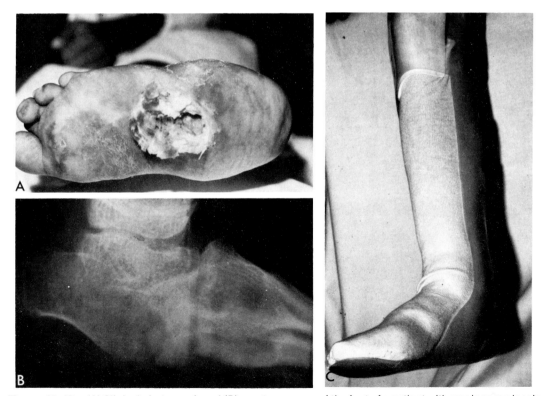

Figure 45–18. *(A) Clinical photograph and (B) roentgenogram of the foot of a patient with meningomyelocele and a neuropathic foot. A large amount of callus was debrided, and the ulcer was closed with a split-thickness skin graft. (C) Protection with a T.R.I. polypropylene splint with polyethylene foam padding and extra-depth shoes. The partial anterior shell of the splint helps unload the foot.*

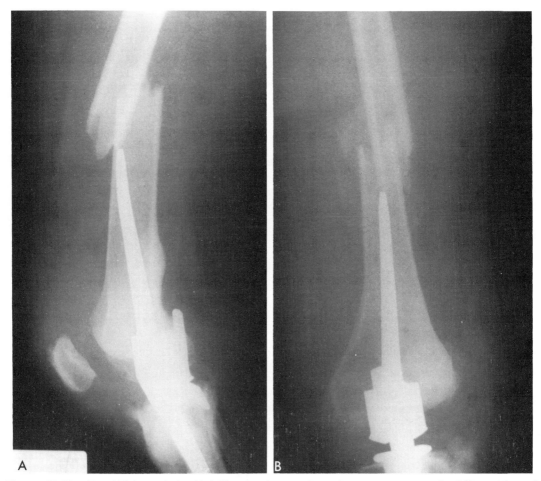

Figure 45–19. *(A and B) A constrained total knee replacement was done on an unrecognized Charcot knee. A spontaneous fracture occurred above this level. Poorly conceived surgery on Charcot joints can lead to major complications.*

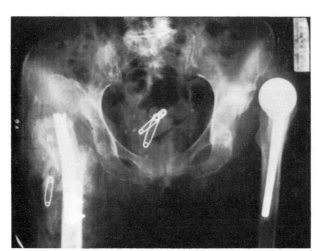

Figure 45–20. *Bilateral unstable Charcot hips in a luetic. An osteotomy and an Austin-Moore replacement were obviously not the answer.*

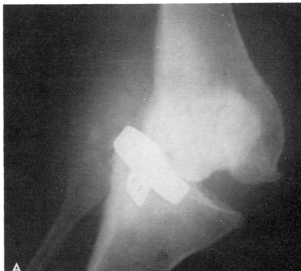

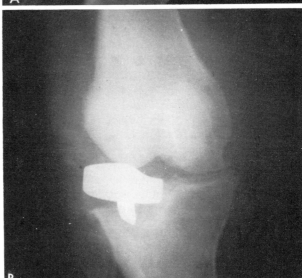

Figure 45–21. *(A and B) A hemiarthroplasty was not the correct form of treatment for this (luetic) Charcot knee.*

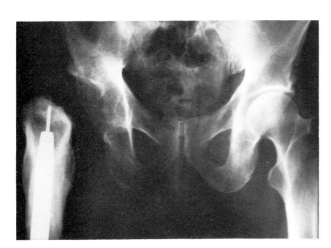

Figure 45–22. *An osteotomy of this Charcot hip was not the solution for this luetic patient.*

Attempts at joint replacement will often end with disintegration and dislocation. These results may be serviceable in terms of function, but offer no improvement over the preoperative status. Only the most optimistic would call them "successful."

More recent experience has shown that, with the proper case selection and meticulous care, surgery can be accomplished successfully. An important factor in achieving a successful result lies in quieting the injury and repair process as much as possible preoperatively. Johnson[10] recommends immobilization in plaster for however long it is necessary to bring the extremity into the healing phase (diminished swelling and erythema, decreased local temperature). Injuries have a chance to consolidate, and fractures to heal. A maximum of good, usable stock and the best soft tissues for repair are obtained. The treatment is thus, to this point, the same as for cases in which no operative intervention is contemplated.

Our most frequent indication for surgery on Charcot feet (other than for mal perforans ulcers or infection, as discussed in Chapter 50) is that of unacceptable deformity. The deformity is usually caused by hindfoot valgus or varus due to ankle joint and/or subtalar involvement. An equally common deformity is that of increasing lateral deviation of the forefoot because of involvement of Chopart's and/or Lisfranc's joints. In almost all instances, this degree of deformity would not have occurred had early protective immobilization been instituted and continued. In almost all of these cases as well, the active process can be quieted by immobilization, even though unacceptable deformity exists. Opinion can vary as to what is unacceptable, but consideration should center around difficulties in shoeing, susceptibility to ulceration, and likelihood of progression (when deformity is such that further weight bearing serves to accentuate and exacerbate the defect).

We treat large numbers of patients with neuropathic joint disease. The effectiveness and value of preventive methods of immobilization can be emphasized by noting that we rarely need to operate on Charcot joints (other than to control infection, as already mentioned). Any type of surgery should be undertaken only with caution and after warning the patient of the many possible pitfalls. The potential for untoward results is well known for other areas of the body (Figs. 45–19 to 45–22), and the foot is no different!

The literature is not replete with series analyzing the results of surgery of this type on Charcot feet and ankles. Most reports, as well as our own experience, are limited and anecdotal.

Reports of amputation are fairly common.[2, 3, 8, 12, 16] This is usually for control of infection after increasing deformity and ulceration. As mentioned, both deformity and ulceration are often arrested by conservative treatment and debridement; amputation may then be unnecessary. Infinite patience and meticulous daily care are often the deciding factors in salvage. With this in mind, the physician need not end with Hobson's choice in treatment!

Steindler[19] reported a successful supramalleolar osteotomy of the ankle in one luetic patient and a successful subtalar fusion in another.

Burman[3] reported three successful fusion operations — a fusion of the long arch of the foot, an ankle fusion, and a triple arthrodesis. Heiple and Cammarn[7] also reported a successful triple arthrodesis, whereas Holt's[8] report of amputation was after a failed triple arthrodesis.

Cleveland[5] reported a successful ankle fusion. Interestingly enough, Cassagrande and associates[4] performed ankle denervation procedures on three patients for painful arthritic changes, but none developed Charcot joint changes.

In 1951, Parsons and Norton[14] reported on two diabetics with Charcot changes in their feet. They claimed that both showed improvement after lumbar sympathectomy. Despite explanation, the rationale for this procedure in this circumstance remains obscure. Sheppe[17] tried the same treatment, also in a diabetic, without success. The possibility that sympathectomy might increase blood flow and at least aid in healing ulcers is decreased by the observation that many diabetics have at least a partial autosympathectomy as a consequence of their disease. In any event, the operation has not been widely performed for this indication, nor is it currently suggested for treatment of bone changes.

Whatever the type of operation (usually

a fusion), several "minor" points increase the probability of a favorable outcome. At the time of surgery, every effort should be made to end with freshly bleeding tissue. Obviously, two opposing sclerotic joint surfaces with thickened avascular joint capsule surrounding them do not stand the chance of fusion that is possible with raw, bleeding bone and fresh surrounding soft tissue. Whenever possible, combined external (cast) and internal fixation should be used. In the case of ankle fusion, we usually run two heavy threaded pins up through the heel into the distal tibia and combine this with a cast. This has been more successful in our hands than the Charnley compression method. The pins are left in for about six weeks.

Prolonged postoperative immobilization is a must, and this should be continued until it is obvious by roentgenogram that no further healing will occur. Immobilization may need to be two to three times longer than that required for a patient without neuropathic joint disease. Prolonged immobilization alone may make the difference between failure and success of fusion.

The failure of a fusion operation does not necessarily mean the total failure of the proposed treatment. If major deformity be corrected, fibrous ankylosis can be a very satisfactory result. Pain will not usually be a major factor, and a stable extremity in a neutral position can be serviceable, especially when protected with an orthosis.

Various forms of joint replacement have been proposed for patients *without* neuropathy. Total ankle replacement has not yet proved to be a completely satisfactory operation in the general population, and some think ankle fusion remains a better operation. Neuropathic joint disease is stated to be a definite contraindication for total ankle replacement, but it will doubtless receive some trial. The most frequent forefoot joint replacement operation in our experience has been the Swanson hemiarthroplasty of the first metatarsophalangeal

joint (we do not have experience with his new *total* replacement). There seems to be no good indication for this procedure in neuropathic forefeet. We have done the simple Keller bunionectomy on many neuropathic forefeet without untoward consequences.

REFERENCES

1. Barth, P.: Histologische Knochenuntersuchung bei tabischer arthropathie. Arch. f. klin. chir., 69:174, 1903.
2. Bolen, J. G.: Diabetic Charcot joints. Radiology, 67:95, 1956.
3. Burman, M.: The weight-stress in Charcot disease of joints: Charcot's disease of the foot and ankle. J. Int. Coll. Surg., 28:183, 1957.
4. Cassagrande, P. A., Austin, B. P., and Indeck, W.: Denervation of the ankle joint. J. Bone Joint Surg., 33A:723, 1953.
5. Cleveland, M.: Surgical fusion of unstable joints due to neuropathic disturbance. Am. J. Surg., 43:580, 1939.
6. Curtiss, P. H.: Changes produced in the synovial membrane and synovial fluid by disease. J. Bone Joint Surg., 46-A:873, 1964.
7. Heiple, K. G., and Cammarn, M. R.: Diabetic neuroarthropathy with spontaneous peritalar fracture–dislocation. J. Bone Joint Surg. 48-A:1177, 1966.
8. Holt, E. P.: Bilateral trophic changes of the foot in diabetics. J.A.M.A., 91:959, 1928.
9. Horowitz, T.: Bone and cartilage debris in the synovial membrane: its significance in the early diagnosis of neuroarthropathy. J. Bone Joint Surg., 30-A:579, 1948.
10. Johnson, J. M. T.: Neuropathic fractures and joint injuries. J. Bone Joint Surg., 49-A:1, 1967.
11. King, E. J. S.: On some aspects of the pathology of hypertrophic Charcot's joints. Br. J. Surg., 18:113, 1930.
12. Lister, J., and Mandsley, R. H.: Charcot joints in diabetic neuropathy. Lancet, 2:1110, 1951.
13. Milgram, J. E.: In Ghormley, R. K. (ed.): The Arthropathies in Orthopaedic Surgery. New York, Thomas Nelson and Sons, 1938, pp. 375–384.
14. Parsons, H., and Norton, W. S.: The management of diabetic neuropathic joints. N. Engl. J. Med., 244:935, 1951.
15. Potts, W. J.: Pathology of Charcot joints. Am. Surg., 86:596, 1927.
16. Shands, A. R.: Neuropathies of the bones and joints. Arch. Surg., 20:614, 1930.
17. Sheppe, W. H.: Neuropathic (Charcot) joints occurring in diabetes mellitus. Ann. Intern. Med., 39:625, 1953.
18. Steindler, A.: The tabetic arthropathies. J.A.M.A., 96:250, 1931.
19. Steindler, A.: Postgraduate Lectures on Orthopaedic Diagnosis and Indications. Vol. IV. Springfield, Ill., Charles C Thomas, Publisher, 1952 (Lecture V, pp. 281–300).

CHAPTER 46

THE INSENSITIVE FOOT (INCLUDING LEPROSY)

Paul W. Brand, M.D.

Feet may become insensitive or hyposensitive from a variety of causes. The subsequent ulceration and tissue breakdown of the foot are often attributed to the disease that caused the neuropathy. Leprosy has been said to result in a "rotting away" of fingers and toes. Ulcers of the foot in diabetes are referred to as "diabetic ulcers," as though the metabolic background were directly responsible for tissue breakdown. In most cases the actual or immediate cause of the foot problems is mechanical. Disease robs the patient of the pain sensibility that would have protected him from injury, and mechanical stress does most of the rest. The disease that causes the neuropathy may also affect the foot in other ways. High spinal injury causes insensitivity of the feet, but it also causes gross motor paralysis that may confine the patient to a wheelchair. Therefore, the foot is spared the trauma of walking and often remains intact. Spina bifida and low meningomyelocele may cause more limited paralysis, so that the patient can still walk but may be unable to plantar flex his foot. Thus, it is common for ulceration to occur under the heel, where the stress of weight bearing is concentrated. In diabetes and leprosy the plantar flexors are usually normal, but the intrinsic muscles may be weakened. Therefore, the claw toes may suffer shear stresses dorsally, and ulcers may also occur under the metatarsal heads, where vulnerability to stress is increased by the clawing of the toes. Radicular sensory neuropathies commonly occur without motor weakness or imbalance. Patients with these disorders are often very active and expose themselves recklessly to all sorts of stress without any inhibition from pain. They suffer gross ulceration and destruction of the feet, often including neuropathic tarsal joints and ankle joints, but there is no predictable pattern of damage because there is no limitation to their activity.

LEPROSY

Leprosy, at least in Asia and Africa, is the most common cause of loss of sensation of the feet. The disease occurs in a number of forms that range from *lepromatous* leprosy, which is found in people who have no natural resistance to the disease, to *tuberculoid* leprosy, which occurs in those who have good resistance but still not enough to prevent infection altogether. The lepromatous patients have masses of bacilli (*Mycobacterium leprae*) in and under the skin and in the bones of the foot. However, these bacilli rarely cause any ulceration or destruction of skin or gross damage to bone, at least in patients who are under treatment. Radiographs will sometimes show a patchy rarefaction of the cancellous part of the bones and some loss of trabeculae. The nutrient foramina of

1266

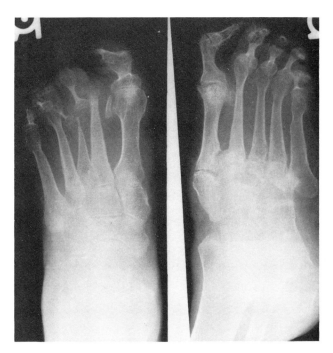

Figure 46–1. *Neuropathic feet in a patient with leprosy. The right foot shows an old healed infection at the third metatarsophalangeal joint, with concentric absorption of the bones, and an acute infection of the second metatarsophalangeal joint, with an open ulcer and subluxation of the joint. On the left foot, there is a neuropathic bone and joint collapse of the first ray in the cuneiform-navicular region.*

long bones are sometimes enlarged. During periods of acute exacerbation, the feet may be hot, swollen, and tender. If stress is placed on the foot during this acute stage, there may be collapse of bones, especially at the metatarsal head and neck and sometimes in the tarsal area (Fig. 46–1). These truly lepromatous bone changes probably result in damage in only about 1 per cent of cases of leprosy. In most cases the bone rarefaction is followed by recalcification and the foot returns to normal. During phases of swelling and acute exacerbation and radiographic change, patients either should be off their feet or should use a total-contact molded sandal made of thick, soft Plastazote. They should also take short steps and walk as little as possible. If actual bony collapse occurs, a plaster cast will be needed. Subsequently, the bones will usually heal and become strong again.

In contrast to the rarity of bone damage due directly to the disease, the effect of nerve damage in leprosy is common. This occurs in both the lepromatous and the tuberculoid forms.

Patients with tuberculoid leprosy have so few *M. leprae* bacilli that most tissue sections will show none at all, and the diagnosis may be missed. However, the diagnosis can be confirmed by the clinical finding of patchy loss of sensation associated with thickened nerves. (The ulnar, tibial, and peroneal nerves; superficial branches of radial nerve on the hand; and posterior auricular nerve in the neck may all be easily palpated.)

In tuberculoid leprosy as well as the other forms, the loss of peripheral sensation and paralysis of peripheral muscles cause the lower limb problems. In tuberculoid leprosy the disease is localized and may affect only one limb or part of a limb. In other forms, both limbs will be equally affected. Gradual loss of sensation, beginning on the dorsum of the foot and spreading to the sole and the leg, will be followed by loss of intrinsic muscles and sometimes later by footdrop and peroneal paralysis. The plantar-flexing muscles and tibialis posterior are not paralyzed in leprosy.

Along with loss of sensation there is a loss of sympathetic nerve function. This results in dry skin, which predisposes to cracks in the keratin layer. Keratin loses all flexibility and elasticity when dry, so it is very important to teach patients to soak their feet in water for 20 minutes every day and then rub petroleum jelly over the skin to prevent evaporation.

ULCERS OF THE INSENSITIVE FOOT

No matter what the disease or primary cause, all ulcers of the insensitive foot are similar in quality, if not in site. An exception is that in some diabetics the vascular component may dominate and result in gangrene, even in the absence of mechanical stress. However, in most cases of diabetic foot ulcers and in all other ulcers that occur in insensitive feet, mechanical stress is responsible for the tissue breakdown. There are important variables that condition the vulnerability of tissues to mechanical stress. One is the degree of insensibility, another is the level and type of stress, and a third is the time factor.

Degree of Insensibility

It is my observation that of all patients who suffer neuropathic ulceration, at least half develop their first lesion before they are aware of their loss of sensation. At that time the physician may test for gross sensibility and report the result as normal. Really careful observation and testing will almost always demonstrate a change in the threshold of sensation, and often a qualitative loss, e.g., a loss of pain and temperature in the local area. Weddel determined that 50 per cent of nerve endings in the skin may be destroyed before the patient is aware of any loss at all (unpublished report). However, the threshold of sensation will be altered, and that may be enough to increase the vulnerability of the skin.

Level and Type of Mechanical Stress

There are at least three different levels of stress that may result in breakdown of the skin of the foot. Each causes damage in a different way, depends on different time relationships, and results in totally different pathology. The ability of a physician to prevent and correct the damage depends on a thorough understanding of these stress relationships. Since the patient has to live with the danger of breakdown of tissue of the feet, he or she also must be helped to understand the nature

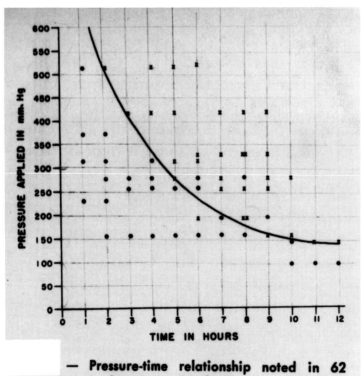

Figure 46–2. Kosiak's classic experiment showing how there is an inverse relationship between the pressure and the time it takes to cause ischemic necrosis. (From Kosiak, M.: Arch. Phys. Med. Rehabil., 40:66, 1959.)

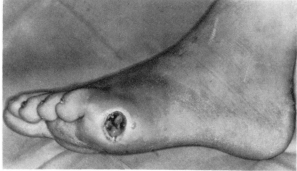

Figure 46–3. *Pressure necrosis at the lateral border of an insensitive foot due to the wearing of a tight shoe all day.*

of the danger and the principles of prevention.

Three levels of stress — low, high, and moderate — may cause problems, and different pathomechanics are associated with each.

Damage from Low Stress

Pressures of 1 or 2 lb/inch^2 are so low that they are not noticed, even by people with normal sensation. However, capillary blood flow may be blocked by these small pressures, and normal people feel the discomfort of ischemia after an hour or two. Actual ischemic gangrene takes several hours to occur and is due to deprivation of oxygen and nutrients (Fig. 46–2). For this reason the pressure must be continuous. Thus, ischemic gangrene of the foot is rarely due to the pressures of weight bearing, which are usually intermittent. This form of gangrene is almost always caused by the pressure of a shoe that is too tight. It is quite rare for pressures in a shoe to exceed 5 lb/inch^2 when the foot is off the ground because it would be difficult to force a foot into a shoe as tight as that. At that degree of pressure no permanent dam-

age is likely before five hours, but might occur in the ten hours or so that a pair of shoes may be worn continuously in one day.

Site of Damage. Since the pressure is due to the tightness of the shoe, it usually occurs either at the medial or the lateral border of the foot (Fig. 46–3), This is because the pressure results from the tightness (tension) of a flexible circumferential band (the shoe). The *tension* in a flexible tight shoe is equal all around any given circumference, but the *pressure* that results from the tension is inversely proportional to the radius of the curve at any given point. The transverse section of a forefoot may be bounded by three different convex curves and one flat or concave side (Fig. 46–4). The sole is either flat or concave and thus will not receive any pressure from circumferential tension. The dorsum may be part of a very large, gentle curve and will experience some pressure. The medial and lateral borders are parts of much smaller circles and will thus receive much more pressure from the same tension. The presence of a bunion adds to the risk of ischemic ulcers since there is a curve in two planes, transverse and longi-

Figure 46–4. *Cross section of a forefoot showing that the dorsum is part of a large curve radius (R_1), the medial border is part of a smaller curve radius (R_2), and the lateral border has the smallest curve radius (R_3). The pressures from a single circumferential band of equal tension all around will be slight on the dorsum (P_1), greater on the medial side (P_2), and greatest on the lateral border (P_3). When the tension is equal, $R_1P_1 = R_2P_2 = R_3P_3$.*

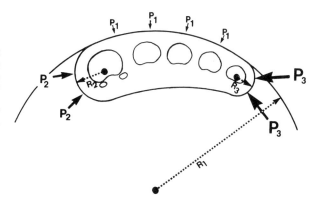

tudinal, to concentrate pressure. When the fabric of a shoe is semirigid, the situation may be more complex. In the case of leather shoes, compliance to the curves and prominences of the foot may be achieved over a period of time. Therefore, old leather shoes may be much less hazardous than new shoes.

Prevention of Damage. Damage from continuous low pressure (ischemic ulcers) can be prevented by:

1. *Selection of shoes.* It is very difficult to measure the pressures inside the shoe on the borders of the feet. A more practical procedure is to advise the use of soft, compliant leather for shoe uppers and to feel the foot through the shoe to make sure it is wide enough across the ball of the foot. Leather shoes may be moistened and then stretched to accommodate local prominences on the foot.

2. *Breaking-in of shoes.* No person who has insensitive feet should ever wear new shoes for more than two hours at a time. The shoes are then removed and the skin examined for redness (reactive hyperemia), local heat, and marks caused by the fabric of socks. Old shoes are worn for the rest of the day. If no problems develop, the new shoes are worn for progressively longer periods each day.

3. *Daily change of shoes.* Even with old shoes, it is wise to keep two pairs in current use and change them at noon each day. One pair of shoes can be kept at work or school, and a midday change becomes routine. A further change to slippers on return home in the evening will usually result in three five-hour periods of shoe-wearing per day. Thus, no shoe, even if a little tight, will ever be worn long enough to cause ischemic problems.

4. *Beware of dressings.* If a wound occurs on an insensitive foot, there is a danger that a dressing may be applied and held in place with padding and a bandage. If the patient then puts his foot back into a previously well-fitting shoe, it may be too tight because of the new bulk of dressings (Fig. 46–5). I have seen actual gangrenous ulcers caused by exactly this sequence of events.

Damage from High Stress

Low stress takes hours to cause damage, but a wound may be caused in a fraction of a second by stepping on broken glass or a projecting nail. This type of injury is caused by high stress concentrated on a small area (Fig. 46–6).

Pressure and shear stress are both directly related to force and inversely related to the area through which the force is applied. A person has little control over the amount of force that is transmitted through his foot. Each foot is bound to accept the whole weight of the body at each step. If that force is transmitted onto a narrow edge or a sharp point, the pressure becomes high:

$$\text{Pressure} = \frac{\text{Force}}{\text{Area}}$$

Yamada[13] quotes experiments to show that human skin is very variable in its threshold for failure under tension or shear stress, depending on the age of the subject and the part of the body involved. However, a figure of 1 kg/mm^2 (1200 lb/inch^2) for ultimate tensile strength seems about average. A 200-lb man would probably suffer a wound if he stepped barefoot on the end of a rod ½ inch in diameter. He would then be experiencing pressure of

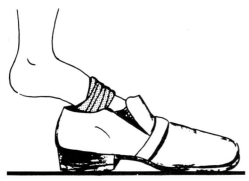

Figure 46–5. *Bulky dressings should be avoided in a well-fitting shoe.*

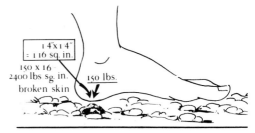

Figure 46–6. *Barefoot walking is good for the feet, but only if they are sensitive enough to respond to pressure.*

800 lb/inch² plus some shear stress at the edge of the rod. By contrast, the same person, if walking in shoes, would rarely be placing his weight on an area of less than 5 inch², or 40 lb/inch².

Prevention of Damage. Almost any type of shoe or slipper will protect the foot from high localized stress, except that rarely a person may step on a projecting nail that will penetrate the sole of a shoe. However, walking barefoot is a real hazard to people with loss of sensation. I have known patients to step on a thumbtack and carry it in their foot all day. Thus, the only rule that needs to be followed to prevent high-stress injuries is "never walk barefoot and always shake out your shoes before you put them on."

Damage from Moderate Stress

This is by far the most frequent cause of injury to the insensitive foot and the least commonly understood.

Figure 46–7 shows a tracing of the pressures under various parts of a normal foot during normal steps on three different floor surfaces. No part of the foot experienced more than 5 kg/cm² (75 lb/inch²) of pressure, even when the individual was walking barefoot on a cement floor. On a leather pad, like the sole of a shoe, the peak readings were less than 50 lb/inch², and on microcell rubber they were less than 25 lb/inch². Thus, a foot in a regular shoe is subjected to pressures less than one tenth of that which would cause direct injury or breakdown of the skin. These pressures of normal walking in a shoe are about a quarter of what is needed to produce pain in a sensitive foot. I have found that the loss of peripheral sensation in the absence of motor defect does not greatly affect the range of pressures on the sole during walking unless some skeletal abnormality is present.

In spite of this apparent ten to one margin of safety, insensitive feet commonly do break down and ulcerate, even though shoes are worn and prolonged ischemia is avoided (Fig. 46–8). This would seem to point to a basic weakness of denervated tissues (so-called "trophic change") that makes them more fragile than normal tissues. Our own experiments have shown that a small but real difference exists between denervated and normal skin that may account for a marginal degree of extra vulnerability. However, there is no way in which it could account for the ten to one difference between the theoretical threshold for damage and the peak pressures of normal walking. At this point there seems to be a gap in our understanding of the causes of tissue breakdown. This gap has now been bridged, at least in part, as a result of our study of long-term repetitive stress.

Repetitive Moderate Stress. There are three sets of experiments that, taken together, help clarify the problems of the management of insensitive feet. All experiments are based on a small machine we call a "walking simulator," or traumatizer. It is designed to apply a measured force repetitively on a small area of palm

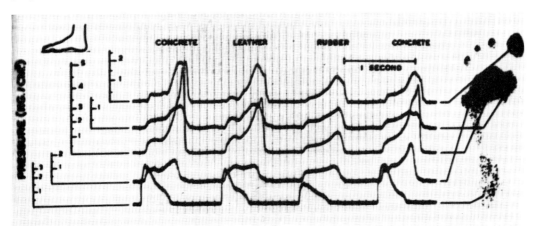

Figure 46–7. *Pressure tracings of a normal foot on three different surfaces. Note how the use of resilient, compliant materials results in equalization of pressures. (From Brand, P. W.: J. Bone Joint Surg., 45B:659, 1963.)*

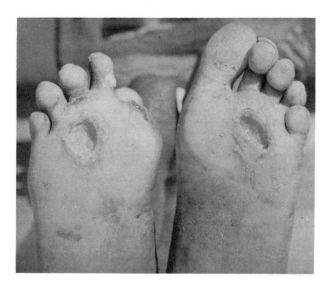

Figure 46–8. *Typical trophic ulcers on the areas of maximum stress from normal walking.*

or sole. We have used pressures of 20 to 30 lb/inch² and repetitions of 8000 and 10,000 "steps" per day. Most of the experiments have been done on the footpads of rats, but a few at the same pressures, have been done on our own fingertips. On our fingers we have found that we can tolerate a few hundred beats at 25 lb/inch² with no discomfort at all. After 1000 repetitions or so the process becomes painful and then intolerable. When the finger is removed from the machine, it is red, and its surface temperature may be 5° C or more higher than that of the other fingertips. The pain soon wears off and the temperature returns to normal. If the process is repeated the next day on the same finger, pain develops much sooner, fewer repetitions can be tolerated, and the temperature of the finger rises to a higher level and stays hot for a longer time. Using the same machine on the footpads of rats, it is possible to study the histologic changes in the tissues and also to carry the experiment further. Using pressures of 20 lb/inch² and 10,000 repetitions per day, we have found that a progressive inflammation develops in the soft tissues of the sole and that by the third day localized concentrations of polymorphonuclear leukocytes, lymphocytes, and macrophages occur. Small areas of necrosis develop and blisters appear in the epidermis. By the eighth day the areas of necrosis have coalesced and the epidermis is destroyed. A true ulcer has thus occurred as a result of repeated mechanical stress of a very moderate degree. The exact

mechanism of tissue damage has not been worked out, but it must be related to the mass of inflammatory cells. Perhaps further mechanical irritation of these cells releases enzymes that result in autolysis.

Integrating the experiments on our own fingers and on the rat footpads, we get a picture of the sequence of events in response to repetitive moderate stress in both normal and insensitive feet.

In normal feet, moderate stress repeated thousands of times results in a mild inflammation that seems to lower the threshold to pain. If the normal subject continues walking in spite of discomfort, the inflammation becomes more intense and the tissues become more vulnerable to damage from further stress. At this stage the tissues become really painful, and the subject begins to limp or stops walking. This allows the condition to subside over the next few days.

The person with an insensitive foot may walk or run with much the same gait and may experience the same stress. The inflammatory change in the tissues will occur in the same way, but perhaps a little sooner. The patient, however, does not experience discomfort or pain. He does not limp. He goes on walking until necrosis and ulceration occur. The repetitive stress that results in the final breakdown of the skin may be of the same degree as it was on each previous day for a period of some weeks. *It is the tissue that has changed, not the stress.* When the patient sees blood on his socks and a fresh ulcer on his foot, he first tries to remember some special incident or trauma that may have caused it. Failing to recollect any trauma, he concludes that "it just came by itself." He attributes the findings to his diabetes or his leprosy or his spina bifida, and concludes that there is nothing he can do to keep the problem from recurring.

The duty of the physician is to take time to explain the condition to the patient. It is a lifelong problem, and the patient has to accept responsibility for his own foot, or he will lose it. He must recognize the role of repetitive force and must realize that his tissues change from day to day. If he has sensitive hands, he should be taught to feel his feet all over to identify warm spots that may indicate inflammation. If a warm spot develops on his foot in the evening after walking during the day, he should feel the area again in the morning after a night's rest. Localized high temperature that persists overnight is an indication for some change in the amount of walking or in the type of shoe being worn. The patient must accept the self-discipline of controlling his gait and the amount of his walking as determined by the response of his feet, e.g., temperature, redness, calluses, and so forth (Fig. 46–9).

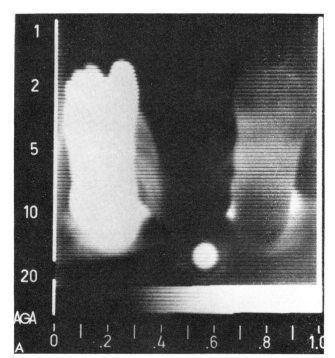

Figure 46–9. *(A) Thermogram showing the temperature contrast between a damaged and undamaged foot. The temperature scale at the bottom spans 10° C. (B) Clinical photograph of the feet in (A).*

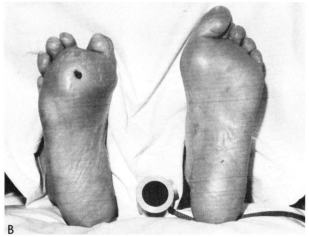

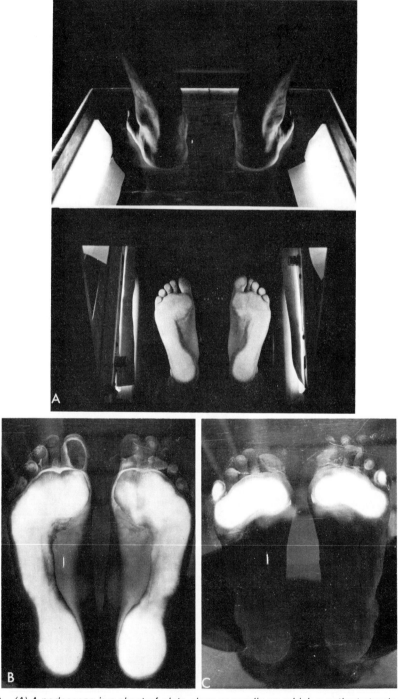

Figure 46–10. *(A) A podoscope is a sheet of plate glass or acrylic on which a patient stands while a mirror angled at 45 degrees underneath displays his weight-bearing pattern. (B) When the plate glass is illuminated only through its edge, the light scatters in proportion to local areas of pressure. (C) The increased brilliance of the forefoot when the heels are raised demonstrates the changed pressure pattern.*

There are three major variables that are under the patient's control and that determine the ultimate safety or destruction of the foot: (1) the length of the stride, (2) the number of steps per day, and (3) the texture and shape of the shoe.

LENGTH OF THE STRIDE. The patient has to understand that he cannot do much to vary the *force* that each foot accepts at each step, as this is related to his total weight. (Of course, reducing excess weight is good, but is usually only a modest gain for the foot). However, it is not total force but local pressure and shear that actually damage the foot, and both of these are related to the area of the skin and bone through which the force or load is exerted. When the foot is flat on the ground, the area of weight bearing is large; consequently, the pressure is small (Fig. 46–10A,B). Therefore, a shuffling gait with short steps causes only small pressures. When the stride is a little longer, the heel is lifted only 20 or 30 degrees at each step, the underside of the metatarsal heads share the weight, and the pressure is moderate (Fig. 46–10C). Thus, walking with rather short steps results in moderate pressures. When the heel is lifted more than 60 degrees, the weight and thrust are taken on the ends of the metatarsals (often on the ends of only the longest metatarsals), and the pressures are very high. Since long strides also indicate hurry, the shear stresses are also high and so is the deceleration and shear at heel strike. Therefore, fast walking with long strides is dangerous.

To avoid the need to walk fast and hurry, the patient needs to plan his day and use forethought and discipline. This will be accomplished only if the patient is convinced of its importance, and it is the job of the physician to convince him. A demonstration of pressure footprints, which will be discussed later, at different stride lengths may be effective.

NUMBER OF STEPS PER DAY. A patient's "quota" of walking depends on the state of his feet. Previously uninjured feet, even though insensitive, can usually accept normal amounts of walking, but long or fast walks (hikes or long periods of jogging) must be avoided. Patients who have previous ulceration and deformity must plan carefully to limit their walking.

In the absence of good mass transit systems, a car or bicycle is an obvious need. It may be good for the patient to wear a pedometer at his hip to help set numerical standards for himself. At the end of the day, if he has a hot spot on his foot and his pedometer reads five miles, he may decide that tomorrow he must restrict his walking to two miles.

SHOE DESIGN AND TEXTURE. As mentioned previously, all shoes for insensitive feet should be of leather and have snug heels and free room for toes. In addition, the sole or walking surface may need to be (1) soft, (2) molded, and (3) rocking.

Soft Insole. A soft insole helps to spread the stress of walking. Figure 46–7 shows the difference between the peak pressures under the third metatarsal head of a person with a normal foot as he strode barefoot over three different textured floor pads. The tracing (third line) shows the pressures on cement, leather, and microcell rubber. These were approximately 75, 45, and 20 lb/inch^2, respectively. A patient could probably walk safely six times as far at 20 lb/inch^2 as he could at 75 lb/inch^2.

When a foot is in a delicate state, such as when it is inflamed (hot) or just recently healed from an ulcer, walking only on a sandal made of deep, soft material such as soft microcell rubber or soft Plastazote is preferable. In a sandal such soft material may be 1 inch or more in depth. However, in a shoe a deep, soft insole results in too much up-and-down movement in the shoe, resulting in blisters on the sides of the foot or heel. Thus, in a regular shoe a layer of $\frac{1}{8}$ inch of Spenco or similar soft insole may be used. In an extra-depth shoe, a soft insole of $\frac{1}{4}$ inch or a little more is permissible. The undersole may be made of soft crepe and, if the patient's heel presents a problem, the heel of the shoe may be made of soft material with a hard layer underneath, such as the solid ankle cushioned heel (SACH). (See Figure 46–11.)

All these modifications are easy, but give only moderate help, suitable for a relatively normal foot.

Molding. When the sole of the shoe is molded to the foot, the forces of walking are spread much more evenly and pressures are therefore lower (Fig. 46–12). The danger of molding for an insensitive foot is that it may be done incorrectly, and the

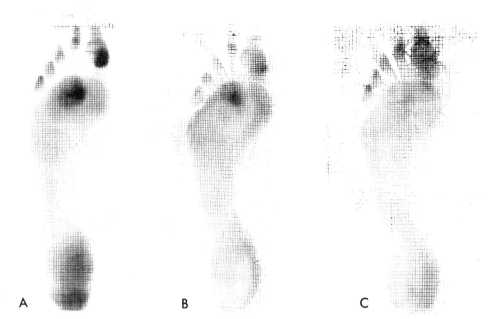

Figure 46–11. *Harris footprints of patient striding (A) barefoot on a hard floor, (B) on thin, soft insole material, and (C) on thick, soft insole material. Note that in C, the metatarsal high-pressure spots are no longer significant. The toes are doing more work.*

patient cannot feel when the bumps and hollows of the sole do not fit the bumps and hollows of his foot. I have known cases in which ulcers have been caused directly by misplaced "correction" such as a scaph-

![Insole of molded Plastazote]

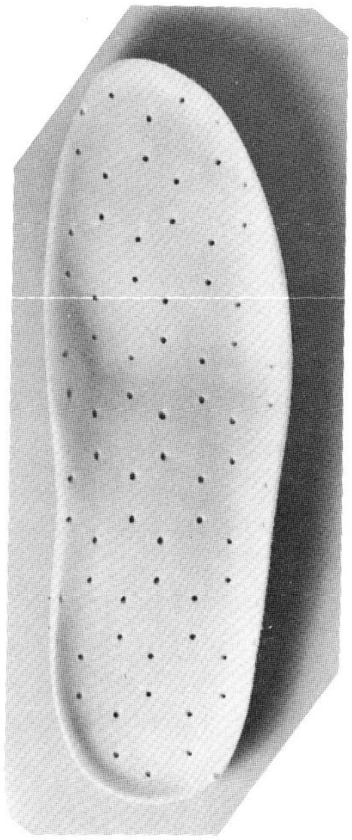

Figure 46–12. *Insole of molded Plastazote heat-formed over the patient's foot or a plaster model of the foot.*

oid pad or a metatarsal bar. Note that a metatarsal bar, although placed under the sole, functions by molding the sole upward; thus, it is classified as a form of molding, just as though it were inside the shoe.

For insensitive feet, insoles must be molded either on the foot iself or on a plaster model of the foot (using Plastazote or other closed-cell polyethylene foam such as Pelite or Alimed). If molding is done by guesswork in an intact shoe, it must be checked by in-the-shoe evaluation using a Harris mat or other pressure sensing device (see later discussion).

To provide room for a molded insole, the patient will need an extra-depth shoe such as the P. W. Minor "Treadeasy," the Alden shoe, the Miller shoe, or the Drew shoe.

In our own practice, we often use a double layer of insole. The inner layer is of heat-moldable polyethylene and a deeper layer of microcell rubber or neoprene is bonded to the polyethylene to give durability and resilience (Fig. 46–13). An innermost layer of horsehide or nylon helps to diminish friction and shear.

Rocking. Even with a soft molded insole that spreads pressure evenly over the entire heel and sole, there is always a

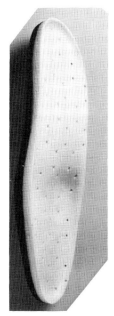

Figure 46–13. *Molded Plastazote insole backed by microcell rubber.*

moment of high pressure under the metatarsal heads when the heel is lifted and the other foot is in the swing phase of gait. This high peak pressure is the cause of most recurrent ulcers in the distal third of the foot, because the proximal part of the foot does no weight bearing when the heel is up.

We recommend a rigid sole and a rocker for the few patients who have recurrent ulceration, even after molded insoles are used. Some authors use the term "rocker" to refer to a metatarsal bar; however, we never use the word unless the shoe is rigid from heel to toe, like a clog (Fig. 46–14B,C). A child's seesaw is a rocker. It rocks on a central pivot and its arms or levers are rigid. If the seesaw were made of rubber, it would sag on both sides of the pivot at the same time, like a leather shoe does around a metatarsal bar. Because a metatarsal bar makes a bump on the inside of the shoe, it is very important that the bar be placed in exactly the right position behind the metatarsal heads (Fig. 46–14A). Because the rocker bar is under a rigid sole, it does not alter the shape of the molded insole; therefore it does not matter exactly where the rocker bar is placed. The farther back the rocker is placed, the more effective it is. However, the shoe beyond the rocker bar must not touch the floor or take any weight, even at the toe-off end of gait (Fig. 46–14B,C). Thus, the rocker must be high enough so that the toe does not touch the ground (Fig. 46–15). The farther back the bar is placed, the higher it must

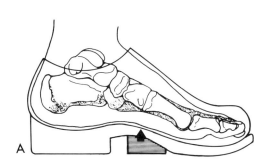

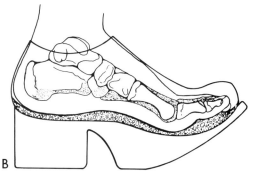

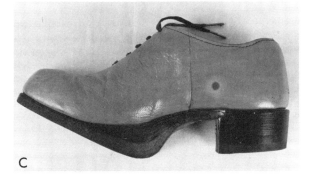

Figure 46–14. *Metatarsal bar. This is used only when the sole is flexible. It must be placed behind the metatarsal heads. (B) Rocker shoe. The rigid sole acts like a seesaw. (C) Rocker shoe.*

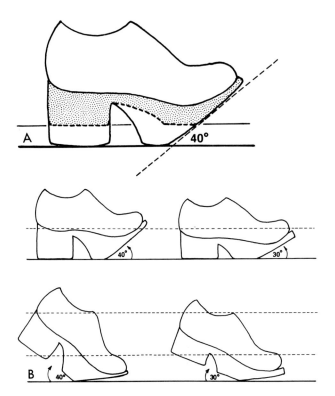

Figure 46–15. *(A) A 40-degree rocker will allow the shoe to be tilted 40 degrees without any weight being borne in front of the rocker bar. The stippled part of the sole shows low 40-degree rocker placed forward. The outline sole shows higher 40-degree rocker placed further back. It would be useless to place a low rocker further back, because when the shoe tilts, the forefoot would take the thrust.*
(B) Top row: A high 40-degree rocker placed correctly and a 30-degree rocker placed correctly at about the same position. Bottom row: A 40-degree rocker allows a 40-degree tilt of the shoe without weight bearing in front of rocker. The 30-degree rocker also relieves forward weight bearing, but only if the shoe is not tilted more than 30 degrees. Therefore, if the patient insists on long strides and a high tilt, he must have steep rocker or none at all.

be for the toe to be clear. But the higher it is, the less acceptable it becomes for the patient, who is more likely to wear another pair of shoes with no correction in them.

Thus, a rocker bar must be far enough forward so that it is low enough to be acceptable to the patient. Better to have a low, forwardly placed rocker bar that the patient wears than a high middle-of-the-shoe rocker that the patient keeps in the closet.

This principle of the rocker shoe is totally different from that of the metatarsal

bar and must be so understood by physician, shoemaker, and patient; otherwise it should not be prescribed. The design of many wooden clogs is close to the rocker shoe concept and can be readily modified to be acceptable for high-risk insensitive feet (Fig. 46–16).

Damage from Infection

Although the skin of the insensitive foot may be damaged and broken by various forms of mechanical stress, these wounds will heal almost as well as similar wounds that may occur in normal feet. The reputation of nonhealing that often attaches to the ulcers in leprosy and diabetes is due almost entirely to misuse of the wounded foot. No person with normal sensation could force himself to walk on a wounded septic foot. A person with loss of sensation will get his foot dressed, will take his antibiotic, and will then stride out of the physician's office and go back to work without even a limp. The infected tissues are squeezed like a sponge and bacteria are forced out into new uninfected areas. Osteomyelitis, septic arthritis, tenosynovitis, and spreading cellulitis occur in spite

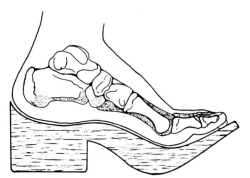

Figure 46–16. *A wooden clog is a very good compromise between a true rocker and a roll-over rigid sole. A molded insole may improve this clog.*

of antibiotics — all because of lack of rest to the damaged part.

It is not enough to tell the patient to rest or even to give him crutches. Even intelligent, cooperative patients will forget or minimize the problem when they compare it with the need to fulfill an urgent appointment.

Any acute wound or ulcer in an insensitive foot must be treated by bed rest (*total bed rest with the foot elevated*) plus medication. When the condition has become less acute and the swelling and discharge are diminished, perhaps after three or four days, a plaster cast may be applied and the patient may begin to walk.

I usually leave a first plaster cast on for about a week and then apply a new one because swelling subsides so rapidly when the foot is in plaster that the cast becomes loose and may cause trouble by movement and friction.

The purpose of a cast is partly to immobilize the foot and partly to distribute the

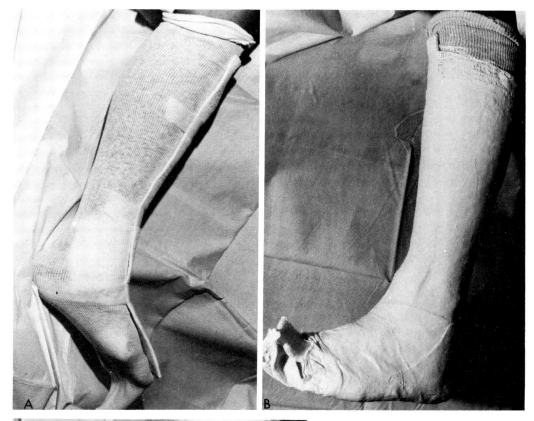

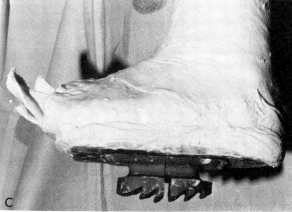

Figure 46–17. *(A) Stockinette and felt applied as a lining for a total contact cast. (B) The first layer of plaster of Paris is molded around the leg and is allowed to set before reinforcement slabs are added. (C) The plaster cast is almost complete; a plywood sole and rubber rocker are ready to be incorporated into it.*

weight bearing all over the foot and up the leg. The calf is conical and will accept weight, but only if the cast is unpadded.

A total contact cast is applied as follows: The patient lies prone on a plinth with knee flexed and foot horizontal. The ulcer is dressed with a few layers of gauze fixed with adhesive. The toes may be covered with a layer of felt or foam. A saddle of felt or foam padding is placed across both malleoli crossing the front of the ankle and is fixed with adhesive. A strip of felt is then placed down the length of the tibia and dorsum of the foot to serve as protection from the oscillating saw that will eventually cut the plaster off. All felt pads have beveled edges. A single layer of stockinette may then cover the leg from knee to toes (Fig. 46–17A). No other padding is used.

One single, fast-setting plaster bandage of good quality, such as Gypsona, is wrapped lightly around the lower leg and foot and then repeatedly rubbed until it has set (Fig. 46–17B). This eggshell-thin layer of plaster must conform to all contours and is the secret of the safety and success of a total-contact plaster. It is most important that, while it is setting, the shell is rubbed firmly into the hollows of the sole, such as the instep. No padding must be allowed between the skin of the sole of the foot and the plaster sole, except for a small dressing over the ulcer. No window should ever be left in a plaster cast on the lower extremity. Edema always results in a window bulge. The edge of the bulge is traumatized, and wounds heal poorly when edematous. If there is profuse discharge, either the patient must be kept in bed a little longer before applying the cast or the cast must be changed frequently. Continued profuse discharge often means that bone is involved, and surgical intervention may be needed.

Once the inner eggshell layer of plaster has set, a full walking cast is rapidly completed. I like to use a layer of plywood between the plaster and the rubber heel to avoid the danger of a crack in the sole caused by the localized pressure of the heel (Fig. 46–17C). People with insensitive feet cannot tell when local pressures from such cracks have occurred.

After one full day without weight bearing in such a cast, a patient may return to home and work so long as neither involves much walking. As soon as the patient feels that his cast is becoming loose, it must be changed.

The Newly Healed Ulcer

Ulcer recurrence is most common within one month of healing. This is because some inflammation still exists and there are friable adhesions between the new skin and deeper tissues or bone. If a new shoe is not ready for the patient before the plaster comes off, a temporary sandal of molded Plastazote may be needed so that the foot may be protected while it is especially vulnerable. The patient must be warned to take short steps and hold his walking to a minimum until the tissues harden and a plane of mobility opens up between the skin and bone. Here also temperature is a good test of healing. Newly healed vulnerable tissues will be warm but will cool off over a few weeks as they become better able to take more stress.

Specific Ulcer Situations and the Role of Surgery

Surgical intervention in the insensitive foot may be necessary for one or more of three reasons: (1) to restore muscle balance and make the foot plantigrade, (2) to remove dead bone or bony prominences that cause local pressure, and (3) to provide skin and soft-tissue cover.

A special warning is needed about operations in the presence of infection. Insensitive feet are very prone to ulcers and infections, and sometimes these infections produce minimal physical signs. Surgeons may be tempted to perform reconstructive surgery too soon after the healing of an ulcer and then find their work ruined by infection. Minor surgery through an ulcer wound is sometimes justifiable to remove or remodel infected bone, but such wounds need to be packed widely open afterward.

The Plantigrade Foot

Any deviation from normal foot balance will tend to place excessive stress on an edge of the foot or on one or the other end of the foot. Corrective action should be taken only after full evaluation and usually only if it can be shown that an actual problem exists, as evidenced by heat pattern or previous ulceration. Many people have variations from average gait that have developed over time to compensate for some earlier problem that will reappear if the compensating irregularity is "corrected."

Claw toes or hammer toes often need correction either because of excess stress on the tip of the toe or dorsal knuckle or simply because gross clawing increases the vertical height of the toes and makes it impossible to use normal shoes with an insole, since the toes alone require a high toe-box.

We usually correct mobile claw toes with a tendon transfer, stiff claw toes with an interphalangeal arthrodesis, and stiff dorsiflexed toes with a diaphysectomy as practiced by Jahss.[10]

The great toe often develops an ulcer at the medial side of the base of the terminal phalanx. This tends to occur in a pronated foot. The condition calls for a careful molding of insole to fill in the angle between the sole of the shoe and the side of the terminal phalanx (the angle causes shear stress) and to give smooth support to the toe distal to the vulnerable area. If this is not enough, it may be necessary to excise the bony prominence and perhaps fuse the interphalangeal joint. With recurrent great toe ulceration, there is great temptation to amputate the toe. This should usually be resisted because after amputation the problem is transferred, in a more intractable form, to the first metatarsal head.

Footdrop

Footdrop often results in improper stress on the forefoot and should be corrected, usually by tendon transfer or by a brace.

Correction of Footdrop. Tendon transfers for the correction of footdrop have not been used as often as they should be because it is widely believed that it is not possible to re-educate the antigravity and progravity muscles of the leg to exchange functions. Thus, a plantar-flexing muscle could not become a dorsiflexor.

We have performed many hundreds of footdrop corrections by tendon transfer and prefer it to any bony block or arthrode-

sis in most cases. The following points should be noted:

1. Re-education of a leg muscle, to change its phase in gait, is more difficult than re-educating an upper limb muscle.

2. Therefore, more time and care need to be taken. A physical therapist should teach the patient (a) to isolate the muscle before operation and learn to contract it on command and (b) to isolate it after operation and learn to dorsiflex the foot by using it in a non-weight-bearing mode for at least one week before he begins to walk.

3. For the first week of weight bearing, the patient must walk only while he is thinking about his transferred muscle. It is helpful to have some device, such as an electromyographic-operated buzzer, which will tell him when he is contracting this muscle.

4. Children and young people re-educate well. Middle-aged and older people may never learn to change phase completely.

5. Even in older people, a tendon transfer out-of-phase may correct the foot drop and allow fairly normal gait. This may still be better than triple arthrodesis because of the strains on joints produced by the latter.

THE OPERATION. We usually use the tibialis posterior transferred to the dorsum of the foot.

The tendon is divided behind the ankle. The interosseous membrane is divided near the tibia, using a vertical incision along the entire middle third of the leg lateral to the anterior border of the tibia. The end of the tendon is grasped in a long, curved tendon forceps and passed back up its own pathway to appear beside the tibia anteriorly. The tendon is pulled upon in the anterior wound. It will subsequently pull its lower muscle fibers into the wound and will then twist the interosseous membrane laterally so that part of the body of the muscle comes to lie between the membrane and the tibia. This happens because the tibialis posterior takes origin from the back of the membrane.

The tendon is split and half of it is attached, by interweaving, to the tendon of tibialis anterior. The other half is then attached, also by interweaving, to the tendons of the extensor digitorum. This second half should be under slightly higher tension than the first. Both attachments should be made with the foot dorsiflexed. A tendo-Achillis lengthening may be necessary to allow full passive dorsiflexion.

To support the medial arch after the transfer of tibialis posterior, we sometimes divide the flexor digitorum at the same level as the tibialis posterior and attach the proximal stump of the digitorum to the distal stump of tibialis, while the distal stump of flexor digitorum is attached to the side of the flexor hallucis.

The foot is immobilized for four weeks in about 10 degrees of dorsiflexion. The cast is then bivalved and removed only during the daily sessions of non–weight-bearing exercises for another two weeks.

Weight bearing under supervision is then started and continued until the patient is in control of his gait pattern.

In cases in which the tibialis posterior is weak, a strong peroneus or flexor digitorum may be used for transfer. The flexor hallucis has too much low muscle bulk to allow for easy transfer.

A Lambrinudi type of triple arthrodesis may help to compensate for footdrop if no suitable muscles are available.[12] However, patients will need to wear boots to help support the foot both from the residual foot drop and from accidental lateral or medial strains at the ankle, which are much more serious in the absence of a mobile subtalar joint.

Lateral Border of the Foot

Inversion of the foot is very prone to result in ulceration of the lateral border of the foot under the fifth metatarsal base (Fig. 46–18A). No attempt should be made to correct such inversion by external pressure created by a build-up on the lateral part of the sole of the shoe, which only increases the tendency to pressure ulceration. The deformity must be either accommodated or corrected by surgery.

Accommodation of the deformity involves making a shoe that is fully molded to the uncorrected position of the foot, with the sole of the shoe being parallel to the ground while the leg is in the standing position. This may sometimes result in the line of weight bearing falling lateral to the axis of deviation of the ankle or subtalar joint, thus making it likely that the foot will turn over and dislocate. To avoid this, the sole of the shoe should be extended outward laterally to provide a broader base on the side of the instability (Fig. 46–18B).

The surgical correction usually involves a triple arthrodesis or a wedge osteotomy to bring the foot squarely under the ankle.

If the subtalar joint has to be arthrodesed, the patient with insensitive feet should be warned to avoid walking on rough or irregular ground, since the loss of lateromedial mobility at the subtalar level transfers all lateral stresses to the ankle joint. Without pain sensation at that level, ankle fracture-dislocation becomes much more probable.

If at any time problems occur at the lateral border of an insensitive midfoot, the outlook is serious and an early decision must be made between very special footwear and surgery, as described above.

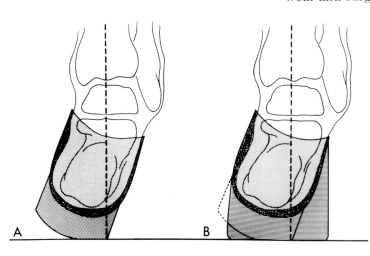

Figure 46–18. (A) A foot in varus position takes stress on the lateral border. There is danger of progressive deformity and rupture of the collateral ligaments because the line of weight bearing is very close to the edge of heel. (B) If the deformity is not to be corrected surgically, it must be accommodated, not corrected, by modification of footwear. The heel is made plantigrade and flared to act as a strut to the lateral side of the shoe.

Forefoot

Sometimes ulceration has occurred and recurred so often under the metatarsal heads that the residual bones are covered only by scar and further recurrence seems inevitable, even with good footwear.

In such cases it may be helpful (1) to perform osteotomies across the foot at the metatarsal neck level to place more thrust proximally; (2) to excise the metatarsal heads, for the same reason; or (3) to perform a transmetatarsal or Lisfranc amputation.

Any one of these procedures will give a period of freedom from tissue breakdown. However, it is the duty of the surgeon to make it very clear to the patient that the same sequence of events will occur at the new proximal level of thrust unless new habits of walking and footwear are adopted. I refuse to use these palliative procedures unless I feel that the patient understands and agrees to take more care in the future. In particular, it is very dangerous to wear a long (normal) shoe on a shortened foot. The leverage may double the pressure on the new site of thrust. If the patient must wear a long shoe, it should be extremely flexible, so that the distal part transmits no force, or, better, it should be completely stiff and roll over a proximal rocker.

The Heel

The heel has fewer problems than the forefoot when muscle balance is normal.

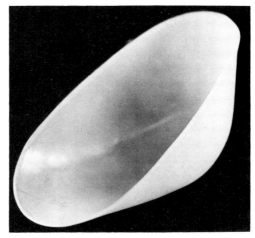

Figure 46–19. *Heel cup to prevent the soft tissues under the heel from spreading.*

However, when plantar flexors are weak, as in spina bifida, heel ulcers are common.

The secret of conservative management of the vulnerable insensitive heel is to use side-to-side support in the form of a heel cup (Fig. 46–19). If this is properly fitted, it will give firm lateral support so that the soft-tissue heel pad does not spread but is kept under the bone. Another method is to remove the heel of the shoe and place a bar under the instep so that the "heel-strike" phase of gait takes place further forward (Fig. 46–20). For healing of an open heel ulcer, a total contact plaster cast, well molded around the heel, will usually be satisfactory.

A surgical approach is to lift half the heel

Figure 46–20. *(A) To reduce the pressure at heel-strike and spread it further forward, a heel rocker is used. Here it is combined with a roll-over clog-type rigid sole. (B) Gait with heel rocker and clog sole.*

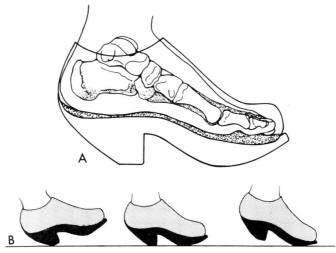
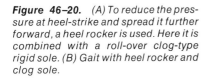

pad off the os calcis through a lateral, non–weight-bearing incision. Dissection must be strictly in the skeletal plane. The edges of the ulcer are then excised and the ulcer is closed with deep figure of eight sutures. The wound is drained through the lateral incision while the plantar wound heals. After this type of surgery, weight bearing must be delayed until the heel pad is well healed and the discharge from the lateral wound has ceased.

A similar operation may be performed if a heel ulcer has already healed, but has left a scar that is vulnerable because of lack of a fat pad. Through a lateral incision the heel pad is lifted off the bone by sharp dissection in the skeletal plane. The old scar is excised and the pad moved across. The lateral defect is then grafted with split skin.

Evaluation of Pressure and Shear Stress

However much care is taken in the fitting of shoes and in modification of soles and insoles, errors sometimes occur. Patients with normal sensation will complain about the shoe. They will say, for example, that the metatarsal bar that was intended to relieve pressure under the metatarsal

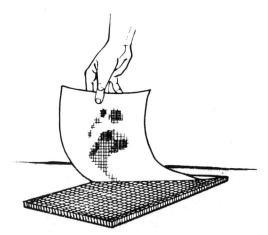

Figure 46–21. *The Harris footprint mat in use.*

heads has actually made it worse. Only then are careful measurements made, and the bar is found to be too far forward. The patient with insensitive feet accepts the altered shoe without complaint and develops an ulcer at the site of pressure.

Thus, objective evaluation of pressures inside the shoe are important. The Harris footprint mat (Fig. 46–21), which gives very good impressions of pressure distribution in barefoot walking, may also be used for evaluating pressure inside the shoe. Some of the thinnest types of Harris

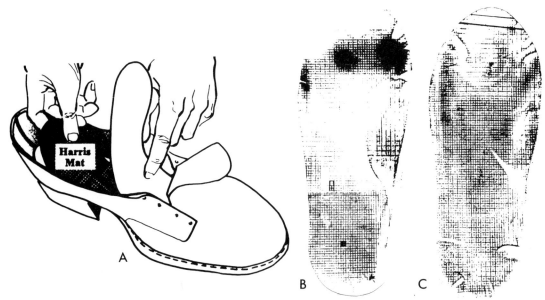

Figure 46–22. *(A) The thinnest variety of Harris mat is cut into insole-shaped pieces and used to test shoes. (B) An example of an unacceptable in-shoe footprint when a simple soft insole was used. (C) A second footprint in the same shoe after a molded insole and rocker bar were used.*

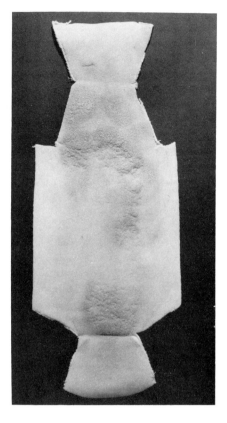

Figure 46–23. *The Carville microcapsule slipper sock, shown opened out here, gives an in-shoe footprint that marks pressure by color.*

mats are cut into various insole shapes and kept ready for testing. They may be used over and over again. A piece of mat is inked with a roller and covered with paper cut to the same shape and placed in the shoe (Fig. 46–22A). The shoe is opened widely and the foot eased gently in. The shoe is firmly laced, and the patient stands and takes about three bold strides. The shoe is then opened widely and the foot eased out. The paper will now show heavy markings where pressure has been high (Fig. 46–22B,C). The Carville microcapsule slipper sock gives a similar read-out of pressure (Fig. 46–23).

Neither method evaluates the effect on the foot of the pressure in the shoe. Thus a careful temperature scan, taken after a shoe has been worn for a few hours, will often provide the most useful evaluation of the total suitability of a shoe. Thermistor probes (skin thermometers) or radiometers or thermograms may be used to show the temperature differentials between areas of skin that have and have not been under stress. I find that my own hand gives a very good evaluation of the pattern of temperature around a foot. By gently passing my hand across the sole and around the dorsum of the foot, the temperature gradients are quickly appreciated. Localized hot spots are easily defined by repetitive stroking. Once the location of a hot spot is defined, it is marked with ink, and its precise temperature is taken, using a thermistor probe or a radiometer. The temperature of a neutral area (mid-tibia for example) is also taken and the temperature differential is recorded ($\Delta T \,^\circ$). The process is repeated after the patient has worn corrected shoes and again at intervals on check-up visits. A significant rise in temperature differential will sometimes mean that the shoe modifications are inadequate. It may also mean that the patient has not been wearing the prescribed shoes. Some of my patients keep a skin thermometer by their bedside at home, and check their own pressure points at night when they go to bed. This helps them to learn what type of activity and what type of shoe are dangerous and what are safe. It also helps them to accept responsibility for controlling their own lives. For a lifetime problem like loss of sensation, this is the key to success.

REFERENCES

1. Bauman, J. H., and Brand, P. W.: Measurement of pressure between foot and shoe. Lancet, *1*:629, 1963.
2. Bauman, J. H., Girling, J. P., and Brand, P. W.: Plantar pressures and trophic ulceration. J. Bone Joint Surg., *45-B*:652, 1963.
3. Bergtholdt, H. T., and Brand, P. W.: Thermography: An aid in the management of insensitive feet and stumps. Arch. Phys. Med. Rehab., *56*:205, 1975.
4. Bergtholdt, H. T., and Brand, P. W.: Temperature assessment and plantar inflammation. Leprosy Rev., *47*:211, 1976.
5. Brand, P. W.: Insensitive Feet: A Practical Handbook on Foot Problems in Leprosy. London, The Leprosy Mission, 1977.
6. Brand, P. W.: Pathomechanics of diabetic (neurotrophic) ulcer and its conservative management. *In* Bergan, J. J., and Yao, J. S. T. (eds.): Gangrene and Severe Ischemia of the Lower Extremities. New York, Grune & Stratton, 1978, pp. 117–130.
7. Brand, P. W.: Pathomechanics of pressure ulceration. *In* Fredericks, S., and Brody, G. S. (eds.): Symposium on the Neurologic Aspects of Plastic Surgery. Vol. 17. St. Louis, C. V. Mosby Co., 1978, pp. 185–189.
8. Enna, C. D., Brand, P. W., Reed, J. P., Jr., and Welch, D.: The orthotic care of the denervated foot in Hansen's disease. Orthot. Prosthet. *30*:33, 1976.
9. Harris, J. R., and Brand, P. W.: Patterns of disintegration of the tarsus in the anaesthetic foot. J. Bone Joint Surg., *48-B*:4, 1966.
10. Jahss, M. H.: Diaphysectomy for severe acquired overlapping fifth toe and advanced fixed hammering of the small toes. *In* Bateman, J. E. (ed.): Foot Science. Philadelphia, W. B. Saunders Co., 1976, pp. 211–221.
11. Kosiak, M.: Etiology and pathology of ischemic ulcers. Arch. Phys. Med. Rehab., *40*:62, 1959.
12. Lambrinudi, C.: New operation on drop foot. Br. J. Surg., *15*:293, 1927.
13. Yamada, H.: Strength of Biological Materials. Baltimore, Williams and Wilkins Co., 1970.

CHAPTER 47

REFLEX SYMPATHETIC DYSTROPHY SYNDROME

Kenneth A. Johnson, M.D.

In this chapter, the *reflex sympathetic dystrophy syndrome, transient painful osteoporosis syndrome, causalgic syndrome,* and *massive osteolysis syndrome* are described. These are properly termed "syndromes" because each represents a group of symptoms commonly occurring together so as to constitute a distinct clinical entity. Each of these conditions can involve the foot, and each has in common the rather loose association of pain and osteoporosis. Although poorly understood, these syndromes are clinically important.

REFLEX SYMPATHETIC DYSTROPHY SYNDROME

For many years, multiple independent descriptions of a painful condition involv-

TABLE 47–1. Alternate Terminology of the Reflex Sympathetic Dystrophy Syndrome

Acute inflammatory bone atrophy[1]
Acute bone atrophy[2, 3]
Post-traumatic pain syndrome[4]
Minor causalgia[5]
Post-traumatic osteoporosis[6]
Post-traumatic dystrophy of the extremities[7, 8]
Post-traumatic painful osteoporosis[9]
Reflex sympathetic dystrophy[10–13]
Sympathetic dystrophy[14]
Post-traumatic sympathetic dystrophy[15–17]
Post-traumatic vasomotor disorders[18]
Sympathetic reflex dystrophy[19]
Sudeck's atrophy[20]
The reflex sympathetic dystrophy syndrome[21, 22]

ing the lower extremities have been reported. In naming this condition, each observer has focused on his particular bias (Table 47–1). Nevertheless, a review of these reports reveals clinical similarities of a *syndrome* whose recognition allows planning of a proper treatment program.

Clinical Aspects

Evidence of a *neurovascular disorder* associated with *dystrophic changes* is characteristic of this syndrome.[12] Pain in the extremity[21] is the most common neurovascular finding (Fig. 47–1A), being present in 96 per cent of the patients in one large series.[17] The pain is usually described as burning, aching, or throbbing and is not confined to a dermatome or peripheral nerve distribution, but rather to a region of an extremity. Hypesthesia, hyperesthesia or paresthesia, swelling, and stiffness and hyperhidrosis are also frequently encountered. Dystrophic changes include thinning of the skin, demineralization of the bones, a decrease in the amount of subcutaneous tissue, and a decrease in muscle volume with attendant diminished motor function. When bone demineralization seems to be the predominant dystrophic change, the condition is frequently referred to as Sudeck's atrophy.[1] These changes have been described as occurring sequentially.[8] Initially, a severe burning pain at the site of injury is associated with warmth, edema, and hypertonic muscles. Later, the edema may spread, and the warm and flushed appearance gives way to a firm, cyanotic, and cool extremity, with increasingly stiff joints. Finally, the pain involves a larger area, and dystrophic changes predominate. In actuality, no such specific sequence seems to frequently occur. Because of overlap and variations in the severity of symptoms and signs, the only recognizable sequence seems to be that neurovascular symptoms begin soon after the inciting trauma and that after a period the dystrophic changes begin to appear.

The reflex sympathetic dystrophy syndrome may become manifest after a number of different types of injuries, such as sprains, soft-tissue wounds, fractures of varied severity, surgical procedures, and infection. A striking feature of this syndrome is that the neurovascular and dystrophic changes are increased out of proportion to the initial trauma. In addition, the changes do not gradually decrease along with tissue healing but tend to persist or increase long after the inciting traumatic episode. A severe injury of fracture seldom gives rise to this syndrome.[7]

Some patients demonstrate a response that is between the normal response of an extremity to trauma and a definite reflex sympathetic dystrophy syndrome.[7, 11] This intermediate response is probably the most common presentation of the reflex sympathetic dystrophy syndrome and one that is frequently overlooked; it subsides spontaneously and sometimes slowly.[2]

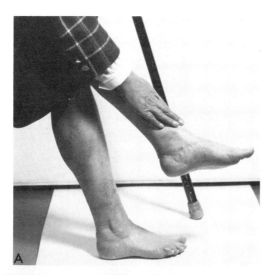
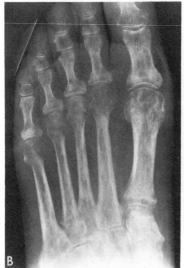
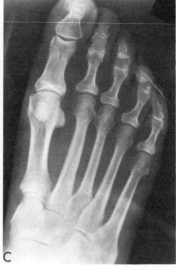

Figure 47–1. This 57-year-old woman had severe pain in the distal lower extremity 10 months after a twisting injury to the ankle. She was unable to fully bear weight on that foot and had diffuse tenderness and swelling with joint stiffness. (B) Roentgenogram shows diffuse spotty osteoporosis involving the entire left foot. (C) Roentgenogram of the unaffected right foot. Hospitalization for 10 days with bupivacaine paralumbar sympathetic blockade every other day and physical therapy measures provided relief of pain.

Awareness of this possibility allows early detection and proper treatment of this "forme fruste" of the reflex sympathetic dystrophy syndrome. As Homans has observed: "There are serious cases and mild ones, and it is the serious ones which have made the mild ones understandable."[5]

The roentgenographic manifestations of the reflex sympathetic dystrophy syndrome are seen most frequently in the short bones of the extremity.[9, 21] The early changes give the bone a mottled or patchy appearance (Fig. 41–1B,C). Later, the irregular areas of rarefaction disappear, and the bone becomes diffusely and sometimes markedly demineralized. During the long period of bone reconstruction, there is a gradual reappearance of calcium, although complete recalcification may never take place. Symptomatic relief will usually occur before evidence of recalcification, as seen on the standard roentgenogram, is very far advanced. Fine-detail roentgenograms as well as scintigraphy, however, demonstrate bone changes early in the juxta-articular regions, and these changes seem to reflect the clinical course of the disease.[22]

Multiple alternate diagnoses must be considered in the evaluation of the patient with the reflex sympathetic dystrophy syndrome. Although some authors believe that transient painful osteoporosis[13] and the causalgic syndrome[15, 21] are only variants of the reflex sympathetic dystrophy syndrome, these conditions seem to be so disparate on a clinical basis as to justify separate discussions.[14, 23] Osteoporosis associated with immobilization secondary to disuse or neuropathy[20, 24] and collagen vascular disease such as rheumatoid arthritis[19] and scleroderma may need to be differentiated from the reflex sympathetic dystrophy syndrome. The relationship of a psychiatric disorder (e.g., malingering, hysteria, psychoneurosis) and its differentiation from the reflex sympathetic dystrophy syndrome have been mentioned often in the literature.[4, 5, 7, 10, 12, 14-16, 19, 25, 26] These psychiatric disturbances may just as well be the result of a prolonged painful condition as the cause. There is an ever-present tendency to try to explain on a psychiatric basis a diagnosis such as reflex sympathetic dystrophy syndrome, the pathogenesis of which remains essentially unknown.

In 1948, it was hopefully expressed that sympathetic dystrophy "is a term that may be rightfully discarded within a few years when a better understanding of the syndrome is obtained."[14] Twenty-nine years later, this same syndrome was said to be one of a "poorly understood nature."[13] Many theories seem to relate the situation to the initiation and excitation of abnormal neural reflexes.[4, 13, 15] Empirically, on the basis of clinical signs and responses to therapy, the sympathetic nervous system seems to be closely involved in the pathogenesis of the syndrome. The exact nature of this association, however, remains obscure.

Some authors believe that the primary physiologic alteration is in the vascular regulation of the involved extremity.[8, 27] The sympathetic nervous system is a major factor in the regulation of body heat by varying the peripheral vascular bed capacity, with both vasoconstriction and vasodilation being sympathetic functions.[28] Whether vascular alterations are causally related to the reflex sympathetic dystrophy syndrome, however, also remains unknown,[14] and observations such as dystrophic softening of bones when damp cold is applied to the skin[29] still await explanation.

Treatment

Prevention of the reflex sympathetic dystrophy syndrome by the proper treatment of the inciting injury,[7, 18] followed by functional mobilization, is the most satisfactory approach.[2] For the established reflex sympathetic dystrophy syndrome, however, treatment taxes the physician's expertise. Sympathy and understanding are those intangible qualities of the physician that, along with specific effects of other therapy, seem to be especially important in the treatment of the established case of the syndrome.[26] Explaining the protean manifestations of the syndrome to the patient, along with reassurance and relief of anxiety, is mandatory.[25] Ascertaining the patient's "state of mind"[7] and its participation in the diseased condition may sometimes reveal that formal psychiatric support is advisable, but a psychiatric approach alone is generally disappointing.[19] Settlement of any litigation associated with the inciting cause should be encouraged.[7, 8]

Specific early therapy should include the use of mild analgesics and tranquilizers to relieve pain and anxiety.[17] Physical therapy measures include local application of heat, contrast baths, manual massage, normal-range exercises, graded use, and occupational therapy.[12] Casts,[6] braces, or forceful manipulations[2, 3, 25] should not be used. For the early reflex sympathetic dystrophy syndrome,[3, 7, 8, 25] the aforementioned measures should be sufficient and relief of symptoms should be expected.[2, 3, 15] Generally, the earlier the syndrome is recognized, the better the results of treatment should be.[11, 25, 28] With more severe symptoms, usually later in the course of the syndrome, more aggressive treatment with hospitalization becomes necessary.[26] If a localized area of tenderness is present, repeated local anesthetic injections may be helpful.[4] Periarterial sympathectomy, a stripping of the soft adventitia from the major vessels entering the painful area, has also been used, with satisfactory results.[6, 8, 29] The primary treatment of the late reflex sympathetic dystrophy syndrome remains, however, interruption of the sympathetic nervous system. Initially, this can be done by injections of local anesthetics in and about the spinal canal.[28, 30] If satisfactory relief of symptoms occurs with anesthetic injection but the symptoms return with the loss of sympathetic blockade, surgical sympathectomy can be considered.[8, 16, 17]

Occasionally, multiple or continuous sympathetic blockades[28, 30] may give adequate symptomatic relief that persists even after the anesthetic has worn off, and surgical sympathectomy can thereby be avoided.[10, 19] Newer local anesthetics with a prolonged duration of action, such as bupivacaine, may make techniques such as the use of an indwelling catheter for multiple anesthetic administrations unnecessary.

Surgical sympathectomy is designed to permanently interrupt the sympathetic nervous system to a region,[16] and good results have been reported.[10, 11, 14, 15] The untoward effects of surgical sympathectomy, such as postsympathectomy neuralgia, and the risks inherent in any surgical procedure make this approach undesirable until less invasive procedures have been found to be ineffective.

If the reflex sympathetic dystrophy syndrome is severe and has been present for a prolonged period, there may be a self-perpetuating painful condition of the higher central nervous system now not directly dependent on the initially painful region.[19] When this occurs, even complete spinal block anesthesia for the region will not relieve the pain, and more involved neurosurgical procedures (e.g., tractotomies and frontal lobotomies) may have to be considered, because sympathetic ablation would be ineffective.[10, 19]

The regional intravenous use of guanethidine has been reported to give prolonged relief of pain by its sympathetic blockade action of displacing norepinephrine from the sympathetic nerve endings.[31] In isolated cases, propranolol hydrochloride has apparently been efficacious in relief of symptoms,[32] as has the oral administration of glucocorticoids.[33] Calcitonin may also be useful in treating the osteoporosis associated with the reflex sympathetic dystrophy syndrome.[24]

TRANSIENT PAINFUL OSTEOPOROSIS SYNDROME

A syndrome of transient painful osteoporosis involving the bones of one or more joints of the lower extremities has been described.[23] Other authors have described a similar condition under the names of *transitory demineralization,*[34] *migratory osteolysis,*[35] *transient osteoporosis,*[36-38] *regional migratory osteoporosis,*[39-42] and *transient regional osteoporosis.*[33]

Clinical Aspects

Characteristically, this syndrome affects a person of good general health, without an unequivocal cause such as trauma or disease, and results in a painful and sometimes tender joint in the lower extremity. The hip is the most common joint affected, but involvement of the knee, ankle, and foot also occurs. In each affected joint, the pain lasts for three to nine months, after which spontaneous resolution occurs. The attacks may be overlapping; that is, a second joint can become painful before the

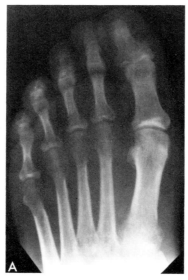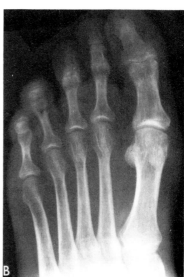

Figure 47–2. (A) Roentgenogram of spotty osteoporosis in the foot of a 53-year-old man two months after onset of pain and tenderness. During the previous few years, this patient also had transient painful osteoporosis involvement of the hip and both knees. (B) Roentgenographic appearance of same foot 17 months later, with restitution of normal appearance and no pain.

pain in the initially involved joint subsides completely, so that the patient has two or more painful joints at one time.[23] The time periods, sequences, and distribution of joint involvement, therefore, are extremely variable. A similar cycle of symptoms may recur a few years later. Lequesne has pointed out the discrepancy between severe functional disability and only moderate pain.[36] Both men and women are affected by the syndrome, usually in the third to sixth decades of life. Signs of inflammation, such as erythema, warmth, and swelling, are often present but minimal and tend to resolve before pain decreases. An association of this syndrome with pregnancy has been described.[34, 37]

Laboratory values, including the erythrocyte sedimentation rate, are almost always within normal limits. Roentgenograms show a diffuse or patchy osteoporosis about the involved area, developing three to six weeks after the onset of pain (Fig. 47–2A). Periosteal elevation with a line of calcification above the normal level of the cortex can occur.[39] The bone density returns to nearly normal over a period of a few years, but the trabecular pattern tends to remain coarser and more irregular than that in the unaffected joints (Fig. 47–2B). The osteoporotic changes are often still apparent when recovery is clinically complete, and no narrowing of the joint space occurs. Biopsy of the bone shows nonspecific changes of osteoporosis consisting of thin, viable trabeculae,[35, 42] and surface resorption and formation studies show evidence of increased bone turnover. Only minimal inflammatory changes are occasionally seen, with no evidence of angiomatosis or granulomatous inflammation.

Bone scanning after radionuclide administration may demonstrate an abnormally increased uptake about the joint even before roentgenographic changes are

TABLE 47–2. Comparison of Transient Painful Osteoporosis and Reflex Sympathetic Dystrophy Syndrome

	TRANSIENT PAINFUL OSTEOPOROSIS SYNDROME	REFLEX SYMPATHETIC DYSTROPHY SYNDROME
Antecedent injury	No	Yes
Pain characteristics	Diffuse aching on weight bearing	Burning, throbbing, constant
Skin dystrophic changes with decreased joint motion	No	Yes
Spontaneous recovery without permanent pain and disability	Yes	No, sometimes severe residuals
Multiple episodes	Yes	No
Knee and hip involvement	Common	Unusual

evident,[43] and this increased uptake remains after clinical resolution of symptoms.[40]

The differential evaluation of pain in a joint with periarticular osteoporosis includes immobilization osteoporosis, monoarticular arthritis, rheumatoid arthritis, gout, sarcoidosis, infection, neoplasia, and massive osteolysis.[38] Although an association with the reflex sympathetic dystrophy syndrome has been claimed by some authors,[36, 38] this syndrome seems to differ enough in significant ways (Table 47–2) that it can be differentiated from the reflex sympathetic dystrophy syndrome.[23, 33, 35]

Treatment

Because transient painful osteoporosis syndrome is a self-limiting condition, treatment should consist of a conservative program of physical therapy with protection of the joint against full weight bearing because of the possibility of fracture. Mild analgesics and anti-inflammatory agents, along with reassurance of the benign course of the disease, are helpful. In severe cases of the disease, corticosteroids may be used,[35, 39, 40] but it is not yet certain that such treatment hastens resolution of the disease.

CAUSALGIC SYNDROME

In 1864, Mitchell, Morehouse, and Keen described a painful syndrome of the extremities that occurred after a gunshot wound directly involving the main nerves.[44] Three years later, Mitchell adopted the term "causalgia" from the Greek roots *kausos* (heat) and *algos* (pain).[45] Since that time, some confusion has developed; some authors place the syndrome described by Mitchell and associates with the reflex sympathetic dystrophy syndrome.[5, 15, 46] The causalgic syndrome, although perhaps related to the reflex sympathetic dystrophy syndrome, is such a specific clinical entity as to justify its separate description.[47, 48]

Clinical Aspects

The pain of the causalgic syndrome was adequately described in 1920 by the Nerve Injuries Committee of the British Medical Research Council as (1) spontaneous; (2) hot and burning, intense, diffuse, persistent, but subject to exacerbations; (3) excited by stimuli that do not necessarily produce a physical effect on the limb; and (4) tending to lead to profound changes in the mental state of the patient.[49]

Kirklin and associates stated:

We consider causalgia to be a clinical syndrome associated with a lesion of a peripheral nerve containing sensory fibers, manifested by pain in the affected extremity; this pain is usually of a burning character and is usually located in an area corresponding in general to the cutaneous distribution of the involved nerve. An integral characteristic of this pain, one whose presence is necessary in order to make the diagnosis, is its accentuation by certain disturbing features in the affected individual's environment.[50]

These definitions are as precise as possible and are consistent with the vivid description of Mitchell and coworkers:

As the pain increases, the general sympathy becomes more marked. The temper changes and grows irritable; the face becomes anxious and has a look of weariness and suffering. The sleep is restless, and the constitutional condition, reacting on the wounded limb, exasperates the hyperaesthetic state, so that the rattling of a newspaper, a breath of air, another's step across the ward, the vibrations caused by a military band, or the shock of the feet in walking gives rise to increase of pain. At last the patient grows hysterical, if we may use the only term which covers the facts. He walks carefully, carries the limb tenderly with the sound hand, is tremulous, nervous, and has all kinds of expedients for lessening his pain.[44]

The causalgic syndrome, as described, is uncommon and is usually secondary to a missile injury involving the brachial or lumbosacral plexus or the median or sciatic nerve. In contradistinction is the common but less precise reflex sympathetic dystrophy syndrome, which usually does not involve a direct injury to a major nerve. Trophic changes can be part of the causalgic syndrome, but the intense pain and its characteristics are so remarkable as to become paramount and to make the observation of such a patient an unforgettable experience. Walters correctly differentiates the hyperpathia associated with such conditions as peripheral neuritis, herpes zoster, or tic douloureux from the causalgic syndrome.[47]

Much remains to be explained about the pathogenesis of the causalgic syndrome. Granit and associates described motor-to-sensory cross stimulation in injured areas of mixed nerves,[51] which is an attractive correlation of the necessary direct nerve injury with the pain. In addition, the sympathetic nervous system seems to be intimately involved either as a pathway for pain impulse conduction or as a source of pain, because its interruption invariably leads to relief of pain.[50]

Treatment

Sympathectomy is so effective and dramatic in the relief of the causalgic syndrome that failure to achieve relief of pain by this procedure makes the diagnosis questionable.[15, 16, 46] There are some reports of spontaneous resolution of the causalgic syndrome as well as of increasing pain with time, but the most common situation is an onset of pain shortly after the nerve injury, which persists unchanged for many years or until sympathectomy is accomplished. As in the reflex sympathetic dystrophy syndrome, when multiple or continuous local anesthetic sympathetic blockade relieves the symptoms only temporarily, surgical sympathectomy should be done.[16] Kleiman has described a patient in whom not only ipsilateral but also contralateral sympathectomy was necessary in order to give complete relief of symptoms.[52]

The nerve lesion itself may infrequently require resection and neurorrhaphy.[50] Such a procedure may sometimes be followed by relief of the causalgic syndrome and, therefore, should probably be done before sympathectomy.

MASSIVE OSTEOLYSIS SYNDROME

In 1954, Gorham and associates defined a rare condition that generally affected children or young adults in which osteolysis of bone occurred.[53] The osteolysis has affected virtually every area of the body and may involve a single bone or may spread to involve adjacent bones. Sponta-neous abatement of the slowly enlarging lesion usually occurs without bone reformation, or its growth may cause death by encroachment on vital structures. Benign-appearing angiomatosis is the pathologic abnormality associated with the osteolysis,[54, 55] but whether or not this angiomatosis is the primary abnormality is uncertain.[56] Treatment involves local resection or amputation. At least four patients with foot involvement have been reported,[56-59] and therefore, this condition should be considered when osteolysis of the foot is present.

REFERENCES

1. Sudeck, P.: Ueber die acute entzündliche Knochenatrophie. Arch. Klin. Chir., 62:147, 1900.
2. Noble, T. P., and Hauser, E. D. W.: Acute bone atrophy. Arch. Surg., 12:75, 1926.
3. Henderson, M. S.: Acute atrophy of bone: report of an unusual case involving the radius and ulna. Minn. Med., 19:214, 1936.
4. Livingston, W. K.: Post-traumatic pain syndromes: an interpretation of the underlying pathological physiology; division I, division II. West. J. Surg., 46:341; 426, 1938.
5. Homans, J.: Minor causalgia: a hyperesthetic neurovascular syndrome. N. Engl. J. Med., 222:870, 1940.
6. Herrmann, L. G., and Caldwell, J. A.: Diagnosis and treatment of post-traumatic osteoporosis. Am. J. Surg., 51:630, 1941.
7. Miller, D. S., and de Takats, G.: Post-traumatic dystrophy of the extremities: Sudeck's atrophy. Surg. Gynecol. Obstet., 75:558, 1942.
8. De Takats, G., and Miller, D. S.: Post-traumatic dystrophy of the extremities: a chronic vasodilator mechanism. Arch. Surg., 46:469, 1943.
9. Herrmann, L. G., Reineke, H. G., and Caldwell, J. A.: Post-traumatic painful osteoporosis: a clinical and roentgenological entity. Am. J. Roentgenol., 47:353, 1942.
10. Evans, J. A.: Reflex sympathetic dystrophy: report on 57 cases. Ann. Intern. Med., 26:417, 1947.
11. Casten, D. F., and Betcher, A. M.: Reflex sympathetic dystrophy. Surg. Gynecol. Obstet., 100:97, 1955.
12. Pak, T. J., Martin, G. M., Magness, J. L., and Kavanaugh, G. J.: Reflex sympathetic dystrophy: review of 140 cases. Minn. Med., 53:507, 1970.
13. Williams, W. R.: Reflex sympathetic dystrophy. Rheumatol. Rehabil., 16:119, 1977.
14. Holden, W. D.: Sympathetic dystrophy. Arch. Surg., 57:373, 1948.
15. Drucker, W. R., Hubay, C. A., Holden, W. D., and Bukovnic, J. A.: Pathogenesis of post-traumatic sympathetic dystrophy. Am. J. Surg., n.s. 97:454, 1959.
16. Bergan, J. J., and Conn, J.: Sympathectomy for pain relief. Med. Clin. North Am., 52:147, 1968.
17. Kleinert, H. E., Cole, N. M., Wayne, L., et al.: Post-traumatic sympathetic dystrophy (abstr.). J. Bone Joint Surg., 54:899, 1972.
18. Abramson, D. I.: Post-traumatic vasomotor disorders [Sudeck's atrophy]. Heart Bull., 10:118, 1961.
19. De Takats, G.: Sympathetic reflex dystrophy. Med. Clin. North Am., 49:117, 1965.
20. Andrews, L. G., and Armitage, K. J.: Sudeck's atrophy in traumatic quadriplegia. Paraplegia, 9:159, 1971–1972.

21. Genant, H. K., Kozin, F., Bekerman, C., et al.: The reflex sympathetic dystrophy syndrome: a comprehensive analysis using fine-detail radiography, photon absorptiometry, and bone and joint scintigraphy. Radiology, 117:21, 1975.

22. Kozin, F., Genant, H. K., Bekerman, C., and McCarty, D. J.: The reflex sympathetic dystrophy syndrome. II. Roentgenographic and scintigraphic evidence of bilaterality and of periarticular accentuation. Am. J. Med., 60:332, 1976.

23. Langloh, N. D., Hunder, G. G., Riggs, B. L., and Kelly, P. J.: Transient painful osteoporosis of the lower extremities. J. Bone Joint Surg., 55:1188, 1973.

24. De Bastiani, G., Nogarin, L., and Perusi, M.: Pig calcitonin in the treatment of localized osteoporosis. Ital. J. Orthop. Traumtol., 2:181, 1976.

25. Steinbrocker, O., and Orgyros, T. G.: The shoulder-hand syndrome: present status as a diagnostic and therapeutic entity. Med. Clin. North Am., 42:1533, 1958.

26. Pulvertaft, R. G.: Psychological aspects of hand injuries. Hand, 7:93, 1975.

27. Hartley, J.: Reflex hyperemic deossification (Sudeck's atrophy). J. Mt. Sinai Hosp. N.Y., 22:268, 1955.

28. Betcher, A. M., Bean, G., and Casten, D. F.: Continuous procaine block of paravertebral sympathetic ganglions: observations on one hundred patients. J.A.M.A., 151:288, 1953.

29. Pavlov, I. P.: Cited by Gantt, W. H.: A medical review of Soviet Russia. III. Scientific work. Br. Med. J., 2:533, 1924.

30. Lund, P. C., and Cwik, J. C.: The role of peridural blocks in the pain clinic. Z. Prakt. Anaesth. Wiederbeleb., 8:83, 1973.

31. Hannington-Kiff, J. G.: Relief of Sudeck's atrophy by regional intravenous guanethidine. Lancet, 1:1132, 1977.

32. Simson, G.: Propranolol for causalgia and Sudek's atrophy (letter to the editor). J.A.M.A., 227:327, 1974.

33. Arnstein, A. R.: Regional osteoporosis. Orthop. Clin. North Am., 3:585, 1972.

34. Curtiss, P. H., Jr., and Kincaid, W. E.: Transitory demineralization of the hip in pregnancy: a report of three cases. J. Bone Joint Surg., 41:1327, 1959.

35. Duncan, H., Frame, B., Frost, H. M., and Arnstein, A. R.: Migratory osteolysis of the lower extremities. Ann. Intern. Med., 66:1165, 1967.

36. Lequesne, M.: Transient osteoporosis of the hip: a non-traumatic variety of Sudeck's atrophy. Ann. Rheum. Dis., 27:463, 1968.

37. Hunder, G. G., and Kelly, P. J.: Roentgenologic transient osteoporosis of the hip: a clinical syndrome? Ann. Intern. Med., 68:539, 1968.

38. Swezey, R. L.: Transient osteoporosis of the hip, foot and knee. Arthritis Rheum., 13:858, 1970.

39. Duncan, H., Frame, B., Frost, H., and Arnstein, A. R.: Regional migratory osteoporosis. South. Med. J., 62:41, 1969.

40. O'Mara, R. E., and Pinals, R. S.: Bone scanning in regional migratory osteoporosis: case report. Radiology, 97:579, 1970.

41. Steiner, R. M., and McKeever, C.: Regional migratory osteoporosis. J. Can. Assoc. Radiol., 24:70, 1973.

42. Gupta, R. C., Popovtzer, M. M., Huffer, W. E., and Smyth, C. J.: Regional migratory osteoporosis. Arthritis Rheum., 16:363, 1973.

43. Hunder, G. G., and Kelly, P. J.: Bone scans in transient osteoporosis (editorial). Ann. Intern. Med., 75:134, 1971.

44. Mitchell, S. W., Morehouse, C. R., and Keen, W. W., Jr.: Gunshot Wounds and Other Injuries of Nerves. Philadelphia, J. B. Lippincott Company, 1864.

45. Mitchell, S. W.: On the diseases of nerves resulting from injuries. In Flint, A. (ed.): Contributions Relating to the Causation and Prevention of Disease, and to Camp Diseases. New York, United States Sanitary Commission Memoirs, 1867.

46. Doupe, J., Cullen, C. H., and Chance, G. Q.: Post-traumatic pain and the causalgic syndrome. J. Neurol. Neurosurg. Psychiatry, 7:33, 1944.

47. Walters, A.: The differentiation of causalgia and hyperpathia. Can. Med. Assoc. J., 80:105, 1959.

48. Richards, R. L.: Causalgia: a centennial review. Arch. Neurol., 16:339, 1967.

49. Nerve Injuries Committee, British Medical Research Council: The diagnosis and treatment of peripheral nerve injuries. Med. Res. Counc. Spec. Rep. Series, No. 54:1, 1920.

50. Kirklin, J. W., Chenoweth, A. I., and Murphey, F.: Causalgia: a review of its characteristics, diagnosis, and treatment. Surgery, 21:321, 1947.

51. Granit, R., Leksell, L., and Skoglund, C. R.: Fibre interaction in injured or compressed region of nerve. Brain, 67:125, 1944.

52. Kleiman, A.: Causalgia: evidence of the existence of crossed sensory sympathetic fibers. Am. J. Surg., n.s. 87:839, 1954.

53. Gorham, L. W., Wright, A. W., Shultz, H. H., and Maxon, F. C., Jr.: Disappearing bones: a rare form of massive osteolysis; report of two cases, one with autopsy findings. Am. J. Med., 17:674, 1954.

54. Gorham, L. W., and Stout, A. P.: Massive osteolysis (acute spontaneous absorption of bone, phantom bone, disappearing bone). J. Bone Joint Surg., 37:985, 1955.

55. Halliday, D. R., Dahlin, D. C., Pugh, D. G., and Young, H. H.: Massive osteolysis and angiomatosis. Radiology, 82:637, 1964.

56. Tilling, G., and Skobowytsh, B.: Disappearing bone disease, morbus Gorham. Acta Orthop. Scand., 39:398, 1968.

57. Sage, M. R., and Allen, P. W.: Massive osteolysis: report of a case. J. Bone Joint Surg., 56:130, 1974.

58. Simpson, B. S.: An unusual case of post-traumatic decalcification of the bones of the foot. J. Bone Joint Surg., 19:223, 1937.

59. Sauve, M.: Ostéolyse du pied. Mém. Acad. Chir., 62:501, 1936.

CHAPTER 48

NEUROSURGICAL SALVAGE OF THE INTRACTABLY PAINFUL, "FAILED" FOOT

Reuben Hoppenstein, M.D., F.A.C.S.

When everything that a foot surgeon can do has been done and the patient still complains of intractable foot pain, there is one last measure that may afford relief — microsurgical dorsal root rhizotomy, provided that selective differential spinal nerve blocks are performed prior to the operative procedure in order to correctly determine which nerves have been damaged.

The differential diagnosis of pain emanating from the foot or originating in the nerve proximally is usually obvious. Local tenderness, exacerbation of pain by joint movement, throbbing, and constant pain that can be increased by local pressure are usually the hallmarks of foot disorders. In addition, constant burning, gnawing, or occasional throbbing pain (which can be well localized and can also be intensified by local pressure) should not be ignored, since this kind of pain might indicate a nerve damaged locally, at a distance, or anywhere along its intraspinal or extraspinal course.

The spinal nerve roots that supply the sensory function of the foot are the L3 to S2 nerves, but primarily the fourth and fifth lumbar roots and the first and second sacral roots (Fig. 48–1). It cannot be overemphasized that there are four groups of nerves that innervate the structures of the foot. They consist of the nerves that supply the skin, muscles, and joints, as well as those that supply the vasculature via the autonomic nervous system. Vascular lesions producing pain may not be alleviated by lumbosacral differential blocks, so that an attempt to provide relief should then be directed to the nerves from T10 to L1 (i.e., the autonomic afferent pathway). Muscles and nerves that cross joints also participate in the innervation of those joints. It cannot be assumed that because the pain is localized to the lateral aspect of the ankle, the S1 nerve root is responsible. Differential blocks may localize the involved nerve as being the L5 or S2 nerve root.

A dorsal root rhizotomy should be a last resort. Nevertheless, chronic pain can be devastating to the individual and his family, and in desperation, they will seek help from anyone who promises even a remote chance of relief. Individuals with an organic cause for their pain, with several

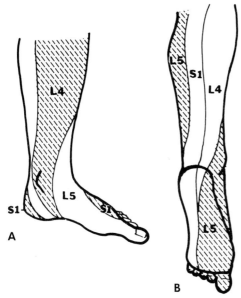

Figure 48–1. *A composite diagram of dermatomes mapped by pinprick sensation in two patients after dorsal rhizotomy. (A) Note the L4 dermatome crosses the ankle and ends on the sole. The S1 dermatome also supplies the entire heel, whereas in B it supplies only the lateral half of the heel. In A, both the L4 and S1 sensory roots were cut, whereas in B, the L5 sensory root was severed on the right and the L4 sensory root on the left. It is important to note that even when identical nerves were cut bilaterally, the resulting areas of hypesthesia were not mirror images.*

surgical scars attesting to an original disorder, should not be directed to psychiatric therapy.

DIFFERENTIAL SPINAL NERVE BLOCKS

The dermatomes depicted in Figure 48–1 do not indicate the innervation of the muscles and joints beneath these areas but do give an indication of the nerve root that is likely to be involved. If the pain is in the region of the L5 dermatome, it is preferable to block this nerve first, as in the majority of patients it will prove to be the offender. Nerves that cross a joint usually supply that joint; this also applies to muscles and vessels and readily explains the necessity of blocking other nerves if the first, second, and even the third nerve blocks fail.

The patient is given no pain medication for 12 hours prior to the nerve blocks and, consequently, is uncomfortable and in pain when brought to the radiology department or operating room. An image intensifier is necessary for the procedure.

With the patient in the prone position, a surgical marking pen with a metallic tip is used to mark the inferior edge of the pedi-

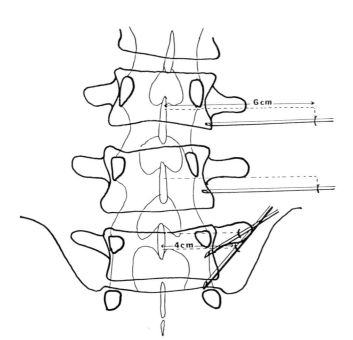

Figure 48–2. *Technique of differential spinal nerve blocks. (See text.)*

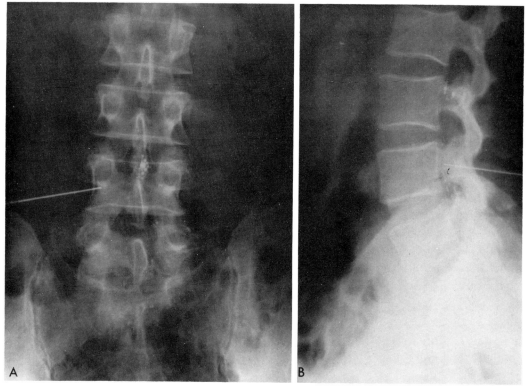

Figure 48–3. (A and B) Placement of needle for left L4 nerve block that relieved pain in a patient complaining of intractable pain in the heel. A hemilaminectomy of L5 on the right and dye droplets from a previous myelogram are visible. Proper placement of the needle must be visualized roentgenographically both on the anteroposterior and lateral views.

cle of the L4 and L5 vertebral bodies. The lower extremities are left undraped to permit testing for decreased sensation in the appropriate dermatome. This confirms which nerve has been blocked. At a point 6 cm from the midline at the level of the skin markers and 0.5 cm inferior to this point, a 20-gauge disposable lumbar puncture needle is introduced at an angle of 30 degrees from the vertical and directed toward the appropriate pedicle. This procedure is done under fluoroscopic control (Fig. 48–2).

Image intensification is *mandatory*. Counting spinous processes and believing that the needle is accurately placed can often be misleading. The needle tip may be either one space higher or lower than desired and could lead to severing of the incorrect nerve root. (See Figure 48–3.)

No anesthesia is used for the skin when the needle is introduced; the patient is forewarned that the first prick is for the local anesthetic and will sting momentarily. The needle is introduced steadily until

the foramen is reached. Correct selection of the injection site may cause the patient to experience a shooting pain into the lower extremity. If this occurs, the radiation of this pain cannot be accurately localized by the patient, and the needle is withdrawn a few millimeters. Only 0.5 ml of local anesthetic is introduced, and a period of five minutes is allowed to elapse before the dermatome is checked with a safety pin. The patient is also asked to confirm if the pain has been alleviated. If movement or pressure produced pain prior to the block, it is repeated; a pain-free response confirms that the correct nerve root has been anesthetized. Failure to produce relief of pain warrants the blocking of the next appropriate nerve root. The S1 nerve root can easily be blocked within the L5–S1 foramen by directing the needle just superior to and 2 mm medial to the S1 pedicle (see Figure 48–2).

Once the appropriate nerve has been found, the spinous process on the vertebra immediately above it is marked. For the

L5 nerve root, the L5 vertebral spinous process should be marked, and this is accomplished with 0.25 ml of methylene blue injected along the lateral surface of this spinous process and onto its tip. This facilitates surgical exposure and avoids unnecessary intraoperative radiography to confirm the vertebral level.

The technique of microsurgical dorsal root rhizotomy has been fully described previously.[1]

CLINICAL STUDIES

In this section, the cases of six patients, all of whom had undergone unsuccessful foot surgery, will be discussed (see Table 48–1). All of these individuals complained of constant pain, usually described as burning or gnawing. However, in one case of incisional neuroma following surgery for removal of the sesamoids, the patient complained of shooting pains, confirmed by a positive Tinel sign. This patient underwent microsurgical exploration with only superficial local anesthesia. When the neuroma was found, additional anesthesia was used, and the nerve was coagulated and severed. Electrocoagulation will destroy the neuronal tubules and reduce the chance of recurrence; the nerve should not be clipped, as this may lead to ulceration in a weight-bearing area.

Three patients who suffered crush injuries to the foot and subsequently underwent multiple operations for excision of neuromas, fusions, and skin grafting presented with a constant burning pain. One had undergone a lumbar sympathectomy that had been unsuccessful. After differential spinal nerve blocks, a single dorsal root was cut in two patients, whereas severing of both the L5 and S1 dorsal roots was necessary in the third.

A 52-year-old diabetic who complained of a constant burning, gnawing pain in the big toe and the head of the first metatarsal associated with intense hyperesthesia was found to have no local pathology and had good peripheral pulses. Roentgenograms were negative. Although the vast majority of diabetic neuropathies are self-limiting and require no drastic therapeutic measures, this patient had endured seven months of agony with no lessening of the intensity of the pain and requested amputation, if that would help. A single spinal nerve block at the L5 level produced immediate relief, and this nerve was subsequently severed by dorsal root rhizotomy.

In a sixth patient, causalgia in the lateral aspect of the foot due to a sciatic nerve injury from an accidental shooting responded well to dorsal rhizotomy of the S1 nerve root. Exploration of the sciatic nerve was contraindicated, since it was felt that the burning causalgic pain would not be relieved by neurolysis. The patient had previously undergone lumbar sympathectomy after lumbar paraspinal sympathetic block. I am convinced that the retroperitoneal space was flooded with local anesthetic and that the patient's symptoms were alleviated not by the sympathetic block but by the anesthetic effects on the lumbosacral plexus in the pelvis. Only minimal amounts of anesthesia should be used for any nerve block under fluoroscopic control.

Discussion

The six patients just described underwent surgery. Four fall into the "failed" foot category (Table 48–1). The other two patients, namely the diabetic and the one with causalgia, are included to remind the reader that the nerve damage is not necessarily local and can occur at a distance or within the spinal canal. Patients with nerve damage in the spinal canal will not be discussed in this section but have been dealt with elsewhere.[1] Nevertheless, discogenic disease at the L4–L5 and L5–S1 levels can present with pain localized to this region, without back pain, especially in patients with the failed back syndrome.[1] (See Figure 48–3.)

Crush injuries can obviously involve more than one nerve, which can become entrapped within the scar tissue (Cases 2, 3, and 4). Transected nerves can develop neuromas, as sometimes occurs after elective surgery (Case 1). The bullet wound of the sciatic nerve (Case 6) and the diabetic neuropathy (Case 5) will be discussed together, since they essentially represent damage to the nerve at a distance from the foot. The former patient presented with causalgia that had not responded to sympathectomy, whereas the diabetic had an

TABLE 48–1.

CASE	ETIOLOGY	SURGERY	RESULT°
1	Incisional neuroma	Local excision of neuroma	Excellent
2	Crush injury of foot	Dorsal rhizotomy L5	Excellent
3	Crush injury of foot	Dorsal rhizotomy L5 and at second surgery the S1 nerve root	Excellent
4	Crush injury of foot	Dorsal rhizotomy S1	Failed
5	Diabetic neuropathy	Dorsal rhizotomy S1	Excellent
6	Causalgia—bullet injury to sciatic nerve	Dorsal rhizotomy S1	Good

°Key: Excellent—Patient is off all medication.
        Good—Patient is pleased with results of surgery; pain medication is reduced.
        Failed—Patient is unhappy and says there is no relief at all.

infarction of the nerve that failed to resolve spontaneously. Excellent results were obtained in both cases after dorsal rhizotomy.

Surgical procedures are not always followed by excellent results, however, as demonstrated by Case 4. I know of no foolproof screening technique to avoid surgery on psychologic cripples. Most patients with intractable chronic pain present as neurotic, angry, unstable individuals, and there is a natural tendency to avoid attempting further surgery on them. All of the patients in this short series, except the diabetic, had undergone psychotherapy for varying periods prior to definitive surgery. None of the patients have resumed that therapy since surgery, although I believe that the patient of Case 4 would benefit from a second course of therapy.

The view has been expressed that if the L5 nerve root is severed, the S1 nerve root should be left intact and vice versa, since the main nerve supply to the foot is provided by these two nerves (see Figure 48–1). However, Echols[2] and White[3] describe cases in which they severed both the L5 and S1 nerve roots, and the only disability that followed was a tendency on the part of the patient to twist the ankle, which persisted for a few months after surgery and thereafter corrected itself. One case was followed for 21 years without evidence of ulceration, joint destruction, or difficulty in wound healing. Nevertheless, I am still reluctant to advocate the severance of both nerves, even though I have done this in seven out of 60 patients who have undergone dorsal root rhizotomy for other reasons.[1] These seven patients have not been followed for more than three years; however, in one patient, there is no defect

detectable on pinprick examination, and position sense is absent only in the toes.

It should be stated that after dorsal root rhizotomy, absolute anesthesia does not occur. Immediately after surgery, the denervated area can be mapped by pinprick. The patient can discern that the sensation is sharp, but it is not painful. This persists for two to six weeks. After three to six months, it is almost impossible to find an area of decreased sensation. This also occurred in the patients who underwent both the L5 and S1 rhizotomies.

In Case 3, a patient whose crush injury originally responded well to severance of the L5 nerve root subsequently complained of even more intense pain in the region of the first and second metatarsals. A second blocking procedure was performed. Needles were placed in the mid-metatarsal region so that periosteal pain could be evoked (Fig. 48–4). The sclerotomes of the first and second metatarsals were shown to be innervated by the S1 nerve. A study is now in progress at the Orthopedic Institute of the Hospital for Joint Diseases to further map out the sclerotomes of the foot.

The classic experiments of Eloesser[4] in 1917 proved conclusively that complete denervation of a joint alone does not produce a Charcot joint. Sensory denervation of the heel following fractures of the os calcis with intractable pain was described by Sallick and Blum,[5] and denervation of the ankle joint for similar reasons was reported by Casagrande and associates.[6] Both reports deny the development of Charcot joints.

In view of the cited literature and my own limited experience, if the pain is not markedly relieved by a single L5 or S1 nerve block, the patient is informed that

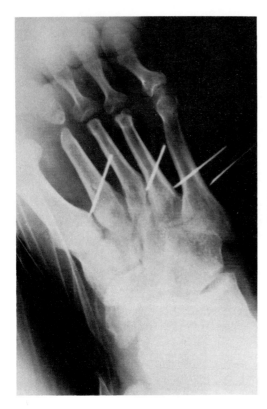

Figure 48–4. *Testing for periosteal pain (sclerotomal innervation). Note the excision of the second to fourth metatarsal heads.*

there is the slight possibility that he may develop a neuropathic joint or may experience difficulty in wound healing in the denervated region and is advised that the dorsal roots of both nerves should be severed.

REFERENCES

1. Hoppenstein, R.: A new approach to the failed back syndrome. Spine, 5:371, 1980.

2. Echols, D. H.: Sensory rhizotomy following operation for ruptured intervertebral disc. J. Neurosurg., 31:335, 1969.

3. White, J. C.: Posterior rhizotomy: a possible substitute for cordotomy in otherwise intractable neuralgias of the trunk and extremities of non-malignant origin. Clin. Neurosurg., 13:20, 1965.

4. Eloesser, L.: Neuropathic affections of the joints. Ann. Surg., 66:201, 1917.

5. Sallick, M. A., and Blum, L.: Sensory denervation of the heel for persistent pain. J. Bone Joint Surg., 30A:209, 1948.

6. Casagrande, P. A., Austin, B. P., and Indeck, W.: Denervation of the ankle joint. J. Bone Joint Surg., 33A:723, 1951.

CHAPTER 49

VASCULAR DISEASES OF THE FOOT

Allastair Karmody, M.D.,
and Richard L. Jacobs, M.D.

The foot that is compromised by vascular pathology is frequently encountered by physicians of all specialties. A brief examination of our referral patterns shows that patients have come with equal frequency from general practitioners, internists, cardiologists, endocrinologists, dermatologists, plastic surgeons, orthopaedic surgeons, and general surgeons. The recognition and proper management of this problem, therefore, transcends all aspects of present-day organized medicine. This is a swiftly increasing aspect of clinical practice. In 1970, our institution carried out over 200 operations for foot salvage, but by 1978, this number had risen to 500, i.e., a 250 per cent increase in eight years. The reason for this lies entirely in the new approaches to the diagnosis and management of vascular diseases, which allow 98 per cent of such conditions to be handled successfully. This chapter will outline the recognition and management of the common and some of the rarer conditions that are encountered in clinical practice. The aspects of vascular disease that are common to nondiabetics and diabetics will also be covered, although specific aspects of the treatment of the diabetic foot will be discussed in Chapter 50.

VASCULAR PHYSIOLOGIC EXAMINATION

Until very recently, the preoperative evaluation of patients with vascular disease of the foot consisted of a history and clinical examination, followed by "diagnostic" contrast angiography. However, this sequence of events commonly fell short of the therapeutic mark because of a failure to correlate the physiologic capacity of the foot with the clinical and angiographic data. Indeed, most arterial angiograms stopped at the ankle[56] and thus failed to identify intrinsic lesions of the foot. The most rewarding approach to these problems is presented in Table 49–1.

The history and clinical examination are not to be denigrated, however, and their descriptions and importance are best discussed with each separate clinical entity. Nevertheless, a simple and yet very effective clinical test that is generally overlooked should be mentioned here, i.e., measurement of the walking distance. The physician should be able, under most circumstances, to work out a short walking course that he has previously measured accurately. The patient is simply asked to walk this distance at his own pace until symptoms in the foot appear. This is taken as the maximum walking distance

TABLE 49–1. Method of Approach for Vascular Diseases of the Foot

Preoperative Evaluation
Vascular Physiology
Angiography
Reconstruction
Rehabilitation

and is a useful measure of the function of the arterial inflow. In general, walking distances of over 400 meters represent quite adequate inflow, whereas those less than 50 meters point to a very low and suspect degree of arterial supply. These simple parameters, therefore, give the clinician reasonably competent guidelines for his initial assessment. This subject will be discussed further in the section on Noninvasive Exercise and Hyperemic Testing. This test plus a detailed history will allow a fairly close appreciation of how limiting the physiologic effects of a given lesion are for each patient. However, the description of symptoms by the patient and their interpretation by the physician are very subjective; furthermore, no objective or quantitative measurements are provided by the raw history, no matter how detailed. Physical examination will allow some objectivity, but even this is notoriously fallible when it is considered that several experienced observers will commonly differ in their detection and grading of pulses and their diagnosis of venous thrombosis. It will be mentioned here and stressed later that arteriography is not a diagnostic test. The physician should be well aware of the nature and effects of the lesion that is present long before arteriography is performed. In modern practice, this highly invasive examination should not be used as a primary diagnostic test.

The approach to peripheral vascular disease should, therefore, be designed to find and treat physiologic rather than anatomic problems. It is often the case that disease can be widespread with little physiologic effect whereas very sharply localized lesions can cause severe problems even in the presence of an otherwise almost normal vasculature. For these reasons, which are well documented in clinical practice, the physician who is concerned with these patients must concentrate on the physiologic effects of the detected anatomic lesions.

The detection and quantitative measurement of all stages of peripheral vascular disease is of key importance in understanding the factors that affect the further progression of the disease as well as in the assessment of the efficacy of preventive and therapeutic measures. It is possible to define the characteristics that can be applied to all methods of instrumentation used for physiologic testing of vascular disease of the foot. In general, any method that is to be useful and have wide application should have the following characteristics: (1) simplicity, (2) safety, (3) accuracy, (4) sensitivity, and (5) reproducibility. In addition, the method should be inexpensive and quantitative, provide "hard copy," and be capable of being taught to and carried out by paramedical personnel. A number of approaches are available and in use, although each vascular laboratory has its own preferences and relies on a variety of equipment that is now commercially available. However, all noninvasive vascular laboratory examinations perform one or all of three functions:[106]

1. Flow detection.
2. Segmental pressure measurements.
3. Production and analysis of pressure wave forms.

These tests have been derived from considerable investigation into all aspects of the hemodynamic spectrum, including pulsation volume, total limb blood flow, local skin blood flow, arterial flow velocity, arterial pressure changes, pulse wave velocity, and arterial wall imaging. An extensive range of instruments and techniques have been designed over the last 15 years for laboratory examination of vascular disease of the foot.[32, 50, 116, 129, 143] Continuous-wave Doppler ultrasound devices, however, are most widely used because they fulfill most of the above criteria and are particularly easy to use, since any accessible artery can be examined.[49, 126, 139] A number of these devices are shown in Figure 49–1. They range from small, portable instruments to table-mounted instruments that provide directional flow information. The most common use of Doppler ultrasound in the peripheral vascular system is to determine the presence or absence of blood flow (Fig. 49–2). In addition, the qualitative sounds that are heard can be interpreted by an observer with a moderate amount of "learning" and can be read as normal or partially or totally obstructed. However, the quality of these signals depends on the absolute velocity presented to the probe, and this itself depends on the angle between the probe and the blood vessel being examined.

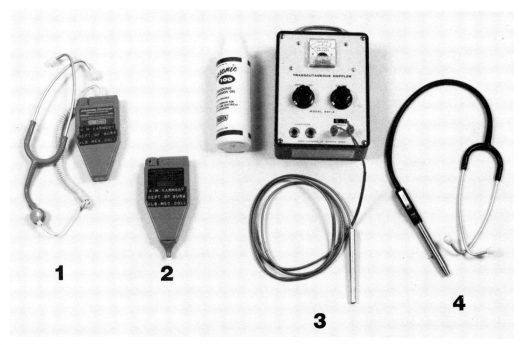

Figure 49–1. *Some of the more commonly used Doppler ultrasound instruments.*

1. Medsonics Model BF4A (5 mHz). This is the best all-purpose model on the market in our view. It has a wide angle of view, is portable, and has a spring switch that prevents undue battery wear.

2. Medsonics BF5A (9 mHz). The probe in this model is smaller, as is the angle of view and the depth of penetration. It is useful for detection of smaller vessels, such as those of the dorsal or plantar arch or the digital vessels. The headset from 1 is also used with this instrument.

3. Parks Transcutaneous Doppler (9.7 mHz). The probe that is shown has the great advantage of being sterilizable for use intraoperatively. Not shown with this model are the headphones that fit into sockets along the side of the probe. This makes the instrument extremely cumbersome and suitable for use only in a static situation. Batteries also appear to run down quickly. Note the container of coupling gel.

4. Physiocontrol Doplette (10 mHz). This is one of the "pocket" probes. The 10 mHz feature makes it suitable for use only on small superficial arteries, and its performance is of average quality.

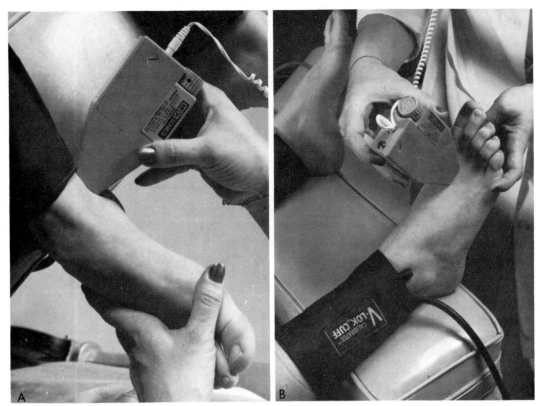

Figure 49–2. *(A) Use of the ultrasound probe over the posterior tibial artery. Notice that the operator is holding the probe at a right angle to the artery and that the foot is slightly inverted to allow relaxation of the artery and better positioning. (B) The probe is being used here over the confluence of the dorsal and plantar arterial arches between the first and second metatarsal heads. If flow cannot easily be detected in either the posterior tibial or dorsalis pedis artery, this is a useful point at which a check could be made.*

Ideally, the instrument should be held at a right angle to the axis of the vessel being examined (Fig. 49–2), but this angle may be difficult to achieve with a hand-held probe. With practice, however, most observers will quickly find a reasonably satisfactory point of examination on a given vessel.

In contrast, the measurement of blood pressure in an artery is a specific quantitative measurement, and the ultrasound probe is a vital instrument in this regard. The method by which this is done is shown in Figure 49–3 and consists simply of the application of pressure by means of a pneumatic cuff until the ultrasound signal disappears and release of the pressure until the sound reappears. These two values can be averaged, but they usually correspond very accurately to within 5 mm Hg. This is a very reliable type of measurement and, in general, should form the

basis of all vascular examinations.[23] This pressure can be expressed diagnostically as degrees of mercury[107] or can be converted into ankle-brachial index, as advocated by Yao.[143] These are the most common uses of ultrasound in clinical practice, and the tests that have been described can be performed under all settings (e.g., office or bedside). Another advantage of Doppler ultrasound flow detectors is their ability to be electronically connected to simple strip recorders, e.g., an ECG recorder, so that the electronic signals are converted into wave forms. This provides quite reasonably accurate wave forms for analysis, and many laboratories are equipped to do this.

The use of wave-form analysis began with the commonly used plethysmographic device, the Collins oscillometer. This is a simple, portable, and inexpensive instrument. However, it has the

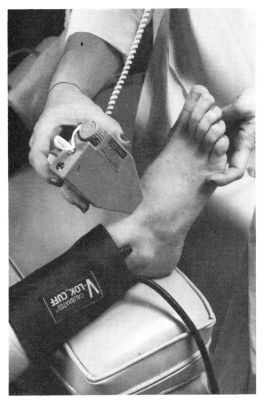

Figure 49–3. *The operator is checking the flow over the dorsalis pedis artery. The cuff at the ankle will be inflated for measurement of the systolic pressure, and a mean will be taken of the disappearance of the systolic signal during inflation and its reappearance during reinflation of the cuff. The correspondence of these two values is usually within 5 mm Hg.*

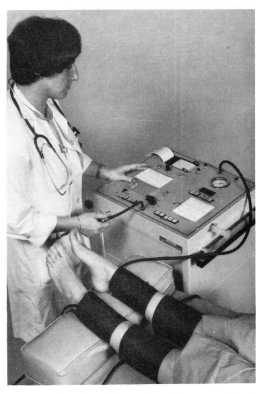

Figure 49–4. *Use of the pulse volume recorder to obtain tracings from the calf and ankle of both legs. The cuff is inflated to 65 mm Hg on the manometer on the upper right-hand corner of the machine. The strip recording is made on standard recording paper on the upper left-hand corner.*

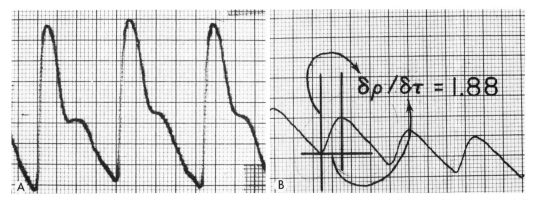

Figure 49–5. *(A) Normal PVR tracing. Notice that the up-slope is almost a straight line and the down-slope falls rapidly with a dicrotic notch. (B) Method of analysis of PVR tracing using a dampened tracing for reference. In practice, this mathematical formula is not often used since pattern recognition is learned swiftly.*

serious disadvantages of being nonstandardized, with poor sensitivity and frequency response, and of providing no "hard copy" wave form for analysis. This instrument is no longer in use in modern vascular centers. Because of recent advances in electronics, more complete understanding of peripheral hemodynamics, and vigorous and rigid development of clinical criteria, the use of quantitative segmental plethysmography has become an important component in the routine evaluation of peripheral vascular disease.[125] One instrument that has been extensively developed and has been in constant use by us for the past five years is the Pulse Volume Recorder (PVR)*[32, 106] (Fig. 49–4). The type of tracings obtained and their analysis are shown in Figure 49–5. With this device, examination of the pulse wave with reference to its contour and amplitude can be examined serially in a given patient, and pattern recognition is soon learned by the observer. In addition, segmental pressures can be taken using the first appearance of pulsatile flow on the chart or, more accurately, by using Doppler ultrasound in conjunction with pressure inflation.

Noninvasive Exercise and Hyperemic Tests

It has been shown by Yao[140, 141] and others that arterial occlusions or high-grade stenoses will produce pressure differences in the limb at rest. However, smaller degrees of stenosis, which may nevertheless be clinically significant, may not show such differences in the resting foot, particularly when they occur at the aortoiliac level. The pressure differences in the feet of such patients will only be demonstrated when the collateral bed is fully dilated by the induction of hyperemic response. This can be achieved noninvasively in one of two ways. The first is by the application of a thigh blood pressure cuff and the production of total ischemia by pneumatic compression for five minutes. Upon release of the cuff, there is usually marked hyperemia, and a pressure

difference can then be measured.[16] This test is somewhat painful and uncomfortable for most patients, however, and the physiologic production of hyperemia is preferable.[24, 128] This can be accomplished either by have the patient walk for a measured distance until symptoms appear or, more easily, in the laboratory by controlled walking on a low-speed treadmill (1 to 3 mph with a 10 to 15 per cent gradient) (Fig. 49–6) (Table 49–2). Exercise on the treadmill can be carried out either to the point at which symptoms appear or for a measured interval of time. At the end of the period, the tracings are again recorded, and the pressure is remeasured as previously described.[107] In addition, the brachial pressure should be measured to obviate any changes in the systemic circulation. The recording form that is used for these purposes is shown in Figure 49–7. On this form, relevant clini-

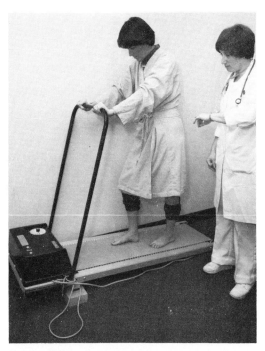

Figure 49–6. Hyperemic exercise testing on a treadmill. The treadmill is elevated on a block to 15 degrees and the operator is timing the subject's walking. The time of maximum tolerated walking is used, or alternatively, a standard time of 5 to 10 minutes is taken before repeat tracings are obtained. Note that the cuffs are left in place so that the hyperemic response is obtained as soon as possible after exercise.

---

*Life Sciences Incorporated, 270 Greenwich Avenue, Greenwich, Connecticut 06830.

TABLE 49–2. Physiologic Measurements

1. Walking Distance
2. Ultrasound Flow and Pressure
3. Electronic Oscillometry
4. Limb Blood Flow

cal data, as well as samples of the tracings and the pressures that are obtained both at rest and after exercise, are recorded. It should be noted that in many instances, it is unnecessary to perform an exercise test, since the tracings and resting pressures may be so grossly abnormal that no further diagnostic maneuvers are required. Other noninvasive tests of circulation are available — for example, radionuclide isotopic clearance[90, 91] and venous occlusion plethysmography[27] — but these are more cumbersome and more difficult to perform in an office or at the bedside. It is not yet possible to obtain relatively simple or well-standardized methods for the measurement of total limb blood flow, although this is, of course, the ideal measurement[130] (Table 49–2). However, on most occasions, the relationship between pressure and flow is sufficiently accurate.[132]

The information that has been obtained from this approach is very useful to the vascular surgeon in his evaluation of the jeopardized foot. However, for most physicians, the extraction and evaluation of these data from the diagnostic forms may be quite cumbersome. It has fortunately been possible to extrapolate a series of easy-to-follow ground rules from this information, which enable accurate decisions to be made about the management of the patients with threatened viability of the foot because of ischemia. An example of the type of data that are possible is set out in a simple form in Table 49–3. It will be noted that the information is expressed in absolute pressures. In practice, this appears to be a satisfactory method of evaluation.[21] Other laboratories use ankle-arm systolic ratios, but there is excellent correlation between the two approaches. At any rate, for the clinician who is not involved in the full-time practice of vascular surgery, the measurement of the ankle pressure can be used straight from the table to work out almost any prognostic end point in a given patient.[58, 135] In the evaluation of post-exercise data, it is useful to point out

here that with a normal arterial inflow, maximum vasodilatation has little effect on either systolic or limb blood pressures. In fact, the pressure at the ankle may actually rise some 10 to 15 mm Hg over the brachial pressure level. However, a posthyperemic fall in systolic pressure of 10 to 15 per cent of the resting level is suggestive of a significant proximal lesion, which should be investigated before any attempt is made to restore pulsatile flow more distally.[130]

The type of data supplied by noninvasive measurements provides a foundation of preoperative physiologic information, aids in making intraoperative judgments, and allows firm conclusions to be made about the immediate results of vascular reconstructive procedures. Equally important is that these noninvasive measurements are easily repeated, and the data obtained from each patient are very consistent when tests are performed exactly the same way.[72] The great advantage of this is that in the postoperative period, reconstructive follow-up is made much simpler, since much of the guesswork is taken out of a subjective interpretation of the clinical examination and the patient's symptoms. It is known that reconstructive deterioration does occur and that there may be progression of disease both proximally and distally. Early detection of signs of inflow and outflow failure is therefore a real clinical advance. In addition, the patient who is being treated conservatively (see Chronic Ischemia, Conservative Management) can be followed serially by means of these tests and the type and level of progression noted. This will help in further decisions about the continuation of conservative management or the need for surgical intervention.[59]

Invasive Measurements of Hemodynamic Physiology

The most well-known methods of invasive measurement of vascular capacity are those that are used during vascular reconstructive procedures. The direct measurement of arterial flow is most commonly performed by square-wave electromagnetic flowmeter.[80] The technical aspects of the use of this instrument do not require com-

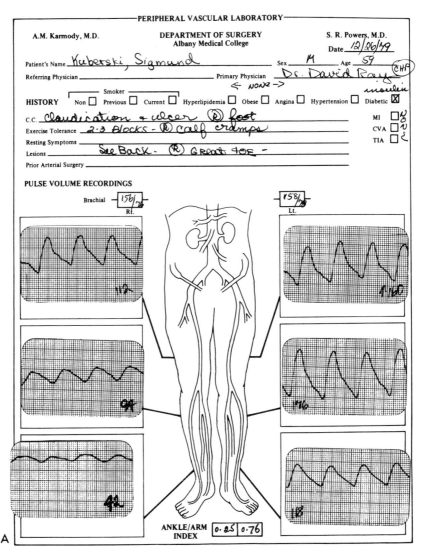

Figure 49–7. (A) Front of the chart used for recording tracings. Tracings have been taken from the thigh, calf, and ankle regions, and if necessary, transmetatarsal and digital readings can also be obtained. On the left side, the tracings are almost normal at the thigh and calf level but are dampened at the ankle level. On the right side, the tracing at the calf level is dampened and the tracing at the ankle level is very sinusoidal, and the pressure is recorded at 42 mm Hg.

Illustration continued on opposite page

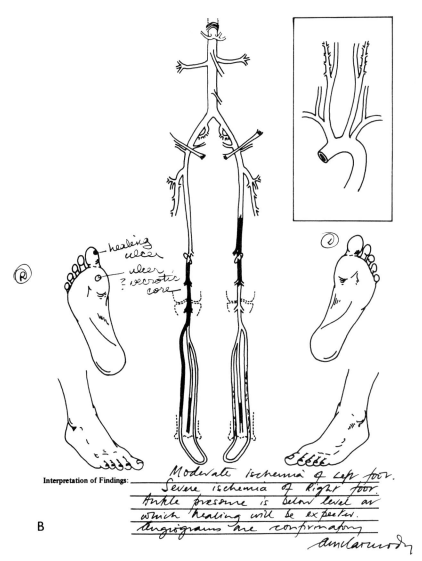

Figure 49-7 *Continued. (B) The back of the recording form shows a correlation between the angiograms that are subsequently obtained. There is excellent correlation between the wave tracings and the anatomic lesions. The lesions of the foot are also recorded on this side so that a permanent record of all the problems of the foot is obtained.*

TABLE 49–3. Correlation Between Ankle Pressures and Clinical States

THERAPEUTIC RESULT	REST PAIN	LESION HEALING
Unlikely	> 80	< 80
Probable	50–80	80–90
Likely	< 55	> 90

plete elaboration here, but in general, these instruments are not easy to use and remain research tools rather than routinely used ones.[11, 12] More consistently useful is direct measurement of intra-arterial pressure by transducer. This is done mainly to check the efficacy of a given inflow source. It is not uncommon to detect angiographically lesions proximal to the site of a proposed arterial graft. If the hemodynamic significance of these lesions is in doubt, the simultaneous measurement of the upstream and downstream pressure of the lesions will readily identify any existing pressure gradients in most cases. This can be done with two arterial punctures or by means of a catheter passed above and through the lesion. Even if no gradient can be identified at rest, induction of hyperemia by arterial cross-clamping or intra-arterial injections of papaverine will reveal any hidden physiologic gradient.[16] In practice, any gradient that is greater than 15 mm Hg or 15 per cent of the simultaneously measured systolic pressure is representative of a significant proximal lesion.

As a corollary to the aforementioned, the catheters that are commonly introduced percutaneously for angiography should also be used routinely for the determination of "pull-back" pressures and wave tracings at successive levels of the arterial tree (Fig. 49–8). For this reason, all angiographic suites should be equipped to measure intra-arterial pressures at all times. This information is frequently of considerable use to the vascular surgeon. Intraoperatively, a reliable estimate of qualitative flow can be obtained by direct application of an ultrasound flowmeter probe to the arterial conduit.[74] Sterilizable probes are available for this purpose (see Figure 49–1).

ARTERIAL OCCLUSIVE DISEASE

Ischemia of the foot because of diminished arterial inflow is sharply divided into two categories: acute or chronic. The effect of any given arterial occlusion depends on the interaction of two factors: (1) the rate of occlusion and (2) the location of the occlusion.[73, 82, 137] The influence of the rate of occlusion on the outcome of the foot depends on the available collateral pathways. Acute occlusion will obviously throw a sudden burden of limb support on the collateral network. Curiously, older individuals may fare better in this regard than the young, because pathologic nar-

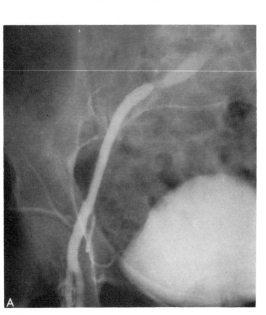

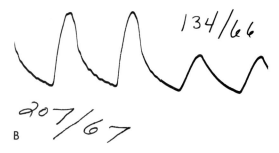

Figure 49–8. *(A) Femoral angiogram showing a well-marked stenotic lesion at the junction of the common and external iliac arteries. (B) Pull-back tracing from an angiographic catheter passed across this lesion shows that the pressure in the common iliac artery is 207/67, with a normal wave form that drops sharply to a sinusoidal form across the stenosis with a 73 mm Hg drop in systolic pressure at this point.*

rowing of the major arterial conduits may have already resulted in development of parallel flow systems. Slower chronic occlusion obviously allows concomitant collateral takeover, and the final occlusive event of the main arterial conduit usually goes completely unnoticed by both the patient and the physician. The location of the arterial occlusion also influences the final effect on the foot, because there is a marked gradation in collateral capacity with progression distally along the anatomic scale. Chronic aortic and iliac occlusions are best tolerated because of the tremendous collateral crossovers available within the trunk. The lower half of the body can be easily supplied from the upper half, and each side will readily support the other. These arrangements become steadily poorer with distal anatomic progression, and occlusions at the level of the foot have the worst possible prognosis (Fig. 49–9).

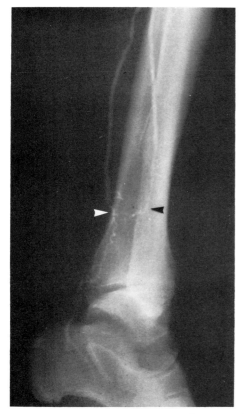

Figure 49–9. *Arrows show sharply defined arterial obstructions of the tibial vessels. There is some collateral flow beyond, but this is of poor quality.*

Arterial Embolism

The most dramatic of all acute occlusive disorders is the displacement of an arterial embolus into the distal circulation. The most common etiologic factors that create emboligenic sources are rheumatic valvular heart disease and myocardial infarction followed by the formation of ventricular mural emboli arising from the diseased arterial walls. In practice, there are two distinct types of emboli — macroemboli and microemboli.

Macroemboli

Thrombi within the heart are especially apt to become dislodged during episodes of cardiac irregularity, for example, upon conversion of a normal sinus rhythm to atrial fibrillation or vice versa, i.e., during some period of pronounced cardiac instability. However, advances in the field of open heart surgery have eliminated some of these problems, and the eradication of rheumatic mitral heart disease has almost completely removed this as a source of arterial emboli. At the present time, therefore, the predominant source of macroemboli is mural thrombosis of the left ventricular wall forming on infarcted myocardium.[31] Macroemboli are 5 to 10 mm or greater in diameter. They tend to lodge where the arteries taper and become reduced in caliber (Fig. 49–10). This ordinarily occurs at points of bifurcation, which also happen to be the sites of major narrowing by pathologic obstructive processes. The common areas of embolic lodgment that affect the foot or feet are the terminations of the aortic, common iliac, common femoral, and popliteal arteries. When embolic impaction occurs, acute ischemia supervenes, rapidly threatening the viability of the foot. The onset of ischemia is particularly rapid and severe when there has been no significant previous obstructive disease of the limb, so that efficient channels are not in place for support of the foot. The patient experiences excruciating pain and notices pallor and paralysis of the foot. In addition, the physician observes paresthesia (Table 49–4). The ischemic foot is pale with blue mottling, rapidly assumes the ambient temperature, has greatly diminished sensation, and may

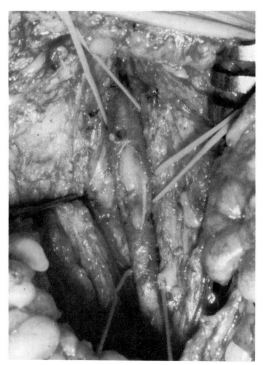

Figure 49–10. *Junction of the common superficial and superficial femoral arteries. The arteries have been opened and a pearly-white embolus is seen impacted at the bifurcation. Notice that the obstruction is so complete that no clamps have been required to prevent blood egress.*

even be anesthetic. It is usually very weakly mobile or totally paralyzed. The pulses immediately distal to the point at which the embolus lodged cannot be obtained, and flow signals may be extremely difficult or impossible to elicit by ultrasound. An obstructive "snap" may also be heard at the site of embolic impaction. PVR tracings distal to the point of embolization are usually flat (Fig. 49–11) (see Vascular Physiologic Examination). The profound ischemia has its primary effect

on somatic muscle, which rapidly undergoes ischemic myositis. One of the more important errors of clinical diagnosis that can be made during acute arterial ischemia is mistaking ischemic muscle that is swollen and tender for the site of venous thrombosis (see Venous Thrombosis). This important distinction between acute arterial occlusion and acute venous occlusion is commonly overlooked, and the patient with acute ischemia may have treatment delayed for several hours before the real diagnosis becomes evident. A particularly important sign is the complete fixation of the ankle joint and other joints of the foot to such a degree that even the strongest applied external pressure will not elicit movement of these joints. This is rigor mortis, and when it occurs, the foot is, in effect, dead and beyond salvage by any means whatsoever. The usual time allowed for this stage to be reached is six hours. However, this figure is based on a World War I experience of injuries of the superficial femoral artery and does not fit all categories of acute ischemia. It is a common experience that irreversible changes in the foot may occur within three hours in some patients or may in fact take up to 12 hours. This determination of ischemic tolerance is entirely dependent on the capacity of the collateral circulation and the site of lodgment of the embolus. In general, the more distal the embolus, the greater the chance of rapid and irreparable harm. It is for this reason that macroembolization to the popliteal artery unquestionably carries the highest rate of limb loss.

Microemboli

Microembolization is a less dramatic but equally important phenomenon that has recently received clinical recognition.[68] These emboli are most commonly formed in ulcerated atheromatous plaques of the major arteries of the affected foot. In 70 per cent of instances, they arise from the superficial femoral artery (Fig. 49–12) or the proximal popliteal artery. Other causes of emboligenesis are stenotic lesions of the iliac vessels or unsuspected abdominal aortic aneurysms. Occasionally, a popliteal aneurysm will be the source of a single microembolus, but a more common pat-

TABLE 49–4. Signs and Symptoms of Acute Ischemia of the Foot (the Five P's)

SYMPTOMS
Pain
Paresthesia (or anesthesia)
Paralysis

SIGNS
Pallor
Pulselessness

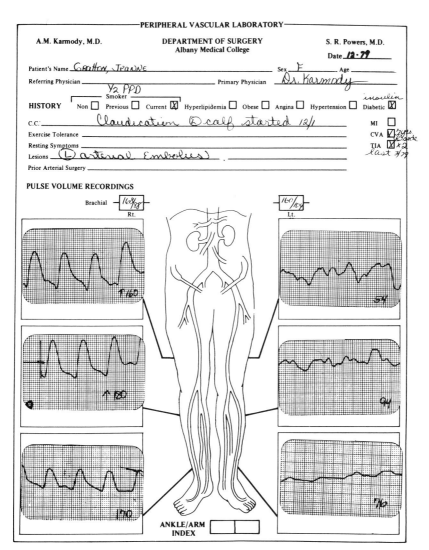

Figure 49–11. *PVR tracings from patients of Figure 49–10. The left foot shows profound ischemia as a result of the embolic occlusion.*

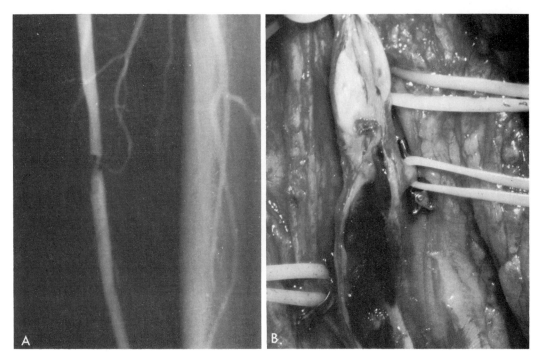

Figure 49–12. *(A) Stenotic lesion of the superficial femoral artery. (B) Same lesion opened surgically. Note the fibrinoplatelet material accumulated at this site. This was the source of digital microemboli.*

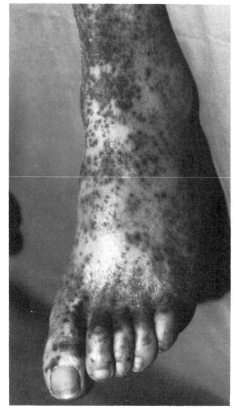

Figure 49–13. *Shower of cutaneous microemboli from a popliteal aneurysm.*

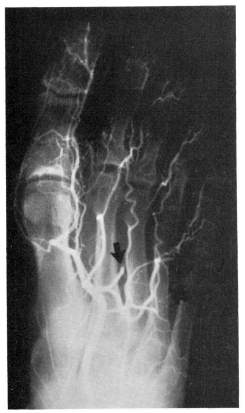

Figure 49–14. *Digital arteriogram. Arrows show that the digital vessel to the fifth toe is not visualized and that the digital vessel to the third toe is abruptly occluded.*

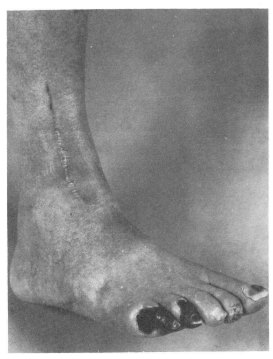

Figure 49–16. *The result of unrecognized and untreated confirmed microembolization to lateral toes. These started as typical "blue-toes," but the significance was overlooked. A second episode has resulted in gangrene. Note the incision through which ill-advised embolectomy was also attempted.*

tern is the release of a large shower of microemboli[14] (Fig. 49–13). The material is usually of a fibrinoplatelet nature, and the embolus most commonly lodges in a digit-

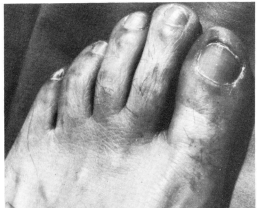

Figure 49–15. *Typical blue, painful, cyanosed great toe after microembolic impaction in the digital arteries.*

al arterial bifurcation, causing embarrassment of the circulation to one or, at the most, two digits (Fig. 49–14). This usually presents as a painful cyanosed toe (Fig. 49–15). The clinical picture may be bewildering because of the presence of palpable pulses in the usual anatomic location in the foot. This represents the condition referred to as the "blue toe" syndrome. The importance of recognizing this as a microembolic problem is that if the source of the microembolus is not located and eradicated, further microemboli will inevitably occur and result in irreparable harm or loss of the foot (Fig. 49–16).

Acute Arterial Thrombosis

The most common cause of acute arterial thrombosis is the final pathologic event of a gradual but severe narrowing of the artery by arteriosclerosis obliterans.[78] In this situation, the collateral circulation develops parallel with the narrowing of the vessel, so that the final thrombotic and occlusive event usually causes little or no recognizable symptoms, except for the possibility of a transient painful episode, which lasts only for a few minutes or hours.[82] Apart from the disappearance of a known weak pulse or a change in ultrasound signal from a pulsatile to an obstructive form, the observer may find very little on clinical examination. The PVR tracings may likewise show only minimal change in wave amplitude, although the ultrasound pressure in the foot may fall (see

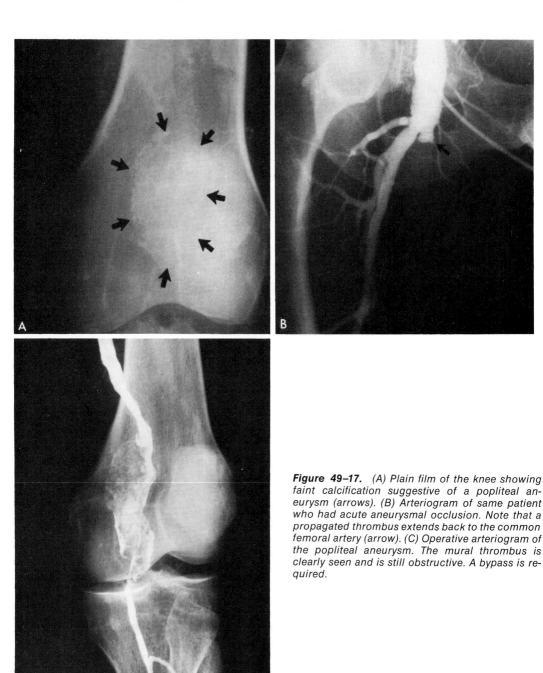

Figure 49–17. *(A) Plain film of the knee showing faint calcification suggestive of a popliteal aneurysm (arrows). (B) Arteriogram of same patient who had acute aneurysmal occlusion. Note that a propagated thrombus extends back to the common femoral artery (arrow). (C) Operative arteriogram of the popliteal aneurysm. The mural thrombus is clearly seen and is still obstructive. A bypass is required.*

Vascular Physiologic Examination). In contrast, sudden thrombosis of an apparently normal channel through which pulsatile flow is taking place will have the same dramatic effect as that which occurs in acute arterial embolism. However, this is an unusual event and is characterized by the presence of a serious underlying disease or condition. This may be a low flow state because of poor cardiac drive or widespread pathologic deterioration of the arterial intima allowing intraluminal thrombogenesis, as is seen in some collagen diseases (e.g., systemic lupus erythematosus) or in widespread metastatic carcinomatosis. Another important cause of acute arterial thrombosis is polycythemia rubra vera, which in its primary state is, in effect, a low-grade malignant condition of the red cells. An abnormally high hematocrit may also be caused by underlying respiratory or renal disease (secondary polycythemia). Although these are rare clinical events, they nevertheless have disastrous implications for the patient, from both a local and a systemic point of view. In general, these situations are completely irreparable with all known methods of therapy.

In most instances, however, arterial thrombosis occurs slowly, and the femoropopliteal arterial segment is most commonly involved. The patient is usually unaware of the gradual loss of this conduit and only slowly recognizes that his walking distance is impaired or that his foot has become cooler and less comfortable over a period of time. Acute arterial thrombosis of

this type is thus an integral part of chronic ischemia, the implications of which may be almost nonexistent or very profound over a long-term period. In contrast, one reasonably common situation assumes quite different proportions. This is the propensity of popliteal aneurysms to undergo a sudden thrombotic occlusion. It has already been mentioned that popliteal aneurysms may present with microembolic showers into the foot, but this is, in fact, the least common type of their acute symptomatology. The most common acute presentation of popliteal aneurysms is that of intrasaccular thrombosis by shift of the thrombotic laminae. Pulsatile flow into the lower extremity is suddenly cut off, and the foot is promptly compromised. Since in this situation pulsatile flow has always been maintained and there is no real obstructive element, the occlusion is very poorly tolerated by the foot. The untreated condition of acute popliteal aneurysm thrombosis will therefore have at least a 75 per cent incidence of loss of the foot. Most patients are unaware of the existence of a popliteal aneurysm within their limbs, and physicians generally do not recognize the necessity for searching for them during routine physical examinations. This represents a statistical danger to the limb that exceeds the dangers to life from abdominal aortic aneurysms simply because the level of physician awareness is so much lower in the search for popliteal aneurysm formation. In addition, once this incident occurs, it is usually considered to be caused by an arterial embolus, and the wrong approach

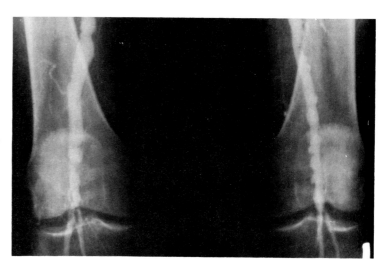

Figure 49–18. Fusiform popliteal aneurysms that are bilaterally placed above the popliteal fossae, thus making clinical detection difficult. The presence of "easily felt" popliteal pulsation should alert the clinician's suspicions.

to surgical therapy may be attempted for some time before the definitive treatment is carried out, because the episode usually presents with great suddenness, and arteriography is rarely used as a diagnostic test in acute arterial embolism. In addition, even if arteriography is performed, the arterial block will only be identified at the midfemoral level because of proximal propagation of a thrombus, and the popliteal aneurysm itself is almost never visualized (Fig. 49–17). The only potential diagnostic clue is the palpation of a nonpulsatile mass in the popliteal fossa, but if the aneurysm is present in the upper popliteal artery, it is buried within the muscles of the thigh, and this sign becomes unavailable to the observer (Fig. 49–18). The only other sign that may be useful is the palpation of a popliteal aneurysm on the opposite leg, since these lesions are frequently bilateral. This may raise the index of suspicion of the observer.

Popliteal Entrapment

Entrapment of arteries by abnormal anatomic structures is a rare but potentially serious condition, particularly for young athletic men. The most common site of entrapment is unquestionably the popliteal fossa. The popliteal artery is usually sandwiched between abnormally inserted heads of the gastrocnemius or plantaris muscles. Acute popliteal thrombosis usually occurs during exertion, although a distal embolism from poststenotic aneurysmal dilation may occasionally herald the existence of this problem.

ARTERIAL DISOBLITERATION

Early Embolectomy

The surgical method of arterial embolectomy was revolutionized by the introduction of the balloon embolectomy catheter in 1963.[45, 46] Until that time, the success of extraction of emboli by forceps, "milking" of the leg, and the application of suction by thin-walled glass "suckers" was at best uncertain.[31] This precarious state of affairs existed even when emboli were easiest to extract, i.e., from healthy arteries of young people who had mitral valvular disease

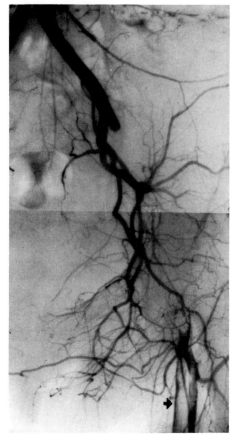

Figure 49–19. *Arteriogram from young woman with mitral valvular disease. Embolic obstruction of the common femoral artery has occurred, with propagated thrombus to the external iliac, superficial femoral, and profunda femoris arteries (arrow).*

(Fig. 49–19). The balloon catheter has, however, made extraction of emboli possible even from very diseased vessels at all locations in the lower limb. The catheters are produced in graded stalk and balloon sizes. This enables clearance of arteries from 1 to 25 mm in diameter.

The essential mechanism of the instrument is based on the pathologic finding that emboli and associated propagated thrombi tend to be soft and that the instrument can be passed through the occluding plug into unobstructed vessel (Fig. 49–20). Beyond the embolus, the balloon is inflated manually to a snug fit on the vessel wall and withdrawn along the arterial walls toward the arteriotomy site, bringing the embolus and any propagated thrombus with it, while wiping the wall clean (Fig. 49–21). This can be accom-

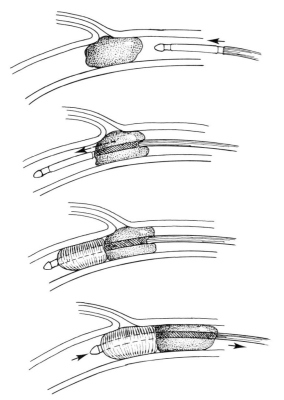

Figure 49–20. *Mechanism of use of a balloon catheter. Note that the catheter tip readily passes through and not around the soft thrombus. When the balloon is inflated, the thrombus is easily extracted with it.*

plished either with arterial flow or against arterial flow. A number of passes (wipes) may have to be made before all the embolus and the propagated thrombus have been extracted, but the final expulsion of the occlusion material should be made in each case by the arterial pressure or by extraction with forceps at the arteriotomy site, i.e. the balloon should not be dragged back in its inflated state through the arteriotomy because of the risk of uncontrolled tearing at the angles of the arterial incision.[47] The type of arteriotomy used depends on the size of the artery in which it is made. It is preferred to use as large an artery as possible so that a longitudinal arteriotomy can be made. This certainly provides a greater surgical opening through which the catheter can be manipulated, but it risks narrowing of the vessel by subsequent closure. On the other hand, when smaller vessels are being used, a transverse arteriotomy provides less working area but will help to prevent narrowing during subsequent closure. Closure of the arteriotomy should be performed with great care. Longitudinal arteriotomies can generally be closed by a running suture of 6-0 suture material, and it is most accurate to close transverse arteriotomies with interrupted sutures inserted while the vessel wall is under tension.

Choice of Artery for Early Embolectomy

Since the introduction of the balloon embolectomy catheter, it has become almost traditional to use the common femoral artery for embolectomy in all acute occlusive situations affecting the foot and

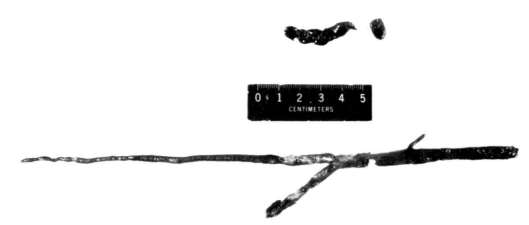

Figure 49–21. *A typical example of extracted thrombus. Note that the profunda femoris artery as well as the inferior epigastric artery has been cleared. This is the material that was in the occluded arteries shown in Figures 49–12B and 49–19.*

at all levels of actual occlusion. For example, the aortoiliac bifurcation can be cleared of emboli by a bilateral approach from the common femoral artery. In addition, the superficial femoral and posterior tibial arteries can be cleared through this approach, certainly as far as the ankle. In over 90 per cent of instances, the common femoral artery will be used primarily and will prove to be very satisfactory in the vast majority of cases. Furthermore, this operation can be performed entirely under local anesthesia usually within 60 minutes, which is an advantage in poor risk patients. However, it is clear that when very distal emboli are being retrieved, alternative anatomic approaches should be considered. When the source of ischemia is embolic impaction in the anterior tibial orifice or artery, it is necessary to approach this directly, because the embolectomy catheter is straight and will not negotiate the right-angled origin of the anterior tibial artery except by a rare accident. In this situation, it is necessary to open the popliteal artery in such a manner that the anterior tibial orifice is exposed, so that a catheter can be passed into the artery. This is a more technical and demanding embolectomy. In addition, from this approach, the catheter may also be passed selectively into the posterior tibial artery and may be induced down the peroneal artery. When it is passed into the posterior tibial artery, a catheter of suitable size (2 or 3 French) may actually be passed into the plantar arch. However, the passage of a balloon catheter into the anterior tibial artery is limited by the downward course of its terminal branch between the first and second metatarsal heads. The catheter usually impinges on this point and cannot be passed further. It is rare that the posterior tibial or dorsalis pedis arteries have to be opened for catheter passage in the foot itself, but when this is done a 2-Fr catheter is chosen because of the size of the vessels that are being manipulated. It must be stressed that great care must be taken with all of these maneuvers, since it is very easy to perforate small arteries and to cause traumatic thrombosis or arteriovenous fistulas. In addition, when working with the distal popliteal and tibial vessels, it is usually necessary to close the arteriotomy by means of a vein patch to insure that pathologic narrowing does not occur.

TRAUMATIC INJURIES OF VASCULAR SUPPLY TO THE FOOT

In most medical centers, there has been a continuous increase in the number of traumatic vascular emergencies that threaten the viability of the foot and sometimes even the patient's life. Although this trend is undoubtedly a result of a greater number of road and industrial accidents, it also represents the increasing awareness of the ability of the vascular surgeon to successfully deal with these problems.[101] Although prompt diagnosis and competent initial management are important, early reconstruction of the involved vessels is a key to success, and optimal results will be obtained only when modern methods of rapid transportation are used to take advantage of those institutions that are best equipped to handle these complex problems. It is frequently better to accept a short delay for transportation than to make an abortive attempt at reconstructive surgery that will result in loss of the time, which is vital in treating these cases.

Traumatic injuries usually cause vascular occlusion because of severe crushing damage, but if the applied force is great enough to disrupt the vascular wall, rapid bleeding may occur. In addition, injuries caused by edged instruments will cause severance of the vessels, resulting in bleeding. The laceration of a major artery in the region of the foot will allow surprisingly rapid blood loss. This is of serious consequence to the patient, threatening not only the foot but also the patient's life, both immediately and within a period of hours to days. Complete avulsion or transection of an artery is usually followed by retraction of the open ends and reduction or cessation of bleeding. Paradoxically, however, incomplete transection of the vessel wall will cause prolonged bleeding, because retraction of the cut edges will increase rather than decrease the size of the vascular wound. External examination is helpful, particularly if both entry and exit wounds can be identified. The direction of the track may give an accurate picture of the anatomic structures that are liable to be involved. This clinical information may be augmented by radiographic studies when radiopaque fragments are likely to have dislodged. The history and physical examination will establish the presence of arterial injury in most patients. However, it is important to note that in a small but significant percentage of patients, there are few or no clinical signs when serious injury has, in fact, occurred.[113] A high index of suspicion must be maintained when there has been any penetrating wound in the region of the neurovascular bundles.

An adequate history of the events that took place at the time of the injury will be very useful. If the patient is unable to provide this, information obtained from eyewitnesses, other individuals injured, police, and ambulance attendants may be very helpful. Particular attention should be given to the degree and the character of blood loss. When hemorrhage occurs from laceration of a major artery, the patient or bystanders will offer a description of bright red blood spurting with considerable violence from the wound. Blood loss in these instances is usually profuse, and the patient and the surroundings usually show strong evidence of this extravasation. Rapid blood loss of one liter or more will almost always cause some signs of hypovolemic shock, i.e., a fall in blood pressure and a rise in pulse rate. It is important to ascertain these facts as soon as possible. Profound shock will occur when the losses are great or continuous, but the immediate physiologic adjustment may be sufficient to provoke a false sense of security by measurement of reasonably normal values when the patient is first seen. This is particularly true of young patients, who are unfortunately more prone to these injuries. In the area of the foot, venous bleeding is less profuse and forceful than arterial bleeding and is generally of little clinical significance.

When an artery is completely transected, pulsatile flow distal to this point usually disappears. However, it is widely recognized that partial transection of an artery will, in many instances, allow sufficient transmission of pulsatile flow for palpation of distal pulses. Therefore, when there has been a wound in the vicinity of a major artery, the presence of distal pulses does not permit complete confidence about the integrity of the pulsatile flow. Failure to recognize this may cause not only renewed bleeding at a later stage but an incidence of traumatic arteriovenous fistula formation, which can be a very difficult problem to deal with at a later date. However, the use of Doppler ultrasound and other methods of determining arterial flow make it possible to differentiate accurately between pulsatile, obstructive, or no flow distal to the point of injury.

Vascular injuries of the foot are often associated with injuries of adjacent nerves. When the signs of specific nerve interruption can be elicited in the presence of excessive bleeding, this is good evidence that there has been injury of the entire neurovascular bundle. In most instances, the patient with external hemorrhage will have received some means of hemorrhage control in the form of firmly applied dressings or even pneumatic tourniquets, It is rare that rapid hemorrhage will be occurring when the patient is first seen. Usually, rapid hemorrhaging will have been stopped either by the first aid measures or as a result of hypotension attendant upon blood loss. Bleeding may, however, resume when the hemostatic measures are dismantled for wound examination or when the blood pressure rises in response to resuscitative measures. It is important to stress that vigorous resuscitation to bring the blood pressure back to "normal" may result in a further brisk hemorrhage because of dislodgement or "blowout" of a poorly attached thrombus that was restraining free arterial bleeding.

In the vast majority of cases, external hemorrhage can be stopped by accurately placed digital pressure. The most effective control is achieved by direct compression over the bleeding point. In all venous and most arterial wounds of the foot, this will immediately stop the blood loss. However, in those rare instances in which arterial bleeding is inadequately controlled by direct pressure, digital compression of the artery proximal to the wound will result in slowing of the hemorrhage until a reasonably stable fibrin clot has been formed. If this fails, a pneumatic tourniquet should be placed at the calf level. This measure will, however, very rarely be necessary and is associated with the obvious dangers of ischemia from prolonged application. In such instances, no time should be lost before the patient is transferred for definitive surgical control. Attempted application of hemostatic clamps in non–operative room settings must be thoroughly discouraged. It is difficult or impossible to securely clamp a retracted vessel in the depths of a wound without surgical exposure. Blind attempts are usually unsuccessful or, worse yet, damage nearby vessels or nerves. Once hemorrhage has been controlled, firm wound packing with sterile gauze dressings will almost always maintain hemostasis until the patient can undergo surgical exploration and control.

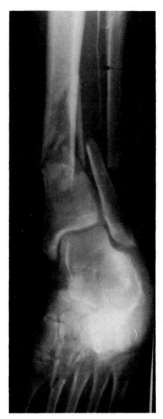

Figure 49–23. *Severe comminuted fracture above the ankle joint. The only artery visualized on the angiogram is the peroneal artery, which terminates abruptly above the fracture. The posterior tibial and anterior tibial arteries are not seen. In this patient, a vein graft was used to bridge a crushed segment of the posterior tibial artery.*

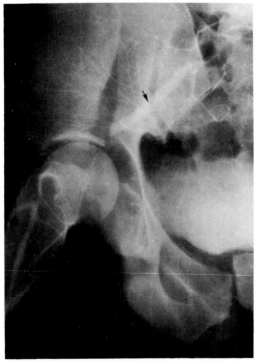

Figure 49–22. *Obstruction of the external iliac, common femoral, and superficial femoral arteries as a result of a severe crush fracture of the pelvis. Note that the fracture extends through the acetabulum and that the pubic symphysis is disrupted. The external iliac artery is faintly visualized, with complete obstruction at the inguinal ligament (arrows). The profunda femoris artery is visualized, but the common femoral and superficial femoral arteries are not seen. Severe ischemia of the foot was reversed by excision of the damaged arteries and replacement by saphenous vein graft.*

In most situations, however, trauma will cause acute arterial occlusion, which will jeopardize the viability of the foot. Acute traumatic occlusion can take place at any level from the common iliac artery (Fig. 49–22) to the tibial arteries (Fig. 49–23) and will have the same effect on the foot.[111] However, occlusion after injury occurs most commonly in the superficial femoral, popliteal, and tibial arteries. Blunt trauma is the usual cause of arterial occlusion because of intimal fracture and intraluminal thrombosis, but complete arterial transection by sharp trauma may also have the same effect. The resulting symptoms and signs of acute ischemia have already been described (see Table 49–4). Objective methods of evaluation should also be employed to confirm this clinical diagnosis.

Ideally, this will include the use of a plethysmograph and a Doppler flow detector. These instruments should be used to elicit three types of information in this situation:

1. Presence or absence of flow.
2. Character of the flow as determined by ultrasound, i.e., pulsatile versus obstructive.
3. Measurement of the pressure within the available arteries.

The first two observations can be determined by both ultrasonic and plethysmographic examination. The third, pressure measurements, can be obtained by the use of a simple blood pressure cuff and a Doppler flow detector. This is a simple and very rewarding test. If these instruments are unavailable, an arteriogram can be utilized to define the level of obstruc-

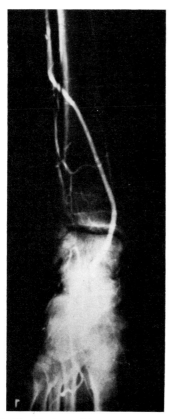

Figure 49–24. *Patient with a severe crush fracture of the os calcis and occlusion of all the arteries crossing the ankle. A vein graft has been placed between the anterior tibial and dorsalis pedis arteries under a bridge of intact skin. Function is still satisfactory after four years.*

tion, but it should be the investigative measure of last resort and should rarely be used under these circumstances.

The treatment of hemorrhage consists of its operative control and repair of the vessel. Above the popliteal termination, repair should consist of control of the bleeding vessels by vascular clamps, trimming of the lacerated edges, and closure with monofilament suture material. If the vessel is badly lacerated or occluded by a thrombus, the damaged portion should be resected back to normal artery and continuity restored by end-to-end anastomosis or an interposition graft, preferably with autogenous vein. If the adjacent vein is also injured, it too should be repaired at this time.[109] When a single tibial artery is the source of hemorrhage, it can be safely ligated only if it can be ascertained that other arteries are functioning satsifactorily. However, if adequate skills are available, it is preferable that microvascular repair be done, so that anatomic continuity is restored. This will clearly protect the patient to some extent against further injuries of other vessels (see Replantation of the Foot). If all the tibial vessels are damaged or occluded, repair of at least one artery is mandatory for survival of the foot (Fig. 49–24). This will usually mean placement of an interposition vein graft, and these vessels, which are usually no larger than 2 mm in diameter, would almost always require microvascular surgical skills for optimal function.

Reperfusion Syndrome

Successful restoration of arterial circulation after acute occlusions is always accompanied by edema of the soft tissues of the lower leg and foot. In general, the degree of tissue swelling is in direct proportion to the length of time of the acute ischemic episode. Of all soft tissue, the skeletal muscle is particularly affected by this process. When the muscle lies within rigid osseofascial compartments (e.g., the anterior compartment of the leg), a small degree of swelling will cause a tremendous rise in compartment pressure. This increase is frequently sufficient to cause secondary circulatory embarrassment by disruption of capillary exchange, with eventual cessation of venous then arterial flow. This swelling can frequently be quite dramatic and may occur rapidly within a few minutes after the arterial flow is first restored. If the muscle is not decompressed with equal rapidity, irreversible necrosis will eventually occur. This problem is so serious that a maxim exists to the effect that if the surgeon even thinks about this possibility in a given patient, measures to effect decompression are probably already necessary. The signs that are most ominous are rapid swelling, inability of the patient to move the foot freely or to have sensation restored completely, or loss of movement or sensation after initial recovery. In addition, the gastrocnemius-soleus muscle, in particular, assumes a very firm texture and will be quite tender.

The most efficient method of decompression is fasciotomy. In closed fasciotomy, the rigid subcutaneous fasciae of the affected compartment(s) are split longitudinally throughout the length of the leg through a small skin incision that allows for the insertion of a pair of long scissors.[97] This has the advantage of leaving the skin cover intact. However, the open fasciotomy is more certain and efficient and is accomplished by the incision of both skin and fascia to allow the muscle to completely emerge from the compartment. Although the muscle will usually require coverage by a split-thickness skin graft, this is a preferable method of fasciotomy when uncertainty exists about the efficacy of closed fasciotomy or the swelling is particularly severe. We have been using hypertonic mannitol along with elevation of the limbs in the management of this condition, as a result of experimental work on and clinical observations of this syndrome.[4] These measures are promptly instituted at the time of restoration of arterial flow and are usually very successful in preventing closed compartment swelling and obviating the need for subsequent fasciotomy.[117, 118]

CHRONIC ISCHEMIA OF THE FOOT: ARTERIOSCLEROSIS OBLITERANS

The most common of all arterial disorders are the chronic obliterative arterial diseases and by far the most common of

TABLE 49-5. Characteristics of Arteries of Conduit and Supply

CONDUIT	SUPPLY
Large diameter	Small diameter
Few or no branches	Many branches
Between tissue planes	Imbedded in muscle

these is arteriosclerosis obliterans. This occurs more commonly in men than women, in the elderly rather than the young, and in the diabetic as opposed to the nondiabetic.[4] Although it is rarely seen in individuals under 50 years of age, it is a well-documented clinical experience that the earlier in life this disease appears, the more pessimistic is the ultimate prognosis. This is particularly true of young women who develop the disease before the age of 40. In all individuals, the arteriosclerotic process is a diffuse one, affecting arteries throughout the body.[15] In these patients, concurrent disease of the coronary and intracranial arterial systems represents the greatest threat to life. In particular, the death rate from coronary artery occlusion in patients of this type is extremely high. Fortunately, this diffuse disease process is characterized by areas of very extensive but localized disease, affecting only relatively small segments of an artery or arteries. The arteries that are particularly affected are those of conduit rather than supply. The difference between these vessels is summarized in the Table 49-5. Arteries of conduit are larger, with few or no branches. The disease process in these arteries tends to be quite sharply localized and makes them amenable to surgical treatment, which is necessary because no form of medical or drug therapy has yet been developed for the eradication of this disease.[26]

Arterial obstructions resulting from arteriosclerosis obliterans, which have a material effect on the foot, may occur at all levels from the infrarenal aorta to the digital arteries. However, the most commonly affected sites, in statistical order of frequency, are the femoropopliteal segment in the region of the adductor muscle hiatus, the aortoiliac bifurcation, the common iliac bifurcation, and the common femoral bifurcation.[51] In addition, in diabetics who demonstrate the aforementioned patterns of disease, the tibial arteries may be seriously and extensively involved. As stated previously, segmental occlusions or stenoses are the rule, but the collateral circulation, which depends on the arteries of supply, generally develops in parallel with the development of these obstructions and tends to be able to keep pace with the disease.[57] However, the blood supply provided by the collateral pathway rarely, if ever, attains the same flow rate or efficiency as that of the original artery of conduit with its provision of pulsatile flow. Unfortunately, it is frequently the case that two or more obstructive lesions at different levels will develop in relation to the same arterial inflow pathway to a particular foot. The combination will inevitably lead to severe ischemia of the foot. In the presence of a recognized single lesion, a careful search for a more proximal or distal lesion should be undertaken before any treatment program is initiated.

Although many theories have been developed regarding the pathogenesis of arteriosclerosis, the fact remains that the single most important factor in the progression of arteriosclerosis is tobacco (nicotine) smoking. The vasoconstrictor effect of a single cigarette may be profound, and measurements of skin temperature have shown that a lowering of temperature will last for four to six hours after the smoking of a single cigarette. Although it is therefore true that the greater the number of cigarettes smoked, the more profound the arteriolar effect, it is also true that a very small number of cigarettes may have a long-lasting vasoactive effect. Smokers tend to develop arteriosclerotic lesions five times more frequently than nonsmokers and to progress poorly or have a poor result from reconstructive surgery at a rate five times greater than nonsmokers. It is also known that in clinical practice, nonsmokers, with the exception of very long-standing diabetics, are almost never found to have a degree of arterial obstruction that will eventually require reconstructive surgery.

Clinical Symptoms

Because of the usual obstructive pattern involving the arteries above the tibial arteries, intermittent claudication is usually the earliest sign of diminution of blood supply to the foot. Typically, the patient develops pain of a cramping nature in the calf after walking for a distance of 100 meters or less. With continued exercise, this pain rapidly becomes so crippling that walking must be stopped. The painful cramping sensation then disappears within two minutes, and the patient is able to resume walking but for an even shorter distance. This pattern of walking, with a continual decreasing of distances, persists until a long halt of five minutes or more is required to alleviate the pain and restore the metabolic equilibrium. This diminished exercise response can be demonstrated by PVR examination (Fig. 49–25). In the less severe stages of occlusive disease, the foot remains relatively unaffected, but as the disease progresses and the blood supply continues to diminish, the poor exercise response of intermittent

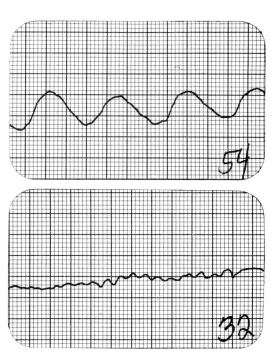

Figure 49–25. *Pre-exercise and post-exercise pulse volume recordings of a patient with unstable claudication. The pre-exercise recording (top) shows diminished but recognizable wave forms at the calf level. However, the post-exercise tracing (bottom) shows that these wave forms completely disappear at the end of the exercise period, indicating that the collateral capacity is unable to respond to the demands of exercise.*

claudication is generally accompanied by sensory changes in the foot. Usually, there is a feeling of intense cold in the foot and toes, and inspection of the foot at this stage usually reveals a blanched, white appearance and marked coolness. Pins and needles may also be a sensory accompaniment at this stage. A period of rest usually restores both color and warmth to the foot, and the paresthesia gradually resolves as well. Sensory relief will also be hastened by keeping the foot in the dependent position.

With disease of the iliac vessels, the muscle groups affected include the buttock and thigh. The maximum walking distance is governed by pain in these muscle groups as well as in the calf. In rare instances (mainly in diabetics), when the occlusive process is most severe below the popliteal arteries, the muscles of the foot itself will be affected more than the calf muscles, and the cramp-like, constrictive sensations may occur with some severity in the intrinsic muscles of the foot. As ischemia becomes more profound, the walking distance becomes considerably decreased, and it is not unusual to find patients who are unable to walk for more than 30 meters. With such short walking distances, exercise symptoms of the foot are the rule rather than the exception. Shortly thereafter, with very little further progression, although the entire lower limb is usually affected, continuous pain appears even at rest and is centered almost exclusively in the foot. This is the symptom of rest pain. At this stage, ischemia is profound and the risk of subsequent tissue loss and loss of the foot exceeds 80 per cent within six months. This pain is always present, although somewhat abated during the day and when the limb is dependent. At night, however, when the leg is both warmed by the bedclothes and horizontal, the demands of the foot for an increase in blood supply cannot be met. The resulting severe burning pain awakens the patient after a few hours of sleep. The usual remedy is quickly discovered by the patient and consists of either sitting on the edge of the bed with the feet dependent or walking around the room until the pain is relieved. In more severe instances, the patient is forced to sleep in the sitting position with the legs on

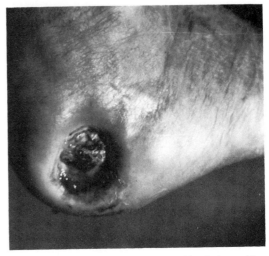

Figure 49–26. Sharply demarcated heel ulcer with a necrotic base. The os calcis is exposed. There is no sign of any healing, and the edges of the ulcer are darkened and very unhealthy.

the floor, which generally results in considerable dependent edema.

The final stage of profound ischemia of the foot is the appearance of lesions of tissue death. These consist either of nonhealing ulcers or gangrene. Nonhealing ulcers are spontaneous ulcerations that do not heal despite careful conservative therapy and show little or no tendency to granulate. In addition, they are usually very painful. The bases of the ulcers are usually whitish gray, with clean, "punched-out" edges (Fig. 49–26). These ulcers usually extend slowly, and the darkened edges of the skin are evidence of continuing tissue death. These ulcers cause a type of pain similar to the burning type experienced in rest pain, which has already been described, and they quickly communicate with structures such as tendons, bones, and joints. Apart from the spreading necrosis, they serve as portals of entry for bacteria, which will inevitably overwhelm the foot, already rendered indefensible by the lack of blood supply. The ulcers most commonly appear in the region of the great toe or over the head of the fifth metatarsal, but frequently they appear in the region of the heel as a result of pressure during recumbency or over the medial and lateral malleoli for similar reasons (Fig. 49–27).

Gangrene is usually defined as "an obviously dead, blackened area of the foot"

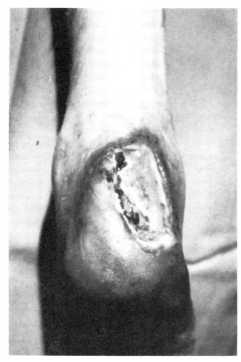

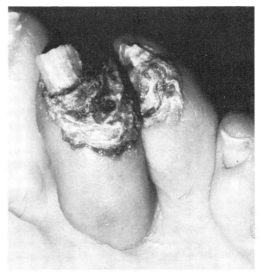

Figure 49–28. *Gangrenous tips of the toes indicative of severely compromised digital circulation.*

Figure 49–27. *Heel ulcer in the typical position resulting from pressure during sleep. In these patients, the skin of the heel is unstable and is very liable to be damaged by degrees of pressure that ordinarily would cause no harm.*

and most commonly begins with one or more toes. The patient first notices increased pain in the infected digit and observes that it rapidly progresses to a blackened structure (Fig. 49–28). The edges of the dead area are not clearly defined, shading insensibly into what appears to be normal tissue. In addition to the digits, gangrenous patches may occur on the skin at any part of the foot (Fig. 49–29). As well as being a site for nonhealing ulcers, the skin of the heel is frequently the site of a large gangrenous patch of skin (Fig. 49–30). The appearance of either or both of these lesions on the foot is a sign of impending death of the entire foot. In the absence of any specific treatment, it can be expected that the lesions will progress inexorably and will also inevitably serve as portals of entry for bacteria. Infection will thereafter spread rapidly to the tendon sheaths and plantar spaces or may even extend into the intermuscular spaces

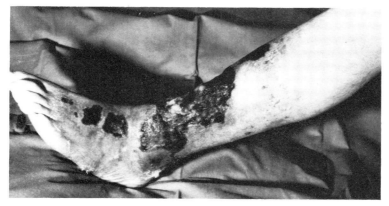

Figure 49–29. *Gangrenous patches of skin extending from the foot well into the lower leg. This is a somewhat unusual distribution but is fairly common.*

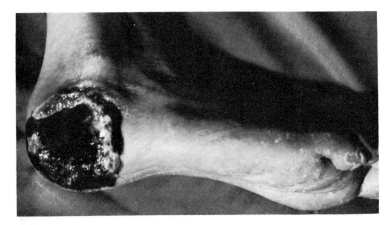

Figure 49–30. *Gangrenous area of the heel that occurred spontaneously without any history of pressure necrosis. Note the very scaly and unhealthy appearance of the skin of the rest of the foot.*

in the calf[67] (Fig. 49–31). Attempts to cure these lesions by surgical excision are doomed to failure in the vast majority of instances and will lead to even more extensive nonhealing areas with the attendant consequences (Fig. 49–32). Rest pain, nonhealing ulcers, and gangrenous changes in the foot are extremely serious signs, indicating very profound ischemia with an overwhelming chance of loss of the foot within three months of onset[66] (Fig. 49–33).

Clinical Signs

Traditionally, the ischemic foot is white and cold, with shiny skin and absence of hair growth. The pulp spaces below the toes are also decreased, and the foot may be painful to the touch or even to light stroking, presumably because of an element of ischemic neuropathy. However, these signs occur only in feet that have been the site of very long-standing rest pain, usually of a duration of six months or more (Fig. 49–34). It is very unusual at present to see feet of this nature, because patients tend to seek the help of their physicians at a much earlier stage. Therefore, although coldness and some discomfort on pressure are usually present, the signs of atrophic, shiny skin and lack of hair growth are generally absent in

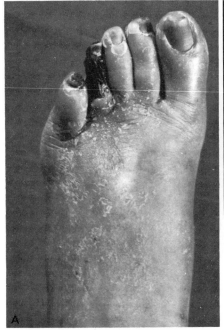

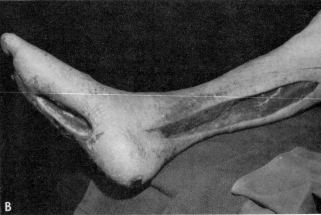

Figure 49–31. *(A) Gangrene of a single digit. The forefoot is swollen. Note the pitting after digital pressure. This was caused by dependent edema as a result of sleeping in a chair. (B) The swelling was found to be caused by tracking of infection along the tendon sheaths both anteriorly and posteriorly into the plantar space and into the compartments of the calf muscles. Extensive draining as well as a reconstructive vascular procedure was required before these abscesses were cured.*

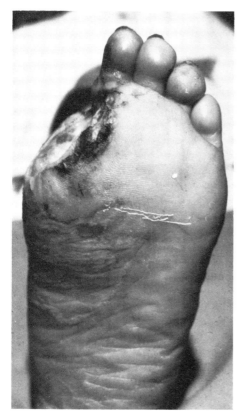

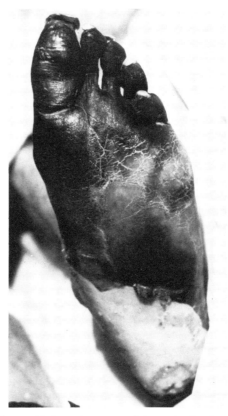

Figure 49–32. Failure of amputation to heal because of poor blood supply. This illustrates that amputation of gangrenous tissue before arterial supply is restored to a level necessary to heal the resulting wound will lead in most instances to an even worse problem.

Figure 49–33. Gangrene of the entire forefoot that started with a single toe. This condition is completely unsalvageable.

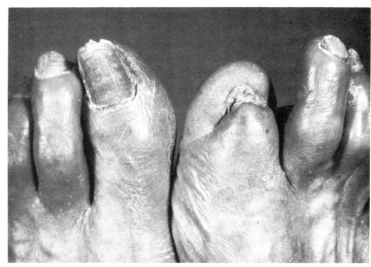

Figure 49–34. Classic appearance of feet that are the site of a long period of chronic ischemia. Note that the skin is very tense and shiny, there is no hair growth, the nails are very brittle, and there has been a subungual infection involving the right great toe.

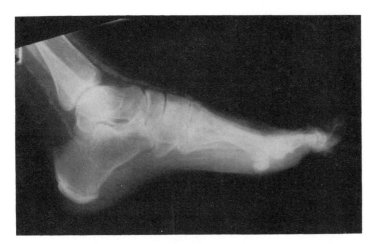

Figure 49–35. A plain x-ray film shows very extensive calcification along the course of the dorsalis pedis and posterior tibial arteries. This calcification extends into the plantar arch and indicates a very extensive degree of arterial occlusive disease, which means that arterial reconstruction is very unlikely to be successful at these levels.

today's patient. Pulses that are usually present behind the posterior malleolus and between the first and second metatarsal rays are always absent. The presence of a clearly ischemic toe when pulses can be felt should lead to the suspicion of a microembolic source at a more proximal point on the arterial tree[102] (see Figure 49–15). (See also Arterial Embolism.)

Sensation to pinprick may also be diminished, but caution should be used in the use of a sharp pin, since the small puncture wounds may act as portals for bacterial entry. The absence of vibration, as well as position senses and tendon reflexes, should lead to investigation of the possibility that the patient is diabetic. Obviously, the presence of nonhealing ulcers and gangrenous areas will be readily apparent to the examiner. However, even when these lesions are not easily seen, careful inspection of the heel and the web spaces between the toes should be made. Cracks, fissures, or small ulcers can often be discovered in these areas and will have been unsuspected by the patient because of his or her preoccupation with the intense discomfort of the foot. All pulses proximal to the foot should be checked by palpation on both sides. The popliteal pulses are generally difficult to elicit, but with practice, it is possible to feel this pulse, if it is present, even with the patient lying on his back with both legs in the horizontal position. Flexion at the knee greatly improves the ability to feel the pulse, and there seems little need to resort to turning the patient onto his abdomen and flexing the knee to a right angle to feel pulses in the popliteal

arteries. The femoral pulse should be sought at the exact midinguinal point. If there is doubt about the presence of this pulse, the inguinal ligament should be formally demarcated between the anterosuperior iliac spine and the pubic tubercle, and the midpoint should be accurately determined and marked. A common error in feeling for the femoral pulse is to seek for it too laterally; this is particularly true in obese patients. A stethoscope should be used to elicit bruits over the common femoral and superficial femoral arteries, although at the common femoral region, injudicious pressure on the artery during auscultation can result in the production of a bruit that is spurious. Plain x-ray examination will frequently show calcification along the course of the pedal arteries especially in diabetics, (Fig. 49–35). This can generally be considered as a sign of advanced arterial disease. The noninvasive and angiographic examinations of the ischemic foot have already been described.

Conservative Management

The foot that is ischemic as a result of chronic obliterative arterial disease demands very careful nonsurgical treatment if reconstructive arterial surgery is unnecessary or technically infeasible. In this program, the education of the patient is vital, and some time should be spent to insure that the patient understands all the principles that will be used in his subsequent treatment. First, it should be emphasized that the measures that will be adopted will be lifelong rather than short-term. Abstinence from tobacco smoking should be advised in the strongest possible terms. This measure is mandatory in patients with thromboangiitis obliterans. Patients who find it difficult to stop smoking should be referred to one of the many clinics that help people to control or discontinue smoking. If this fails, the most innocuous form of smoking should be considered. This is probably the use of a pipe with an efficient filter, which tends to reduce the amount of smoke that is inhaled and lessens the vasoconstrictive effects. Patients' weight should be reduced as much as possible to the ideal height-weight ratio. Cessation of smoking commonly causes an increase in appetite and a gain in weight. This weight gain should be avoided by explaining the problem to the patient and by using the aid of nutritionists and other methods of planning diets to insure adequate nutrition while weight is being lost. Decrease in weight not only reduces the burden on the foot but also has a direct effect on cardiac output, increasing it by increasing the supply of whole blood per kilogram of body weight per minute.

Patients should be taught to examine their feet with care on a daily basis and to take extraordinary measures to ensure that the skin cover is intact (Fig. 49–36). Washing the feet with soap and water and careful drying, followed by examination of the interdigital and web spaces, are important not only for cleanliness but also as a practical method of actually seeing every part of the foot. Nails should be trimmed carefully and in such a way as to minimize the hazard of developing ingrown toenails and prevent incisions into the adjoining soft tissue, which would produce portals for bacterial entry. Patients should at least inform their physicians about what appear to be minor difficulties with the feet rather than pursue time-wasting attempts and potentially dangerous homespun or proprietary remedies. Seemingly trivial lesions such as calluses, fissures, and shallow ulcers may eventually lead to loss of parts of the foot, if not promptly treated.

Footwear should be loose but sturdy and as waterproof as possible. Socks should be thick rather than thin, and even for women, thick socks are better footwear than thin stockings. Thick socks will allow the warmth of the foot to be maintained, which is important because ischemic feet are very susceptible to cold and will rapidly develop frostbite. Therefore, patients who live in climates with seasonably cold variations should be particularly careful to habitually institute protective measures before venturing outdoors during the colder months. These patients should be advised to walk as much as is comfortably possible for the foot and to persist with a steady program of walking, even though the pace may be very slow. This remains the best known method of developing and maintaining adequate collateral circulation.[61, 127]

Existing diabetes should be kept under

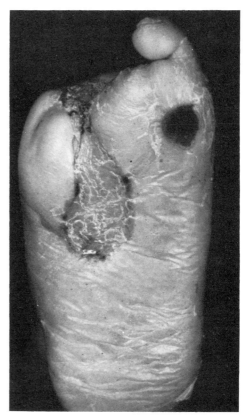

Figure 49–36. *This photograph illustrates the importance of daily care and inspection of the foot. This diabetic patient had a reconstructive procedure that allowed most of the foot to be salvaged. He failed to notice this gangrenous patch for many days because of lack of daily inspection. It was caused by walking on a small pebble inside the shoe with an insensitive foot.*

rigid control, although it is as yet uncertain whether even the most excellent control of the biochemistry of the diabetic state will circumvent the development of arteriosclerosis. Regardless of this rigid control of the diabetic state, it is certainly very necessary to prevent wild fluctuations of the glucose level in the blood, which predispose to the development and rapid spread of local infections when the level of blood sugar is high. The cardiac state should be carefully evaluated and maintained as best as possible at all times. In some patients, rest pain can be relieved simply by improvement of cardiac output, particularly if congestive cardiac failure can be reversed and brought under control.

STANDARD SURGICAL APPROACHES TO ELECTIVE VASCULAR RECONSTRUCTION AFFECTING THE FOOT

Elective reconstruction of the arteries that directly affect the survival and well-being of the foot can be performed for either relative or absolute indications. The relative indications are the presence of an abdominal aneurysm that may threaten the patient's life or, less frequently, will threaten the foot because of distal embolization, or socially or economically pressing reasons. The absolute indications refer to those conditions already mentioned, i.e., rest pain, nonhealing ulcers, or gangrene, which, when present, indicate that survival of the foot is seriously threatened within a short period of time. In addition, some conditions, such as popliteal or femoral aneurysms, may in fact be considered absolute indications for reconstructive surgery, since their complication rate is extremely high, as has been noted.

This section will consist of a brief description of the operative procedures and materials that are available for elective reconstruction from the infrarenal aorta to the arteries of the foot itself and the results that can be obtained with these operations.

Aortoiliac Reconstruction

The patient should be placed in the prone position on the operating table, with the legs slightly extended and the knees slightly flexed. This has the advantage of lifting the heels from the pressure of the table and also allows for slight pooling of blood in the calf muscles, which is useful as a source of autotransfusion immediately before declamping. For these types of procedures, the entire abdomen should be prepped from the nipples to the knees, with the knees being prepped circumferentially. The cleansing solution of choice is 2 per cent iodine, and provided it is freshly made up and has not evaporated to a higher concentration, removal of the iodine with alcohol is not necessary. However, care should be taken not to touch the genitalia with this solution, and preliminary cleansing of the genitalia with a water-soluble povidone-iodine mixture is both helpful and protective. A small catheter (12 or 14 Fr) should be placed within the bladder to monitor the urine output during the procedure and to prevent enlargement of the bladder, which may expose the structure to damage by retractors and also severely limits exposure during the operation.

The incisions appropriate for exposure of individual arteries are shown in Figure 49–37. For exposure of the upper part of the aorta from the intrarenal area to the bifurcation of the iliac arteries, a long midline incision is preferable. This area can also be reached through a retroperitoneal incision on the left side, but this incision requires extension into the thorax by excision across the costal margin and mobilization of the spleen, left kidney, and pancreas. In general, therefore, the transperitoneal approach is more commonly used and provides a reasonable working area. If the aortic control is only required distal to the inferior mesenteric artery, a long, muscle-cutting, oblique extraperitoneal approach is also excellent, although the exposure of the aorta itself is not as good as that obtained transperitoneally. However, the physiologic disturbance is less, and the iliac vessels can be exposed in their entirety from the bifurcation of the aorta to the inguinal ligament.[67] The right common iliac artery can be dissected and manipulated from a left retroperitoneal aortic approach, but accurate surgery on this vessel is not possible through this incision. Operations utilizing a left-sided extraperitoneal approach must therefore be confined to a reconstructive procedure on this side on its own or combined with a cross-limb bypass through the extraperitoneal space of Retzius to the right-sided arteries (Fig. 49–38).

The aortoiliac system lends itself very comfortably to endarterectomy, since the vessels are of considerable size and have much operative tolerance. This operation has the benefit of excellent long-term patency and eliminates the necessity for

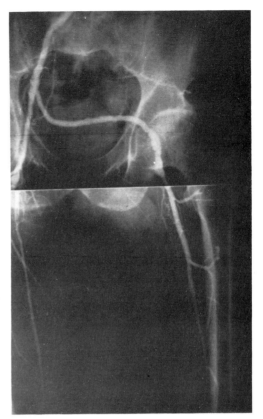

Figure 49–38. *Crossover vein bypass from the right common iliac artery to the left profunda femoris artery. The vein graft has been passed in the retroperitoneal space behind the symphysis pubis.*

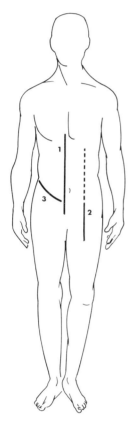

Figure 49–37. *Incisions commonly used during aortoiliac surgery.*

(1) A long midline incision extending from the xiphoid process to the symphysis pubis. Through this incision, exposure of the area from the infrarenal aorta to the common iliac bifurcation is easily obtained, but the external iliac artery is not readily exposed by this approach.

(2) A femoral incision, with a dotted line showing the possibilities of extension across the inguinal ligament into the retroperitoneal space. The iliac artery on either side can be exposed in this way as far as the bifurcation of the aorta.

(3) The more commonly known oblique incision for retroperitoneal exposure of the iliac artery from the aortic bifurcation to the inguinal ligament.

placement of an artificial graft.[138] However, artificial grafts, particularly those of external velour construction, now have a long-term patency that is comparable to that of endarterectomized vessels, and improvements of the graft composition now allow the formation of a new intimal surface that carries a very low thrombogenicity.[115] Most surgeons therefore favor the use of grafts, since they are more expeditious and do not involve the time-consuming and admittedly tedious maneuvers required for endarterectomy.[38] In addition, the use of grafts, particularly to replace the left common iliac conduit, will prevent disturbance of the nervi erigentes, which cross the left common iliac artery and are responsible for potency in the male.[92]

It is usually possible by careful study of the preoperative angiogram to decide whether aortoiliac reconstruction will be performed intra-abdominally or whether the reconstructions will need to extend as far as the femoral vessels. However, on a number of occasions, what appear to be simple aortoiliac operations will necessarily have to extend to the femoral vessels. For this reason, preparation of the skin for possible operative intervention below the inguinal ligament is a vital preoperative measure. The long-term patency of aortoiliac reconstructions, particularly in patients with superficial femoral thrombosis, will be considerably influenced by the integrity of the outflow tract, i.e., the profunda femoris artery. This vessel must be carefully evaluated preoperatively by means of anteroposterior and oblique arteriography[81] (Fig. 49–39). In the presence of such lesions, orifice profundaplasty should also be performed, since this will afford considerable long-term postoperative protection for the graft (Fig. 49–40). In the performance of aortofemoral graft placement, the graft can be extended into the profunda femoris artery, thus obviating a separate patching procedure at this orifice.[70]

It is our current practice to use intra-operative antibiotic coverage. Cephaloridine, 1 or 2 gm, is given by intravenous bolus at the start of the operation, with 1 gm or more continued intravenously throughout the operation, depending on the patient's weight. By using meticulous surgical technique and preventing hematoma formation around the graft, the infection rate for the placement of arterial grafts has been reduced to less than 1 per cent over the last 10 years. This is considerably enhanced by reperitonealization of the artery or graft when a transperitoneal approach has been done, although large-caliber grafts may take up so much retroperitoneal space that the peritoneum cannot be closed over it. This problem does not, of course, arise when the operation is performed in the retroperitoneal space in the first instance. The abdominal wall itself is closed with No. 2 Ethilon with loose approximation, so that the muscle and fascia are not strangulated by tension on the closure. Femoral wounds should be closed in two layers with 4-0 monofilament suture material, approximating the fascia overlying the artery and clos-

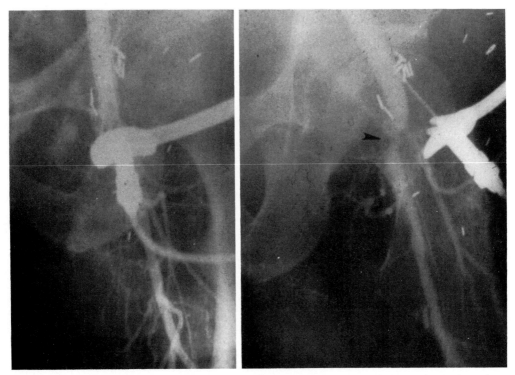

Figure 49–39. *Anteroposterior and oblique angiograms showing a lesion of the profunda femoris artery obscured in the anteroposterior view and clearly defined (arrow) in the oblique view.*

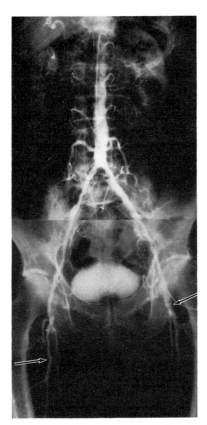

Figure 49–40. *A patient with severe iliac occlusive disease on both sides and rest pain of both feet. The arrows indicate lesions extending into the profunda femoris artery, which constitutes the main run-off pathway in both legs. The operation of aortoiliac endarterectomy was extended to the common femoral and profunda femoris arteries as far as second perforators on both sides.*

ing the immediate subcutaneous fat and skin thereafter. In the performance of aortic surgery in particular, it has been found that there is increased cardiac output and oxygen transport following preoperative and intraoperative isovolemic hemodilution.[119] This measure has a number of advantages, not the least being that the patient's own blood can be used for retransfusion in the event of operative blood losses.

Infrainguinal Arterial Reconstruction

Common Femoral and Profunda Femoris Reconstructions

As previously mentioned, in the presence of occlusion of the superficial femoral

artery, the profunda femoris artery becomes the main and unquestionably the most important outflow tract for the iliac and common femoral arteries. Lesions of the orifice of this artery (Fig. 49–41) and even more distally along its length have been identified since angiography became useful for the visualization of the arteries in extremities with peripheral vascular disease.[99] It is only relatively recently, however, that specific attempts have been made at surgical reconstruction of these arteries. The advantage of this procedure is that it may, on many occasions, obviate the need for a longer, more complex operation to the distal part of the leg, achieving a desirable result with a simple procedure that can often be done under local anesthesia.[39, 73] The reason for this is that the profunda femoris is an artery of supply rather than of conduit, and the technical demands of its reconstruction are subse-

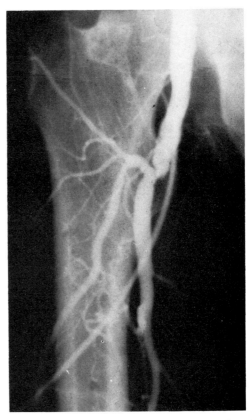

Figure 49–41. *Clearly defined lesion of the orifice of the profunda femoris artery. Notice that the superficial femoral artery is absent because of complete occlusion.*

quently much greater than usually required. However, a careful approach to this problem, which necessitates the maintenance of patency of the main branches of this artery, provides excellent surgical results (Fig. 49–42). We have found, for example, that the procedure of orifice or extended profundaplasty will provide for limb salvage, will relieve symptoms in all patients with rest pain, and will also allow healing of lesions in 70 per cent of patients with ischemic loss of tissue of the foot. This procedure therefore lends itself admirably to use in elderly patients who may be deemed less suitable for the more distal and time-consuming reconstructive procedures. In patients who are at particular risk, the femoral artery of one side can also be used as an inflow source by means of a subcutaneous graft placed across the pubic symphysis to the opposite femoral or profunda vessel. This operation can be performed in large part under local anesthesia and has an acceptable patency rate under

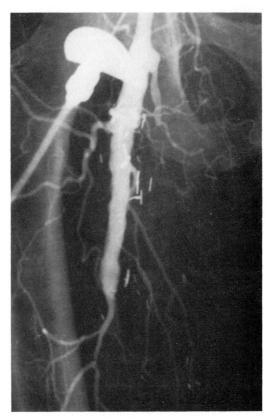

Figure 49–43. *Same artery as in Figure 49–42 extended profundaplasty. Notice that the profunda femoris artery is considerably widened by means of a vein patch and that intregity of all the branches is well preserved by extension of the profundaplasty into each orifice of each branch.*

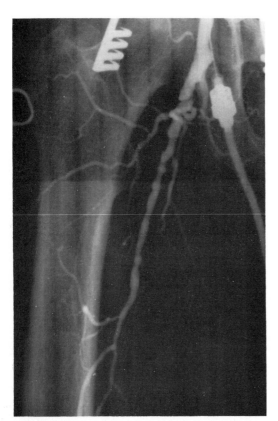

Figure 49–42. *Extensive disease of the profunda femoris artery as far as its termination.*

the circumstances for which it is being used[17] (Fig. 49–43).

Infrainguinal Arterial Bypasses

Although it is now well known that autogenous vein grafts were used before arterial replacement during World War II, their popularity as a therapeutic mode for the treatment of occluded arteries really started after publication of the report of Kunlin, to whom credit is given by most surgeons for the introduction of this concept.[75] Autogenous vein grafts are now the most well known and traditionally time-honored method of reconstruction for salvage of the ischemic foot. The femoral artery is exposed in the groin, usually by means of a longitudinal incision extending downward from the inguinal ligament

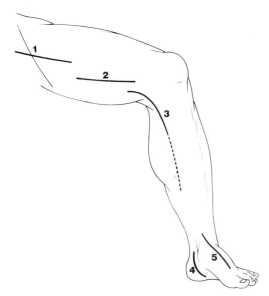

Figure 49–44. *Surgical approaches used for reconstructive operations on arteries below the inguinal ligament.*

(1) Incision for exposure of the common femoral, superficial femoral, and profunda femoris arteries.

(2) Incision for exposure of the midfemoral and upper popliteal arteries in the subsartorial and adductor canals.

(3) Incision for exposure of the lower popliteal arteries. The dotted line shows the extension of this incision downward, through which the posterior tibial and peroneal arteries can be exposed.

(4) Incision for exposure of the posterior tibial artery behind the ankle and the medial malleolus.

(5) Incision for exposure of the dorsalis pedis artery in the foot.

(Fig. 49–44). In patients with infections of the feet, the lymph nodes in the infrainguinal area are usually very large and easily damaged, and bacteria can be cultured from their damaged or cut surfaces. When this situation is encountered, the dissection should be carefully carried around the lymphatic tissue, so that a "lymphatic flap" is lifted to expose the artery. In this way, the lymph nodes are not transected, which would contaminate the field with the bacteria infecting the foot. This is particularly important when a nonautogenous graft is going to be used for a more distal reconstruction. The appropriate antibiotic as determined by culture and sensitivity tests of these bacteria should be used both systemically and in irrigation of the wound to provide a high level of antibiotic coverage in the area of the graft, thus decreasing its contamina-

tion and the potential for subsequent infection as much as possible.

Figure 49–44 illustrates the surgical approaches to the popliteal artery. Whenever it is to be used above the knee, it is found in the subsartorial canal by means of a medial approach. It is generally easier and physiologically more satisfactory to use the popliteal artery below the knee whenever possible. In this region, it is found by downward reflection of the medial head of the gastrocnemius muscle and is dissected in the popliteal space before the soleal arch is encountered. In making both of these incisions, care should be taken to avoid damage to the saphenous vein, which may be directly in the path of the incisions. The most difficult area for exposure of the popliteal artery is between these two points, i.e., in the region of the knee joint itself. In this area, the medial head of the gastrocnemius muscle will require division, as will the tendons of the semimembranosus, semitendonosus, gracilis, and sartorius muscles. The amount of dissection required for this midpopliteal exposure is therefore greater than any of the previous approaches and has a somewhat greater degree of postoperative morbidity.

From a pathologic standpoint, it is preferable to insert the bypass from the common femoral artery to the distal popliteal artery, since pathologic and angiographic studies have shown that these two areas remain relatively free from atheromatous degeneration, although they are certainly not immune by any means, particularly in diabetics.[82] In clinical practice, however, a number of departures from this ideal are used because of certain practical considerations. It is not uncommon to use the upper end of the superficial femoral artery as an inflow source if it can be identified preoperatively and intraoperatively as being relatively free of disease. On the other hand, the upper popliteal artery may be used as the distal site of entry of the bypass, particularly when there is difficulty in obtaining a suitable length of adequate graft. This refers almost exclusively to the graft material that is most commonly used, which is ipsilateral autogenous saphenous vein. In general, this vein is meticulously dissected free from its bed; all its branches are securely ligated;

and the vein is reversed, so that the valves face downward and do not provide a mechanical obstruction to arterial blood flow. Preparation of the vein is extremely important. It has been well shown that warm ischemia of the vein grafts causes endothelial sloughing and degeneration of the myofibrillae.[1] The best method of preservation of such excised reversed veins is therefore their placement in and manipulation with cold heparinized autologous blood.

Although this system has been used in the vast majority of infrainguinal bypasses with saphenous veins, there are certain problems with it. The most obvious difficulty is the mechanical discrepancy between the size of the upper end of the saphenous vein and its lower end. The upper end is usually 6 to 8 mm in size; the lower end will vary at the knee level from 2 to 4 mm in size. Reversal of the vein, therefore, causes the smaller end to be fitted into the larger femoral artery, whereas the large end of the vein is fitted into the smaller popliteal artery. The flow characteristics in such a conduit are therefore hydrostatically very abnormal, and extensive research into this problem now indicates that 4 mm is the lowest acceptable size for the lower end of the reversed saphenous vein. It is possible that as many as 30 per cent of all saphenous veins will not meet this criterion and will therefore be ineligible for use in distal infrainguinal bypass.[133] It is therefore preferable to find a method in which the large end of the saphenous vein is inserted into the common femoral artery and the smaller end is inserted into the distal artery of choice. There are two methods of doing this: (1) utilization of the nonreversed, valve-excised saphenous vein, which is obtained by removal of the saphenous vein from its bed, removal of its valvular obstruction, and its replantation as an arterial graft and (2) the in-situ method of vein bypass in which the vein is left completely in its bed and the valves are excised or rendered incompetent.[77] The latter is a much more suitable and ideal method, since the vasa vasorum are preserved in the living saphenous vein and there is no warm ischemia time. This allows not only for the use of a nonischemic venous conduit but also for the use of veins that are 3 mm or

smaller in size and for insertion into the popliteal artery at the ideal position below the knee (Fig. 49–45). When the reversed saphenous vein is being used, it is generally placed between the heads of the gastrocnemius muscle and follows the natural course of the artery in the subsartorial space. In contrast, the in-situ bypass is left in the subcutaneous position, and the lower free end is rotated in to reach the artery of choice. Although this requires a greater length of mobilized vein, it appears to have no significant effect on the long-term results of this procedure.

Although it is best to place the lower end of the bypass in a popliteal artery, which is continuous with one or more tibial vessels, in many instances, particularly in diabetic patients, the popliteal artery is not continuous with the tibial vessels and its patency is maintained by the genicular arteries (the isolated poplite-

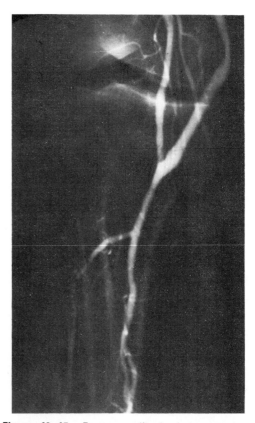

Figure 49–45. *Femoropopliteal vein bypass placed in the optimal position below the knee. Notce that the anterior tibial artery is irregular in its origin and that the tibioperoneal trunk and other arteries appear to be relatively healthy.*

al segment). In other instances, it will simply be so extensively occluded that its use cannot even be considered. In the first situation, it is possible to use the isolated popliteal artery for the lower end of the bypass, and in the second, it will be necessary to use one or more of the tibial or peroneal arteries if these can be visualized angiographically in the infrapopliteal region. Isolated popliteal bypasses will work reasonably well, particularly when used solely for the relief of rest pain. This is because the increase they provide in the vascularity of the foot is obtained by collateral vessels, i.e., the pathway is indirect as opposed to the more direct route of a tibial or peroneal bypass (Fig. 49–46).

With respect to the use of the tibial arteries, the posterior tibial artery is the simplest to use when possible, because it is easy to expose and has the most direct

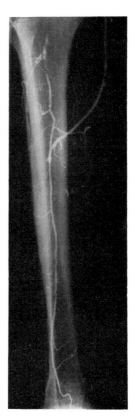

Figure 49–47. *In-situ peroneal bypass. The origin of the peroneal artery from the tibioperoneal trunk was obstructed, and a vein graft was placed in the mid-peroneal position where exposure of the artery is easiest. Notice that the vein graft is about the same size as the peroneal artery, i.e., 2 mm in diameter.*

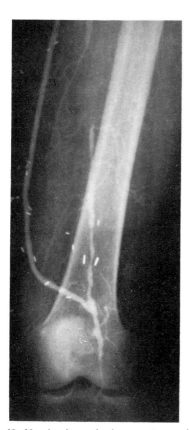

Figure 49–46. *In-situ vein bypass to an isolated popliteal segment. Notice that the artery is irregular and that its outflow tract consists entirely of geniculate and muscular branches. Nevertheless, rest pain was completely relieved by this procedure.*

communication with the deep plantar arch. It is approached by an extension of the medial incision used to expose the popliteal artery and is usually found by retraction of the medial head of the gastrocnemius muscle, division of the medial half of the soleal arch, and detachment of the soleus muscle fibers from the tibia. The artery will then be seen to be traversing or lying on the soleus muscle bed. The peroneal artery is more deeply imbedded in the lower leg but can also be readily exposed through this incision (Fig. 49–47). The peroneal neurovascular bundle lies in the same "arterial plane" as the posterior tibial artery, although it is located 2 to 3 cm more laterally.

The surgical principles governing anterior tibial bypass have been described by us,[69] and in general, anterior tibial by-

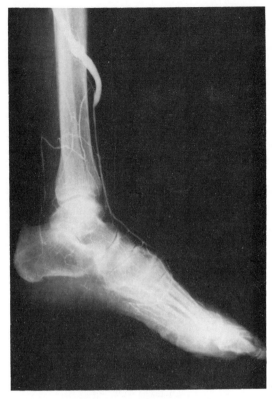

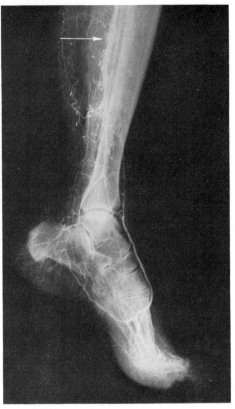

Figure 49–48. Bypass of the anterior tibial artery in the lateral compartment of the leg. This bypass was carried out just above the ankle. The plantar arch is well visualized in the operative angiogram. This patient required two ray resections but has a viable and very functional foot.

Figure 49–49. A distal peroneal bypass. The bypass (arrow) is placed just above the bifurcation of the peroneal artery, which communicates with the plantar arch by means of abundant collateral vessels.

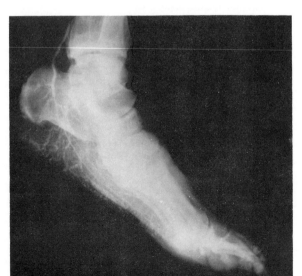

Figure 49–50. Operative angiogram of the posterior tibial artery behind the malleolus. Notice that the deep plantar arch is well filled with contrast material, which represents a very satisfactory outflow tract for distal tibial bypass.

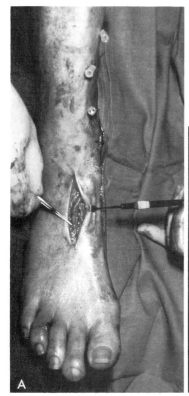

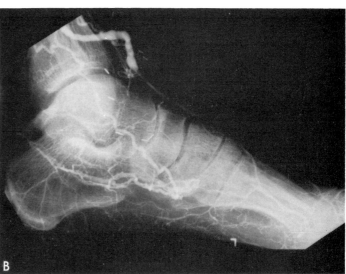

Figure 49–51. (A) Completion of a bypass to the dorsalis pedis artery. The anastomosis is shown by the forceps. Notice the needles inserted in the skin, which act as a grid for operative angiography and the interdigital ischemic ulcer between the third and the fourth toes, which necessitated the bypass. (B) Operative angiogram of this bypass showing communication of the dorsalis pedis artery with the deep plantar arch via its terminal branches.

pass is best carried out into the lateral compartment of the leg (Fig. 49–48). Both anterior and posterior tibial arteries generally become easier to expose as one proceeds distally on the limb, but this is not true of the peroneal artery, which may be quite difficult to expose above the ankle because the tendinous structures do not allow easy retraction for dissection of the artery (Fig. 49–49). In the foot itself, the posterior tibial artery is readily exposed behind the medial malleolus and can be tracked easily as far as the first calcaneal branch (Fig. 49–50). The dorsalis pedis artery will be found on the dorsum of the foot, lying behind the extensor hallucis longus tendon and beneath the extensor retinaculum (Fig. 49–51). The peroneal artery disappears above the ankle and is generally not represented in the foot itself. All of these arteries are arteries of supply, with many small, easily torn branches. Particular care is necessary to preserve these branches, which are important because they provide the run-off for these vessels and are a troublesome source of bleeding if torn.

Some appreciation of the communication of the artery being used with the plantar arch is usually desirable, at least from a prognostic point of view. It has been stated that angiographic demonstration of communication between the tibial or peroneal artery and the plantar arch of the foot is not only desirable but necessary,[56, 64] but we now have experience with a small number of documented cases of bypasses that have been inserted into tibial arteries without direct communication to the plantar arch. These have functioned well and provide sufficient flow into the foot to heal small lesions or to sustain minor amputations (Fig. 49–52).

The size of these tibial vessels is usually about 2 mm or less, and it is in this situation that valve-excised veins with ends that are more closely matched to the size of the tibial artery become most important (see Figure 49–47). Because of the size of these vessels, magnification is mandatory for performing accurate anastomoses. This can usually be obtained with three- to four-power loupes or with six-power magnification on the operating microscope.

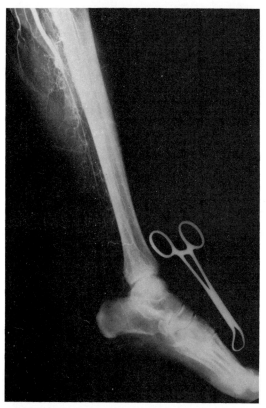

Figure 49–52. *Bypass to the posterior tibial artery that shows no communication to the plantar arch. However, this bypass has continued to function for three years, and the patient is still free of rest pain.*

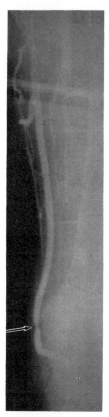

Figure 49–53. *Operative angiogram showing well-marked stenotic lesion in a vein graft (arrow), which required intraoperative correction. Discovery of these lesions intraoperatively and their correction will save subsequent and less rewarding re-explorations of arterial reconstructions.*

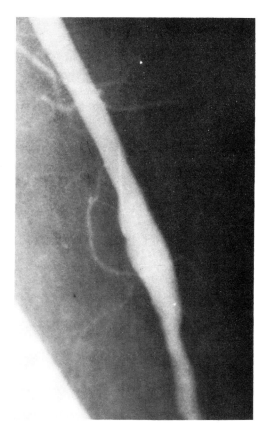

Figure 49–54. Result after femoropopliteal thromboendarterectomy and a vein patch. This is the same artery as in Figure 49–12A.

Needless to say, technical errors are most common during these procedures, and it is here that the routine use of intraoperative angiography is most important[30] (Fig. 49–53). It has proved to be better to spend the extra time at the initial operation to insure the maximum possible reconstructive result than to have to return to the operating room at a later date to perform increasingly less rewarding and more risky attempts at further revisions.[30] Because of the size of the superficial femoral and upper popliteal arteries, and the usual extent of their occlusions when the patient first presents, the opportunities for local endarterectomy or reconstructions are limited. However, when these are present, relatively minor operations will often result in very worthwhile improvements in arterial inflow to the foot. One such example is shown in Figure 49–12, and the completed thrombointimectomy and vein patch graft is shown after its completion in Figure 49–54.

Nonautogenous Materials in Infrainguinal Arterial Surgery

As indicated previously, the saphenous vein either may be present but unsuitable because of size or extensive phlebitic change or may not be present because of previous operative procedures, e.g., stripping of the varicose vein or previous use for bypass. Under these circumstances, when local endarterectomy of the profunda femoris, superficial femoral, or popliteal arteries is not possible, some form of arterial substitute will be required for bypass grafting. A number of prosthetic materials have been used for this purpose. The theoretical principles involve the creation of a graft material whose surface thrombogenicity most closely approaches that of healthy saphenous vein.[144] Dacron has been used extensively but has essentially been abandoned because it functions very poorly below the knee and the very poor results of tibial bypass almost totally exclude its use. It does have a limited use in above-the-knee popliteal bypasses, however. The Sparks mandril device[124] has also been tried but has not found great use. At present, attention is turned almost exclusively to the use of human umbilical vein[29] or to tubes of expanded polytetrafluorethylene (PTFE).[22] There is now an expanding literature on the use of these materials and a regrettable tendency to abandon the use of excellent saphenous veins in favor of them. It is clear, however, that the saphenous vein still remains the material of choice, although these other materials do provide acceptable results as well. It is not yet clear which material will finally prove to be the most satisfactory type of replacement for arteries at the below-the-knee level and size when saphenous vein is not available.

In many patients with aortoiliac disease of one or both sides, the patients' condition or previous operation may make them unsuitable for an intra-abdominal or retroperitoneal procedure. Under these circumstances, the use of long, subcutaneous arterial grafts becomes the procedure of choice.[13] The axillary arteries usually provide the inflow source for these grafts. The right artery is better than the left because of the propensity of the left subclavian artery for stenotic disease. However, grafts have also been led subcutaneously from the carotid arteries and from the aortic arch for this purpose. The placement of these grafts has become increasingly more common because of the observation that the high flow rates that are produced by simultaneous operation from one axillary artery to both femoral arteries provide considerable protection from subsequent platelet deposition within the grafts and their thrombotic occlusion. Nevertheless, it remains true that all grafts in subcutaneous positions are more amenable to mechanical misadventure (e.g., compression during sleeping) than the intra-abdominal or retroperitoneal grafts. However, this approach does provide a very worthwhile alternative to direct aortoiliac reconstruction.

In addition, if the axillary arteries are not available for this use, and the aortoiliac segment has previously been operated on, it remains possible to use the visceral arteries, in particular the celiac axis or superior mesenteric artery, as an inflow source for the femoral or profunda femoris arteries. Much longer lengths of artificial graft are prone to more rapid thrombotic occlusion because of the large area of graft that is exposed to platelet adherence along the surface.

RESULTS OF RECONSTRUCTIVE ARTERIAL SURGERY

Extensive longitudinal prospective studies have now clearly shown the value of arterial reconstructive surgery in salvage of the chronically ischemic foot in which survival is threatened. This holds true both for diabetic and nondiabetic patients. With relatively normal femoral vessels to serve as the distal run-off for aortoiliac reconstruction, the patency rate and foot survival rate of reconstruction starting in the aorta or iliac vessels and terminating in the femoral or profunda femoris vessels should exceed 90 per cent over a five-year period. This figure should stand regardless of the technique used, i.e., endarterectomy or synthetic grafts.[38]

In general, the statistical results become progressively less in terms of five-year survival of the foot as one proceeds distally. Our experience with orifice and extended profundaplasty shows that patients with rest pain symptoms are completely relieved and that the limb and foot survival rate is 90 per cent over a five-year period. However, in patients with ischemic lesions, particularly infected lesions in diabetic patients, the limb and foot survival rate after extended profundaplasty falls to 75 per cent over this period of time. DeWeese and others have shown that autogenous vein bypass grafts continue to function in 70 per cent of instances up to five years[36, 65] and that even after failure, survival of the foot is still assured because of the slow rate of progression of the disease for development of collateral circulation. The results of femorotibial bypass was indicated in the largest series to be about a 50 per cent survival rate of the grafts over two years, with a slightly higher survival rate of the feet themselves after graft failure.[42] Baird and associates have shown that vein bypass grafts functioned well even when inserted into the arteries of the ankle and foot,[3] and these procedures are very worthwhile to insure salvage of the ischemic foot. However, our experience with bypasses inserted to this level indicates that even better results can be obtained when the saphenous vein is used "in situ." With today's technical expertise, therefore, it is possible to perform arterial reconstruction from the infrarenal aorta to the ankle or the foot. In many instances, reconstructions of this extent need to be performed. They can readily be staged. We have previously presented data that allow determination of whether a proximal reconstruction should or should not be followed by more distal reconstruction, as judged by the ultrasound pressures that are obtained after the initial proximal operation. In general, it can be stated that small increments of arterial flow are sufficient for the relief of rest pain, but much larger increments are required to provide for lesion healing, particularly when they are open, infected lesions in patients with long-standing diabetes.[72]

When the reconstructions are successful, the relief of rest pain is immediate.

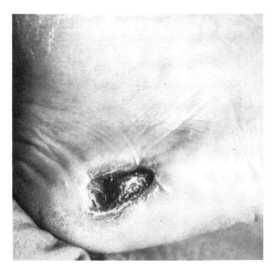

Figure 49–55. *Almost healed and greatly contracted lesion three weeks after femoropopliteal bypass. This is the same patient as in Figure 49–26.*

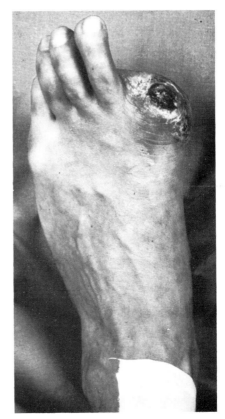

Figure 49–57. *This is the same patient as in Figure 49–32. The lesion healed in spite of injudicious removal of the toe.*

Healing of gangrenous or ulcerated lesions of the foot should start almost immediately and will generally be complete within six weeks. Figure 49–55 shows the same patient as in Figure 49–26 with marked healing and contraction of the nonhealing ulcer three weeks after a femoropopliteal bypass. Figure 49–56 is a two-year follow-up of a patient whose foot was shown in Figure 49–30. The gangrenous area is fully healed after a femorotibial bypass. This patient required excision of half of the os calcis and a skin graft to the underlying bone. Figure 49–57 shows the healed lesion resulting from amputation of the toe depicted in Figure 49–32. A femoropopliteal patch graft was used, and the lesion is almost fully healed two months later. Figure 49–58 shows a large, nonhealing ulcer just above the ankle, which healed following isolated popliteal bypass. Note that in three weeks, the lesion is greatly contracted, and healthy granulations are beginning to appear within the ulcer bed. Figure 49–59 illustrates an important point. On the right side an ischemic lesion is clearly present and a femoropopliteal in-situ bypass has been performed to insure healing of this lesion. Note, however, that on the left great toe, there is a healed area of skin

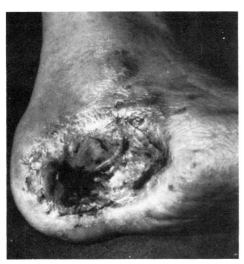

Figure 49–56. *This is the same patient as in Figure 49–30. This extensive gangrenous area required removal of half of the os calcis and a skin graft of the subsequent granulating bed. The lesion has remained healed and stable for four years.*

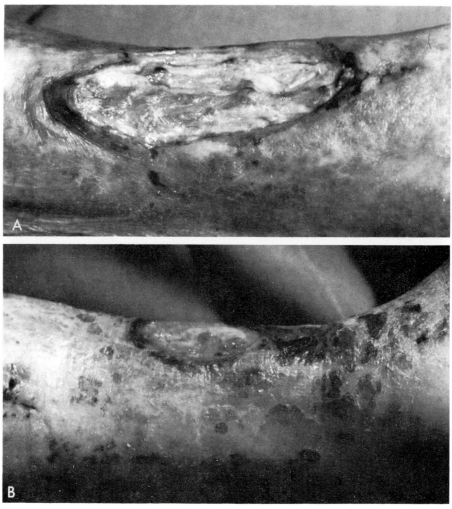

Figure 49–58. (A) Large nonhealing ischemic ulcer just above the foot. This has been present for six months, and many attempts at local treatment were unavailing. (B) Same lesion two weeks after arterial reconstruction. The lesion is considerably shrunken and shows signs of healthy granulation. It finally healed one month later with placement of a skin graft.

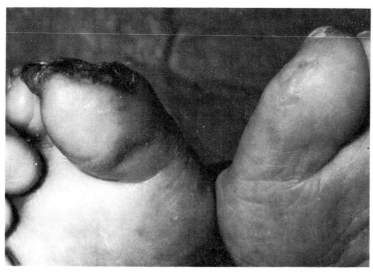

Figure 49–59. The right great toe is obviously the site of an ischemic ulcer which was healed by an in-situ femoropopliteal bypass. Note, however, that the left toe shows a healed area, which was identical to the lesion on the right six months previously and which also required an in-situ femoropopliteal bypass. This case illustrates the propensity for ischemic lesions to appear on the opposite foot with great frequency within 12 months of the original onset of recognizable clinical ischemia.

that represented an identical lesion that was present six months previously and for which an in-situ bypass was also performed. It is a well-known clinical observation that in patients with ischemic lesions of one foot, the chances of the limb-threatening condition affecting the other foot exceeds 30 per cent within 12 months of the onset of the original lesion. These experiences underline and re-emphasize the need for continued and careful follow-up of these patients by both the surgeon and the family practitioner and by the patients themselves in their education and training to recognize what might be rapidly developing or potential problems in their feet.

EDEMA OF THE FOOT AFTER PROXIMAL ARTERIAL RECONSTRUCTION

Edema of the lower leg and foot is common after bypass procedures involving the femoral and popliteal arteries. Although this would at first appear to be caused by venous trauma that occurs during the surgical procedure, careful venographic studies have shown that this is not so. It is much more likely that surgical lymphatic disturbance is responsible for this edema, which can be very pronounced in some patients. It is particularly important to preserve the lymphatic channels during dissection as much as possible. This is not the sole explanation for the edema, however. In some patients in whom very little anatomic disturbance of the lymphatic channels has occurred, swelling perists because of an altered hemodynamic state of the capillary walls during a long period of chronic ischemia. Under these circumstances, the capillary wall is so permanently damaged by the ischemia that leakage of proteinaceous material occurs through the basement membranes when the arterial pressure is increased. This material accumulates in the extravascular space and is not recovered via the capillary wall or cleared by the lymphatic circulation. The management of this problem is by the use of pressure-graded external support and continued active exercises of the foot, which seem to help in relieving the edema over a period of weeks.[104]

THROMBOANGIITIS OBLITERANS

Thromboangiitis obliterans was first described by Buerger in 1908 and occurs with far less frequency than does arteriosclerosis obliterans. Thromboangiitis obliterans is a disease that is rarely seen, even by surgeons who exclusively practice vascular surgery. The diagnosis is made far more commonly than the incidence of the disease warrants, and it is frequently confused with Raynaud's phenomenon and vasospastic conditions caused by other diseases. It was originally thought to occur exclusively in the Jewish population, but it is now known to affect people of all ethnic backgrounds.[63] It occurs predominantly in males under the age of 40. Females are much less commonly affected. Although the lower extremities are affected primarily, the upper extremities may become involved as well in time. This is a marked difference from the natural history of arteriosclerosis.[88] In a substantial number of patients, there is a premonitory history of superficial migratory phlebitis, and the disease quite frequently first presents with this complaint.

The cause of thromboangiitis obliterans is not known. However, the relationship of this disease to tobacco smoking is extremely pronounced. Tobacco (nicotine) smoking causes the most rapid and rampant progression of this disease, and many authorities consider this disease to represent early malignant arteriosclerosis, which is either caused by or is extremely sensitive to tobacco (nicotine) smoking. Many of the patients who contract this disease are not necessarily heavy smokers, but it is a common finding that patients with this disease who have stopped smoking will maintain a reasonable level of circulation, which deteriorates noticeably within a few days of resumption of cigarette smoking. However, it is also curious that only a minority of all cigarette smokers ever develop this particular syndrome.

Microscopically, the disease affects the smaller arteries and arterioles, but it will eventually involve the larger vessels at the tibial level. The pathologic findings are those of a noninfective panvasculitis associated with a proliferation of intimal cells and cellular infiltration, particularly around the vasa vasorum and adventitial

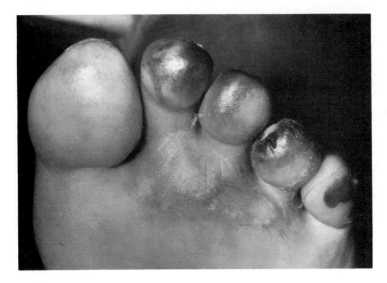

Figure 49–60. *Appearance of the toes in a patient with early thromboangiitis. Four of the toes show small areas of gangrenous skin, and two of the toes have small ulcers at the tips.*

layers. In almost all instances, there is a highly organized obstructive thrombus. In general, this disease is more rapidly progressive than arteriosclerosis, and the major amputation rate is considerable despite all attempts at treatment. Unlike arteriosclerosis, the clinical symptom pattern usually starts as intermittent claudication affecting the small muscles of the foot rather than the gastrocnemius-soleus muscle. This occurs because the digital arteries and the plantar arch are first involved by the disease. At this stage, the dorsalis pedis and posterior tibial pulses may still be felt by the observer. However, transmetatarsal PVR tracings will show lack of pulsatile flow at this level,[135] and this coupled with failure to find Doppler signals in the digital arteries will usually provide the first clue to the onset of thromboangiitis obliterans. Claudication of the calf muscles is less pronounced, although as the disease extends more proximally it may also appear. However, by this time the foot will already be showing advanced and quite severe ischemia, and one or more of the toes will have died or been amputated (Fig. 49–60).

Recurrent episodes of quite painful superficial thrombophlebitis may also occur in conjunction with these symptoms in short segments of apparently normal veins of the upper and lower extremities. It is at this stage that thromboangiitis obliterans is most often confused with other disease processes. The differential diagnosis is usually fairly simple, since Raynaud's disease usually affects the hands of young females, and vasospastic disorders do not generally progress to threatened tissue loss except in patients with collagen diseases (e.g., scleroderma). Radiographic evidence of calcification of the digital arteries appears to be reasonable evidence that the lesions are atherosclerotic rather than thromboangiitic, since calcification is almost never seen in this condition. The arteriographic findings are typical enough of this disease and will provide good evidence of the diagnosis by a demonstration of sharply defined occlusions in the digital or tibial vessels and their replacement by many fine collateral vessels classically in a corkscrew configuration. The site where these vessels are best demonstrated is in the region of the ankle (Fig. 49–61). The arterial walls of any patent vessels usually appear to be quite undiseased, as opposed to those in patients who have diffuse arteriosclerosis. The course of the disease in patients with thromboangiitis obliterans is greatly influenced by their ability to stop smoking completely and permanently. Even in patients who smoke as little as five cigarettes a day, continued progression of the disease is the rule, and major amputations of the foot and even the limb at very high levels will be the inevitable result. Gangrene usually begins at the tips of the toes, extends onto the forefoot, and then inexorably involves the ankle and calf muscles. Even though the patient may have stopped smoking, the digits are still very sensitive to minor degrees of trauma

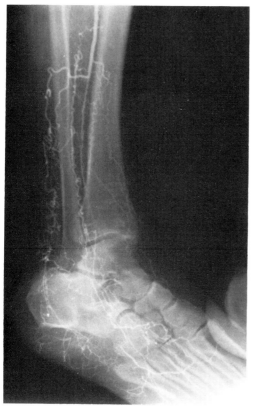

Figure 49–61. *Angiographic appearance of thromboangiitis. The anterior tibial artery stops abruptly, and there are numerous fine, corkscrew, collateral vessels around the ankle. The plantar arch is poorly developed.*

and may ulcerate or become gangrenous with relative ease. The rate of limb loss in this disease, as stated previously, is extremely high, but curiously, these patients appear to have a normal life span as compared with those with arteriosclerosis. The cause of this is unknown, since the coronary arteries may reasonably be expected to suffer the same fate as the smaller arteries in the limbs. In some instances, very large arteries, such as the superior mesenteric artery, may become acutely obstructed and life-threatening, although this is a rare occurrence.

Treatment (See also Chronic Ischemia, Conservative Management)

The fundamental basis of treatment of this disease is the avoidance of inhalation of tobacco smoke in any form whatsoever.

This not only applies to direct smoking of cigarettes, cigars, or pipes, but also encompasses the inhalation of smoke exhaled by other tobacco smokers. The patient must be told with considerable firmness about this, and no opportunity should be lost for re-emphasizing the absolute necessity for avoidance of smoking and inhalation of smoke for the rest of his life.[114] Local lesions of the foot should be treated according to well-recognized surgical principles, that is, small abscesses should be drained, necrotic tissue should be removed, and local infection should be treated by the application of a non–tissue-toxic material that is bacteriostatic, e.g., povidone-iodine. The chances for vascular reconstruction for salvage of the foot in these patients are small to nonexistent. Vasodilating agents have been tried in many instances but are generally ineffective. In some patients, lumbar sympathectomy may be of use in the healing of lesions of the skin, but its effect is not long-lived. In any event, it cannot and will not overcome the effects of continued tobacco smoking.

RAYNAUD'S PHENOMENON AND COLD SENSITIVITY

Raynaud's phenomenon is defined as episodic attacks of vasoconstriction of the smaller arteries (mainly digital) of the hand and foot when they are exposed to cold environmental conditions. The attacks can be recognized clinically by successive color changes, which first take the form of extreme pallor, followed by a bluish discoloration or cyanosis and then a deep red flush.[108] When this condition occurs in patients with no other associated diseases, it is referred to as Raynaud's disease, and when it occurs in association with other diseases (mainly of the collagen variety), it is referred to as Raynaud's phenomenon. However, it is uncertain whether a pathologic entity such as primary Raynaud's disease actually exists, since many patients with this condition will eventually show clear evidence of widespread collagen disease such as scleroderma or dermatomyositis. The intense vasoconstriction caused by exposure to cold is due to sudden severe spasm of their arteries and arterioles, which become dilated after a short interval because of an accumulation of anoxic metabolic products. Although it has been very difficult to demonstrate that there is specific sympathetic overactivity, much circumstantial evidence appears to indicate that the basic abnormality is that of a markedly increased sympathetic reaction to cold. Porter and associates have also demonstrated arteriographically this immediate and prolonged reaction of arterial spasm after exposure to cold water and have shown that there is a high titer of autoantibody formation and reduced levels of complement in these patients.[105] They suggest that a cold-stimulated antibody may be responsible for the peripheral arterial spasm and that this is the reason why sympathectomy is not totally effective in the treatment of this condition. However, it is clear that no single explanation will cover all the findings and that there is a range of cold sensitivity from subjective feelings of discomfort to excruciating pain because of total cessation of arterial flow for a period of time.

Raynaud's disease occurs almost exclusively in young adult females. The problem is almost universally bilateral and will affect males as well as females when collagen diseases are the underlying cause. There is no ethnic preference. In some patients, it is hard to document this disease, and the attack may have to be induced by deliberate exposure to cold before the examiner can be totally convinced. Furthermore, in some patients, the prolonged ischemic episodes will lead to small skin ulcerations, which will generally occur on several digits simultaneously. The nail bed is very frequently affected, and nail growth is subsequently impaired. The other clinical signs of collagen diseases should be sought, and investigations for these signs should be a matter of routine. Even though these investigations may prove negative initially, it is a common experience that over 80 per cent of these patients will eventually show other signs of collagen diseases (e.g., esophageal stricture in scleroderma). However, one of the simplest tests is repeated measuring of the sedimentation rate, elevation of which points to some form of generalized systemic disorder. Oc-

casionally, if the disease appears to have a nerve distribution, conduction velocities of that particular nerve should be measured, since this may represent a simple and relatively easily curable form of nerve entrapment rather than Raynaud's disease. In doubtful cases, measurement of the digital temperature recovery time is useful. In this test, after stabilization of the foot temperature in a warm room, a thermistor probe is used to measure digital temperature immediately after insertion of the foot in an ice water mixture. In most normal people, skin temperature will return to the normal level within 10 minutes, but if skin temperature has not fully recovered after 20 minutes, this is good presumptive evidence of Raynaud's disease. Arteriography is not usually used for diagnosis of this condition, but it should be performed whenever there is doubt about whether other disease processes may be present.

Treatment

The treatment of patients with this disease is careful avoidance of exposure to cold. In most patients this will suffice, and they soon learn to identify the conditions that cause some of their greatest problems. In cool conditions, the use of comfortable gloves may be necessary, even while working indoors. Such simple adjustments will prevent most attacks and reduce the possibility of skin loss because of temporary ischemia. Surgical sympathectomy has generally been disappointing, since the condition tends to recur within six months if no other precautions are taken. The best results are obtained from the use of drugs that decrease the transmission of sympathetic impulses. Prolonged improvement has been obtained with intra-arterial reserpine, but the need for intra-arterial puncture greatly limits the usefulness of this form of therapy. The oral administration of alpha-receptor-blocking drugs will help most patients who cannot be cured by simple avoidance of cold. Guanethidine and phenoxybenzamine appear to offer the best results. The use of immunosuppressive drugs has been tried sporadically, but sufficient clinical information is not yet available.

Cold Sensitivity Following Cold Injury

Many patients will suffer from persistent cold sensitivity of the foot after recovery from prolonged exposure to severe cold with or without the development of frostbite. In these patients, feelings of numbness persist even when the foot is warm, and the toes become particularly painful, with an unhealthy bluish discoloration when exposed to cold again. The reason for this increase in sensitivity to cold is not known, but it is presumed to be a causalgic phenomenon. In this condition, surgical sympathectomy has had better results than in Raynaud's disease, but the oral alpha-blocking drugs will provide quite reasonable relief for the majority of patients.

VENOUS DISORDERS OF THE FOOT

Venous Thrombosis

The form of venous thrombosis traditionally considered to be clinically most important is that which occurs in the deep veins of the foot, calf, and thigh. In this context, "deep" is used to distinguish these veins from the subcutaneous or superficial veins of the lower limb. The mechanisms that initiate venous thrombosis are still largely speculative, although a number of causes are clearly recognizable. There is usually a background of inactivity because of confinement to bed or to a seat, such as in an automobile or an airplane during long travel. Surgical operations and chronic congestive cardiac failure are also well-known contributory causes. Indeed, autopsy studies have shown that fully three fourths of patients who died after more than one week of confinement to bed had identifiable premortem thrombi within the veins of the soleal sinuses or tibial veins. These studies have been confirmed by ^{125}I-labeled fibrinogen examinations, which have indicated that, at least in surgical patients, thrombi have been found to begin developing on the operating table. The most common site of occurrence of venous thrombosis is unquestionably in the soleal sinuses and paired tibial veins, but the iliofemoral venous segment, consisting of the common femoral, external iliac, and common iliac veins, is also frequently affected and constitutes a much greater threat to both life and limb.[83] Just how any of these events cause or initiate venous thrombosis is largely unknown. Stasis occurs after surgical operation both because of the patient's relative immobility and because flow studies have demonstrated that there is an absolute reduction in the speed of venous return following operations on the abdomen or lower limb. However, despite these well-authenticated observations, the clinical symptoms and signs of deep venous thrombosis do not generally appear for seven to 10 days following operation. Thus, there appears to be some discrepancy between the time of initiation of the process and the time of appearance of the clinical symptomatology.

Other disease conditions are also known to be associated with deep vein thrombosis. The incidence increases in patients with all forms of thrombocytosis, particularly polycythemia rubra vera, or after splenectomy for hemotologic or reticuloendothelial disorders. There is a clear association with certain malignant neoplasms, especially those of the bronchus, pancreas, and kidney, and, in fact, massive venous thrombosis may first herald the appearance of very small neoplasms of these types that are difficult to detect. Thrombophlebitis migrans has already been mentioned as part of the symptom pattern in thromboangiitis obliterans. It is also clear now that estrogen administration, whether for therapeutic reasons (e.g., for cancer of the prostate or breast) or in the form of a contraceptive pill, creates a statistically significantly greater risk of venous thrombosis. It has been shown that this form of therapy usually produces a drop in the antithrombin concentration, thus predisposing patients even more to thrombosis.[43]

Since the calf veins are the best known site of thrombotic initiation, relation of this event to other thrombotic processes has been the subject of intense investigation. Bauer has shown angiographic evidence that calf vein thrombosis may extend from the tibial veins into the popliteal veins and then into the femoral veins.[9] It has also been suggested from time to time that the plantar veins of the foot may be the site of incipient thrombosis, which extends into the tibial veins and then propagates to the larger veins of the lower limb.[94] This theory has never gained support because it has never been fully examined by isotope or venographic studies. In addition, ultrasound examination of the veins of the foot has never supported this concept, and although autopsy studies of the pedal veins are uncommon, premortem thrombosis has never been noticed as a feature in these examinations.

Symptoms and Signs of Deep Venous Thrombosis

The traditional sign of deep venous thrombosis is mild pain or tightness in the calf that is constant, especially when the patient is walking. The patient may also notice swelling of the foot and calf area. Swelling of the calf is particularly evident when the thrombotic process has occluded the femoral venous outflow tract. The classic signs that are used in the diagnosis of this condition are tenderness of the gastrocnemius-soleus muscle, cyanotic discoloration of the foot, distention of the superficial veins, and pitting edema of the foot and ankle. It is now abundantly but belatedly clear, however, that many of these signs are simply those of any inflammatory process in this area and can be reproduced by many other common conditions. For example, they will be present in all instances of intramuscular hematoma, true infection, or even rupture of the plantaris tendon of which the patient was unaware.

The clinical diagnosis of venous thrombosis of the calf veins is therefore fallible in at least 50 per cent of instances.[28] It is also apparent that when thrombi are present in large proximal veins but are not completely obstructive, they may not be recognized clinically at all. It is apparent, therefore, that the diagnosis of venous thrombosis can no longer be based on clinical appreciation alone but must be confirmed by a more objective diagnostic measure.[131] This will be discussed subsequently. In two conditions, however, clinical diagnosis will be very accurate. The first condition is acute iliofemoral venous thrombosis. In this condition, the entire limb is swollen from the inguinal ligament to the foot and has a bluish discoloration, with distention of the superficial veins and subcutaneous venules. The foot is usually severely swollen, with stiff, pitting edema. The femoral vein can commonly be felt as a tender cord-like structure just below the inguinal ligament because it is solidly packed with a soft thrombus, which generates a small inflammatory component. The saphenous vein is frequently patent from the foot to the groin, and this can usually be confirmed by Doppler ultrasound. The second condition that is easily recognizable clinically is progressive saphenous phlebitis. The finding of a solid subcutaneous venous cord is usually indicative of saphenous vein or superficial thrombophlebitis. This, incidentally, is almost the only true "phlebitis," and for this reason, the condition is quite painful. In addition, the saphenous nerve, which is adjacent to the saphenous vein, is also considerably irritated by this process and is another source of discomfort. However, the inflammatory adherence of the thrombus to the vein wall usually prevents its disruption and proximal embolization. The proximal involvement of this vein can be mapped on a daily basis by both the patient and the physician. The "tongue" of a thrombus always extends more proximally than the clinical signs of redness or tenderness. Therefore, when the process can be clinically detected in the upper thigh, the probability of extension into the common femoral vein is high. In addition, there may be coexistent, nonocclusive thrombosis of serious pathologic significance within the common femoral vein itself.[48]

In general, therefore, when the diagnosis of venous thrombosis is being considered, some means other than clinical examinations must be employed for confirmation of this diagnosis. Venous impedance plethysmography is a relatively simple, noninvasive test but has its greatest accuracy when the thrombotic occlusions are in the femoral vein.[93] Isotope venography with technetium-99m has also been used but has not found much popularity. In contrast, development of the use of radioisotope-labeled fibrinogen in the detection of venous thrombosis is well advanced.[53] This examination, which is now done almost exclusively with ^{125}I-labeled fibrinogen is very accurate in the detection of tibial vein thrombosis. For example, studies have shown that 30 per cent of patients develop venous thrombi at the time of or within 24 hours of surgery.[124] However, the vast majority of these thrombi are clinically silent and, indeed, clinically insignificant. This test, therefore, appears to be too sensitive for routine use.[85] It also has the serious disadvantage of having to be administered before thrombi

actually begin to form or during the period of active thrombogenicity.[76] Nevertheless, venographic examination with radioactive iodinized fibrinogen has provided considerable insight into the pathogenesis of venous thrombosis in the lower leg and must still be regarded as the most important examination in the investigative and scientific study of this problem.

The Doppler ultrasound stethoscope is of great bedside and laboratory value for

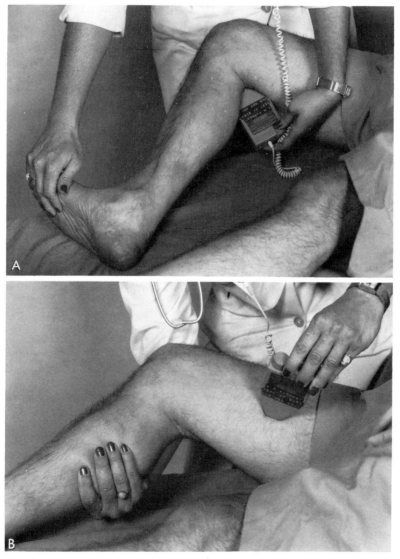

Figure 49–62. (A) Optimum position for ultrasound examination of the veins of the lower limb. The knee is slightly flexed and the hip is externally rotated. The popliteal veins of the foot and calf are accentuated by passive motion of the foot through the full range of the ankle joint. (B) Further details of the technique. The midfemoral vein is being examined, and flow waves are produced by the technique of alternating manual compression and relaxation of the calf muscle. The signals are heard and interpreted by the observer.

the evaluation of obstructive lesions of the venous circulation from the popliteal vein[7] to the common femoral vein.[142] Careful studies that have compared clinical and Doppler ultrasound evaluations of lower extremity venous thrombosis confirmed by venography show that the Doppler ultrasound stethoscope is of excellent diagnostic value when compared with both clinical and radiocontrast venographic examinations. Ultrasound examination is much less predictive when used in the detection of tibial vein thrombosis,[121] and the signals are very difficult to interpret over the veins of the plantar and dorsal venous arches. However, with continuing experience and the use of more sensitive instruments (9 to 10 mHz), quite reasonable information can be obtained even from the veins of the foot. The patient is usually examined in the supine position with the lower limb completely relaxed, the hip externally rotated, and the knee slightly flexed (Fig. 49–62A). This gives excellent access to all veins, including the greater saphenous vein at the ankle. Normal signals are low-pitched with a variable range of frequencies, particularly during respiratory movements. Venous flow induced by distal muscle compression and flexion and extension of the ankle (Fig. 49–62B) usually produces a "windstorm" effect, which sounds like air being expelled from an inflated balloon. When the probe is placed over a totally obstructed vein, there is no signal, even with these means of flow augmentation. Placement of the probe over a vein distal to an obstructive lesion will generally provide a continuous signal unaffected by the respiratory phases. This occurs particularly when the resultant venous hypertension is at such a level that it is not affected by changes in intra-abdominal or intrathoracic pressure.

However, despite these advances in the noninvasive diagnosis of acute venous thrombosis, the best of all diagnostic methods continues to be the radiologic contrast venogram because of its ease of performance, relative lack of invasiveness, and accuracy. New techniques of venography and the use of anteroposterior and lateral projections have also improved the diagnostic information from this study to a point of high accuracy (Fig. 49–63). Some problems are still experienced with venog-

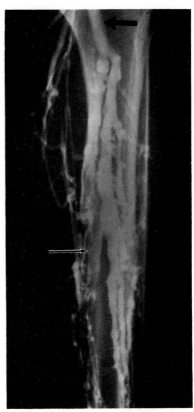

Figure 49–63. *Venogram of the tibial veins. The small arrow points to one of the paired posterior tibial veins, which is filled with thrombus and shows "ghosting" of the contrast material within its walls. This suggests that the thrombus is unattached and is capable of embolic dislodgement. The larger arrow indicates the popliteal vein that is free of thrombus.*

raphy in the calf area because of the overlap of tibial veins and because of the difficulty of determining whether the filling defect is acute or of longer duration (Fig. 49–64). However, in general, venographic confirmation is much to be desired whenever there is any diagnostic suspicion of venous thrombosis. In practice, therefore, a practical method of diagnostic approach is the use of Doppler ultrasound either at the bedside or in the laboratory, with radiologic contrast venographic confirmation thereafter.

Management of Acute Venous Thrombosis

At present, the management of lower limb deep venous thrombosis consists of strict bed rest, with elevation of the legs to

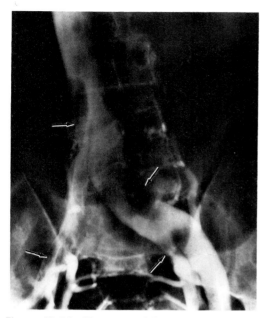

Figure 49–64. *Venogram of the common iliac veins and the inferior vena cava. The arrows point out areas of translucency, which appear to be thrombi within these vessels. This venogram was performed by contrast injection from veins in the dorsum of the foot and represents a greatly increased ability to obtain detailed information of the entire venous tree through a relatively noninvasive procedure.*

45 degrees. The knees should be slightly bent for maximum patient comfort. This position has been shown by radiosodium studies to more than double the speed of venous return to the limb, thus effectively obviating the role of stasis in further formation of thrombi (Fig. 49–65). This will be considerably assisted by regular activation of the calf muscle "pump," which is best achieved by training the patient to move the foot through the maximum range of ankle joint motion for specific intervals of time, for example, 10 minutes every hour. It is our experience that in the vast majority of instances, this mode of therapy will be extremely effective in producing swift resolution of the symptoms and signs of acute venous thrombosis.

The presently accepted therapeutic norm is the systemic delivery of heparin in addition to the measures just enumerated.[10] This can be given by intermittent intramuscular injection (100 units per kilogram body weight every four to six hours) or by constant infusion by pump. Both regimens should provide for a reasonably steady elevation of partial thromboplastin time (PTT) of two to three times normal levels. In most institutions, however, the hemorrhagic complications of heparin therapy are forcing further examinations of the routine use of this drug by a series of measurements on healthy medical students as well as on patients on carefully controlled continuous and pump infusion of heparin. We have found that there are severe and unpredictable fluctuations of PTT, which daily exceed the desired therapeutic levels on many occasions (pre-

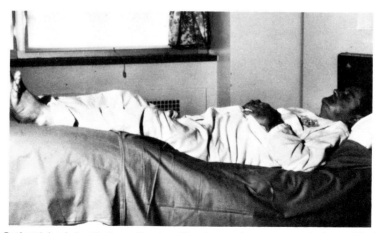

Figure 49–65. *Patient lying in bed in the optimal position for maximum venous drainage. The trunk is parallel to the floor, the thigh is raised 45 degrees, and the break at the knee joint enables the patient to lie comfortably without jeopardizing the most efficient venous drainage from the limb.*

sumably bleeding can and will occur during these unwelcome peaks of anticoagulant activity). Heparin is, however, of unquestioned use in patients with known pulmonary emboli and iliofemoral venous thrombosis in whom the risk of embolic dislodgment is great.

Subsidence of the swelling of the foot and leg signals that the venous collaterals are developing and that the thrombi are becoming organized and adherent to the vein walls. Patients can then be gradually mobilized, wearing efficient pressure-graded below-the-knee elastic stockings. Heparin therapy should be converted to oral anticoagulation after seven days, and this should be continued for three months and then discontinued if there are no further signs of development of venous thrombi. During this time, the stringent use of pressure-graded elastic support must be maintained, because the prevention of subcutaneous edema is of primary importance until stabilization of the collateral pathways is obtained. The prevention of chronic subcutaneous edema is of profound pathologic and prognostic significance for the foot. Uncontrolled persistence of swelling of the foot for a period of weeks will allow the ingrowth of fibrous tissue into the subcutaneous tissue. This will strangulate the microlymphatic circulation, thus leading to chronic and intractable lymphedema in association with any degree of venous hypertension already present. The skin becomes brawny and indurated, and its nutrition is then permanently disturbed. The undrained lymphatic pools provide an excellent substrate for bacterial growth, and the foot proceeds to suffer from serial attacks of low-grade noninvasive infection, usually of a streptococcal nature. Each infectious episode inflicts further damage on the lymphatic drainage, and the course of the disease is a continuous downhill spiral that leads to the development of chronic irreversible subcutaneous edema. Therefore, vigorous treatment in the first instance to prevent and control swelling of the foot will be considerably beneficial later. Within a period of three months, these rigid measures can be relaxed considerably, because by then, the collateral, venous, and lymphatic pathways will be fully established. With moderation of the patient's living and exercise habits, control of swelling becomes relatively simple. In most instances, physician time is not taken up with this stage, provided that patient education is instituted promptly and forcefully from the time of the first episode.

Chronic Venous Insufficiency

Chronic venous insufficiency is the pathologic state that ensues when venous outflow from the foot is severely and permanently impaired because of extensive obstruction of the tibial and/or popliteal and femoral veins or when valvular incompetence induced by intravascular diseases becomes so severe that venous outflow is permanently impaired. As a result of one or both of these pathologic events, the venous pressure in the deep veins of the foot[6] rises precipitously and is not reduced by exercise, as occurs in the normal physiologic state. In fact, in many instances, the effect of exercise causes such an increase in venous pressure that the systolic arterial pressure can commonly be exceeded.[103] These changes have also been observed during acute venous thrombosis but are resolved when treatment has been properly instituted.[5] When these changes of chronic venous insufficiency become fixed, it is clear that there will be considerable disturbance of Starling's equilibrium in the tissues of the foot. This therefore "sets the stage" for the permanent brawny edema of both subcutaneous and deep tissues that is so uncomfortable for the patient and so difficult for the physician to eradicate. Tissue of this type is particularly susceptible to ongoing attacks of low-grade streptococcal infection, which increases the inflammatory tissue, leading to the deposition of fibrous tissue and strangulation of the lymphatic circulation. This further compounds the already disordered physiology of fluid transfer in the tissues of the foot (Fig. 49–66).

Another equally common result of chronic venous insufficiency and venous hypertension is the development of stasis dermatitis and ulceration. Characteristically, this occurs in the lower third of the leg around the malleoli, and the area just above the medial malleolus is most affected. Because of the severe, chronic disturb-

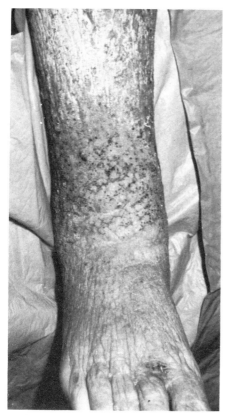

Figure 49–66. *Long-standing brawny edema of the foot due to chronic venous insufficiency. The speckled area is indicative of epithelial breakdown and is a potentially ulcerative area. The wrinkles have occurred after a period of maximum venous drainage, which allows the edema to subside. This is not to be confused with chronic lymphedema.*

venous insufficiency and stasis ulceration is compounded by an ischemic component, thus exposing the patient to the worst of both conditions. Treatment of this problem must be pursued in the same manner as previously described. Elevation of the leg to prevent further edema and to promote venous drainage must be regularly maintained not only during the hours of sleep, but also as much as possible during working and ambulant hours. External support of the leg with elastic stockings or with Unna boot paste bandages, which provide better support, together with simple dressings (e.g., povidone-iodine), is absolutely necessary to maintain bacteriostasis of the ulcer surface and to promote healing. When these measures are working well, the ulcer quickly granulates

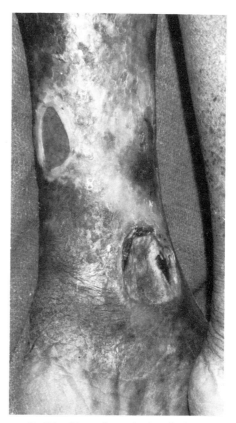

Figure 49–67. *Clean, "punched-out" ulcers on the medial aspect of the leg just above the medial malleolus. The white areas of skin are the end result of a chronic, low-grade, subcutaneous streptococcal infection that has caused the formation of a great deal of fibrosis in the skin. (Compare these ulcers with those shown in Figure 49–26.)*

ances of dermal nutrition, subcutaneous fat is slowly lost over this area, so that the skin becomes closely approximated to the bone. In addition, the breakdown of red cells leads to the deposition of hemosiderin in the skin, producing an irreversible dark-brown pigmentation. Because of the loss of subcutaneous tissue, the shape of the ankle becomes considerably narrowed at this point and has the appearance of an inverted bottle. With continued breakdown of the skin, a chronic stasis ulcer then develops. This ulcer is shallow, with an irregular shape and a granulating base with rounded edges. It is not as clearly "punched out" as an ischemic ulcer and is not associated with the degree of pain of an ischemic ulcer (Fig. 49–67). In a few instances, the problem of chronic and will either heal completely or accept skin grafts readily. Once the ulcer has healed, continuation of the prophylactic measures to prevent further ulceration and stabilization of this permanently unstable area must continue for the rest of the patient's life. If incompetent perforators can be demonstrated by ultrasound[6] or venography, consideration should be given to ligation of these vessels, which will materially aid in short- and long-term healing. If rapid healing does not occur within six weeks, the arterial circulation should be evaluated. In the presence of obstructive arterial disease, surgical attempts should be made to restore distal pulsatile inflow, since it is our experience that this promotes very rapid healing.[73]

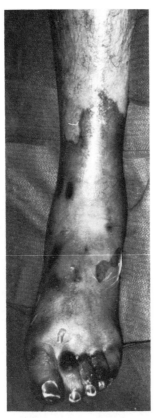

Figure 49–68. *Rare clinical entity of venous gangrene following phlegmasia cerulea dolens. Despite massive swelling and demarcating skin changes in this foot, arterial signals could be heard with great clarity even at this stage. A below-the-knee amputation was eventually required.*

Phlegmasia Cerulea Dolens

Iliofemoral venous thrombosis, previously described, refers to massive interference of the venous outflow from the foot and lower limb because of proximal venous obstruction in the iliofemoral venous segments.[83] Although this is an uncomfortable situation, it very rarely progresses to such an extent that it compromises the arterial circulation of the foot.[18] However, in a few instances the venous obstruction becomes so profound that arterial inflow is brought to a virtual halt by the total lack of venous outflow.[123] At this point, the viability of the foot is clearly threatened. This condition is extremely difficult to treat and more often than not leads to loss of the foot (Fig. 49–68). It is in this situation that venous thrombectomy should be strongly considered, although the results of this procedure in salvage of the foot are disappointing because of the inability to clear the smaller tibial channels on which venous outflow from the foot depends.[84]

REPLANTATION OF THE FOOT

The biologic advances in whole organ transplantation during the 1960's and the technologic advances of several surgical specialties have expanded the application of the surgery of small blood vessels in many directions. With the rapid advancement of microsurgical knowledge, few systems or organs have not been restored, repaired, or improved by microsurgery. The application of microsurgical techniques in the reconstruction of severely injured and amputated lower extremities has also been extremely successful.

To date, opportunities for replantation of the lower extremity and foot have been sparse. The Chinese have reported some of these cases, and four of their attempts have been briefly examined by English-speaking physicians and described in the literature. McDowell has seen a replantation at the ankle level.[86] O'Brien[95] and Roth[112] have also described above-the-ankle replantations seen in Peking. In one of these patients, because of the severe soft-tissue damage at the mid-leg level of the right leg and at the ankle on the left leg, a formal below-the-knee amputation was carried out on the right side, but the undamaged right foot was attached to the left leg. A similar cross-leg replantation of the foot that was performed in Shanghai has also been described.[95] We have replanted two transtarsal amputations and have reported them with sufficient documentation for clinical study.[54, 55, 60] We have also performed one successful above-the-ankle replantation.[89] Although the number of these cases is not sufficient for statistical analytical conclusions, certain principles regarding replantation of the foot have clearly emerged from these experiences.

Theoretical Considerations

When a foot has been amputated, replantation should be considered in every circumstance. As in many areas of surgical endeavor, the expertise of the replantation team and the quality of their decisions are directly related to their experience. Although it is acknowledged that infants and children sustain injuries that lend themselves more easily to replantation and demonstrate better return of function, candidacy for replantation should be based on physiologic rather than chronologic criteria.

Because of the experience gained in replantation of upper extremities and digits, guidelines can now be set down for amputated parts of the lower extremities. It seems clear that replantation of one or more toes would be indicated only in the more unusual circumstances. Function of the foot in the absence of one or all of the toes is satisfactory in all age groups.

In contrast, however, traumatic midtarsal, Chopart's, and above-the-ankle amputations should always be considered for replantation because of the potential for restoration of significant and worthwhile function. As O'Brien has noted, the preservation of even a partially sensitive foot is far superior to a prosthetic device and justifies these replantation efforts.[96] All total foot and lower leg amputations should also be considered for replantation, although our experience has shown that the higher the level of amputation, the greater the force required to separate the member from the body, and this is always reflected in a more extensive degree of soft-tissue and osseous damage. (The replantation team must practice restraint, as short, mismatched replants do not function well and are cosmetically unacceptable.)

It seems appropriate to restore function in the lower extremity with the same vigor and enthusiasm demonstrated in restorations of the upper extremity. As stated previously, restoration of even limited sensation and motor function to a foot is preferable to a nonsensitive prosthetic device, despite the advanced state of the art of prosthetic design.

Surgical Considerations

The following case reports illustrate the surgical considerations involved in replantation of the foot.

Case Report 1

A two-and-a-half-year-old boy slipped on wet grass and thrust his right foot under the deck of a rotary lawn mower, sustaining a clean amputation at the level of Chopart's joint (Fig. 49–69A, B). The forefoot was placed in a clean plastic bag and surrounded by ice for transportation to the hospital. Radiographic examination of the lower extremity and the amputated forefoot revealed the bony extent of the traumatic amputation (Fig. 49–69C). The proposed replantation and its guarded prognosis were discussed in detail with the child's parents.

Ninety minutes after the injury, general anesthesia was instituted, and debridement begun. The skin and subcutaneous tissue margins were debrided back to clean, normal tissue. The dorsalis pedis artery was identified. The posterior tibial vessels were explored but were found to have been severed across the plantar arch. To provide adequate bone shortening for tension-free vascular anastomoses, the cartilaginous articular surfaces of the cuneiforms and the cuboid were excised. Complete debridement of the soft tissue and articular surfaces of the talus and calcaneus finally produced a total shortening of the foot of 2 cm.

Bone stabilization was achieved with Kirschner wires, which were introduced obliquely, with both surfaces held in alignment. Ankle joint motion was prevented by a calcaneotibial Kirschner wire. The posterior tibial vessels, severed at the plantar arch, were technically unsuitable for repair. The proximal dorsalis pedis artery was cleared with a 2-Fr balloon catheter and heparinized. The distal artery was gently perfused (50 mm Hg) with chilled heparinized Ringer's lactate solution for "core" cooling and tissue preservation. The arterial edges were debrided, and end-to-end anastomosis was performed with interrupted sutures of 10-0 monofilament nylon under the microscope (magnification ×6). The saphenous vein and a dorsal pedal vein were anastomosed in a similar fashion. Circulation was re-established approximately four hours after injury. When diminished arterial flow was noted, the extensor retinaculum was released proximally and distally, restoring adequate flow. Tendon and nerve repairs were deferred because of the proximity of the vascular repairs on the dorsum and soft-tissue destruction in the porta pedis. The dorsal skin was loosely approximated over the vascular repairs for protection. Elsewhere, the skin edges were left open to permit free exit of accumulated venous blood and lymph. Intravenous low–molecular-weight dextran was given for 12 hours, followed by intravenous heparin, which was continued until secondary skin closure. Administration of cephalothin was begun in the operating room and was continued every eight hours for 14 days.

Wound care consisted of normal saline dressings, which were changed every 12 hours. Initially, there was much lymphatic

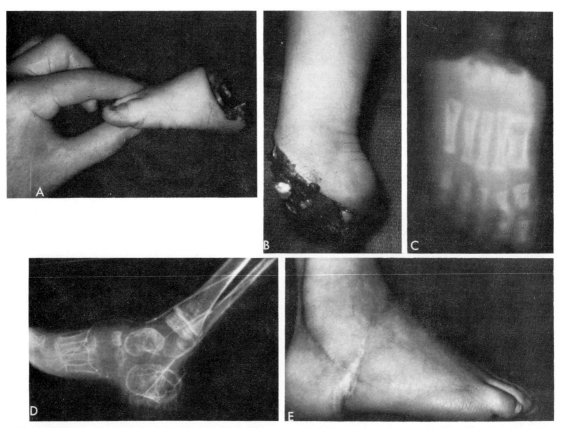

Figure 49–69. *(A and B) Transection of the foot of a two-year-old boy at the transproximal level by a lawn mower blade. (C) A radiograph of the amputated foot shows that the ossification centers in the tarsus were divided during this accident. (D) A femoral angiogram done five months after the injury shows the anastomosis of the dorsalis pedis artery with the anterior tibial artery. The plantar arch is well filled with contrast material, but there is an avascular zone near the entry of the posterior tibial artery into the plantar arch. (E) Five years after replantation, the contour of the foot is normal and function is excellent. The varus deformity is slight. Sensation is not perfect but is remarkably good, and the child appears to have no disability whatsoever.*

fluid loss, but by the fifth postoperative day, the rate of the loss had begun to decrease considerably. By the seventh day, lymph seepage was small enough to allow coverage of the open areas with biologic dressings. These dressings were replaced by autogenous split-thickness skin grafts on the twelfth post-operative day. All wounds healed primarily. The left foot and leg were immobilized in a bulky plaster cast that suspended the foot free and restricted motion, but the forefoot was exposed for frequent inspection. The calcaneotibial Kirschner wire was removed on the twenty-seventh postoperative day and the transmetatarsal wires after six weeks. Plaster cast immobilization continued for three months. When unprotected weight bearing was permitted, the insensitive forefoot was protected by an Aliplast boot. At six months, the patient was permitted full activity in normal shoes. His parents supervised skin care and daily activities. Five months after the injury, the necessity for restoration of sensation for the protection of the skin of the plantar surfaces of the foot dictated a secondary neurorrhaphy, through a counter incision, into the porta pedis. A femoral arteriogram documented patency and identified collateral circulation (Fig. 49–69D). Secondary repair of the medial and lateral plantar nerve branches was done. Adequate return of protective sensation has been confirmed by absence of any skin damage in the course of the normal activities of a five-year-old child.

At this time, evaluation of his gait revealed strong active inversion of the foot and weak eversion, but no clawing of the toes was noted. These findings suggested a dynamic tenodesis of the anterior and posterior tibial tendons at the level of amputation. It was assumed that the peroneal tendons were also tenodesed. To correct this imbalance, a Z-plasty of the peroneus brevis and longus tendons at the level of the ankle was also performed. Over five years, it appears that satisfactory foot balance has been achieved, but a slight varus deformity persists (Fig. 49–69E).

Growth measurements 15, 26, and 36 months after replantation indicate a definite discrepancy in length (Table 49–6), but this is small and does not appear to be of functional importance. However, it

TABLE 49–6. Foot Growth After Replantation

DATE	HEEL-TO-TOE LENGTH		MAXIMUM FOOT WIDTH	
	Right	*Left*	*Right*	*Left*
5/12/75	14.0	14.5	5.5	6.0
2/25/76	14.3		5.9	
8/20/76	14.8		6.4	
2/8/77	15.0		6.8	
7/25/77	15.2	15.3	6.7	6.9
7/27/78	15.5	16.7	6.9	6.9
6/11/80	16.1	17.2	7.1	7.0

appears to be of greater importance that the foot has continued to grow and shows normal ossification.

Case Report 2

A 24-year-old white male was struck with a snowplow, which transected his lower leg 10 cm above the medial malleolus (Fig. 49–70A, B). The anterior compartment of the leg was severely contused, and the lateral anterior lower leg skin was degloved from the level of the amputation site to the proximal third of the lower leg. A similar degloving was present on the medial anterior aspect of the lower leg.

The tibia was shortened by resecting the irregular transverse fracture with a Stryker saw.

One and a half centimeters were removed from the distal part of the tibia, and 3.5 cm were removed from the proximal part. The fibula was shortened in a similar fashion. A large butterfly fragment was present on the lateral aspect of the tibia and was attached to the proximal tibia. A rod was then placed in the tibia to provide skeletal stabilization, and another rod was inserted in the fibula to provide further stabilization and to eliminate the use of metal fixation in the operative area where arterial, venous, neural, and soft-tissue repair would be critical across the fracture site (Fig. 49–70C).

The dorsalis pedis artery was identified distally and proximally and was debrided to uninjured tissue. The foot was then "core cooled" with Ringer's lactate solution at 4° C. Approximately 10 cm of vessel were removed, and a vein graft was taken from the dorsum of the left foot, reversed,

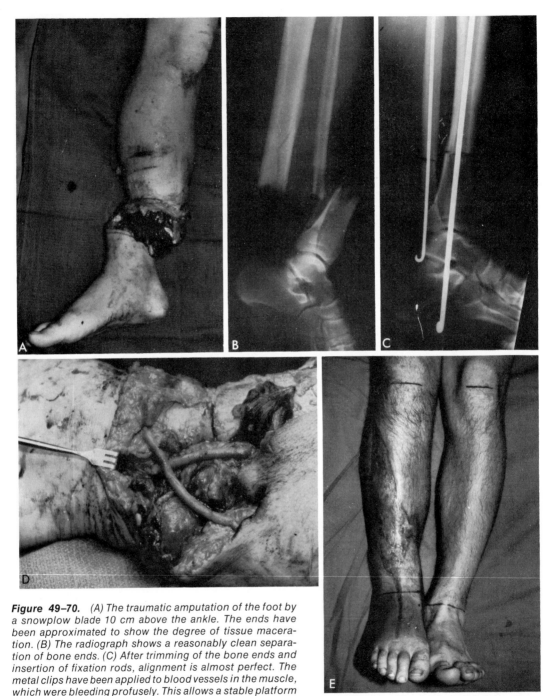

Figure 49–70. *(A) The traumatic amputation of the foot by a snowplow blade 10 cm above the ankle. The ends have been approximated to show the degree of tissue maceration. (B) The radiograph shows a reasonably clean separation of bone ends. (C) After trimming of the bone ends and insertion of fixation rods, alignment is almost perfect. The metal clips have been applied to blood vessels in the muscle, which were bleeding profusely. This allows a stable platform for revascularization of the foot. (D) One arterial and one venous graft in place. The most superficial graft runs from the dorsal venous arch to the saphenous vein and the deeper graft bridges the gap in the posterior tibial artery that resulted after debridement had been performed on normal vascular tissue both proximally and distally. (E) Final result 18 months after injury. Skin grafts have been used to cover the areas where skin was lost. Note the long, relaxing skin wound made over the dorsum of the foot. The lines show that the leg is now 2 cm shorter than the other. However, sensation has been well maintained and gait compensates well. No further reconstructive procedures are planned at this time.*

and used to bridge the defect. Proximal and distal anastomoses were performed, anastomosing the dorsalis pedis artery to the vein graft just proximal to the extensor retinaculum. The anterior tibial artery was anastomosed to the vein graft, proximal to the reduced tibial fracture. An unreversed vein graft was used between the dorsal venous arch and the anterior tibial vein. Circulation was then restored to the foot (Fig. 49–70D). The total ischemic time (warm and cold) was five hours.

A second venous channel was then established between the greater saphenous vein in the foot and in the leg. The posterior tibial artery was then reconstituted in similar fashion. All anastomoses were done with 9-0 monofilament sutures under magnification. A crushed area just below the level of the medial malleolus was exposed through a longitudinal split of the skin down to the subcutaneous tissue. A similar split of skin was made on the dorsum of the foot. This permitted satisfactory venous return through the superficial venous drainage system. The deep peroneal nerve was identified as it entered the extensor retinaculum on the ankle. The proximal end was located and, after appropriate debridement, was anastomosed to the distal end with interrupted 8-0 nylon sutures. The posterior tibial nerve was identified and had been transected proximal to its bifurcation into the medial and lateral plantar nerves. The severely contused ends were resected and anastomosed with interrupted 6-0 nylon sutures.

All the muscles at the transection level were contused and were appropriately debrided. The gastrocnemius was debrided where indicated, and a portion of its aponeurosis was used with the adjacent soleus as a muscle flap to cover the posterior tibial venous and arterial anastomoses. The tibialis anterior, extensor hallucis longus, and peroneus longus were rotated over the anterior tibial and dorsalis pedis venous and arterial anastomoses. Extensive fasciotomies of the anterior and posterior muscle compartments of the leg were performed proximally. The degloved lateral anterior flap of proximal skin and subcutaneous tissue was sutured back into position.

Bulky dressings were applied and radiographs were taken to confirm an accurate reduction. A long-legged posterior plaster cast was then applied. The limb was immobilized for six months. After final coverage of all raw areas with skin grafts, the patient's limb is now completely functional, although it is 2 cm shorter (Fig. 49–70E) 18 months after the injury.

Discussion

As a result of continuing experience in digital and limb replantations, certain basic principles of replantation surgery have evolved. Bone shortening is mandatory in most instances to allow tension-free vascular anastomoses. However, bone stability must be achieved prior to any attempt at anastomosis of the vascular structures. This is easily done with currently available orthopaedic techniques.

The degree of debridement is also learned by experience, but it must be thorough and meticulous. This may produce sufficiently large arterial and venous defects to frighten the uninitiated. However, autogenous vascular grafting has become a very refined method of "bridging" these defects. The saphenous vein works well in the arterial system but is generally too thick-walled and prone to spasm for service as a venous conduit. For tibial vein replacement, therefore, tibial vein grafts from the other leg are preferred. Although one arterial and one venous channel are theoretically sufficient, it is wise to repair at least two of each, if technically possible, although this greatly increases the margin of technical error, and the possibilities of further reconstruction.

Our experience with the use of primary and secondary wound coverage has been satisfactory.[40] Lymphatic drainage may be quite profuse, and in this event, fluid replacement, which may sometimes be quite vigorous, will be required. Antibiotic coverage is employed to help infection of these contaminated wounds. Frequent wound inspection is necessary for adequate assessment of the wound. In the upper extremity, complete repair of all structures, including tendons, is technically feasible in most instances, but this does not appear to be an absolute requirement in the foot. Thus, mass tenodesis appears to be sufficient in the foot, and the provision of protective sensation is the most important consideration.

Near-Total Amputations

Devascularized but not amputated lower extremities present an entirely different set of theoretical, surgical, and ethical problems. It has been said that it is far easier to replant an amputated part than to decide to complete the amputation of a nearly severed extremity. However, the application of the principles and experience gained from foot replantations has allowed us to undertake several successful surgical ventures that would not have been considered a short time ago. Severely traumatized but unamputated feet have now been salvaged by the application of microsurgical and standard reconstructive procedures.

Cold perfusion of the amputated foot appears to be very beneficial in reducing the effects of ischemia. The experience of renal preservation for transplantation has shown that vessel flushing can be done without significant initimal damage when this is performed with a low perfusate pressure in vessels of sufficient size. "Core cooling" reduces the metabolic rate of muscle and other soft tissue, thus affording increased protection until the circulation is restored. Therefore, we believe that it is a useful adjunct to cool and perfuse amputated parts containing muscles and other significant soft-tissue structures in order to minimize the effects of warm ischemia.

AMPUTATIONS

Many standard textbooks are available to detail techniques for amputation at various levels. Just as germane as these "basics" are modifications that allow amputation to be done at the lowest level consistent with function. The whole patient and all circumstances should be considered. A textbook procedure should not be indiscriminately applied. A discussion of some of these relevant circumstances follows.

Is An Amputation Actually Necessary?

1. One of the most common reasons for amputation is vascular insufficiency. An extremity may have major vascular disease, with threatened or actual loss of soft tissue as a consequence. These cases are often amenable to salvage by means of current vascular surgical techniques. These techniques are discussed more completely elsewhere in this book. Noninvasive as well as arteriographic techniques can clearly establish the nature of such problems, and arterial surgery may well insure survival of all or a major portion of the threatened limb. This is equally true for the diabetic with peripheral vascular disease of major vessels; a pessimistic prognosis based on small vessel disease should not be a valid consideration.

2. Traumatic amputations also deserve special consideration. If there has been loss of only one or two toes, simple revision and closure are surely best. With greater loss, replantation procedures should be considered. Avulsed or massively traumatized extremities are not suitable for replantation. Relatively clean, sharp amputations have the greatest

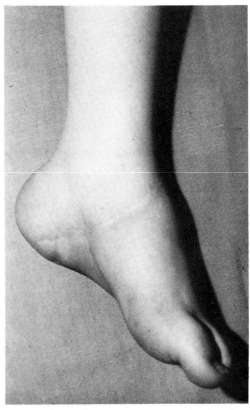

Figure 49–71. *Replanted forefoot.*

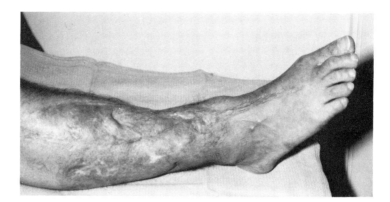

Figure 49–72. *Replanted leg.*

chance of being successfully replanted. Two functional examples of successful replantation are shown in Figures 49–71 and 49–72.

3. Diabetic patients may present with massive pyoderma gangrenosum, another condition that, at first glance, might seem to warrant amputation. This full-thickness gangrene may be circumferential or patchy. If the foot remains viable, salvage is obviously indicated. If sufficient time is taken and appropriate antibiotic coverage given, the dead tissue can be repeatedly debrided until a clean bed is obtained. This is facilitated by use of organic iodine and then sterile saline dressings while granulations are forming. With subsequent application of split-thickness skin grafts, the limb can usually be salvaged. Successful grafting was just completed on the patient shown in Figure 49–73; much larger defects are still amenable to treatment.

The aforementioned are just a few examples of cases in which no amputation at all is necessary. In keeping with this thought of maximum conservation of functional tissue, what of cases in which some amputation *is* necessary? Again, the intent should be to maintain or restore the best function with the least loss of tissue.

Conservation of Tissue in Amputations

1. Textbook pictures of flap formation in amputation should be used only as guidelines to follow in the ideal situation, which will rarely be seen. If rigidly adhered to, these methods will often lead to amputation at higher levels than necessary, simply because the tissue required for classic flap formation is not available at lower levels. Instead, the initial incision should be carried down directly to bone through the most distal margin of skin in a circum-

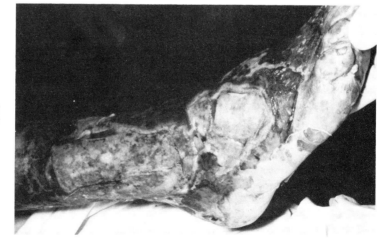

Figure 49–73. *Foot and leg after split-thickness skin grafts for pyoderma gangrenosum.*

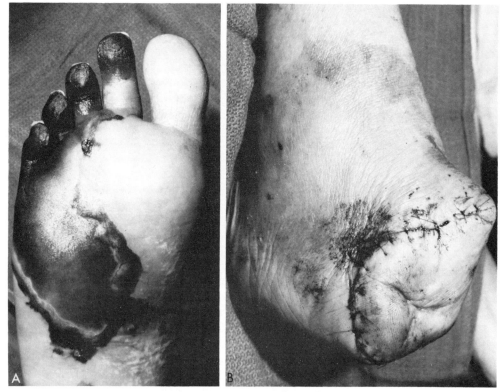

Figure 49–74. *(A) Gangrene of the entire lateral side of the foot. The medial soft tissue is intact. (B) After a Lisfranc amputation with atypical flaps.*

ferential manner, regardless of how irregular the flaps may be. The viable soft tissues and skin are reflected from the bone proximally, and the bone is sectioned at a level sufficient to allow soft-tissue closure of the foot. For instance, there may be a gangrenous change of the entire lateral side of the forefoot (Fig. 49–74A). With the usually described flaps, the most that could be hoped for would be a successful Syme amputation. Instead, the viable soft tissue and skin of the medial side of the foot can be swung laterally to produce a very functional Lisfranc amputation (Fig. 49–74B). To do this, a tourniquet should never be used. One must be able to judge the viability of retained tissue, and this is difficult with occluded circulation. Furthermore, there must be an additional risk factor in adding tourniquet ischemia to an already ischemic foot!

Another instance in which nonstandard flaps were used was after a freight train crushed and mangled all of the toes of a child's foot and also avulsed a large patch of skin from the dorsum of the foot. Superficial debridement of the dorsal aspect of the metatarsal heads left them largely intact. The dangling plantar skin flaps that remained from the toes were turned up over the top of the foot to give good closure (Fig. 49–75). Several small skin grafts from the redundant skin of the toes were used to close uncovered gaps. The result, in effect a five-toe amputation, was certainly better than a higher transmetatarsal amputation at "the site of election."

A final pair of examples of patients with necrosis of the entire plantar surface of the foot will now be presented; only the skin on the dorsum of the foot, along with small patches of skin over the malleoli and heel cord, remained viable in each patient. A patient need not be a candidate for below-the-knee amputation, even though the *usually* described Syme procedure is not possible. The bone portion of the amputation can still be done at the Syme level, through the plafond. The conserved soft tissue and skin from the dorsum of the foot,

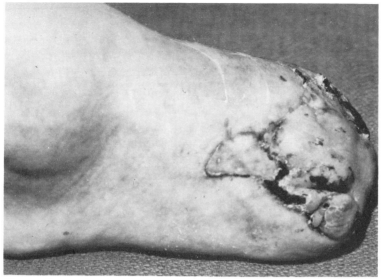

Figure 49–75. *Atypical flaps and skin grafts for closure of a railroad injury.*

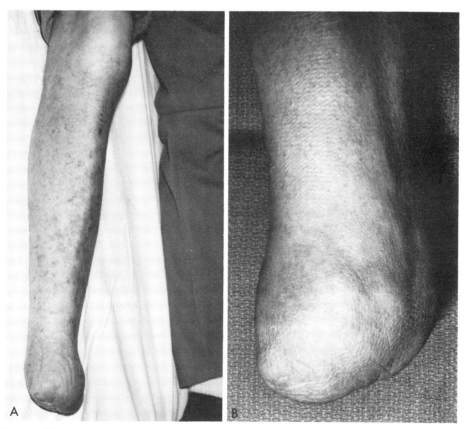

Figure 49–76. *(A) A modified Syme amputation. The heel pad was necrotic and atypical flaps were used. (B) Another modified Syme amputation.*

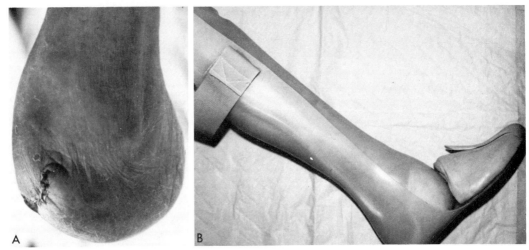

Figure 49–77. *(A) A Chopart amputation with percutaneous lengthening of the heel cord. (B) Chopart amputation prosthesis (fabricated by Richard LaTorre, LaTorre Orthopedic Laboratories, Schenectady, New York).*

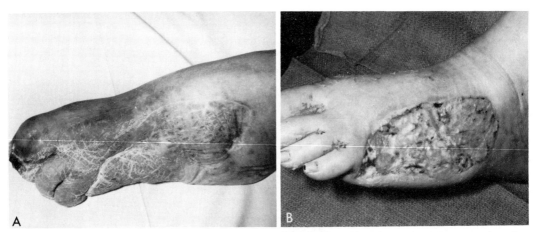

Figure 49–78. *(A) Amputation of two rays. Closure was with split-thickness skin grafts. (B) Amputation of one ray and excision of gangrenous skin from the dorsum of the foot. Closure was with split-thickness skin grafts.*

the malleoli, and the heel cord can be arranged over the end of the stump and closed in the most geometrically satisfactory manner. This "modified" Syme amputation was, in fact, mentioned and used in some instances by Syme. These two patients, an auto mechanic (Fig. 49–76A) and a housewife (Fig. 49–76B) have been fitted with standard Syme amputation prostheses and do not suffer because the cover of their stumps is not as thick or resilient as the heel fat pad would be. These prostheses aim toward total contact, and the situations are not those of complete end weight bearing.

2. Some levels of amputation have been unjustly condemned. As discussed more completely in the chapters on insensitive and diabetic foot problems (Chapters 46 and 50, respectively), Chopart and Lisfranc amputations can give very satisfactory results if the heel cord is percutaneously sectioned (to prevent equinus and ulceration) and if suitable prostheses are provided. *Without* these two requisites, these amputations are unsatisfactory. The patient shown in Figure 49–77A who underwent a Chopart amputation and heel-cord lengthening can comfortably wear a special prosthesis (Fig. 49–77B).

3. Coverage with split-thickness skin grafts may enable major functional components of the foot that would otherwise be sacrificed to obtain soft-tissue closure to be salvaged. A common example of when this would be applicable is after resection of one or two lateral rays of the foot. Usually, not enough skin can be swung up from the sole of the foot to obtain complete closure. Rather than turning to transverse amputation at a higher level, the open area can simply be recovered with split-thickness skin grafts primarily, or later after sustaining granulations have formed. The patients in Figure 49–78 were left with functional medial rays of the foot. An insole with filler for the lateral rays of the foot will enable a standard shoe to be worn.

4. Do not be hasty in determining the success or failure of an amputation. In some ischemic feet, one of the flaps may die or appear to die and turn black and hard. As long as infection does not supervene, such a condition can be expectantly watched for a reasonable period of time. In some flaps, the basal layers of the skin

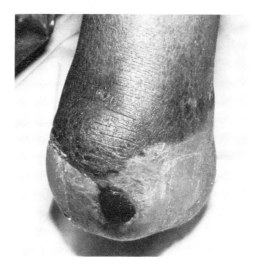

Figure 49–79. *A Chopart amputation. A small part of the eschar remains; much more has already been shed.*

survive and the eschar is eventually shed, leaving intact skin beneath. In the patient shown in Figure 49–79, a small portion of the originally large flap eschar is yet to be shed, months after the original Chopart amputation and heel-cord lengthening. In another use, a wedge of the plantar flap necrosed in an instance of Lisfranc amputation (Fig. 49–80A). Because of continuing serous drainage and evidence of deep necrosis, administration of antibiotics was continued, and the area was sharply debrided on several occasions. Debrisan was used to promote granulation (Fig. 49–80B), and the defect was then successfully closed with split-thickness grafts (Fig. 49–80C). Another important effect of ischemia is the slowness of healing. A patient with severe ischemia underwent a Chopart amputation (Fig. 49–81). Postoperatively, she had continuing serous drainage from one small spot along the suture line. The flaps gradually shrunk, and a small bit of collagenous tissue (extensor tendon) was seen protruding from this sinus. This tendon was grasped with rongeurs, pulled down, and divided. This left a draining sinus that never became infected but took seven months to close. Holes in incision lines do not close readily, and this is one good reason why we do not place drains in this position. It also demonstrates why it is important to debride all such avascular tissue as fascia or tendon from wound

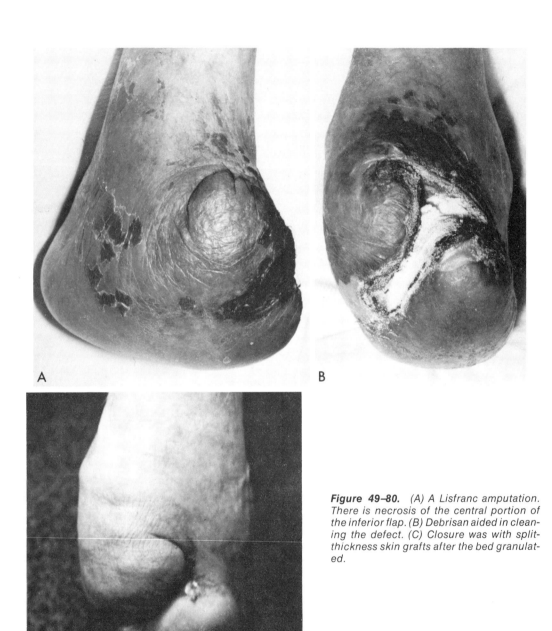

Figure 49–80. *(A) A Lisfranc amputation. There is necrosis of the central portion of the inferior flap. (B) Debrisan aided in cleaning the defect. (C) Closure was with split-thickness skin grafts after the bed granulated.*

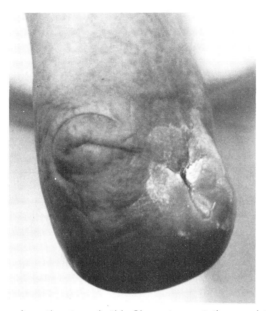

Figure 49–81. *Drainage from the stoma in this Chopart amputation persisted for seven months.*

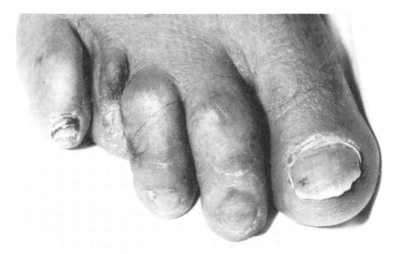

Figure 49–82. *Only the fourth toe was dead in this patient with drug gangrene of the second, third, and fourth toes. Eschar covered the viable second and third toes.*

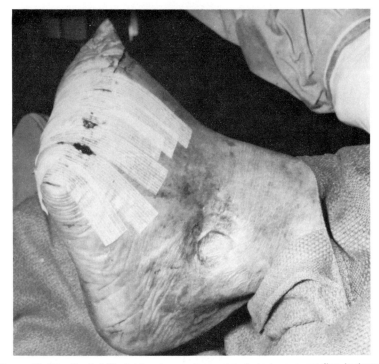

Figure 49–83. *Partial Steristrip closure is used to help to prevent flap ischemia.*

margins before closure. Ischemic feet can and do heal but take a prolonged time to do so. Do not be in a hurry, and do not give up too soon!

5. Toes can be a special case, and the discussion that follows is actually an extension of what has already been said about flap eschars. In some patients with vascular disease, one or more toes may become black, hard, and obviously involved with "dry gangrene." At the time of surgery, nothing is lost by prying away at the edges of the eschar to see if it will separate before an actual amputation is done. There will be some surprises. The patient shown in Figure 49–82 had dry gangrene of the second, third, and fourth toes as far back as the middle of the proximal phalanx. It was possible to pry away a "thimble" of hard, black skin, including the toenail, from the second and third toes, which were intact beneath. The fourth toe was totally necrotic and was amputated just distal to the metatarsophalangeal joint. Flaps were made from a small margin of viable skin beneath the eschar. When possible, an amputation at this level has less surface area to heal and is functionally just like a disarticulation.

6. As mentioned, all the amputations are done without use of a tourniquet. After suturing of the flap is complete, blanching of the skin around one or more stitches is sometimes seen. This cannot be allowed to remain, as the blanched portion of the flap will surely die. One or more of the stitches are removed. If the blanched areas become pink, Steristrips (Fig. 49–83) can be used to complete the closure. If the flap remains blanched, revision is needed before closure. Closure should never be done under tension.

Perhaps the major lesson to be learned here is to use common sense. Exercise just a little creativitiy and *do not* be bound by standard textbooks. If some variation seems reasonable, it may be well worth a try.

REFERENCES

1. Abbott, W. M., Wieland, S., and Austen, W. G.: Structural changes during preparation of autogenous venous grafts. Surgery, 76:1031, 1974.
2. Allen, V. E., and Brown, G. E.: Raynaud's disease: a critical review of minimal requisites for diagnosis. Am. J. Med. Sci., 183:187, 1932.
3. Baird, R. J., Tutassaura, H., and Miyagishima, R. T.: Saphenous vein bypass grafts to the arteries of the ankle and foot. Ann. Surg., 172:1059, 1970.
4. Barner, H. B., Kaiser, G. C., and Willman, V. L.: Blood flow in the diabetic leg. Circulation, 43:391, 1971.
5. Barnes, R. W., Collicott, P. E., Mozersky, D. J., et al.: Noninvasive quantitation of maximum venous outflow in acute thrombophlebitis. Surgery, 72:971, 1972.
6. Barnes, R. W., Collicott, P. E., Mozersky, D. J., et al.: Noninvasive quantitation of venous reflux in the postphlebitic syndrome. Surg. Gynecol. Obstet., 136:767, 1973.
7. Barnes, R. W., Kinkead, L. R., Wu, K. K., and Hoak, J. C.: Incidence of venous thrombosis in suspected pulmonary embolism: detection by Doppler. Circulation, 49–50 (Suppl.):299, 1974.
8. Barnes, R. W., Shanik, G. D., and Slaymaker, E. E.: An index of healing in below-knee amputation: leg blood pressure by Doppler ultrasound. Surgery, 79:13, 1976.
9. Bauer, G.: A roentgenological and clinical study of the sequels of thrombosis. Acta Chir. Scand., 86 (Suppl. 74):1, 1942.
10. Bauer, G.: Venous thrombosis: early diagnosis and abortive treatment with heparin. Lancet, 1:447, 1946.
11. Bernhard, V. M., Ashmore, G. S., Rodgers, R. E., and Evans, W. E.: Operative blood flow in femoral-popliteal and femoral-tibial grafts for lower extremity ischemia. Arch. Surg., 103:595, 1971.
12. Bernhard, V. M.: Intraoperative monitoring of femoro-tibial bypass grafts. Surg. Clin. North Am., 54:77, 1974.
13. Blaisdell, F. W., et al.: Aorto-iliac arterial substitution utilizing subcutaneous grafts. Ann. Surg., 172:775, 1970.
14. Bouhoutsos, J., and Martin, P.: Popliteal aneurysms: a review of 116 cases. Br. J. Surg., 61:469, 1974.
15. Boyd, A. M.: Natural course of arteriosclerosis of lower extremities. Proc. R. Soc. Med., 53:591, 1962.
16. Brener, B. J., Raines, J. K., Darling, R. C., and Austen, W. G.: Measurement of systolic femoral arterial pressure during reactive hyperemia. Circulation, 49–50(Suppl.):259, 1974.
17. Brief, D. K., Brener, B. J., Alpert, J., and Parsonnet, V.: Crossover femorofemoral grafts followed up five years or more. Arch. Surg., 110:1294, 1975.
18. Brockman, S. K., and Vasko, J. S.: The pathologic physiology of phlegmasia cerulea dolens. Surgery, 59:997, 1966.
19. Browse, N. L.: The ^{125}I-fibrinogen uptake test. Arch. Surg., 104:160, 1972.
20. Browse, N. L., and Thomas, N. L.: Source of nonlethal pulmonary emboli. Lancet, 1:258, 1974.
21. Buckley, C. J., Darling, R. C., and Raines, J. K.: Instrumentation and examination procedures for a clinical vascular laboratory. Med. Instrum., 9:181, 1975.
22. Campbell, C. D., Goldfarb, D., and Roe, R.: A small arterial substitute. Expanded microporous polytetrafluoroethylene: patency versus porosity. Ann. Surg., 182:138, 1975.
23. Carter, S. A.: Clinical measurement of systolic pressures in limbs with arterial occlusive disease. J.A.M.A., 207:1869, 1969.
24. Carter, S. A.: Response of ankle systolic pressure to leg exercise in mild or questionable arterial disease. N. Engl. J. Med., 287:578, 1972.
25. Clagett, G. P., and Salzman, E. W.: Prevention of venous thromboembolism in surgical patients. N. Engl. J. Med., 290:93, 1974.
26. Coffman, J. D., and Mannick, J. A.: Failure of vasodilator drugs in arteriosclerosis obliterans. Ann. Intern. Med., 76:35, 1972.
27. Cranley, J. J., Gay, A. Y., Grass, A. M., and Simeone, F. A.: A plethysmographic technique for the diagnosis

of deep venous thrombosis of the lower extremities. Surg. Gynecol. Obstet., *136*:385, 1973.

28. Cranley, J. J., Canos, A. J., and Sull, W. J.: The diagnosis of deep venous thrombosis. Arch. Surg., *111*:34, 1976.

29. Dardik, H., Ibrahim, I. M., and Dardik, I. I.: Glutaraldehyde-stabilized human umbilical cord vein as a vascular prosthesis. *In* Dardik, H. (ed.): Graft Materials in Vascular Surgery. Miami, Florida, Symposia Specialists, Inc., 1978, pp. 279–295.

30. Dardik, I. I., Ibrahim, I. M., Spayregen, S., et al.: Routine intraoperative angiography. An essential adjunct in vascular surgery. Arch. Surg., *110*:184, 1975.

31. Darling, R. C., Austen, W. G., and Linton, R. R.: Arterial embolism. Surg. Gynecol. Obstet., *124*:106, 1967.

32. Darling, R. C., Raines, J. K., Brener, B. J., and Austen, W. G.: Quantitative segmental pulse and volume recorder: a clinical tool. Surgery, 72:873, 1972.

33. Dean, R. H., Yao, J. S. T., Thompson, R. G., and Bergan, J. J.: Predictive value of ultrasonically derived arterial pressure in determination of amputation level. Am. Surg., *41*:731, 1975.

34. DeCamp, P. T., Schramel, R. J., Roy, C. J., et al.: Ambulatory venous pressure determinations in postphlebitic and related syndromes. Surgery, 29:44, 1951.

35. DeWeese, J. A., and Rogoff, S. M.: Phlebographic patterns of acute deep venous thrombosis of the leg. Surgery, 53:99, 1963.

36. DeWeese, J. A., and Rob, C. G.: Autogenous venous bypass grafts five years later. Ann. Surg., *174*:346, 1971.

37. Douglas, A. S., and Ogston, D.: Anticoagulant and thrombolytic therapy. Clin. Hematol., 2:175, 1973.

38. Duncan, W. C., Linton, R. R., and Darling, R. C.: Aortoiliofemoral atherosclerotic occlusive disease; comparative results of endarterectomy and Dacron bypass grafts. Surgery, 70:974, 1971.

39. Dundas, P., and Hillestad, L. K.: Profunda revascularization. The early postoperative effect upon calf blood flow. Scand. J. Thorac. Cardiovasc. Surg., 5:275, 1971.

40. Elliott, R. A., Jr., and Hoehn, J. G.: Use of commercial porcine skin for wound dressings. Plast. Reconstr. Surg. 52:401, 1973.

41. Evans, D. S.: The early diagnosis of deep vein thrombosis by ultrasound. Br. J. Surg., 57:726, 1970.

42. Evans, W. E.: Femorotibial bypass in patients with popliteal aneurysms. Am. J. Surg., *122*:155, 1971.

43. Fagerhol, M. K., Abildgaard, U., Bergshe, P., and Jacobsen, J. H.: Oral contraceptives and low antithrombin III concentration. Lancet, *1*:1175, 1970.

44. Flanc, C., Kakkar, V. V., and Clarke, M. B.: The detection of venous thrombosis of the legs using ¹²⁵I-labeled fibrinogen. Br. J. Surg., 55:742, 1968.

45. Fogarty, T. J., Cranley, J. J., Krause, R. J., et al.: A method for extraction of arterial emboli and thrombi. Surg. Gynecol. Obstet., *116*:241, 1963.

46. Fogarty, T. J., Dennis, D. L., and Drippaehne, W. W.: Surgical management of iliofemoral venous thrombosis. Am. J. Surg., *112*:211, 1966.

47. Foster, J. H., et al.: Arterial injuries secondary to the use of the Fogarty catheter. Ann. Surg., *171*:971, 1970.

48. Galloway, J. M. D., Karmody, A. M., and Mavor, G. E.: Thrombophelebitis of the long saphenous vein complicated by pulmonary embolism. Br. J. Surg., 56:360, 1969.

49. Gosling, R. G.: Continuous wave ultrasound as an alternative and complemented to x-rays in vascular examinations. *In* Gosling: Cardiovascular Applications of Ultrasound. Northville, MI, Holland Press, 1974.

50. Greenfield, A. D. M., Whitney, R. J., and Mowbray, J. F.: Methods for the investigation of peripheral blood flow. Br. Med. Bull., *19*:101, 1963.

51. Haimovici, H.: Patterns of arteriosclerotic lesions of the lower extremity. Arch. Surg., 95:918, 1967.

52. Haller, J. A., Jr.: Effects of deep femoral thrombophlebitis on the circulation of the lower extremities. Circulation, *27*:693, 1963.

53. Hobbs, J. T., and Davies, J. W. L.: Detection of venous thrombosis with ¹³¹I-labelled fibrinogen in the rabbit. Lancet, 2:134, 1960.

54. Hoehn, J. G., Jacobs, R. L., and Karmody, A. M.: Replantation of the foot. Surgical Rounds, January 1978, pp. 53–60.

55. Hoehn, J. G., Jacobs, R. L., and Karmody, A. M.: Replantation of the lower extremity. *In* Textbook of General Microsurgery.

56. Imparato, A. M., Kim, G. E., Madayag, M., and Haveson, S.: Angiographic criteria for successful tibial arterial reconstruction. Surgery, 74:830, 1973.

57. Imparato, A. M., Kim, G. E., Davidson, T., and Crowley, J. G.: Intermittent claudication: its natural course. Surgery, 78:795, 1975.

58. Jacobs, R. L., Karmody, A. M., and Wirth, C.: The team approach to management of diabetic extremities. *In* Nyhus, L.: Surgical Annual. New York, Appleton-Century-Crofts, 1977.

59. Jacobs, R. L., and Karmody, A. M.: Management of the diabetic foot. Instructional Course Lectures, American Academy of Orthopedic Surgeons, 28:118, 1979.

60. Jacobs, R. L., and Karmody, A. M.: Reimplantation of the amputated foot in a 2 year old. Presented before the American Orthopaedic Foot Society, San Francisco, 1978.

61. Joh, H. T., and Warren, R.: The stimulus to collateral circulation. Surgery, 49:14, 1961.

62. Johnson, W. C., Patten, D. H., Widrich, W. C., and Nebseth, D. C.: Technetium 99m isotope venography. Am. J. Surg., *127*:424, 1974.

63. Juergens, J. L.: Thromboangiitis obliterans (Buerger's disease). *In* Juergens, J. L., Spittell, J. A., Jr., and Fairbairn, J. F., II (eds.): Allen, Barker, Hines Peripheral Vascular Diseases 5th ed. W. B. Saunders Company, Philadelphia, 1980, p. 469.

64. Kahn, S. P., Lindenauer, S. M., Dent, T. L., et al.: Femorotibial vein bypass. Arch. Surg., *107*:309, 1973.

65. Kaminski, D. L., Barner, H. B., Dorighi, J. A., et al.: Femoropopliteal bypass with reversed autogenous vein. Ann. Surg., *177*:232, 1973.

66. Kammel, W. B., and Shurtleff, D.: The natural history of arteriosclerosis obliterans. Cardiovasc. Clin., 3:1, 1971.

67. Karmody, A. M., and Jacobs, R. L.: Salvage of the diabetic foot by vascular reconstruction. Orthop. Clin. North Am., 7:77, 1976.

68. Karmody, A. M., Powers, S. R., Monaco, V., and Leather, R. P.: Blue toe syndrome — an indication for limb salvage surgery. Arch. Surg., *111*:1263, 1976.

69. Karmody, A. M., Powers, S. R., and Leather, R. P.: Surgical guidelines for direct anterior tibial bypass. Am. J. Surg., *134*:301, 1977.

70. Karmody, A. M., Shah, D. M., and Leather, R. P.: The distal profunda femoris artery. Its use in limb salvage. Clin. Res. 25:651, 1977.

71. Karmody, A. M., Leather, R. P., and Shah, D. M.: Extended profundaplasty. Am. J. Surg., *136*:359, 1978.

72. Karmody, A. M.: A study of clinically necessary arterial pressure levels in the management of ischemic diabetic feet. Presented before the American Orthopaedic Foot Society, San Francisco, 1978.

73. Karmody, A. M., and Leather, R. P.: Guidelines for vascular surgery in geriatric patients: an update. Geriatrics, *34*:45, 1979.

74. Keitzer, W. F., Lichti, E. L., Brossart, F. A., and DeWeese, M. S.: Use of the Doppler ultrasonic flowmeter during arterial vascular surgery. Arch. Surg., *105*:308, 1972.

75. Kunlin, J.: Le traitement de l'artérite oblitérante par la greffe veineuse. Arch. Mal. Coeur, 42:371, 1949.

76. Lambie, J. M., Mahaffy, R. G., Barber, D. C., Karmody, A. M., et al.: Diagnostic accuracy in venous thrombosis. Br. Med. J., 2:142, 1970.

77. Leather, R. P., and Karmody, A. M.: A reappraisal of the 'In-situ' bypass. Its use in limb salvage. Surgery, 86(3):453, 1979.

78. Lindbom, A.: Arteriosclerosis and arterial thrombosis in the lower limb: a roentgenogenological study. Acta Radiol., Suppl. 80:1, 1950.

79. Louw, J. H.: Splenic-to-femoral and axillary-to-femoral bypass grafts in diffuse arteriosclerotic occlusive disease. Lancet, 1:1401, 1963.

80. Mannick, J. A., and Jackson, B. T.: Hemodynamics of arterial surgery in atherosclerotic limbs. I. Direct measurement of blood flow before and after vein grafts. Surgery, 59:713, 1966.

81. Martin, P., Frawley, J. E., Barabas, A. P., and Rosengarten, D. S.: On the surgery of atherosclerosis of the profunda femoris artery. Surgery, 71:182, 1972.

82. Mavor, G. E.: The pattern of occlusion in atheroma of the lower limb arteries. The correlation of clinical and arteriographic findings. Br. J. Surg., 43(180):352, 1956.

83. Mavor, G. E., and Galloway, J. M. D.: Iliofemoral venous thrombosis: pathological considerations and surgical treatment. Br. J. Surg., 56:45, 1969.

84. Mavor, G. E., Galloway, J. M. D., and Karmody, A. M.: The surgical aspects of deep vein thrombosis. Proc. R. Soc. Med., 63:126, 1970.

85. Mavor, G. E., Walker, M. G., Dhall, D. P., et al.: Peripheral venous scanning with ^{125}I-tagged fibrinogen. Lancet, 1:661, 1972.

86. McDowell, F.: Get in there and replant! Plast. Reconstr. Surg., 52:562, 1973.

87. McLachlin, A. D.: Venous disease of the lower extremities. Curr. Probl. Surg., 3:44, 1967.

88. McPherson, J. R., Juergens, J. L., and Gifford, R. W., Jr.: Thromboangiitis obliterans and arteriosclerosis obliterans: clinical and prognostic differences. Ann. Intern. Med., 59:288, 1963.

89. McShane, R. H., Jacobs, R., and Karmody, A. M.: Replantation of the lower leg with primary muscle flaps. International Congress of Microsurgery, Brescia, September 1979.

90. Moore, M. F., Flesh, L., Karmody, A. M., and Shah, D. M.: Evaluation of aortoiliac aneurysms by ultrasound and radionuclide angiograms. Clin. Res., 26:604, 1978.

91. Moore, M. F., Shah, D. M., and Karmody, A. M.: Radionuclide angiography. A preliminary experience. Clin. Res., 26:604,, 1978.

92. Mozersky, D. J., Sumner, D. S., and Strandness, D. E.: Long-term results of reconstructive aortoiliac surgery. Am. J. Surg., 123:503, 1972.

93. Mullick, S. C., Wheeler, H. B., and Songster, G. F.: Diagnosis of deep venous thrombosis by measurement of electrical impedance. Am. J. Surg., 119:417, 1970.

94. Nicolaides, A. N., Kakkar, V. V., Fields, E. S., and Renney, J. T. G.: The origin of deep venous thrombosis. A venographic study. Br. J. Radiol., 44:653, 1971.

95. O'Brien, B.: Replantation surgery in China. Med. J. Aust., 2255, 1974.

96. O'Brien, B.: Microvascular Reconstructive Surgery. Edinburgh, Churchill, Livingstone, 1977, p. 140.

97. Patman, R. D., and Thompson, J. E.: Fasciotomy in peripheral vascular surgery. Arch. Surg., 101:663, 1970.

98. Peabody, R. A., Tsapogas, M. J., Karmody, A. M., et al.: Altered endogenous fibrinolysis and biochemical factors in atherosclerosis. Arch. Surg., 109:309, 1974.

99. Pearse, H., and Warren, S.: The roentgenographic visu-
alization of the arteries of the extremities in peripheral vascular disease. Ann. Surg., 94:1094, 1931.

100. Peking Hospital of Workers, Peasants and Soldiers, and Peking Chishueit'an Hospital: Autotransplantation of severed foot, Report of Case. Chin. Med. J. (Engl. sect.), 6:74, 1973.

101. Perry, M. O., Thal, E. R., and Shires, G. T.: Management of arterial injuries. Ann. Surg., 173:403, 1971.

102. Philip, P. K., Goldman, M., Sarrafizadeh, M., Karmody, A. M., et al.: The ulcerated plaque of the femoropopliteal artery: a contraindication to transluminal angioplasty. The Radiological Society of North America, November, 1979.

103. Pollack, A. A., and Wood, E. H.: Venous pressure in the saphenous vein at the ankle in man during exercise and changes in posture. J. Appl. Physiol., 1:649, 1949.

104. Porter, J. M., Lindell, T. D., and Lakin, P. C.: Leg edema following femoropopliteal autogenous vein bypass. Arch. Surg., 105:883, 1972.

105. Porter, J. M., Snider, R. L., and Bardana, E. J.: The diagnosis and treatment of Raynaud's phenomenon. Surgery, 77:11, 1975.

106. Raines, J. K., Jaffrin, M. Y., and Rao, S.: A noninvasive pressure pulse recorder: development and rationale. Med. Instrum., 7:245, 1973.

107. Raines, J. K., Karling, R. C., Buth, J., et al.: Vascular laboratory criteria for the management of peripheral vascular disease of the lower extremities. Surgery, 79:21, 1976.

108. Raynaud, M.: De l'asphyzie locale et de la gangrene symétrique des extrémités, Paris, 1862. Rignoux. In Selected Monographs (translated by Thomas Barlow). London, The New Sydenham Society, 1888.

109. Rich, N. M., Hughes, C. W., and Baugh, J. H.: Management of venous injuries. Ann. Surg., 171:724, 1970.

110. Rosenberg, D. M. L., Glass, B. A., Rosenberg, N., et al.: Experiences with modified bovine arteries in arterial surgery. Surgery, 68:1064, 1970.

111. Rosenthal, J. J., Gaspar, M. R., Gjerbrum, T. C., and Newman, J.: Vascular injuries associated with fractures of the femur. Arch. Surg., 110:494, 1975.

112. Roth, R. B.: Letter: Replantation in China. J.A.M.A., 230:1127, 1974.

113. Rutherford, R. B.: Peripheral Vascular Injuries. The Management of Trauma. Philadelphia, W. B. Saunders Company, 1973.

114. Rutherford, R. B.: The nonoperative management of chronic peripheral arterial insufficiency. In Vascular Surgery. Philadelphia, W. B. Saunders Company, 1977.

115. Sauvage, L. R., Berger, K. E., Wood, S. J., et al.: Interspecies healing of porous arterial prostheses observations 1960–1974. Arch. Surg., 109:698, 1974.

116. Schenk, W. B., Jr., and Dedichen, H.: Electronic measurements of blood flow. Am. J. Surg., 114:111, 1967.

117. Shah, D. M., Karmody, A. M., Newell, J., et al.: Blood flow and resistance changes during reperfusion syndrome in dogs. Clin. Res., 25:654, 1977.

118. Shah, D. M., Rosenberg, M., and Karmody, A. M.: Hypertonic mannitol in the management of the revascularization syndrome following acute arterial ischemia. Clin. Res., 27:569, 1979.

119. Shah, D. M., Drichard, M. N., Newell, J. C., Karmody, A. M., et al.: Increased cardiac output and oxygen transport following intraoperative isovolemic hemodilution in patients with peripheral vascular disease. Arch. Surg., 115:597, 1980.

120. Sigel, B., Poply, A., Wagner, D., et al.: Comparison of clinical and Doppler ultrasound evaluation of confirmed lower extremity venous disease. Surg. Gynecol. Obstet., 127:339, 1968.

121. Sigel, B., Felix, W. R., Jr., Poply, G. L., and Ipsen, J.: Diagnosis of lower limb venous thrombosis by Doppler ultrasound technique. Arch. Surg., 104:174, 1972.

122. Skinner, J. S., and Strandness, D. E.: Exercise and intermittent claudication. I. Effects of repetition and intensity of exercise. Circulation, 36:15, 1967.

123. Snyder, M. A., Adams, J. T., and Schwartz, S. I.: Hemodynamics of phlegmasia cerulea dolens. Surg. Gynecol. Obstet., 125:342, 1967.

124. Sparks, C. H.: Silicone mandril methods for growing reinforced autogenous femoro-popliteal artery grafts in situ. Ann. Surg., 177:293, 1973.

125. Strandness, D. E., Jr., and Bell, J. W.: Peripheral vascular disease. Diagnosis and objective evaluation using a mercury strain gauge. Ann. Surg., 161 (Suppl.):1, 1965.

126. Strandness, D. E., Jr., Schultz, R. D., and Sumner, D. S.: Ultrasonic flow detection — a useful technique in the evaluation of peripheral vascular disease. Am. J. Surg., 113:311, 1967.

127. Strandness, D. E.: Collateral Circulation in Clinical Surgery. Philadelphia, W. B. Saunders Company, 1969.

128. Strandness, D. E., Jr.: Exercise testing in the evaluation of patients undergoing direct arterial surgery. J. Cardiovasc. Surg., 11:192, 1970.

129. Strandness, D. E., Jr., and Sumner, D. S.: Ultrasonic velocity detector in the diagnosis of thrombophlebitis. Arch. Surg., 104:180, 1972.

130. Strandness, D. E., Jr., and Sumner, D. S.: Hemodynamics for Surgeons. New York, Grune and Stratton, 1975.

131. Strandness, D. E., Jr., and Sumner, D. S.: Acute venous thrombosis. A case of progress and confusion. J.A.M.A., 233:46, 1975.

132. Sumner, D. S., and Strandness, D. E.: The relationship between calf blood flow and ankle pressure in patients with intermittent claudication. Surgery, 65:763, 1969.

133. Szilagyi, D. E., Elliott, J. P., Hagemen, J. H., et al.: Biologic fate of autogenous vein implants as arterial substitutes. Clinical, angiographic, and histopathologic observations in femoropopliteal operations for atherosclerosis. Ann. Surg., 178:232, 1973.

134. Tsapogas, M. J., Peabody, R. A., and Karmody, A. M.: Incidence and prevention of postoperative venous thrombosis. Arch. Surg., 103:561, 1971.

135. Verta, M. J., Jr., Gross, W. S., van Bellen, B., et al.: Forefoot perfusion pressure and minor amputation for gangrene. Surgery, 80:729, 1976.

136. Voorhees, A. B., Jaretski, A., III, and Blakemore, A. H.: Use of tubes constructed of Vinyon-N cloth in bridging arterial defects. Ann. Surg., 135:332, 1952.

137. Warren, R., Gomex, R. L., Marston, J. A. P., and Cox, J. S.: Femoropopliteal arteriosclerosis obliterans — arteriographic patterns and rates of progression. Surgery, 55:135, 1964.

138. Wylie, E. J., Olcott, C. O., IV, and String, S. T.: Aortoiliac thromboendarterectomy. In Varco, R. L., and Delaney, J. P. (eds.): Controversy in Surgery. Philadelphia, W. B. Saunders Company, 1976.

139. Yao, S. T., Hobbs, J. T., and Irvine, W. T.: Pulse examination by an ultrasonic method. Br. Med. J., 4:555, 1968.

140. Yao, S. T., Hobbs, J. T., and Irvine, W. T.: Ankle systolic pressure measurements in arterial disease affecting the lower extremities. Br. J. Surg., 56:676, 1969.

141. Yao, S. T.: Hemodynamic studies in peripheral arterial disease. Br. J. Surg., 57:761, 1970.

142. Yao, S. T., Gourmos, C., and Hobbs, J. T.: Detection of proximal-vein thrombosis by Doppler ultrasound flow-detection method. Lancet, 1:1, 1972.

143. Yao, S. T.: New techniques in objective arterial evaluation. Arch. Surg., 106:600, 1973.

144. Yates, S. G., II, Nakagawa, Y., Berger, K., and Sauvage, L. R.: Surface thrombogenicity of arterial prostheses. Surg. Gynecol. Obstet., 136:12, 1973.

CHAPTER 50

THE DIABETIC FOOT

Richard L. Jacobs, M.D.,

and Allastair Karmody, M.D.

About 5 per cent of the population of the United States suffers from either juvenile-onset or maturity-onset diabetes. Although many cases are mild, this is a major public health problem, and one that will be seen in its protean manifestations by most physicians. About 50 per cent of all major lower extremity amputations are in diabetics. Sir William Osler once said "He who knows syphilis knows medicine." With changing disease patterns, perhaps the same statement can now be made in regard to diabetes.

HISTORICAL PERSPECTIVE

Clinical advances in understanding and treating diabetes have been neither successive nor rapid. Rollo described diabetic neuropathy as early as 1790.[13] Charcot[4] described similar neuropathy and musculoskeletal changes in syphilitics in 1868, but no one apparently recognized the parallels to be found in patients with diabetes mellitus. In that era, before insulin was discovered, most diabetics did not survive long enough to develop many of these chronic complications. By the early 1900's, Williamson[22-26] wrote a series of classic papers further describing diabetic neuropathy, but it remained for Jordan[10] (in his classic paper of 1936 describing neuropathic joint changes in diabetic feet) to start us toward a real understanding of the many problems faced in diagnosis, treatment, and care of the diabetic foot. The resistance to these new ideas was to persist for many years. Even to this day, there is often a failure to appreciate some of the basic concepts in this complicated disease.

PATHOPHYSIOLOGY

Diabetic neuropathy can affect both the peripheral nerves and the central nervous system. At least 35 per cent of all diabetics will develop a degree of neuropathy that can be detected on gross clinical examination. It was long assumed that these neurologic changes were secondary to changes in the vasa nervorum, until Thomas and Lascelles[20] found that there are rarely changes in the local vascular supply of nerves. Ischemic infarction is sometimes seen, but this generally presents as a rapid-onset mononeuropathy, not as the more diffuse pattern usually seen in diabetics.[7]

Most recent studies[5] demonstrate that the peripheral neuropathy of diabetics is more likely the result of an intrinsic metabolic abnormality of the Schwann cell. This almost certainly involves more than one enzyme system, but which, if any, of these defects is primary is purely speculative at the present time.

Standard textbooks of medicine often discuss the "stocking" type of hypesthesia in diabetics, but the true picture is more often one of patchy change in specific peripheral sensory nerves of the foot. The usual changes that can be elicited on routine physical examination are of impairment of sensation (light touch, heat, cold, pain), proprioception, and pallesthesia. This impairment of protective sensation can permit recurrent soft tissue, bone, and joint injuries, which will be discussed later.

It has been stated that there seems to be no rhyme or reason to diabetic neuropathy; some patients with severe disease and poor control apparently never develop neuropathy, whereas others with maturity-onset diabetes and very mild disease can develop a rather serious neuropathy. It is likely, however, that such observations are anecdotal rather than statistical. Some studies[12, 19, 21] indicate that patients with diabetic neuropathy often improve after hyperglycemia is controlled. Nonetheless, prevention of neuropathy by diabetic control is not as unequivocal as is prevention of vascular complications by such control.

Although sensory involvement is usually more severe than motor involvement in diabetic neuropathy, some stigmata of increasing motor imbalance are difficult to miss in diabetics. Thus, frequent findings are progressive claw toe and bunion deformity.

Circulatory Problems

Impaired circulation can be a major limiting factor in maintenance of the diabetic foot. Angiopathy and nephropathy are almost certainly related to control of the diabetes. The Joslin Clinic Study[12] showed this quite clearly. Patients with best control developed the least vascular complications. The impairment of microcirculation in diabetics has been stressed. The basement membrane changes of these small vessels are often mentioned, and most physicians are well aware of the extra-valuable information that can be obtained from examining the vascular patterns of the patient's eyegrounds. This emphasis on small vessel disease in diabetes has doubtless led to undue pessimism when problems of ulceration, infection, or gangrene do arise. The feeling is expressed that even if something is done for disease involving the larger vessels, these surgical efforts will be of little benefit because of circulatory impairment at the capillary level.

This has not been our experience. Ther-

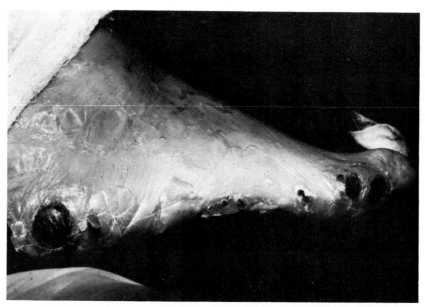

Figure 50–1. An elderly diabetic previously developed gangrenous changes in the other foot, necessitating amputation of the lateral two rays. Similar changes and ulcerations now developed on this foot. After bypass surgery, these early changes were reversed, and the ulcers crusted and healed.

apy designed to increase circulation in larger vessels often brings sufficient increment in pressure and flow to the distal circulation to ensure healing and survival of an otherwise doomed extremity, even if there are microscopic changes in the capillary bed. In fact, despite these microscopic changes, Goodson[8] claims that there is actually a normal or *increased* permeability in diabetic skin and muscle capillaries.

Atherosclerotic changes occur with increased frequency in the larger vessels of the diabetic. The evaluation and treatment of such peripheral vascular disease in diabetics differ in no significant way from evaluation and treatment of similar disease in nondiabetic patients. This is discussed in greater detail in Chapter 49. We have been impressed by the favorable results of bypass surgery in augmenting peripheral blood flow when arteriography indicates lesions amenable to such therapy. This is mirrored in the reversal of distal ischemic changes that previously failed to heal with bed rest and conservative local treatment. Indolent ulcers may heal, and chronic

deep infections are often controlled or eradicated for the first time. Progressive skin changes in what appeared to be a doomed foot may well be reversed (Fig. 50–1).

Charcot Joints

Neuropathic arthropathy was first recognized in patients suffering from tertiary syphilis. Since that time, this disease pattern has been recognized in at least 20 other systemic diseases, the most common being diabetes, syphilis, and syringomyelia. The common denominator is loss of protective pain sensation.

A diabetic with impaired pain sensation may go for many years with no difficulties caused by this defect. Then, however, he may sustain injury to the foot of any degree from very minor to major. An individual with normal pain sensation would limit activities until the injury healed or would seek appropriate medical care. However, because of varying degrees of impairment of protective pain sensation, the diabetic

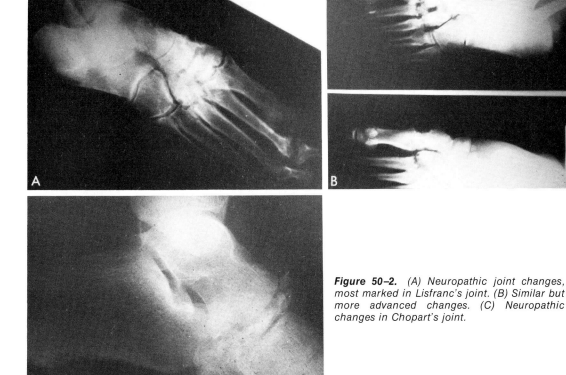

Figure 50–2. (A) Neuropathic joint changes, most marked in Lisfranc's joint. (B) Similar but more advanced changes. (C) Neuropathic changes in Chopart's joint.

may not even realize that an injury has occurred and may continue with full weight bearing. The bone or joint trauma never has a chance to heal appropriately, and still further injuries are superimposed. The end result of this remorseless cycle of continuing trauma can be the equivalent of a severe but painless traumatic arthritis that may be rapidly progressive (Fig. 50–2). There may also be (spontaneous) fractures of any of the various bones in the foot. Because of continuing injury and repair reaction, the foot may become tremendously swollen and erythematous (Fig. 50–3). Local temperature will also be increased. It may be difficult for one inexperienced in the care of neuropathic feet to distinguish this from deep infection. Indeed, the gross changes of destruction and fragmentation of bone and joints seen by roentgenogram may "confirm" the casual diagnosis of "osteomyelitis"!

When the diabetic foot is infected, the usual portal of entry is through a local skin defect, usually a mal perforans ulcer. Until late in the course of the disease, the infection of bone at this site seems to involve the soft tissues *around* bone along with the surface layers of bone. This is *not* the usual bloodborne osteomyelitis with pus in the *medullary cavity* and devitalized bone. Were it otherwise, the local debridements, partial amputations, and various salvage procedures used would rarely be successful. This empirical observation is one noted by most physicians handling any large volume of diabetic foot problems.

Structural changes of valgus or varus deformity may develop as neuropathic joint disease progresses and new bony prominences become weight bearing. This may lead to ulceration through the overlying soft tissues and is discussed in greater detail in Chapter 44.

Skin Changes

Thirty per cent of diabetics manifest cutaneous signs of the disease during the

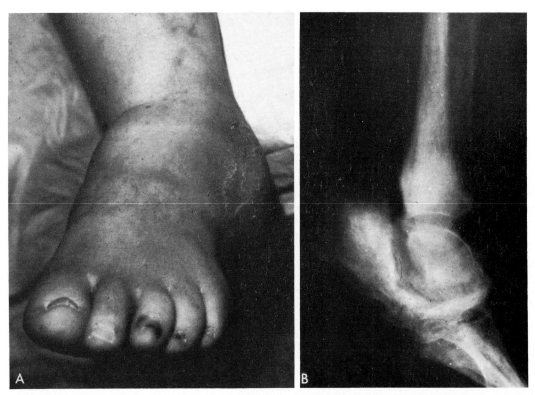

Figure 50–3. *(A) Increasing varus deformity and erythema of the lateral side of the foot. The patient experienced relatively little pain, and there was no elevation of temperature or of white count. Good chemical control of the diabetes — a Charcot foot. (B) Advanced roentgenographic changes of destruction in the subtalar and (to a lesser degree) the ankle joint.*

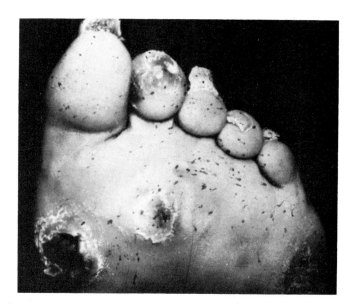

Figure 50–4. *Plantar corns and calluses. A purulent, infected ulcer was found beneath the second metatarsal head.*

course of their illness. Among the more common problems are necrobiosis lipoidica diabeticorum, diabetic dermopathy, skin infections, xanthomas, carotenemia, pruritus, idiopathic bullae, and granuloma annulare.[16, 17]

One of the major problems is the tendency of diabetics to form excessive corns and calluses (Fig. 50–4). No satisfactory explanation has ever been given for this phenomenon, but it has been demonstrated that the stratum corneum in denervated extremities does not absorb water to nearly the same extent as that in normal extremities. Dense, hard deposits of cornified tissue subsequently accumulate.

Wound Healing

Goodson[8] studied wound healing in rats treated with streptozotocin, a drug that selectively kills pancreatic β-cells. Hyperglycemic animals developed appreciably less tensile strength in experimental wounds and also developed less scar tissue in implanted chambers. These changes reverted to normal when the animals were treated with insulin. Apparently, healing is of poor quality in the diabetic state, and this impairment is at least partially responsive to insulin treatment.

Leukocyte Changes

Defective phagocytosis and decreased mobilization of leukocytes are described

in diabetic patients. These are equally important mechanisms in diminishing resistance to infection.[1, 18]

PHYSICAL EXAMINATION

Every patient with diabetic foot problems requires a thorough initial physical examination. These patients are often referred specifically for care of their foot problems, but it is surprising how often other systemic manifestations of the disease have not been considered. Most surely, initial examination should pay special attention to organs such as the eyes. As renal and cardiovascular complications are responsible for approximately 75 per cent of deaths in diabetics,[11] these systems also need special attention.

Examination of the foot should, whenever possible, include quantitative data. Circumferential measurement of the foot at the level of Chopart's or Lisfranc's joints and circumferential measurement of any affected toes can give baseline values. The dimensions of ulcerations of the foot are likewise recorded. The temperature of the foot is determined by palpation; the human hand can detect temperature contrasts of 2° C. More accurate measurements can be obtained with use of thermistors (skin thermometers). Thermography is the most accurate method but, because of expense, is usually done only in research applications.[3] Early loss of sensation is sometimes detected only by loss of vibratory sense in the toes, using a 128-c.p.s. tuning fork.

A quantitative measure of the blood pressure at the level of the ankle can be obtained with a Doppler apparatus (see Chapter 49). Diabetic ulcers heal better with ankle pressure of at least 90 mm Hg,

although we have often found that, with prolonged care, such lesions will heal with appreciably lower pressure than this.[15]

The Harris foot mat provides a permanent graphic record of areas of excessive loading of the foot (Fig. 50–5). This demonstrates spots of high pressure, and such a record can be made both before and after

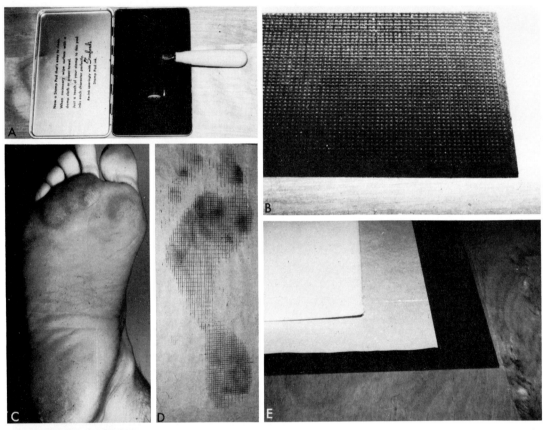

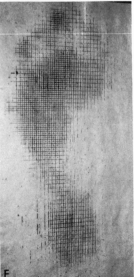

Figure 50–5. *(A) An inked roller is used to prepare the Harris mat. (B) The Harris mat — a soft rubber pad with rectangular ribs of varying height. The greater the pressure, the more ribs in contact with the impinging surface and the heavier the printing. (C) This foot shows varying thicknesses of callosities beneath the metatarsal heads. (D) Paper is placed over the inked mat, and a single print is made as the patient walks over the mat. Notice that the most dense areas of the print are beneath the great toe and the medial metatarsal heads. These are the areas of greatest pressure on weight bearing. (E) The mat is inked, and a sheet of paper and then a sheet of Aliplast of the thickness proposed for protective insoles are placed over it. (F) Another walking step is made onto this "sandwich." The print now shows more even distribution of weight bearing and elimination of high-pressure areas.*

appropriate padding is added to the shoes. An instantaneous evaluation of whether such areas have or have not been unloaded is obtained. We routinely take multiple pictures of damaged feet, and high quality 35-mm color slides are easily obtained with an electronic flash unit.

In the presence of infection, a smear is made of the exudate draining from any open lesion or of material aspirated from closed lesions.

Gram stains help to select appropriate antibiotics provisionally until the results of culture and sensitivity testing become available. The foul odor of anaerobic infections may be obvious clinically, but, in any event, cultures for anaerobic organisms should always be taken.

Appropriate anteroposterior, lateral, and oblique films of the feet are always worth obtaining, not only to detect pathologic changes but to serve as a baseline for continuing care of the patient. Weight-bearing films may demonstrate instability that is not shown on routine films.

TREATMENT OF THE DIABETIC FOOT

Diabetic patients should be examined as a preventive measure before they actually experience any difficulties with their feet. The ideal situation is to educate the patient in foot care and maintenance before he has problems. The physiology of diabetic foot problems is explained and repeated on subsequent visits until the patient is quite aware of potential problems and is well versed in continuing prophylactic care of his own feet. Good foot hygiene is required, but excessively warm bathing water must be avoided, especially in the foot with marginal circulation. The patient should inspect his own feet every night and seek medical care for any variation from the normal (local cuts or bruises, infected ingrown toenails, ulcerated calluses, local swelling). He should avoid walking barefoot because of the possibility of injury. Direct trauma to unshod feet may cause injuries as simple as subungual hematomas, but we occasionally see full-thickness necrosis of toe-tip skin from such trauma. This can lead to ulceration of the tips of the toes and can be a portal of entry for infection.

Special care should be exercised in buying new shoes. Shoes with a deep toe-box should be selected. New shoes should be removed at frequent intervals and the feet checked for pressure areas.

The patient should have corns and calluses periodically debrided to avoid later development of pressure areas. As will be discussed, we usually apply insoles to the shoes to lessen shear forces and more evenly distribute pressure.

It is always difficult to alter smoking patterns, but this becomes a crucial matter in diabetics. It is an often repeated truism that circulation in the feet is decreased about 50 per cent during smoking; this can literally kill the diabetic foot. We have seen foot lesions in hospitalized diabetic patients finally heal only after cigarettes were withdrawn.

Bunions and Claw Toes

Structural abnormalities such as bunions or claw toes often should be surgically corrected before local pressure difficulties develop, especially in the young diabetic (Fig. 50–6). This is decided on an individual basis, as the peripheral circulation must be adequate to sustain the foot after surgery. Undue trauma is always avoided during these operations, and skin edges are not handled with forceps. Sharp dissection and minimal development of tissue planes help minimize trauma.

Our most frequent operation for claw toes has been resection of the base of the proximal phalanx along with proximal interphalangeal joint fusion. These toes are stabilized by intramedullary Kirschner wires extending into the metatarsal heads. The wires are removed about three weeks after surgery. Syndactylization has not been necessary. In the same manner, a modified Keller bunionectomy can be done by resecting the base of the proximal phalanx of the great toe through a straight *dorsal* incision. The dorsal incision is carried directly down to the base of the proximal phalanx, and the base is delivered by sharp dissection rather than by use of an elevator. This toe likewise is stabilized with an intramedullary Kirschner wire after surgery. No attempt is made to imbricate the soft tissues on the medial aspect of the joint, as this may occasionally compromise circulation to the toe. We have

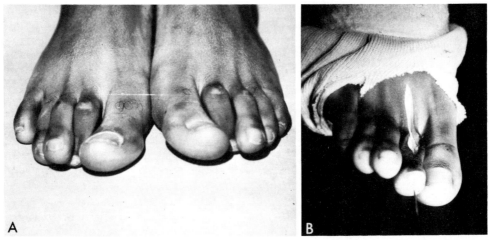

Figure 50–6. *(A) Congenital claw-toe deformities in this young diabetic should be corrected before complications can occur at a later age. (B) The claw toe is corrected with sharp dissection. The pin is left in place for three to four weeks. The proximal interphalangeal joint may heal with bony or fibrous union, but recurrent deformity is not a common problem.*

encountered no problems of untoward deviation in the great toe because of this failure to reef tissues medially.

These prophylactic operations are advantageous for two reasons. By correcting deformity in the claw toes, these procedures eliminate the dorsal callosities and possible areas of ulceration over the proximal interphalangeal joints. Even more important, surgery will often aid in the control of callosities beneath the metatarsal heads. As these toes go into a clawed position, they draw the plantar fat pad from beneath the metatarsal heads to a position anterior to the metatarsal heads.

As the metatarsophalangeal joint is decompressed, this fat pad can once again fall beneath the metatarsal head, and the callosities will usually disappear spontaneously. Less frequently, we resect all the metatarsal heads through a dorsal approach, as described by Clayton[6] for patients with rheumatoid arthritis.

Another advantage of these prophylactic operations is that feet after such corrections require much less frequent debridement of corns and calluses.

It must be stressed that any surgery on the diabetic foot be done with the greatest deliberation and caution and only for valid

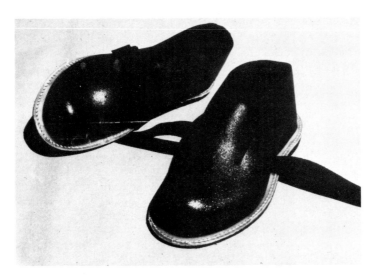

Figure 50–7. *Various brands of "healing shoes" are available to protect damaged feet during the healing phase.*

indications. Careful circulatory evaluation is necessary, and the patient must be informed of the additional risks of surgery.

Special "healing shoes" (Apex Co.) (Fig. 50–7) are sometimes of value in postoperative care after dressings are no longer needed. These help avoid further trauma or blistering of the foot during the healing period. The shoes are not durable and cannot be expected to be suitable for long-term use.

Charcot Joints

See Chapter 45 for treatment.

Mal Perforans Ulcers

The most common cause of mal perforans ulcers is the formation of plantar corns and callosities (Fig. 50–8). When a patient with normal plantar sensation develops a corn, he limps because of pain. As a result, the area is effectively unloaded. The diabetic patient does not have normal pain sensation and continues about his normal activities with full, unprotected weight bearing. As the corn grows in depth and density, it behaves as a hard foreign body fixed to the foot directly beneath the bone prominence. This ulcerates through the dermis. Initially, there is no change in the external appearance. The superficial layers of the skin are completely intact, and there is no evidence of violation of the protective dermis. If routine hygiene is practiced at this time and the corns are debrided, the ulcer is demonstrated. Following this relief of pressure, the ulcers will often heal with no further treatment. More commonly, the patient continues to walk on the painless corn. Serous exudate then undermines the corn and burrows its way to the surface. The patient may notice serous drainage and often seeks medical attention. Equally common, the drainage is ignored until infection develops in the soft tissues through this portal of entry. In each of these instances, it is helpful to obtain permanent record of these areas of excessive weight bearing, using a Harris footprint mat. A roller is used to distribute ink over the surface of the ribbed mat, and the mat is placed on the bare floor with no underlying rug and is overlain with a sheet of paper. The patient is instructed to take one normal step on the paper as he walks across the room. Because of the compliant nature of this rubber grid, the areas of heaviest weight bearing will demonstrate the greatest density of print, and a permanent record will be obtained of the points of maximum pressure.

For small ulcers that are obviously not infected, the combination of debriding the corns and fitting the patient with protective shoes may be all that is needed. Extra-depth shoes are ordered. These are simple laced oxfords with an extra-high toe-box to accommodate the thickness of insoles that may be placed in the shoe. For insole material, we usually use polyethylene sheet (Aliplast, Plastazote, Pelite) of quarter-inch thickness.* This unloads the ulcers by providing a "total contact" type of insole and also relieves shear forces. Although some authors have recommended heating this material in an oven and making molded insoles, we have found this to be unnecessary. With weight-bearing stress, the material tends to adapt and mold to the foot within several days. We have not encountered problems with blistering of the feet as the insole material packs down. The patient is instructed to bathe the feet daily and then to apply a few drops of organic iodine solution until the ulcer heals. With this regimen, and sometimes with repeat debridement of the corn, most small ulcers will heal rather rapidly. We have not had experience with topical application of insulin to the wound, a technique that has been suggested may speed healing. Once the ulcers heal, the less durable polyethylene foam is replaced by neoprene rubber foam (see listing for supplies) to prevent recurrence. For larger ulcers that are still not obviously infected clinically, the plantar callosities are debrided and the patient's extremity is immobilized in a short-leg cast. A layer of polyethylene sheet is used as an insole in this cast. A total-contact plaster cast is applied with an absolute minimum of padding (mainly around the malleoli), and a felt strip is placed along the anterior aspect overlying the tibia. When the cast is to be removed, it is cut along this felt strip. This total-contact cast not only unloads the foot but also prevents push-off. The cast is usually changed at weekly intervals. If

---

*A list of materials and manufacturers is provided at the end of this chapter.

there is a great deal of serous drainage, we sometimes use a Fiberglas cast (Lightcast II). This is more expensive than the plaster cast but does permit the patient to cleanse the foot periodically in a whirlpool bath. We have come to use plaster almost exclusively in more recent years, however.

If the ulcer heals following this treatment, we then use the extra-depth shoe with the appropriate insole material. The insoles are often composite, with a top layer of polyethylene for total contact and shear relief and bottom layer of neoprene for durability.

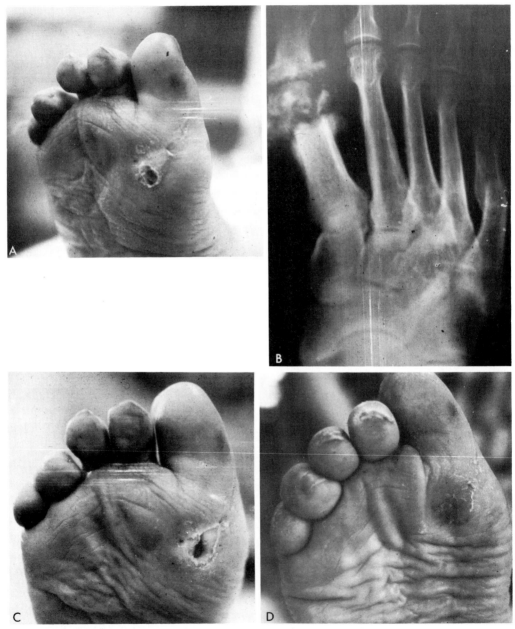

Figure 50–8. *(A) A diabetic with a corn beneath the first metatarsal head. There was no pain on weight bearing. (B) The first metatarsophalangeal joint was destroyed. This was a Charcot joint, not "osteomyelitis," which is a common misdiagnosis. (C) When the corn was sharply debrided away, a full-thickness ulcer was found. (D) After three weeks in a weight-bearing cast with an Aliplast insole, the ulcer healed. Extra-depth shoes with Aliplast insoles were prescribed.*

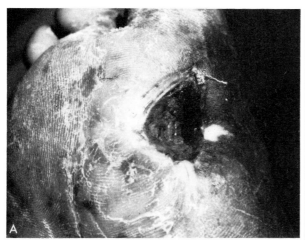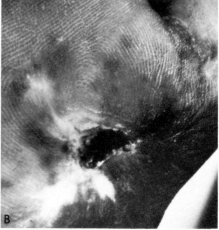

Figure 50–9. *(A) A large, undermined ulcer of long duration was widely debrided, and split-thickness grafts were applied after a clean bed with granulations was obtained. A practically 100 per cent "take" was obtained. (B) The split-thickness graft contracts. This is an advantage — surrounding soft tissues are drawn in and a smaller defect is obtained.*

For larger ulcers, the patient is hospitalized for bed rest and daily debridement (Fig. 50–9). When a good granulating tissue bed is obtained, split-thickness skin grafts are applied. These are carefully checked three days after surgery, and any serum beneath the graft is expressed by a rolling motion using cotton swabs. The dressing is then reapplied, with a Telfa pad being applied directly over the graft and fluff dressings over this. It is next checked at one week and periodically thereafter. The patient is not allowed to go to full weight bearing until the graft has had a chance to mature. Again, protective shoes are prescribed for these patients. Proposed insole combinations are checked with the Harris footprint mat. Paper is placed on the inked mat, and a sheet(s) of insole material of the proposed thickness(es) is placed over this. The patient then prints with a walking step. If the insole material is adequate, the new footprint will show the area of high-density print to be effaced.

Some may criticize use of split-thickness grafts in weight-bearing areas. We have found them to be quite durable, as (contrary to general belief) they thicken up and do *not* "wipe away."

Another criticism of split-thickness grafts is their tendency to contract as they mature (Fig. 50–10). However, in this form of ulcer repair, such contraction is an absolute virtue. Deep cavities shrink to a fraction of their former size as surrounding soft tissue is drawn in. Large ulcers often shrink to 25 per cent or less of their former area — an altogether desirable outcome. We frequently use multiple pinch grafts instead of split-thickness grafts, especially with smaller ulcers (Fig. 50–11). These are also helpful in closing small areas that have been missed earlier with split grafts.

On occasion, the ulcers may extend down to the metatarsal head, and the metatarsophalangeal joint may be grossly infected. In such instances, we resect the metatarsal head through a short longitudinal dorsal incision. All necrotic tissue is debrided, and the dorsal wound is closed. The ulcer usually closes spontaneously within a very short time (Fig. 50–12).

Secondary infection in the forefoot can develop through the portal of entry of mal perforans ulcers. Such patients will characteristically have plantar abscesses involving the central space of the foot. Swelling and erythema occur in the region of the longitudinal arch, and there may be lymphangitic streaks up the leg. The infection may dissect along the flexor tendons, behind the medial malleolus, and up into the calf of the leg — a true surgical emergency. Materials for appropriate smears and cultures are obtained (by aspiration if necessary), and provisional intravenous antibiotic therapy is started based on results of the smear.

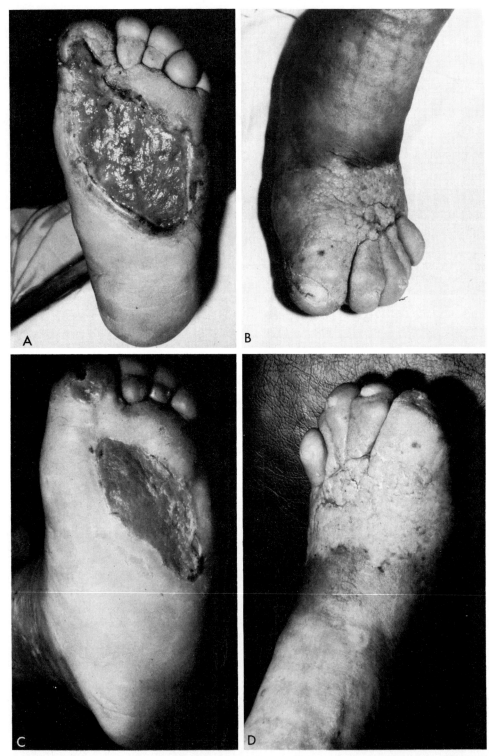

Figure 50–10. *(A) A diabetic with an old, large ulceration on the sole of his foot. (B) There were advanced lymphedematous changes in the forefoot. (C) A split-thickness graft had a 100 per cent "take," and the dimensions of the ulcer contracted rapidly. Extra-depth shoes with Aliplast insoles, tested by a Harris mat, protected the result. This graft, on the sole of the foot, progressively thickened and did not "rub" away. (D) The lymphedematous changes subsided, but at a much more gradual rate.*

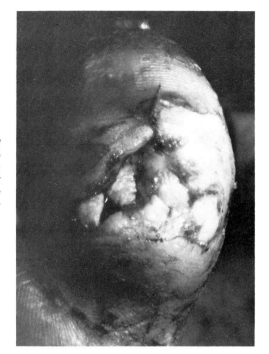

Figure 50–11. *An ulcerated great toe. A lidocaine-filled syringe with No. 25 needle was used to raise wheals on the anterolateral aspect of the thigh. With the needle still in place, each wheal was excised and placed as a pinch graft onto the clean, granulating ulcer. This can be done in the patient's room with a minimum of bother to close small defects.*

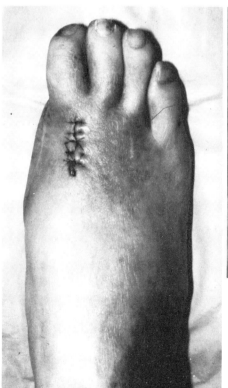

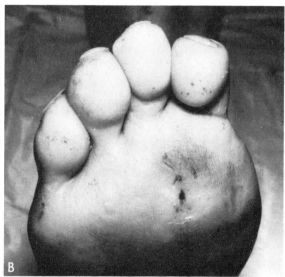

Figure 50–12. *(A) This patient had a previous amputation of the great toe. He wore no protective shoes and has now developed an ulcer beneath the second metatarsal head (a common occurrence). Because of gross infection and copious purulent drainage from the joint itself, the second metatarsal head was excised through a dorsal incision. The wound was thoroughly debrided, as were the margins of the ulcer. The wound was sutured; the ulcer was left open. The wound was clean and cool after two weeks. (B) The ulcer rapidly closed as edema subsided. Two weeks postoperatively it was closed. Extra-depth shoes with protective neoprene rubber insoles were prescribed to prevent recurrence of ulceration under the remaining lateral metatarsal heads.*

The patient is taken to the operating room and the foot is debrided without the use of a tourniquet (Fig. 50–13). A longitudinal plantar incision is made overlying the area of maximum fluctuance. This should be long enough to thoroughly debride the foot. All necrotic tissues are debrided, and this may include part or all of the flexor tendons. Only bleeding, viable tissue is left. The distal leg is "milked" downward in the direction of the plantar incision. Seropurulent exudate may express into the wound along the course of the flexor tendons at the level of the porta pedis. If there is evidence of such proximal spread, separate incisions are made behind the medial malleolus up into the calf of the leg to debride and drain necrotic tissue. Small catheters are then placed into the depths of the wounds, and each is secured to the skin surface with one suture. The wounds are then loosely packed open over the catheters, which are led out through the external dressing to the surface. Organic iodine solutions (Betadine or Pharmadine) are introduced into the catheters three or four times a day to keep the depths of the wounds saturated with these antimicrobial solutions. Dressings are changed in the patient's room by the physician every other day under sterile conditions. These relatively infrequent dressing changes evolve from the teachings of Orr and Trueta. As they noted years ago, frequent dressing changes add nothing, and introduce the possibility of superinfection. Let the wound, with your occasional help, clean itself! During these infrequent dressing changes, further debridement can usually be done without causing the patient any appreciable pain. This is continued until the wound is clean and has begun to granulate.

We have not found any rationale for the use of topical enzymes in wound debridement. Dressing changes help with debridement. This, combined with further mechanical debridement at each change,

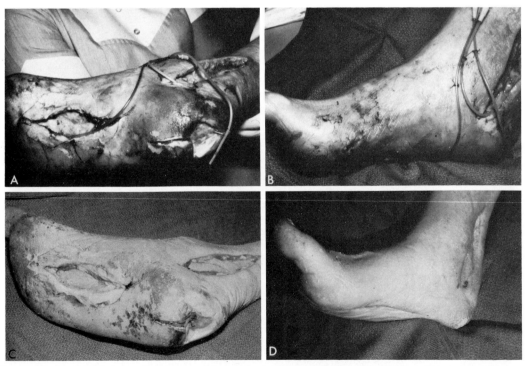

Figure 50–13. *(A) First dressing change. A large plantar abscess as well as an accumulation along the flexor tendons above the ankle was drained. The posterior aspect of the heel also had a large ulceration. Plastic catheters for irrigating solution are seen to lead into each wound. (B) The drainage incision behind the medial malleolus. (C) After repeated debridement, the wound granulated and split-thickness grafts were applied. At the first dressing change, the grafts are in good position and the wounds are clean. (D) Complete coverage with the grafts and a successful result. Protective shoes are now mandatory.*

serves the same purpose as topical enzymes.

As mentioned, the use of topical insulin to aid in wound healing, especially of ulcers, has been suggested for diabetic patients. We have not had sufficient experience to give a statistical comment on its effectiveness.[14]

A new product, Debrisan (Pharmacia AB, Sweden), has been marketed recently. These microscopic, porous, hydrophilic beads are composed of a dextran polymer and are sugar-like in appearance. Poured directly into the wound, they swell and absorb the wound exudate. Changes two or three times daily are claimed to clean wounds rapidly, reduce edema, dry up wounds, and promote granulation.[9] We have limited experience with this product thus far, but early trials after surgical debridement in plantar abscesses have been promising.

On occasion, the whirlpool bath is used to speed debridement. We often found, however, that this caused the granulations to become pale and hypertrophic. This was interpreted as edema secondary to the hypotonicity of the whirlpool solutions. When table salt was added to the solution to a concentration to make it physiologic (0.9 per cent), these changes were less obvious. Still, the whirlpool is not used frequently.

When the wound has begun to granulate, the patient is returned to the operating room and split-thickness skin grafts are applied. These are quickly and easily obtained with a Davol battery-powered dermatome. The grafts are applied in patches rather than in one continuous sheet. They are carefully laid in place and equally carefully covered with Betadine-saturated Telfa pads. Xeroform gauze is used as the next layer of packing, followed by fluff dressings held in place by a circumferential roller bandage. When the grafts are checked after two or three days, the dressing is easily removed down to the Xeroform level. The Xeroform is then carefully removed. The Telfa pads are saturated with sterile saline and teased away from the wound surface. Exudate is expressed from under the grafts by a rolling motion using cotton swabs, and the wound is redressed in the same manner. After several dressing changes, "take" of the grafts is completed. On occasion, one or two pinch grafts are used as "fillers" in still-open areas.

We have found that prolonged debridement and dressing changes before grafting will add little to the ultimate result. When the wound has been debrided, purulent exudate has diminished, and surrounding cellulitis has begun to respond to antibiotic therapy, it is time to think of grafting. We often graft wounds that still appear slightly "dirty." They are once again debrided down to clean tissue, and packed until bleeding stops. Split-thickness skin grafts are then applied. We do not feel that porcine grafts are nearly as valuable as is the early definitive application of human skin.

The situation may not lend itself to complete salvage, e.g., when gangrene of one or more toes is present. In these cases, we combine debridement and drainage with excision of all dead tissue at the most distal possible site that will still provide good bleeding tissue.

After completion of this debridement, it is possible to determine what tissue is left to form a weight-bearing surface. For example, it may be necessary to resect the lateral two rays of the foot. This may leave the patient with a defect that is too large to be closed without tension (Fig. 50–14). If everything else is favorable, we have often applied split-thickness skin grafts immediately to close the remaining skin deficiency. In other cases, further shortening of bone will allow the skin flaps to be closed completely without tension. At still other times, skin grafts can be applied several days later on a newly granulating tissue bed.

In any event, we have often successfully partially or totally closed such wounds at the time of primary surgery when it appeared the wound was *totally and well debrided*. Closure is loose, using several deep chromic sutures to close dead space and widely spaced loose nylon skin sutures. Infrequent dressing changes are done. We do not take the wound down unless there is evidence of spreading infection or grossly purulent drainage. This may be contrary to usual teaching, but with *loose* closure such wounds can drain and, given sufficient time, *do* heal.

In any of these cases, skin stitches are left in for much longer than usual. Healing can be quite slow in diabetics, for the

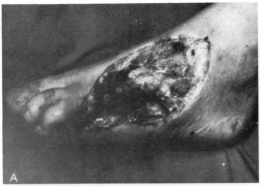
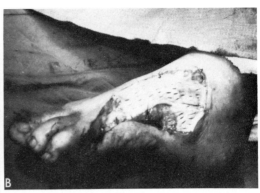
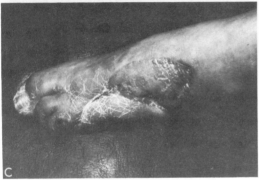

Figure 50–14. *(A) Gangrene of the lateral side of the foot. The lateral two rays and all necrotic skin and deep tissue have been resected. (B) Split-thickness grafts were applied on the raw, bleeding, freshly debrided surface. Multiple stab wounds were made in the large grafts to allow any exudate to escape. (C) Good closure of the wound was obtained. The help of a skilled orthotist-prosthetist is needed to maintain the result.*

reasons already discussed. (One has to see only one dehiscence of a clean wound when sutures are removed at, say, three weeks after surgery to realize the truth of this statement!)

In some cases, the entire forefoot may be gangrenous and infected with no hope of salvage. Conventional wisdom in such cases has been to do a Syme amputation or even a below-the-knee amputation. Most textbooks mention Chopart or Lisfranc amputations only to condemn them. There are two major factors behind these statements. First, after such amputations, patients tend to go into a marked equinus position because of unopposed pull of the heel cord. This fixed position often causes ulceration of the tip of the stump, and the patient never can ambulate properly. Second, there has always been difficulty in shoeing patients after the amputations. If they are merely fitted with high-laced shoes, the shoes soon disintegrate. In addition, blisters and calluses develop at various areas on the stump because of "pumping" action of the stump within the shoe.

Cutting the heel cord alleviates some of these problems (Fig. 50–15). When a Lisfranc or Chopart amputation is done, a transverse percutaneous tenotomy of the heel cord is also performed. The hindfoot can easily dorsiflex beyond the right angle when the division is complete; the gap is palpable. After amputation and heel cord lengthening, the foot is placed in a dorsiflexed position and immobilized with a posterior plaster splint. When this is done and section of the heel cord has been completed, we have seen no problems with equinus deformity or ulceration.

The forefoot amputation is done with maximum conservation of tissue. Using a marking pencil, a line is drawn around the entire forefoot at the level of the most distal viable tissue. This is *not* drawn with regard to the conventionally described flaps (Fig. 50–16). Rather, it is drawn in whatever irregular manner is needed to excise necrotic and inflamed skin and leave viable tissue for the closing flaps (Fig. 50–17).

The initial incision is made down to bone along this line, with no development of planes. When this circumferential incision is completed, the soft tissue is sharply dissected from the bone back toward the hindfoot. Care is taken not to handle the skin edges with forceps, and retraction is gentle. Dissection is carried back to the most distal level at which it appears that the available skin flaps will be able to

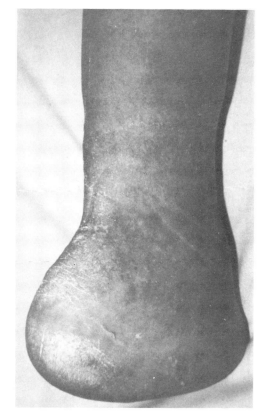

Figure 50–15. *Percutaneous transverse section of the heel cord in a patient with a Chopart's amputation. (The heel is to the left — note the "dimple" at the site of tenotomy.) The remaining stump is broad, durable, and plantigrade.*

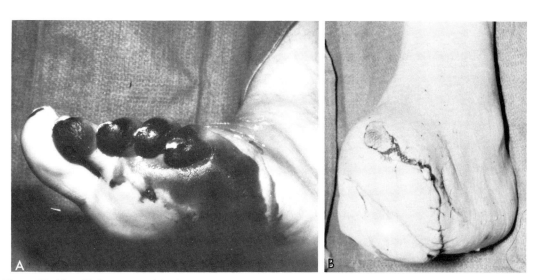

Figure 50–16. *(A) Gangrene of the lateral four toes and sole of the foot. The skin of the great toe and the medial side of the foot does not show changes. (B) Amputation is done, preserving all possible viable tissue. The flaps are then trimmed for optimum closure. Here, the skin of the medial side of the foot forms the flap. A small free graft from the great toe covers a defect at the superior end of the wound.*

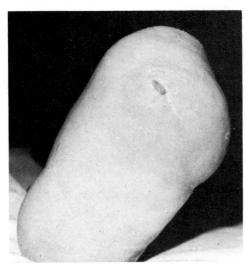

Figure 50–17. *A further illustration of flap geometry. In a Lisfranc's amputation, the skin of the medial side of the left foot has been turned to cover the anterior and lateral aspects of the stump.*

cover without tension in closure. This may be transmetatarsal, Lisfranc's, or Chopart's level. The metatarsals are divided with a sharp osteotome or the disarticulation is completed with sharp dissection, and the necrotic forefoot is discarded. The wound is frequently irrigated with topical antibiotic solution and is now sharply debrided. Tendons are avascular structures and can interfere with healing if infection develops in their vicinity. Visible tendons are pulled down and severed at the highest possible level.

Any flap edges that do not seem to have at least minimal bleeding or appear inflamed are trimmed back to better tissue. The flaps are then tested in any of several possible arrangements to give the best and most tension-free closure. Appropriate trimming of the flaps for best closure is now done, taking care not to narrow the base of the flaps. We often find that the major flap ends up being from the medial side of the foot. If any residual small areas are not closed, we often thin out portions of the viable edges trimmed from the graft and apply them as split-thickness grafts.

A tourniquet is *not* used at any time. Suction drainage tubes are used only if there is apparent dead space. This is infrequent and every care is taken to avoid it.

Again, we realize that Lisfranc and

Chopart amputations have been considered to be of only historical interest, but we find them of value.

The key to our success in subsequent ambulation of such patients is a polypropylene prosthesis that was designed by Richard LaTorre. A plaster cast is taken of the patient's extremity, and a positive plaster mold of the extremity is made from this. An anterior polypropylene shell is fabricated over the mold and lined with Pelite. A similar posterior shell is fabricated over the same mold; the plantar surface is a complete foot plate of the normal foot size. A lightweight polyethylene foam forefoot is affixed to this foot plate of the posterior shell. When this prosthesis is worn, the amputation stump is firmly gripped, and there is no pumping in the shoe. The flexibility of the sole of the prosthesis simulates normal push-off in gait, and the prosthetic forefoot prevents excessive wear-and-tear changes in the shoe and gives further stability (Fig. 50–18). Many advantages can be listed for these types of amputations:

1. Full length of the extremity is preserved.

2. A broad weight-bearing surface, including the undisturbed plantar fat pad of the heel, is preserved.

3. There are remarkably few problems as a result of motion within the prosthesis, and calluses are rare.

4. The enclosure does tend to increase the local temperature in the stump, and skin color often improves remarkably after wearing this for short periods of time.

5. Regular street shoes can be worn and changed.

6. The prosthesis is lightweight.

A corollary is, of course, that a skilled prosthetist is needed to make these amputations work satisfactorily.

SUMMARY AND CONCLUSIONS

In closing, why all the emphasis on maximum preservation? It is simply that we *now* know that, with painstaking care, we can use these various techniques with a high degree of success. Modern prosthetic and orthotic techniques help preserve results and optimize functional results.

Twenty years ago, every medical stu-

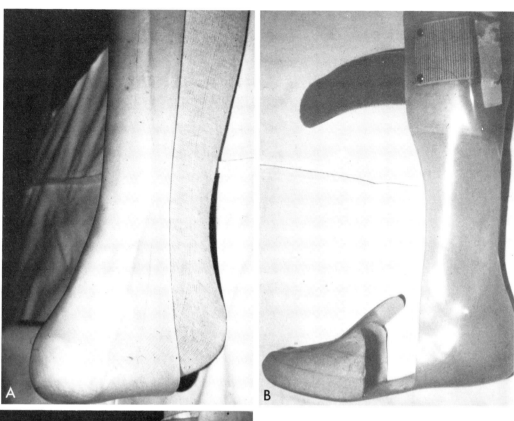

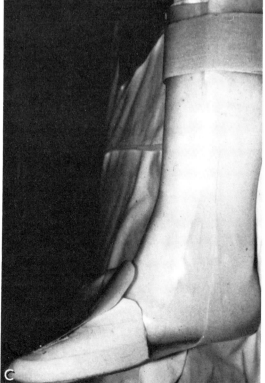

Figure 50–18. (A) The LaTorre prosthesis. The anterior polypropylene shell is placed on the limb (Lisfranc's amputation, in this instance). A protective lining of Pelite can be seen shining through the polypropylene. (B) The posterior shell. Notice the foam filler for the front of the shoe. The flexible sole simulates normal push-off in gait. (C) The prosthesis in situ. A variety of different shoes may be worn with this lightweight, well-fitting prosthesis.

Insole Materials and Footprint Mats*

PRODUCT	MANUFACTURER
Polyethylene Sheet-Bulk	
Aliplast 4E, 1/8, 1/4, 3/8, 1/2 inch	AliMed
Aliplast 6A, 1/8, 1/4 inch (greater density)	172 W. Newton Street
Use 6A for double-layer insoles along with 4E	Boston, Massachusetts 02218
Plastazote, 1/8, 1/4, 1/2 inch (similar to Aliplast 4E)	Knit-Rite
	1121 Grand Avenue
	Kansas City, Missouri 64106
Pelite (firm), 3/16, 3/8, 1/2 inch	Fillauer Orthopedic
Pelite (medium), 3/16, 3/8 inch	936 E. Third Street
	Chatanooga, Tennessee 37401
Platazote (plain and nylon covered), all thicknesses	Apex Foot Products
Moldene #6—same as Pelite (firm)	118 W. 22nd Street
	New York, New York 10011
Microcellular Rubber-Bulk	
Neoprene R-425-N	Rubatex Corporation
Neoprene R-431-N (slightly more dense)	Bedford, Virginia 24523
Both in 1/8 and 1/4 inch thickness	
Fabric-Covered	
Spenco insole material, blue, 1/8 inch	Knit-Rite
	1121 Grand Avenue
	Kansas City, Missouri 64106
	and
	Spenco Medical Material Co.
	P.O. Box 8113
	Waco, Texas 76710
Footprint Mats	
Harris foot mats	Down Surgical, Inc.
3 mm thickness, 1/8 inch	655 73rd Street
1 mm thickness, 1/32 inch	Niagara Falls, New York 14304

These companies will send bronchures upon request. Knit-Rite and Apex also carry a pre-fabricated "healing shoe."

*From a similar list, with the kind permission of Dr. Paul Brand, Carville, Louisiana.

dent was taught that diabetics with infected feet "deserved" above-the-knee amputations. Everyone "knew" that lower amputations simply did not heal. Patients should not be subjected to successive "futile" operations! About ten years ago it was discovered that most below-the-knee amputations in diabetics *could* heal. Now, many investigators are finding that healing can be achieved with even less sacrifice of tissue.

Consider the axiom that, within three years of amputation, one third of all diabetics come to amputation of the other limb. It is rare for bilateral above-the-knee amputees to ambulate with prostheses in a continuing manner. When one above-the-knee and one below-the-knee amputation has been done, only about 50 per cent of diabetics will avoid use of a wheelchair.

With these figures as an incentive, *every* effort should be made to salvage these limbs. The next episode could end with the patient confined to a wheelchair. The savings can be great, both in an economic sense and in maintaining the quality of life for a large group of patients.

REFERENCES

1. Bagdade, J. D., Neilson, K., Root, R., and Bulger, R.: Host defense in diabetes mellitus: the feckless phagocyte during poor control and ketoacidosis. Diabetes, *19*:364, 1970.
2. Bradley, R. V.: Debridement and amputations. *In* Levin, M. E., and O'Neal, L. W. (eds.): The Diabetic Foot. St. Louis, C. V. Mosby, 1973, p. 182.
3. Brand, P.: Repetitive Stress on Insensitive Feet. Leaflet from the U.S. Public Health Service Hospital, Carville, La., 70721.
4. Charcot, J. M.: Sur quelques arthropathies qai paraissant dépdndre d'une lesion du cerveau on de la moelle epinere. Arch. Physiol. Norm. Pathol., *1*:161, 1868.

5. Chapra, J. S., Hurwitz, L. J., and Montgomery, D. A. D.: The pathogenesis of sural nerve changes in diabetes mellitus. Brain, 92:391, 1969.

6. Clayton, M. L.: Surgical treatment of the rheumatoid foot. Giannestras, N. J. (ed.): *In* Foot Disorders. 1st Ed. Philadelphia, Lea and Febiger, 1967, p. 319.

7. Ellenberg, M., and Krainer, L.: Diabetic neuropathy. Diabetes, 8:279, 1959.

8. Goodson, W. H.: Studies of wound healing in experimental diabetes mellitus. J. Surg. Res., 22:221, 1977.

9. Jacobsson, S., Rathmou, U., Arturson, G., Ganrot, K., Haeger, K., and Juklin, I.: A new principle for the cleaning of infected wounds. Scan. J. Plast. Reconstr. Surg., 10:65, 1976.

10. Jordan, W. R.: Neuritic manifestations in diabetes mellitus. Arch. Intern. Med., 57:307, 1936.

11. Locke, S.: The nervous system and diabetes. *In* Marble, A., et al. (eds.): Joslin's Diabetes Mellitus. 11th Ed. Philadelphia, Lea and Febiger, 1971.

12. Marks, H. H., and Krall, L. P.: Onset, course, prognosis and mortality in diabetes mellitus: *In* Marble, A., et al. (eds.): Joslin's Diabetes Mellitus. 11th Ed. Philadelphia, Lea and Febiger, 1971, p. 214.

13. Martin, M. M.: Involvement of autonomic nerve fibers in diabetic neuropathy. Lancet, 1:560, 1953.

14. Paul, T. H.: Treatment by topical application of insulin of an infected wound in a diabetic. Lancet, 2:575, 1966.

15. Raines, J. K., Darling, R. C., Buth, J., Brewster, D. C., and Austen, W. G.: Vascular laboratory criteria for the management of peripheral vascular disease of the lower extremities. Surgery, 79:21, 1976.

16. Roenigk, H. H.: Diabetic skin disease. Consultant, June, 1976, p. 76.

17. Stawiski, M. A.: Cutaneous signs of diabetes mellitus. Cutis, 18:415, 1976.

18. Tan, J. S., Watanakunakorn, C., and Phair, J. P.: Differentiation of defective phagocytosis from impaired intracellular killing by neutrophils with the use of lysostaphin. Tenth Interscience Conference on Antimicrobial Agents and Chemotherapy, Chicago, October 18, 1970.

19. Terkildsen, A. B., and Christensen, N. J.: Reversible nervous abnormalities in juvenile diabetics with recently diagnosed diabetes. Diabetologia, 7:113, 1971.

20. Thomas, P. K., and Lascelles, R. G.: The pathology of diabetic neuropathy. O. J. Med., 140:489, 1966.

21. Ward, J. D., Bornes, C. G., and Fischer, D. J.: Improvement in nerve conduction following treatment in newly diagnosed diabetics. Lancet, 1:428, 1971.

22. Williamson, R. T.: Changes in the posterior column of the spinal cord in diabetes mellitus. Br. Med. J., 1:398, 1894.

23. Williamson, R. T.: On the knee jerks in diabetes mellitus. Lancet, 2:138, 1897.

24. Williamson, R. T.: Note on the tendo achillis jerk and other reflexes in diabetes mellitus. Rev. Neurol. Psychiatr., 1:667, 1903.

25. Williamson, R. T.: Changes in the spinal cord in diabetes mellitus. Br. Med. J., 1:122, 1904.

26. Williamson, R. T.: The symptoms due to peripheral neuritis or spinal lesions in diabetes mellitus. Rev. Neurol. Psychiatr., 5:550, 1907.

CHAPTER 51

INFECTIONS OF THE FOOT

Ambrose James Selvapandian,
B.Sc., M.S., F.A.C.S.

Yaws

Donald M. Qualls, M.D.

INTRODUCTION

The feet are the most used part of the body and for this reason the most misused. Unlike the hands, they are perhaps protected from casual trauma and subsequent infections because they are confined in shoes.

In tropical countries, the customs and socioeconomic and climatic conditions are such that walking barefoot or use of open footwear is preferred to constant wearing of closed shoes. Therefore, the foot can be the site of inflammation due to trivial trauma or acute or chronic infections. Unless the patient seeks medical advice because of pain, the usual tendency is to pay less attention to foot conditions than to other disorders. This results in an advanced state of disease because of neglect.

Pain is the important symptom that draws attention to any minor injury or commencing infection. Superficial pain is caused by irritation of the skin. Deep pain is usually due to tension within deeply situated structures such as tendon, fascia, bursa, bone, or joint following inflammation caused by trauma or infection.

Pain caused by any acute infection or trauma to the foot enforces rest, as the patient is unable to bear weight or to walk on the affected foot. Rest and elevation constitute an important aspect in the treatment of these conditions, along with local treatment of the affected part. However, in chronic disorders such as granulomatous infections, pain may not be a major disabling factor, and the patient retains a reasonable degree of function of the inflamed foot. Hence, such an infection may be neglected by the patient until other symptoms appear. Trophic or perforating ulcers are known for their nonhealing nature because of interference with the sensory nerves and blood supply. Loss of sensation, including pain sensation, allows the infection to involve the deeper tissues before medical attention is sought. This happens in disorders such as leprosy, diabetes, congenital sensory neuropathy, and peripheral nerve injuries. The absence of pain is the most characteristic feature of these conditions and leads to delay in diagnosis, neglect, and subsequent delay in healing of the infection. Also, the chance of recurrence of trophic ulcers is very high. With every subsequent infection the residual destruction and loss of tissue substance increase, resulting in grotesque deformities and altered patterns of weight bearing. The latter predisposes to further ulceration and infection of the unprotected foot.

ROUTES OF INFECTION

Infection reaches the foot by discontinuity in the covering skin caused by trauma or by the hematogenous route (Fig. 51–1).

Most pyogenic infections develop following contamination of open wounds of varying degrees. Occasionally, pyogenic infection of the foot is a local manifestation of septicemia with other foci of infection. In such cases the causative organism reaches the foot by the hematogenous route. Some of the organisms causing granulomatous lesions, such as fungi, enter the foot through openings due to unrecognizable trauma to the skin or through fissures that are already present. Other organisms responsible for granulomatous infections, such as those causing tuberculosis, syphilis, leprosy, and sarcoidosis, are blood-borne. In guinea worm infestation, the worm traverses the fascial planes to reach the skin (see Figure 51–22).

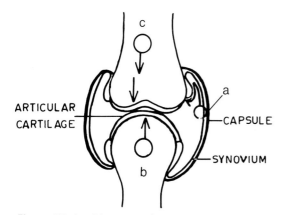

Figure 51–1. *Diagrammatic representation of the hematogenous spreading of infection. (a) From synovium to articular cartilage. (b) From osseous intra-articular lesion to articular cartilage. (c) From osseous extra-articular lesion to articular cartilage.*

Anatomy of Skin of the Foot

The skin of the foot (Fig. 51–2) resembles the skin over the rest of the body in most histologic aspects except for the greater thickness and the absence of hair follicles on the sole. Even in the fetus, the skin of the sole is appreciably thicker than the skin over other areas. Continuous friction and pressure during postnatal life lead to further adaptive thickening of the skin of the sole. There are two main layers in the skin of the sole — the outer layer, or epidermis, and the inner layer, or dermis.

Epidermis. The epidermis consists of several layers of stratified squamous epithelial cells and is about 1.4 mm thick. Four layers can be distinguished. The deepest of these is the stratum malpighii, which is subdivided into (1) the stratum germinativum (stratum basale), the layer of cells in contact with the dermis, and (2) the stratum spinosum (prickle cell layer), a layer of variable thickness above the stratum germinativum. The next deepest layer is the stratum granulosum, or the granular layer; then comes the stratum lucidum, or the clear cell layer. The most superficial layer is the stratum corneum, or the horny layer. The superficial keratinized portion of the epidermis consists of stratum corneum and stratum lucidum.

The cells of stratum germinativum adjacent to the dermis are cuboidal to columnar and have their cell axis perpendicular to the basal lamina. As the cells move up into the stratum spinosum, they assume a flattened polyhedral shape, with their long axis parallel to the surface and their nuclei elongated in this direction. The cells of this layer have short processes that are attached to similar projections from adjacent cells. The stratum granulosum consists of three to five layers of flattened cells containing conspicuous, irregularly shaped granules that stain deeply with basic dyes. These are keratohyaline granules. The stratum lucidum is formed of several layers of flattened, closely packed eosinophilic cells. In section, the stratum lucidum appears as a clear, wavy strip. The nuclei of the cells in this layer have disappeared. The stratum corneum consists of many layers of flat cornified cells without nuclei and with cytoplasm replaced by keratin. In the most peripheral layers (stratum disjunctum), these cells are dry and horny and are constantly being desquamated.

Dermis. The dermis of the sole is 3 mm or more in thickness. The outer surface of the dermis, in contact with the epidermis, is usually uneven and is composed of papillae that project into the concavities of the ridges on the deep surface of the epidermis. This layer is called the papillary layer; the main deep portion of the dermis is known as the reticular layer.

These two layers cannot be clearly differentiated.

The reticular layer consists of dense connective tissue with collagenous fibers in bundles running in various directions, most of which are parallel to the surface. A few bundles are almost perpendicular to the rest. The papillary layer consists of loose connective tissue with much thinner collagenous fibers. The cells of the dermis are more abundant in the papillary than in the reticular layer and are similar to those

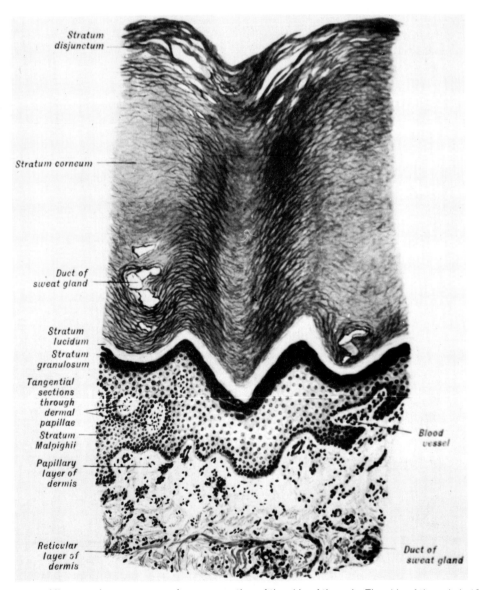

Figure 51-2. *Microscopic appearance of a cross section of the skin of the sole. The skin of the sole is 10 times thicker than other areas of the body, mainly because of the stratum corneum. (From Bloom, W., and Fawcett, D. W.: A Textbook of Histology, 9th ed. Philadelphia, W. B. Saunders Company, 1968, p. 482.)*

of the subcutaneous layer (see following paragraph) except for the relative lack of fat cells.

Beneath the dermis is a looser subcutaneous layer consisting of connective tissue. This is the superficial fascia, or the hypodermis, which is largely subcutaneous adipose tissue. Its fibers are directly continuous with those of the dermis and also run in all directions, most of them parallel to the skin. This layer is penetrated by large blood vessels and nerves and contains many nerve endings.

Anatomy of Spaces of the Foot

The foot is divided by the plantar aponeurosis into superficial and deep plantar spaces (Fig. 51–3). The superficial plantar space is further divided into web spaces, corresponding to the position of the webs of toes; interdigital spaces; and the heel space, corresponding to the calcaneus. Web spaces are four triangular regions between the dorsal and plantar skin filled with loose fat that bulges between the divisions of the plantar fascia. Interdigital spaces are subcutaneous areas that lie between the five digital slips of the plantar aponeurosis. The shafts of the metatarsals border the spaces on the sides.

The deep plantar space is divided into central, medial, and lateral spaces by vertical fibrous intramuscular septa arising from the borders of the central part of the plantar aponeurosis. The space between the medial and lateral intramuscular septa is the central deep plantar space. It is further divided by the four layers of plantar muscles. The space medial to the intramuscular septum is the medial deep plantar space and those lateral to the lateral intramuscular septum are the lateral deep plantar spaces. Fibrous septa extend from the phalanges to the medial and lateral aspects of each toe.

ACUTE INFECTIONS OF THE FOOT

Whenever the body is injured, typical changes occur in the affected part. The inflammatory changes are recognized as the area becomes warm, red, painful, and swollen. These changes denote tissue destruction, which occurs in direct proportion to the extent of trauma.

Blister

A blister usually arises following irritation of the skin, frequently due to improperly fitting footwear. It is characterized by a swelling without breakdown of skin and contains clear fluid. The superficial layers of the epidermis are raised away from the deeper layers. The fluid contains chemicals produced as a result of reaction that vary in toxicity according to the duration of the blister.

Removal of the local external irritant, aspiration of the fluid, and resting the foot will lead to healing of the blister. If infection supervenes, particularly when the blister breaks down, healing is delayed.

Abrasion

If irritation of the skin persists, the horny layer wears off and the source of irritation is in direct contact with the stratum granulosum, causing an abrasion. In such cases, the danger of infection is much greater.

Treatment consists of preventing further irritation and avoiding or eradicating infection by use of a local antibiotic cream dressing until the abrasion epithelializes.

Ulcer

If the irritation is severe and continuous, the abrasion proceeds to form an ulcer. The entire thickness of the skin is dam-

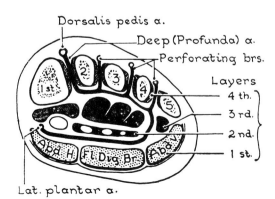

Figure 51–3. *A cross section of the foot illustrating the fascial spaces.*

aged and subcutaneous tissues are exposed. An ulcer can also result following neglect of an infected abrasion. Sometimes vital structures may be exposed in the floor of the ulcer, e.g., tendons of extensors of the toes in an ulcer on the dorsum of the foot. The tendons may slough off and have to be removed. In cases in which bone lies close to the subcutaneous tissue, the danger of spread of infection to the underlying bone is real. The skin is indurated and brawny around infected ulcers.

Treatment consists of eradicating the infection and healing the skin defect. Rest, elevation of the affected part, and regular application of local dressings are essential to heal the ulcer. In instances in which the ulcer overlies a joint, it is often necessary to immobilize the foot in a plaster splint. If infection is present, appropriate antibiotics, both systemic and local, must be covered with a split-thickness Thiersch graft.

Ulcers over the weight-bearing part of the foot are difficult to treat, as the skin graft tends to break down under the strain and shearing forces of weight bearing.

Wounds

These are caused by severe mechanical violence that results in the rupture or division of true skin and deeper tissues. Wounds are classified into crush, puncture, or degloving injuries, according to the degree of violence.

Crush Injury. Such injury is generally caused by the foot being crushed between two objects or by a heavy object falling on the foot. Varying degrees of damage and loss of skin, subcutaneous tissue, and sometimes bone occur. Usually the wound is contaminated by foreign bodies, dirt, or grease acquired from the crushing object.

A crush injury must be treated as a surgical emergency. Thorough preparation of the wound and surrounding skin followed by strict surgical debridement to remove foreign bodies and necrotic tissue is essential to prevent infection. Initially, the wound is left open in preparation for a delayed primary or a secondary closure. Sometimes, a Thiersch skin graft is essential to close the skin defect.

Puncture Wound. Stepping on needles, nails, or other sharp objects produces this type of wound. In a puncture wound,

the external injury to the skin is minimal, whereas the deeper tissues are more severely damaged. Hence, there is a real danger of failing to recognize the extent of the wound. Also, the drainage in such a wound is inadequate.

Treatment consists of surgical exploration of the wound followed by removal of devascularized and necrotic tissue and establishment of adequate drainage.

Degloving Injuries. These are caused by accidents in which a heavy object runs over the body, e.g., motor vehicle accidents. The skin loss can be extensive and difficult to restore. In some cases skin may still be attached to the edges of the wound.

Treatment consists of immediate surgical debridement of the wound and later skin coverage. In cases in which skin overhangs the edges of the wound, there is a temptation to preserve and sometimes suture the skin. However, before retaining any of the degloved skin, its viability and vascularity must be confirmed. If the skin appears normal and its edges bleed freely, it is probably viable and may be retained. In wounds in which a flap of skin is distally based, the chances of skin survival are poor and the flap must be excised.

Inappropriate or inadequate primary care will lead to infection and subsequent delay in healing.

Callus

A callus, or callosity, is formed as a result of repeated intermittent pressure that is usually caused by improper footwear. It is also seen on deformed feet with inherent structural defects, such as neglected clubfeet in which the weight bearing is on thinner portions of the skin of the foot. The callus is also seen in areas where the skin is soft, e.g., the outer border of the foot. The pressure occurs over a small surface area.

A callus consists of thickening of the keratinized area of the skin that is produced by proliferation of cells of the stratum basale. It appears as a thickening of the skin and is painful on weight bearing and tender on pressure.

The ill-fitting footwear causing the callus must be discontinued. Keratolytic agents may be applied locally. In cases in which the cause is an inherent deformity of the foot, weight bearing must be prevented until the deformity is corrected and weight bearing is thus transferred to more normal areas.

Corn

A corn is produced by repeated intermittent pressure. It is seen on areas of the foot where the skin is thick (e.g., the sole) and where the area exposed to the abnormal pressure is large. Corns are usually seen on the heel and under the metatarsal heads.

The corn consists of a conical wedge of keratinized tissue with the apex of the wedge pointing toward the subcutaneous surface. Usually the apex is in contact with the nerve fibers in subcutaneous tissue, and this can make the corn extremely tender.

Treatment consists of rest and enucleation of the wedge of keratinized tissue without causing tissue injury. Following healing, modifications are made either in the footwear or in the pattern of weight bearing. The insole of the shoe must be padded with soft rubber with a "cutout" over the area of the corn. In cases of recurrence of corns on the sole, under the metatarsal heads, the metatarsal heads are relieved of weight bearing by using a metatarsal bar on the sole of the shoe or a metatarsal pad on the insole.

Fissure

A fissure is a deep crack in the epidermis. It is commonly encountered between the toes, in flexor creases of the toes (Fig. 51–4), or around the back of the heel. A fissure is always slow to heal. It is associated with dry hyperkeratinized skin, e.g., the heel, or in areas where the skin is moist and structures are deformed, e.g., the flexor creases of the toes in cases of flexion contracture of the interphalangeal joints.

When fissures are associated with dry hyperkeratotic skin, the excess skin must be removed with a scalpel and the raw area treated with 5 to 15 per cent silver nitrate solution. In cases in which the skin is moist and the toes are deformed, the incidence of infection is higher. In such cases, the skin should be dried and the fissure debrided and treated with appropriate antibiotics. Recurrence is prevented by correction of the deformity.

Chronic Plantar Ulcers (Figs. 51–5 and 51–6)

Healing of an acute infection of the foot is usually assured in a normal person because the pain reflexes compel him to rest until healing results. If a plantar ulcer has not healed for some time, neurotrophic causes such as leprosy, congenital absence of pain, or diabetes are suspected. In older

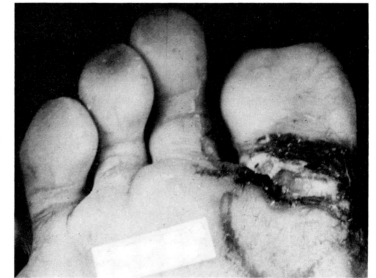

Figure 51–4. Infected fissure along the flexor crease of the hallux.

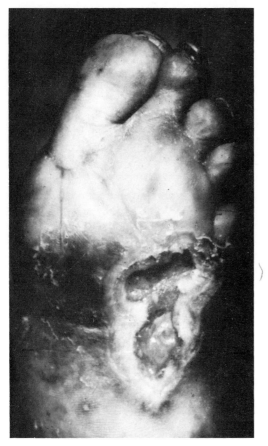

Figure 51–5. *A chronic plantar ulcer along the lateral border of the sole.*

people, vascular disorders are frequently the cause of slow healing.

In less developed countries, the majority of people in rural areas prefer to walk barefoot and subsequently develop an unusually thick sole. The thickness of the sole is due to accumulated cornified epithelium. This, in fact, protects the sole of the foot from casual injuries such as blister or abrasion. However, the skin is liable to develop cracks and fissures, usually at the edges and creases of the toes. When such cracks or fissures become infected, healing does not readily occur.

Chronic Ulcers Over Bony Prominences

Ulcers develop over bony prominences of the foot (Fig. 51–7) following constant pressure of a shoe or splint. The common areas of occurrence are the malleoli and the back of the heel.

Removal of the causative factor, rest, and regular dressing of the ulcer lead to cure. Neglect of such ulcers permits infection to reach the underlying bone and cause osteomyelitis.

Of special importance is the ulcer over the back of the heel. The skin over the back of the heel is very thin and devoid of subcutaneous tissue. Ulceration of this

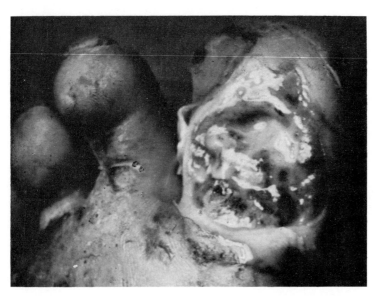

Figure 51–6. *A chronic plantar ulcer on the plantar aspect of the hallux demonstrating necrosis of the skin and sloughing of the underlying soft tissue.*

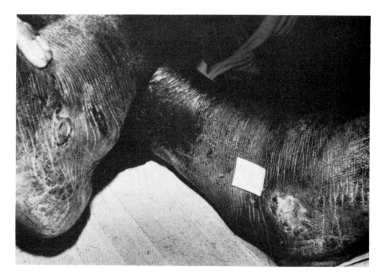

Figure 51–7. *Malleolar ulcers following application of a plaster cast.*

skin is commonly seen in bedridden patients and paraplegics because of constant contact and irritation by bedclothes. It also follows inappropriate application of plaster splints with inadequate padding. As the tendo Achillis and calcaneus lie just under the skin, they are usually exposed if the ulcer deepens. This can lead to sloughing of the tendon and calcaneal osteomyelitis.

Treatment consists of early recognition, removal of the pressure, rest, and dressings.

Tenosynovitis

Inflammation of tendon sheaths of the tibialis posterior, tibialis anterior, and, occasionally, the peronei occurs spontaneously following nonspecific inflammation. It is occasionally a manifestation of generalized rheumatoid disease.

A well-defined fluctuant swelling is seen along the course of the tendon. Active contraction of the muscle produces pain, as does passive stretching of the affected tendon.

Treatment consists of anti-inflammatory drugs, local heat, rest, and application of a plaster splint.

Painful Heel

Inflammation of the skin and subcutaneous tissues behind the heel is common in babies and toddlers who wear shoes. The skin is red and swollen, the subcutaneous tissues are thickened, and a bruise may form superficial to the insertion of the tendo Achillis. Discontinuation of the use of shoes, rest, and anti-inflammatory drugs are curative.

Purulent Infections of the Foot

Infected Blister. An infected blister is one of the most common foot infections. If the patient's temperature is normal but the blister appears questionably purulent, it is aspirated and the aspirate is sent for bacteriologic examination. If the blister is frankly purulent, it must be incised and drained.

Treatment includes dressings, bedrest, and appropriate antibiotics.

Paronychia. Paronychia of the great toe is common and often occurs as a complication of an ingrowing toenail. Abrasion of the eponychium by using a contaminated scissors is also a known cause. Suppuration occurs and is confined to the base of the nail by the adherence of the eponychium to the base. Pus tracks form around the nail, and later the pus extends beneath the nail and lifts it off.

In early cases, adequate rest and antibiotic therapy can abort the infection. Once pus has formed, it has to be expressed surgically. At operation, the eponychium is stripped gently and completely from the base of the nail, and loose cuticle is cut away. If there is a pocket of pus under the corner of the nailfold, a wedge of overlying skin is removed to ensure healing from below. The loose eponychium is then excised with sharp scissors. When pus has extended beneath the nail, the undermined part of the nail must be excised with fine, strong scissors. If the pus has extended beneath 50 per cent or more of the width of the nail, the proximal third of the nail is excised. Appropriate antibiotic therapy and rest ensure healing.

Infection of Adventitious Bursae. Infection of adventitious bursae beneath corns can lead to suppuration. Treatment includes drainage, rest, and antibiotics.

Infection of the Pulp Space. Pulp space infection, although uncommon, is sometimes seen in the great toe. Surgical drainage, rest, and antibiotics lead to healing.

The fibrous septa in the toes prevent the infection from spreading to the dorsum of the toe, but there is a great danger of the infection spreading along the synovial sheath of long flexor tendons to the deep plantar space.

Infection of the Web Space. Infection of the plantar aspect of the web space of the foot commonly presents with extension of abscesses to the dorsal aspect as well. The adjacent toes are widely separated, with gross swelling and inflammation of the plantar and dorsal aspects of the web space.

Surgical drainage through a small diamond-shaped incision on the plantar aspect of the web space must be done. If the pus extends to the dorsum, a corresponding incision should be made on that aspect also. Occasionally the infection spreads to the adjacent web space, which should be drained separately. Adequate rest and appropriate antibiotics are essential.

Infection of the Plantar Interdigital Subcutaneous Space. Infection in these spaces is seen commonly in people who walk barefoot. Increasing pain occurs between the shafts of the metatarsals that bound the space, and exquisite tenderness located over the infected space is diagnostic. Pus may decompress itself between the two bones into the dorsal subcutaneous space.

Incision for drainage is similar to that for web space infection. A sinus forceps is

introduced through this incision and directed to the pus-filled cavity, which is opened. Drainage must be followed by antibiotics and rest.

Infection of the Heel Space. This infection is intradermal in one third of the cases, and a few of these are a "collarstud" extension from a deeper plane. The remaining cases are due to infection of the fat pad of the heel, which is situated in the subcutaneous portion of the posterior third of the sole. The usual portal of entry is a crack in the overlying calloused skin.

The pain is of the steadily increasing, throbbing type and usually interferes with sleep. Swelling of the soft tissues covering the sides of the calcaneus is present. Occasionally, edema develops around the ankle. Tenderness over the heel space is diagnostic.

Drainage is through an incision in the medial or lateral side of the heel, so that the scar does not lie on the weight-bearing part of the heel. Fibrous septa within must be broken through and accumulations of pus allowed to drain. The lips of the incision must be trimmed elliptically to prevent premature closure of the skin. Drainage is followed by rest and antibiotic therapy until healing occurs.

Deep Plantar Space Abscesses. The central deep plantar space abscesses present deep to the plantar aponeurosis. This space resembles a house with four stories. Infection of the various floors becomes increasingly less common as one proceeds deeper and upward.

Drainage is through an incision parallel to and just above the medial border of the foot in close proximity to the instep. Following drainage, the foot must be rested adequately and antibiotics administered.

Infection of the Dorsum of the Foot. The dorsal subcutaneous space is usually infected by extension from a subcutaneous interdigital or web space infection, whereas the dorsal subaponeurotic space is infected either by a direct puncture or by extension from the deep plantar space.

To drain a dorsal subcutaneous space abscess, the incision is placed distal to the dorsal venous arch in line with the digital vessels and nerves. Prior to draining the dorsal subaponeurotic space, the space is first aspirated. If pus is obtained, the incision is made longitudinally alongside the needle. Antibiotics and rest are advocated following drainage.

CHRONIC INFECTIONS OF THE FOOT

Chronic infections of the foot are commonly of the granulomatous variety. Few of the chronic infections are nongranulomatous. Granulomatous disorders include tuberculosis, mycosis, syphilis, sarcoidosis, and leprosy; whereas nongranulomatous disorders are caused by either pyogenic infection or parasitic infestation.

Granulomatous Infections

Tuberculosis

Tuberculosis of the foot and ankle is the most common form of granulomatous lesions seen in the tropics. It is always a secondary tuberculous lesion, as is any other form of musculoskeletal tuberculosis. The primary tuberculous focus is in the lung or lymph nodes.

Tuberculosis may involve the ankle joint, tarsal bones, metatarsals, phalanges, or synovial sheaths of tendons. The most common form is tuberculous arthritis of the ankle.

Tuberculous lesions reach the foot by the hematogenous route, and the disease starts in the soft tissue–like synovium of tendons and joints or in osseous foci within the bones. If untreated, the synovial lesions spread beyond the limits of the synovial membrane to the articular cartilage in the form of tuberculous granulation (Fig. 51–8). This pannus extends on the superficial and deep surfaces of the articular cartilage and erodes it. Similarly, intra-articular osseous lesions expand and then break into the neighboring joint, thereby destroying it. Extra-articular osseous tuberculous lesions expand and erode the cortex and involve the surrounding soft tissue. The tuberculous detritus, in the form of tuberculous pus, forms a cold abscess in the overlying tissue or tuberculous granulation around the bone. If the tuberculous abscess bursts, an indolent sinus develops over the site of breakthrough. Occasionally the lesion spreads locally along the skin, producing a tuberculous ulcer. Multiple sinuses are usually seen in chronic tuberculous lesions of the foot.

Chemotherapy for any form of tuberculosis of the foot must be given for a period of at least 18 months. The usual regimen is daily streptomycin injections with oral isonicotinic acid hydrazide (INAH) and para-aminosalicylic acid (PAS) for a period of three months followed by INAH and PAS for the next 15 months. The dosage in children is streptomycin, 40 mg/kg/day;

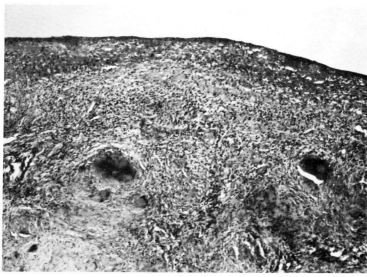

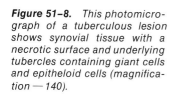

Figure 51–8. *This photomicrograph of a tuberculous lesion shows synovial tissue with a necrotic surface and underlying tubercles containing giant cells and epitheloid cells (magnification — 140).*

INAH, 15 mg/kg/day; and PAS, 250 mg/kg/day. The adult dosage is streptomycin, 1 gm/day (0.75 gm/day in older patients or 1 gm on alternate days until a total of 90 gm is administered; INAH, 300 to 400 mg/day; and PAS, 4 gm three times a day.

Pyridoxine, 50 mg daily, should be given as a supplement to antituberculous therapy.

Tuberculosis of the Ankle. This form of tuberculosis usually starts as synovitis with gross thickening and hypertrophy of the synovial membrane (Fig. 51–9). The synovium feels boggy on clinical examination, and x-ray studies reveal a generalized osteoporosis of the ankle joint. No specific lytic lesions are seen in the bones. In early cases, in which the disease is limited to the synovium, the cartilage space of the ankle retains its normal width. However, as the disease progresses from the synovium to the articular cartilage, narrowing of the joint space occurs, and subsequent erosion of the joint surface and late collapse with destruction of the joint surface are seen. If unchecked, the tuberculous process involves periarticular structures and breaks through the skin, resulting in a tuberculous sinus. Secondary infection of such a sinus alters the clinical, radiologic, and histopathologic picture of the disease.

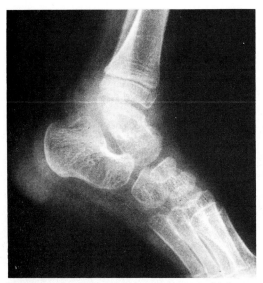

Figure 51–9. *Radiographic appearance of tuberculous synovitis of the ankle. Note the diffuse soft-tissue thickening and osteoporosis of the tarsal bones.*

In the osseous form of tuberculosis of the ankle joint, the lesion develops first in the talus, lower end of the tibia, calcaneus, navicular, or cuboid bone. Findings include local pain and tenderness and signs of inflammation in the skin overlying the bony lesion. The radiograph shows discrete osteolytic lesions within the bones, which are associated with a fair amount of generalized osteoporosis of the surrounding bones. As the disease progresses, the osteolytic lesions expand and involve the joint surface and cartilage. In cases in which the lesion begins in the calcaneus or other tarsal bones of the foot (except the talus), the disease process usually involves the subtalar and midtarsal joints before involving the ankle. As the disease progresses, the joints become more and more painful, and the patient develops equinus contracture at the ankle and is unable to bear weight on the foot because of the pain. Following erosion of the articular surfaces, fibrous tissue develops between the articulating bones, resulting in a painful fibrous ankylosis of the ankle joint. For the reasons mentioned, tuberculous involvement of the ankle is commonly seen in association with involvement of other bones and joints of the foot.

In the synovial form of disease, complete healing and return to normal function of the ankle can be expected. Treatment is either conservative (involving rest, a plaster splint, and adequate chemotherapy) or operative (involving a synovectomy followed by adequate rest and chemotherapy). During synovectomy, the joint surfaces are inspected and cleared of any tuberculous granulation tissue.

Once the disease has involved the articular surface and the articular cartilage shows signs of destruction, restoration of normal function is impossible. Treatment includes arthrodesis of the ankle in neutral position using Charnley's compression clamps (Fig. 51–10).

Tuberculosis of the Tarsal Bones. Tuberculous osteitis of the tarsal bones is seen in the calcaneus, talus, navicular, and cuboid in descending order of incidence (Fig. 51–11). Usually, tuberculosis of the navicular or the head of talus leads to the involvement of the talonavicular joint. Treatment consists of adequate rest and chemotherapy. When the disease has ex-

Figure 51–10. Radiographic appearance of old tuberculosis of the ankle following arthrodesis and healing of the lesion.

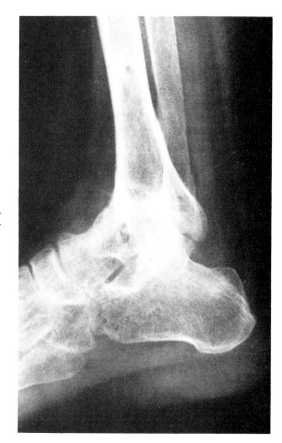

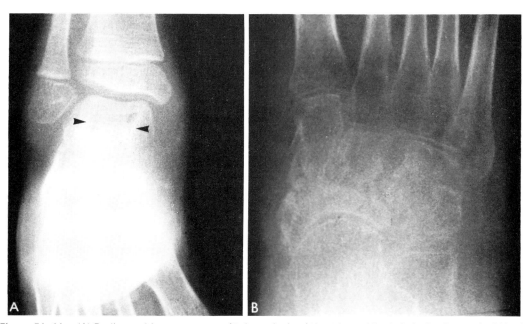

Figure 51–11. (A) Radiographic appearance of tuberculosis of the talus, with a lytic lesion (arrows) within the talus. (B) Radiographic appearance of tuberculosis of the navicular, with destruction of the naviculocuneiform joints. Note the extensive osteoporosis, which is typical of tuberculosis without secondary infection.

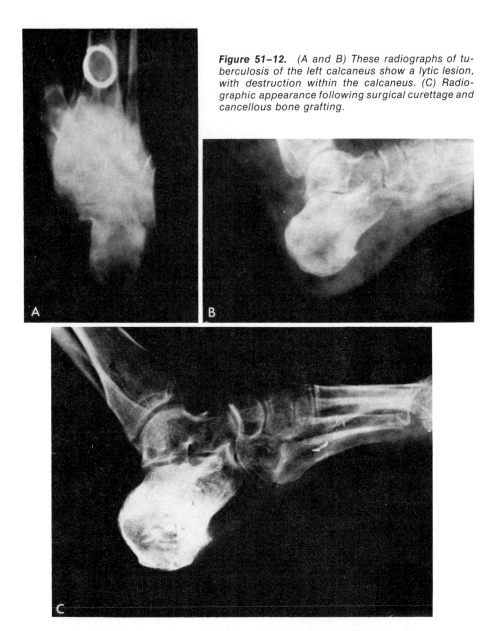

Figure 51–12. (A and B) These radiographs of tuberculosis of the left calcaneus show a lytic lesion, with destruction within the calcaneus. (C) Radiographic appearance following surgical curettage and cancellous bone grafting.

tended to the neighboring joint and produces pain on movement and walking, surgical intervention is warranted. Curettage of the affected tarsal bone with arthrodesis of the neighboring affected joint is carried out. In large bones such as the calcaneus, an extensive tuberculous lesion is curetted, and the cavity is filled with cancellous bone graft (Fig. 51–12).

Tuberculous Dactylitis (Spina Ventosa). Tuberculous dactylitis is seen only in early childhood. Phalanges are involved

more often than metatarsals, and other foci of skeletal tuberculosis are usually detectable. Thickening and spindling of the involved digit are also present. Within the bone, the marrow cavity is replaced by tuberculous granulations. The cortex appears thin and expanded and may be perforated in places. Some periosteal bone formation may be seen. Following perforation of the cortex, the disease enters the surrounding soft tissue, and a sinus forms. Later, the disease involves the epiphyseal cartilages at the ends of the bone, with subsequent retardation of growth and shortening of the toe.

Tuberculous Tenosynovitis. Tuberculous tenosynovitis is seen most commonly in the flexor sheath at the ankle. Usually there is evidence of the other forms of tuberculosis in such a patient. Treatment consists of thorough surgical excision of the infected tendon sheath, adequate chemotherapy, and rest.

Mycosis

Involvement of bones and joints by fungal infections is not usual, although when this does occur, the foot is the most common site for this type of infection (Figs. 51–13 to 51–17).

Fungi enter the foot through breaks in the skin. This occurs most commonly in tropical countries where people walk barefoot. The fungus may be present in the soil and enters through cuts and fissures in the sole (e.g., Madura foot), or the organism reaches the foot as a blood-borne infection (e.g., blastomycosis). In such cases, the lesion in the foot is a local manifestation of systemic disease. The primary lesion is commonly seen in the lungs. Occasionally more than one variety of fungus is responsible for the infection.

Mycetoma. This condition is a chronic granulomatous fungal infection that most often affects the feet (mycetoma pedis). The terms Madura foot and maduromycosis are used to emphasize the high prevalence of the condition in Southern India, although it is found in other parts of the world as well. Rarely this infection can involve hands and arms.

Mycetoma pedis is caused by a variety of organisms, which are classified into two main groups: (1) false fungi, or higher bacteria (actinomycetes) and (2) true fungi, or higher fungi (Table 51–1).

After the fungus enters the sole, an indurated nodule develops at the site of entry. The nodule gradually enlarges and breaks down, producing numerous sinuses with raised margins. There may be associated secondary infection as well (Fig. 51–18). The infection spreads to the subcutaneous tissue, capsule, and periarticular structures. The bone and the joints of the foot are involved subsequently, and the

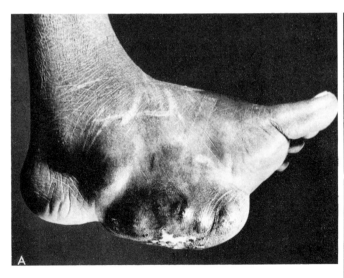
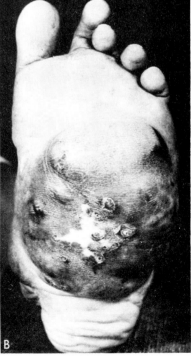

Figure 51–13. *(A and B) Madura mycosis. Granulomatous mycotic abscess with multiple sinuses on the sole of the foot.*

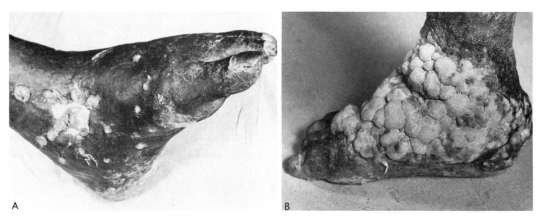

A   B

Figure 51-14. *(A and B) Madura mycosis with extensive involvement of all of the tissues of the foot, multiple sinuses, and exuberant granulation tissue.*

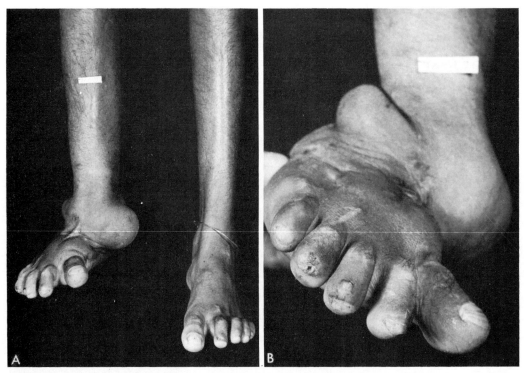

A   B

Figure 51-15. *(A) Mycetoma of the right foot and ankle, with extensive destruction and collapse of the tarsus and residual shortening and deformity. (B) Close-up view.*

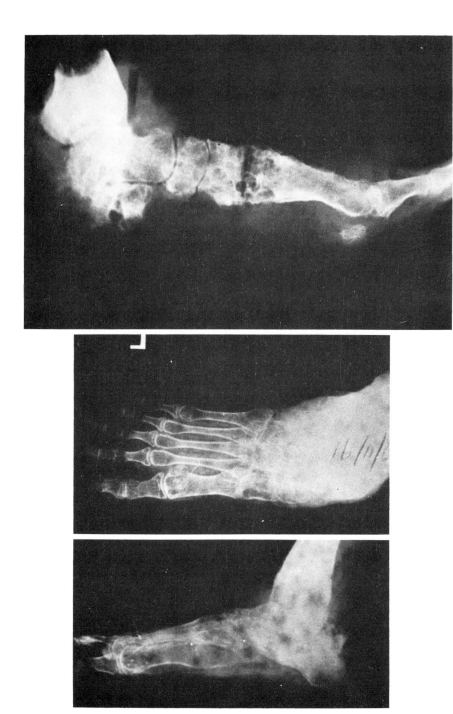

Figure 51–16. *Radiographic appearance of Madura mycetoma. Note the extensive involvement of all the bones of the foot, with multiple "punched-out" osteolytic lesions.*

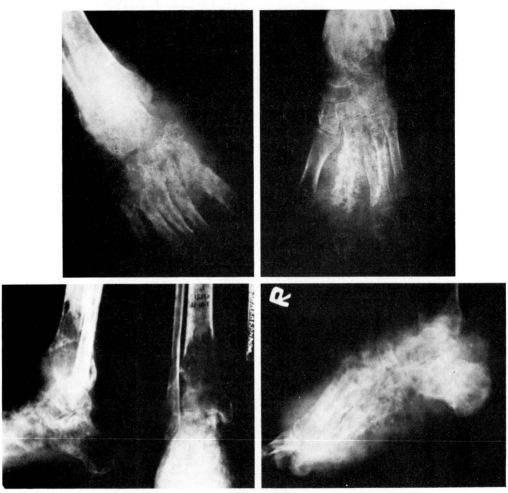

Figure 51–17. *Radiograph of Madura mycetoma showing extension of the disease to the bones of the leg with osteolysis and destruction of the lower end of the tibia.*

TABLE 51–1.   Causes of Mycetoma Pedis

FALSE FUNGI (HIGHER BACTERIA)	TRUE FUNGI (HIGHER FUNGI)
Streptomyces madurae	*Madurella mycetomi*
S. pelletieri	*M. grisea*
S. somaliensis	
	Aspergillus
Nocardia brasiliensis	
N. caviae	*Allescheria boydii*
	Phialophora jeanselmei
	Cephalosporium sangelensis
	Leptosphaeria

entire foot may be disorganized following destruction and collapse of the bones. The discharge contains granules. There is little or no pain, the lymph nodes are not enlarged, and there is no general dissemination of the disease.

Early radiologic changes include multiple "punched-out" osteolytic lesions. Periosteal reaction is not generally seen. However, following progression of the condition and secondary bacterial infection, periosteal new bone and osteosclerotic lesions appear and confuse the roentgenographic picture. As healing progresses, the affected bone regains its normal radiologic appearance.

Prior to institution of treatment, it is essential to identify the causative fungus (Fig. 51–19). A Gram stain of the discharge from the sinus is helpful. If gram-positive, the causative organism is a false fungus (higher bacteria). If gram-negative, the causative organism is a true fungus. This difference is important, as the former responds to high doses of penicillin, sulfa drugs, and dapsone (diamino diphenylsulfone, DDS), whereas the latter does not respond to any form of chemotherapy. Additional subclassification can be made by microscopic examination of the discharge.

Surgical management is as follows: Local excision of the soft tissue lesion is indicated in the early stages in the absence of bone involvement. Occasionally, surgical drainage of abscesses and curettage of the involved bones afford temporary relief of symptoms. Conservative treatment and chemotherapy must be continued until the foot allows weight bearing and retains an acceptable degree of function. In advanced cases with involvement of bone and soft tissue, there is gross functional impairment, leaving no choice other than amputation of the affected foot.

Cryptococcosis. *Cryptococcus neoformans* is a yeastlike fungus that usually has a predilection for the central nervous system but may also infect lungs, other organs, bones, and joints. In the literature, the pelvis, femur, spine, and tibia were

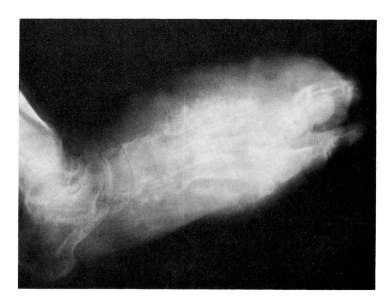

Figure 51–18. Radiographic appearance of long-standing Madura mycetoma with secondary infection showing new periosteal bone formation in response to the secondary bacterial infection.

among the most common sites of skeletal cryptococcosis.

The initial symptoms and signs are pain associated with swelling and tenderness of soft tissues overlying the affected part of the bone.

The radiographic appearance is one of extensive bone destruction with osteolytic changes and destruction of joint spaces.

Coccidioidomycosis. The causative agent is the fungus *Coccidioides immitis*, which is a spherical, thick-walled organ-

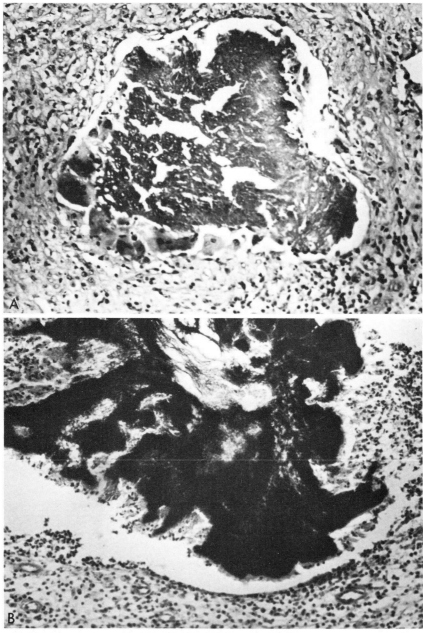

Figure 51–19. *Photomicrographs of Madura mycetoma. (A) True fungal mycetoma demonstrating foreign-body giant cell reaction and a true fungal granule that is pigmented and has spores (magnification — 320). (B) False fungal mycetoma demonstrating polymorphonuclear reaction around a large fungal granule composed of filaments that stain with hematoxylin (magnification — 320).*

ism filled with endospores. In the United States the incidence of this disease is highest in the Southwest.

Clinical manifestations are either localized or disseminated, according to the distribution of the lesion. The disease is primarily and most commonly a pulmonary disorder and appears similar to pulmonary tuberculosis or pulmonary histoplasmosis. The skeletal lesions affect the articular ends of a number of bones, and lead to destruction of the joints. This can also occur as chronic synovitis (involving the joints most commonly). In the foot the lesion is seen in the tarsal bones.

Chemotherapy involves intravenous infusions of amphotericin B, diluted form, 1 mg/kg body weight per day, for a total dose of 1 to 10 gm.

Blastomycosis. The causative organism in blastomycosis (Fig. 51–20) is *Blastomyces dermatitidis*, which is a budding yeastlike fungus, spherical and thick-walled. This is a granulomatous infection involving the skin, internal organs, bones, and joints. Usually the primary infection is

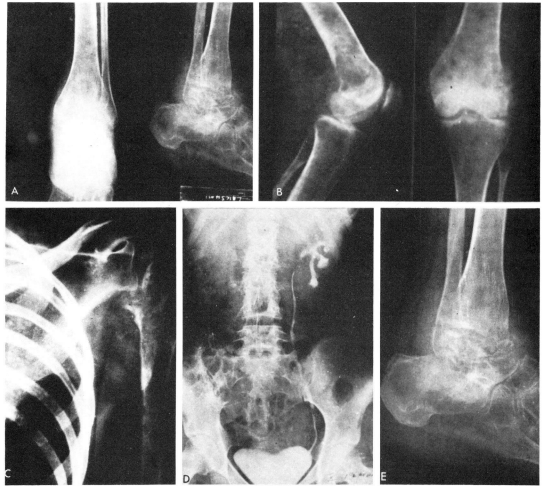

Figure 51–20. *Radiographs of a patient with concomitant systemic blastomycotic and coccidioidomycotic infections. (A) Left foot and ankle showing involvement and destruction of the talus. (B) Right knee showing multiple "punched-out" lesions of the lower end of femur and destruction in the region of the lateral epicondyle. (C) Right shoulder showing destruction of the head of the humerus. (D) Intravenous pyelogram showing nonfunctioning right kidney and lytic lesions of the right ilium adjacent to the right sacroiliac joint. The patient also had consolidation of the upper part of the right lung and bony ankylosis between L1 and L2 and between L3 and L4. (E) Magnified view of A.*

seen in the lungs. Bone lesions can occur without cutaneous or pulmonary manifestations, which can lead to a diagnostic problem. Patients between the ages of 20 and 50 are most often affected. The route of infection is by inhalation of spores that contaminate the soil. From the lungs, the infection spreads by the hematogenous route to other parts of the body. Skeletal involvement may be seen in six or seven bones concurrently. The tarsus is one of the common sites of involvement, the other sites being vertebrae, ribs, tibia, and carpus. Radiologically, the tarsal lesions show areas of osteolysis and bone destruction without any new bone formation.

Treatment consists of intravenous infusions of amphotericin B in highly diluted form, maximum daily dose 75 to 100 mg, for a total dose of 1 gm.

Syphilis

The bones of the foot are infected by *Treponema pallidum* in both the congenital and the acquired forms of syphilis. Syphilitic dactylitis of the phalanges of the toes is seen in patients over 14 years of age as a late manifestation of congenital syphilis. The dactylitis is one of the skeletal manifestations of the disease. The affected digit is swollen and spindle-shaped. Radiologically, increased radiolucency of the distended cortex is seen. A certain amount of periosteal reaction and periosteitis occurs, and healing is associated with the appearance of periosteitis and hyperosteitis.

Dactylitis is seen much less often in the acquired form of syphilis. Phalanges and metatarsals of the various toes may be involved. The dactylitis is attributed to gummatous periosteitis or gummatous osteomyelitis of the involved bone; sometimes both factors are known to occur together. Dactylitis seems to be caused by local extension of gummatous lesions of the overlying soft tissue to the bone. Gummatous periosteitis occurs more often in the acquired form, whereas gummatous osteomyelitis is seen commonly in the congenital form.

Congenital syphilis is treated with benzathine penicillin G, 50,000 units/kg body weight, in one single dose intramuscular-ly. For the acquired form, benzathine penicillin G, 1.2 million units, is given intramuscularly into each buttock.

Sarcoidosis

Sarcoidosis of the bones of the foot occurs more often in young adults. There is a slight male predominance. The proximal and middle phalanges are commonly involved, and less often the terminal phalanges and the metatarsals. The tarsal bones are rarely involved. Infection of the bones of the toes is heralded by reddening of the skin, diffuse swelling, aching pains, and low-grade fever. The acute changes regress to a certain degree but recur after a period of time. Eventually the affected toes show signs of lupus pernio. Trophic disturbances occur at times. In extreme cases, mutilation of the toes results, whereas in the mild cases, swelling and thickening of the toes are gradual and painless.

On hematologic examination, there is anemia, a mild eosinophilia, and hypoproteinemia (with reversal of the albumin/globulin ratio). The Kveim test is diagnostic of sarcoidosis.

The radiograph shows radiolucent foci, especially in the phalangeal heads. No periosteal new bone formation is seen, but "punched-out" lesions are occasionally noted. Extension to joints is rare.

Histologically there are discrete hyperplastic tubercles composed mainly of epithelial cells, lymphocytes, and Langhans' giant cells with no caseation.

Leprosy

Specific leprous lesions of the foot are seen in patients with Hansen's disease. Infection usually spreads from the dermal or mucosal surfaces to the underlying bone. Such an infection of the bone presents in the form of periostosteitis. Sometimes the leprous lesions develop in the bones of the foot in the absence of superficial skin lesions. They occur as small osteolytic foci in the ends of bones, which show diffuse infiltration. The spongy trabeculae within the bone absorb, and cortical bone may later become perforated. Destruction of osseous tissue is very slow and does not provoke much reactive proliferation of the new bone. Leprous lesions of the bone are slow to develop in the absence of secondary infection.

Specific leprous arthritis is common in the ankle. Articular involvement is usually the result of the extension of a disease focus in the bone to the articular surface or the extension of periarthritic disease to the synovial membrane. Occasionally, infection occurs in the synovial membrane, leading to arthritis of the ankle.

Leprous lesions of the foot are aggravated and the clinical picture and prognosis altered by secondary infection and neuropathy. No specific treatment for the leprous involvement of bones and joints is necessary, except for continuation of dapsone therapy.

Nongranulomatous Infections

Pyogenic Infections

Pyogenic infection of the bones of the foot occurs most often from extension of infection from the overlying soft tissues. Occasionally, it may occur as an individual localization of multifocal infection, the infection being deposited in the foot by a hematogenous route. Infection may also spread to the underlying bone from an overlying infected ulcer (which may be traumatic or infectious). Osteomyelitis of the bones and arthritis of the joints of the

foot then develop. Occasionally, infection spreads to the bones and joints from an abscess in the foot, leading to chronic osteomyelitis with multiple sinus formation.

Pyogenic infection is associated with copious periosteal reaction and new bone formation with sequestration of bone.

The most common causative organism is *Staphylococcus aureus*, which is responsible for 90 per cent of infections. Beta-hemolytic and nonhemolytic streptococci account for 3 per cent of cases. The hemolytic variety is seen more often than the nonhemolytic type. Other causative bacteria are *Pseudomonas, Escherichia coli, Salmonella,* pneumococci, and gonococci.

Treatment consists of surgical drainage of abscesses, removal of sequestrae, appropriate systemic antibiotic therapy, and immobilization of the foot in a plaster splint. In severe intractable infections, an amputation of the foot may occasionally be required.

Rarely, a squamous cell epithelioma develops in an ulcer or sinus associated with chronic osteomyelitis of long standing (Fig. 51–21). Amputation of the foot will be essential in such a case.

Gonococcal infection of the foot requires special mention. It is commonly seen in the ankle joints and is most often bilateral and symmetric with concomitant tenosynovitis. Synovial involvement is the most common lesion. Gonococci can be isolated

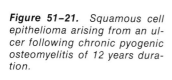

Figure 51–21. Squamous cell epithelioma arising from an ulcer following chronic pyogenic osteomyelitis of 12 years duration.

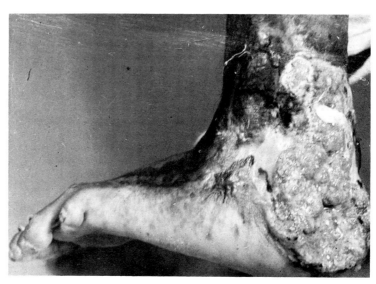

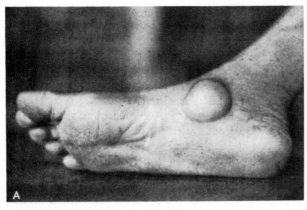
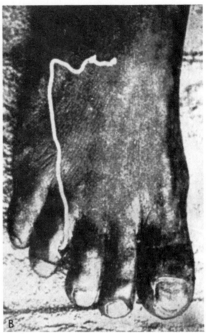

Figure 51–22. *Dracunculus medinensis. (A) Guinea worm blister on the medial aspect of the foot. (B) An adult female guinea worm being extruded through a ruptured blister. (From Craig, C. F., and Faust, E. C.: Clinical Parasitology. Philadelphia, Lea and Febiger, 1945–48, p. 387.)*

from the joint aspirate. The lining cells of synovium remain undisturbed. Polymorphonuclear leukocytes, lymphocytes, and plasma cells are seen in the deeper layers. Later, articular surfaces are covered by granulation. Finally, the articular cartilage is destroyed and infection spreads to the cortical bone. Treatment includes appropriate chemotherapy and surgical debridement of the foot.

Parasitic Infestations

Guinea worm *(Dracunculus medinensis)* infestation occurs by drinking water contaminated by a small crustacean *(Cyclops)* that carries the infecting larvae. Following

completion of its life cycle in the human host, the adult female worm escapes through the skin of parts of the body most commonly in contact with water. (For example, in endemic areas of rural India, where the source of water is step wells, the foot is in contact with the water for a considerable length of time.) The adult female worm finds its way through the subcutaneous tissues of the foot and forms a blister on the skin (Fig. 51–22A). The blister later bursts when in contact with water and the worm comes out through the skin to discharge its eggs (Fig. 51–22B).

Administration of oral metronidazole and extraction of the worm through the skin are recommended.

YAWS

Donald M. Qualls, M.D.

Yaws (bouba, pian frambesia) is a disease caused by the spirochete *Treponema pertenue*. It is contagious, infectious, and nonvenereal. Morphologically yaws cannot be distinguished from pinta *(Treponema carateum)* or syphilis *(Treponema pallidum)*.

Hudson[14] believes that yaws originated in Africa, possibly because of spirochetes

from decaying vegetable matter becoming invasive to man. He recognizes only *Treponema pallidum* and states that the other groups are indistinguishable intraspecific strains.

Hackett[11] disputes this. He believes that pinta is the progenitor of treponematosis and is probably transmitted by animal infection. Hackett thinks that yaws developed as a mutant of pinta about 15,000 BC and that endemic syphilis developed from yaws about 7000 BC. Despite the dispute, Bahr[2] states that clinically and epidemiologically there are differences in spirochetal diseases. Although treatment is the same for all, prevention is not.

Adams and MacGrath[9] state that yaws is a disease of the nonurban tropical countries but that distribution is not even. It is found in North and Equatorial Africa, India, Thailand, northern South America, the West Indies, Burma, Malaysia, Indonesia, the Philippines, Panama, Sri Lanka, Mexico, and northern Australia. While a member of the medical staff of Firestone Plantation Hospital, Harbel, Liberia, from 1948 to 1952, Qualls did a survey and clinical examination of 1000 patients, representing a cross section of all tribes. The Kahn test and the Mazzini test were also done. At that time the incidence of yaws was 34 per cent.

In regions in which yaws is endemic, the disease is of primary concern to orthopaedic surgeons, as, because of its musculoskeletal manifestations, this differential diagnosis must always be kept in mind.

Yaws is usually acquired in childhood. Transmission is by direct contact, believed to be through broken skin. Person-to-person contact in overcrowded areas represents the environment best suited for spread.

The diagnosis of yaws may be made by clinical findings. The presence of spirochetes in a darkfield preparation and positive serologic test results further support clinical diagnosis.

Differentiation of yaws into primary, secondary, and tertiary stages is the accepted method of classification.[12] Turner[15] described the principal tissue reaction in treponematosis as an exudate with infiltration of lymphocytes, plasma cells, and macrophages; proliferation of fibroblasts; and endarteritis. The primary lesion (Fig. 51–23) develops after two to eight weeks of incubation and appears at any site. Since the pathology is granulomatosis, the primary lesion is a granuloma papule, which is raspberry-like in appearance. (The French word for raspberry is *framboise*; hence, the term frambesia.) Systemic response, temperature elevation, and gener-

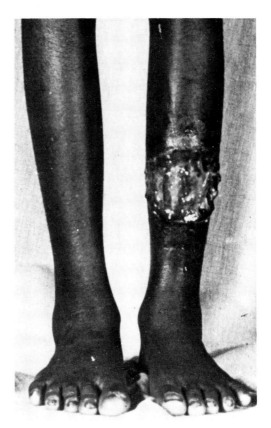

Figure 51–23. *A lesion in the primary stage of yaws —a large, sharply margined ulcer that extends down to the fascia, with heaped-up granulomatous tissue.*

alized bone and joint aching appear. The secondary stage (Fig. 51–24) is characterized by multiple skin lesions of granuloma-papillary type. This stage may continue for years. Therefore, the grading into a tertiary stage in migratory populations, who are difficult to follow closely, makes for clinical controversy. The secondary stage is also characterized by osteitis and periosteitis with focal rarefaction and, in general, nondestructive lesions (Fig. 51–25).

The tertiary phase presents with subcutaneous nodules (Fig. 51–26); ulceration with deep, irregular configuration; and gumma formation (Fig. 51–27). Hyperkeratosis of the palms and soles of feet with ulcers and deep fissures may also appear (Fig. 51–28). "Crab" yaws (plantar hyperkeratosis), one of the most common manifestations of late yaws, is illustrated in Figure 51–29 (also note papules of the right fourth toe and left first toe). Figure

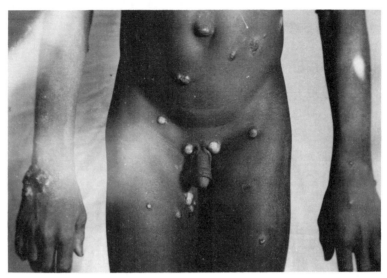

Figure 51–24. *Lesions in the secondary stage of yaws — multiple papillary granulomas of the skin.*

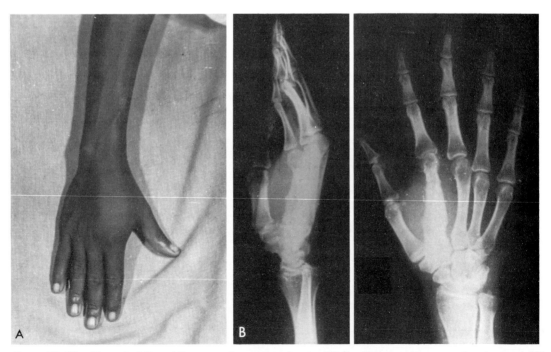

Figure 51–25. *Characteristics of the secondary stage of yaws. (A) Swelling over the second metacarpal. (B) Note the osteitis and periostitis of the second metacarpal.*

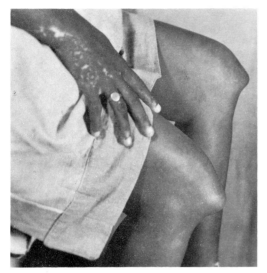

Figure 51-26. *Juxta-articular nodules over knees in the tertiary phase of yaws.*

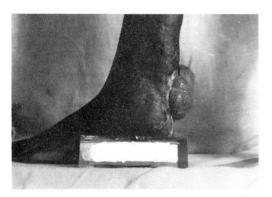

Figure 51-27. *Large granuloma over the Achilles tendon in the tertiary phase of yaws.*

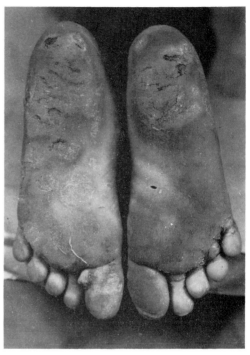

Figure 51-29. *Plantar hyperkeratosis. Also note the papillomas on the left hallux and right fourth toe.*

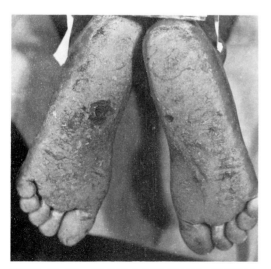

Figure 51-28. *Plantar hyperkeratosis, fissuring, and ulceration in the tertiary stage of yaws.*

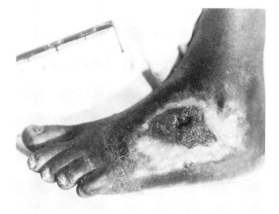

Figure 51-30. *Healing of a large granulomatous ulceration over the dorsum of the foot.*

51–30 shows a healing ulceration granuloma of the dorsum of the foot. Other
tertiary findings are bone destruction and
saber shin (anterior tibial bowing) (Fig.
51–31) (note severe stress on the foot and
ankle due to malalignment of the tibia).
Goundou is the term used to indicate in-

volvement of the nasal bones, producing a
tumor-like mass (Fig. 51–32). I removed
the large left goundou shown in Figure
51–32, as it was obstructing the patient's
vision. Gangosa, another of the late lesions
of yaws, produces destruction of bone and
cartilage, resulting in total structural loss

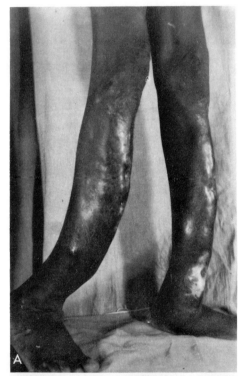

Figure 51–31. (A–C) Severe saber shins in
the tertiary stage of yaws.

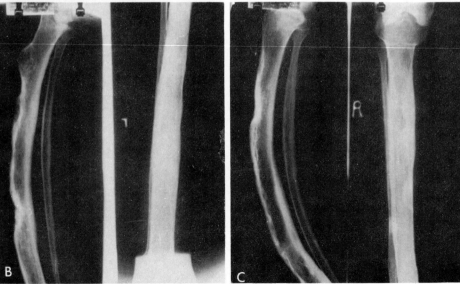

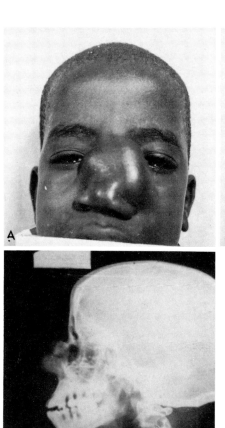
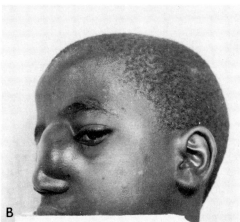
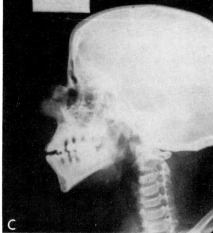

Figure 51-32. *(A–C) Goundou. Note the periosteal bone proliferation. It arises from the superior maxillary bone.*

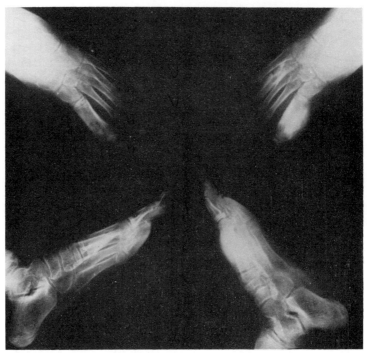

Figure 51–33. *Tertiary lesions of the first metatarsal bilaterally. Note the destruction, expansion, and periosteal cortical proliferation.*

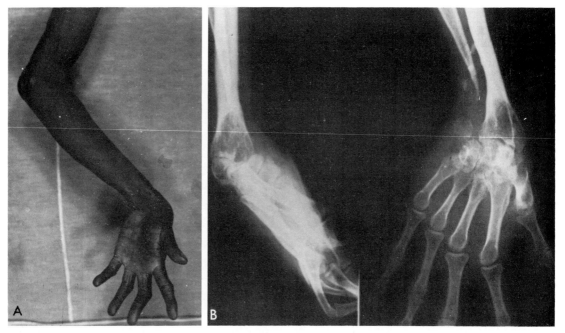

Figure 51–34. *(A and B) Destruction of the wrist and secondary contracture in the tertiary phase of yaws.*

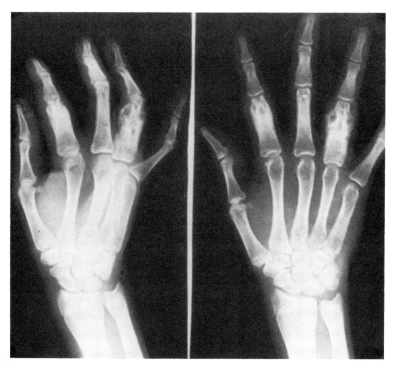

Figure 51–35. *Destruction and expansion of the proximal phalanges of the second and fourth fingers.*

of the nose. The cardiovascular and central nervous systems are not affected in yaws, as they are in syphilis.

The tertiary bone lesions of the hands and feet (Figs. 51–33 to 51–35) show thickening with expansion of metacarpals, metatarsals, and phalanges and varying degrees of destruction associated with periosteal cortical proliferation.

The treatment of choice is procaine penicillin in 2 per cent aluminum monostearate (PAM). Doses of not less than 1.2 million units for adults and proportionately less for children are recommended for treatment of usual cases. The minimal total dosage of PAM recommended by the World Health Organization (WHO) in 1960 is as follows: For patients under 15 years of age — 0.6 megaunit for early and late active cases and 0.3 megaunit for late cases and contacts; for patients 15 years of age and older — 1.2 megaunits for early and late active cases and 0.6 megaunit for late cases and contacts. A single intramuscular injection may be given. Penicillin

reactions should be watched for, and emergency treatment should be available.

Late yaws may require longer treatment. A dosage of 0.6 megaunit of PAM given daily or twice weekly for 15 to 20 doses has been suggested, corresponding to the treatment of late syphilis. Other antibiotics are effective, i.e., chlortetracycline, oxytetracycline, tetracycline, and chloramphenicol. The use of bismuth, oxophenarsine (Mapharsen), and neoarsphenamine has been discontinued.[10]

The local treatment of yaws lesions should not be neglected. Appropriate cleansing and care will hasten healing of lesions and prevent secondary infection. Control of yaws requires all modalities of management of infectious disease, good hygiene, adequate nutrition, treatment of infectious stages, and follow-up care of breakout cases. Shoes or sandals prevent some of the trauma to feet while plantar lesions are healing. Treatment with penicillin is very effective. Yaws requires mass therapy to prevent breakout of disease, especially in highly endemic regions. To keep incidence down, ongoing repeated treatment programs are necessary in these endemic areas.

REFERENCES

Infections of the Foot

1. Bloom, W., and Fawcett, D. W.: A Textbook of Histology. 9th ed. Philadelphia, W. B. Saunders, 1968, p. 482.
2. Chatterjee, K. D.: Human Parasites and Parasitic Diseases. Calcutta, Sree Sarawswatty Press, 1952, p. 619.
3. Craig, C. F., and Faust, E. C.: Clinical Parasitology. Philadelphia, Lea & Febiger, 1945, p. 387.
4. Das, K.: Clinical Methods in Surgery. 8th ed. Calcutta, 1968, p. 142.
5. Grant, J. C. B., and Basmajian, J. V.: Grant's Method of Anatomy. 7th ed. Baltimore, Williams & Wilkins, 1965, p. 425.
6. Jaffe, H. L.: Metabolic, Degenerative and Inflammatory Diseases of Bones and Joints. Philadelphia, Lea & Febiger, 1972, pp. 907, 1004, 1058.
7. Pratt, C. A.: The Essentials of Chiropody. London, H. K. Lewis & Co., Ltd., 1945, p. 78.
8. Rains, A. J. H., and Ritchie, H. D.: Bailey and Love's Short Practice of Surgery. 16th ed. London, H. K. Lewis & Co., Ltd., 1975, p. 188.

Yaws

9. Adams, A. R. D., and MacGrath, B.: Clinical Tropical Diseases. 6th ed. Oxford, Blackwell Scientific Publications, 1976, p. 552.
10. Bahr, C. W.: *In* Manson, P. E. C. (ed.): Manson's Tropical Diseases. 19th ed. Baltimore, Williams & Wilkins, 1972, pp. 563, 579.
11. Hackett, C. J.: Clinical course of yaws in Lango, Uganda. Trans. Roy. Soc. Trop. Med. Hyg., 40:206, 1946.
12. Hackett, C. J.: Bone Lesions of Yaws in Uganda. Oxford, Blackwell Scientific Publications, 1951.
13. Hackett, C. J.: On the origin of the human treponematoses (pinta, yaws, endemic syphilis and venereal syphilis). Bull. WHO, 29:7, 1963.
14. Hudson, E. H. Non-venereal Syphilis: A Sociological and Medical Study of Bejel. Edinburgh, Churchill Livingstone, 1958.
15. Turner, L. H.: Notes on the treponematoses with an illustrated account of yaws. Bulletin, Institute for Medical Research, Federation of Malaya, 9:1, 1959.

CHAPTER 52

PSYCHIATRIC ASPECTS OF FOOT PROBLEMS

Monroe W. Spero, M.D., and Earl Schwartz, M.D.

FOREWORD

One of the most frustrating problems encountered by the practicing orthopaedist relates to patients who have chronic nonanatomic pains about their feet and ankles without any corroborating objective evidence of organic disease. Their foot hypersensitivity may reach such a degree that even putting on silk stockings causes discomfort. The orthopaedist is only too aware of these patients, who walk into his office with a huge bag filled with arch supports, shoes, and shoe corrections. It goes without saying that any foot surgery performed on such patients, even for minor deformities, will not result in any subjective relief.

The purpose of this chapter is to give the practicing physician some insight into how to "spot" these patients, how best to gain rapport with them, and how to refer them for psychiatric help, along with understanding the psychiatric basis of their symptomatology.

Melvin H. Jahss

INTRODUCTION

The orthopaedic surgeon is often confronted with a patient seeking help whose history has been a long series of therapeutic disappointments and whose physical work-up reveals no clearly defined organic pathology and indicates no specific therapeutic regimen. However, illness behavior and symptom communication may be significantly influenced and sometimes determined by psychosocial as well as organic factors.[1]

The goal of other chapters of this book is to help the orthopaedist in the diagnosis and treatment of organic pathology. The goal of this chapter is to aid the orthopaedist in understanding, treating, or appropriately referring for psychiatric consultation those patients whose symptoms are not associated with definite physiologic or anatomic pathology or whose symptoms for no apparent reason are unresponsive to indicated medical treatments or surgical procedures. In this chapter, hysteria, psychophysiologic disorders, hypochondriasis, and malingering will be discussed. Chronic pain, the most frequent psychosomatic complaint among orthopaedic patients, will also be considered. The orthopaedist will be helped to better understand and treat the chronic pain patient. Then the psychiatrist's role in assisting both the orthopaedist and the chronic pain patient will be outlined.

FUNCTIONAL DISORDERS OF THE FOOT

It has been estimated that functional foot disorders account for perhaps as much as 5 to 20 per cent of all foot problems seen by the orthopaedic physician and others who treat such problems in outpatient settings. However, accurate statistical data and epidemiologic information are lacking, and it is difficult to present exact figures.[2]

Functional disorders can present (1) without a relevant or organic lesion, either in the present or the past; (2) with related physiologic or structural abnormalities; or (3) as a continuation of the symptoms of an organic lesion that is no longer acute or has even healed.[3, 4] Hysterical symptoms frequently appear at the site of former lesions that had produced symptoms. A diagnosis may be difficult to establish, as conversion hysteria may frequently simulate organic disease. Often the difficulty in diagnosis will depend upon the medical sophistication or lack of sophistication of the patient, as conversion symptoms will conform to the patient's knowledge and ideas about a certain illness or disease. This may be done in a crude manner, or a medically sophisticated patient may unconsciously simulate a very complicated disease such as multiple sclerosis, myasthenia gravis, or a cyst of the third ventricle.[5]

Pain may also frequently continue as an hysterical conversion symptom well after the physical lesion that originally produced the pain has healed. The question of chronic pain and the physician–patient relationship in such a situation is an important area that many physicians find full of pitfalls and difficulties. This will be dealt with in more detail in the discussion of the physician–patient relationship and the evaluation and treatment of the chronic pain patient.

THE CHRONIC PAIN PATIENT

Description

A chronic pain patient is one whose pain is resistant to indicated medical treatments and surgical procedures or is not associated with any physiologic or anatomic disorders.[6] When encountering a chronic pain patient, the physician may repeat the same treatment or prescribe a different treatment, based on the assumption that the pain will eventually respond to therapy. Alternatively, the physician may repeat or expand the diagnostic evaluation, based on the assumption that the pain is associated with an undiscovered physiologic or anatomic disorder. However, if the assumptions prove to be invalid, the patient often feels that the physician has failed the patient, and the physician often feels the same about the patient. The patient may accuse the physician of diagnostic and therapeutic incompetence, and the physician may accuse the patient of faking pain and duping the physician. Unfortunately, both physician and patient may have been operating on incomplete assumptions, i.e., that the pain is always associated with a specific physical disorder, that the pain is proportionate to the pathology, and that the pain will diminish in accordance with the pathology's response to treatment. However, psychologic factors may affect the pain to the point that medical and surgical assumptions are not sufficient to diagnose and treat the problem. Pain experience and pain communication may be significantly influenced and sometimes determined by cognitive, emotional, and interpersonal factors. Prior to the initial encounter between patient and physician, the patient has often formulated ideas, experienced emotional distress, and established relationship expectations, all of which may be affecting the pain experience and communication.

The patient has usually contemplated one or more diagnoses, etiologies, treatments, and prognoses. For example, the patient may fear, suspect, or firmly believe that the diagnosis is cancer. The patient may be blaming others for causing or exacerbating the pain; e.g., the father who beat the patient on the same part of the body, the mother who suffered from the same disorder and from whom the patient believes the disorder was inherited, the spouse with whom the patient argued prior to driving the car into a tree, the employer who failed to heed the patient's repeated warnings about safety precautions, or the previous physician whose treatment the patient considers not only failed to alleviate but rather exacerbated the pain. Less frequently, the patient may blame himself or herself and believe the pain is a punishment for transgressions, as well as an expiation of guilt. Prior to the initial visit to the physician, the patient may have formulated a treatment plan that definitely includes or excludes surgery and may have established the prognosis as definitely terminal or instantly curable.

Emotional factors may also be affecting the pain experience and pain communication. The emotional distress may be related to the pain experience and to the contemplated diagnoses, etiologies, treatment, and prognoses. For example, the patient may feel guilty for having failed him- or herself or others, angry at those blamed for causing or exacerbating the pain, fearful of the possible treatment, or ashamed of how he or she imagines that others perceive the distress and disability. In addition, the patient often experiences intense emotional distress over the marital, sexual, parental, familial, social, educational, occupational, and financial problems that have, in fact, developed or worsened since the pain or that the patient fears will develop. Furthermore, the patient may have had or developed a specific emotional disorder such as an anxiety disorder or depression. The association between chronic pain and depression is so frequent that the physician should be alerted to the following symptoms of depression as described by Beck[7]: sadness, pessimism, sense of failure, dissatisfaction, guilt, expectation of punishment, self-dislike, self-accusations, suicidal ideas, crying, irritability, social withdrawal, indecisiveness, body-image change, work retardation, insomnia, fatigability, anorexia, weight loss, somatic preoccupation, and loss of libido.

In addition to cognitive and emotional factors, interpersonal factors may influence the patient's pain experience and communication. Pain communication includes not only the verbal complaint but also nonverbal behavior such as moaning, crying, yelling, grimacing, or limping. The patient expects to elicit help from the receiver of the pain message. A person in acute pain often succeeds in eliciting help, but the patient in chronic pain often fails because in time the expected helper feels ineffectual over the failure to alleviate the pain and angry about the repeated implicit demands of the chronic pain patient. Both the patient in pain and the expected helper may become locked into recurrent, mutually reinforcing patterns of behav-

ior. The pain may be utilized as a source of power and means of aggression. The patient can demand assistance and then attack the helper for exacerbating or failing to relieve the pain. The patient may then also assume a dependent, irresponsible role to avoid the obligations that he or she felt incapable of fulfilling prior to the pain or now feels incapable of fulfilling because of the pain and associated disability. The patient may not attempt to succeed in order not to face the possibility of failing in the attempt. He or she may seek to legitimize the pain and disability for the purpose of justifying the dependent, irresponsible role and obtaining specific pain payoffs, such as financial compensation. The assumption of the dependent, irresponsible position often leads to self-dislike, sense of failure, dissatisfaction, somatic preoccupation, and pessimism, which may develop into depression. Also, the patient with chronic pain may become angry at those upon whom he or she depends. The expected helper who eventually feels ineffectual and angry may retaliate by accusing the patient of irresponsibility and frustrating the various needs of the patient. Moreover, the expected helper may unconsciously sabotage attempts the patient makes toward independence and responsibility, with the result of maintaining the patient in what the helper considers the subordinate position. The relationship may then crystallize into a pattern in which neither patient nor helper finds it easy to listen to, understand, negotiate about, or attempt to satisfy the needs of the other.

Physician–Patient Relationship

As just described, the quality of the physician–patient relationship has an important influence on the patient's cooperation with the orthopaedist in working together toward a successful therapeutic outcome. Orthopaedists are frequently dissatisfied with their chronic pain patients; chronic pain patients are frequently dissatisfied with their orthopaedists. Physician and patient satisfaction can be promoted best by a mutual understanding of each other's needs and expectations.

Encumbered with recurrent cognitive, emotional, and interpersonal distress, the chronic pain patient visits the physician with the belief that the primary (if not the only) problem is physical and with the hope (if not the demand) that the physician will perform the indicated procedure to relieve the pain and extricate the patient from his or her life's problems. The patient considers these problems to be a result of the pain and expects them to disappear when the pain is cured. The physician's initial task is to establish a working relationship on the basis of a mutual understanding of each other's expectations; otherwise, the patient will quickly feel that the physician has become part of the problem rather than part of the solution.

The patient needs to be listened to, and the physician needs to listen to understand the patient's concerns. The physician can listen attentively, ask clarifying questions when necessary, and express understanding of the patient's thoughts and feelings. Unfortunately, the chronic pain patient usually has difficulty in expressing emotional suffering and emotional needs, as opposed to ease in expressing physical suffering and the need for immediate pain relief. The physician's attention toward and acceptance of the emotional distress can immeasurably aid emotional expression. During the medical evaluation the physician can explore preconceived ideas about diagnoses, etiologies, treatments, and prognoses; feelings, including fear, anger, sadness, and guilt; interpersonal effects of pain; and expectations of the physician. Questions similar to the following may be asked at appropriate times:

1. How are you feeling emotionally? physically? How do you feel about the pain?

2. What do you think is the cause of the pain?

3. What do you think is going to happen to the pain?

4. How has pain affected your life? your relationships?

5. When you become very upset, how is the pain affected? In what way do you become upset?

6. How would you like me to help you?

The physician is not expected to perform an exhaustive psychiatric evaluation, but is capable of eliciting and understanding enough of the patient's thoughts, feelings, and expectations to establish a working, caring relationship. In communicating therapeutically, the physician may help the patient to feel that the former is a warm, genuine, empathic person who nonjudgmentally cares about and accepts the patient as a person. Furthermore, the physician can explain the medical findings and recommendations, the possible beneficial and adverse consequences of the recommended treatment and any alternative treatments, and the probable consequences of no treatment. In contributing such information (even if not specifically requested, although generally expected, by the patient), and in granting the opportunity to give or refuse informed consent, the physician is not only complying with the rules of informed consent but is sharing responsibility. In discussing etiology, the physician can relieve guilt and anger; in stating a diagnosis, the physician can correct misbeliefs; and in planning treatment and predicting prognosis, the physician can dispel fear and engender hope. The physician can more effectively do these things if he or she understands the patient's guilt, anger, fear, and misbeliefs. The physician is able to monitor the patient's verbal and nonverbal responses, especially emotional responses, to his or her statements. At appropriate times the physician may simply ask, "How do you feel about what I just told you?"

It is also important that the patient understand the expectations of the physician. The physician, despite numerous technologic advancements, is neither omniscient nor omnipotent. The physician requires cooperation in all phases of diagnosis and treatment, especially in chronic illness. The patient must assume some responsibility for the therapeutic outcome, as he or she chose when, how, and what to relate to the physician; was involved via informed consent in deciding upon the treatment; and determined the degree of cooperation. Furthermore, a definitive diagnosis and indicated treatment plan cannot always be easily established. Indeed, the patient and/or physician can undermine the efforts of the latter by demanding a physiologic or anatomic disorder to be associated with the pain.

Thus the physician has the opportunity to listen to and understand the patient's cognitive, emotional, and interpersonal distress. The physician can then utilize such understanding in creating an effective working relationship, establishing a complete diagnosis, synthesizing a treatment plan, granting the opportunity for informed consent (which the patient will more readily give), partially relieving emotional distress, correcting misbeliefs, and making expectations more realistic. By fostering the patient's independence, responsibility, and awareness of thoughts, feelings, and expectations, the physician promotes hope and also trust and confidence in him- or herself, with resulting increased cooperation and usually improved therapeutic outcome. In brief, the physician is a therapeutic instrument. The goal of therapeutic communication is the satisfaction of both physician and patient in the process and outcome of their relationship.

Psychiatric Consultation

The patient needs to understand that the physician may require one or more consultations, including psychiatric, to assist in establishing a complete diagnosis and formulating a treatment plan. Consultations, especially psychiatric, are more easily accepted in the context of a satisfactory physician–patient relationship, in which the physician explains the current findings and indications for consultation and discusses the possible benefits from the consultation. A psychiatric consultation that is advised because of positive indications rather than the absence of physical findings is also more easily accepted. For example, the physician might state that he or she understands how depressed the patient is and wants the patient to visit a psychiatrist to help evaluate the depression and recommend a specific treatment. Some patients feel that a physician's request for a psychiatric consultation is tantamount to a denial of the patient's pain experience, a total psychiatric explanation for the pain, and an abandonment of the patient by the physician. Very helpful would be an explicit statement by the physician accepting the subjective reality of the pain, explaining the possible psychiatric aspect of the pain, and planning for the continuation of the physician–patient

relationship, if possible. When possible, the chronic pain patient would benefit from discussing the findings and recommendations with both the psychiatrist and the physician, so as to synthesize a combined therapeutic approach to both the medical and psychologic problems.

If the physician advises and the patient accepts referral, what can they expect from the psychiatrist? The psychiatrist, utilizing individual and family interviews and possibly psychologic testing, will assess the psychosocial factors involved in the onset, development, and maintenance of the pain behaviors and will explore psychophysiologic, hysterical, and hypochondriacal pain mechanisms. The psychophysiologic mechanism is the production of a functional or anatomic change that is influenced by emotional distress and mediated by the autonomic nervous system or by the involuntary somatic nervous system, which regulates muscle tension. The hysterical mechanism is the defense mechanism of somatization, whereby a distressing emotion or emotional conflict is repressed from awareness but may be expressed in symbolic body language. The repressed emotions may be any combination of sexual, angry, sad, fearful, or guilty feelings. These repressed emotions may be conflictual and indicative of ambivalent feelings toward significant others. For example, the death of a mother whom the patient both loved and hated intensely may engender overwhelming guilt, sadness, and anger, which the patient may repress and unconsciously convert into a symbolic physical symptom. The unconscious choice of physical symptom may be influenced by identification with the lost person or by the patient's own body image. If the mother died of diabetes involving chronic foot pain, the patient may then convert the repressed emotional conflict over the death into foot pain. This pain may not only represent identification with the bodily suffering of the mother but may also be a punishment in expiation of the guilt experienced by the patient over hating as well as loving the mother.

Body Image

The patient's own body image is an important factor in the choice of symbolic

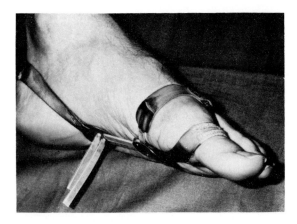

Figure 52–1. *A schizophrenic patient thought this leather brace on his foot supported his spine, which would crumble without it. (Courtesy of Melvin H. Jahss, M.D.)*

body language in hysterical mechanisms and in hypochondriacal mechanisms leading to the development of pain and maladaptive responses to pain. Hypochondriacal responses to pain include somatic preoccupation with the pain, exaggerated fear of the pain and its potentially disabling consequences, and, in the extreme, somatic delusions (e.g., a fixed, irrational belief in cancer) to account for the pain. It is important to remember that the schizophrenic may initially present at times with what first appears to be hypochondriacal preoccupation or bizarre somatic delusions (Fig. 52–1).

The body image, upon which hysterical and hypochondriacal mechanisms depend, is composed of the thoughts about, feelings toward, and expectations of one's body, which have developed out of the patient's body experiences, from birth until death. As defined by Cath and associates,[8] the body image is:

. . . that composite picture which the individual has of his own body. This picture is a multiply determined, continuously developing and therefore constantly changing, condensed representation of the individual's current and past experiences of his own body. It has both conscious and unconscious aspects and it exerts profound influences not only on the individual's behaviour but on his perception of his evironment as well.

The patient may consider the entire body or specific parts especially vulnerable or invulnerable, or may feel proud, sad, ashamed, fearful, angry, or loving toward the body or specific parts. The patient may overvalue or devaluate certain body parts and may expect too much or too little function, particularly after a physical change introduced by trauma or disease. Injury to the limbs is especially damaging to the person's image and psychologic integrity. Such patients frequently make use of the psychologic mechanism of denial. This may be seen in the phenomena of the phantom limb and phantom pain and in denial of limitation of function after trauma or surgery. For most patients the body has been a significant source of self-esteem and social esteem, such as that derived from sexual, athletic, or occupational activities.

The body image is very sensitive to other people's responses to one's body. Specifically, the patient's pain body image (composed of thoughts, feelings, and expectations in reference to pain that have developed out of pain experiences) is very sensitive to the responses of others to one's pain communications. For example, as a child or adolescent, did one's parents demonstrate caring for the patient only when he or she was ill and communicated pain? Or were the patient's most significant pain experiences a result of parental beatings as punishment for misbehavior? What were the parental responses to the patient's crying out in pain during the beatings? When impaired, the body image may adversely affect both self-image and social image, leading to the potential for a generalized social, behavioral, cognitive, and emotional regression as a result of damage, loss of function, or actual loss of specific body parts.

Psychiatric Treatment

Hopefully, the psychiatric assessment of body image; psychophysiologic, hysterical, and hypochondriac mechanisms; and cognitive, emotional, and interpersonal factors will imply specific, effective treatments. The therapeutic armamentarium of the psychiatrist ranges from the somatic therapies of psychotropic medication and electroconvulsive therapy; to the psychosomatic therapies of hypnosis, biofeedback, and relaxation therapy; to individual, family, and group psychotherapies based on psychoanalysis, transactional analysis, gestalt therapy, and behavior therapy.

The psychotherapeutic aspect of many multidisciplinary pain programs is founded on the operant conditioning approach to chronic pain, as fully described by Fordyce.[9] This is essentially a direct attempt to change behavior by the establishment of new, realistic, progressive expectations by the patient, the family, and the medical staff. The goal is improvement in physical, emotional, and social functioning, with expected concomitant improvement in body image, self-image, and social image.

The behavioral analysis of chronic pain for operant conditioning begins with a description of the pain behavior. Fordyce[9] writes (page 12):

. . . verbal statements about pain are one kind of behavior, and the other visible and audible methods by which the problem is communicated to the environment are another. For the moment they will be distinguished as verbal and nonverbal pain behaviors. The latter group includes nonlanguage sounds (such as moans and gasps), body posturing and gesturing (limping, rubbing a painful area, grimacing), and displaying functional limitations or impairment (reclining excessively to rest or staying home from work because it hurts too much).

The effects of the pain behaviors are then evaluated. The pain behavior may result in positive consequences or in avoiding negative consequences. Key questions to be asked of both patient and partner include: What are you or your partner doing now that you did not do before the pain? What are you or your partner not doing that you did before the pain? What would you or your partner do differently if the pain diminished? The answers to these questions assist in determining the gains the patient and partner have achieved despite the pain and the costs the patient and partner would incur if the pain were to be reduced. A therapeutic

program is then defined with the goal of decreasing or eliminating pain behavior and increasing well behavior, such as physical exercise and occupational activities, which the patient may have been avoiding. A progressive, graduated behavioral improvement plan is prepared with the patient. Similarly, family members and health professionals are instructed and rehearsed in responding with attention and praise to behavioral improvements and in ignoring behavioral regressions.

Whatever behavioral improvements have been achieved in the multidisciplinary pain clinic must be generalized and maintained by helping the patient gain access to reinforcers in his or her natural environment. As recognized by Fordyce,[9] the family is obviously an integral component of the natural environment.

To focus solely on the patient is to ignore a major set of highly influential factors. There are many implications to the preceding point. One is that once a pain problem has become chronic, it also has become a family affair. Inevitably, patient-family interactions will be playing significant roles in the maintenance of pain behavior or the failure to reinforce or support well behavior or both. It follows that diagnosis and treatment almost certainly need to involve the family as well as the patient (page 8).

Although instruction and rehearsal in rewarding of well behavior and ignoring of pain behavior may be helpful, instituting and maintaining improvements in interpersonal behavior may depend on more than simply decreased pain communication and increased social activity. Marital and family therapy may be indicated to promote effective and responsive communication, fair negotiation and decision-making, cooperative behavior, functional roles, appropriate marital and parental coalitions, and well-defined intergenerational boundaries, all of which may have been influential antecedents or consequents of pain behavior.

Individual, group, or family therapy may be recommended to foster understanding of and change in cognitive, emotional, and interpersonal pain factors. Psychotropic medication and electroconvulsive therapy have been used successfully not only in treating specific psychiatric disorders, such as depression associated with chronic pain, but also the chronic pain itself. Both phenothiazines and tricyclic antidepressants, either separately or in combination, have ameliorated chronic pain.

Interpersonal, cognitive, and emotional pain factors must be evaluated and treated in patients with chronic pain and probably in those with any chronic illness. Family members may play an important role in the development and maintenance of the chronic pain. Moreover, the relationships among physicians, psychiatrists, and other health professionals with each other and with their patients and patients' families are important determinants of everyone's satisfaction in the course and eventual outcome of the therapeutic process.

The following clinical history is of a chronic pain patient. It contains excerpts from the patient's diary that illustrate the difficulties encountered when a patient is fitted with various orthopaedic appliances and, if unfortunate enough, subjected to questionable surgery in an attempt to alleviate a problem that is basically no longer morphologic or physiologic. The patient is a 49-year-old woman, intelligent and "medically unsophisticated," but with a long history of episodic hypochondriacal preoccupation. This is her view at time of psychiatric referral:

At the present time I have extremely painful conditions in both feet in various areas: the small toes and an area comprising the tailor bunion area — the area under the tailor bunion, the end of the fifth metatarsal bone, and top of the foot near the tailor bunion. For the past ten years since I had my small hammer toe operated upon, they have been very sensitive. I do not recall when I started to have pain in the tailor bunion area. My condition has generally worsened for the past two years. It is impossible for me to walk more than three or four blocks at a time, to stand for any length of time, to wear orthopaedic shoes for more than a few hours a day, and my feet also pain me when I sit or lie down. I cannot carry on my normal activities or interests. I have felt painful side effects due to tension and pain, which in effect have made me a cripple, and have affected me both mentally and physically. I have consulted with and followed the recommendations of orthopaedic doctors and podiatrists and am told by them that my foot problems are due to the following:

1. I pronate, thereby throwing my feet out of balance, putting too much pressure on certain areas and rolling on the outside of my feet.

2. Because of the operation on my small toes, they have been shortened and turn up, and the

pressure they ordinarily would take is now absorbed by other areas of my feet. My small toes hurt even though I wear cut-away shoes or sandals which do not touch them.

3. Pinched nerves from scar tissue.

4. Gout (not confirmed later).

The doctor who did my hammer toe surgery recommended soft, loose shoes to keep as much pressure off this area as possible. I gradually reduced the type of shoe I wore to a rubber-thong sandal at home, and over-sized soft leather moccasins outside the house. He also suggested my wrapping lamb's wool around my small toes. After wearing a stiff platform sandal for about a week, I had severe pains in the tailor bunion area and went back to my moccasins and the pain gradually subsided to the usual state.

I then saw another physician who told me my pain was caused by my feet not being balanced (pronating and short small toes) and he thought that if I wore moulded shoes to balance my feet, I would be comfortable. He sent me to an orthopaedic shoemaker who made five pairs of moulded shoes, trying in various ways to keep pressure off my tailor bunion area. The pain became more severe and I was unable to wear the first three pairs. Not having results anticipated from the shoes I then tried acupuncture three or four times without results.

My physician then operated on both feet. Besides removing additional bone from the small toes, he explored to see if there was a neuroma between the fourth and fifth toes, but did not find any. I believe that he said he also blocked some nerves in contact with the bones. The operation provided no relief, the pain continued in the same area, becoming worse. A new platform moulded arch was then prescribed and made. After a good try, I stopped wearing them, as they did not improve my condition and I went back to the previous shoes. Valium was prescribed, which only depressed me terribly and had no other effect on my feet. Over a period of time I have taken a whirlpool bath for my feet once or twice a day, without any effect.

Next a podiatrist tried to relieve pressure on the sore area with a bandage, but it did not work and neither did the injections he tried in each foot. The foot pain produced a side effect, I felt pain in my jaws. My dentist found I was having spasms in that area, which he attributed to the stress and pain. All the doctors I have seen, as well as orthopaedic shoe specialists, have been surprised that I have had so much pain despite the fact that I pronate and have reduced small toes. To correct my pronating problem, to keep me from rolling when I walk, three pairs of appliances have been made, two temporary, on which various adjustments were made, and a permanent pair which can be altered. My doctor is not satisfied that he has found the correct adjustment as yet, and says that will take time. I have continued pain in the tailor bunion area, at times very severe, and in the small toes whether walking, standing or sitting, with or without shoes.

Because of the painful areas in my feet and the size of the appliances I wear, I have not been able to find shoes that do not irritate or cause pain to some part of my feet and I am wearing men's sneakers cut away on the sides to avoid contact with sensitive areas of the foot and which can be laced to hold appliances. Another orthopaedic physician refused to deaden or cut nerves and thought that there was the possibility of a tarsal tunnel syndrome. However, a nerve conduction test was negative.

Still concerned with my lack of progress and increasing pain, I saw another orthopaedic physician for his ideas on my problem. After examination, he pointed out that a combination of very loose joints, rigid arches, and an improper alignment of legs and feet have caused my problems, which he assures me are not insoluble, but will require the attention of someone who knows and is interested in foot problems.

Orthopaedic examination prior to psychiatric referral revealed supple feet, multiple fine scars, normal metatarsals, unremarkable peripheral vascular status, and normal ankles and subtalar motion. Vibration sense was negative, and knee jerk and ankle jerk responses were 2+ bilaterally. Internal rotation was 40 degrees and external rotation 15 degrees. There were multiple surgical scars of the fifth toe bilaterally, as well as the third and fourth web spaces, both bilaterally. Multiple surgical procedures for ingrown toenail, especially on the left, had been performed. The patient came to the physician's office with a three-suiter valise full of dozens of shoes and appliances (Fig. 52–2).

After examination, the patient was told that her problem could not be helped by any further orthopaedic treatment, and she was referred for psychiatric consultation, which she accepted after some reluctance. Psychiatric examination revealed a woman who had used repression and denial in response to emotional problems and who would develop functional complaints and illness when under emotional stress. In therapy, emphasis was placed on helping the patient to establish contact with her feelings and at times their connection with her pain and symptoms. After a year of treatment her foot pain diminished greatly as she became more mobile, and she managed without any additional orthopaedic

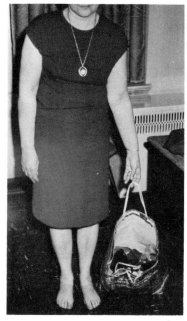

Figure 52–2. *A chronic pain patient with her collection of shoes and appliances. (Courtesy of Melvin H. Jahss, M.D.)*

or specific foot care other than soft shoes without appliances. In this case, individual psychotherapy with some contact and consultation with family members was the treatment of choice.

THE HYPOCHONDRIACAL PATIENT

Hypochondriasis, according to the American Psychiatric Association's manual on nomenclature, the *Diagnostic and Statistical Manual of Mental Disorders, 3rd ed. (DSM-III)*[10] is defined by the following diagnostic criteria:

A. The predominant disturbance is an unrealistic interpretation of physical signs or sensations as abnormal, leading to preoccupation with the fear or belief of having a serious disease.

B. Thorough physical evaluation does not support the diagnosis of any physical disorder that can account for the physical signs or sensations or for the individual's unrealistic interpretation of them.

C. The unrealistic fear or belief of having a disease persists despite medical reassurance and causes impairment in social or occupational functioning.

D. Not due to any other mental disorder such as schizophrenia, affective disorder, or somatization disorder.

The hypochondriacal patient reacts to physical sensations or pre-existing somatic illness as if the body and self were in imminent danger. This patient presents quite differently from the hysterical patient. The hysteric classically presents with "belle indifference," a lack of concern that is theoretically based upon the anxiety having been converted into the somatic symptom; i.e., the psyche has produced or exacerbated a physical symptom. On the contrary, the hypochondriac presents with intense anxiety and fear over the symptom and is committed to searching for a physician who will diagnose what has eluded all other physicians and who will save the patient from further suffering and possibly from death itself.

How can the orthopaedist recognize the hypochondriacal patient? The patient's complaints may be vague, diffuse, multiple, variable, shifting, generalized, exaggerated, and improbable or impossible on the basis of anatomic structure or pathophysiology. The patient is unclear and unspecific in describing the symptom, has difficulty in pointing to a specific symptomatic area, and refers to multiple locations and organic symptoms. The chief complaint may vary with time or may shift from one location to another. Generalized complaints, such as weakness, tiredness, or fatigue, are common. The patient's descriptions may be overstated, magnified, and unverifiable. For example, the patient may bitterly complain of foot swelling, which on physical examination is undetectable or insignificant compared with the patient's description.

The complaints to the physician, or anyone else who will listen, are marked by anxiety, fear, urgency, and anger. The patient does not calmly present a symptom for diagnosis and treatment, but rather anxiously and fearfully complains of a symptom or an array of symptoms that he or she believes would lead to a serious diagnosis requiring immediate treatment — if the orthopaedist only cared enough. Anger is directed toward physicians who have failed to discover the obvious underlying disorder and toward anyone else who refuses to accept the complaint and heed the warning.

The patient attempts to convince the orthopaedist of the validity of the complaints by forcefully presenting a detailed, prolonged account of chronic symptoms, incomplete work-ups, incorrect diagnoses, failed treatments, and uncaring, rejecting, disbelieving physicians. In order to verify the complaints the patient may use medical terminology and medical "facts" learned from multiple office visits. Some patients may also produce a large collection of orthopaedic shoes and appliances, attesting to their suffering and frustration. The patient's life and interactions with others revolve around the somatic symptoms and the search for diagnosis and cure. He or she explains many of life's problems as a direct or indirect effect of the illness. Indeed, the orthopaedist may wonder about what and how the patient would talk to other people if the symptoms were not present.

The physician–patient relationship is revealing. The patient often suggests and complies with multiple diagnostic techniques and therapeutic procedures, about which he or she may be initially grateful and hopeful, until the work-up reveals little or nothing and the therapy fails to improve or even exacerbates the symptoms. Despite open disagreement with the choice of diagnostic and therapeutic procedures, the patient often remains ambivalently attached to the physician, unless and until the physician rejects the patient by essentially denying his or her complaints. A most important clue is the orthopaedist's feelings of frustration in attempting to diagnose and treat the patient and annoyance at the patient's continuing dissatisfaction with and yet attachment to the orthopaedist.

At times, chronic pain patients may present with a combination of hysterical and hypochondriacal characteristics. Some patients may present with symptoms and characteristics that may overlap and change with time, making psychologic diagnosis all the more difficult.

CONVERSION REACTIONS (HYSTERICAL NEUROSIS, CONVERSION TYPE)

History

In antiquity, the ancient Egyptians (from as early as the fourteenth century BC) and then the Greeks and Romans in turn were all cognizant of hysterical phenomena.[11] This was felt to be a disorder of women caused by abnormal movements of a discontented uterus, which the Greeks believed could wander through the body. The Greek term *hysteria* is derived from the Greek word for uterus, *hystera*. The Middle Ages, with its spiritual emphasis, explained phenomena such as hysterical symptoms as being the result of demonic possession and witchcraft. However, in the late seventeeth and early eighteenth centuries, as clinical medicine again began to focus on physical phenomena and the physical universe, physical symptoms were again related to physical pathology. Sydenham (1681) first stated that almost all known physical diseases could be simulated by hysterical phenomena. In 1837, Brodie, an English surgeon, expanded the concept of hysteria to include somatic symptoms such as arthralgias that had no apparent organic basis. In France, in the last half of the nineteenth century, Charcot, a neurologist at the Salpêtrière, was the first to attempt a systematic study and clarification of hysterical manifestations. However, he considered them to be a hereditary degenerative disease of the nervous system due to precipitating trauma, often minor in nature. This concept was held even though his goal was to identify hysterical disease and separate it from its organic counterparts.[12] Nevertheless, Charcot was not completely unaware of the psychologic origin of hysteria. He was the first to demonstrate that by the use of hypnosis such symptoms could be both reproduced and removed in hypnotizable subjects. This was confirmation of their psychologic origin.

Pierre Janet, a pupil of Charcot, was later to contribute the concept of dissociation, i.e., ideas are not in conscious awareness but operate autonomously and appear as sensory and motor manifestations of hysterical symptoms.[13]

In 1894 Freud formulated the mechanism of conversion. Freud had studied in Nancy, France, and also at Paris with Charcot, but he was greatly influenced by the Nancy School of Lebeault and Bernheim, which was theoretically opposed to Charcot. This school supported the idea of the psychologic nature of hysteria, believing that all symptoms of hysteria were the result of suggestion. Freud's concept of conversion held that if a psychic trauma is not expressed emotionally, these affects are dissociated from consciousness and converted into the formation of physical symptoms. These symptoms in turn have a symbolic meaning and protect the patient from a conscious awareness of unacceptable fantasies, affects, or ideas.[14]

Definition

Today the term *hysteria* has three principal meanings:

1. Briquet's hysteria, first described by him in 1859. This is essentially a disease of women (only 5 per cent incidence in men), which usually starts before the age of 30 and is principally characterized by multiple physical complaints that may involve various organic systems. These women are apt to be emotionally unstable and tend toward the histrionic, but are not of any specific personality type. As noted, they have records of multiple physical complaints that result frequently in a complicated history with numerous hospitalizations, diagnostic work-ups, and often polysurgery. Conversion symptoms may be present at times but are not essential for the diagnosis.[15]

2. Conversion reaction or conversion hysteria. This disorder is characterized by physical symptoms, usually suggesting neurologic disease, but of a nonorganic basis. There is no sign of nervous system disease or morphologic or physiologic pathology. The signs that are present cannot be produced by nervous system dysfunction. The symptoms of "patterns of disorder arise from mental disposition" to "reflect the subject's notions about his bodily arrangements and functioning."[16] The patient is convinced of their somatic and organic origin. Thus, for a diagnosis of conversion reaction there must also be a psychiatric evaluation that will substantiate that the reaction is psychologically possible and based on psychologic mechanisms. The *Diagnostic and Statistical Manual of Mental Disorders* has the following definition of conversion reaction or hysterical neurosis, conversion type:

A. The predominant disturbance is a loss of

or alteration in physical functioning suggesting a physical disorder.

B. Psychologic factors are judged to be etiologically involved in the symptom, as evidenced by one of the following:

1. There is a temporal relationship between an environmental stimulus that is apparently related to a psychologic conflict or need and the initiation or exacerbation of the symptom.

2. The symptom enables the individual to avoid some activity that is noxious to him or her.

3. The symptom enables the individual to get support from the environment that otherwise might not be forthcoming.

C. It has been determined that the symptom is not under voluntary control.

D. The symptom cannot, after appropriate investigation, be explained by a known physical disorder or pathophysiologic mechanism.

E. The symptom is not limited to pain or to a disturbance in sexual functioning.

F. Not due to somatization disorder or schizophrenia.[17]

3. The last meaning of hysteria refers to the hysterical personality or hysterical character, which is a characterologic disorder. In this form, there is no sensory or motor disturbance of a psychogenic etiology. This definition is also frequently used as a pejorative term for patients, especially women, who show emotional lability with shallowness of affect, are vain and histrionic, and although seductive and sexually provocative, are most often anorgasmic. They may be very dependent and demanding in their interpersonal relationships.[18] The hysterical personality may occasionally be a male but is generally a female. This may be due in large part to the historical development of the concept of hysteria, as in Charcot's time it was almost universally held that hysteria could only be a female illness or disease.

Current Theories and Findings

Modern concepts of conversion hysteria recognize that such symptoms may be found in a variety of personality types and not always as monosymptomatic and discrete clinical entities. Frequently, minor trauma or a frightening physical accident that resulted in little bodily injury can produce hysterical symptoms as a circumscribed clinical entity. However, the hysterical conversion symptom may often be only one symptom in a mixed collection of various clinical manifestations or part of a psychoneurotic constellation of depression, anxiety, and obsessions. Purtell and associates[19] compared 50 women with "hysteria" with 50 healthy women and found that back pain, joint pain, pain in the extremities, and paresthesia was 4 to 20 times more common in "hysterics" than in controls. In addition, paralysis of the extremities was present in some form in 33 per cent of the "hysterical" women but was absent in controls. The illness was always found to be polysymptomatic, with no patient having fewer than 11 symptoms and the mean being 23 symptoms. However, some authors, such as Guze,[15] seek to define terms more restrictively. They state that conversion symptoms are always individual symptoms, whereas hysteria or Briquet's syndrome is a polysymptomatic disorder. Another important finding was that the conversion symptom most often encountered clinically was pain. Ziegler and associates[5] also remarked that conversion symptoms, especially pain, frequently mask an underlying depression. They also felt that conversion reactions may be another defense against overt depression. As a result, the depression may be covert and difficult to recognize. A conversion reaction may also be a defense against neurotic anxiety. It often occurs in adolescents with anxiety and difficulty due to deficient ego development associated with adolescent conflicts.

Conversion hysteria is seldom found in men, except when there are work-related compensation or insurance factors or obvious secondary gain, as in military service. Luck[20] found that psychogenic musculoskeletal symptoms were diagnosed in 11.1 per cent of patients in a military orthopaedic hospital during wartime. In addition, more than 25 per cent of patients in the orthopaedic outpatient department presented with psychogenic musculoskeletal symptoms. The findings most often encountered were circumferential hypalgesia, hysterical paralysis, and coarse intention tremors along with anxiety.

Various authors give different male-to-female ratios of conversion hysteria, but females are always greatly in the majority. However, Chodoff and Lyons[18] believe that there may well be a question of "semantic distortion." They state that the hysterical personality is more common in women but that conversion reactions are readily found in both men and women. The latter may possibly be even more common in men, as a result of work-related compensation and post-traumatic cases.

Newer models and concepts of conversion hysteria add another dimension, as these do not see conversion symptoms serving principally or only to relieve unconscious conflict. Instead, hysterical conversion reactions have been conceptualized as a form of nonverbal communication or a protolanguage conditioned by the physician–patient interaction and relationship. This communication model means that the symptoms of many patients are better understood, as Chodoff[21] states, "within the context of role and game theory" and not uniquely in medical terms. Thus, the symptom becomes a communication rather than a defense and "it is useful as an instrument in negotiating interpersonal transactions."[22] The patient therefore communicates distress in nonverbal ways.

This is especially true in regard to pain, which is the conversion symptom most often encountered clinically. It frequently represents the somatization of an affect and a verbalized appeal for help.[5, 19] The conversion symptom, especially pain, frequently masks an underlying depressive affect, as both may coexist. The depression may be hidden or clinically evident.

In our review of hysterical symptoms we will not discuss hysterically altered states of consciousness or dissociative reactions. These reactions, such as seizures, amnesia, fugue states, and syncope, may accompany conversion reactions and are important and not altogether rare hysterical symptoms.

Hysterical Motor Disorders

Hysterical motor disorders are varied and may be manifest as either paralyses or abnormal movements.

Paralysis or paresis is most common and is manifest usually as hemiplegia, monoplegia, or paraplegia. These may be either spastic or flaccid, if the weakness is total. Hysterical paralysis or weakness does not conform to known or anatomic distribu-

tion, but will conform to the patient's conventional ideas of anatomy. The foot will be paralyzed from the ankle down or from the knee, and the weakness will fluctuate and is inconsistent on repeated examinations.

Suggestion can also play an important role in the inconsistency, and it may appear to the examiner that the patient displays excessive effort while withholding strength. There is no Babinski's reaction and no true clonus, and electrical conduction tests are within normal limits. Tendon reflexes are usually present and, if so, are suggestive of a disorder of psychogenic origin, especially in the case of flaccid motor weakness. However, in some spastic forms of paralysis the deep reflexes may be exaggerated. The hysterical leg is dragged inertly instead of being swung by circumduction from the hip, as in neurogenic hemiplegia or crural monoplegia. If lifted by the examiner, the leg is light and if suddenly relaxed, it does not fall heavily but in a more orderly fashion. The hysteric very seldom injures him- or herself — no matter what the disability (e.g., hysterical gait) and no matter how bizarre the movements. The movements depend upon the patients' conception of their motor disability. Also, if hysterical, the weakness will be most pronounced at the proximal part of the extremity, rather than at the distal portion. This is the opposite of what happens in neurologic impairment of the central nervous system.

Testing for the contraction of agonistic and antagonistic muscles can help in the diagnosis of hysterical paralysis or paresis. By suddenly increasing or withdrawing resistance there is an observable response based upon physiologic principles, as illustrated by the Hoover test. This test of unilateral leg paresis detects associated pressure if the paralysis or weakness is hysterical in origin, but not if it is of organic etiology. It is summarized by Walshe[23] as follows:

In the case of an hysterical hemiplegia or crural monoplegia . . . if the patient, lying on her back, be asked to press the heel of the paralysed leg down upon the observer's hand which lies under it, no effort but a feeble one is made. If now the observer's hand be retained in this position and the patient be asked to elevate the sound leg forcefully, the heel of a formerly

Hoover Test

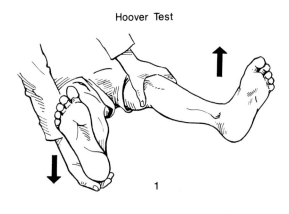

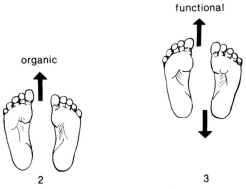

Figure 52–3. *The Hoover Test. (1) When the patient is asked to raise his sound limb the examiner's hand placed beneath the heel of the "paralyzed" leg feels a reciprocal downward pressure from the "paralyzed" leg. (2) In organic paralysis, the sound limb is elevated without the downward pressure of the "paralyzed" leg. (3) In functional or hysterical paralysis, the heel of the "paralyzed" leg presses down by reciprocal pressure as the sound leg is raised. (Adapted from Weintraub, M.I.: Hysteria: a clinical guide to diagnosis. CIBA Clinical Symposia, 29:22, 1977.)*

paralysed leg will be felt to press down on the observer's hand with force equal to that of the elevation of the sound limb, because to perform the latter movement strongly against resistance is possible only when the fellow limb is equally strongly pressed in the opposite direction (Fig. 52–3).

Tremors may vary greatly in nature and can also present as choreiform or clonic movements. These may involve the hand or foot. They are usually seen when the extremity is activated, but may occur, although less intensively, when the extremity is at rest.

Contractures are not uncommon, and hysterical contracture of the foot may at times be present in equinovarus.

The following clinical case history illustrates many of the salient features of this disorder. These features were described in essence in the classic literature of the last century by authors such as Richter[24] and Janet,[25] among others. However, conversion reactions, as expressed in major sensory and motor disorders, have decreased and changed in many ways during the past 100 years. This is due to social, cultural, and economic changes in our society that affect both patient and physician.

Case Report

The patient, a 31-year-old woman, was seen in psychiatric consultation 30 months after she slipped and fell on an icy sidewalk while walking. She fell on her left knee, stood up, and fell backwards, landing on her back. She was released from the emergency room of a nearby hospital with the diagnosis of "a sprained left ankle," but was hospitalized two weeks later for continued and increased pain in her ankle, knee, and back. The patient had been unable to walk since the accident or to put any weight on her left leg and foot, and she supported herself on crutches. After two weeks of cervical and pelvic traction, she was placed in a below-the-knee walking cast for six weeks, but continued unable to put pressure on her foot. When the cast was removed, she states that her leg was "swollen and immediately turned in" and that she was unable to "turn it out." However, the pain had disappeared, to be followed by "no pain sensation from the knee to the ankle along the outside" of her leg, while "only a small part of the inner leg was sensitive to pain." Afterwards, several casts were applied, and traction was used between each period of casting. Upon removal of each cast, however, the foot always returned to its abnormal position. During this period an initial electromyogram (EMG) was abnormal, but two subsequent EMG's were completely normal. Two myelograms were negative, and there was no evidence of Sudeck's atrophy. Neurologic examinations were negative, and repeated courses of physiotherapy and traction were of no help during extensive work-ups. Six or seven casts were applied before her short-leg brace became permanent, as the patient claimed that without it she could not lift her foot or turn her foot out. She sleeps wearing the short-leg brace and attached shoe, as she claims it is too difficult to reposition her foot in the morning and reapply her brace if she sleeps without it.

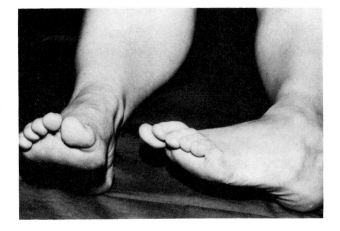

Figure 52–4. *Patient with hysterical conversion "contracture" (equinovarus) of the left foot. (Courtesy of Melvin H. Jahss, M.D.)*

Orthopaedic examination just prior to psychiatric consultation revealed the following: No intrinsic foot atrophy, circulation normal, left calf 15 inches compared with 16⅛ inches on the right. Knee jerks 2+ bilaterally and ankle jerks 3 to 4+ bilaterally, whereas Babinski's reactions were negative bilaterally. Minimal thickening of the skin under the fifth metatarsal, an indication that the patient is not putting particular amount of weight on the foot. No clonus. Patient using mainly her tibialis posterior for the inversion deformity. However, in testing the patient for muscle power, all the muscles appear weak, although the tibialis posterior is working at maximum. Alleged zero power of her toes. Vibratory sense absent in her left foot, which is a nonanatomic finding. There is numbness of her left leg up to the mid-tibia, which is also a nonanatomic finding.

The patient was felt to have a purely functional paralysis and conversion reaction and was referred for psychiatric evaluation and treatment (Fig. 52–4).

Mental status examination showed no evidence of psychotic thinking or psychotic thought content in a young woman of average intelligence. She was cooperative and superficially pleasant but guarded about revealing herself. "I'll talk about most things but not sex." She appeared to be a rigid individual who held a perfectionist view of herself and was unable to recognize or acknowledge that she had personal difficulties, viewing psychologic maladjustment as a character weakness. She had a need to be strong and invulnerable and to deny anxiety or worry.

The patient was the middle of five children. Her childhood had been traumatic and difficult, as she had an alcoholic, violent father who disappeared when she was six years old. The mother, a strict, controlling woman, struggled to support the family and bring up the five children. After high school graduation the patient joined the army for three years and received an honorable discharge after attaining the rank of sergeant as a technician. Her work history prior to the accident had been regular, and there was no history of alcohol or drug abuse. Medical and surgical histories were essentially negative. The patient described herself as being very athletic, participating in many sports, and having no personal problems. She refused to see her disability in psychologic terms and insisted that it had to be organic, although several physicians had also told her previously that her problem was possibly of psychologic origin. However, she accepted her disability and deformity quite blandly, without expressing much emotion or intense affect. Thus, a minor trauma precipitated this severe disability. The intensity and depth of the patient's denial of psychologic origin and conflict precluded her recognizing the psychologic basis for her need for psychiatric treatment.

Hysterical Sensory Disorders

Hysterical sensory disturbance most frequently occurs in the extremities, although it may be found in any area or distribution. Findings consist of anesthesia, paresthesias, hypesthesia, dysesthesia, and hyperesthesia. Again, hysterical anesthesia, like hysterical motor disturbance, does not follow sensory nerve distribution, but rather the patient's idea of body anatomy and sensory distribution. Thus, one frequently finds the characteristic "glove and stocking" anesthesia, which stops at obvious and readily defined margins. Anesthesia may be overlooked and not noticed, as patients often do not include this in their list of complaints, although these sensory disturbances are frequently associated with hysterical motor abnormalities.

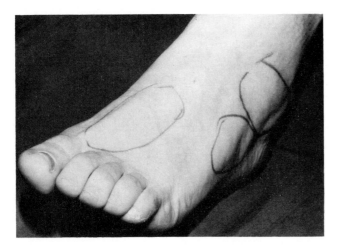

Figure 52–5. *Nonanatomic areas of hyperesthesia (circled with crayon by the patient). (Courtesy of Melvin H. Jahss, M.D.)*

In hysterical hemianesthesia all modalities are involved, and lack of sensation extends exactly to the midline; whereas in neurologic disease this loss is never strictly on the midline, and a small amount of sensation is preserved on the affected side of the midline. Hysterical anesthesia of the foot will show a single level of loss at the ankle for touch, pain, and temperature, whereas an organic lesion would produce a dissociation of the sensory modalities at different levels. As previously noted, pain is perhaps the conversion symptom most frequently encountered clinically. It may often be associated with hyperesthesia of a certain area of the skin (Fig. 52–5).

SELF-INFLICTED INJURIES

Dermatitis Artefacta (Factitial Dermatitis)

There are self-inflicted, psychologically determined skin lesions and eruptions produced uniquely by the patient, often in an unconscious manner and at times while sleeping.[26] These disorders are infrequent in young children (except for the mentally retarded), and most often are seen in women (adolescents and young adults) and occasionally in an older person. Often the artifact may be superimposed on another process, but it is still self-inflicted and no longer has any causal relationship to the associated process.[27]

The self-inflicted lesions of factitial dermatitis are produced by a variety of imaginative and ingenious techniques, such as caustic chemicals, hot coins, glass, knives, fingernails, or burning with a cigarette. Thus, the lesions vary considerably in both their distribution and morphology; however, the site is always accessible to the patient's hands. These lesions are bizarre in outline and configuration and do not conform to any known pathologic condition. Their perfect roundness may be unnatural, or else their irregular rectilinear or angular, sharp margins do not form natural-looking outlines. There is usually either intense denial or rationalization by the patient. However, at times it may be difficult to evaluate the unconscious element. These patients are different from malingerers who consciously and deliberately produce their lesions either for material gain or to avoid an undesired activity. There are also patients who may surreptitiously prevent the healing of wounds.

In neurotic excoriation, which includes nail- or toe-picking, scratching, and some cases of neurodermatitis, as well as more serious disorders, the patient seldom denies causing the lesions, but is unaware of his or her reason for producing them (Fig. 52–6). The majority of such cases are seen in women.[28] These excoriations are again found in easily accessible areas and are usually scooped-out in shape or saucerized.

Mentally retarded and senile patients also produce self-inflicted lesions and trauma at times, but in these groups the problem is based essentially on physiologic rather than functional pathology. A hereditary organic syndrome such as familial dysautonomia, or Riley-Day syndrome, results in more blunt trauma. This is due to a combined defect of somatic sensory and autonomic motor function, which is

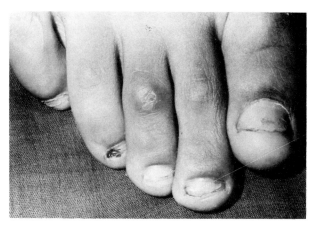

Figure 52–6. *Neurotic excoriation of the toenails. (Courtesy of Melvin H. Jahss, M.D.)*

thought to result from an imbalance of autonomic nervous function. Because of this sensory loss, multiple skin abrasions are common, and some of these children are mentally retarded.[29] In the Lesch-Nyhan syndrome, found only in males, there is an almost complete deficiency of hypoxanthine-guanine phosphoribosyltransferase (HGPRT). The onset is usually by the age of 10 years from renal failure. There is self-mutilation, mental deficiency, cerebral palsy, hyperuricemia, and uricaciduria.[30]

Narcotics addicts, especially heroin users, may utilize the veins of the foot for injecting or "mainlining" narcotics after other veins have become sclerosed and useless for self-injection.

Malingering

Malingering, which is the conscious control and simulation of disease, pain, or disability, must be distinguished from conversion hysteria and psychogenic pain, which it most resembles. However, malingerers are usually evasive and inconsistent in their history, and the potential for gain appears to be more obvious. Such gain may be in the form of compensation or the avoidance of an unpleasant or threatening situation. In malingering a minor injury may be exaggerated, or a prior disability may be attributed to a subsequent and more recent accident. The hysteric cannot control his or her symptoms, whereas the malingerer may even produce physical signs and other symptoms, no matter how bizarre or difficult.[31, 32]

Hysterics, if paralyzed, will not move their paralyzed limbs when alone, whereas malingerers will do so if they believe that they are not being observed. This fact corresponds to the unconscious enacting of the sick role by the patient with a hysterical conversion reaction. As a group the malingerers are quite heterogeneous and range from being mildly mentally disturbed to being severely disturbed.

MAJOR AND MINOR CAUSALGIA (REFLEX SYMPATHETIC DYSTROPHIES)

Causalgia (hot pain), although not a hysterical or malingering disorder, is also manifested by hyperesthesia, as well as hyperalgesia and autonomic and atrophic changes that especially affect the peripheral portion of the extremities. The condition was described and the term first used by S. Weir Mitchell regarding wounded Civil War soldiers.[33] This post-traumatic condition may follow either a major or a minor injury to an extremity. "Major causalgia" results from partial injury to a peripheral nerve (especially the sciatic or median nerve) or arterial or perivascular injury and sympathetic nerve dysfunction.[34] There is diffuse, continuous, burning pain that can be exacerbated by apparently insignificant stimuli such as a draft, air motion, sound, or emotional stress. The hyperpathia can be so severe that the patient cannot move the involved extremity or allow it to be touched. Although psychogenic etiology is not an initial factor, these patients often become depressed, anxious, and debilitated, and some may develop hysterical features, severe personality changes, and psychotic behavior. Because of the intense emotional agitation often found, a mistaken diagnosis can be made of a primary psychogenic illness. If compensation is involved, this can become an added complicating factor. The pain and vasomotor and sympathetic nerve changes are not well understood, but early treatment is essential, starting with local anesthetic infiltration. If this is not successful, sympathetic nerve block, repeated if necessary, may give temporary or permanent relief. If temporary but not permanent relief is obtained, surgical sympathectomy is often indicated. Both tranquilizers and psychotherapy have been reported to be of value at times.[35]

"Minor causalgia" is a less painful condition, is seen chiefly in civilian practice, and may occur subsequent to even minor injury and nonpenetrating wounds without any apparent gross nerve injury. This condition is also called reflex dystrophy, post-traumatic painful osteoporosis, or Sudeck's atrophy if there is osteoporosis that is sudden and acute in onset and is accompanied by intense pain, tenderness, swelling, and vasomotor changes, such as sweating of the surrounding soft tissues. A fracture is not necessary, and joints are frequently involved. An example of these lesser precipitating injuries would be a dog bite with subsequent infection; lacerations; and blows. Treatment is the same as with major causalgia. The emotional reaction to chronic pain (discussed previously) may, in turn, stimulate sympathetic nerve activity, which may hinder treatment and reinforce the pathologic condition by affecting pain perception. Because of their withdrawal, depression, personality change, and possibility of secondary gain, these patients need emotional support as part of a comprehensive program in their physical treatment and rehabilitation.[36]

PSYCHOLOGY OF THE FOOT AND SHOE

Symbolism

In many cultures and throughout history the foot has had a symbolic and communicative significance. As we have seen, the patient may utilize foot symptoms to communicate both physical and emotional suffering. A person may also develop an excessive attachment to the foot, either consciously and unconsciously, as an object of adornment or symbolic sexual meaning. Menninger[37] notes the various meanings of the foot throughout history: speed, vitality, power, domination, foundation, and health. The foot of a woman has especially been a symbol of fecundity in various cultures and also a connection between the life-giving earth and the gods or goddesses. Women were thought to obtain their procreative powers through foot contact with the earth. Such beliefs are to be found in the folklore and mythologies of most cultures and nations that have associated the foot with sexual ideation and phallic symbolism. In some cultures, including our own in the not too distant past, it was disgraceful for a woman to expose her feet. In other cultures, a woman exposing her feet may be more disgraced than if she exposed her genitals.

Foot Binding

Chinese foot binding is one example of the foot's erotization. This custom, which lasted over a thousand years, was part of a complex cultural and sexual orientation that was well described by Levy.[38] The bound foot, or lotus foot, was of prime erogenous importance, almost as important as the vagina as a center of erotic stimulation and pleasure. Body deformation has existed in most cultures, including our own, and is especially true of the foot, with the shoe as a contributing factor. Fashion is seldom functional and footwear is usually purchased for its stimulant and erotic value, in part as a substitute for the foot itself. Most women will wear uncomfortable shoes, either too small or with high heels, for narcissistic pleasure and not for comfort. Women past a certain age or women fearful of giving a "wrong impression" will not wear such shoes. These shoes with various nonfunctional modifications can only be explained by their contribution to the psychosexual stimulation of the male. Rossi[39] traces the sexual roots of all shoe styles for both women and men and their "erotic communication."

Fetishism

In our society one finds the fetishist, almost always a male, who can obtain sexual satisfaction only if he is looking at or touching a special and specific object. It is estimated that a quarter to a third of such fetishists choose as objects the foot and/or shoes as their source of erotic gratification.[39] It is necessary for the fetishist to have this article or object present, as he cannot become sexually excited or potent without it. This object may be sufficient to itself or a precondition for "normal" intercourse. The person cannot become sexually excited otherwise.

Fetishism is described in the early sexual and psychoanalytic literature by authors such as Krafft-Ebing, Binet, Havelock Ellis, Freud, Jung, and Stekel among others. Stekel[40] even describes two cases of shoenail fetishism, in which the individual had a need to observe the feet of women in order to see if their shoes had nails in the soles or not.

Footnote. Although the orthopaedist will see few foot or shoe fetishists, he or she is very likely to be visited by patients with considerable emotional investment in their feet. Such patients will be extremely sensitive to foot symptoms and diagnostic and therapeutic procedures. Any disfigurement or surgical scar that may alter their foot image and how they think others may respond to them and their feet will create difficulties in treatment. Indeed, such patients may have great difficulty in accepting prescribed appliances, comfortable shoes, or what they consider unflattering orthopaedic shoes, despite continued suffering and disability.

These patients must be carefully evaluated before surgery. Their expectations of surgery and their psychologic needs may be so unrealistic that no matter how successful the procedure may be from the surgeon's point of view, the patient will be disappointed and perhaps even worse after therapeutic intervention. Although this is also true with many "pain patients," on the contrary some functional conversion patients will improve and even be "cured" after surgical exploration or biopsy has proved negative. This is especially true in adolescents and children.

REFERENCES

1. Reading, A.: Illness and disease. Clin. North Am., 61:703, 1977.
2. Ziegler, F. J.: Hysterical conversion reactions. Postgrad. Med., 47:175, 1970.
3. Nemiah, J. C.: Hysterical neuroses, conversion type. In Freedman, A. M., Kaplan, H., and Sadock, B. (eds.): Comprehensive Textbook of Psychiatry. 2nd ed. Baltimore, Williams and Wilkins Co., 1975, pp. 1208–1220.
4. Clawson, D. K., Bonica, J. J., and Fordyce, W. E.: Management of chronic orthopaedic pain problems. In American Academy of Orthopedic Surgery: Instructional Course Lectures. Vol. XXI. St. Louis, C. V. Mosby Co., 1972, Chapter 2.
5. Ziegler, F. J., Imboden, J. B., and Meyer, E.: Contemporary conversion reactions: A clinical study. Am. J. Psychiatr., 116:901, 1960.
6. Engle, G. L.: "Psychogenic" pain and the pain-prone patient. Am. J. Med., 26:899, 1959.
7. Beck, A. T.: Depression: Clinical, Experimental and Theoretical Aspects. New York, Harper and Row, 1967, pp. 333–335.
8. Cath, S. H., Glud, E., and Blane, M. T.: The role of the body image in psychotherapy with the physically handicapped. Psychoanal. Rev., 14:34, 1957.
9. Fordyce, W. F.: Behavioral Methods for Chronic Pain and Illness. St. Louis, C. V. Mosby Co., 1976.
10. American Psychiatric Association: Diagnostic and Statistical Manual of Mental Disorders. 3rd ed. Washington, D.C., American Psychiatric Association, 1980, p. 25.
11. Vieth, I.: Hysteria: The History of a Disease. Chicago, University of Chicago Press, 1965, p. 3.
12. Woolsey, R. M.: Hysteria: 1875 to 1975. Dis. Nerv. Syst., 37:379, 1976.
13. Janet, P.: Etat Mental des Hysteriques — Les Accidents Mentaux. Paris, Rueff et Cie., 1892, p. 30.
14. Breuer, J., and Freud, S.: Studies on hysteria. In Strachey, J. (ed.): Standard Edition of the Complete Psychological Works of Sigmund Freud. Vol. 2. London, Hogarth Press, 1955, p. 3.
15. Guze, S. B.: The validity and significance of the clinical diagnosis of hysteria (Briquet's syndrome). Am. J. Psychiatr., 132:138, 1975.
16. Walshe, F.: Diagnosis of hysteria. Br. Med. J., 11:1451, 1965.
17. American Psychiatric Association: Diagnosis and Statistical Manual of Mental Disorders. 3rd ed. American Psychiatric Association, Washington, D.C., 1980, p. 247.
18. Chodoff, P., and Lyons, H.: Hysteria, the hysterical personality and "hysterical" conversion. Am. J. Psychiatr., 114:374, 1958.
19. Purtell, J. J., Robins, E., and Cohen, M. D.: Observations on clinical aspects of hysteria: Quantitative study of 50 patients and 156 control subjects. J.A.M.A., 146:902, 1951.
20. Luck, J. V.: Psychosomatic problems in military orthopaedic surgery, J. Bone Joint Surg., 28:213, 1946.
21. Chodoff, P.: The diagnosis of hysteria: an overview. Am. J. Psychiatr., 131:1073, 1974.
22. Ziegler, F. J., and Imboden, J. B.: Contemporary conversion reactions. II. A conceptual model. Arch. Gen. Psychiatr., 6:279, 1962.
23. Walshe, F.: Diseases of the Nervous System. 2nd ed. Baltimore, Williams and Wilkins Co., 1970, p. 352.
24. Richter, P.: Etudes sur la Grande Hysterie ou Hystero-Epilepsie. Paris, Delahaye et Lescrosnier, 1885, p. 950.
25. Janet, P.: Etat Mental des Hysteriques — Les Accidents Mentaux. Paris, Rueff et Cie., 1892, p. 113.
26. Mustaph, H.: Aggression and symptom formation in dermatology. J. Psychosom. Res., 13:257, 1969.

27. Rook, A., and Wilkinson, D. S.: Psychocutaneous disorders. *In* Rook, A., Wilkinson, D. S., and Ebling, F. (eds.): Textbook of Dermatology. Philadelphia, F. A. Davis Co., 1968, pp. 1587–1592.

28. Fisher, B. K.: Neurotic excoriations. Can. Med. Assoc. J., *105*:937, 1971.

29. Carins, R. J.: The skin and the nervous system. *In* Rook, A., Wilkinson, D. S., and Ebling, F. (eds.): Textbook of Dermatology, Philadelphia, F. A. Davis Co., 1968, p. 1583.

30. Thorn, et al. (eds.): Harrison's Principles of Internal Medicine. 8th ed., New York, McGraw-Hill Book Co., 1977, p. 648.

31. Spiro, H.: Chronic factitious illness. Arch. Gen. Psychiatr., *18*:569, 1968.

32. Peterdorf, R. C., and Bennett, I. L., Jr.: Factitious fever. Ann. Intern. Med., *46*:1039, 1957.

33. Mitchell, S. W., Morehouse, G. R., and Keen, W. W.: Gunshot Wounds and Other Injuries of Nerves. Philadelphia, J. B. Lippincott Co., 1864.

34. Homans, J.: Minor causalgia: a hyperesthetic neurovascular syndrome: New Engl. J. Med., *222*:870, 1940.

35. Sternschein, M. D., Meyers, S. J., Frewin, D. B., and Downey, J. A.: Causalgia. Arch. Phys. Med. Rehab., *56*:58, 1975.

36. Bonica, J. D.: Pain in the extremities. Northwest Med., *69*:570, 1970.

37. Menninger, K. A.: The Human Mind. 3rd ed. New York, Alfred A. Knopf, 1966, p. 298.

38. Levy, H. C.: Chinese Foot Binding. New York, Walter Rawls, 1966.

39. Rossi, W. A.: The Sex Life of the Foot and Shoe, 1st ed. New York, Saturday Review Press/E. P. Dutton & Co., Inc., 1976, p. 83.

40. Stekel, W.: Sexual Aberrations: The Phenomena of Fetishism in Relation to Sex. Vol. 2. New York, Liveright Publishing Co., 1940, p. 82.

Part VI

TRAUMA TO THE FOOT AND ANKLE

CHAPTER 53

INJURIES OF THE FOREFOOT AND TOES

William H. Blodgett, M.D.

Injuries of the toes and forefoot include contusions; crush injuries; avulsions of toenails; sprains; lacerations; fractures; dislocations; chemical, thermal, and electrical burns; and snake bite injuries. A patient may present with more than one type of injury, which may greatly modify the treatment plan.

A *contusion* of the foot is a soft tissue injury that does not cause a break of the skin and is the result of a direct blow or a compression force. Usually there is a subcutaneous hemorrhage, which together with ensuing edema, adds to the tissue damage.

A rough estimation of the forces involved is useful in the evaluation and treatment, as the degree of initial pain may be unreliable for such purposes. It is obviously worse to have a foot run over by an automobile wheel than by a bicycle.

The presence of fractures and ligamentous or tendon injuries must be excluded, as must the possible presence of limited blood clotting ability, either primary or drug-induced. When these have been excluded, the treatment varies according to the degree of injury and the desire of the

patient to continue uninterrupted activity (e.g., sporting events).

The spectrum of therapy progresses from reassurance, to limited cooling with a few ice cubes or ethyl chloride spray, to a compression bandage and return to activity. However, if the contusions are more severe, adequate elevation, compression bandaging, cold applications, and sedation are indicated. If required, medical treatment for coagulation defects or hypo-osmolality should be instituted.

Contusions of the toes may result in painful subungual hematoma. The severity of the pain under the nail characteristically increases as the pressure of the hematoma builds up. Pain is relieved by puncturing the nail to release the hematoma. This is done by drilling or by burning with a hot, blunt wire.

If return to function has not occurred after several days, re-check x-ray examination should be considered to exclude an occult fracture that had been missed in the initial studies.

Ligamentous sprains of the adult forefoot are rare because the usual shoe protects against the torsion forces that produce such injuries. Swelling, local tenderness, and pain on motion in the absence of roentgenographic evidence of fracture confirm the diagnosis.[17, 30]

Elastic bandage forefoot support, reduced weight bearing, and elevation yield early return to function. Circumferential forefoot support and metatarsal insole support may be required for several weeks.

Avulsion of a toenail is painful and is usually incomplete. Unless the avulsion is minimal, the nail will be lost and sometimes should be excised under appropriate anesthesia.[8, 10] A nonadherent dressing should be used together with an anesthetic ointment, as the exposed subungual tissue is very sensitive for a few days. About nine months are required to completely regrow the nail of a great toe.

A *crush injury* of the foot is a severe contusion that occurs when the foot has been subjected to a very heavy weight. The degree of soft-tissue damage is much more extensive than in a simple contusion, arteries and veins are obliterated, and multiple fractures are present. Varying degrees of tissue necrosis result.

Partial early realignment of the fractures by skeletal traction and countertraction help to improve the circulation.[17, 22] Surgical release of fascial planes may be necessary to decompress the foot as swelling develops.

In treating crush injuries, multiple pins with external fixation devices, as the Roger Anderson or Hoffman units, are applicable, so that the soft tissue damage can be assessed and cared for.

The patient's circulatory status is important, as is the presence or absence of diabetes. The degree and type of contamination and foreign body implantations are additional factors in the treatment outline.

Massive doses of intravenous antibiotics are used. Repeated cultures are necessary to determine the choice of antibiotics.

When viability of the foot is in doubt and weight-bearing function is improbable, in my opinion, early amputation may be preferable to months of protracted treatment with failure always imminent.

COLD INJURIES

The extent of tissue damage to the foot by cold temperatures is related to the de-

gree of cold and the duration of exposure. Exposure varies with the type of footwear and the type and thickness of stocking material. Other factors are the activity of the individual, the wetness of the feet, and the competence of the circulation.

Trench foot is a cold injury that occurs when the individual is subjected to periods of subfreezing weather while walking activities are limited, as when soldiers are confined to foxholes for several days. Removing the boots, massaging the feet, and changing the socks are of help in delaying tissue damage.

Dusky cyanosis and blanching of the foot develop first, followed by superficial blisters. The foot is painful and, as the process continues, toe motion is lost, sensation is absent, and apparent gangrene may develop.

Hundreds of American soldiers who had been pinned down in foxholes by a German counterattack were treated for trench foot in the United States Army Hospital in Paris during World War II during the winter days of December 1944.

The demarcation between viable and thermally destroyed tissue may take weeks to determine. The processes of repair are so much more effective in the younger individual with cold injuries than in an older person that the physician is often surprised by the return of viability of the young person's foot.

Immersion foot is a term that had its origin in World War II. It identifies a cold injury that is caused by long periods of immersion in cold water, as happens to individuals escaping from sinking ships or downed aircraft. Maceration of the skin and edema of the foot and leg are greater than that seen in trench foot. The treatment program consists of elevation, cooling of the extremity, antibiotics, and debridement, when necessary. The time required for healing is the same as that for trench foot.

Frostbite, especially of the forefoot, occurs in cold climates. Alcoholics who are unduly exposed to cold are very susceptible, as are persons during wartime and concentration camp victims. There may be distal necrosis, late deformities, and, in milder cases, persistent vasomotor instability, such as excess sweating and burning. Treatment consists of slow thawing, with temperatures not to exceed 40°C (104°F).

ELECTRICAL BURNS

Electrical burns destroy tissue in proportion to the electrical force and the duration of the electrical energy. Tissue necrosis inside the skin is usually much more extensive than is suggested by the skin destruction, and this should be kept in mind when planning therapeutic management. Debridement of subcutaneous necrotic tissue may require extensive skin incision because the skin may be viable while subcutaneous structures are destroyed.

FRACTURES AND DISLOCATIONS OF THE FOREFOOT AND TOES

General Considerations

The structural strength of the concave plantar aspect of the foot is much greater than that of the dorsal or convex side. The combination of the strong plantar ligaments, the strong tendons of the toe flexors, and the posterior tibial and peroneus longus tendons of the plantar aspect are the anatomic reason for the differences in force resistance of the plantar and dorsal sides of the foot. A force that seeks to flatten the arch from heel to toe is resisted much more effectively than one that tends to increase the heel to ball arc.[1, 29]

The tarsal bones of the forefoot include those distal to the talus and calcaneus, i.e., the navicular, cuboid, and three cuneiforms. The metatarsotarsal joints or the "joints of Lisfranc" have some important anatomical features that relate to the results of trauma and the treatment of injuries of this area.

The French surgeon Jacques Lisfranc was graduated in medicine in 1813. He immediately joined the armies of Napoleon as a medical officer. His biographer in the *Dictionnaire des Sciences Médicales* describes him as "a man of fiery nature and hard working with rigorous precision in operative technique." His advocacy of amputation of the forefoot through the metatarsotarsal joints has resulted in these joints retaining his name. It was said that Lisfranc could perform the amputation in one minute!

Important anatomic features of Lisfranc's joint include the following: The proximal end of the second metatarsal is mortised between the first and third cuneiforms. The medial structural support is more secure than the lateral support. The first metatarsal articulates with the medial cuneiform, the second with the middle cuneiform, and the third, fourth, and fifth metatarsals share contacts with the lateral cuneiform and the cuboid. Longitudinal ligaments pass across the metatarsotarsal joints. There are ligaments placed transversely between the proximal ends of the metatarsals, except between the first and second metatarsal;[1, 29] in this instance, a ligament is found from the second metatarsal to the medial cuneiform (Fig. 53–1). This structural ligamentous configuration results in less security of the bases of the first and second metatarsals to each other than is present between the bases of the other metatarsals.

The insertion of the anterior tibial tendon on the medial side of the proximal first metatarsal and the proximal lateral insertion of the peroneus longus tendon to the base of the first metatarsal are factors in both the security and the displacement of

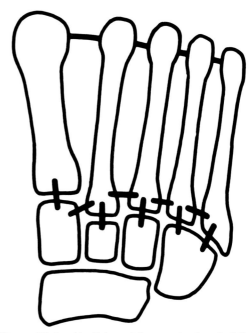

Figure 53–1. *Mortising of the proximal end of the second metatarsal between the first and second cuneiforms and the configuration of the ligaments at the base of the metatarsals. Note that the bases of the first and second metatarsals are not secured to each other as are those of the other metatarsals. (From Wiley, J. J.: J. Bone Joint Surg., 53B:473, 1976.)*

the first metatarsocuneiform joint. These features are factors that may block anatomic reduction.

Dislocations of the Forefoot Joints

Traumatic dislocation of the tarsal navicular and of the cuboid does occur. These are usually in conjunction with fractures or other dislocations of the joints of the foot. The presence of the other fractures may lead one to overlook the dislocation. Such dislocations should be confirmed by multiple projection x-ray studies, which may need to be compared with similar projection roentgenograms of the opposite foot. Early reduction of these dislocations is essential to prevent excessive swelling, circulatory embarrassment of the foot, and possible aseptic necrosis of the cuboid or navicular.

Dislocation of the first metatarsal on the medial cuneiform is usually concomitant with dislocation of the first metatarsal from the base of the second metatarsal.[29] This is related to the ligamentous anatomy, since the proximal ends of the first and second metatarsals are not tethered to each other by ligaments.

Dislocation of the metatarsotarsal joints (Lisfranc's joint) are, as a rule, accompanied by fractures of the base of the second metatarsal and often of the base of the fifth metatarsal.[1, 5, 13, 22, 24, 29] These displacements are almost always dorsal and lateral, consequent to the flexion force on the forefoot and the ligamentous configuration (Fig. 53–2). Severe displacement may occur following what seems to have been trivial trauma — such as missing the final step of a stair (see Figure 53–4A, B).

There are two basic types of Lisfranc fracture-dislocations (Fig. 53–3). The most common consists of lateral dislocation or subluxation of all the metatarsals on the tarsus. The minor subluxations are frequently overlooked. The second type consists of a divergent dislocation with the first two metatarsals being separated. In these cases, there may also be an associated fracture of the navicular with separation of the medial and middle cuneiforms. Vascular compromise may occur in the more severe cases, but this is relatively rare.

Following such an injury, the patient is unable to bear weight, and there is de-

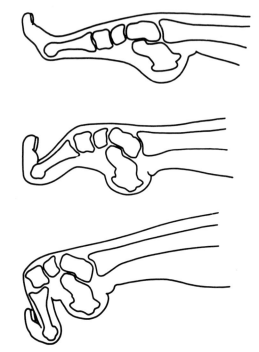

Figure 53–2. *Diagram of the changes that develop as forefoot equinus force progresses beyond the point of resistance. Subsequent to dorsal displacement, lateral displacement of the proximal metatarsals may occur. (From Wiley, J. J.: J. Bone Joint Surg., 53B:473, 1971.)*

formity of the foot consisting of a forefoot equinus, forefoot abduction, prominence of the medial tarsal area, and early and marked swelling.

When this fracture-dislocation is the result of a serious automobile or motorcycle accident, it may be overlooked because of other visceral, head, or skeletal injuries that demand immediate life-saving treatment.[1, 3]

Closed reductions of fracture-dislocations of Lisfranc's joint may be difficult, incomplete, and insecure.[1, 13, 22, 24, 31] Open reduction is often necessary when closed reduction is blocked by bone fragments or soft tissue, e.g., the insertion of the anterior tibial or the peroneus longus tendon. Fixation by transfixation Kirschner wires as well as external immobilization is often necessary (Fig. 53–4). This is because of both the initial insecurity of the reduction and the subsequent loss of position that may develop when decrease of swelling invalidates the adequacy of external fixation. Late loss of reduction may develop

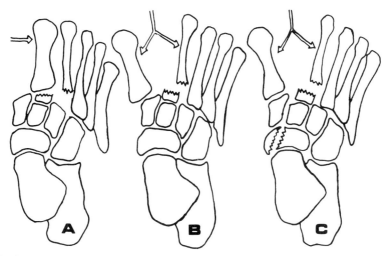

Figure 53–3. *Displacements that occur with a fracture-dislocation of Lisfranc's joint. Common to all three is a fracture of the base of second metatarsal, which is the hallmark of this fracture. When the force is applied purely laterally all of the metatarsals are displaced lateral to the tarsals (A). If the force separates the first and second metatarsals (B, C), the medial displacement of the first ray may dislocate the first metatarsal–cuneiform joint, or the first and second cuneiforms separate and the navicular fractures (C). (From Aitkin, A. P., and Poulson, D.: J. Bone Joint Surg., 45A:250, 1963.)*

when weight bearing is instituted too early.

When a fracture-dislocation of Lisfranc's joint is inadequately reduced, an unsightly malfunctioning foot results (Fig. 53–5). The forefoot is abducted and rigid. There are bony prominences of the distal tarsal bones both superiorly and inferiorly, and a painful weight-bearing area develops under the plantar surface of the tarsal navicular. Shoe fitting is difficult, and distortion of the shoe shortens the shoe life.

The nonoperative treatment involves attempts at redistribution of the weight on the plantar surface of the foot. This includes molded arch supports, shoe modifications, and individualized shoes built to a custom last. However, one pair of specially constructed and expensive shoes may be comfortable, whereas the next pair may be intolerable!

Excision of weight-bearing bony prominences offers some amelioration, but never complete relief of walking discomfort.

Isolated fractures and fracture-dislocations of the anterior tarsal bones are uncommon, except for small avulsion fractures of the proximal lateral edge of the cuboid that are associated with inversion sprains. These fractures are best seen on anterior tangential roentgenographic views. Treatment consists of simple strapping for two to three weeks.

Occasionally, a forceful dorsiflexion injury will produce a transverse fracture of the navicular (Fig. 53–6). Early open reduction with threaded Kirschner-wire fixation is advised, since the head of the talus tends to approximate the cuneiforms, making late reduction extremely difficult.

One rare type of injury recently described is a splitting apart of the bases of the first and second metatarsals. The separation may extend between the medial and middle cuneiforms (Fig. 53–7). Treatment consists of a compression bandage followed by plaster immobilization for five to six weeks. Mild "separation" between the medial and middle cuneiforms may occasionally be seen on normal roentgenograms.

Fractures of the proximal end or styloid of the fifth metatarsal are the most common of metatarsal fractures.[22] Usually the patient experiences sudden pain during an unexpected inversion of the foot. This type of injury frequently is encountered by basketball players or by individuals experiencing an unexpected inversion during other games or civilian activities. The fracture is ascribed to sudden overpull of

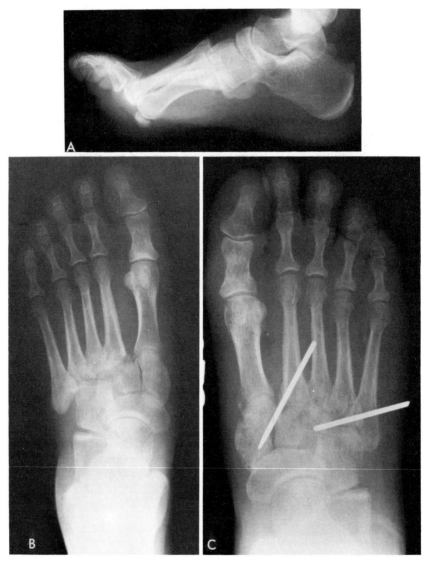

Figure 53–4. See legend on opposite page

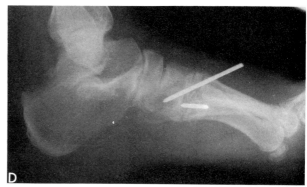

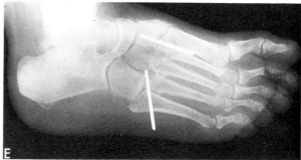

Figure 53–4. *(A–E) Roentgenograms of the foot of a 52-year-old woman who injured her right foot when she slipped down a few steps, landing with the foot in equinus. She sustained the fracture-dislocation of Lisfranc's joint, as seen. Attempts at closed reduction failed, even when skeletal traction was used. At open reduction, it was found that reduction was blocked by loose bone fragments. Kirschner-wire fixation was used, as well as plaster immobilization. The wires were removed after seven weeks; partial weight bearing was begun in a week, and full weight bearing at ten weeks. The early function was good.*

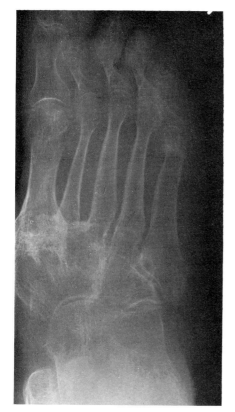

Figure 53–5. *Roentgenogram of the forefoot of a 68-year-old female who was severely injured in an automobile accident 12 years previously. The injury to the foot was unrecognized. The foot was painful, limiting the patient's walking and distorting her shoes for 12 years. Six months after an osteotomy of the shaft of the fourth metatarsal and partial condylectomy of the fifth metatarsal, the foot was comfortable but markedly limited in mobility.*

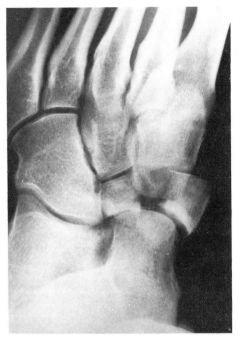

Figure 53-6. *Three-week-old transverse fracture of navicular in a 26-year-old male. Open reduction was required. (Courtesy of Melvin H. Jahss, M.D.)*

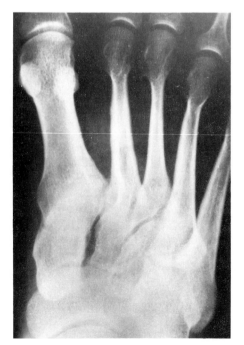

Figure 53-7. *Mild separation of the first and second rays, with pain, swelling, and local tenderness. (Courtesy of Melvin H. Jahss, M.D.)*

the peroneus brevis tendon. If this is indeed the mechanism of injury, it seems strange that further separation of fragments is not the rule!

The patient experiences both local pain on weight bearing and swelling, with progressive symptoms as swelling increases.

The cardinal signs on examination are local swelling and tenderness with pain on full passive inversion or attempts at active eversion. Dorsoplantar and oblique roentgenographic studies reveal the fracture, which is usually oblique but may be comminuted or transverse. The transverse fractures are seen when direct trauma to the area has occurred.

A sesamoid bone, the os vesalianum, may occur in this area and can mimic a fracture of the proximal fifth metatarsal. This can be distinguished from such a fracture by the smooth edges of the fragment and by the fact that it is usually present on the roentgenogram of the opposite foot.

The physician has a choice of treatment in the undisplaced fracture of the proximal portion of the fifth metatarsal. Many of these patients do very well with adhesive strapping together with an Ace bandage and crutches for a few days. The patient should be advised of the advantages of this treatment as compared with plaster fixation, as many patients are convinced by friends or tradition that all fractures must be immobilized by plaster.

When the fracture is particularly symptomatic or unusually displaced, a walking boot for four to six weeks is indicated. This is followed by a period of wearing an Ace bandage to protect against inversion. A nonunion of a proximal fragment may be treated by excision and reinsertion of the peronus brevis tendon at the proximal portion of the fifth metatarsal.

Fracture through the neck of the metatarsals is subsequent to a direct blow or jam and twist forces in the forefoot. Realignment of the head on the shaft is important because the weight-bearing functions of the involved metatarsal are decreased or increased by malposition. Metatarsalgia is a late complication and may require corrective osteotomy to relieve the pain experienced on weight bearing.

Manipulation during traction with a Chinese finger trap usually can accomplish reduction. External fixation will usually be adequate. When position is not maintained by these means, Kirschner-wire fixation is required.[5, 6, 10, 11, 15, 22]

Interpretation of postreduction lateral or slightly oblique roentgenograms taken through plaster as to detail of head-shaft position may be difficult and thus deceiving. When there is doubt concerning accuracy of reduction, a tomogram is helpful. A "Cutter" cast with almost no radiopacity is a useful aid in obtaining diagnostic roentgenographic evaluation.

Shatter fractures of the metatarsal head are usually the result of crush injuries or bullet or shell fragment wounds. This fracture is best treated by maintained traction.[17, 22, 25] This can be by skeletal traction with transverse Kirschner through the proximal or middle phalanx of the toe or by pulp wire transfixation. The traction force is slight and is obtained by a rubber band attached to an outrigger on a below-the-knee cast.

The traction must be maintained for about 7 weeks with limited weight bearing on the forefoot for 10 to 12 weeks; only limited metatarsophalangeal flexion can be expected.

March fracture is a stress fracture of a metatarsal shaft that may develop with increased walking activity or decreased strength of the bone.[1, 6, 10, 22, 26] An atavistic first metatarsal, i.e., when the first metatarsal is shorter than the second metatarsal, is a factor in the stress fracture of the second metatarsal. Recurrent march fractures have been reported under these circumstances. March fracture of the second metatarsal is occasionally seen following the Keller operation as a result of weakened first ray function. March fractures are also frequent in Charcot forefoot arthropathy secondary to diabetic neuropathy.

Typically the patient is not aware of any specific trauma, develops increasing metatarsal pain with normal weight bearing, and experiences progressive disability. The examination may be negative initially except for some tenderness at the stress fracture level. There is no instability of the metatarsal shaft. The roentgenogram is often entirely negative at first and in some cases fails to suggest a fracture line or evidence of fracture healing for up to six weeks. The orthopaedist must rely on the history and minimal findings to institute therapy.

Treatment is symptomatic, in that displacement of the fragments does not occur. Some patients respond to a metatarsal bar or to a metatarsal pad and a longitudinal arch support applied to a firm soled shoe, whereas others require a plaster walking boot.

Fractures and Dislocations of the Toes

Fractures of the toes have been rather casually described in orthopaedic and fracture textbooks. This subject usually occupies the final pages or paragraphs of the text.

Except for the great toe, the range of motion of an interphalangeal joint or metatarsophalangeal joint is not of much functional significance. However, malunion at a fracture site of a toe may be a source of persistent discomfort while wearing a shoe.

Fracture of Proximal Phalanx of the Fifth Toe

Perhaps the most common, but unheralded, fracture of the toes is the "night walker" fracture of the proximal phalanx of the fifth toe. Typically, the patient has been walking in the dark in his own home. Inadvertently a piece of furniture is struck by the fifth toe and is followed by immediate local pain, disability, subsequent swelling, ecchymosis, and subsequent increased pain with shoe constriction.[6, 10, 22]

Many such patients suffer because of self-care following such an injury. X-ray examination demonstrates varying degrees of dorsal angulation of the fractured proximal phalanx of the fifth toe, at times with comminution.

Adhesive strapping to secure the fifth toe to the forefoot and to the fourth toe can be of great symptomatic relief. Lamb's wool or cotton between the two toes prevents maceration of the skin. Adequate elevation and a shoe cut-out over the fifth toe are therapeutic adjuncts. Some swelling may persist for months.

Fractures of the proximal phalanx of the second to fourth toes are subject to plantar angulation. This deformity at the fracture site is consequent to the combined forces of the toe extensor and flexor muscles working together with the interosseous and lumbrical muscles.

If the angulation is allowed to persist with subsequent malunion, painful plantar pressure areas develop under the toe and may require operative correction.

Management of fractures of the proximal phalanx of the small toes may require aggressive treatment to prevent deformity. This may be immobilization in flexion with Kirschner-wire fixation or traction, which can be skin traction, pulp traction, or skeletal traction through the middle or distal phalanx.

When multiple comminution occurs, the overall alignment of the toe and fixation with a small piece of plaster or adhesive secured to adjacent toes is all that is required. This is because the group of bones is held in alignment by the tubular construction of the toe and full recovery of

joint motion is not required for full return of walking function and shoe wearing. Rarely, after healing, a misaligned fragment that is symptomatic may require surgical removal.

Crush fractures of the terminal phalanx of the great toe are more frequent than those of the smaller toes. The associated soft-tissue trauma results in swelling and pain, which require more care than does the bone displacement. Adequate elevation, ice applied locally, and analgesics represent the initial treatment, followed by a cut-out shoe with a stiff sole.

Traumatic Dislocations of the Toes

Dislocations of the toes include those of the metatarsophalangeal joints and the interphalangeal joints. The history of trauma, immediate pain, obvious deformity,

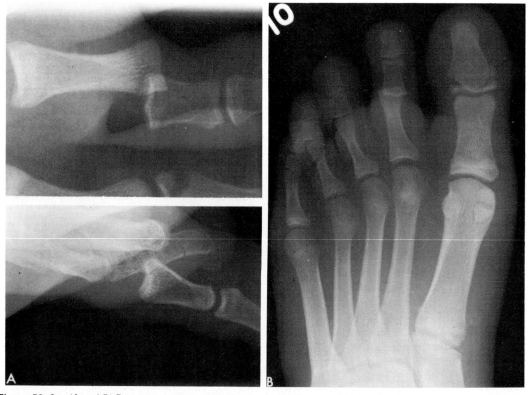

Figure 53–8. (A and B) Roentgenograms of the forefoot of a 16-year-old boy whose foot was struck by a motor that fell from a table in a school mechanics shop. An undisplaced comminuted fracture of the distal phalanx of the great toe and dorsal displacement of the middle phalanx of the second toe are demonstrated. Reduction could not be accomplished in the Emergency Room with Valium sedation or later with heavy traction under ankle block anesthesia. Two days later, under general anesthesia, an open reduction was performed. The proximal end of the middle phalanx was found to be extruded through the capsule, which blocked replacement during traction. Division of the capsule allowed for easy reduction.

and palpable displacement make the diagnosis evident.

A "complex" or, as Watson-Jones calls it, a "button-hole" dislocation,[30] cannot be distinguished clinically or roentgenographically from a simple dislocation except by the fact that it fails to reduce by the usual means (Fig. 53–8).

In this type of injury either the distal element or the proximal element of the dislocation tears through the capsule of the joint. The capsule then blocks replacement or reduction. The usual methods of reduction fail even in the most experienced hands. Open reduction is required, during which the opening of the capsule is enlarged so that reduction is not prevented by the capsule. Replacement is then easily accomplished.

MISCELLANEOUS INJURIES OF THE FOREFOOT AND TOES

Blast injuries of the foot, such as occur when a land mine has exploded, are associated with other life-threatening injuries to the body. The first requirement in the treatment of the foot is the debridement of obviously destroyed tissue and the second is to try to maintain the viability of the remaining structures. Swelling may be intense and may require release of the edema pressure in the several closed spaces of the foot to limit further tissue necrosis.

Immobilization to reduce pain during nursing care, prevention or control of infection, secondary debridement, alignment of bone contours, skin closure, and skin grafting are all factors in effective treatment.

Amputations must be considered at any stages of treatment, as the surgeon weighs the immediate threat to the patient's life, function of the foot, and the eventual quality of life for the patient.

Tennis toe is a term used to describe pain of the great toe that is localized at the base of the toenail. It commonly results from recurrent trauma caused by sudden stops on the tennis court. The foot slides forward in the shoe, and the great toe repeatedly strikes the end of the shoe. This traumatizes the nail bed, and pain develops with even normal walking. Tenderness and some swelling are found over

the nail bed, with normal range of motion of the interphalangeal joint. At times there is evidence of subungual hemorrhage. Onychomycosis may be present, which, because of thickening or loosening of the nail, facilitates the development of symptoms.

Treatment consists of advice about keeping the toenail short without rounding the corners and obtaining adequate fit of the tennis shoe about the forefoot and adequate length of the shoe beyond the toes. Adding a piece of felt under the tongue of the shoe may help, as may double stringing the upper two grommet holes of the shoe with the laces. As is true in treating many injuries of sports enthusiasts, the last resort may be omitting tennis.

The terminal portion of one of the small toes, usually the second or third, may be subject to *recurrent trauma associated with a hammer-toe deformity*. The distal two phalanges are squeezed between the sole and the top of the shoe, and a painful callus develops at the tip end of the toe. This may be complicated by the bending of the nail over the end of the toe. When this occurs, the terminal callus is modified and may be more painful. The toenail becomes thickened and so closely related to the underlying epithelium that it is virtually impossible to trim with the usual home equipment.

Treatment involves increasing the depth of the forefoot of the shoe or hollowing out the sole of the shoe at the area under the toe and stretching the upper structure of the shoe. Most of these patients eventually require surgical correction of the hammer toe.

SESAMOIDITIS

Diseases of, and especially injuries to, the sesamoids have become much more common with the increasing popularity of ballet, jogging, and long-distance running.

The medial and lateral sesamoids of the great toe underlie the head of the first metatarsal. They are invested by the tendons of the short flexor of the great toe and are joined to each other by a strong, short transverse ligament. Each has a concave articulating surface that contacts the plantar aspect of the first metatarsal head and provides a gliding surface for the weight-bearing functions of the first metatarsal. Incomplete coalition of the primordial calcification centers may result in a bipartite or tripartite configuration, which may be confused with fractures in roentgenograms of the foot. Bipartite sesamoids are often bilateral; therefore, the presence of a divided sesamoid on the contralateral side helps in establishing a correct diagnosis.

Painful motion of the sesamoid on the metatarsal head may be the result of old fracture or degenerative articular cartilage changes of the sesamoid. The medial sesamoid is more frequently involved. The patient often has the history of habitually wearing high heels, being a dancer, or having a cavus foot or short heel cord. Consistent and localized tenderness over the individual sesamoid is diagnostic.

Nonoperative treatment involves reduction of weight bearing by the sesamoids. This may be accomplished by cutting out a localized area of the shoe, placing a Spenco insert in the shoe, or using a metatarsal bar. A program to stretch the heel cord may effectively reduce the forefoot stress during walking.

If symptoms persist after conscientious conservative treatment, removal of the sesamoid is required.[5, 8, 10, 15, 17] There are those who believe that excision of both sesamoids should always be carried out because of subsequent degenerative changes of the remaining sesamoid. This has not been my experience. Removing both sesamoids may risk invalidating the function of the short flexor of the great toe, with subsequent flexion deformity of the interphalangeal joint, dorsal callosities, and subsequent need for interphalangeal fusion or transfer of part or all of the long flexor tendon.

Removal of a sesamoid of the great toe is tedious and at times exasperating. The tendon attachments must be cut using sharp dissection with a constant effort to limit the dissection to an area close to the sesamoid in order to avoid dividing the short flexor.

Earl McBride told me, when discussing this meticulous little piece of surgery, that the secret was to divide the strong ligament between the sesamoids as early as possible. This permits easier mobilization and removal. My preference is to excise the medial sesamoid through a medial incision, taking care to avoid the plantar medial nerve of the great toe, and to excise the lateral sesamoid through a plantar approach, taking care to avoid the lateral plantar nerve to the great toe. The lateral sesamoid is often removed during bunion procedures. In this surgical situation a dorsal intermetatarsal approach is employed because additional purposes are served during this procedure.

Hypertrophic additions to the sesamoids may be seen on roentgenograms of the feet of older patients. Symptoms are variable, and frequently these changes are an incidental asymptomatic finding.

Calcific tendinitis of the short flexor has been described.[13] I have had no experience with this condition. Kelekian recommends "irrigation, injections and needling and occasional surgical evacuation."[15] I interpret this to mean irrigation with an anesthetic solution and steroid instillation.

VENOMOUS SNAKE BITE OF THE FOOT AND ANKLE

With the increasing popularity of wilderness camping and off-the-road recreational vehicles, venomous snake bites of the foot and ankle can be anticipated. Ten per cent of the 3000 species of snakes are poisonous to man. Almost all of the venomous snake bites in the United States are by rattlesnakes, which are found in all of the contiguous states. These snakes occur in several sizes. They have a triangular-shaped head and a diamond pattern of the skin of the back. This design, however, is shared by a number of other nonvenomous snakes. The series of rounded, beadlike linear pods of the tail of the rattlesnake is the most individual identification. Some rattlesnakes do not bear rattles at all times of the year.

The venom of the rattlesnake is a very complex substance,[9] the components of which are only partially understood. Subsequent to envenomation, a wide variety of responses may occur, including local tissue necrosis; hematologic changes caused by lysis of red cells, modification of clotting mechanisms, and subsequent hemorrhage; pulmonary edema; renal damage; and neurotoxic changes. Local effects may include severe pain at the site, dusky cyanosis and edema of the extremity, dysesthesia, areas of anesthesia, reduced motor function, severe pain on muscle stretch, and marked tenderness.

An initial consideration in treating snake bite victims is to establish, if possible, the identity of the snake and whether in fact envenomation has occurred. Even though fang marks are present, it is estimated that in 20 to 30 per cent of these cases actual injection of toxic venom does not occur.

The immediate first aid treatment of venomous snake bites is accepted without disagreement by the experts. Subsequent hospital treatment causes divergent opinions, particularly as to the presence or absence of compartment pressure syndromes and thus the need for surgical treatment.

The immediate treatment of a venomous snake bite is directed toward reducing the amount of venom that reaches the local tissue and the body as a whole.[9] A constricting band is applied around the extremity proximal to the fang marks. The compression should be limited to that which will constrict the superficial venous and lymphatic return but will not obstruct the deep venous return or the arterial input flow.

Within 45 minutes of the attack,[9] some of the venom may be released from the local tissue by incision and suction. The depth of the incisions should be three quarters of the distance between the fang marks. On the foot or ankle the incisions should be longitudinal, even if two incisions are required, because a novice may divide important anatomic structures with a transverse incision.

Suction is applied either by mouth or by a suction device to increase the release of fluids. Mouth suction should not be done by anyone with open lesions of the mucous membranes of the oral cavity because of the danger of absorption of the toxins. Considerable suction can be developed when the neck opening of a heated jar is applied to the skin area and allowed to cool while pressure of the jar mouth is maintained on the skin to keep it airtight as it cools.

The victim should then be transported to the nearest hospital while being kept as calm as possible. The affected limb should be elevated slightly, but cooling with ice is not advised. The hospital staff should be alerted as to the expected arrival of the patient.

On arrival at the hospital, blood type and cross matching with donor blood, bleeding and clotting profiles, complete blood count, electrolyte evaluation, and renal function tests are indicated. Horse serum sensitivity tests should be done at once to anticipate the initiation of intravenous antivenom treatment.

The polyvalent antivenom is prepared by developing an antibody response in a horse by increasing increments of parenteral venom. In the United States polyvalent antivenom is manufactured by Wyeth Laboratories, Inc., Box 8299, Philadelphia, Pennsylvania, 19101. It is marketed under the trade name of Antivenin *(Crotalidae)* Polyvalent and comes in 10-ml vials for reconstruction, together with disposable needles and syringes.

When the horse serum response is negative, the initial adult dose of antiserum is four to five vials in 500 ml of saline or five per cent glucose. Three to four vials may be repeated in three hours. Ten to fifteen vials may be required for treatment of an adult. An infant or small child requires more antiserum because of the different ratio of venom to weight. The initial dose may have to be eight to ten vials; a total of twenty vials may be required. However, the fluid vehicle has to be much less to avoid fluid overload. Broad-spectrum antibiotics are also used intravenously for children and adults.

The signs of envenomation of an extremity may be identical to those of increased compartment pressure syndrome. Rowland,[23] in describing 20 cases of snake bite treatment, advocates early fasciotomy. Garfin and coworkers[9] urge that evaluation of compartment pressure by wick catheter should be carried out and demonstrated to be elevated, approaching 30 mm Hg, before compartmental fasciotomy is justified. The saline and needle technique of Whitesides and associates[27] can be used to measure compartment pressure if a wick catheter is not available.

Since Garfin and associates[9] have been measuring muscle compartment pressures, fasciotomy in snake bite has not been required in their patients. They also fear that tissue damage may already be irreversible when the decision for such procedures hinges on evidence of reduced arterial flow or peripheral nerve damage. The surgeon must decide which of the four compartments of the leg are involved as well as the exact type of release to be performed.

REFERENCES

1. Anderson, L. D.: Injuries of the forefoot. Clin. Orthop. Rel. Res., *122*:18, 1977.
2. Böhler, L.: The Treatment of Fractures. 4th English ed. Baltimore, William Wood and Co., 1935.
3. Cassebaum, W. H.: Lisfranc fracture-dislocations. Clin. Orthop. Rel. Res., *30*:116, 1963.
4. Clayton, M. L.: Surgery of the forefoot in rheumatoid arthritis. Clin. Orthop. Rel. Res., *16*:136, 1960.
5. Crenshaw, A. H. (ed.): Campbell's Operative Orthopaedics. 5th ed. St. Louis, C. V. Mosby Co., 1971.
6. DePalma, A.: The Management of Fractures and Dislocations. Vol. 2. Philadelphia, W. B. Saunders Co., 1959.
7. Dickson, F. D., and Diveley, R. L.: Functional Disorders of the Foot. 3rd ed. Philadelphia, J. B. Lippincott Co., 1953.
8. DuVries, H. L.: Surgery of the Foot. 1st ed. St. Louis, C. V. Mosby Co., 1959.
9. Garfin, S. R., Mubarak, S. J., and Davidson, T. M.: Rattlesnake bites — current concepts. Clin. Orthop. Rel. Res., *140*:50, 1979.
10. Giannestras, N. J.: Foot Disorders, Medical and Surgical Management. Philadelphia, Lea and Febiger, 1973.
11. Goldstein, L. A., and Dickerson, R. C.: Atlas of Orthopaedic Surgery. St. Louis, C. V. Mosby Co., 1974.
12. Hauser, E. D. W.: Diseases of the Foot. Philadelphia, W. B. Saunders Co., 1950.
13. Jeffreys, T. E.: Lisfranc's fracture dislocation. J. Bone Joint Surg., *45-B*:546, 1963.
14. Jones, R., and Lovett, W.: Orthopaedic Surgery. New York, William Wood and Co., 1923.
15. Kelikian, H.: Hallux Valgus, Allied Deformities of the Forefoot and Metatarsalgia. Philadelphia, W. B. Saunders Co., 1965.
16. Kidner, F. C.: The pre-hallux (accessory scaphoid) and its relation to flatfeet. J. Bone Joint Surg., *11*:831, 1929.
17. Klenerman, L.: The Foot and Its Disorders. Oxford, Blackwell Scientific Publications, 1976.
18. Lewin, P.: The Foot and Ankle. 4th ed., Philadelphia, Lea and Febiger, 1959.
19. Mubarak, S. J., Hargens, A. R., Owen, C. A., Garetto, L. P., and Akeson, W. H.: The wick catheter technique for measurement of intramuscular pressure. J. Bone Joint Surg., *58-A*:1016, 1976.
20. Mubarak, S. J., and Owen, C. A.: Double incision fasciotomy of the leg for decompression of compartment syndromes. J. Bone Joint Surg., *59-A*:184, 1977.
21. Reneman, R. S.: The anterior and the lateral compartmental syndrome of the leg due to intensive use of muscles. Clin. Orthop. Rel. Res., *113*:69, 1975.
22. Rockwood, C. A., and Green, D. P.: Fractures. Philadelphia, J. B. Lippincott Co., 1975.
23. Rowland, S. A.: Early fasciotomy in the treatment of snake bite. J. Bone Joint Surg., *55-A*:1314, 1973.
24. Sel, J. M.: The surgical treatment of tarso-metatarsal fracture dislocations. J. Bone Joint Surg., *37-B*:203, 1955.
25. Speed, K.: Fractures and Dislocations. 2nd ed. Philadelphia, Lea and Febiger, 1928.
26. Turek, S. L.: Orthopaedic Principles and Their Application. 2nd ed. Philadelphia, J. B. Lippincott Co., 1967.
27. Whitesides, T. E., Jr., Haney, T. C., Moritomo, K., and Harada, H.: Tissue pressure measurements as a determinate for the need of fasciotomy. Clin. Orthop. Rel. Res., *113*:43, 1975.
28. Whitman, R.: Orthopaedic Surgery. 8th ed. Philadelphia, Lea and Febiger, 1927.
29. Wiley, J. J.: The mechanism of tarso-metatarsal joint injuries. J. Bone Joint Surg., *53-B*:473, 1971.
30. Wilson, J. N. (ed.): Watson-Jones Fractures and Joint Injuries, 5th ed. New York, Longman, 1976.
31. Wilson, P. D.: Management of Fractures and Dislocations. Philadelphia, J. B. Lippincott Co., 1928.

CHAPTER 54

INJURIES TO THE TALUS AND MIDFOOT

Marvin L. Shelton, M.D., and Walter J. Pedowitz, M.D.

The talus is normally subjected to extremely large stress forces during walking and running. Despite this vulnerability, injuries to it are uncommon, accounting for less than 1 per cent of all fractures. The resistance to injury is due in part to the great strength of the dense cancellous bone composing the talus. The compression force required to break the talus is reported to be twice that needed to fracture the calcaneus and navicular bones.[64] Extreme nonphysiologic forces — mainly vertical compression, extreme dorsiflexion, pronation, and supination — are required to fracture the talus or disrupt its ligamentous articulations. In addition to its important weight-bearing function, the talus is the link connecting the talocrural, subtalar, and midtarsal joints, which allow the hinge movements of the ankle and rotation of the foot.

Injuries to the talus are often spectacular and have fascinated surgeons since the first account of talar dislocation by Fabricius of Hilden in 1608. In 1919, Anderson called attention to the frequent association of aircraft accidents and talar injuries and coined the term "aviator's astragalus."[1] Further interest was generated by Coltart after World War II, when he reported on 228 talar injuries among 25,000 fractures and dislocations treated by the orthopaedic units of the Royal Air Force.[12] Although flying accidents accounted for 43 per cent of the total group of talar injuries, and 70 per cent of the serious injuries in this group, the remaining 57 per cent demonstrate that nonflying hazards to the talus are also common.

The talus may be injured by (1) transchondral (dome) fractures, (2) dislocation of the subtalar joint, (3) dislocation of both the subtalar and talocrural joints (total talar dislocation), (4) talar neck fractures, (5) body fractures including fractures of the lateral process, and (6) midtarsal joint injuries. Many of the injuries occur together, producing a fascinating array of possible combinations.

TRANSCHONDRAL (DOME) FRACTURES OF THE TALUS

Transchondral fractures of the talar dome are produced by a force transmitted from the articular surface of a contiguous bone across the joint and through the articular cartilage to the subchondral trabeculae of the fractured bone.[4] They generally occur along the midlateral or posteromedial portion of the dome, but are often missed on initial examination because of "reportedly negative" radiographs and more obvious soft tissue damage.[1, 9, 29, 55] These fractures are commonly associated with other more obvious injuries to the malleoli and adjacent ligaments, which tend to obscure their detection.[2, 4, 74, 82]

Rendu (1932) is credited with the initial description of interarticular fracture of the dome of the talus.[67] Subsequent to this, many case reports appeared discussing "osteochondritis dissecans" of the ankle, "chip fractures of the talar dome," and "loose bodies of the ankle."[9, 14, 66, 68] Approximately 300 transchondral fractures have been reported to date, but long-term follow-up studies are still needed.[2, 76]

In 1959, Berndt and Harty first elucidated the mechanism of injury and classified the fractures according to degrees of displacement.[4] Based on anatomic studies of amputated limbs, they investigated the sequence of injury and demonstrated that the common denominator is inversion injury to the ankle. Midlateral dome fractures are produced by inversion injury and dorsiflexion, causing impaction and compression of the anterolateral aspect of the talus against the articular surface of the fibula. However, with the foot in plantar flexion, the narrow posterior half of the talar dome now occupies the mortise, and forceful inversion accompanied by medial rotation of the tibia on the fixed foot leads to posteromedial talar impaction. Isolated case reports of lesions with no antecedent history of trauma appear in the literature from time to time, but there is overwhelming agreement that the majority of these fractures are post-traumatic in nature.[79]

Classification. The fractures are classified according to the degree of displacement[4] (Fig. 54–1):

Stage I — this represents a small area of compression of subchondral bone, causing microscopic damage to the bony trabeculae. No damage may be evident on superficial examination of the talus.

Stage II — the osteochondral fragment has now become partially detached, and fissuring is now evident on the radiograph.

Stage III — complete detachment of the osteochondral fragment from its underlying bed has now taken place, but the fragment remains in anatomic position.

Stage IV — the detached osteochondral fragment has now become inverted in the fracture bed or lies displaced elsewhere in the joint.

Clinical Findings. In most reported series, athletic males in the second and third decades are affected much more frequently than are females.[14, 69, 82] Medial lesions are often seen in women after sustaining inversion injuries while wearing high heels, whereas men often sustain the injury subsequent to landing on the toes associated with a torsional inversion component, as in basketball, football, or a fall from a height.

Clinically, the patient frequently gives a history of having severely twisted his ankle and having heard something "pop." There is marked tenderness over the lateral aspect of the ankle, and the lateral ligament injury may initially overshadow the osteochondral fracture.

In midlateral lesions, pain and tenderness to local palpation often occur in the area between the talus and the tibiofibular syndesmosis. In the posteromedial lesions, tenderness presents behind the medial malleolus.

If initially missed, the lesion will progress to a chronic stage. In Stages I, II, and III there will often be freedom from pain with the joint at rest. However, with increased demands on the joint, symptoms of chronic pain between the talus and the tibiofibular syndesmosis, recurrent swelling, grating sensation, and the feeling of a "weak ankle" should alert the clinician to the possible presence of an osteochondral fracture. In Stage IV there may actually be intermittent locking of the joint.

Radiographic Assessment. Accurate diagnosis demands meticulous radiographic study since the fracture may initially be difficult to visualize, and delay may lead to chronic irreversible disability. Indeed, delays in diagnosis averaging nine months are commonly reported.[2, 4, 53, 55, 76, 82]

Initial roentgenograms should include an anteroposterior view of the ankle with the foot internally rotated 10 degrees, as well as lateral and oblique views.[2, 4, 53] When a fracture is suspected, additional internal rotation mortise views should be obtained with the ankle in plantar flexion, neutral position, and dorsiflexion to profile the talus in different planes. Accurate reading is critical, because slight overlapping of normal bony structures may obscure a bone fragment.[29, 55, 76]

If pain persists despite initial negative

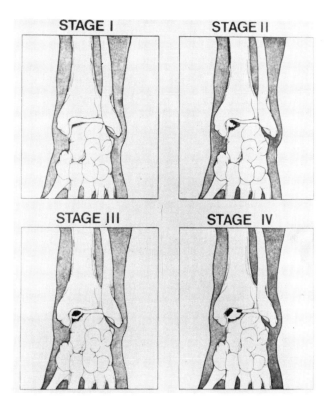

Figure 54–1. Classification of dome fractures of the talus. (From Mukherjee, S. K., and Young, A. B.: J. Bone Joint Surg., 55B:319, 1973.)

films, x-ray studies should be repeated at appropriate intervals. Inasmuch as these symptoms are also consistent with a functionally unstable ankle, stress views in inversion and eversion should be done to ascertain the competency of the medial and lateral ligamentous structures.

Several of these lesions have been reported in association with subchondral cysts of the talus and impaction fractures of the tibial plafond, so their presence should prompt the surgeon and radiologist to search carefully for a talar dome fracture.[76, 81]

"Air contrast" tomography is extremely helpful in these situations and should be done in all cases considered for operative intervention to further help delineate the pathology.[76] It should be remembered that the fragments are invariably larger than they appear on the roentgenograms, in which the articular component is not visualized. Arthrograms may also be useful in helping to delineate defects in the joint surface.[55, 76] Arthroscopic visualization would be very helpful for all stages.

Treatment. Appropriate staging and prompt treatment offer the best chance for a good result. In order for healing to take place, capillaries must bridge the fracture line. Whether or not this happens is directly dependent upon the degree of initial trauma, the age of the patient, and the promptness and duration of adequate immobilization. If immobilization is inadequate, the repetitive frictional effect of an uneven joint surface will cause the fracture to proceed through the various stages of delayed union to established nonunion. The ability of the cartilage of the ankle joint to withstand this irregularity is limited; therefore, late osteoarthritic changes will occur in some cases.[2, 52, 55, 75, 76]

Undisplaced fractures in Stages I, II, and III without signs of established nonunion (marked sclerosis, grossly uneven joint surfaces, or osteoarthritic changes) are best treated conservatively by a short leg non–weight-bearing plaster cast until union is demonstrated radiographically.[2] Stage IV displaced fractures, large or small, are best treated by surgical removal of the fragment in order to prevent further deterioration of the ankle joint (Fig. 54–2).[2, 75, 76] In advanced Stage IV fractures with associated severe osteoarthritic

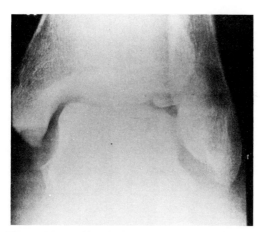

Figure 54–2. *Chronic Stage IV lateral dome fracture with 180-degree rotation of the fragments.*

changes, mere removal of the loose body will usually be inadequate and ankle fusion should be considered.

Hopefully, a satisfactory resurfacing type of total ankle replacement will be developed in the future that will allow preservation of function.

SURGICAL TECHNIQUE. Lateral lesions can often be reached through an anterolateral arthrotomy. Division of the anterior fibulotalar portion of the collateral ligament is usually necessary. If more exposure is needed, fibular osteotomy via a modification of the Gatellier technique (as described by Davidson and associates[14]) affords complete exposure.[25]

A long oblique skin incision is made from below and is directed backward and upward, beginning at the tip of the malleolus. The periosteum of the distal 4 inches of the fibula is carefully elevated to include the anterior tibiofibular and anterior talofibular ligaments. A hole is drilled through the lower fibular fragment into the tibia, and proper position is confirmed by roentgenograms. A self-tapping screw is inserted and then partially withdrawn. The screw is subsequently utilized, along with hook retractors, to externally rotate the fibular fragment after the bone is divided. Care must be taken to protect the peroneal tendons, which are also retracted backward.[25]

Some medial lesions can be reached via arthrotomy alone. However, osteotomy of the medial malleolus at the level of the ankle joint (with pre-insertion of a self-tapping screw to aid anatomic reposition-

ing) greatly facilitates the exposure (Fig. 54–3).

Once inside the joint, inspection should be meticulous. Probes or forceps tips may be used to palpate the joint surface, and areas of depression, softness, or color change are sought.

Large fractures, as described by Mukherjee and Young[52] and Smillie,[75] are actually body fractures involving the articular dome and should be accurately reduced and internally fixed in order to preserve congruity of the joint surface. Small fractures are delineated and debrided with curettes and fine gouges. The cartilage is cut vertical to the joint surface, thus creating a pit, and the underlying sclerotic bed is perforated with multiple fine drill holes, using a narrow-gauge Kirschner wire. Saucerization of the defect should be avoided, because this only increases the size of the lesion and prolongs the postoperative morbidity.[58]

Postoperative Care. Early resumption of motion and partial weight bearing at two weeks postoperatively are recommended for those patients treated by simple arthrotomy, curettage, and drilling. Malleolar osteotomy requires bone union prior to weight bearing (usually about six weeks postoperatively), but active range of motion is usually possible at two weeks. The screw fixing the fibula to the tibia should be removed after union of the osteotomy and before institution of weight bearing. In patients treated by internal fixation of dome fragments, no weight bearing is allowed until fracture union is demonstrated radiographically.[53, 79]

Prognosis. Because the diagnosis is so frequently missed on initial examination, there is ample clinical evidence that if this fracture is left untreated, it certainly can progress to incapacitating degenerative arthritis of the ankle joint.[9, 14, 52, 55, 69, 76, 82] The rate and severity of the arthritic deterioration will vary owing to factors such as size of the lesion, location (lateral lesions are more symptomatic than medial lesions), weight and activity status of the patient, and associated ligament laxity (which leads to repetitive injury). Twenty-five per cent of patients in Davidson and associates' series required arthrodesis of the ankle joint.[14]

Conservative treatment of the early non-

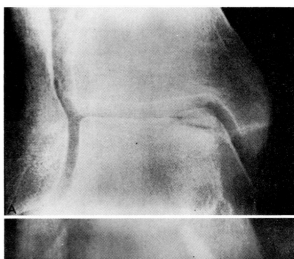

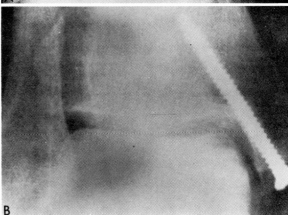

Figure 54-3. (A) Stage III medial dome fracture. (B) Fracture after excision through osteotomy of the medial malleolus.

displaced fracture (Stage I) has shown good results in about 75 per cent of cases.[2, 24, 69, 76] Stage II and III lesions treated conservatively show satisfactory result in only 15 to 25 per cent of cases.

No large series with prolonged follow-up after operative intervention have been reported in the literature to date. Early operation in the displaced or chronic lesion seems the best method of preserving a joint that is at risk for late degenerative arthritis.

DISLOCATIONS OF THE SUBTALAR JOINT

Peritalar Dislocations of the Foot

Peritalar dislocation of the foot describes the simultaneous dislocation of the talocalcaneal and talonavicular joints while the tibiotalar relationship is maintained. A torsional force that is secondary to a fall or jump from a height, athletic injury, or automobile accident is the usual causative factor, and the injury is labeled in terms of the direction taken by the foot in relation to the talus: medial, lateral, posterior, or anterior.

Peritalar dislocation of the foot is often referred to as subtalar or subastragalar dislocation. It was first reported in the literature by Judcy and Dufaurest in 1811.[36] Although originally thought to be a rare injury, more than 300 cases have now been reported.[8, 11, 20, 24, 28] They make up 15 per cent of the injuries of the talus in Pennal's series[60] and approximately 1 per cent of all dislocations seen in active trauma services.[42, 77] Patients vary in age from 10 to over 60 years, and men are affected from three to ten times more frequently than women.

Anatomically, a fibrous capsule attaches the adjacent articular margins of the three talocalcaneal facets. This is reinforced by a formidable interosseous talocalcaneal ligament in the sinus tarsi. Medially and laterally the superficial portion of the deltoid ligament and the calcaneofibular ligament buttress the talus, and the weak talonavicular capsule adds support distally. All these structures must be broached in order for peritalar dislocation to occur. In addition, the contoured congruous surface of the subtalar (talocalcaneal) joint affords a significant amount of stability,[8] particularly to anteroposterior displacement independent of the ligaments and joint capsules. Fractures of the lateral and posterior tubercles of the talus represent failures of the stabilizing forces to resist anterior and posterior subluxation.

Medial Dislocation

This is overwhelmingly the most frequent type of peritalar dislocation reported in the literature.[3, 8, 13, 28, 65] A violent inversion force (with its component plantar flexion, adduction, and supination) uses the sustentaculum tali as a fulcrum, causing initial dislocation of the talonavicular joint and rotary subluxation of the talocalcaneal joint. Further force causes the complete dislocation.

The patient gives a history of severe trauma to the foot, with marked deformity and pain about the hindfoot. On physical examination there is tenderness over the talar head, which now lies between the extensor hallucis longus and the long toe extensors. The heel is noted to be displaced medially in relation to the long axis of the leg.

Anteroposterior, lateral, and oblique roentgenograms are the minimum required x-ray studies (Fig. 54–4). The lateral view may be misleading, and Barber[3] recommends a superoinferior view of the foot, which will clearly demonstrate the absence of the head of the talus in the cup of the navicular (Fig. 54–5).

The roentgenograms should also be carefully scrutinized for associated fractures, which are usually masked by the obvious deformity. Fractures of the malleoli, talar articular margins, fifth metatarsal, and navicular are frequently reported.[3, 8, 30, 47, 60]

Treatment. Reduction should be carried out as soon as possible under general or spinal anesthesia for complete muscle relaxation. The foot is grasped while an assistant applies countertraction to the flexed thigh. The deformity is accentuated slightly, and the mechanism of injury is reversed, i.e., pronation, abduction, and dorsiflexion.

If reduction cannot be accomplished easily with closed methods, the foot should be immediately opened. Impaction of the lateral side of the navicular onto the medial side of the head of the talus (Fig. 54–6), buttonholing of the talar head through the extensor retinaculum (Fig. 54–7) or muscle belly of the peroneus brevis, and entrapment by the peroneal tendons have been described as obstacles to closed reduction.[8, 30, 42]

The surgical incision should be made laterally parallel to the long axis of the foot over the talar head, which is palpated subcutaneously. The extensor retinaculum is partially divided and retracted dorsally. The talus is gently levered back into the cup of the navicular, using a periosteal elevator. This should also reduce the talocalcaneal joint. The torn calcaneofibular ligament, seen in the proximal portion of the wound, should also be repaired at this time.

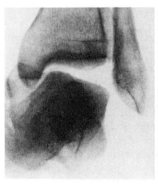 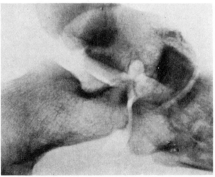

A   **B**

Figure 54–4. *(A) Anteroposterior view of the ankle and (B) lateral view of the foot showing medial peritalar dislocation.*

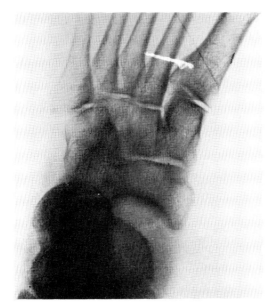

Figure 54–5. *Superoinferior view of a foot with a medial peritalar dislocation showing clearly the absence of the talar head in the cup of the navicular.*

The reduction should be stable, so that no internal fixation is necessary.

Whether reduction is open or closed, the foot is immobilized in a non-weight-bearing short leg plaster cast, and post-reduction roentgenograms are taken. At

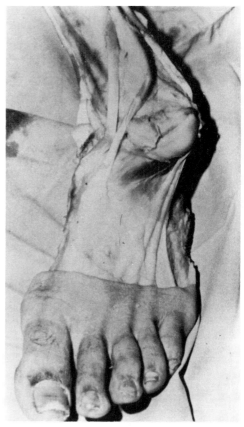

Figure 54–7. *Buttonholing of the talar head through the extensor retinaculum preventing closed reduction of a medial peritalar dislocation. (From Leitner, B.: J. Bone Joint Surg., 36A:299, 1954.)*

two weeks the cast is changed, and immobilization is carried out for an additional four weeks. Weight bearing is then begun as tolerated.

Lateral Dislocation

This type is the next most frequent form of peritalar dislocation, accounting for approximately 30 per cent of all such injuries.[28] At the time of injury the foot is everted (pronated, abducted, and dorsiflexed), and, with the anterior calcaneal process acting as a fulcrum, the head of the talus is forced through the talonavicular capsule and the calcaneus is dislocated laterally[40] (Fig. 54–8).

The foot is painful, swollen, and deformed, with the heel lying lateral to the long axis of the leg. The prominent talar head can be palpated medially.

Anteroposterior, lateral, and oblique

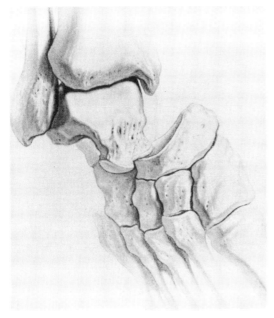

Figure 54–6. *Impaction of the medial aspect of the talar head preventing closed reduction of a medial peritalar dislocation. (From Leitner, B.: J. Bone Joint Surg., 36A:299, 1954.)*

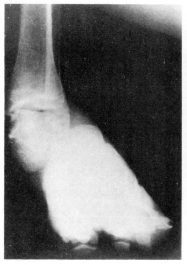
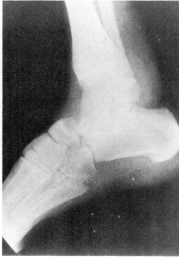

A   **B**

Figure 54–8. (A) *Anteroposterior and (B) lateral views of a lateral peritalar dislocation.*

roentgenograms must be taken and, again, carefully examined for the commonly associated lateral malleolar and talar articular margin fractures. The lateral view will be misleading and should be compared with the superoinferior view in order to demonstrate absence of the talar head in the cup of the navicular.[3]

Treatment. Closed reduction should be carried out as soon as possible under general anesthesia with good muscle relaxation. The foot is grasped by the surgeon while the assistant applies traction to the flexed thigh. Traction reduces the talocalcaneal joint, and the talonavicular position is restored by manual pressure with the foot held in pronation.[26, 42]

If closed reduction is not easily accomplished, the cause is probably due to a slipping of the talar head between the tendons of either the tibialis posterior (Fig. 54–9) or the flexor digitorum longus around the talar neck or to an interlocking of articular marginal fractures on the adjacent talus and navicular.[8, 42] Böhler's method of extreme dorsiflexion and medial displacement of the foot may assist in freeing the posterior tibial tendon.[6, 42] If not, open reduction should be carried out immediately.

We prefer an oblique anterolateral incision over the sinus tarsi, from the long extensor tendon sheath to the peroneal tendon sheath. The subtalar and midtarsal joints are exposed, and the neck of the talus is freed of all obstacles. Reduction is then carried out, and the torn calcaneofibular ligament is repaired.

A medial incision over the talus head would be inviting skin necrosis and is not recommended. Postreduction x-ray studies are mandatory.

A short leg plaster cast is applied and changed at two weeks. Immobilization is

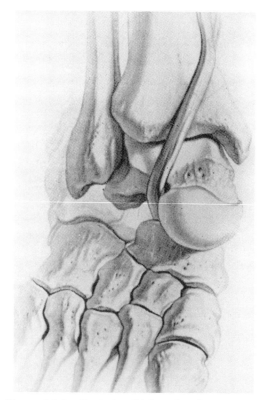

Figure 54–9. Posterior tibial tendon displaced and trapped lateral to the talar head and neck, preventing closed reduction of a lateral peritalar dislocation. (From Leitner, B.: J. Bone Joint Surg., 36A:299, 1954.)

continued for an additional four weeks, at which time ambulation is begun.

Posterior Dislocation

Posterior dislocations are rare and constitute 6 per cent of the reported cases in Grantham's review.[28] This type of injury is reported to occur as a result of a fall from a height onto an outstretched foot in the plantar flexed position. The posterior edges of the joint surfaces between the talus and calcaneus act as a fulcrum.[40] The posterior tubercle of the talus, which normally prevents displacement in this direction, should be carefully examined for fracture.

Clinically, the forefoot is shortened and the heel projects posteriorly, but the normal longitudinal axis of the foot appears to be maintained. The lateral roentgenographic view is diagnostic (Fig. 54–10).

Treatment. Closed reduction under general anesthesia should be carried out as follows: The forefoot is plantar flexed, thus releasing the neck of the talus from the upper edge of the navicular. The heel is then pulled plantarward, and the entire foot is drawn dorsally.

If closed reduction is not possible, an incision is made under the lateral malleolus, and the talus and calcaneus are separated by an elevator. Careful postreduction roentgenograms must be obtained. Internal fixation is usually not required.

The reduction is quite stable, and a short leg non–weight-bearing plaster cast is worn for six weeks.

Anterior Dislocation

Anterior dislocation is the least frequently reported and occurs secondary to a fall from a great height onto the dorsiflexed foot, with the anterior portions of the talus and calcaneus acting as a fulcrum. The heel is flattened and the foot appears extended, but it maintains its longitudinal orientation.[40]

Lateral roentgenograms are again diagnostic and should be examined for fractures of the talar neck, which may accompany the dislocation.

Treatment. Closed reduction under general anesthesia is done by drawing the foot distally so that the posterior surface of the calcaneus is free of the talar sulcus. The foot is then directed backward to effect the reduction. If closed reduction is blocked, open reduction is carried out, as with posterior dislocation. Good postreduction films should be obtained in the operating room. A short leg non–weight-bearing plaster cast is worn for six weeks.

Complications and Prognosis of Peritalar Dislocations

In general, a satisfactory result is to be expected with early recognition and proper treatment of the injury. Delay in reduction can lead to severe blistering and subsequent sloughing of the skin and to neurovascular compromise of the distal foot.

Late complications include talonavicular arthritis, talocalcaneal arthritis, osteoporosis, limitation of eversion and inversion, and persistent swelling and pain of the midfoot.[49, 66] Young, active patients have fewer complications. Dislocations with associated marginal fractures or compounding wounds have a poorer prognosis. Some degree of subtalar arthritis usually develops after subtalar dislocation, even without associated fracture.[19] Fortunately, the symptoms are relatively mild and the accompanying limitation of subtalar mo-

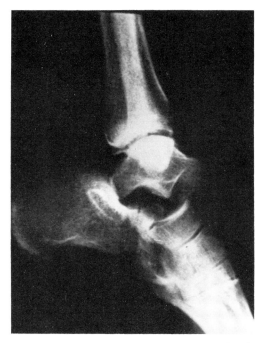

Figure 54–10. *Lateral roentgenogram showing posterior peritalar dislocation.*

tion may not be noticed except when walking on uneven ground or doing high-performance athletics.

Blood supply is abundant via the main arteries of the leg through a periosteal vascular network. Blood is also supplied by two discrete vessels; i.e., the artery of the tarsal sinus from the dorsolateral arteries and the artery of the tarsal canal from the posterior tibial artery.[40] In these dislocations only the blood supply of the inferior tarsal canal is lost.[31] Avascular necrosis of the talus is a rare occurrence with this injury and seems to occur only in cases of open dislocation, infection, or severe associated trauma.

Persistent incapacitating post-traumatic subtalar pain, despite an adequate trial of physical therapy and anti-inflammatory medication, is an indication for triple arthrodesis.[3] The resulting stiff subtalar joint is well tolerated in the young individual and can be well compensated by the use of a stiff shoe and molded arch support. Triple arthrodesis in patients over 40 should be carefully considered because of the prolonged postoperative convalescent time.[24]

TOTAL DISLOCATION OF THE TALUS

Total dislocation of the talus is characterized by complete disruption of the ankle and subtalar joints. This is certainly one of the most serious talar injuries. Fortunately, considerable force is required to produce this injury and it occurs infrequently. Many surgeons have never personally treated a case, so the literature on this topic is meager. Nevertheless, there are many controversial aspects such as the mechanism of injury, the primary treatment, the incidence and treatment of avascular necrosis, and the ideal reconstruction procedure for the collapsed or infected talus.

Many of the problems that accompany this injury begin with the soft tissues. Open wounds and late sloughing of skin from pressure of displaced bone, excessive skin tension from massive swelling, and vascular compromise from direct injury create a profound surgical dilemma. The evaluation of different treatment protocols

is difficult because of the many variables. Infection and avascular necrosis with collapse of the talus are the major causes of severe disability. Frequently both complications are present.

Incidence. Coltart described nine cases of total dislocation occurring in 228 major talar injuries among the Royal Air Force units in World War II.[13] Six of these were open injuries, and all occurred in aircraft accidents. In 1969, Detenbeck and Kelly reported on nine cases seen at the Mayo Clinic over a nine-year period.[15] Seven of these were open injuries. This lesion occurs in no more than 10 per cent of major talar injuries, and is more often than not an open injury.

Mechanism of Injury. Leitner reviewed 42 cases of subtalar dislocation and found six patients with a concomitant subluxation of the ankle joint[43] (see Figure 54-4).[43] Four had medial subtalar dislocations in which the talus was inverted or supinated in the mortise and displaced forward. Two patients had lateral subtalar dislocations in which the talus was inverted or pronated in the mortise and displaced forward. Leitner felt that the incidence of concomitant subluxation of the ankle joint in subtalar dislocations would be higher if roentgenographic stress views of the ankle were obtained routinely. He also felt that dislocation resulted from excessive supination first displacing the talus laterally or excessive pronation displacing the talus medially. A first-degree supination or pronation injury caused subtalar dislocation (Fig. 54-11A,D). A second-degree injury caused subtalar dislocation and ankle subluxation (Fig. 54-11B,E). A third-degree injury caused subtalar dislocation and ankle dislocation, i.e., total dislocation of the talus (Fig. 54-11C,F). This seems to explain the radiographic and clinical picture in most instances. The isolated case of complete posterior dislocation of the talus reported by Pinzur and Meyer in 1977 was obviously caused by a different mechanism.[65] This injury was accompanied by a wide diastasis of the mortise and fracture of the anterior process of the calcaneus and was probably produced by severe dorsiflexion and forward displacement of the foot onto the leg.

Treatment. Because of the forces required to produce the dislocation and the

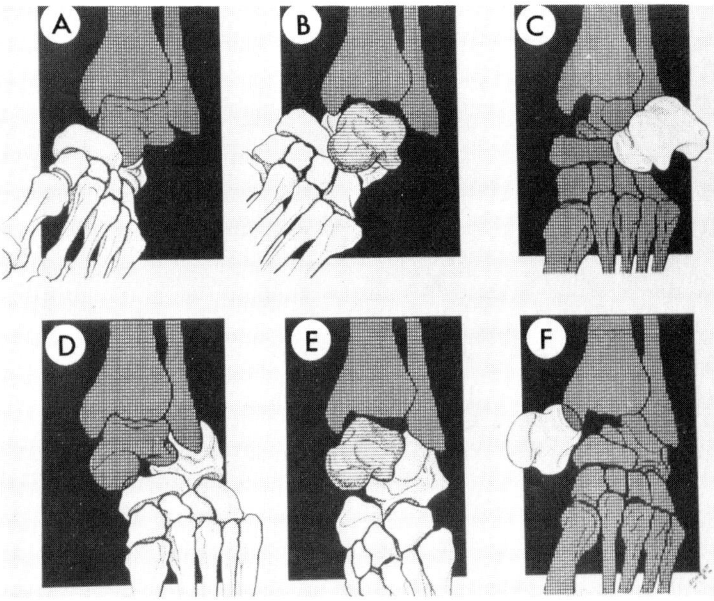

Figure 54–11. Sequential subtalar dislocation, ankle subluxation, and total talar dislocation in first-, second-, and third-degree supination injuries (A–C) and first-, second-, and third-degree pronation injuries (D–F). (From Leitner, B.: J. Bone Joint Surg., 37A:89, 1955.)

resultant displacement, compounding is present in at least 75 per cent of the cases.[15] The open wound is usually a bursting-type laceration from within that follows the direction of the skin lines and folds. These are not parallel to the longitudinally oriented vascular and lymphatic structures. The margins of the wounds are relatively ischemic, and wound slough leading to deep wound infection is a serious threat. Torn capsular structures, ligaments, and tendons afford very poor cover for the underlying cartilage and bone. The skin cannot be shifted by undermining or by creation of flaps, and the opportunity to transfer local muscles by rotation on a pedicle is virtually nonexistent, especially on the lateral aspect of the foot.

Total dislocation of the talus implies rupture of all major vascular connections, so that the talus is avascular. Incomplete dislocations, especially at the ankle joint, can spare ligamentous vessels, especially in the deltoid ligament, and may be the reason why avascular necrosis does not occur in all cases.[50, 56, 74]

This injury demands immediate reduction to take the pressure off the skin margins, open patent circulatory channels, and decompress and realign any vascular connections that might remain. The open injury must be thoroughly cleaned immediately and covered to prevent sepsis. The

paucity of soft tissue that can be sacrificed and the critical articular cartilage that covers three fourths of the talus make debridement difficult (much as in hand injuries). A Water Pik is a valuable aid to performing an atraumatic but thorough debridement, without unnecessary sacrifice of tissue. Delayed treatment invariably results in skin slough, wound infection, osteomyelitis, and a higher rate of avascular necrosis of the talus. The neurovascular bundles to the foot may be compromised by the dislocation, leading to amputation because of ischemia secondary to thrombosis.[15]

Closed reduction by forefoot and heel traction, with countertraction on the leg and direct pressure on the displaced talus, has been successfully done for closed injuries. Initial radiographs from the Emergency Room are usually inadequate, and additional views of the foot and ankle, as well as careful inspection and palpation, are required prior to carrying out the manipulation. Complete muscle relaxation is mandatory. Skeletal fixation with Steinmann pins through the os calcis and distal tibia has been helpful in achieving the distraction of the ankle joint space required to allow closed reduction of the talus.[50, 56, 60] A clear understanding of the talar displacement is necessary to effect closed reduction.

Closed reductions are usually stable and

complete. It would be dangerous to make a skin incision to attempt ligamentous repair, even though this would be advantageous, especially in repairing the deltoid ligament. Revascularization following dislocation of the talus is slow because of the large articular area that limits access to vascular structures. The medial attachment of the deltoid ligament is an important primary route of vascularity, and several authors have noted that revascularization of the talus begins from the medial aspect.[15, 39, 60]

Open reduction is of course indicated when the dislocation is open and will usually require extension of the compounding wound. Preliminary skeletal traction on the calcaneus or forefoot is helpful. Capsular repair aids in covering the exposed joint surfaces, since marginal skin necrosis is to be expected. Leaving the skin open for delayed primary closure is helpful in minimizing skin necrosis, especially if the underlying joint can be covered. If the wound is closed primarily, suction drainage is indicated to prevent hematoma and to collapse the dead space between the skin and the deep tissue. When closure cannot be anticipated within five days, plastic surgery consultation to plan the application of a delayed cross-leg pedicle or direct myocutaneous flap by microsurgical anastomosis is indicated. Wounds left open more than seven days usually become clinically infected. Because the joint is usually not closed, septic arthritis and possibly osteomyelitis will almost certainly occur when skin coverage is not achieved quickly.

Postoperative Care. Postoperative care after open or closed reduction consists of immobilization in a well-padded, bent-knee, long leg cast with the ankle in neutral position. The cast should be bivalved immediately and the limb elevated. Intravenous antibiotics should be continued until cultures are negative and the wounds are healed.

Complications. Continuous elevation of the leg is essential to prevent swelling. We have found that low doses of heparin given subcutaneously hasten resolution of massive swelling of the leg and foot. Immobilization should be continued for four weeks in a long leg cast followed by further immobilization in a short leg cast. At six weeks, vascularity of the talus is usually discernible. Failure of the development of subchondral radiolucency at the dome of the talus (Hawkins' sign) indicates avascular necrosis[34] (see Figure 54–22). Revascularization can be expected, but requires about two years. Protection against weight-bearing forces has been shown to be reasonably effective in preventing talar collapse. This protection can be achieved and still allow ambulation by using a patellar–tendon-bearing foot-ankle orthosis.[60, 65, 74] Preservation of the talus is definitely preferable to sacrificing talar motion by fusion or excision.

Primary excision of the talus was formerly the treatment most generally used. When done as simple talectomy, the resultant varus deformity, weakness, and pain were generally unsatisfactory to both patient and surgeon.[15, 60] Primary talar excision with tibiocalcaneal arthrodesis gives much better results than simple talectomy, especially when compression clamps or plates are used.[15, 60] As shortening is objectionable, the best result is achieved when the talus is preserved, even if pantalar arthrodesis is required later for post-traumatic arthritis.

Avascular necrosis without collapse, even with moderate pantalar arthritis, is compatible with a fair to good clinical result.[34, 49, 50, 60] Post-traumatic arthritis occurs primarily in the subtalar joint, just as it does after simple subtalar dislocation. The extent of talocrural arthritis depends mainly on the degree of revascularization of the talus and the amount of collapse of the talar dome.

In summary, even though total dislocation of the talus is a serious injury, if deep infection can be avoided and if adequate protection against weight bearing is afforded the revascularizing talus, a surprisingly good functional result can be achieved without resorting to excision or fusion. Salvage of infected feet is difficult. Adequate excision of infected bone and closure of dead space with cancellous bone grafts or arthrodesis under compression plus expert antibiotic therapy for prolonged periods may salvage a functional foot. In many cases, a below-the-knee amputation or a Syme amputation is the only solution for the frustration of both the surgeon and the patient.

FRACTURE OF THE TALAR NECK

Mechanism of Injury. Fractures of the talar neck are usually caused by motor vehicle accidents, aircraft accidents, and falls from heights.[1, 10, 13, 21, 27, 34, 38, 39, 72] These injuries were first attributed to excessive dorsiflexion of the ankle causing impaction of the talar neck against the anterior margin of the tibia, which acted like a fulcrum.[13] However, the frequent lack of damage to the anterior margin of the tibia and cervical cortex of the talus casts some doubt on this simplistic explanation.[72] Typical fractures of the talar neck were not produced experimentally by simple forced dorsiflexion, but only by eliminating ankle joint motion and fixing the talus as a cantilever between the tibia and calcaneus.[68] Under these conditions, a pendulum blow to the sole of the foot produced a fracture of the talar neck in six of nine consecutive tests. Other studies of combined talar and ankle injuries suggest that supination may play an important role in producing talar neck fractures.[21, 78] One per cent of ankle fractures are associated with major talar fractures.[10]

Classification. Although various classifications have been put forward, the most accepted is that of Hawkins, which represents a clarification of the patterns noted by Coltart.[13, 14]

Group I — Vertical fracture through the neck of the talus without displacement (Fig. 54–12).

Group II — Vertical fracture of the neck of the talus with displacement of the body from the subtalar joint but not from the tibiotalar joint (Fig. 54–13).

Group III — Vertical fracture of the neck of the talus with displacement of the body of the talus from the subtalar joint and the tibiotalar joint (Fig. 54–14).

A fourth group with Group III features plus a dislocation of the talonavicular joint was recently added by Canale and associates.[10] The main shortcoming of Hawkins' classification is the failure to differentiate slight subluxation from frank dislocation of the subtalar and tibiotalar joints or to recognize a momentary subluxation that reduces itself prior to the initial x-ray studies and can be diagnosed only on stress films. An injury comprising a displaced fracture of the neck of the talus, a subluxed subtalar joint, and a dislocated talonavicular joint falls between the classifications (Fig. 54–15).

Group I fractures occur in approximately 20 per cent of cases, Group II fractures in approximately 45 per cent of cases, and Group III fractures in 35 per cent of cases in most reported series.[34, 38, 63]

To some extent, all types threaten the abundant but vulnerable vascular supply of the talus (Fig. 54–16). Peterson and associates[61, 62] found the ascending branches of the tarsal sinus and the tarsal canal arteries torn in each instance of experimentally produced fracture of the talar neck. Branches from the dorsalis pedis were

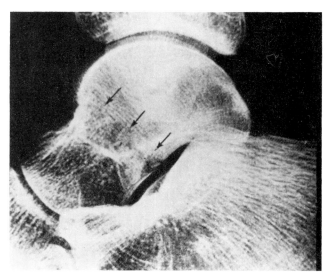

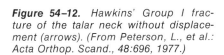

Figure 54–12. Hawkins' Group I fracture of the talar neck without displacement (arrows). (From Peterson, L., et al.: Acta Orthop. Scand., 48:696, 1977.)

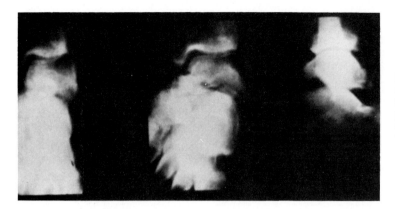

Figure 54–13. Hawkins' Group II fracture of the talar neck with anterior subtalar dislocation. (From Canale, S. T., and Kelly, F. B.: J. Bone Joint Surg., 60A: 143, 1978.)

disrupted if the fracture was displaced. Several excellent anatomic studies have elucidated a rich interosseous blood supply to the talus from adjacent bones through capsular and ligamentous vessels.[32, 54] In Group I fractures, the interosseous collaterals from the adjacent tibia, calcaneus, and navicular are spared, accounting for the low incidence of avascular necrosis and nonunion. In Group II injuries, interosseous collaterals from the calcaneus are disrupted, but those from the tibia and navicular are preserved. Nonunion is not a problem, but the incidence of avascular necrosis increases significantly.

In Group III injuries, all vascular sources to the body of the talus are in jeopardy. Some vessels to the body may miraculously survive, accounting for the occasional reports of uncomplicated healing after this serious injury.[39,60]

Treatment. Group I injuries (undisplaced fractures of the talar neck) present few problems or controversy in management. Simple immobilization in a short leg, non–weight-bearing plaster cast until union occurs, usually in eight to ten weeks, is the treatment recommended by most authors (Fig. 54–17). Nonunion has not been reported. Avascular necrosis has been

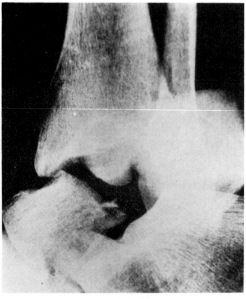

Figure 54–14. Hawkins' Group III fracture of the neck of the talus with subtalar dislocation and posterior dislocation of the body of the talus. (From Peterson, L., et al.: Acta Orthop. Scand., 48:696, 1977.)

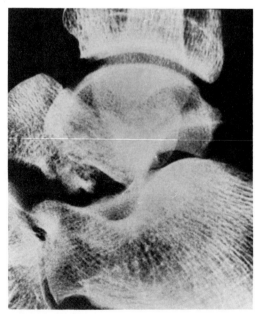

Figure 54–15. Roentgenogram showing a fracture of the talar neck, subluxation of the subtalar joint, and dislocation of the talonavicular joint. This illustrates the problem of any classification including all possible presentations of any injury.

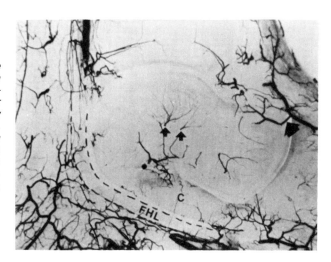

Figure 54–16. *Sagittal section of ankle specimen injected with contrast medium showing intraosseous vessels and interosseous anastomosis of the talus. The contour of the calcaneus (C) is partly obliterated by the tendon of the flexor hallucis longus (FHL). The large arrow indicates the branch from the dorsalis pedis entering the talus. The small arrows indicate the continuation of the penetrating branches from the ramus deltoideus. (From Peterson, L., and Goldie, I. F.: Acta Orthop. Scand., 46:1026, 1975.)*

reported only in rare instances, and these injuries may be occult Group II lesions that have reduced spontaneously. Open wounds are unusual and, if present, are usually not extensive, so that osteitis is uncommon.

Group II injuries (displaced fractures of the talar neck with subtalar dislocations) require prompt, accurate reduction of the subtalar dislocation and talar neck fracture. Open fractures necessitate prompt, meticulous soft-tissue debridement, followed by anatomic reduction and internal fixation. Skin closure is usually a problem. Primary suturing has the advantage of protecting the joints and bone from secondary infection but increases the risk of skin slough from hematoma and edema. We recommend leaving the skin wounds unsutured

initially. Early plastic surgery consultation is indicated in these cases. Skin slough leading to wound infection places the osseous and joint structures at risk of deep infection. Once deep infection is established, it is very difficult to eradicate, and the final result is always poor.[38, 39, 59, 60] The risk of skin slough (75 per cent in one series) and soft-tissue infection and even septic arthritis and osteitis is formidable, according to all the reported series.[27] This problem is related to the severe soft-tissue injury accompanying the fracture, the associated swelling, and the scant soft tissues such as fat and muscle surrounding the talus.

Group II fractures involve subtalar dislocations, usually anterior or medial, which should be reduced without delay under

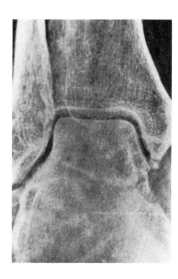

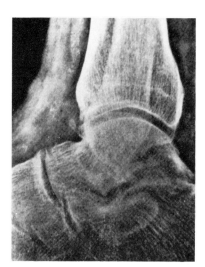

Figure 54–17. *Healed Group I fracture after eight weeks of immobilization in a short leg, non–weight-bearing cast.*

general or spinal anesthesia to ensure complete muscle relaxation. In medial subtalar dislocations, the head of the talus appears laterally between the extensor hallucis longus and the extensor digitorum longus, resting on the cuboid or the tarsal navicular. The foot is adducted. Reduction is carried out by applying traction, plantar flexion, and digital pressure medially against the head of the talus while the forefoot is abducted.

In anterior subtalar dislocations, the talar body is in the equinus position. Closed reduction is carried out by applying traction in the equinus position, followed by posterior displacement of the foot.

In the lateral subtalar dislocations, the head of the talus is prominent medially, whereas the rest of the foot is displaced laterally. Reduction is generally carried out by bringing the foot into adduction. The calcaneus will automatically slip under the talus. Some subtalar dislocations are irreducible by closed manipulation. Their management was discussed earlier in the section on peritalar dislocations. The foot should generally be kept in full plantar flexion to align the talar neck fracture.[21, 26, 34, 60] Eversion is usually necessary for a medial dislocation and inversion for a lateral dislocation. A long leg, padded cast is applied, and roentgenograms of the foot and ankle should be obtained. Only a perfect reduction is acceptable. A special anteroposterior (AP) view of the foot in pronation, as suggested by Canale and Kelly,[10] is helpful in detecting slight varus angulation not seen on routine films. Repeat films in 2 days, 7 days, and 14 days should be obtained because of the tendency of the fracture to re-displace. The cast should be changed under heavy sedation or general anesthesia at the beginning of the fourth week.[13] The foot should be gently manipulated into 5 to 10 degrees equinus and a short leg cast applied for six more weeks.

When closed reduction of the talar neck fracture is unsatisfactory or unstable, open reduction should be carried out as soon as the soft tissues permit an operation. A medial approach through an osteotomy of the medial malleolus is preferred to division of the deltoid ligament.[27] Extensive soft-tissue damage laterally makes skin necrosis and secondary infection a formidable risk. Soft-tissue dissection should be kept

to a minimum. Particular care should be taken to avoid damage to the arterial branches to the talus that are located in the deltoid ligament.[27] The subtalar dislocation should first be stabilized with a smooth Steinmann pin through the calcaneus across the talocalcaneal joint. The talar neck fracture should then be anatomically reduced and fixed, first with two temporary Kirschner wires and then definitively by an interfragmentary compression screw (Fig. 54–18). Cancellous bone from the distal tibial metaphysis can be used to fill any areas of bone loss. Avascular necrosis occurs more often in fractures treated by open reduction but is less common when secure internal fixation is used.[63] Immobilization in a short leg, non–weight-bearing cast with the foot in neutral position is carried out until the fracture unites (8 to 12 weeks).

Group III fractures are obviously serious injuries with almost certain complete disruption of blood supply. Blood to the body of the talus is disrupted from all sources, except possibly the deltoid ligament branches. The body of the talus is usually displaced posteriorly and medially and trapped behind the sustentaculum tali. The medial soft tissues are usually intact, whereas the lateral soft tissues are blanched and stretched. In open injuries, the compounding usually occurs laterally from within. The medial neurovascular bundle usually escapes direct injury but is obviously kinked, stretched, and compressed. Thrombosis of the posterior tibial artery, leading to gangrene and amputation, has been reported when reduction was unduly delayed.[27]

Immediate closed reduction should be attempted first unless there is an open wound that demands debridement. In this case open reduction is undertaken without formal closed reduction. General or spinal anesthesia for muscle relaxation is preferred. Most authors recommend first placing a heavy Kirschner wire or Steinmann pin transversely through the calcaneus.[26, 34, 60] Using this as a handle, the calcaneus is plantar flexed and everted as the joint is distracted. Pressure is applied from behind the body of the talus to force it forward into the mortise. The subtalar dislocation, which is usually medial, should then be reduced by applying traction to the forefoot and lateral pressure to the calca-

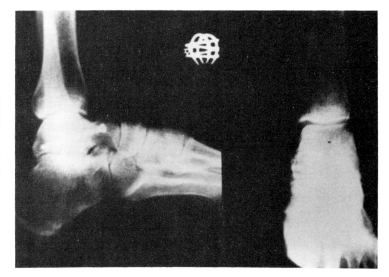

Figure 54–18. Lateral and anteroposterior views of the Group II fracture shown in Figure 54–13 four months after injury showing union of the fracture without avascular necrosis and with perfect reduction of the subtalar joint. (From Canale, S. T., and Kelly, F. B.: J. Bone Joint Surg., 60A:143, 1978.)

neus with the ankle in equinus position. Finally, the talar neck fracture is aligned and the subtalar joint reduced and immobolized in a long leg bent-knee cast with the foot in eversion and equinus (Figs. 54–19 and 54–20).

Group IV fractures require reduction and temporary fixation of the talonavicular joint.[10]

The literature indicates that closed reduction is rarely satisfactory in this difficult injury, but we feel that it should be tried.[27] Frequently, routine postreduction roentgenograms look good, but anteroposterior views of the foot reveal a varus angulation at the site of the talar neck fracture that would lead to delayed union or nonunion.[10] In such instances careful open reduction should be carried out as soon as possible.

A medial approach sparing the deltoid ligament is preferred. The talar body dislocation is reduced, and the subtalar relationship is restored and fixed temporarily. The talar neck fracture is then reduced and fixed internally. An interfragmentary compression screw is ideal for this fixation.

Immobilization should be carried out in a neutral position in a short leg non–weight-bearing cast for three months or until fracture union is demonstrated radiographically. Range-of-motion exercises may begin earlier, after soft-tissue healing in ideal selected cases, but weight bearing should be delayed until fracture healing is complete (about 12 weeks). If the talus is radiographically avascular, further protection of weight bearing with a patellar–tendon-bearing foot-ankle orthosis is indicated for another 6 to 18 months.[34, 38, 60] Although talar collapse sometimes occurs despite non–weight bearing, most authors have found that protecting the talus from excessive weight-bearing forces during the period of revascularization greatly im-

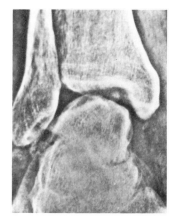

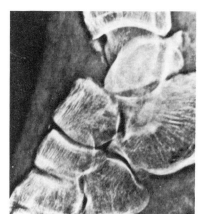

Figure 54–19. (A) Anteroposterior and (B) lateral views of a Group III fracture. This is atypical, as the tibiotalar and subtalar joints are subluxed rather than dislocated.

A   **B**

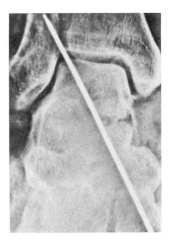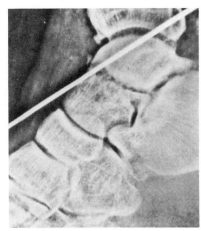

Figure 54–20. Anatomic reduction and internal fixation of the fracture shown in Figure 54–19. Interfragmentary compression of the talar neck fracture with a screw would have been ideal.

proves the prognosis for a functional recovery without further surgery.[34, 38, 39, 49, 60] Several authors have proposed primary or early subtalar fusion for Group III and IV injuries to promote revascularization of the talus.[39, 46, 60] However, long-term studies have not supported the usefulness or effectiveness of this procedure.[34]

Excision of the talus is indicated for comminuted fractures with extensive cartilaginous damage and for infected fractures. The results of simple astragalectomy are unpredictable and are not regarded highly by most authors because of residual pain, varus deformity of the foot, weakness of take-off, and swelling following this procedure.[7, 60, 72] Tibiocalcaneal arthrodesis is preferred by most authors, and the tibio-anterior talar neck fusion of Blair also has several supporters.[5, 10, 51, 60] The combination of tibiocalcaneal arthrodesis and tibio-anterior talar neck fusion is most logical to us. These reconstructive procedures are best done electively after the swelling has subsided and consequences have been discussed with the patient, especially the inch or so of shortening caused by loss of talar height.

Prognosis. Group I fractures carry a very favorable prognosis. Bony union is usually present by the eighth week, and no cases of nonunion have been reported. Avascular necrosis has been noted infrequently (2 per cent incidence), usually only in large series, and there are several authors with considerable experience who have not seen this complication. Children with this fracture have a higher incidence of avascular necrosis and should be managed carefully to prevent talar collapse.[80] Late degenerative changes are responsible

for the 10 to 25 per cent incidence of fair and poor results. These changes may be due to slight malunion caused by comminution of the fracture site and resultant degenerative arthritis of the tibiotalar, talonavicular, and subtalar joints. The more likely explanation is that direct cartilage damage occurred to the tibiotalar and talocalcaneal joint surfaces at the time of injury, which leads to accelerated cartilage wear. The degenerative changes result in loss of motion and radiographic changes, but symptoms may be mild or absent, especially early in the course.

The results reported in long-term studies of Group II injuries are much less favorable than those in Group I injuries.[27, 34, 63, 79] Some reports give a more favorable prognosis when prompt open reduction and internal fixation are done.[38] Many of these fractures are open and are associated with extensive soft-tissue damage, leading to serious problems of wound healing and deep infection. Prompt, expert treatment of the soft-tissue components is of utmost importance. Failure of bony union is never a problem unless overwhelming sepsis supervenes. A delayed union incidence of 15 per cent was reported by Peterson and associates.[63] Delayed union appears to be associated with a higher incidence of poor results.[49] Malunion with dorsal talar neck impingement blocking dorsiflexion and varus angulation can occur, particularly in injuries treated nonoperatively with the foot in equinus position.

As Group III injuries will have nearly a 100 per cent complication rate, their results will be discussed under the following section on complications.

Complications. Avascular necrosis and

degenerative arthritis are two major complications to be anticipated. [5, 10, 13, 21, 27, 34, 38, 47-49, 59, 60] In Hawkins' series, 42 per cent of patients with Group II lesions developed avascular necrosis, even though union of the fracture occurred in all cases[34] (Fig. 54–21). Nine per cent of these subsequently experienced collapse of the body of the talus and developed significant osteoarthritic changes. Fortunately, only a small number of the patients with avascular necrosis will be symptomatic enough to require early surgical treatment. Peterson and associates' series noted avascular necrosis in only 15 per cent of Group II patients, and they felt that collapse of the talar head, especially if it occurred late in the disease, did not have a profound effect on the clinical condition.[63] This was affected primarily by the amount of degenerative arthritis in the tibiotalar and talocalcaneal joints. Ninety-seven per cent of Peterson's patients had varying, and to some extent disabling, functional disturbances due to degenerative arthritis in these joints.[63] Most had difficulties but had adjusted their activities and life style to compensate, and few required secondary reconstructive surgery. The recent careful study by Canale and Kelly revealed that although avascular necrosis occurred in 50 per cent of Group II patients, only one third of these required reconstructive surgery.[10] On the other hand, almost all had significant limitation of subtalar motion due to degenerative arthritis (Fig. 54–21). Both Peterson and Canale have

found the appearance of a subchondral radiolucency in the anteroposterior lateral view at four to six weeks (Hawkins' sign) to be a fairly reliable indicator of vascularity of the talus[10, 39, 63] (Fig. 54–22). When the radiolucency is seen, avascular necrosis is unlikely. This finding is most helpful in deciding when to begin weight bearing.

Group III and IV fractures have the poorest long-term results, primarily because of the 90 to 100 per cent rate of avascular necrosis. This complication was associated with only a 15 per cent chance of satisfactory results in Hawkins' group.[39] However, in Canale's group, 48 per cent of the patients with avascular necrosis had satisfactory results.[10] It would appear that an anatomic reduction achieved by either opened or closed methods and protected during the period of healing and early avascular necrosis (average eight months) can be expected to produce a satisfactory result without requiring a secondary procedure in approximately 50 per cent of cases.

Primary and Secondary Reconstruction Procedures. Talectomy has been mentioned since the time that talar dislocation was originally described by Fabricius in 1608. In some cases, the talus is too comminuted to restore, or it may be left at the scene of the accident. These seem to constitute the only instances when this treatment should be elected in view of the nearly uniform poor functional results reported by many authors. Partial talar excision appears to give better results than simple talec-

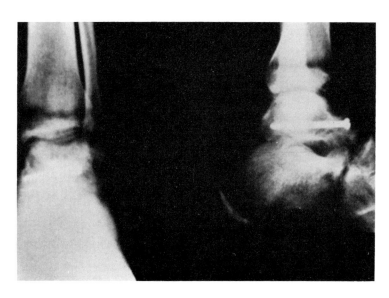

Figure 54–21. *Anteroposterior and lateral views of a Group II fracture of the talar neck showing avascular necrosis of the talar neck and residual subluxation of the subtalar joint.*

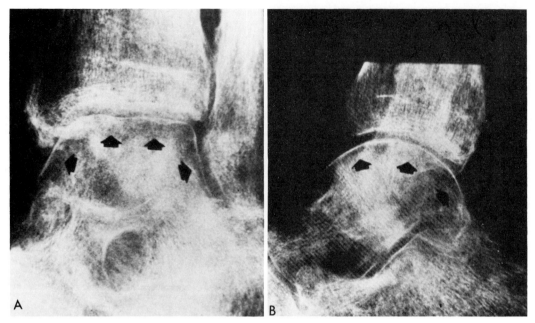

Figure 54–22. *(A) Mortise view of an ankle eight weeks after a Group I fracture occurred shows a complete line of radiolucency beneath the subchondral plate (Hawkins' sign). (B) Lateral view of the same ankle. The fracture is united without avascular necrosis. Weight bearing can begin safely. (From Peterson, L., et al.: Acta Orthop. Scand., 48:696, 1977.)*

tomy. The partial procedure spares the head, which is then fused to the tibia, as suggested by Bonnin and later reported on by Blair.[5, 7, 51] It is a technically demanding procedure requiring good skin coverage and non–weight-bearing immobilization. Retention of the talar head was favored by Bonnin because it preserved the longi-

tudinal arch.[7] This procedure is best suited to the late reconstruction period rather than primary treatment. Its main drawback is late settling with tibiocalcaneal contact that probably accounts for the residual discomfort experienced by some of these patients.

Fusion of the tibia to the calcaneus ap-

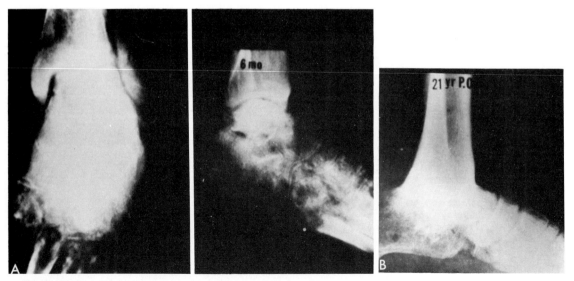

Figure 54–23. *(A) Anteroposterior and lateral views six months after open reduction of a Group III fracture. Infection developed, along with delayed union of the fracture, residual subluxation of the subtalar joint, and narrowing of the ankle joint with severe disability. (B) Lateral view 21 years after reconstruction by talar body excision, tibiocalcaneal arthrodesis, and fusion of the talar head to the anterior tibia.*

pears to be the most reliable reconstruction after severe injury to the talus complicated by avascular necrosis or infection. If it is possible to salvage the head of the talus and fuse it to the tibia, both stability of the medial long arch and overall cosmetic and functional results are improved (Fig. 54–23). This procedure is preferred by us.

Pantalar arthrodesis is indicated in the presence of severe degenerative arthritis of the tibiotalar and subtalar joints without significant avascular necrosis, i.e., when bone scans show good vascularity and the talus is not infected. This procedure is better than tibiocalcaneal fusion because more length is preserved and the foot and ankle have a normal appearance.

Triple arthrodesis is likely to give good results when the degenerative arthritis involves the talonavicular and talocalcaneal joints but spares the tibiotalar joint.

Correction of limitation of dorsiflexion by resection of a residual dorsal step-off on the talar neck after malunion of Group II and III fractures was found to give a high percentage of satisfactory results.

Talocalcaneal fusion to hasten revascularization, as advocated by earlier authors, has not proved helpful in more recent studies.[10, 47] Primary triple arthrodesis alone has been associated with a 10 per cent rate of avascular necrosis of the talus. It certainly would require many months for vascularity to extend all the way across the dense body of the talus. Revascularization without subtalar fusion appears to take place with regularity, although slowly, and, if protection against collapse of the talus can be effected, a satisfactory outcome can be anticipated despite the documented avascular necrosis.

FRACTURES OF THE TALAR BODY

As mentioned earlier, the talus is normally subjected to extremely large stress forces during normal walking and running, and the extremely compact cancellous bone of the talus reflects this marvelous adaptation. Extreme nonphysiologic forces — mainly vertical compression, pronation, and supination — are required to injure the trochlea (body of the talus). The trochlea has an important role in weight bearing as well as in talocrural, subtalar, and midtarsal joint function, which allows hinge movements of the ankle and rotation of the foot.

In 1952 Coltart provided a simple classification of the various fractures and dislocations involving the talus.[13] This was much easier to use and more completely documented by actual cases than the earlier classification by Bonnin in 1940.[7] In Coltart's series, fractures of the body of the talus occurred in 5.7 per cent of 4000 ankle and tarsal injuries. One third of these were associated with subtalar dislocations. It was not until 1977 that Sneppen and associates provided another large series of injuries to the body, or trochlea, and proposed a more detailed classification.[79] They examined 218 cases of fractures of the talus, of which 62 (28 per cent) were major fractures affecting the body of the talus. Other authors reporting large series of talar injuries have noted a somewhat lower incidence. Pennal noted an 11 per cent incidence of fractures of the body of the talus in 98 talar injuries reported in 1963.[60] Kenwright and Taylor noted an incidence of 8 per cent,[38] and Mindell and associates found an occurrence rate of 7 per cent.[49]

Sneppen and associates classified 51 fractures of the talar body into five types: compression, coronal shearing and sagittal shearing, fracture of the posterior tubercle, fracture of the lateral tubercle, and crush fractures[79] (Fig. 54–24). In 21 cases (41 per cent) there were associated fractures of the ankle or foot of the same extremity.

Shearing fractures were the most common type (33 per cent). Displacement or associated subluxation of the talocrural or talocalcaneal joint occurred in 80 per cent of these fractures.

Compression fractures, the next largest group, were always displaced but were not associated with subluxation. The crush injuries were also associated with displacement and subluxation but were relatively uncommon (8 per cent). Fractures of the posterior tubercle accounted for approximately 20 per cent of their cases, as did fractures of the lateral tubercle. Neither type was associated with marked displacement or subluxation.

Compression Fractures

Compression fractures usually involve the medial or lateral aspects of the talus

Types of fracture

 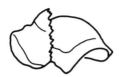

A Compression   **B** Coronal shearing   **C** Sagittal shearing
     fracture   fracture   fracture

Figure 54–24. Classification of fractures of the body of the talus. (From Sneppen, O., et al.: Acta Orthop. Scand., 48:317, 1977.)

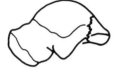

D Fracture in the   **E** Fracture in the   **F** Crush
   posterior tubercle   lateral tubercle   fracture

and are due to compression and either inversion or eversion. Concomitant ankle fractures are not uncommon. The talar fractures are always displaced but are not associated with subluxation of either the ankle or the subtalar joints. There is no threat to the vascularity of the talar body. Even though the fragments of the fracture on the tibiotalar joint side are avascular, union and revascularization can be expected. The major concerns are articular congruity and late post-traumatic degenerative arthritis in the tibiotalar and subtalar joints. Whether these develop or not depends on (1) the percentage of the total area of the talus that is involved; (2) whether the remaining talar dome is congruous, i.e., does not tilt or subluxate; and (3) the presence of fragments that do not unite and become loose bodies. In the series reported by Sneppen and associates, 50 per cent of the patients developed arthritis in the tibiotalar or subtalar joints.[79] Subjective complaints correlated well with the radiographic appearance of the adjacent joints. Those with marked arthritis usually had severe pain that disabled them from their usual occupation or from doing any work at all.[79]

Treatment. Closed reduction will seldom result in improvement of the compression. When loose bodies or tilting is expected, open reduction by osteotomy of the lateral or medial malleolus is recommended. Autogenous bone grafts will be necessary, but internal fixation will be difficult.

Protection of the restored areas by pins in plaster, Hoffman-type external fixation, or calcaneal traction will be necessary to prevent re-collapse. Residual disabling late post-traumatic arthritis is inevitable in some cases owing to talar cartilage damage and may require ankle or pantalar arthrodesis.

Shearing Fractures

Shearing fractures are the most frequent type of talar body fracture. Many are due to supination and have associated ankle fractures. The coronal type resembles a fracture of the talar neck except that the former is located more posteriorly and involves the articular surface of the trochlea. It is frequently displaced, leaving a beak that will block dorsiflexion. The sagittal type somewhat resembles a lateral compression fracture. Comminution is usually not severe, although the majority of fractures are displaced and are associated with joint subluxation, especially of the subtalar joint (Fig. 54–25). There is a 35 per cent chance of avascular necrosis in this group, and about 50 per cent of these patients develop arthritis in the tibiotalar or subtalar joints.[79]

Treatment. The displacement may be improved by closed reduction, but it is difficult to obtain an anatomic reduction by closed means. In the group treated by closed reduction, results were good in slightly over half the cases reported by Sneppen and colleagues.[79] On the other

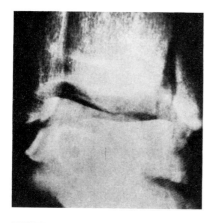

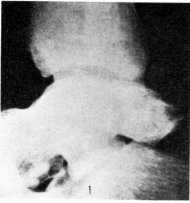

Figure 54–25. *Sagittal-type shearing fracture with subtalar subluxation and a supination fracture of the medial malleolus. (From Sneppen, O., et al.: Acta Orthop. Scand., 48:317, 1977.)*

hand, these fractures lend themselves to a careful open reduction and internal fixation to restore the articular surface and correct joint subluxation. More frequent careful open reductions with internal fixation should improve the prognosis.

The preferred surgical approach for both coronal and sagittal fractures would be by osteotomy of the lateral malleolus, rather than of the medial malleolus. The lateral approach avoids the deltoid ligament, which contains important vascular channels to the talar body, and will also allow good visualization of the talocalcaneal joint. This aggressive approach will minimize the possibility of residual subtalar joint subluxation and dorsal step-off on the upper surface of the trochlea. However, a good result cannot be guaranteed because of damage to the articular cartilage at the time of injury and the risk of at least a localized area of avascular necrosis. Since avascularity of the entire talar body is not as likely as in Group III fractures of the talar

neck, a very poor clinical result due to total collapse of the talus is seldom seen. Late disabling post-traumatic arthritis should be treated by arthrodesis of the involved joints.

Crush Fractures

Crush fractures fortunately are uncommon. They are usually caused by high velocity injuries such as motorcycle accidents and free falls of more than 10 meters. Anatomic reduction is impossible because of comminution and impaction. Avascular necrosis is to be expected, and associated calcaneal and malleolar fractures are frequent.

Treatment. Management should consist of gross alignment of the foot and ankle in a functional position. Primary attention to circulation and the condition of the skin will ensure viable tissue should late reconstruction, such as tibiocalcaneal arthrodesis, be necessary. Amazingly, this injury has commonly resulted in a partial fibrous ankylosis that allows comfortable, although limited, function without formal reconstructive surgery.[79] A molded foot-ankle orthosis is helpful for patients who are not quite symptomatic enough to require arthrodesis.

Fracture of the Posterior Tubercle

Fracture of the posterior tubercle occurred in 20 per cent of the talar body fractures reported by Sneppen and associates.[79] This study is by far the largest documented experience with this injury. The fracture described by the authors is interesting because even though the dorsal aspect of the talus is not completely covered by articular cartilage, the plantar aspect is. This is due to the posterior tubercle's articulation with the posterior facet of the calcaneus (see Figure 54–24). Therefore, it is a weight-bearing part of the talus and is shaped to prevent posterior subluxation of the talocalcaneal joint and to act as a normal bone block to prevent excessive plantar flexion.

The posterior tubercle projects posteriorly beyond the posterior facet of the calcaneus. The groove for the flexor hallucis longus tendon creates a medial prominence to which the deltoid ligament attaches and a lateral prominence to which a fasciculus of the lateral ligament of the ankle attaches. The posterior tubercle may be avulsed in hyper-dorsiflexion or pinched off between the posterior tibial margin and the calcaneus in hyper-plantarflexion. This is a common injury in ballet dancers and soccer players and may be acute or chronic.

It is important to differentiate this injury from an os trigonum. In approximately 70 per cent of children between eight and nine years of age, two secondary centers of ossification develop on the posterior aspect of the talus and fuse within one year.[46] Normally there is a larger lateral projection to which the posterior fasciculus of the lateral collateral ligament attaches. This is separated by a groove for the flexor hallucis longus tendon from a smaller projection to which the posterior fibers of the deltoid ligament attach. These centers may not coalesce with the body of the talus and persist as a separate ossicle known as the os trigonum. The ankle and subtalar joints are not involved. Therefore, degenerative arthritis of the ankle or subtalar joints does not develop. This separation usually causes no symptoms. However, after acute injury or chronic repetitive strain, pain may develop, requiring excision of the os trigonum in active individuals. Good results have been reported.

The injury described in Sneppen's series is quite different because it is a coronal shearing fracture involving a significant articular cartilage–covered portion of the trochlea, some of which articulates with the tibia and which always extends into the subtalar joint. This fracture appears to us as most likely due to hyper-plantar flexion of the ankle joint and posterior subluxation of the subtalar joint combined with vertical compression. It is usually produced by a significant fall or a motor vehicle accident.

Treatment. Anatomic reduction and rigid fixation by open technique followed by early range of motion would be the ideal treatment. However, this has not been reported on and would be technically difficult. Plaster immobilization with non–weight bearing for six to eight weeks until union occurs is the treatment currently being used. Even though displacement is unusual at the time of initial radiographic examination, the finding, on long-term evaluation, that 70 per cent of patients had significant degenerative arthritis in the subtalar and/or tibiotalar joints is not en-

tirely unexpected. Avascular necrosis has not been reported. The residual symptoms have not been severe enough to require late surgical reconstruction in the form of subtalar or plantalar arthrodesis.

Fracture of the Lateral Tubercle

Fractures of the lateral tubercle account for 24 per cent of talar body fractures. Several authors have provided informative articles about this type of fracture.[12, 17, 22, 34, 53, 79] All found that the injury was frequently overlooked initially and that it led to considerable difficulty when improperly treated. There was some confusion as to terminology, as "fracture of the lateral process" and "fracture of the posterior facet" were also used.

Anatomically, the injury involves the posterior lateral aspect of the talus, which forms a portion of both the fibulotalar and talocalcaneal joints.[22] The inferior surface articulates with the posterior facet of the calcaneus. The heavy cancellous bone structure and horizontal orientation of the lateral process support its importance in weight bearing (Fig. 54–26). It serves as a point of attachment for several important ligaments, i.e., the lateral talocalcaneal, cervical, bifurcate, and anterior talofibular ligaments. The function of the lateral tu-

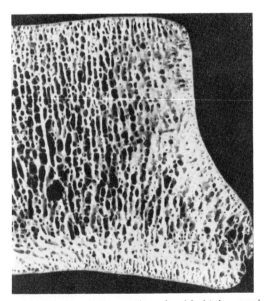

Figure 54–26. *Cross section of a dried talar specimen showing the dense cancellous structure of the lateral process, especially the lateral fibular surface and the inferior calcaneal surface, which supports its importance in weight bearing.*

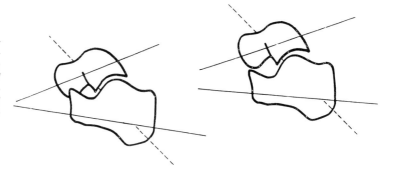

Figure 54–27. Drawings showing the congruity of the posterior talocalcaneal articulation with the heel in neutral (left) and the lack of congruity and concentration of force on the lateral process of the talus when the foot is supinated (right).

bercle in fibulotalar articulation has not been emphasized, but is obviously significant, as this joint is important in hinge movements of the ankle, in stabilizing the ankle mortise, and in the recently appreciated role of the distal fibula in weight bearing.

The calcaneal articulation is an interesting one and has been emphasized by several authors.[12, 17] They point out the incongruity of the posterior talocalcaneal articulation caused by heel inversion and supination. This causes a concentration of weight-bearing forces on the lateral process of the talus, especially when the foot is simultaneously dorsiflexed and supinated[12, 17, 33] (Fig. 54–27).

The mechanism of injury mentioned most frequently is a fall on the inverted dorsiflexed foot.[12, 17, 22, 53, 74] This mechanism is supported by the association of this fracture with the following clinical observations: (1) anterior subtalar dislocations, (2) fractures of the talar neck, (3) adduction-type fractures of the medial malleolus, (4) complete rupture of the lateral collateral ligament, and (5) avulsion fractures of the tip of the fibula.[12, 33] Figure 54–28 shows a vertical load applied to the calcaneus with the heel supinated, dor-

siflexed, and in neutral position, which produced a fracture of the lateral talar process, fracture of the talar neck, and fracture of the calcaneus. Figure 54–29 shows increasing force producing an undisplaced fracture, a displaced fracture, and finally a displaced fracture with subtalar subluxation.

Three types of fractures have been reported: (1) a simple fracture seen best on the anteroposterior view of the ankle and extending from the talofibular articular surface down to the posterior talocalcaneal articular surface of the subtalar joint (Fig. 54–30), (2) a comminuted fracture that involves both the fibular and the posterior calcaneal articular surfaces of the talus and the entire lateral process, and (3) a chip fracture of the anterior and inferior portions of the posterior articular process of the talus. The chip fracture is best seen in the region of the sinus tarsi on the lateral ankle roentgenogram and does not extend to the talofibular articulation. Several normal accessory ossicles occur in the hind- and midfoot and must be differentiated from true fractures[83] (Fig. 54–31).

Treatment. Nonoperative treatment consists of closed reduction with direct pressure on the fragment, if displaced, and

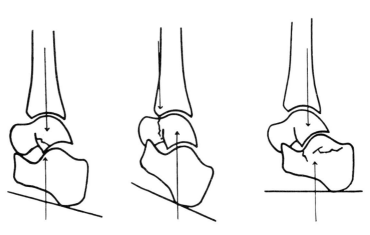

Figure 54–28. Mechanism of fracture of the lateral process of talus, the talar neck, and the calcaneus.

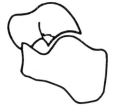 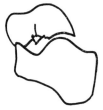 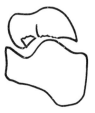

Figure 54–29. *Anterior sub-luxation of the subtalar joint causing displacement of a fracture of the lateral talar process.*

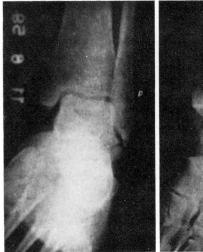 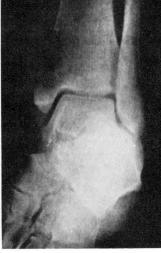 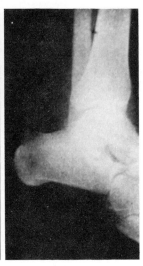

Figure 54–30. *A fairly large displaced fracture of the lateral talar process best seen on the anteroposterior view of the ankle.*

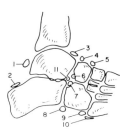

FRACTURES

1. Posterior Malleolar Tip
2. Posterior Tip of Astragalus
3. Dorsum of Astragalus
4. Dorsum of Navicular (proximal)
5. Dorsum of Navicular (distal)
6. Base of Navicular
7. Dorsum of Cuboid
8. Calcaneal Beak
9. Base of Cuboid
10. Base of 5th Metatarsal

ACCESSORY OSSICLES SIMILARLY LOCATED

1. Os Trigonum
2. Accessory Supracalcaneus
3. Os Supratalare
4. Os Supranaviculare
5. Os Infranaviculare
6. Os Tibiale Externum
7. Os Cuboides Secondarium
8. Os Peroneum
9. Os Vesalianum
10. Apophysis of 5th Metatarsal
11. Secondary Calcaneus

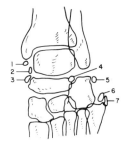

FRACTURES

1. Tip of Medial Malleolus
2. Medial Border of Talus
3. Medial Border of Navicular
4. Proximal Medial Tip of Cuboid
5. Proximal Lateral Border of Cuboid
6. Base of 5th Metatarsal

ACCESSORY OSSICLES SIMILARLY LOCATED

1. Os Subtibiale
2. Accessory Talus
3. Os Tibiale Externum
4. Os Cuboides Secondarium
5. Os Peroneum
6. Os Vesalianum
7. Apophysis of 5th Metatarsal

Figure 54–31. *Differential diagnosis of common avulsion fractures. (After Zatkin, H. R.: Sem. Roentgenol. 5:419, 1970.)*

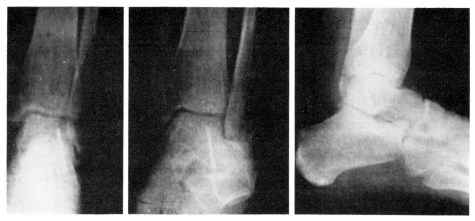

Figure 54–32. *Displaced fracture of the lateral talar process after open reduction and screw fixation. Note the bony union. (From Dimon, J. H.: J. Bone Joint Surg., 43A:275, 1961.)*

immobilization in neutral dorsiflexion and slight eversion in a short leg cast for four weeks without weight bearing and two weeks with weight bearing. Simple fractures that remain displaced should be treated by open reduction and internal fixation using Kirschner wires or preferably small compression screws[53] (Fig. 54–32). Comminuted and chip fractures may be treated by closed reduction or primarily by excision.[17, 22, 53] The results of early excision are far superior to nonoperative treatment and treatment by late excision[2, 53] (Fig.

54–33). Nonunion due to inadequate immobilization is symptomatic and may require excision of the fragments. Overgrowth of the lateral process with painful calcaneal impingement may occur and may require a medial heel wedge or local resection.

Rarely, subtalar arthritis will require subtalar fusion. The key to the management of this fracture appears to be a high level of suspicion and early diagnosis followed by perfect reduction or early excision.

ANALYSIS OF THIRTEEN CASES OF FRACTURE OF THE LATERAL PROCESS OF THE TALUS

Figure 54–33. *Results of treatment of 13 cases of fracture of the lateral talar process. (From Mukherjee, S. K., et al.: J. Bone Joint Surg., 56B:263, 1974.)*

Case number	Age (years)	Sex	Time from injury to operation	Treatment	Follow-up (months)	Results
1	30	Male	1 day	Excision	15	Symptom free
2	54	Male	1 day	Replacement	14	Symptom free
3	20	Male	1 month	Excision	14	Symptom free
4	42	Female	1 month	Excision	10	Symptom free
5	53	Female	1 day	Excision	9	Symptom free
6	49	Male	*	Conservative	35	Subtalar pain, advised fusion
7	35	Male	*	Initially conservative	*	*
8	68	Male	Same day	Replacement	9	Discomfort only
9	20	Male	9 months	Excision and cheilotomy	22	Awaiting subtalar fusion
10	42	Male	10 months	Exploration	18	Discomfort only
11	35	Male	3 weeks	Excision	9	Under treatment for painful scar
12	24	Female	2 weeks	Excision	4	Symptom free
13	54	Female	4 months	Excision	12	Symptom free

* Indicates "details not known"

INJURIES OF THE MIDTARSAL JOINT

The talonavicular and calcaneocuboid joints function as a single unit in movements of the foot and in this discussion will be considered together as the midtarsal joint.[45] This joint occupies a key position in both the medial and the lateral longitudinal arches of the foot.[7, 16] It also acts in unison with the subtalar joint in the important functions of inversion and eversion. Injuries produce dislocations and fractures of the components, i.e., talar head, tarsal navicular, anterior process of the calcaneus, and cuboid bones. Apart from detailed reports of 71 patients with midtarsal joint injuries published by Main and Jowett[45] in 1975 and 10 patients by Kenwright and Taylor[38] in 1970, injuries to the midtarsal joint had previously been described rather briefly in most textbooks[26, 48, 68] and in small reported series of combined talar injuries or as case reports of isolated injuries to the talus, navicular, and cuboid bones.[19, 21, 23, 35, 38, 49, 60, 73]

Diagnosis is difficult because of the rarity of these injuries and the unfamiliarity of most trauma surgeons with the radiographic appearance of the injured foot. Good quality and well-positioned anteroposterior, lateral, and oblique roentgenograms of the foot and ankle are mandatory.[16, 18] Comparison views are helpful, especially in children. A special oblique view centered on the talonavicular joint in the plane of the metatarsals is frequently required to correctly and completely diagnose and classify these rare but potentially disabling injuries[18] (Fig. 54–34). Computerized axial tomography should be extremely useful when it becomes more available. The presence of multiple injuries frequently complicates the clinical picture.

Classification is important, and the best study to date has been done by Main and Jowett, based on the direction of the deforming force.[45] Seventy-one injuries were classified into five types: (1) medial, (2) longitudinal compression, (3) lateral, (4) plantar, and (5) crush. For the first time, a swivel-type rotation injury was described in both the medial and the lateral types. This classification appears to be reasonably easy to apply to most injuries and

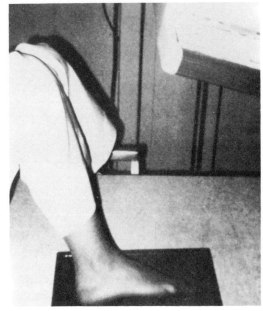

Figure 54–34. *Special oblique view centered on the talonavicular joint in the plane of the metatarsals for diagnosis of midtarsal injuries. (After London, P. S.: Injury, 5:66, 1973.)*

serves as a useful guide for both treatment and prognosis.[45]

Medial Injuries

Medial forces produce fracture sprains, fracture subluxation and dislocation, or swivel dislocations. Inversion and/or adduction is the usual mechanism.[45]

Fracture Sprains. These injuries produce avulsion or flake fractures of the dorsal surfaces of the talar head, navicular, and lateral margins of the cuboid or anterior process of the calcaneus. Since there is no dislocation and the bony fragments are small and minimally displaced, no formal reduction is required. However, these injuries are potentially unstable, especially when untreated. Simple plaster immobilization in a short leg cast with the foot in neutral position for four to six weeks is usually adequate initial treatment. A well-constructed shoe with longitudinal arch support is indicated in the convalescence period. Long-term disability should be minimal.

Fracture Subluxation and Dislocation. This injury results in medial displacement of the forefoot (Fig. 54–35A,B). The mechanism of the injury and the bony pathology

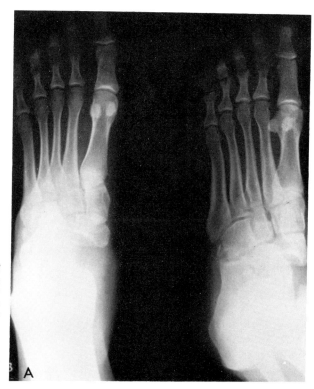

Figure 54-35. *(A) Anteroposterior and oblique views of a medial midtarsal dislocation with a compression fracture of the navicular and an avulsion fracture of the cuboid. (B) Lateral view showing only the subtle overlap of talonavicular and calcaneocuboid joints. (C) Anteroposterior view of same injury four years after closed reduction showing degenerative changes in the midtarsal joints. (D) Lateral view.*

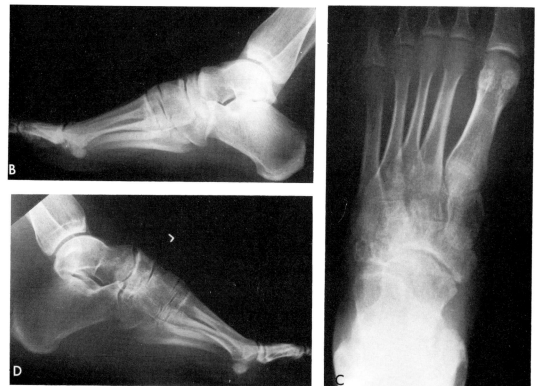

are the same as in the fracture sprain group; however, reduction is required and can usually be accomplished by closed means (Fig. 54–35C,D). Reduction should be absolutely perfect. These injuries tend to be unstable, and careful plaster immobilization and post-reduction roentgenograms are required. Percutaneous Kirschner wire stabilization should be carried out when swelling, circulatory problems, or local skin conditions prevent applications of an adequate plaster cast. Six weeks in a short leg plaster cast and two weeks in a walking plaster cast followed by progressive weight bearing using a molded arch support are recommended. Inaccurate reduction, inadequate immobilization, or articular damage at the time of injury can be expected to lead to midtarsal arthritis and instability (Fig. 54–35C,D). Persistent disability has been treated by midtarsal arthrodesis, but this has not been universally successful, and triple arthrodesis is usually the definitive reconstructive procedure required.

Swivel Dislocations. This injury is usually produced by falls from significant heights. Unlike medial fracture dislocations in which both the talonavicular and calcaneocuboid joints are separated, in swivel dislocations only the talonavicular joint is displaced medially. The forefoot rotates medially and dislocates the talonavicular joint, but leaves the calcaneocuboid joint intact (Fig. 54–36). The interosseous talocalcaneal ligament is intact, and the heel is not inverted or everted, as in a subtalar dislocation. Treatment requires an anatomic reduction, as failure to reduce the fracture will always lead to a poor result. Open reduction is usually required because of interposed soft tissues. The results of closed reduction have been discouraging, in that a triple arthrodesis is usually required because of midtarsal ar-

thritis. On the other hand, prompt open reduction and non–weight-bearing plaster immobilization for six weeks, with or without temporary Kirschner-wire fixation of the talonavicular joint, usually result in satisfactory outcome after this serious injury.

Longitudinal Injuries

Longitudinal forces account for the largest percentage of midtarsal injuries.[45] If the foot is plantar flexed at the moment of impact on the metatarsal heads, the navicular is compressed between the cuneiforms and the head of the talus, resulting in navicular fractures or crushing of the talus. If the forces are along the lateral cuneiforms, there is medial displacement of the forefoot, including the calcaneocuboid joint, in addition to compression fracture of the lateral segment of the navicular and frequently an impaction of the talar head.

If the ankle is less plantar flexed at the moment of impact, a dorsiflexion component is added, resulting in compression of the lower pole of the navicular and the dorsal displacement of the upper pole. This leads to rupture of the talonavicular and/or naviculocuneiform ligaments with dorsal dislocation of the upper pole of the navicular.

Treatment. In the large series by Main and Jowett,[45] 24 of 29 longitudinal injuries were displaced. Simple plaster immobilization for six weeks in a short leg cast was adequate to obtain excellent or good results in undisplaced fractures. Failure to reduce the fractures usually had an unsatisfactory result. Open reductions did not greatly improve the results in their patients, but isolated reports of similar injuries treated by prompt anatomic reduc-

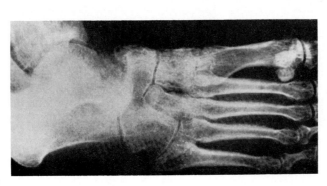

Figure 54–36. Oblique roentgenogram showing a medial swivel dislocation. The talonavicular joint is dislocated medially, but the calcaneocuboid and subtalar joints are intact.

tion and internal fixation showed more encouraging results. Temporary Kirschner-wire fixation of the navicular to the cuneiforms is preferable to fixation of the talus. Condensation on follow-up roentgenograms, indicating avascular necrosis of the navicular, does occur. It is difficult to differentiate this disability from the articular irregularity caused by the fracture. Interestingly, avascular necrosis did not seem to be a significant problem after complete plantar dislocation when prompt open reduction was carried out.

Lateral Injuries

Lateral forces such as occur in falls or automobile accidents that force the forefoot into pronation result in fracture sprains, fracture subluxation, or swivel dislocation.

Fracture Sprains. These injuries produce avulsion of the navicular tuberosity or flake avulsions of the dorsum of the navicular and talus on the medial side. On the lateral side, impaction fractures of the articular margins of the cuboid and/or calcaneus occur. These injuries are not displaced but are potentially unstable. Treatment by plaster immobilization for six weeks appears to be very adequate and usually gives excellent results.

Fracture Subluxations. Such fractures produce subluxations of the talonavicular joint laterally and more comminution of the anterior column of the calcaneus or cuboid, resulting in collapse of the important lateral longitudinal arch. This mechanism probably produces the "nutcracker" fracture of the cuboid and total dislocation (extrusion) of this bone[19, 35] (Fig. 54–37A,B). These are all serious injuries de-

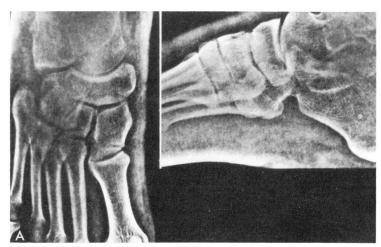

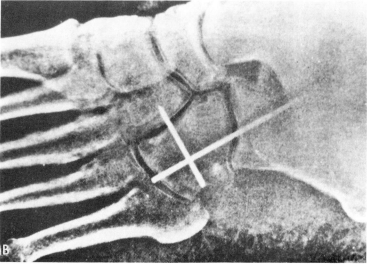

Figure 54–37. (A) Anteroposterior and lateral roentgenograms of a complete dislocation of the cuboid. A variation of the "nutcracker fracture." (B) Anteroposterior view after open reduction and Kirschner-wire fixation. There was no roentgenographic evidence of avascular necrosis.

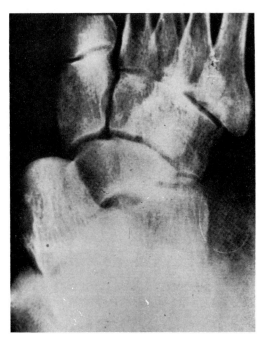

Figure 54–38. *Anteroposterior view of a lateral swivel dislocation. Note the absence of the head of the talus in the cup of the navicular, the lateral deviation of the forefoot, and the intact calcaneocuboid joint. Other views showed the subtalar joint to be intact as well.*

spite somewhat innocuous-appearing initial roentgenograms. None of the patients reported by Main and Jowett had excellent or good results and 50 per cent required triple arthrodesis. Comminution of the calcaneocuboid joint appears to be the major problem. Open reduction may be indicated but cannot be guaranteed to restore a smooth, stable articulation. After a period of plaster immobilization of several months to allow fracture and soft-tissue healing, calcaneocuboid arthrodesis, or formal triple arthrodesis, should be considered.

Lateral Swivel Dislocation. This injury results in lateral dislocation of the talonavicular joint while the calcaneocuboid and talocalcaneal joints remain intact (Fig. 54–38). The heel does not evert and the interosseous talocalcaneal ligament remains intact, which differentiates this injury from lateral subtalar dislocations. Closed reduction gave a good result in the one case reported in the literature.[45]

Plantar Injuries

Plantar forces can result in sprains or fracture subluxation and dislocation. Mo-

torcycle accidents and falls account for most of these injuries.[45]

Fracture Sprains. Such injuries cause avulsion of fragments from the dorsum of the navicular or talus and from the anterior process of the calcaneus. These tend to be stable injuries and respond well to plaster immobilization with some weight bearing for six weeks.

Fracture Subluxation and Dislocation. This results in plantar displacement of the navicular, cuboid, and distal forefoot (Fig. 54–39). Impaction can occur at the calcaneocuboid joint inferiorly. The talocalcaneal joint is undisturbed, as the interosseous talocalcaneal ligament is intact, in contrast to the pathologic findings in posterior subtalar dislocations.

Treatment includes closed reduction and plaster immobilization for six to eight weeks, which can be expected to give good results if there is little comminution. If closed reduction is not possible or if open injuries are present, open reduction and temporary fixation of the talonavicular joint is indicated (Fig. 54–40).

Crush Injuries

Crush injuries are usually due to motorcycle accidents or heavy weights falling

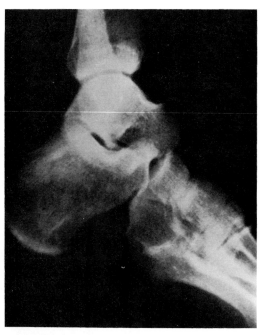

Figure 54–39. *Lateral view of plantar dislocation of the midtarsal (Chopart's) joint.*

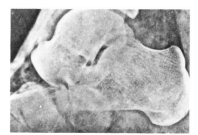 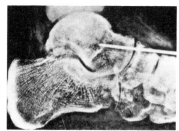

Figure 54–40. *Lateral view of an irreducible Chopart dislocation before and after open reduction and Kirschner-wire fixation of the unstable talonavicular joint.*

directly on the foot. There is no constant pattern and compounding is frequent.

Careful management is required to achieve reduction without compromising skin or distal circulation. Limited open reduction or external skeletal fixation after debridement of open wounds is appropriate, but anatomic fixation of the comminuted fractures will usually not be possible or practical. Malunion and extensive articular incongruity are to be expected. Despite these problems, none of the patients of Main and Jowett required secondary surgery.[45] Midtarsal thickening, loss of motion, tendency to swell, and lowering of the longitudinal arches requiring shoe modifications are usually long-term problems.

REFERENCES

1. Anderson, H. G.: The Medical and Surgical Aspects of Aviation. London, Oxford University Press, 1919.
2. Arcomano, J. P., Kamhi, E., Karas, S., and Moriarity, V.: Transchondral fracture and osteochondritis dissecans of talus. N.Y. State J. Med., December, 1978, p. 2183.
3. Barber, J. R., Brucker, J. D., and Haliburton, R. A.: Peritaler dislocation of the foot. Can. J. Surg., 4:205, 1961.
4. Berndt, A. L., and Harty, M.: Transchondral fractures (osteochondritis dissecans) of the talus. J. Bone Joint Surg., 41-A:996, 1959.
5. Blair, H. C.: Comminuted fractures and fracture dislocation of the body of the astragalus. Am. J. Surg., 59:37, 1943.
6. Böhler, L.: Technik der Knochenbruchbehandlung. Vienna, W. Maudrich, 1943–1944.
7. Bonnin, J. G.: Dislocations and fracture-dislocations of the talus. Br. J. Surg., 28:188, 1940.
8. Buckingham, W. W., Jr.: Subtalar dislocation of the foot. J. Trauma, 13:753, 1973.
9. Cameron, B. M.: Osteochondritis dissecans of the ankle joint. J. Bone Joint Surg., 38-A:857, 1956.
10. Canale, S. T., and Kelly, F. B.: Fractures of the neck of the talus. J. Bone Joint Surg., 60-A:143, 1978.
11. Christensen, S. B., Lorentzen, J. E., Krogsøe, O., and Sneppen, O. Subtalar dislocation. Acta Orthop. Scand., 48:707, 1977.
12. Cimmino, C. V.: Fracture of the lateral process of the talus. Am. J. Roentgenol. Radiat. Ther. Nuc. Med., 90:1277, 1963.
13. Coltart, W. D.: Aviator's astragalus. J. Bone Joint Surg., 34-B:535, 1952.
14. Davidson, C. D., Steele, H. D., MacKenzie, D., and Penney, J. A.: A review of twenty-one cases of transchondral fractures of the talus. J. Trauma, 7:378, 1967.
15. Detenbeck, L. C., and Kelly, P. J.: Total dislocation of the talus. J. Bone Joint Surg., 51-A:283, 1969.
16. Dewar, F. P., and Evans, D. C.: Occult fracture —subluxation of the midtarsal joint. J. Bone Joint Surg., 50-B:386, 1968.
17. Dimon, J. H., III: Isolated displaced fracture of the posterior facet of the talus. J. Bone Joint Surg., 43-A:275, 1961.
18. Dixon, J. H.: Letter to the Editor. Injury, 10:251, 1979.
19. Drummond, P. S., and Hastings, D. E.: Total dislocation of the cuboid bone. J. Bone Joint Surg., 51-B:716, 1969.
20. Dunn, W. A.: Peritalar dislocation. Orthop. Clin. North Am., 5:1, 1974.
21. Fahey, J. T., and Murphy, J. L.: Dislocation and fractures of the talus. Surg. Clin. North Am., 45:70, 1965.
22. Fjelborg, O.: Fracture of the lateral process of the talus. Acta Orthop. Scand., 39:407, 1968.
23. Friedmann, E.: Key graft fixation in mid-tarsal fracture dislocation. Am. J. Surg., 96:81, 1958.
24. Garcia, A., and Parker, J. C., II: Fractures of the foot. *In* Giannestras, N. J. (ed.): Foot Disorders, Medical and Surgical Management. 2nd ed. Philadelphia, Lea & Febiger, 1973.
25. Gatellier, J.: The juxtaretro-peroneal route in the operative treatment of fractures of of the malleolus with posterior marginal fragment. Surg. Gynecol. Obstet., 52:67, 1931.
26. Giannestras, N. J., and Samnarco, G. J.: Fractures and dislocations in the foot. *In* Rockwood, C. A., and Green, D. P. (eds.): Fractures. Philadelphia, J. B. Lippincott, 1975.
27. Gillquist, J., Oretop, N., Stemstrom, A., Reiger, A., and Wennberg, E.: Late results after vertical fracture of the talus. Injury, 6:173, 1974.
28. Grantham, S. A.: Medial subtalar dislocations; five cases with a common etiology. J. Trauma, 4:845, 1964.
29. Gustilo, R. B., and Gordon, J. J.: Osteochondral fractures of the talus. Minnes. Med., 51:237, 1968.
30. Haliburton, R. A.: Discussion — Peritalar dislocation. Orthop. Clin. North Am., 5:1, 1974.
31. Haliburton, R. A., Babber, J. R., and Fraser, R. L.: Further experience with peritalar dislocations. Can. J. Surg., 10:322, 1967.
32. Haliburton, R. A., Sullivan, R., Kelly, P. J., and Peterson, L. F. A.: The extraosseous and intra-osseous blood supply of the talus. J. Bone Joint Surg., 40-A:1115, 1958.
33. Hawkins, L. G.: Fractures of the lateral process of the talus: A review of thirteeen cases. J. Bone Joint Surg., 47-A:1170, 1965.
34. Hawkins, L. G.: Fractures of the neck of the talus. Bone Joint Surg., 52-A:991, 1970.
35. Hermel, M. B., and Gershon-Cohen, J.: The nutcracker fracture of the cuboid by indirect violence. Radiology, 60:850, 1953.
36. Judcy and Dufaurest. Quoted by Straus, D. C.: Subtalar

dislocations of the foot with report of two cases. Am. J. Surg., *30*:427, 1935.

37. Kelly, P. J., and Sullivan, C. R.: Blood supply of the talus. Clin. Orthop., *30*:37, 1963.

38. Kenwright, J., and Taylor, R. G.: Major injuries of the talus. J. Bone Joint Surg., *52-B*:36, 1970.

39. Kleiger, B.: Fractures of the talus. J. Bone Joint Surg., *30-A*:735, 1948.

40. Larsen, H. W.: Subastragalar dislocation (luxatio pedis sub talo). Acta Chir. Scand., *113*:380, 1957.

41. Larson, R. L., Sullivan, C. R., and Jones, J. M.: Trauma, surgery and circulation of the talus — What are the risks of avascular necrosis? J. Trauma, *1*:13, 1961.

42. Leitner, B.: Obstacles to reduction in subtalar dislocations. J. Bone Joint Surg., *36-A*:299, 1954.

43. Leitner, B.: The mechanism of total dislocation of the talus. J. Bone Joint Surg., *37-A*:89, 1955.

44. London, P. S.: Wrinkle corner. A special view for mid-tarsal fracture-subluxation. Injury, *5*:65, 1973.

45. Main, B. J., and Jowett, R. L.: Injuries of the mid-tarsal joint. J. Bone Joint Surg., *57-B*:89, 1975.

46. McDougall, A.: The os trigonum. J. Bone Joint Surg., *37-B*:257, 1955.

47. McKeever, F. M.: Treatment and complications of fractures and dislocations of the talus. Clin. Orthop., *30*:45, 1963.

48. McLaughlin, H. L.: Trauma. Philadelphia, W. B. Saunders Co., 1959, pp. 299–332.

49. Mindell, E. R., Cisek, E. E., Kartalian, G., and Dziob, J. M.: Late results of injuries to the talus: Analysis of forty cases. J. Bone Joint Surg., *45-A*:221, 1963.

50. Mitchell, J. I.: Total dislocation of the astragalus. J. Bone Joint Surg., *18*:212, 1936.

51. Morris, H. D., Hand, W., and Dunn, A. W.: The modified Blair fusion of fractures of the talus. J. Bone Joint Surg., *53-A*:1289, 1971.

52. Mukherjee, S. K., and Young, A. B.: Dome fractures of the talus: A report of ten cases. J. Bone Joint Surg., *55-B*:319, 1973.

53. Mukherjee, S. K., Pringle, R. M., and Baxter, A. D.: Fracture of the lateral process of the talus. J. Bone Joint Surg., *56-B*:263, 1974.

54. Mulfinger, G. L., and Trueta, J.: The blood supply of the talus. J. Bone Joint Surg., *52-B*:160, 1970.

55. Newburgh, A. H.: Osteochondral fractures of the dome of the talus. A report of ten cases. J. Bone Joint Surg., *55-B*:319, 1973.

56. Newcomb, W. J., and Brav, E. A.: Complete dislocation of the talus. J. Bone Joint Surg., *30-A*:872, 1948.

57. Nisbet, N. W.: Dome fractures of the talus. J. Bone Joint Surg., *36-B*:244, 1954.

58. O'Donohugh, D. H.: Chondral and osteochondral fractures. J. Trauma, *6*:469, 1966.

59. Pantazopoulos, T., Galanos, P., Vayanos, E., Mitsou, A., and Hartofilakides-Garofalidis, G. Fractures of the neck of the talus. Acta Orthop. Scand., *45*:296, 1974.

60. Pennal, G. F.: Fracture of the talus. Clin. Orthop. Rel. Res., *30*:53, 1963.

61. Peterson, L., Goldie, I., and Lindell, D.: The arterial supply of the talus. Acta Orthop. Scand., *45*:260, 1974.

62. Peterson, L., and Goldie, I. F.: The arterial supply of the talus. Acta Orthop. Scand., *46*:1026, 1975.

63. Peterson, L., Goldie, I. F., and Irstam, L.: Fracture of the neck of the talus. Acta Orthop. Scand., *48*:696, 1977.

64. Peterson, L., Romanus, B., and Dahlberg, E.: Fracture of the collum tali — An experimental study. J. Biomechanics, *9*:277, 1976.

65. Pinzur, M. S., and Meyer, P. R., Jr.: Complete posterior dislocation of the talus. Clin. Orthop. Rel. Res., *131*:205, 1978.

66. Plewes, L. W., and McKelvey, H. G.: Subtalar dislocation. J. Bone Joint Surg., *26*:585, 1944.

67. Rendu, A.: Fractures intra-articulaire parcellaire de la poulie astraglienne. Lyon Med., *150*:220, 1932.

68. Rockwood, C. A., Jr., and Green, D. P. (eds.): Fractures. Philadelphia, J. B. Lippincott, 1975.

69. Roder, S., Tillegard, P., and Unander-Scharin, L.: Osteochondritis dissecans and similar lesions of the talus: A report of fifty-five cases with special references to etiology and treatment. Acta Orthop. Scand., *23*:51, 1953.

70. Rogers, L. F., and Campbell, R. E.: Fractures and dislocations of the foot. Sem. Roentgenol., *8*:157, 1978.

71. Rosenberg, N. J.: Fracture of the dome. J. Bone Joint Surg., *47-A*:1279, 1965.

72. Schrock, R. D.: Fractures of the foot: Fractures and dislocations of the astragalus. *In* American Academy of Orthopaedic Surgeons: Instructional Course Lectures. Vol. 9. Ann Arbor, Mich., Edwards, pp. 361–368.

73. Seymour, N.: The late results of naviculo-cuneiform fusion. J. Bone Joint Surg., *49-B*:558, 1967.

74. Shahriaree, H., Sajadiiik, A., Silver, C., and Modsavi, A.: Total dislocation of the talus. Orthop. Rev., *9*:65, 1980.

75. Smillie, I. S.: Loose bodies in joints: etiology, pathology, treatment. *In* Osteochondritis Dissecans. Baltimore, Williams and Wilkins, 1960.

76. Smith, G. R., Winquist, R. A., Allan, T. N. K., and Northrop, C. H.: Subtle transchondral fractures of the talar dome: A radiological perspective. Radiology, *114*:667, 1977.

77. Smith, H.: Subastragalar dislocation: Report of seven cases. J. Bone Joint Surg., *19*:373, 1937.

78. Sneppen, O., and Buhl, O.: Fracture of the talus. A study of its genesis and morphology based upon cases with associated ankle fractures. Acta Orthop. Scand., *45*:307, 1974.

79. Sneppen, O., Christensen, S. B., Krogsøe, O., and Lorentzen, J.: Fracture of the body of the talus. Acta Orthop. Scand., *48*:317, 1977.

80. Sullivan, C. R., and Jackson, S. C.: Fracture dislocation of the astragalus in children. Acta Orthop. Scand., *21*:302, 1958.

81. Ywan, H. A., Cady, R. B., and De Rosa, C.: Osteochondritis dissecans of the talus associated with subcondral cysts. J. Bone Joint Surg., *61-A*:1249, 1979.

82. Yvars, M. F.: Osteochondral fractures of the dome of the talus. Clin. Orthop., *114*:185, 1976.

83. Zatkin, H. R.: Trauma to the Foot. Sem. Roentgenol., *5*:419, 1970.

CHAPTER 55

TRAUMA TO THE OS CALCIS AND HEEL CORD

Isaac Stephens McReynolds, M.D., F.A.C.S.

FRACTURES OF THE OS CALCIS

It has been recognized for many years that the end results following severe fractures of the os calcis have been far from what might be desired. Cotton and Henderson concluded that conservative treatment gave incredibly bad results.[1] Bankart felt that "results of treatment of the os calcis are rotten."[2] Mercer was quoted as saying that "fractures of the os calcis are among the most disabling of injuries."[3] McLaughlin likened attempts to maintain reduction of a comminuted os calcis fracture by internal or external means to "nailing a custard pie to the wall."[4] Böhler thought that fractures of the os calcis should be treated like all fractures, i.e., "exact reduction must be made and the reduced fragments must be fixed in position until bony union occurs."[5] Wilson wrote, "The position of the fragments may be improved, but complete reduction, using the term in the sense in which it is employed in speaking of fractures elsewhere, is rarely, if ever, obtained."[6]

In the past, management of fractures of the os calcis has been divided into nonoperative and operative treatment:

A. Nonoperative treatment
 1. Immobilization without reduction
 2. Immediate active exercises without reduction or immobilization
 3. Closed manipulative reduction
 4. Reduction by the use of instruments

B. Operative treatment
 1. Open reduction done from the lateral side of the heel, with internal fixation or bone grafts
 2. Primary subtalar arthrodesis
 3. Triple arthrodesis

It is puzzling that the results claimed by very different methods of treatment are somewhat similar. Giannestras and Sammarco stated: "There are essentially four basic methods of treatment. On careful investigation, we have found that the end results of all these methods yield essentially the same percentage of good, fair, and poor results in our experience."[7]

An excellent result from triple arthrodesis is not the same as an excellent result from another method in which there is normal contour to the heel and excellent motion in the forefoot and in the subastragalar joint.

Parks, in writing on the nonreductive treatment for fractures of the os calcis, said: "The basic simplicity of this method of treatment, the relatively few complications encountered, coupled with the uniformly satisfactory results, lead us to recommend it as a useful form of treatment in the majority of cases of intra-articular fractures of the os calcis."[8]

Widén, in an excellent and very comprehensive paper on fractures of the calcaneus wrote: "The most reliable way to maintain mobility of the subtaloid joint lies in performing as exact a reduction as possible."[9] He felt that conservative treatment should be reserved for fractures with slight or no displacement, and I am of the same opinion.

In England, immobilization of a fracture of the os calcis in a patient over age 50 has not been supported because of resultant stiffnes; Essex-Lopresti thought that open reduction in patients over 50 years of age was definitely contraindicated.[3] In my experience with open reduction in the treatment of fractures of the os calcis, however, 41 per cent of the patients were over age 50.

Closed manipulative reduction of fractures of the os calcis was developed and performed extensively in Boston over a period of about 25 years. Hermann wrote of the conservative therapy for fractures of the os calcis in 1937.[10] Historically, the armamentarium included a weighted 7-lb wooden mallet, the sawed-off upper end of a crutch, ice tongs, a sandbag, and a Forrester clamp. The end results in 152 cases were listed as "73 per cent good; 14 per cent fair; and 13 per cent poor."[10]

One of Pridie's conclusions in proposing excision of the os calcis as a new method of treatment was that "this operation will undoubtedly save many an injured foot from amputation."[11] It was ironic that one of his patients so treated required amputation later. In Pridie's hands, late arthrodesis of the subastragalar joint proved so disappointing that it was abandoned and early arthrodesis was tried. To quote Pridie: "The os calcis was not so much a bone in fragments as a bag of bones. Under such circumstances, the satisfactory removal of the articular cartilage from the subastragalar joint surfaces is a procedure of great difficulty. In fact, the operation is impossible."[11]

Pennal and Yadov reported 75 per cent excellent and very good results with primary subtalar fusions;[12] yet, Pennal told me in 1976 that he no longer used subtalar arthrodesis but did an open reduction from the lateral side of the heel.

Harris summarized: Even the best attempts at reduction seldom restore perfectly the articular surfaces of the os calcis. The late result is a stiff and painful subtalar joint which requires fusion as a secondary procedure to relieve pain. Consequently, the time-saving procedure is immediate reduction of the fracture by skeletal traction and compression, followed within three or four weeks by subtalar fusion by Gallie's technique."[13, 14] Conn condemned subtalar arthrodesis in favor of triple arthrodesis.[15]

Thompson and Friesen feel that as the initial primary treatment of severe, comminuted, displaced calcaneal fractures with peritalar involvement, triple arthrodesis has given extremely gratifying results.[16] In patients so treated, "eighty-four per cent were listed as having obtained excellent results."[16]

In a detailed study of os calcis fractures, Thorén stated his belief that "open reduction in combination with early physiotherapy is probably the treatment of choice in these cases of os calcis fracture with considerable displacement in the posterior articular facet. In comparing a series that had been treated by early triple arthrodesis, it appeared that both early physical therapy and open reduction gave better results than an arthrodesis."[17]

It is difficult to analyze the results reported by Essex-Lopresti with the use of a sagittal pin as originated by Westhues[18] and used extensively by Gissane, but apparently 53.8 per cent of the tongue-type fractures treated with the use of a spike had good results, and 35 per cent were found disabling for recreation or for work, with 2 per cent being severely disabling.[3] Ten per cent of the results were unknown. His results with open reduction of joint depression fractures were 54 per cent good and 34 per cent disabling for recreation or for work, with 2 per cent being severely disabling.[3] The results in 7 per cent of the cases were unknown.

King stated: "In a series of 75 fractures of the os calcis involving the posterior facet, the axial pin fixation technique of Essex-Lopresti was efficacious."[19]

Widén reported 65 per cent excellent

and good results, 19 per cent fair results, and 14 per cent poor results in 56 cases treated by open reduction.[9]

It is difficult to interpret the results in the same manner from Soeur and Remy's report on open reduction and internal fixation with Kirschner wires using a lateral approach.[20] Of the patients treated, 35 per cent had normal subastragalar joint motion, but motion was absent in 20 per cent. Thirteen per cent of the patients did not resume their normal work.

As the preceding discussion unquestionably demonstrates, the treatment of severe fractures of the os calcis is a controversial subject. As long ago as 1938, Goff illustrated 41 methods of treatment of these fractures and had a bibliography of 151 references.[21] Widén listed 173 articles in his bibliography.[9] A review of the surgical literature on the subject should be confusing to the student or the doctor who has had little experience in treating these fractures and must be puzzling to the surgeon who has had considerable experience. The average orthopaedic resident has relatively little exposure to this subject during training. In private practice, few surgeons have the opportunity to treat a great number of cases. Many surgeons may have less scientific curiosity than might be expected in understanding more of the nature of the injury. In general, the pathology of the fracture is not well understood by surgeons.

Fractures of the body of the os calcis involving the subastragalar joint are, at the least, severe and complex injuries, can cause considerable difficulty and marked economic loss, and warrant very careful evaluation in an effort to carry out adequate treatment. They represent a challenge in management. Few fractures require as much in the way of special knowledge for their best treatment. They should be treated by surgeons who are knowledgeable, experienced, and skilled in the management of this type of injury. Treatment of these severe fractures could very well be relegated to a subspecialty.

Causes of Os Calcis Fractures

Most fractures of the os calcis are caused by a fall from a height. Falls or jumps from ladders, scaffolds, and roofs have been the chief causes of this injury. Böhler stated: "A fall from more than one meter should suggest this fracture."[5] Fractures of the os calcis may occur in wartime from explosions below decks or from land mines. They are seen infrequently as the result of automobile accidents, and direct blows may result in some type of fracture of the os calcis. Falls from greater heights are more apt to be associated with other injuries. The frequency of associated or concomitant fractures has varied in different studies, ranging from 8 per cent to more than 20 per cent. Vertebral fractures have long been recognized as a complication of fractures of the os calcis and have been reported to have an incidence of as much as 10 per cent. A patient who lands with most of his weight directly on the heel is more apt to incur a fracture of the os calcis. I have seen one patient who suffered a severe joint depression fracture when he landed on his forefoot in jumping over a ditch. It is difficult for a patient to describe to the surgeon just how he landed in a fall. Such factors as extension of the knee, the position of the foot and ankle in regard to valgus, varus, dorsiflexion, or plantar flexion of the ankle, and the force involved all have a bearing on the type of fracture produced. Fractures of the heel have been overlooked in isolated injuries and are more apt to be overlooked in multiple severe injuries.

Clinical Evaluation

With the history of a fall directly on the heel, accompanied by acute pain and followed by swelling on the medial or lateral side of the heel, acute tenderness on palpation or compression of the heel, pain on attempted elicitation of motion in the subastragalar joint or on attempted weight bearing, and evidence of ecchymosis, the patient is likely to have a fracture of the os calcis. With a fracture of significance involving the cancellous bone, there is fairly rapid swelling and a definite increase in intensity of the pain. Pain is severe because of the marked bleeding from the cancellous bone and the fact that the heel is tightly enveloped by fascia, which prevents rapid extravasation of blood into the subcutaneous tissues. Later, there may be evidence of discoloration of both the medial and lateral sides of the heel from hemorrhage, and hemorrhage may extend up the calf, some distance away from the site of injury. Some days after injury, a small area of hemorrhagic discoloration may be noted in the anterior portion of the sole of the foot. With continued and severe swelling, especially without treatment, there is likely to be bleb formation in the skin over the lateral or medial side of the heel. The swelling extends rapidly to involve the toes. Very acute pain may be present on movement.

Roentgenologic Evaluation

The diagnosis of a fracture of the os calcis is suspected from the history and clinical examination, but it is confirmed by roentgenologic examination. Roentgenograms are the only means by which information about the type and extent of the fracture can be obtained.

Recognition of the deformities present is a prerequisite for successful treatment. Since the roentgenograms are the only source of accurate determination of the pathology involved, high-quality, properly positioned, multiple-view films must be obtained. Proper diagnostic roentgenograms of the os calcis are relatively simple to take; however, even with the present highly advanced state of electronics and with the most sophisticated and expensive x-ray machines and processing equipment that we have ever had, there are entirely too many substandard films. Surgeons and Roentgenology Departments should not continue to accept poor-quality films. If the surgeon accepts a poor-quality film, he may be sorry that he did so at a later date.

The surgeon must interpret the films carefully. Roentgenograms are seldom described in a way that enables a mental picture of the fracture to be formed. Unless there is a routine set of views for evaluation of a fracture of the os calcis, the information that is needed will not be obtained in every case. For this reason, I believe that it is best to have the following views taken routinely:

1. Axial view (tangential or semi-axial) (Fig. 55–1A).
2. Lateral views.
    a. Mediolateral view (taken with

the lateral side of the heel closest to the film) (Fig. 55–1B).
    b. Lateromedial view (taken with the medial side of the heel closest to the film).
3. Anteroposterior view of the ankle.
4. Anteroposterior oblique view of the ankle (Fig. 55–1C).
5. Anteroposterior and medial oblique views of the calcaneocuboid joint (Fig. 55–1D).

In addition, for a proper study of fractures involving the subastragalar joint, special views such as Brodén I (10-, 20-, 30- and 40-degree) views and Brodén II views may be indicated. Giannestras used an axial medial oblique view and an axial lateral oblique view.[7] These views are described adequately by Merrill.[22]

According to Thorén, "Ordinary lateral and semi-axial roentgenograms usually do not reveal in detail the extent of injury in the fractured os calcis."[17] He felt that Brodén's projections I and II provide the most valuable information for clinical evaluation of the fracture, stating that this method is based on the fact that the posterior articular facet constitutes a cone whose axis forms an angle of about 30 degrees with the long axis of the foot. It is my opinion that axial and lateral views are the most important and most necessary views. Evaluation of the fracture is not based on one or two views, but from information furnished or not furnished in a series of views.

Axial View

The axial view (Fig. 55–1A) is the most important one, primarily for demonstrating what I believe to be the most constant and significant deformity of fractures of the body of the os calcis involving the subastragalar joint and which is referred to as "medial displacement and overriding of the superomedial fragment" (see Figure 55–3A). This view demonstrates the fracture that originates in the medial cortex of the os calcis and extends obliquely upward and outward, usually into some portion of the articular surface of the posterior facet. It may demonstrate other fracture lines extending in the long axis of the os calcis. It may also provide some idea of the width of the articular surface on the superomedial fragment as well as of the width of the articular surface of the lateral fragment. It will demonstrate whether or not there is a bulge of the lateral cortex from impaction of bone inside the lateral cortical wall and how much widening there is of the os calcis. It is important to note whether or not there is comminution of the sharp, thin spicules of bone at the inferior distal tip of the superomedial fragment at the fracture site. The axial view

may also demonstrate deformity in fractures involving the posteroinferior tuberosity. (See Figure 55–10A.)

An improperly positioned view may produce excessive shortening (see Figure 55–4A) or lengthening. Unless the foot is in a vertical plane, it will not show the medial contour of the os calcis properly. Ordinarily, I have not obtained very much information of value with regard to the irregularity of the posterior facet from routine axial

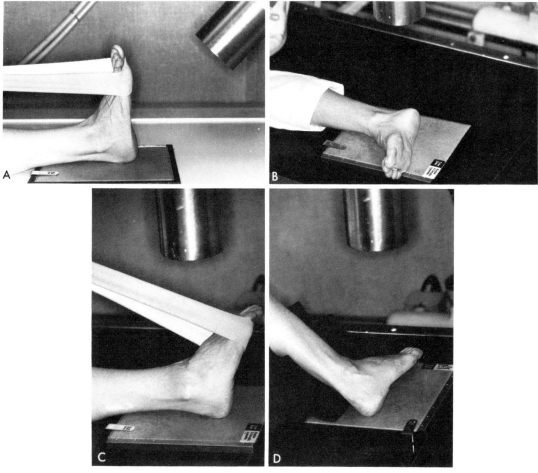

Figure 55–1. *(A) Axial view (plantodorsal projection). The ankle is dorsiflexed to 90 degrees by means of a strip of bandage placed around the ball of the foot. With the foot in a vertical axis to the film, the central x-ray beam is directed at an angle of 45 degrees through the area of the base of the fifth metatarsal and out just proximal to the ankle joint. (B) Lateral (mediolateral) view. The foot is positioned on its lateral surface, with the plantar surface perpendicular to the film. The central x-ray beam is directed vertically to the midportion of the os calcis. (C) Anteroposterior oblique view of the ankle (medial oblique projection, 45 degrees). The extremity is internally rotated 45 degrees medially by elevating the hip, so that the medial side of the ankle and foot rests against a 45-degree foam wedge. The ankle is dorsiflexed to 90 degrees, and the central x-ray beam is directed in a vertical axis to the ankle. (D) Oblique view of the calcaneocuboid joint (lateromedial oblique projection). The medial border of the foot is positioned on a film holder with a 45-degree foam wedge under the medial side of the foot. The central x-ray beam is directed vertically at an area just distal to the external malleolus.*

views. Generally, the tube is tilted at a 45-degree angle for this view. If the subastragalar joint is to be shown, the tube should be tilted to an angle of 55 degrees, and the technical factors relative to the exposure will be changed.

Lateral Views

Mediolateral View. This lateral view (Fig. 55–1B) taken with the lateral side closest to the film is used because the appearance of the foot is more familiar in this view. It will enable the fracture of the body involving the subastragalar joint to be classified as either (1) a joint depression fracture (Fig. 55–2), or (2) a tongue-type fracture (Figs. 55–3 to 55–6). There must be sufficient bone detail to enable one to determine if there is a rotation of a portion of the posterior facet, and if so, to what degree.

In the joint depression fracture, the degree of impaction of the posterosuperior margin of the posterior facet should be noted in those fractures having impaction or depression of most of the facet at the posterosuperior margin. One should also note the presence or absence of linear fracture lines involving the plantar surface of the os calcis anterior to the tuberosity and the site of involvement of the vertical fractures extending from some portion of the plantar surface anterior to the tuberosity upward in an irregular manner to the superior cortex of the os calcis, usually adjacent to the posterior margin of the subastragalar joint. It may show comminution of the superior cortex at the site of exit of the fracture, and the site of exit may involve the cortex at a more posterior location. It may also demonstrate a fracture involving the posterior tip of the astragalus. The mediolateral view may also show extension of linear or longitudinal fracture lines into the articular surface of the os calcis at the calcaneocuboid joint.

In tongue-type fractures, this view demonstrates extension posteriorly of the secondary fracture from the area of the crucial angle, described by Gissane,[3] out through the tuberosity, with tilting up of the long lever arm posteriorly (Fig. 55–5B). More rotation and impaction of the anteroinferior portion of some part of the posterior

facet may be noted near the crucial angle area (Fig. 55–5B).

The roentgenograms should be examined for evidence of extension of fracture lines obliquely from the area of the crucial angle to the plantar surface somewhere anterior to the posterior tuberosity. Again, in any lateral view, the bone detail must be sufficient to delineate the articular surface of the posterior facet so that rotation or impaction can be seen if it is present.

The mediolateral view enables the salient angle, or the tuber angle, described by Böhler,[5] to be measured. This angle is determined by drawing a line from the posterosuperior tip of the tuberosity through the highest point of the os calcis at the posterosuperior margin of the posterior facet, and by drawing a line from the highest point of the os calcis anteriorly through this same point of the os calcis at the posterosuperior margin of the posterior facet (Fig. 55–6C). Böhler referred to this complementary angle as ranging from 20 to 40 degrees in normal heels. The angle does vary, but the tuber angle of the opposite foot in my measurements in unilateral fractures has been close to 35 degrees. A five-degree variation in measurement might at times be within the normal limits of error. The angle is decreased in most fractures involving the subastragalar joint, and in severe injuries, there may be a minus tuber angle of considerable degree (Fig. 55–6B).

Although the tuber angle may be diminished or reversed from some upward displacement or tilting of the tuberosity, it is decreased most often from impaction or depression and rotation of the articular surface of the posterior facet. The superior portion of the displaced superomedial fragment will be one point to measure through (Fig. 55–2B).

Lateromedial View. The lateromedial projection taken with the medial side of the heel in contact with the film holder may possibly provide some indication as to which part of the posterior facet is rotated. There is often considerable rotation of the articular surface of the superomedial fragment. Since the medial side of the heel is closer to the film in this view, it should show rotation of the medial portion of the facet better. This view is used only for that

Text continued on page 1511

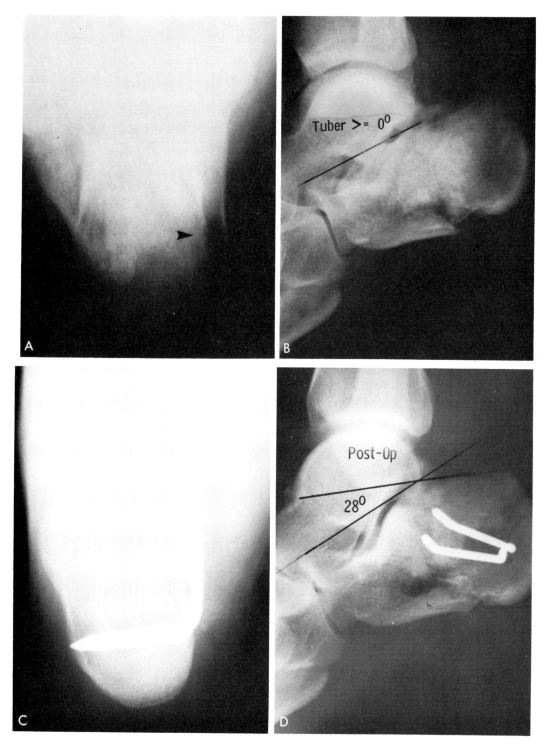

Figure 55–2. *Joint depression fracture of the os calcis. (A) This axial view is of poor quality because of technical factors, but it shows the typical medial displacement and overriding of the superomedial fragment of the os calcis (arrow), which, with the marked lateral expansion, produces a grossly widened heel. (B) The tuber angle is zero. An irregular fracture line extends from anterior to the tuberosity up to the posterior aspect of the subastragalar joint, where there is comminution of the cortex. A segment containing articular cartilage of the posterior facet is rotated and impacted down into the cancellous bone. (C) The postoperative axial view shows a good restoration of the medial contour and a narrowed heel. Two staples gave a more secure fixation. (D) The postoperative lateral view shows a dead space present after elevation of the impacted rotated facet, a tuber angle correction of 28 degrees, good contour of the heel, and good appearance of the subastragalar joint.*

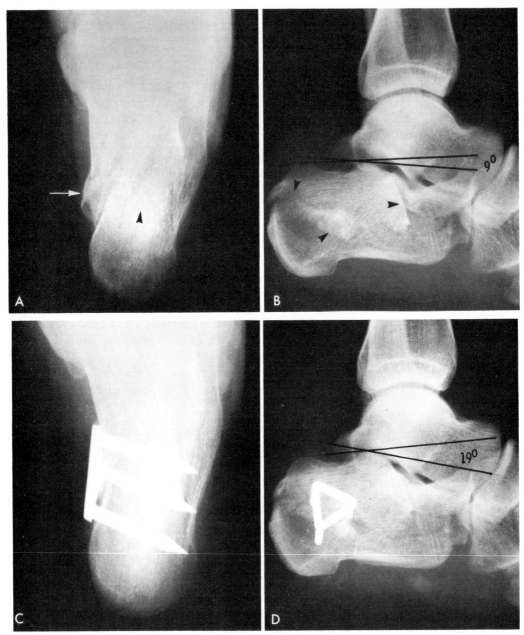

Figure 55–3.   *Tongue-type fracture of the os calcis. (A) There is gross medial displacement and overriding of the superomedial fragment, with comminution of its tip; a long, oblique fracture, extending from the medial cortex into the articular surface of the posterior facet; lateral cortical bulge; widening of the heel; and some impaction (arrow). (B) The lateral view shows displacement and rotation of the articular surface of the posterior facet (arrow); the linear fracture extending from the area of the crucial angle posteriorly through the upper third of the tuberosity (arrow) with some upward tilting of this tongue fragment; increased density from overlap of the superomedial fragment (arrow); and a tuber angle of 9 degrees. (C) The postoperative axial view demonstrates a good reduction of the superomedial fragment and a narrow heel. (D) The postoperative lateral view shows incomplete elevation of the impacted portion of the posterior facet anteriorly, reflected in a tuber angle of only 19 degrees. A triangular staple was used for fixation.*

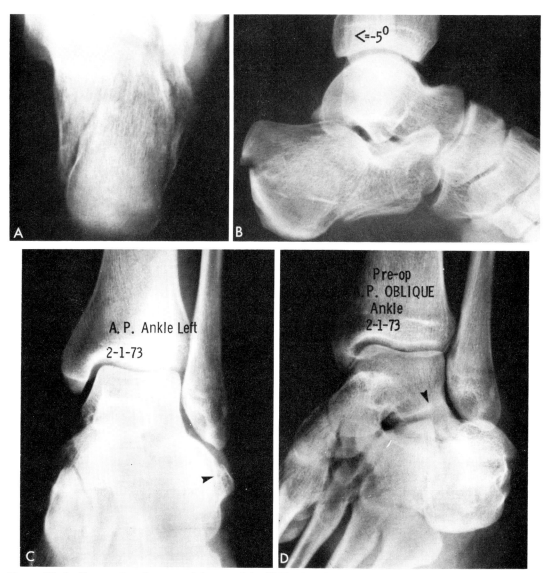

Figure 55–4. Tongue-type fracture of the os calcis. (A) The heel is somewhat shortened because of abnormal angulation of the x-ray tube but shows marked medial displacement and overriding, impaction of cancellous bone, and lateral cortical bulge. Some of the impacted bone trabeculae are directed laterally to accent the lateral cortical bulge. (B) The tongue fragment is displaced posteriorly and tilted upward; the articular surface is tilted downward, but sufficient bone detail is not shown. A linear fracture is present anterior to the plantar surface of the tuberosity. The tuber angle is reduced to minus 5 degrees. (C) The anteroposterior view of the ankle shows lateral cortical bulge (arrow) low on the os calcis below the fibula. (D) The anteroposterior oblique view of the ankle demonstrates the gross displacement, impaction, and rotation of the lateral 7 mm of the articular surface of the posterior facet (arrow).

Illustration continued on following page

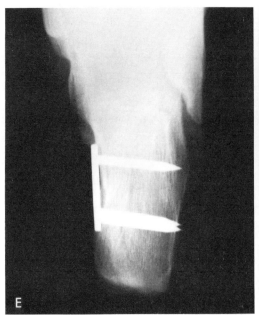

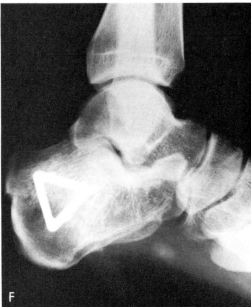

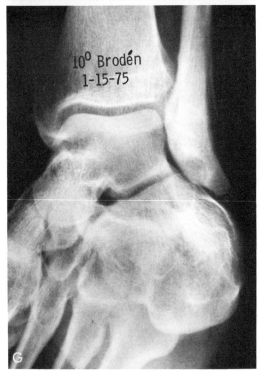

Figure 55–4 Continued. (E) and (F) The fractures have healed. The contour of the heel is excellent. The tuber angle is 25 degrees, a correction of 30 degrees. Subastragalar joint motion is normal. (G) Because of the patient's age (33), the staple was removed after union of the fracture. The 10-degree Brodén I projection taken two years after injury and after removal of the staple shows a level articular surface of the posterior facet when compared with D. No hypertrophic changes are present. The patient wears cowboy boots with no problem.

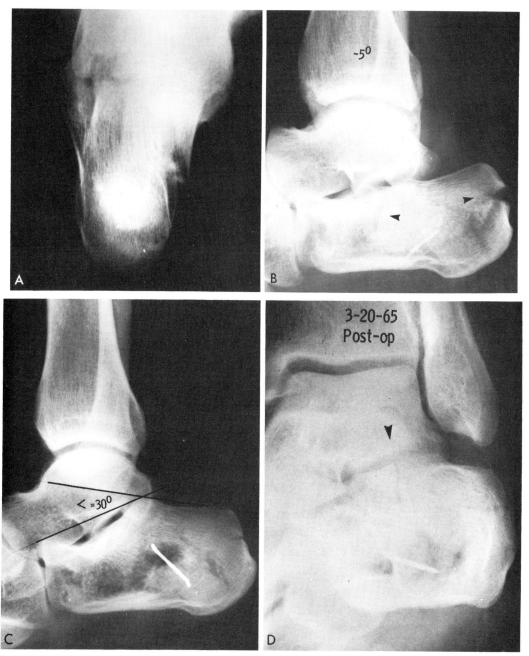

Figure 55–5. *Tongue-type fracture of the os calcis. (A) The tip of the superomedial fragment is comminuted, displaced medially, and overriding. Impaction is noted in the tuberosity. The heel is widened. (B) The long lever arm is tilted up posteriorly (arrow), with rotation and impaction anteriorly near the crucial angle (arrow), creating a minus-5-degree tuber angle. (C) Following open reduction of the superomedial fragment on the day of injury, there is excellent reduction of the rotated segment of the articular surface of the posterior facet and long lever arm. There is a definite dead space after reduction. The fixation staple is too small in diameter. The tuber angle has been increased from minus 5 degrees to 30 degrees. (D) A postoperative anteroposterior oblique view of the ankle shows a level articular surface at the site of the fracture (arrow).*

Illustration continued on following page

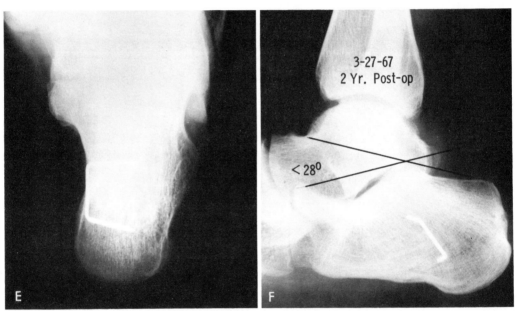

Figure 55–5 *Continued. (E) and F) Two years after injury, there is normal subastragalar joint motion and excellent contour of the heel, and the patient had no particular complaints. Physical activity was unrestricted. The patient returned to regular work three months after the operation.*

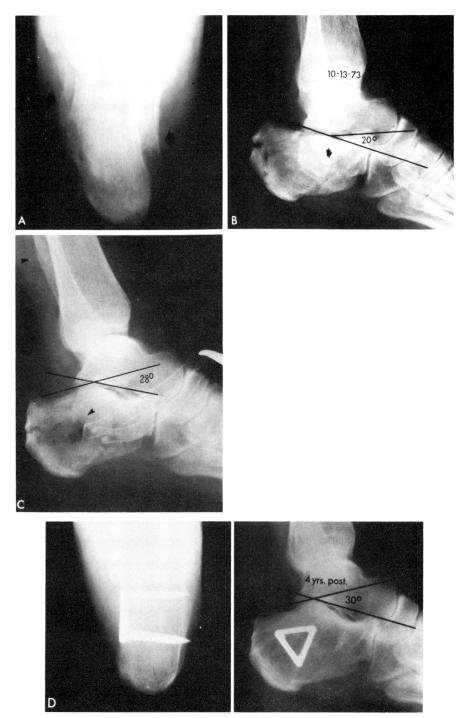

Figure 55–6. *Tongue-type fracture of the os calcis. (A) The axial view demonstrates expansion laterally of thin cortical bone and medial displacement and overriding of the superomedial fragment (arrows) to produce shortening and widening of the heel. (B) There is rotation and impaction of the articular surface shown less desirably (arrow) and tilting upward posteriorly of the long lever arm to produce a minus-20-degree tuber angle. (C) A postoperative lateral roentgenogram taken during surgery shows the pattern of involvement of the medial cortex in tongue-type fractures (arrow). After reduction of the superomedial fragment, there is a 28-degree tuber joint angle, a correction of 48 degrees. The rubber dam drain about the vascular plexus shows its location in relation to the fracture. Concomitant injuries were fractures of the fibula (arrow) and lumbar spine. (D) Four years following injury, there is normal contour of the heel, normal subastragalar joint motion, and normal function, and the patient has no complaints.*

Illustration continued on following page

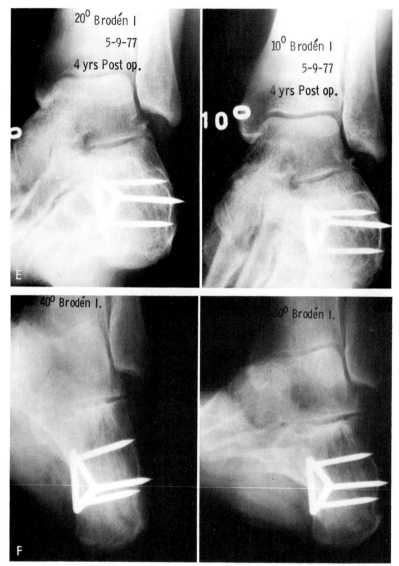

Figure 55–6 *Continued.* *(E) Ten- and 20-degree Brodén I views show very little in the way of changes in the lateral portion of the subastragalar joint four years following operative treatments. (F) The 30- and 40-degree Brodén I views show no hypertrophic lipping at the lateral margin of the subastragalar joint.*

purpose and in an effort to possibly obtain a little more information about the fracture.

Anteroposterior View of the Ankle

This view is made only for the supplemental information that may be obtained about the presence or the degree of lateral cortical bulge or expansion of the lateral cortex of the os calcis (Fig. 55–4C).

Anteroposterior Oblique View of the Ankle

This view (Fig. 55–1C), taken with the leg internally rotated 45 degrees and with the central x-ray beam directed just distal and anterior to the lateral malleolus, is a simple view to obtain and will demonstrate, through the superimposed astragalus, the articular surface of the posterior facet in most instances and will show the site of involvement of the oblique fracture. It will demonstrate irregularity of the articular surface laterally where there is rotation and impaction of the lateral portion of the posterior facet. It is a necessary and informative view that is to be taken both preoperatively and postoperatively (Fig. 55–4D).

Anteroposterior and Medial Oblique Views of the Calcaneocuboid Joint

Since there are linear fracture lines that sometimes extend anteriorly into the calcaneocuboid joint in fractures of the body of the os calcis that involve the subastragalar joint, it is best to have an anteroposterior view centered over the calcaneocuboid joint and a lateromedial oblique projection of the joint, in addition to the lateral view of the os calcis (Fig. 55–1D).

Special Views

Brodén Projections I and II. The technique for these projections, according to Brodén (1949) and as presented by Thorén, is as follows:

Projection I: The patient supine. Leg and foot are turned 45 degrees inwards with right angle flexion at the ankle joint. The central ray is directed against a point 2–3 cm. caudoven-

trally to the lateral malleolus. Four pictures are taken with the tube angled 40, 30, 20, and 10 degrees, respectively, towards the head.

The picture taken with the tube angled 40 degrees shows the anterior part of the talocalcaneal joint, the picture with the tube angled 10 degrees reproducing the posterior part. Some of the pictures (generally those with the tube angled 30 or 20 degrees) make the articulation between the sustentaculum and the talus visible.

Projection II: The patient supine. Leg and foot are turned 45 degrees outwards with right angle flexion at the ankle joint. The central ray is directed against a point 2 cm. caudoventrally to the medial malleolus with the tube angled about 15 degrees towards the head. It is suitable to take 3 pictures with a difference of 3–4 degrees. One of these will, as a rule, be perfect.[17]

In the Brodén projection I, the anterior part of the posterior facet is shown best in the roentgenogram taken with the central x-ray beam in the 40-degree tilt toward the head (Fig. 55–6E,F and Fig. 55–7A,B). The roentgenogram taken with the central x-ray beam in the 10-degree tilt toward the head may demonstrate the posterior part of the facet best.

Classifications

Perhaps one of the reasons why so much difficulty has been encountered in the treatment of fractures of the os calcis involving the subastragalar joint is a lack of understanding of the pathology of these fractures. Numerous classifications of fractures of the os calcis have been made, including those by Böhler,[5] Palmer,[23] Widén,[9] Rowe and associates,[24] Warrick and Bremner,[25] Watson-Jones,[26] Lindsay and Dewar,[27] Allan,[28] Essex-Lopresti,[3] and Soeur and Remy.[20]

Widén wrote: "The temptation arises to subscribe to that much quoted opinion of Cotton's (1916), 'To formulate and classify these fractures is about as useful as classifying cracks in a walnut after the nutcracker is finished with it.' "[9] It is, however, necessary to have a classification — but one that is more uniform and somewhat anatomic or descriptive in nature so that orthopaedic surgeons can readily recognize the type of fracture and can communicate freely in efforts to study and to treat these severe and often disabling fractures

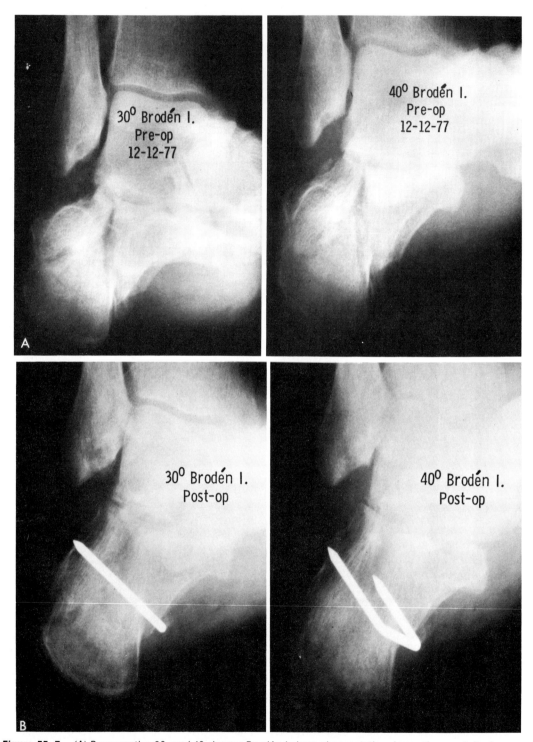

Figure 55–7. (A) Preoperative 30- and 40-degree Brodén I views show rotation, impaction, and displacement of the lateral portion of the posterior facet of the os calcis. (B) The 30- and 40-degree Brodén I views taken two months following open reduction and staple fixation through a medial approach show correction of the deformity.

more effectively. Since it is the os calcis fracture involving the subastragalar joint that presents problems in treatment, classification of these fractures is even more important.

The Superomedial Fragment and the Primary Fracture

In all the classifications just noted, there is no mention of the most constant and significant deformity in fractures of the body of the os calcis involving the subastragalar joint. This deformity consists of medial displacement, overriding, and rotation of what I refer to — because of its anatomic location — as "the superomedial fragment." It consists of the medial portion of the primary fracture, a fracture that originates in the medial cortex posterior to the sustentaculum tali and extends anteriorly obliquely upward and outward, usually into some portion of the articular surface of the posterior facet. This deformity occurs in the majority (almost 90 per cent) of fractures involving the subastragalar joint, in both joint depression and tongue-type fractures (see Figure 55–9A).

From the marked frequency of occurrence of the oblique shearing fracture alone, I would consider it to be the primary fracture. It was considered the primary fracture by Palmer,[23] Widén,[9] Warrick and Bremner in their classification of 300 fractures of the os calcis,[25] and Soeur and Remy in a study of 93 thalamic fractures.[20] Shearing and compression occurred in 98 per cent of the thalamic fractures studied.[20] Widén found a diagonal shearing fracture in more than 90 per cent of 73 fractures through the body of the os calcis, 40 of which were treated by open reduction.[9]

From my observation and study of more than 90 open reductions of fractures of the os calcis, I believe that the oblique shearing fracture is the primary fracture mechanism, in contrast to Gissane and Essex-Lopresti's views that the primary fracture is produced by sudden forceful eversion of the subtalar joint, allowing the sharp lateral spur of the talus to be driven inferiorly into the crucial angle of the calcaneus (described by Gissane), splitting it along the lateral cortex of the bone.[3] Essex-Lopresti stated, "At the moment of greatest compression, the sustentacular half is depressed down to the level of the outer half, but on release, the soft tissue resilience in the foot causes the sustentacular half to be drawn up by its intact attachment to the talus."[3] I do not believe that this is true. What happens is that the sustentacular portion, or superomedial fragment, is sheared off, displaced medially, rotates, and overrides the cortex of the lateral main body at the site of the fracture on the medial cortical surface of the os calcis (see Figure 55–9A). It is impacted in this position, often rather firmly. This impaction is demonstrated to some extent in the post-injury roentgenograms and I have seen it repeatedly in performing open reduction of these fractures through a medial approach. This deformity of the superomedial fragment is considerable.

As the superomedial fragment is displaced medially, rotates, and overrides, the lateral articular surface of the talus exerts a great deal of concentrated force on the part of the articular surface of the posterior facet that lies lateral to the oblique fracture line that goes into the joint; this lateral portion of the posterior facet may be impacted in different patterns, depending on the size of the superomedial fragment, its displacement, and the force exerted. In my opinion, it does not appear that sufficient eversion of the subastragalar joint could occur to allow this fracture to take place as described by Essex-Lopresti until after the superomedial fragment is sheared off and displaced.

The area where the oblique fracture enters the posterior facet varies, but I believe that it is often far more lateral than has been assumed in the past. The superomedial fragment most often contains much more of the articular surface of the posterior facet than the lateral fragment. Little attention has been given to the superomedial fragment, which contains the sustentaculum, probably because it was thought by such a great surgeon as Böhler and by others that the sustentaculum tali remained in position.[5] This explained the use of strong traction in an effort to pull the main lateral fragment down. It was the superomedial fragment that should have been reduced back to the main lateral fragment.

In discussing these fractures, it is well to mention that a small percentage of fractures of the os calcis involving the subastragalar joint in which there is marked impaction of a portion of the lateral part of the posterior facet do not have medial displacement of the superomedial fragment but have a fracture of the medial cortex (see Figure 55–15) and may have oblique fracture lines extending from the area of the tuberosity up to the subastragalar joint.

Joint Depression (Fig. 55–9F) and Tongue-Type Fractures (Fig. 55–9G)

Essex-Lopresti made a definite contribution to the understanding of these fractures when he classified fractures involving the articular surface of the subastragalar joint into (1) joint depression fractures and (2) tongue-type fractures. These designations provide a better mental picture of the fractures than the Type I and Type II designations, respectively, given by Palmer[23] for the same fractures.

Joint depression fractures and tongue-type fractures have much in common. In the vast majority of instances, both are fractures that involve the medial cortex of the os calcis and extend anteriorly and obliquely upward and outward — usually into some portion of the articular surface of the posterior facet. In both, there is usually medial displacement, overriding, and rotation of the superomedial fragment as well as lateral cortical expansion from impaction of cancellous bone or a portion of the articular surface of the posterior facet. There is also widening of the heel, diminution of the tuber joint angle, and irregularities of the articular surface of the posterior facet in both types of fractures.

The pattern of involvement of the medial cortical surface of the os calcis is different in the two fractures. In the joint depression fracture, the fracture line usually extends from the plantar surface anterior to the tuberosity upward in an irregular manner to the superior cortex, just posterior to or adjacent to the posterior margin of the subastragalar joint. The exit of the fracture line may at times be located a little more posteriorly. In the tongue-type fracture, the posteroinferior tip of the superomedial fragment is located more posteriorly on the medial cortex of the os calcis (see Figure 55–6C).

The size of the superomedial fragment influences the type of joint depression present. In those fractures in which the oblique shearing fracture extends far laterally or to the lateral margin of the subastragalar joint, there is likely to be more impaction at the posterosuperior margin of the facet (see Figure 55–14A[R]. In other joint depression fractures, there may be severe rotation and impaction of the lateral portion of the posterior facet so that the impacted fragment faces forward and is literally countersunk (see Figure 55–15A). In some fractures, there may be an irregular, somewhat mosaic pattern of involvement, which cannot be demonstrated roentgenographically (Fig. 55–8).

In tongue-type fractures, there is a distinguishing secondary fracture line that extends posteriorly from the area of the crucial angle out through the upper part of the tuberosity posteriorly. This creates a tongue-like, long lever arm, which may be tilted up posteriorly and down anteriorly, where it contains part of the articular surface of the posterior facet. It was described by Essex-Lopresti as containing the outer half of the articular surface of the posterior facet,[3] but I have noted the articular surface to be much smaller on several occasions (see Figures 55–4D, G and 55–7). There is a significant bony connection between the long lever arm and the superomedial fragment, because open reduction alone of the superomedial fragment through a medial approach has resulted in excellent reduction of the tongue-like lever arm in several instances (see Figure 55–6C).

In tongue-type fractures, the pattern of joint depression is more consistent. It is usually composed of the impaction or depression of the lateral portion of the posterior facet, progressively more from the posterosuperior to the anteroinferior end. Both tongue-type and joint depression fractures may have oblique fracture lines extending from the area of the crucial angle obliquely toward the plantar surface.

In joint depression fractures, there may be linear fractures of the plantar surface of the os calcis, and linear fracture lines may extend anteriorly into the articular surface at the calcaneocuboid joint.

Although considerably more is known

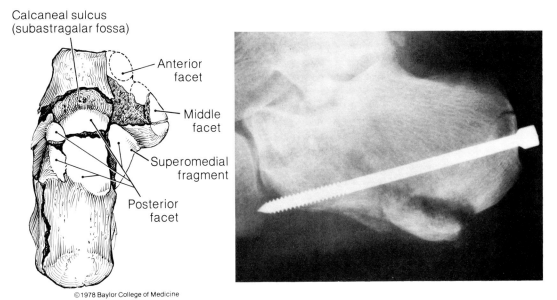

Calcaneal sulcus
(subastragalar fossa)

Anterior
facet

Middle
facet

Superomedial
fragment

Posterior
facet

©1978 Baylor College of Medicine

Figure 55–8. *This joint depression fracture caused by a severe explosion force seen after primary treatment by axial pin reduction was characterized by intractable pain, sloughing of skin over the lateral side of the heel with exposure of cancellous bone, and necrosis of all muscles under the plantar fascia, which resulted in amputation. Continued severe pain following reduction of a fracture of the os calcis may be a bad omen.*

The drawing (left) of the partially united, dissected amputation specimen shows five separate fragments on the articular surface of the posterior facet; a transverse fracture near the sinus tarsi area; comminution of the lateral cortex and lateral cortical bulge; and an incomplete fracture of the middle facet. Part of the sustentaculum tali is missing; it was lost at dissection. The superomedial fragment, smaller than usual, was grossly displaced and could not be replaced in the position shown in the drawing until the axial pin and displaced medial and plantar fragments were removed. The roentgenographic appearance in the lateral view (right) does not suggest the severe deformity that was present.

about joint depression and tongue-type fractures than was previously known, it may be possible to know more when the same fractures that are seen clinically can be reproduced on amputated or cadaver specimens. I have such a project underway.

Treatment

In general, the treatment necessary for fractures of the os calcis is best determined on an individual basis, and each fracture should be considered as an individual problem. First, an accurate determination of the involvement or deformity must be made. Is the deformity sufficient to require treatment? If so, how can it best be accomplished?

Notwithstanding some statements to the contrary, I feel very strongly that the better the reduction or the less the deformity, the greater the likelihood of a better result. Many of the os calcis fractures involving the subastragalar joint are severe, present

problems in treatment, and require considerable expertise in management.

The results from treatment should not be expected to be the same irrespective of the methods used. Methods of treatment that have little prospect of producing real improvement should be discarded in favor of a method that, theoretically at least, has a better chance to improve the deformities. Significant deformities that are likely to produce considerable disability are not accurately reducible by closed manipulative procedures or by the use of pins, spikes, or instruments, and they will require operative treatment if a better reduction and a better result are to be obtained.

Treatment of fractures of the os calcis will be discussed on the following descriptive basis or classification (Fig. 55–9):

1. Fractures of the tuberosity
   a. Posteroinferior (Fig. 55–9B)
   b. Posterosuperior
      i. Beak (Fig. 55–9C)
      ii. Avulsion (Fig. 55–9D)
2. Fractures of the body of the os calcis

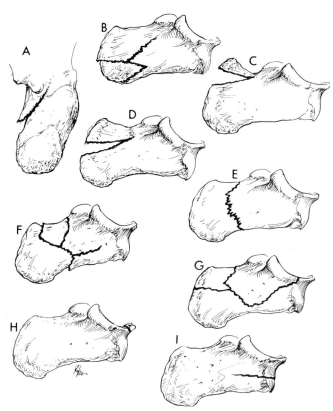

Figure 55–9. *Schematic interpretation of fractures of the os calcis. (A) The axial view shows the oblique fracture that originates in the medial cortex and extends upward and outward as well as anteriorly, usually into some portion of the articular surface of the posterior facet to form the superomedial fragment. There is medial displacement, overriding, and rotation of the superomedial fragment in probably 90 per cent of tongue-type and joint depression fractures; and this is the most constant and significant deformity of these fractures. The oblique fracture usually enters the articular surface of the posterior facet at a point more laterally than shown in this drawing. There is some lateral cortical bulge shown, which is the result of impaction of bone inside the usually comminuted lateral cortex.*

(B–I) Medial views. (B) Fractures of the posteroinferior tuberosity may be associated with an oblique fracture extending up toward the subastragalar joint and often occur as part of a joint depression fracture. The posteroinferior tuberosity fragment is usually displaced medially and may be displaced anteriorly. It usually involves the posteroinferior medial tuberosity. (C) Fractures of the posterosuperior tuberosity occur as a beak fracture and, (D) as an avulsion fracture when the insertion of the tendo Achillis is involved. (E) Fractures of the body of the os calcis without subastragalar joint involvement are not seen frequently. (F) The pattern of involvement of the medial cortex varies in a joint depression fracture. One pattern shown here was drawn from its appearance in the postoperative or postreduction lateral roentgenogram. (G) The pattern involvement of the medial cortex is different in a tongue-type fracture. This drawing was made from a postoperative or postreduction lateral roentgenogram. The fracture of the medial cortex originates more posteriorly than in a joint depression fracture. (H) Fractures of the anterior process or superior tip are seldom seen. They are more like sprain-fractures and are thought to be produced by force exerted on the bifurcate ligament. (I) In joint depression fractures, there may be linear fracture lines extending into the anterior articular surface. Gross displacement is not usually present, and special treatment is seldom necessary. They are not likely to occur as an isolated fracture as shown here.

without subastragalar joint involvement (Fig. 55–9E)

3. Fractures of the body of the os calcis with subastragalar joint involvement
   a. Medial displacement, overriding, and rotation of the superomedial fragment (Fig. 55–9A)
      i. Joint depression fracture (Fig. 55–9F)
      ii. Tongue-type fracture (Fig. 55–9G)
   b. Others
4. Fractures of the anterior end of the os calcis
   a. Anterior process (beak fractures) (Fig. 55–9H)
   b. Linear fractures extending into the calcaneocuboid joint (Fig. 55–9I)

With the exception of fractures of the body of the os calcis involving the subastragalar joint, to which there has been added "medial displacement, overriding,

and rotation of the superomedial fragment," all other portions of the classification may have been referred to by someone else at one time or another and are present to some extent in other classifications.

Fractures of the Tuberosity

Posteroinferior Tuberosity (Fig. 55–9B). These fractures of the posteromedial inferior tuberosity were listed as "vertical fractures of the tuberosity" by Warrick and Bremner and were noted in 31 of the 300 fractures analyzed by them, an incidence of 10 per cent.[25] The diagnosis should be evident from the history, clinical findings, and roentgenograms. Treatment is based on the degree of deformity present. The fracture, if associated with significant displacement, may not be an isolated fracture but rather one associated with fractures or fissure lines involving the body of the os calcis; this can produce a diminished tuber joint angle (Fig. 55–10). Not only may the posteromedial inferior tuberosity be involved, but there can also be associated incomplete impacted fractures of the plantar portion of the tuberosity. I would consider deformity from medial displacement of the fragment to be more significant in women than in men as far as reduction is concerned. If there is significant displacement, I doubt that it is correctable by a snug, molded cast to which the compression is applied. With significant displacement that appears amenable to surgical correction, open reduction through a medial approach and internal fixation are indicated (Fig. 55–10).

Fractures of the posteroinferior tuberosity (Fig. 55–9B) usually involve a fracture of the medial cortex extending obliquely up toward the subastragalar joint. The inferior tuberosity is displaced medially and that, plus the oblique fracture of the medial cortex, is the reason to expose the fracture from the medial side. The medial displacement is noted in the axial roentgenogram. There may be anterior displacement, presumably from the plantar fascia, and anterior displacement is difficult to reduce and maintain. With correction of the medial displacement, staple fixation through the tuberosity and the cortex of the body of the os calcis should afford a stable reduction. It is important to restore the posteroinferior tuberosity to its normal position, because that is the point where the heel strikes in a normal gait. The incision may need to be projected a little lower, posteriorly, in the approach to

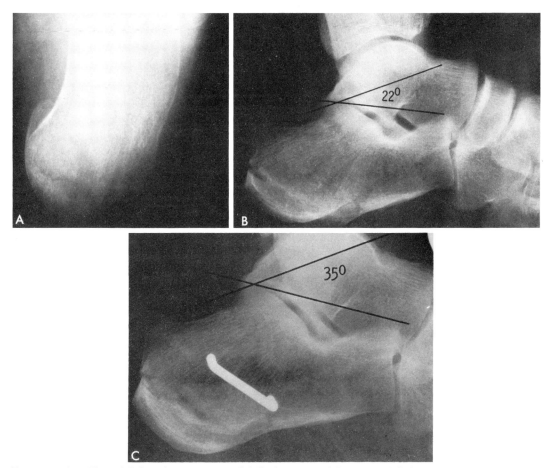

Figure 55–10. *The axial view shows some medial displacement of the posteroinferior tuberosity. (B) The lateral view shows impaction and displacement of the inferior posterior tuberosity and also a fracture immediately posterior to the subastragalar joint, which has reduced the tuber angle to 22 degrees. (C) Following open reduction and staple fixation through a medial approach, the contour of the heel is very much better. There was a linear fracture extending from the tuberosity toward the posterior facet.*

this type of fracture. It is associated with some joint depression fractures. Early weight bearing in a walking cast or a 5-inch top lace-up shoe will expedite recovery by preventing demineralization from non–weight bearing.

Posterosuperior Tuberosity (Fig. 55–9C, D). These fractures have been referred to as horizontal fractures. They are beak fractures when the insertion of the tendo Achillis is not involved and avulsion fractures when the insertion of the tendo Achillis is involved. Fractures of the posterosuperior tuberosity are relatively uncommon. Rowe and associates noted an incidence of 3 per cent;[24] Warrick and Bremner reported a 1

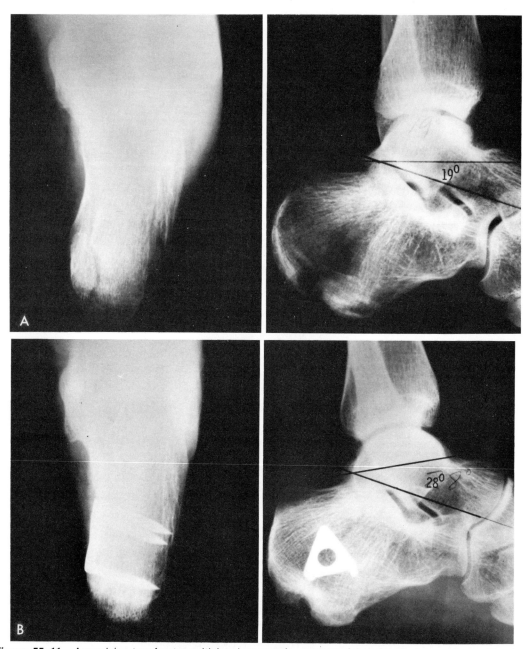

Figure 55–11. *An avulsion-type fracture with involvement of a segment of the posterior tuberosity resulting in a tuber angle of 19 degrees. There is displacement of the medial cortex at the posterior portion. (B) After open reduction and staple fixation, the fracture united with a good medial contour of the os calcis. The tuber angle was not quite corrected. The staple is located well posteriorly.*

per cent incidence.[25] Böhler referred to the open beak fracture as "a typical fracture by direct injury."[5] The lateral roentgenogram is the primary means by which the fracture is assessed.

When gross displacement is present, I believe that open reduction and internal fixation by suitable means are indicated. In the beak fracture, a screw might be a more desirable means of fixation. It has been replaced by the use of sutures.

In the fracture in which there is more of an element of avulsion, open reduction through a medial approach with staple fixation is indicated. With adequate fixation, immediate weight bearing in a walking cast, which is replaced in four weeks by a 5-inch top lace-up shoe, will expedite recovery (Fig. 55–11).

Fractures of the Body of the Os Calcis Without Subastragalar Joint Involvement
(Fig. 55–9E)

I do not have ready statistical information from my own experience relative to the incidence, findings, type of treatment, and results in this classification of os calcis fractures. I would think that it would not be frequently encountered to the degree that it would require special treatment. Warrick and Bremner, however, reported an incidence of 16 per cent.[25] If the tuberosity is displaced significantly, it might very well be pulled down and secured by axial pin fixation. As in any fracture, early weight bearing, when it will not worsen the deformity appreciably, will do much to expedite recovery.

Fractures of the Body of the Os Calcis with Subastragalar Joint Involvement

This classification includes those fractures with medial displacement, overriding, and rotation of the superomedial fragment, i.e., joint depression fractures (Fig. 55–9F) and tongue-type fractures (Fig. 55–9G). In both joint depression fractures and tongue-type fractures in which there is sufficient deformity to require reduction, it is my opinion that open reduction and internal fixation should be performed, because it is not possible to correct the deformity adequately by closed manipulative procedures or with pins or spikes.

When there is roentgenologic evidence of medial displacement, overriding, and rotation of the superomedial fragment, operative treatment utilizing my method of "open reduction and internal fixation with staples, using a medial approach" is indicated. It is my opinion that medial displacement, overriding, and rotation of the superomedial fragment cannot be adequately corrected and maintained by a surgical procedure done from the lateral side of the heel. However, it is possible in a definite percentage of cases to correct or improve the deformities involving the lateral portion of the heel through instrumentation or leverage performed through a medial incision.

If the deformity incident to the depression or impaction and rotation of the lateral part of the posterior facet cannot be adequately corrected from the medial approach, the fracture should be treated through an additional lateral incision.

Open Reduction and Internal Fixation with Staples, Using a Medial Approach

This is a new method of treatment for these fractures of the body of the os calcis involving the subastragalar joint, but I have, in fact, used it since 1958. It is diametrically opposite to the open reduction done through a lateral approach introduced by Morestein in 1902,[29] which has since been used with some modifications. It is diametrically opposite because of the significant and rather constant deformity involving the medial side of the heel, that is, medial displacement, overriding, and rotation of the superomedial fragment. With more medial displacement and overriding of the superomedial fragment, there will be more impaction of the underlying bone (see Figure 55–9A).

The indications for this operative procedure are significant deformity and medial displacement and overriding of the superomedial fragment. Extensive comminution of the medial cortical surfaces of the os calcis makes it very difficult to reduce the fracture, to determine when it is adequately reduced, and to insert fixation that will efficiently maintain position.

Surgery should be carried out as soon as possible following injury, preferably on the day of injury. With immediate surgery, reduction can be accomplished more easily and to a better degree; prompt relief of pain may be obtained; and soft-tissue damage from extreme swelling may be prevented.

The operative procedure is performed through a 2- to 3-inch incision in the midportion of the medial side of the heel, somewhat in line with the longitudinal axis of the os calcis (Fig. 55–12A). The central portion of the incision should be over the site of medial displacement and overriding of the superomedial fragment. Because of the different pattern of involvement of the medial cortex in tongue-type fractures, the incision may be shorter and more posteriorly located for these fractures than for joint depression fractures (see Figure 55–6C). The fascia is incised in the line of the incision, and this is done very carefully in order to avoid injury to the vertical neurovascular plexus that is immediately beneath the fascia and near the

anterior and middle thirds of the incision (Fig. 55–12A). (See also Figure 55–6C.) The vascular plexus is mobilized above and below and is retracted with a rubber dam drain (Fig. 55–12B). The muscle fibers of the quadratus plantae and the abductor hallucis are separated down to the medial cortex of the os calcis, and the medial cortical surfaces of the os calcis adjacent to the fracture are denuded of soft tissue with a small, thin osteotome. This is done sufficiently to reveal the medial displacement, overriding, and rotation at the fracture site. The field of vision in the inferosuperior plane is very limited (Fig. 55–12C).

Reduction is accomplished by first introducing a very small, blunt instrument — a periosteal elevator or joker — obliquely into the oblique fracture line, into the cancellous substance of the os calcis, and cautiously mobilizing the su-

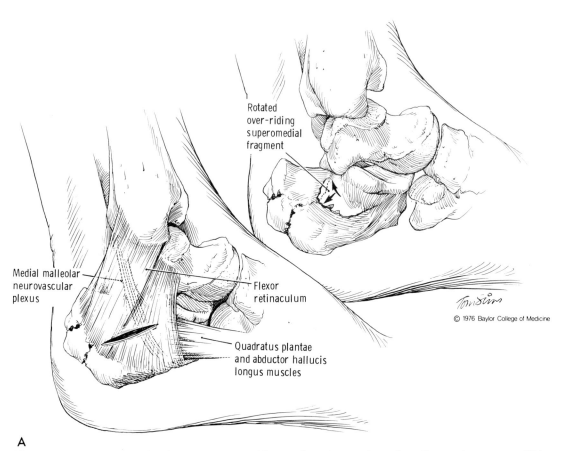

Rotated
over-riding
superomedial
fragment

Medial malleolar
neurovascular
plexus

Flexor
retinaculum

Quadratus plantae
and abductor hallucis
longus muscles

© 1976 Baylor College of Medicine

A

Figure 55–12. *(A) The medial displacement, overriding, and rotation are drawn from the roentgenogram of this tongue-type fracture (arrows). The approximate location of the incision, fascia, and vascular plexus is shown.*
Illustration continued on opposite page

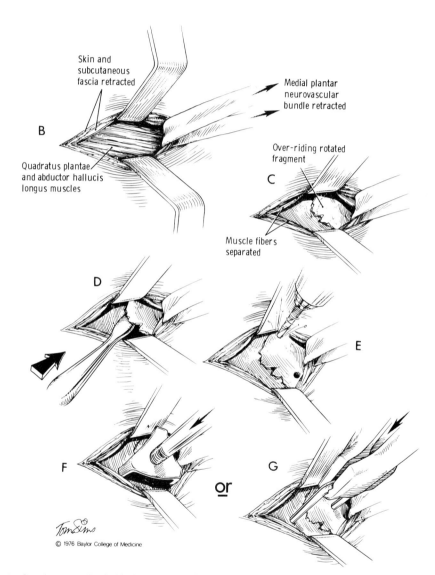

© 1976 Baylor College of Medicine

Figure 55–12 *Continued. (B–G) Various steps of the operative procedure. (C–G) The exposure of the medial cortex in the inferosuperior plane is very limited.*

Illustration continued on following page

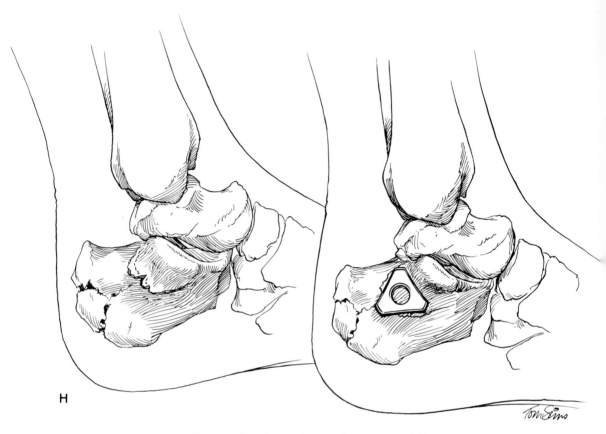

H

Figure 55–12 *Continued. (H) The area of cortical surface on the superomedial fragment where staple tines can be inserted is limited above by the tendon of the flexor hallucis longus and the posterior tibial vessels and nerve crossing in the sulcus and continuing under the middle facet. The subastragalar joint is not exposed.*

peromedial fragment to some extent. A Freer tonsil dissector or a small Cloward periosteal elevator may be used. The fracture is opened up a little bit, so to speak (Fig. 55–12D). The irregular, thin cortical edges of the superomedial fragment are treated gently to avoid breaking a tip that can be used to determine when overriding and rotation have been corrected. At times, it is like fitting a jigsaw puzzle together.

The presence of any impacted or depressed areas of bone or articular cartilage and whether or not this impaction, if present, has caused lateral cortical bulge or expansion must be determined from proper preoperative roentgenograms. The impacted or depressed areas should be elevated, and since the elevation is done blindly, using an instrument for leverage, the type and degree of force is determined from a careful analysis of the preoperative roentgenograms. The small Cloward peri-

osteal elevator is introduced obliquely into the oblique fracture line toward and under the area of impaction demonstrated in the preoperative roentgenograms. If the impacted or depressed segment of bone driven like a wedge down inside the thin lateral cortical wall of the os calcis is elevated adequately, there will be a dead space; the lateral cortical bulge is then corrected by bimanual compression.

Following correction of impacted or depressed areas, the medial displacement, overriding, and rotation of the superomedial fragment are reduced by cautious leverage. Some knowledge of the degree of reduction is obtained from inspection and palpation of the heel, but reduction must be verified by roentgenograms, which at the least should include an axial and lateral view of the heel and an anteroposterior oblique view of the ankle.

Because the reduction might be lost

from positioning of the heel for the re-check roentgenograms, a staple is inserted for partial fixation. Because triangular three-point and four-point staples made to specifications have not been readily available in the past, it has been necessary most often to use two-point staples. The staples should be 7/64 inch in diameter, should have very sharp points for scoring the cortical surface of the os calcis, and should not be more than 3/4 inch in overall width. Wider staples cause technical problems in insertion because of the limited exposure of the medial cortex of the os calcis. The staples should be available in 1-inch, 1⅛-inch, 1¼-inch, and 1⅜-inch lengths.*

The sites of insertion of the staples is influenced by the multiple irregular fracture lines and the roentgenologic appearance of the fractures. In general, the staples should be inserted in an axis that is most likely to be best for prevention of both recurrence of displacement at the fracture site and recurrence of depression of articular surfaces.

The tip of the superomedial fragment is often very thin. The tines of the staple must have adequate purchase in the lateral fragment. If possible, the points of the staple should be well away from the fracture line as far as the superomedial fragment is concerned in order to prevent the cortex from splitting out of the drill hole. The medial cortex only of the superomedial fragment is drilled at a scored point, using a drill point that is usually 1/64 inch smaller or the same size as the staple tine. The size drill selected is a matter of surgical judgment. The tuberosity side of the cortex is drilled with a drill $1/64$ inch smaller than the staple tine (Fig. 55–12E).

After roentgenologic confirmation of a satisfactory reduction in all views (the roentgenograms must be of diagnostic quality), the staple insertion is completed. A special staple holder that does not obscure the field of vision in the operative field is helpful (Fig. 55–12 F,G). A four-point, triangular, or one or more two-point staples may be indicated for fixation. Joint depression fractures may require more

secure fixation from multiple tines or more than one staple. The ordinary "tabletop" staple, the Stone staple, and staples with

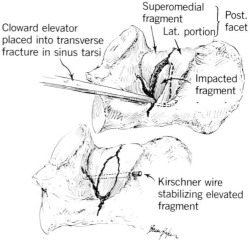

Figure 55–13. *Surgical reduction of a depressed impacted segment of cartilage and bone in the lateral portion of the posterior facet of the os calcis from a lateral approach. This illustration shows the articular surface of the posterior facet and the sinus tarsi area. The superomedial fragment is shown in a nondisplaced position, but in most instances, it is grossly displaced in relation to the articular surface of the facet lateral to the oblique fracture line. Instead of a more central depressed segment, the lateral 5 to 10 mm of the articular surface is usually rotated and impacted.*

The anterolateral portion of the posterior facet and the sinus tarsi area can be shown through a short, slightly oblique lateral incision above the level of the peroneal tendons, but visualization of very much of the articular surface of the superomedial fragment is difficult.

There is usually more impaction and rotation of the depressed segment and/or the lateral part of the articular surface at its anteroinferior portion. Reduction is done preferably by instrument leverage through the transverse fracture in the sinus tarsi area or the anteroinferior part of the articular surface, as shown, rather than by opening the lateral cortex, as has been done by some in the past.

Usually the reduction is not stable and requires some type of fixation. One or two small Kirschner wires have been used. A preferable type of fixation, when it can be used, is insertion of a 1.25-, 7/64-, or 9/64-inch screw in a transverse plane just below the level of the articular surface of the posterior facet in its anterior portion. This gives better fixation. Kirschner wires have a tendency to migrate, and this may result in a loss of fixation and soft-tissue irritation. Iliac bone grafts can be inserted through the transverse fracture under the elevated segment for a strut-like support in the dead space left after reduction.

___
*Specially designed staples manufactured by Howmedica are available on order from Howmedica, 359 Veterans Blvd., Rutherford, New Jersey 07070.

tapered tines are not considered satisfactory for this operative procedure.

Adequate reduction of the impacted, rotated lateral portion of the posterior facet may not be possible through a medial approach in a definite percentage of joint depression fractures; if this should be the case, an additional incision must be made laterally, superior to the peroneal tendons, and the lateral deformity of the posterior facet corrected through the subastragalar fossa area (Fig. 55–13). After reduction, it has to be maintained in a corrected position while a staple is inserted for fixation through the reduced superomedial fragment, which should also transfix the lateral cortex. This is done in the same manner as when the staple is inserted when only the medial incision is used; however, it is technically more difficult. After elevation of the depressed, rotated segment with an instrument introduced through the transverse fracture near the sinus tarsi, it may be necessary to partially transfix the elevated segment in a reduced position by a Kirschner wire or a 7/64-, 9/64-, or 1¼-inch screw inserted from the lateral side, just inferior to the margin of the lateral articular surface, before the partially inserted staple with 1-inch tines is driven in completely from the medial side. Because of technical difficulties in obtaining a level articular surface in the reduction of both the superomedial and the lateral fragments, consideration may be given to placing an iliac cortical and cancellous prop graft under the elevated lateral fragment prior to internal fixation through the superomedial fragment. Failure to reduce the lateral fragment of the posterior facet through a medial approach is less likely in a tongue-type fracture. The lateral view and the anteroposterior oblique view of the ankle made after instrumental manipulation will verify progress of the reduction or confirm reduction. Because the impacted, rotated lateral portion of the posterior facet may be difficult to reduce, the instrumental manipulation should be performed carefully.

Prior to closure, a surgical toilet of the wound, which includes hemostasis of any obvious bleeding points and excision of devitalized tissue, is performed. The wound may be irrigated with an appropriate antibiotic solution. Gentle handling of the tissues is stressed throughout the operation. Needless placement and replacement of retractors and traumatic retraction are avoided.

To insure free drainage from the operative wound, the separated muscle fibers are allowed to approximate without suturing. The fascia is sutured with infrequently placed, loosely tied sutures of 3-0 plain catgut. The skin is closed in the same manner with 4-0 Prolene. Placement of the skin sutures closer to the skin margins produces better coaptation of the skin wound. The wound must drain freely, and it will do so if closed as suggested. A bulky pressure dressing is applied to the foot and lower leg, using several rolls of Kerlex gauze, 6-inch stockinette cut on the bias, and sheet wadding. Two rolls of 6-inch plaster of Paris bandages will generally suffice for immobilization of the foot and ankle. Considerable bleeding from the loosely closed operative wound is expected, and it should contribute to the patient's postoperative comfort and reduce the chance of infection.

The toes should be elevated above the level of the knee in the postoperative period. Active exercises for the toes and extremity are indicated. The bulky pressure dressing can be replaced with a snugly fitting, short leg, walking type of cast seven to ten days following surgery. If there is incomplete healing of the operative wound, the sutures are left in.

Immediate partial weight bearing with a rapid increase to full weight bearing in 10 to 14 days has been instituted after reduction of practically all tongue-type fractures and after reduction of several joint depression fractures. This should not be done for any fracture not demonstrating secure fixation at surgery or in the postoperative roentgenograms or for extremely comminuted fractures. Certain joint depression fractures, particularly those that are vertical fractures that make a large segment of the posterior facet more unstable after reduction, are especially dangerous in regard to postoperative settling. They require longer, special, or multiple staples, and weight bearing should be delayed.

Continuous weight bearing is of great value in the prevention of demineralization or osteoporosis and should be instituted when there are no contraindications, because it definitely expedites recovery. If adequate weight bearing is performed, the walking cast may be replaced by a 5-inch top lace-up shoe in six to eight weeks. Exercises for the toes and extremity are done during immobilization and are performed with renewed vigor after removal of the cast. A program of active use and intensive specific active exercises designed to mobilize the joints of the foot and promote the return of muscle bulk is the therapy necessary for an early return to normal activity. These exercises should include standing on the injured foot alone for balance, tiptoe exercises, and efforts to regain forefoot eversion and inversion as well as motion in the subastragalar joint. Circulatory stasis must be prevented by a lace-up shoe, elastic stocking, and active use.

Because this is a new method for the treatment of these fractures, it is essential to discuss the results so that this method can be adequately compared with other forms of treatment. More than 90 open reductions have been done in private patients but statistics will be confined to the first 51 operations, involving 44 patients, which were reviewed as completely as possible in 1976.

Eighteen of the 44 patients, or 41 per cent, were over age 50. There were 10 bilateral fractures and seven bilateral operations. Six of the patients were females; 38 were males. About 30 per cent of the operations were on tongue-type fractures; and 70 per cent were on joint depression fractures. Medial displacement of the superomedial fragment was present in 50 of the 51 heels, but to a lesser degree than usual in 10 per cent. The patients were followed from one to 19 years (Fig. 55–14).

Many factors were considered in determining the end results, including the appearance of the heel on inspection and palpation, the medial and lateral contour of the os calcis, its roentgenologic appearance as well as that of the subastragalar joint, motion in the subastragalar joint, the tuber joint angle, the patient's ability to resume regular occupational and recreational activities, the presence of a normal heel-toe gait, shoe fit, endurance, and the rapidity of return to work.

Of 11 patients returning to work later than three and a half months after surgery, seven returned at four months (of these, two had bilateral fractures, one had a compound fracture, and one had an isolated fracture of the femur); three returned to work at four and a half months (all had undergone bilateral operations); and one who had had a bilateral operation required six months before returning to work. One patient considered able to work four months after the operation would not attempt to do so.

The end results were graded as excellent, good, good-minus, fair, and poor. *Excellent* was used to designate those cases having an excellent appearance on clinical examination, an excellent or good appearance in the roentgenograms, excellent subastragalar joint motion, no complaints, and excellent function. *Good* was assigned to those cases having a little more deviation from normal than "excellent" on clinical and roentgenologic examinations, but with no complaints of consequence and excellent function. *Good-minus* was used to designate those cases that did not quite measure up to the standard of "good" on roentgenologic or clinical examination, but with no complaints of consequence and very good function. The designation *fair* was given to one patient in whom there was insufficient correction of some portion of the deformities when surgery was attempted 18 days after injury, although function was good. *Poor* was assigned to those patients in whom there was a failure to adequately improve the original deformities, either because of an inadequate reduction or because of a recurrence of the deformity after reduction and fixation, irrespective of function. Classification of results by this method is shown in Table 55–1.

With one exception, all patients, including those rated poor, returned to their regular occupations and activities. The exception, rated poor because of the roentgenologic appearance, was considered able to work but would not do so.

An analysis of the eight cases rated poor because of unsatisfactory roentgenologic appearance indicated that factors responsible for these results were inadequate reduction in three heels, inadequate reduction and fixation in one heel, inadequate fixation in two heels, and inadequate fixa-

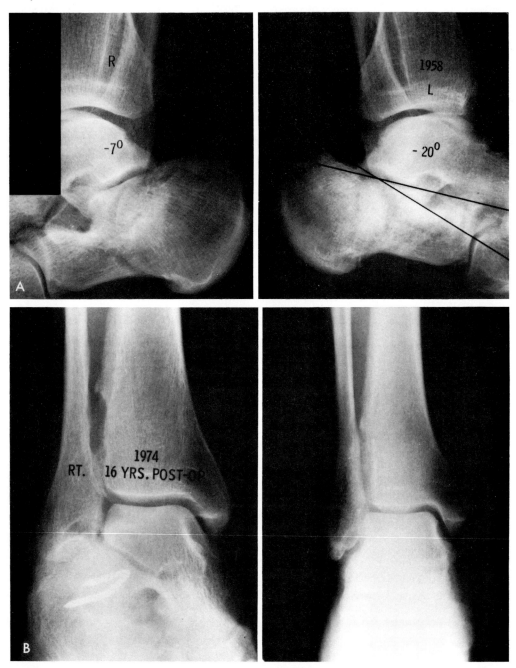

Figure 55–14. *(A) A 19-year follow-up was done on these bilateral joint depression fractures, the first to be treated by open reduction and staple fixation using a medial approach. (B) Sixteen years following reduction, the anteroposterior and anteroposterior oblique views of the right ankle show a good appearance of the articular surface of the posterior facet and no lateral cortical prominence of the os calcis.*

Illustration continued on opposite page

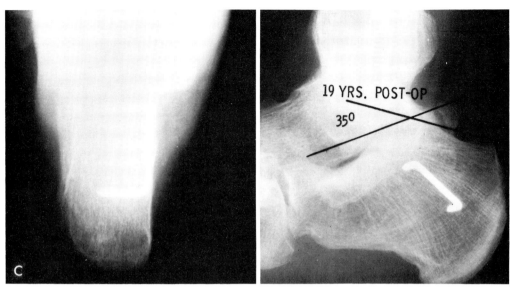

Figure 55–14 *Continued.* *(C) Nineteen years following surgery, there is an approximate 35-degree tuber joint angle of the right ankle, a correction of 42 degrees. The heel has an excellent appearance. Subastragalar joint motion is excellent in the right and left ankles. The patient has a normal gait and unrestricted physical activity and is symptom-free.*

tion plus excessive early weight bearing in two heels.

There are many opportunities for complications to occur with this method or any other method of open reduction in fractures of the os calcis, and preventive measures should be taken to guard against them. In this series, which included one compound fracture and one compound puncture wound, there was no bone infection, and wound healing, which can be delayed, was considered satisfactory. With development of the method, there was an occasional staple extrusion, and in one case, this was responsible for a poor result classification when reduction was lost. Errors in surgical judgment were responsible for a failure to open the fracture laterally, a failure to reduce lateral cortical

bulge, excessive early weight bearing, and attempted reduction 18 days after injury.

It is expected that a definite percentage of cases rated poor because of subastragalar joint irregularities will require additional definitive treatment in the form of subastragalar arthrodesis in order to provide the patient with satisfactory endurance and relief of symptoms in his or her occupational and recreational activities. The need for this treatment will be influenced by the patient's age, physical activity, and type of occupation. In one patient, a prominent lateral mass was excised, and in two patients, secondary subastragalar arthrodesis was performed.

With adequate recognition of the deformities of these fractures and the development of skill in reduction and more

TABLE 55–1 **Results of Open Reduction and Fixation with Staples (Using a Medial Approach) for 51 Os Calcis Fractures Involving the Subastragalar Joint**

GRADE	NUMBER OF PATIENTS	% OF PATIENTS		
Excellent	17	33%	64%	82%
Good	16	31%		
Good-minus	9	18%		
Fair	1	2%		
Poor	8	16%		

satisfactory fixation, the poor results should become fewer. There can be certain expectations with this method to reduce the number of grossly deformed heels with poor functional results that have been too prevalent in the past.

Open Reduction Using a Lateral Approach

Morestein has been credited with originating open reduction of fractures of the os calcis through a lateral approach.[29] This method has been used with some variations since it was introduced in 1902. Some French surgeons used bone grafts with the open reduction, but the use of bone grafts was popularized following an article by Palmer in 1948.[23]

Although this surgical method will allow correction of the depressed, impacted, or rotated portion of the lateral part of the posterior facet of the os calcis, it is my opinion that it will not allow adequate reduction of the medial displacement, overriding, and rotation of the superomedial fragment, which is such a constant and significant deformity in these fractures.

Open Reduction With Bone Grafts. Palmer described his open reduction with bone graft as follows:

A curved incision 6 centimeters in length is made beneath the lateral malleolus. The sheath of the peroneal tendons is incised and the tendons are displaced forward. At the proximal portion of the peroneal sheath, the incision is deepened to divide the middle part of the fibulo-calcaneal ligament and expose the talocalcaneal joint. If the foot is carefully dislocated into a varus position over a wedge, it is possible to look into the joint and to observe and measure the pathological ledge between its facets. A transfixion wire is drilled into the angle between the point of the tuber calcanei and the Achilles tendon and is tightened with a bow. Traction downward and backward will now reduce the lateral block of the shearing fracture without difficulty. An elevator is introduced into the compressed substance under the articular surface and it is used to lever this fragment into position until the intra-articular ledge is level. The reduction is extremely unstable. The compression cavity is filled with an iliac graft slightly larger than the cavity and it is hammered into the cavity by means of a punch.[23]

Palmer stated that transfixion pins are unnecessary. "After closure of the wound, a short leg cast is used, the patient being ambulatory in two to four days on crutches without weight bearing. After twelve weeks, the cast is replaced by a strong shoe with an arch support. Circulatory stasis is avoided."[23] In 23 cases, the patients were back at their previous work in four to eight months after operation. Subastragalar joint motion ranged from one fourth to one half of a normal range. There was one failure and one painful ankylosis in good position.[23]

After this procedure, Maxfield routinely applied a plaster boot for eight weeks and a walking boot for two weeks, and then allowed unrestricted weight bearing.[30] Maxfield and McDermott listed about 68 per cent excellent and very good functional results, 26 per cent fair results, and 1 per cent poor results in 19 patients.[31] It is of interest that they compared this with Geckeler's results of 70 per cent good and 30 per cent fair with arthrodesis.[32] Maxfield accomplished reduction by inserting a periosteal elevator just inside the displaced lateral wall to a position beneath the depressed fragment, so that it could be lifted up. I have introduced a small Cloward periosteal elevator distally through the transverse fracture in the sinus tarsi area, under the anterior end of the depressed fragment, to pry the fragment up, correcting both the rotation and the impaction; a cortical cancellous graft can be inserted under the elevated fragment through the same fracture line.

Maxfield noted instability and the need for fixation of the fragment at times. There was delayed wound healing in some degree in 5 of 40 patients. He also encountered instability in three patients that required a bone peg or screw for fixation, and he felt that the long-term end results were much more satisfactory than he had been able to obtain with other methods of treatment.

Allan used almost the same technique as has been described, but utilized a longer Kocher incision to prevent delay of wound healing.[28] He did not immobilize the foot longer than six weeks, so as to obtain a better range of subastragalar joint motion. Massage and active exercises were used for four more weeks. Weight bearing was then permitted in a sturdy shoe. Excessive broadening of the heel occurred in three of his patients, one of whom required removal of bone beneath the external malleolus.

Widén, in reporting on 92 open reductions done from the lateral side, dissected a way into the bone distal to the tendon sheaths instead of incising the lateral wall of the peroneal sheaths, forcing the sheath and its contents upward with a raspatory.[9] The sural nerve was protected. He used traction through a Kirschner wire in the tuberosity to reduce the lateral main fragment and performed the reduction by introducing a bone lever through the badly fractured wall and lifting the depressed lateral joint fragments. He also tried to raise the depression of the medial fragment. After raising the lateral joint fragment into position, he inserted a bone graft or grafts so that there was conformation of the joint. Widén recognized that a depression of the medial part of the articular surface was usually impossible to see at operation and advised that the reduction be checked roentgenologically. He used a Brodén I projection. If the calcaneus was badly shattered, the bone graft would not have sufficient support at the bottom of the compression cavity. In a few cases, the Kirschner wire was retained for a few weeks. In other cases, pressure was applied to the underside of the calcaneus with the palm of the hand when applying the plaster cast. Some difficulty was encountered with lateral spreading. Following reduction of the fracture, the peroneal tendons were restored to their usual position and the wound was closed. A non–weight-bearing cast was worn for six weeks. After wearing supporting bandages for two to three weeks, a walking cast was applied for six weeks with weight bearing allowed. His program called for no weight bearing without a plaster cast for at least 14 weeks. Widén did not feel that open reduction involved greater risk of infection than did continuous traction or transfixion.[9]

Open Reduction Without Grafts. Soeur and Remy reported on 58 operations done through a lateral approach above the peroneal tendons in which the sinus tarsi was exposed and a metal spatula was inserted into the transverse fracture line anterior to the impacted, rotated lateral portion of the posterior facet, which they referred to as the semilunar fragment of

the thalamic fracture.[20] The spatula engages the semilunar fragment and reduces it by rotation in the opposite direction. The authors mentioned that the semilunar fragment should be properly aligned with the medial fragment or with an intermediate fragment if this is present. The semilunar fragment is fixed to the medial fragment by a transverse Kirschner wire 2 mm in diameter. An anteroposterior wire passing slightly obliquely from the lateral to the medial side completes the fixation. The extremity, which is immobilized in plaster, is elevated for four weeks, at which time the plaster is changed to a walking cast, which is worn for a further eight weeks, for a total of 12 weeks of plaster immobilization. On the average, wires were removed seven months after operation.

Skin grafting of the operative wound was done in five cases. In industrial cases, complete incapacity averaged six months. The authors stated that the articular surface of the subtalar joint was restored in every case, but also indicated that no subtalar motion was present in 12, or 20 per cent, of the cases. They also mentioned that the midtarsal joint was completely ankylosed in four patients, one of whom had had a subtalar arthrodesis. About 14 per cent of the patients did not resume their normal work. Bone grafts were not used. For further information, the article of Soeur and Remy should be reviewed.[20]

I noted that there was residual gross widening of the heel and medial displacement and overriding of the superomedial fragment in one of the few axial postoperative roentgenograms shown in the aforementioned article, and I believe that this is likely to be present frequently with this method. In a small series of cases in which this method was used and which I saw presented by Schein, none had subastragalar joint motion and almost all had gross widening from residual displacement and overriding of the superomedial fragment.[36]

When it is necessary to use open reduction from the lateral side to reduce an impacted, rotated lateral fragment of the posterior facet, it is well to do the reduction as suggested by Soeur and Remy.[20] I feel that an iliac prop graft could be necessary to maintain reduction of the elevated fragment, but I also believe that it is necessary to correct the medial displacement, overriding, and rotation, if present, through a medial approach in order to obtain a more satisfactory result.

The Sagittal Pin Method of Reduction

The use of a sagittal pin for the reduction of fractures of the os calcis was originated by Westhues, a Bavarian surgeon, in 1934. The original article in regard to this was a very brief abstract.[18] References have been made to its use by Böhler and Ehalt. Gissane introduced the method to England and perfected a reduction technique, finding that the method was suitable for use only in tongue-type fractures. He devised a special spike for use in the reduction of tongue-type fractures and another longer one for use in fixation following open reduction of joint depression fractures.[3]

Essex-Lopresti restricted the use of this method to tongue-type fractures in patients under 50 years of age.[3] Following the posthumous publication of Essex-Lopresti's paper in 1952, there was an increased use of this method. Some texts list it as the recommended method of treatment.

Discussion and Evaluation. The one definite aspect of this method is that a pin or spike inserted into the superolateral portion of the long lever arm or tongue fragment and directed toward the lateral side can, with leverage, readily reduce the upward tilting posteriorly of the tongue fragment and can increase the often considerably reduced tuber joint angle. This creates a very much improved roentgenologic appearance in the lateral view of the os calcis as far as the tuber angle is concerned.

There are other aspects of this sagittal pin method of reduction that are not so positive and leave room for questioning. Postmanipulation roentgenograms frequently show the pin or spike bent from considerable leverage or force, with an abnormal tilt of the tuberosity toward the plantar surface and an increase beyond normal of the tuber angle. A warning was given about this by Essex-Lopresti.[3] Exaggeration of the tuber angle does not make a good reduction.

In general, in the postmanipulation axial roentgenograms, I have not seen evidence

of the desired restoration of the medial contour of the os calcis or the desired reduction in the transverse diameter of the os calcis that can and should be obtained in the reduction of tongue-type fractures. This makes it questionable whether the superomedial fragment has been properly reduced and whether the impacted lateral portion of the posterior facet has been elevated sufficiently to allow the lateral cortical bulge to be corrected.

From surgical experience with tongue-type fractures, I know that reduction of the superomedial fragment can, in some instances, in itself, reduce the upward tilt of the long lever arm of the tongue fragment, but I do not believe that reduction of the upward tilt of the tongue fragment by a pin directed toward the lateral side of the foot will result in a proper reduction of the superomedial fragment. Essex-Lopresti reported that in reduction of a total of 74 fractures (39 reductions by spike and 35 open reductions), approximately 30 per cent were unsuccessful.

In my opinion, the most important unanswered question is: What is the articular surface of the posterior facet like following reduction or in the end result? In none of the published papers, material in textbooks relative to the method, or scientific papers by proponents of this method are there any roentgenograms that adequately demonstrate the articular surface of the posterior facet, such as an anteroposterior oblique view of the ankle (see Figure 55–4D) or a Brodén I 10-, 20-, 30- or 40-degree projection (see Figure 55–6E,F and Figure 55–7). These views are necessary to determine whether or not the weight-bearing surface of the posterior facet of the os calcis is level. It cannot just be assumed that it is. I am doubtful that the posterior facet is level in a large percentage of cases; the superomedial fragment is not that easy to reduce.

Essex-Lopresti indicated that only 20.5 per cent of his patients returned to work by three months; an additional 38 per cent returned to work by six months. In the four or five cases treated by others using this method, which I subsequently evaluated, there was not a satisfactory reduction present. In some, it was not much more than a surgical exercise, but these cases were not selected at random.

There is an indication for use of the

sagittal pin method of reduction in fractures of the body of the os calcis that do not involve the subastragalar joint but in which there is upward displacement or tilting of the tuberosity and a marked decrease in the tuber joint angle. The method could be of use in maintaining reduction in some joint depression fractures.

I do not use and do not advise the use of the sagittal pin method of reduction for the treatment of tongue-type fractures. Tongue-type fractures should have a much more precise reduction than can be expected or obtained by closed manipulation with a pin or spike.

Surgical anatomic reduction of the superomedial fragment in itself has, at times, a very important contributing influence on reduction of the long, tongue-like fragment and its tilted articular surface of the posterior facet; and in tongue-type fractures, the surgeon is presented with the unique opportunity to obtain a high percentage of excellent and good results both anatomically and functionally from open reduction using a medial approach, and in some instances an additional lateral exposure.

Sagittal pin reduction of tongue-type fractures is a somewhat primitive type of treatment when compared with a more precise surgical reduction. It served a purpose when it was introduced in that it compared favorably with other methods available at that time. I believe that there is now a rather limited indication for the use of this method.

Triple Arthrodesis

In 1935, Conn was one of the first to advocate triple arthrodesis rather than subastragalar arthrodesis in the treatment of fractures of the os calcis.[15] He was influenced by the feeling of reciprocal function, not only between the subastragalar joint and the astragalonavicular joint, but between the astragalonavicular and the calcaneocuboid joints.

Thompson and Friesen believed "that injury to the talo-calcaneal joint is irreparable and that fusion of this weight bearing joint is necessary. The associated injuries to the two peritalar joints similarly prevent the restoration of their normal function."[16] This was the basis for their recommending triple arthrodesis as the initial primary treatment of these fractures, and they mention the frequency of involvement of the calcaneocuboid joint. Bankart advised triple arthrodesis as a primary measure in crush fractures.[2]

Harris stated, "Though fractures of the os calcis sometimes extend forward to involve the calcaneocuboid joint, this seldom causes trouble. It need not be fused at the time of the subtalar fusion. It seldom requires operation."[13]

I believe that triple arthrodesis as a primary type of treatment is not indicated for the usual joint depression fracture and certainly not for tongue-type fractures. Its use as a secondary or salvage type of procedure is extremely limited. Triple arthrodesis was used considerably at one time, but more satisfactory ways to treat these fractures have largely eliminated the need for triple arthrodesis.

Linear fracture lines extend anteriorly into the area of the articular surface of the os calcis at the calcaneocuboid joint, but involvement of this joint seldom requires surgical treatment.

Subastragalar Arthrodesis

Subastragalar arthrodesis as a treatment for fractures of the os calcis was introduced by Von Stockum in 1912.[33] Wilson used subastragalar arthrodesis in 1927.[34] In 1943, Gallie advised subastragalar arthrodesis in fractures of the os calcis and proposed a posterior surgical approach, cutting a mortise in the subastragalar joint and inserting a tibial graft.[14] Hall and Pennal,[35] as well as Pennal and Yadov,[12] were advocates of subastragalar arthrodesis. In 1963, Harris concluded that "the time-saving procedure is immediate reduction of the fracture by tri-radiate skeletal traction and compression, followed within three or four weeks by subtalar fusion by Gallie's technique."[13]

I used primary subastragalar arthrodesis in the treatment of severe fractures involving the subastragalar joint prior to the development of open reduction through a medial approach. Now, it is infrequently indicated as a primary method of treatment.

In a small percentage of os calcis fractures involving the subastragalar joint, largely joint depression fractures, which are treated by open reduction through a medial approach, there may be considerable or gross irregularity of the articular surface of the posterior facet owing to a failure to reduce and to maintain reduction of the lateral portion of the posterior facet. When it is obvious from roentgenologic findings that this is the case and that it will be disabling for this particular patient, subastragalar arthrodesis, which appears necessary in the long run, should be performed early so as not to delay final recovery of the patient.

End results following subastragalar arthrodesis should be and are better when there is not gross widening of the heel due to uncorrected medial displacement and overriding of the superomedial fragment and uncorrected lateral cortical bulge.

Other Methods of Treatment

In my opinion, closed manipulative methods of treatment based on use of instruments, such as skeletal traction in the os calcis to increase the tuber angle and the use of compression clamps to decrease the transverse diameter of the heel, cannot be expected to produce a satisfactory reduction of the medial displacement, overriding, and rotation of the superomedial fragment or a satisfactory reduction of the impacted, rotated lateral portion of the posterior facet in joint depression and tongue-type fractures. A failure to correct these deformities will produce an incongruous articular surface of the posterior facet, and any improvement in the tuber angle that can be obtained by traction is of relatively little benefit. For these reasons, the Böhler and Hermann methods[5, 10] or a modified Hermann method[7] appear to me to have little to recommend their continued use when compared with other methods available. Skeletal traction may have value in some instances as an adjunct in reduction of these fractures, particularly in those cases with upward displacement of the tuberosity of the body.

Impacted Fractures of the Lateral Portion of the Posterior Facet Without Medial Displacement and Overriding of the Superomedial Fragment

A very small percentage of fractures involving the subastragalar joint will demonstrate considerable impaction or rotation of one or more lateral portions of the articular surface of the posterior facet, but will not have medial displacement and overriding

of the superomedial fragment (Fig. 55–15). These fractures should be treated by open reduction done from the lateral side above the peroneal tendons. The reduction is accomplished by exposing the transverse fracture in the anteroinferior portion and inserting a small instrument such as a Cloward elevator into the distal transverse fracture under the impacted end of the facet and correcting both the impaction and rotation by leverage (see Figure 55–13). In my experience, there may be some springiness or a tendency for recurrence of deformity after reduction, and careful consideration should be given to the type of fixation to be used, whether it is a cortical cancellous iliac graft or Kirschner wire fixation or both, or some type of two-point staple fixation. If staple fixation were used, it would require a special small-diameter staple. A $7/64$-, $9/64$-, or $1\frac{1}{4}$-inch transverse screw can be inserted as a transfixation device just below and parallel with the articular surface and above the peroneal tendons. The transverse screw gives stable fixation, and I prefer it. The lateral fragment must be flush with the articular surface of the medial part of the facet after fixation, and this may be difficult to accomplish. If there is tilting or impaction of the medial portion of the articular surface of the posterior facet, it must be corrected. If there is an undisplaced fracture of the medial cortex, care should be taken to prevent displacement there from manipulation or insertion of the fixation device.

Other fractures under this classification might include isolated fractures of the sustentaculum tali. In my experience, they are extremely rare. It is possible that they occur in association with joint depression or tongue-type fractures and may not be recognized. Fractures of the middle facet might occur in the same manner.

Fractures of the Anterior End of the Os Calcis

These fractures include those of the anterior process (beak fractures) and linear fractures extending into the calcaneocuboid joint. Fractures of the superolateral tip of the os calcis are more like sprain fractures. They occur very infrequently, and treatment is usually conservative (Fig. 55–16). Linear fractures extending into the

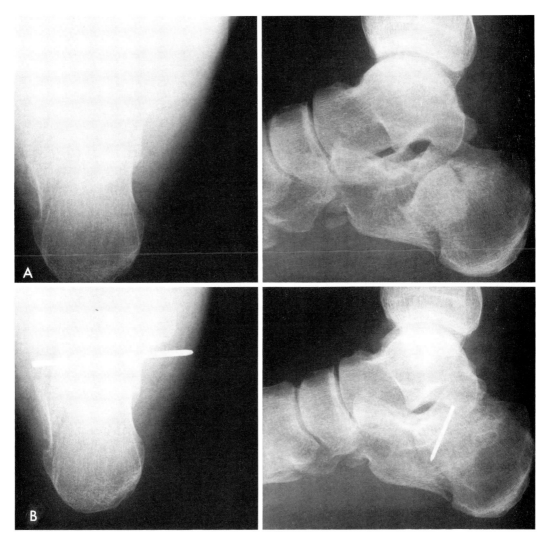

Figure 55–15. *(A) The preoperative axial view shows a fracture of the medial cortex but without significant displacement of the superomedial fragment. There is some lateral cortical expansion from impaction of a segment of the lateral part of the posterior facet. The lateral view shows a severely impacted fragment countersunk beneath the level of the articular surface. (B) The fracture of the medial cortex was not displaced additionally when the impacted lateral portion of the posterior facet was elevated through a lateral incision. The fragment was elevated by an instrument introduced through the transverse fracture in the sinus tarsi areas. An iliac bone graft was inserted through the transverse fracture. A Kirschner wire was used to transfix the fragment.*

Illustration continued on following page

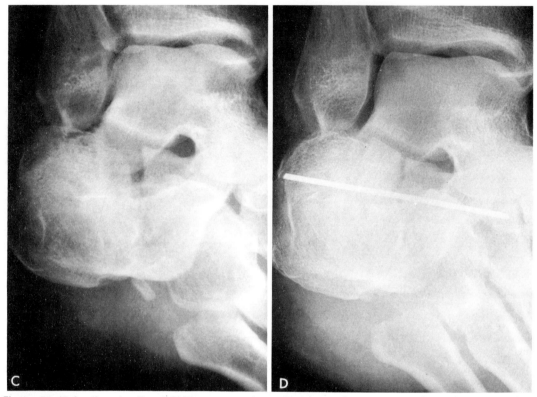

Figure 55–15 Continued.   (C and D) The preoperative and postoperative anteroposterior oblique views of the ankle show the gross deformity of the posterior facet from the impacted segment and the level articular surface of the posterior facet following reduction.

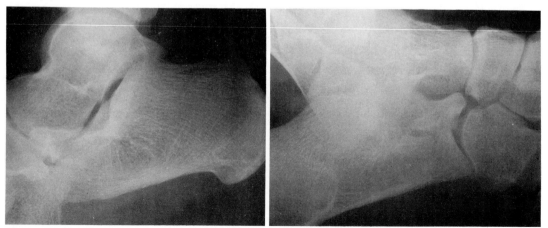

Figure 55–16.   These lateral and oblique views demonstrate a fracture of the superolateral tip of the os calcis. The avulsion-type, large fragment is attached to the bifurcate ligament.

calcaneocuboid joint are rather common. Displacement is usually minimal, and they ordinarily require no special treatment. Residual deformities of the joint, if severe and symptomatic, may require surgical treatment.

Immediate Active Exercises Without Reduction or Immobilization

The nonreductive method of treatment for fractures of the os calcis may have come into being as a result of complications and unsatisfactory results with other methods used. It has been advocated by Barnard,[40] Lance and associates,[41] Parkes,[8] and others and has been used in England and the Scandinavian countries.

Lance and coworkers, in sanctioning this method, stated that "the initial deformity must not be incompatible with good function."[41] They cited the advantages of the method as "mobilization of edema, fluid and hemorrhage with subsequent minimizing of fibrosis and adhesion formation; the preservation of joint mobility; and the prevention of ligamentous contracture; preservation of the optimum condition of uninjured structures; the simplicity and freedom of the paraphernalia; and the negligible opportunity for complications."[41] They referred to operative methods as being complicated in every sixth case and to plaster immobilization as being complicated in every twentieth case.

Parkes wrote that "in our hands, the treatment of intra-articular fractures of the os calcis by elevation, compression and early active motion has, with rare exceptions, led to satisfactory results; patients left the hospital sooner, had no significant complications, regained use of the foot more rapidly, began effective weight bearing sooner and returned to work earlier than with other forms of treatment."[8]

The application of bulky pressure dressings — consisting of Kerlex rolls, Webril or soft rolls, stockinette cut on the bias, elastic bandages, plus continuous suspension of the extremity so that the toes are higher than the knee — will do a great deal to decrease swelling in a fracture of the os calcis. With ice bags and analgesics for pain, active exercises for all joints and muscles of the foot and leg can be started

and continued to tolerance. Physiotherapeutic measures that increase circulatory stasis should be used with caution. With progress in the exercises and with decreased swelling, the patient can begin non–weight-bearing ambulation with crutches and can progress to wearing an elastic stocking and a snugly fitting 5-inch top lace-up shoe to prevent swelling of the foot and leg. With this method of treatment, weight bearing has been allowed in four to six weeks in fractures of the processes, but has been deferred for 10 to 12 weeks in other types of fractures. Undisplaced joint depression fractures of significance are rare but do occur, and early weight bearing in such a case could result in the production of deformity.

Lance and associates stated that the presence of significant clinical deformity or incongruity of the subastragalar joint surfaces, if uncorrected, will predispose to a poor end result; hence, these cases are not suitable for this method of treatment.[41] I am of the same opinion.

Both Lance and coworkers and Parkes claim negligible opportunity for complications or no significant complications as a main feature of the nonreductive method of treatment of os calcis fractures.[8, 41] In my opinion, the advantages of the method seem overstated. The majority of fractures of the os calcis involve the subastragalar joint, and most of these fractures have either medial displacement, overriding, and rotation of the superomedial fragment or impaction and rotation of the lateral portion of the articular surface of the posterior facet, or both. If these deformities are not corrected, a malunion of the fracture will occur, and the result will be undesirable. Malunion can be considered a complication of the method, and the rate of complications will be very high unless the method is used only for cases demonstrating no deformity—which would limit use of the method to a rather minimal number of the fractures that involve the subastragalar joint.

I believe that this method of treatment may be indicated for the elderly or chronically ill patient and that at times it may have to be used in the critically ill patient with multiple major injuries. Ordinarily this method is indicated only when there is no significant deformity present.

Sequelae of Fractures of the Os Calcis

Residual upward displacement of the tuberosity creates a flatfoot. It may be associated with painful abnormal weight bearing over the posterior end of an angulated plantar fragment of the os calcis just anterior to the tuberosity. If severe enough to warrant correction, the plantar fragment can be excised and used as a graft in an opening wedge osteotomy of the body of the os calcis anterior to the tuberosity. It is best to use temporary skeletal traction through the tuberosity during surgery as a means of pulling the tuberosity posteriorly and downward to correct the upward displacement and rotation. A graft in the opening wedge osteotomy helps to maintain correction of rotation and may produce some slight increase in length. A Steinmann pin inserted through the tuberosity into the body serves as fixation to prevent recurrence of the deformity.

So-called plantar fasciitis from a projecting bone fragment may be a manifestation of gross abnormalities in the normal contour and weight-bearing function of the heel.

A flatfooted, shuffling gait and inability to walk on the toes may be helped relatively by repeated exercises. They can be avoided in a rather large percentage of cases by adequate reduction and treatment of the original fracture.

In my experience, distortion of the architecture of the fat pad of the heel and rupture and irregularity of the U systems of fibrous tissue strands have not been significant factors in fractures of the os calcis.[42]

Sensory denervation of the heel, which has been proposed,[43] does not seem to me to be an indicated method of treatment for painful malunited fractures of the os calcis.

Lateral Bony Prominences

When a segment of the lateral part of the posterior facet with its underlying bone is impacted down into the cancellous bone of the os calcis, there is usually rotation of the segment so that its anteroinferior portion is more impacted, and it may be countersunk. This acts like a wedge, which is driven inferiorly and posteriorly inside the thin lateral cortical wall. The wedge produces multiple fractures in the lateral cortex as it spreads or forces the cortical wall of the os calcis laterally to create a lateral bony prominence posterior and inferior to the lower end of the fibula.

If this deformity is not corrected in the reduction of the fracture, a permanent bony prominence is present. It may impinge the peroneal tendons against the fibula. Severe spreading of the cortex may result in lateral displacement, subluxation, or dislocation of the tendons.[37] It has produced limitation of motion in the ankle from a bony block.

It is not likely that the tendons are significantly injured at the time of the fracture. Widén noted evidence of laceration of the tendon sheaths in 12 of 92 open reductions done laterally in fresh fractures.[9] In three of them, the tendons were injured in the fracture. From an examination of 50 old fractures, Deyerle found a total of nine cases in which the peroneal tendons were dislocated anterior to the fibula.[37] These patients had symptoms of instability, and a lack of ability to resist inversion was noted.

Lindsay and Dewar's findings from a review of old fractures indicated no correlation between lateral malleolar impingement and lateral malleolar pain.[27] McLaughlin mentioned peroneal spastic flatfoot as being secondary to chronic stenosing tendovaginitis caused by crowding of the peroneal tendons between the lateral mass and the fibula.[39] He stated that operative resection of the mass should be approached with great caution.

Deyerle stated, "The main correctible disability in severely comminuted and spread fractures of the os calcis is a decompression of the peroneals and, in some cases, their re-routing behind the fibula." He removed a wedge-shaped portion of the mass, with the base of the wedge anteriorly, and used bone wax over the raw bone surface to prevent reformation of bone. Peroneal synoviagrams have been used, but it appears to me that the need for this operation could be determined from clinical findings, which would include the appearance of the lateral cortex of the os calcis in axial roentgenograms and in the anteroposterior view of the ankle.

If the bony mass is large, relative improvement is to be expected with its removal. I have routinely excised portions of the lateral cortical bulge in performing subastragalar arthrodesis on malunited fractures in which there was lateral cortical bulge, but the location of the incision used for the arthrodesis is not as suitable as an incision directly over the mass.

In any patient who has a large, lateral bony mass as a result of a malunited fracture, there is a strong likelihood of intraarticular abnormalities being present, and these should not be overlooked in treatment.

Subastragalar Joint Abnormalities

Controversy exists about the treatment of sequelae of fractures of the os calcis, just as it does about the treatment of fresh fractures, and abnormalities of the subastragalar joint are no exception.

Speed and Stewart stated that the functional results after four or five years are surprisingly good; and that many patients with considerable deformities either have a spontaneous subastragalar arthrodesis or have an almost painless subastragalar joint despite traumatic arthritis.[38] Lindsay and Dewar wrote that a definition of subastragalar joint pain is extremely difficult if not impossible to obtain and that radiologic osteoarthritis of the subastragalar joint is not an indication for fusion. They also stated that a detailed study of their series "has not solved the problem of disability in fractures of the os calcis."[27]

McLaughlin was of the opinion that "a person who has fractured the calcaneus is not likely to reach a point of maximum spontaneous recovery in less than one year and sometimes two years after the injury, and that follow-up studies show that sooner or later, most persons who have fractured the os calcis become able to get around with reasonable comfort, and that gross disorders of the subtalar joint may be quite innocent of pain."[39] Some authors have advised subastragalar arthrodesis, and others triple arthrodesis.

In my opinion, gross irregularities of the articular surface of the posterior facet from a failure to reduce the medial displacement, overriding, and rotation of the superomedial fragment or the impaction and rotation of the lateral part of the posterior facet, or both, will result in degenerative changes involving the joint. These changes will be associated with some degree of limited and painful subastragalar joint motion. Such a joint will have diminished stamina for the extremes of work and physical activity. Although considerable fixation of the joint may occur spontaneously in the long run, bony ankylosis of the subastragalar joint is not likely.

Gross abnormalities such as irregularities of the weight-bearing surface of the posterior facet and degenerative changes in the joint can be readily recognized from a lateral roentgenogram of the heel, an anteroposterior oblique view of the ankle, and Brodén I projections. These views may demonstrate hypertrophic lipping of the lateral margins of the subastragalar joint. Irregularities of the joint surface may cause varus or valgus deformity of the heel.

A solid bony ankylosis of a deranged subastragalar joint functions better than a fibrous ankylosis of this weight-bearing joint. Subastragalar arthrodesis is the indicated method of treatment when there is obvious roentgenologic evidence of deformities and degenerative changes in the joint associated with limited, painful motion and an inability to perform normal or regular occupational work and recreational activities. It may not be indicated in the elderly or in those leading sedentary lives.

When there is roentgenologic evidence of gross deformity involving the posterior facet following adequate efforts to reduce the fracture and which can be expected to be symptomatic in an active worker, subastragalar arthrodesis should be done relatively early so as to reduce the recovery period for the injury, and one should not wait 12 to 18 months to see what sort of function will result. A Gallie-type subastragalar arthrodesis does not allow correction of valgus or varus deformity.[14]

Many malunited fractures involving the subastragalar joint have associated lateral cortical bulge. It is my practice to excise this lateral cortical bulge and to use the bone that is suitable for bone grafts in the arthrodesing procedure. Hypertrophic lateral margins of the joint, which are manifestations of the degenerative changes, are excised. The diminished tuber angle may be increased relatively by inserting a wedge-shaped iliac cortical and cancellous bone graft at the posterior part of the subastragalar joint after resecting the articular surfaces of the joint. Iliac bone grafts are placed in a prepared bed in the subastragalar fossa to expedite the production of a solid bony ankylosis. Care is taken to correct valgus or varus deformity and particularly to prevent varus deformity of the heel. A two-tine staple is inserted across the joint anterior to the fibula for fixation. Partial weight bearing is started in a short leg walking cast about three weeks following operation and is increased rapidly to full weight bearing. After removal of the cast, some eight weeks after surgery, the patient is filled with a 5-inch top lace-up shoe.

The results of subastragalar arthrodesis done under these circumstances have been satisfactory. A better foot results when the subastragalar joint irregularities are not associated with other severe deformities of the fractures. Limited but useful forefoot inversion and eversion may be retained. In my opinion, a lack of complete foot stiffness after this operation makes it much more satisfactory than triple arthrodesis.

The only complication noted was the development of a mildly painful callosity under the head of the fifth metatarsal in one patient, which was presumed to be due to some varus of the heel. One staple was removed after a solid fusion was obtained. No technical difficulties have been noted in the operation. Wound healing has been good.

RUPTURE OF THE TENDO ACHILLIS

Spontaneous rupture of the tendo Achillis is infrequent, and rupture of the tendon from blunt trauma or through an open wound is even less common. The presence of degenerative changes in the tendon has not been consistent. Spontaneous rupture may be due to the application of a stretching force on a muscle already contracted. It occurs when great force is exerted and again when it is not, such as in running, tripping, stumbling, and falling. Individuals with sedentary occupations may be more prone to rupture of the tendo Achillis on vigorous physical activity. It might occur in two stages. Laceration of the ten-

don is usually caused by broken glass or a sharp metal object.

Missed diagnosis has been a problem in that it has occurred in 20 to 30 per cent of cases. It is probably influenced by the lack of a severe injury and the presence of some degree of active power in plantar flexion of the ankle from other muscles. A puncture wound in the area of the tendo Achillis should be viewed with suspicion. Early recognition of the injury is important.

Spontaneous rupture may be accompanied by a sensation of a snap or tear, a variable degree of pain, a sudden feeling of weakness, and some swelling. Tenderness and weakness in plantar flexion may be present. A gap on palpation over the taut tendon is indicative of rupture. Rupture may occur at either the distal end or near the musculotendinous junction. Rupture occurs most often in individuals in the fourth decade.

Treatment of rupture of the tendo Achillis can be surgical or nonsurgical. Results with either method are better when treatment is performed soon after injury.

Lea and Smith, advocates of the nonsurgical or gravity equinus walking cast method, stated,

> The virtues of the method are that the hazards of anesthesia and open surgery are avoided. The complications of infection, skin slough and scar formation do not occur; and the patient is spared the expense of hospitalization. Early return to work is a distinct economic advantage. The functional results are as entirely satisfactory as those from operative repairs; the cosmetic appearance is much better.[44]

They also cite the frustrations of performing surgery on the mop-like frazzled ends of the ruptured tendon.

Inglis and associates advocated surgical repair, believing that patients not treated surgically have less satisfactory subjective and objective results and have a high incidence of re-rupture when compared with surgically treated patients.[45] Of their patients treated nonsurgically, 34 per cent had re-rupture — an incidence three times greater than the 11 per cent incidence of re-rupture in the series of Lea and Smith. Their surgical complications were less than reported by others. Lea and Smith found 105 complications in a review of 255 cases treated surgically.[44] Major complications occurred once in each 5.8 cases and minor complications once in each 4.2 cases.

Ma and Griffith have introduced percutaneous repair of acute closed rupture of the Achilles tendon.[46] It can be performed under local, regional, or general anesthesia without a tourniquet. No complications of significance were present in the 18 patients reviewed. Of the 18 patients, 12 had been followed from 13 to 40 months and demonstrated 86 per cent restoration of power of the injured ankle within 12 months postoperatively. Their report is a preliminary one, but the method shows a great deal of usefulness because of its simplicity, the indicated restoration of strength, and the lack of complications.

As a general rule, the treatment of spontaneous rupture of the Achilles tendon in the elderly or debilitated should be by the gravity equinus walking cast method. In the open-wound laceration rupture, surgical treatment is indicated. In the closed spontaneous ruptures seen early in younger patients, I would consider percutaneous repair after the method of Ma and Griffith.[46]

In the surgical repair, it is well to approximate the frayed tendon ends with absorbable sutures, and the incision should be on the medial side. A pull-out wire suture may be indicated. In any method of treatment, adequate protection of the tendon until there is a firm union at the site of rupture is important.

In the delayed surgical repair of rupture of the tendo Achillis, it may be necessary to weave the plantaris tendon between the ruptured ends of the tendon. The method of Bosworth (Fig. 55–17) may be used, in

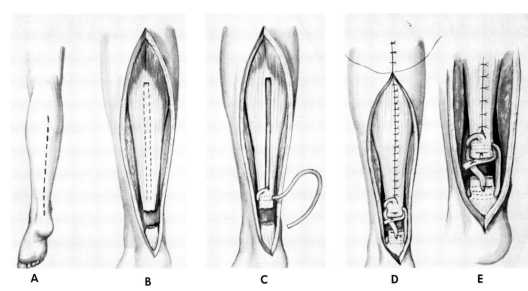

A   **B**   **C**   **D**   **E**

Figure 55–17. *Bosworth method for surgical repair of a ruptured Achilles tendon. (A) Line of incision on the posterior calf. (B) Outline of the area of excision of a 0.5-inch-wide strip of tendon 7 to 9 inches long from the proximal part of the raphe of the tendo Achillis. This extends upward into the lower portion of the calf. The strip is turned downward and left attached below, just above the proximal end of the lacerated tendo Achillis. Fibrous tissue in the defect between the ends of the tendo Achillis has been removed. (C) The tip of the strip of tendon that was turned down has been passed transversely through the proximal end of the lacerated tendo Achillis. This is to prevent its tearing out of the end of the proximal portion of the tendo Achillis. This part of the stitch should be fastened with one or two chromic sutures. (D) After being passed transversely through the proximal end of the lacerated tendo Achillis, the tendon strip has been brought downward and passed transversely through the distal end of the tendo Achillis and then forward through the distal stump, drawn tight, and sutured. It has then been passed upward and again transversely through the proximal end of the tendo Achillis, drawn tight, and sutured; and finally passed downward and sutured to itself. Note that the defect in the posterior raphe on the lower portion of the calf and upper tendo Achillis has been closed with interrupted sutures and the skin is being closed. (E) Enlarged drawing to show the passage of the tendon as it is woven between the two ends of the sutured tendo Achillis, bridging the gap therein. (From Bosworth, D. M.: J. Bone Joint Surg., 38A:112, 1956.)*

which a 0.5-inch-wide strip of the central part of the tendinous raphe is used across the gap between the tendon ends.[47] Hooker found no excellent results, one satisfactory result, and three poor results in operations done more than one year after rupture.[48]

Conservative Treatment

The conservative treatment recommended by Lea and Smith for an acute tendo Achillis rupture is immobilization in a walking plaster cast applied with the foot in a gravity equinus position.[44] Forced equinus is to be avoided. Weight bearing is allowed when the cast is dry. The extremity is immobilized for eight weeks, never for a shorter period. When the cast is removed, the patient is cautioned about falling, and a 2.5-cm heel is worn for four weeks. Active gastrocnemius-strengthening exercises are prescribed, to be used gradually, and the ankle is mobilized gently. Patients are allowed to bear weight on the ball of the foot at 24 weeks, and some then resume sports activities.

Percutaneous Repair of Acute Closed Rupture of the Tendo Achillis as Used by Ma and Griffith[46]
(Fig. 55–18)

Surgery is performed with the patient prone under local, regional or general anesthesia, without a tourniquet. A Number "0" or Number "1" nonabsorbable suture, 12 to 14 inches in length, is threaded with two straight (Keith) needles.

The proximal portion of the ruptured Achilles tendon is palpated 2.5 cm proximal to the defect between the free ruptured ends. At this site, stab wounds are made through the skin on the lateral and medial aspects of the tendon. The wounds pierce the skin and subcutaneous tissue without puncturing the tendon or its sheath. A small, curved hemostat is introduced into each wound between the subcutaneous tissue and the tendon sheath and rotated 360 degrees to free the skin and subcutaneous tissue from the tendon sheath underneath.

Step 1. Starting with the lateral stab wound, the needle and suture are passed transversely through the stab wound, subcutaneous tissue

and tendon, and out the medial stab wound. This creates a skin-to-skin suture that runs transversely lateral-to-medial through the largest anterior-to-posterior diameter of the Achilles tendon. The traversing suture is adjusted so that equal lengths of the free ends of the suture are on the lateral and medial sides of the tendon.

Step 2. The stab wounds from which the free suture ends are exiting are carefully enlarged with a small, curved hemostat as described above. Care is taken not to damage the suture with the hemostat. The straight needles are then inserted through the ipsilateral stab wound, angulated distally 45 degrees to the long axis of the tendon and passed through the tendon and out through the skin on the contralateral side. The needles are not pulled completely through the skin until the new skin puncture wounds are enlarged around the needle using a No. 15 blade and the small curved hemostatic clamp, as described earlier. The site of exit for the angulated needles and sutures is

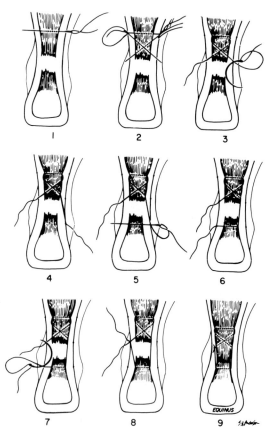

Figure 55–18. Steps 1 to 9 for percutaneous repair of acute closed rupture of the tendo Achillis. (From Ma, G. W. C., and Griffith, T. G.: Clin. Orthop. Rel. Res., 128:248, 1977.)

usually near the proximal edge of the rupture defect gap. At this point, the ends of the sutures are both pulled completely through the skin and traction applied to both suture ends simultaneously tightening the proximal portion of the suture. Undermining around the suture with a clamp minimizes snaring of subcutaneous tissue when the suture is tightened. The straight needle on the lateral suture is replaced with a curved cutting needle

Step 3. The curved cutting needle on the lateral suture is passed distally between the subcutaneous tissue and the tendon sheath (parallel to the tendon) and out through the skin at the level of the midportion of the distal segment of the ruptured tendon, about 1.25 cm distal to the rupture gap.

Step 4. The distal skin exit hole is carefully enlarged around the curved needle (before pulling the suture through the skin) with the No. 15 blade and a small curved hemostatic clamp is used to separate the subcutaneous tissue from the tendon sheath as before. The suture is then pulled through the enlarged curved needle puncture hole.

Step 5. The curved needle is replaced with the straight needle on the lateral suture. The suture is then passed back through the enlarged lateral skin puncture hole and transversely through the tendon, and out through the skin on the medial side. At this point the suture courses transversely through the tendon 1.25 cm distal to the rupture defect.

This medial skin puncture hole is enlarged around the straight needle (before pulling the suture through the skin) with the No. 15 blade and the small curved hemostatic clamp, as described previously.

Step 6. The suture on the medial side is pulled through the enlarged distal medial needle puncture hole and is pulled taut. This flattens the suture against the lateral aspect of both the proximal and distal segments of the tendon.

Step 7. A curved needle again replaces the straight needle on the distal medial suture, and passes the suture back through the distal medial skin puncture hole proximally between the subcutaneous tissue and the tendon sheath (parallel to the tendon), and out through the enlarged medial skin puncture hole at the level of the rupture gap. Thus 2 sutures exit from the skin at the middle hole on the medial aspect of the ankle.

Step 8. Traction is applied to both of the free ends of the suture in a crisscross manner. This traction is applied while the ankle is positioned in maximum equinus, and the ends of the ruptured Achilles tendon are approximated. Once the approximation is felt to be complete, a surgeon's knot is tied, followed by 2

more knots. The suture is cut short and then pushed subcutaneously with the point of the hemostatic clamp.

No skin sutures are required since stab wounds and puncture wound enlargements are limited. The 6 small puncture wounds, 3 medial and 3 lateral, are covered with dry sterile dressings.

Step 9. A non–weight-bearing short leg cast is applied to the injured leg with the ankle in equinus, after the suturing is completed. All patients are treated with a non–weight-bearing equinus short leg cast for 4 weeks postoperatively. After 4 weeks, all patients are treated for 4 additional weeks with a low-heel weight-bearing short leg equinus cast. The patients are then instructed in toe-heel–raising gastrocnemius-soleus exercises, and continue these for 4 weeks. Finally, the patients are given heel-cord stretching excercises for 4 additional weeks. . . .

When performing the procedure, several points are important, including: (1) tying the surgeon's knot on the medial side of the tendon (to avert sural nerve damage. (2) Adequate separation of subcutaneous tissue from the tendon sheath for suture passage (to avert adhesions and skin dimpling). (3) Limitation of the final surgeon's knot to only about 2 further knots (to minimize tender nodule granuloma formation about the knot. (4) Averting damage to the suture material when enlarging skin puncture wounds (damaged sutures will break under tension).[46]

REFERENCES

1. Cotton, F. J., and Henderson, F. F.: Results of fractures of the os calcis. Am. J. Orthop. Surg., *14*:290, 1916.
2. Bankart, A. S. B.: Fractures of the os calcis. Lancet, 2:175, 1942.
3. Essex-Lopresti, P.: Mechanism, reduction technique, and results in fractures of the os calcis. Br. J. Surg. 39:395, 1952.
4. McLaughlin, H. L. (ed.): Trauma. Philadelphia, W. B. Saunders Company, 1959.
5. Böhler, L.: The Treatment of Fractures, 4th English ed. Bristol, John Wright and Sons, 1935.
6. Wilson, P. D.: Management of Fractures and Dislocations. Philadelphia, J. B. Lippincott, 1938.
7. Giannestras, N., and Sammarco, G. J.: Fractures and dislocations of the foot. *In* Rockwood, C. A., and Green, D. P. (eds.): Fractures, Vol. 2. Philadelphia, J. B. Lippincott Co., 1975.
8. Parkes, J. C., II: The non-reductive treatment of fractures of the os calcis. Orthop. Clin. North Am., *4*:193, 1973.
9. Widén, A.: Fractures of the calcaneus. Acta Chir. Scand., Suppl. 188, 1954.
10. Hermann, O. J.: Conservative therapy for fractures of the os calcis. J. Bone Joint Surg., *19*:709, 1937.
11. Pridie, K. H.: A new method of treatment for severe fractures of the os calcis, a preliminary report. Surg. Gynecol. Obstet., *82*:671, 1946.
12. Pennal, G. F., and Yadov, M. P.: Operative treatment of

comminuted fractures of the os calcis. Orthop. Clin. North Am., 4:197, 1973.

13. Harris, R. I.: Fractures of the os calcis: treatment by early subtalar arthrodesis. Clin. Orthop. Rel. Res., No. 30, 1963, p. 100.

14. Gallie, W. E.: Subastragalar arthrodesis in fractures of the os calcis. J. Bone Joint Surg., 25:131, 1943.

15. Conn, H. R.: The treatment of fractures of the os calcis. J. Bone Joint Surg., 17:392, 1935.

16. Thompson, K. R., and Friesen, C. M.: Treatment of comminuted fractures of the calcaneus by primary triple arthrodesis. J. Bone Joint Surg., 41A:1423, 1959.

17. Thorén, O.: Os Calcis Fractures. Copenhagen, Munksgaard, 1964.

18. Westhues, H.: Zur Behandlung der Calcaneus Fraktur. Z. Chir., 39:1438, 1934.

19. King, R.: Axial pin fixation of fractures of the os calcis (method of Essex-Lopresti). Orthop. Clin. North Am., 4:185, 1973.

20. Soeur, R., and Remy, R.: Fractures of the calcaneus with displacement of the thalamic portion. J. Bone Joint Surg., 57B:413, 1975.

21. Goff, C. W.: Fresh fractures of the os calcis. Arch. Surg., 317:744, 1938.

22. Merrill, V.: Atlas of Roentgenographic Positions and Standard Radiologic Procedures, 4th ed. St. Louis, C. V. Mosby Co., 1975.

23. Palmer, I.: The mechanism and treatment of fractures of the calcaneus: open reduction with the use of cancellous grafts. J. Bone Joint Surg., 30A:2, 1948.

24. Rowe, C. R., Sakellarides, H., Freeman, P., and Sorbie, C.: Fractures of the os calcis—a long term follow-up study of one hundred forty-six patients. J.A.M.A., 184:920, 1963.

25. Warrick, C. K., and Bremner, A. E.: Fracture of the calcaneum, with an atlas illustrating various types of fractures. J. Bone Joint Surg., 35B:33, 1953.

26. Watson-Jones, R.: Fractures and Joint Injuries, 4th ed., Vol. 2. Baltimore, Williams and Wilkins Co., 1955.

27. Lindsay, R. N., and Dewar, F. P.: Fractures of the os calcis. Am. J. Surg., 95:555, 1958.

28. Allan, J. H.: The open reduction of fractures of the os calcis. Ann. Surg., 141:890, 1955.

29. Morestein (1902): Quoted by Schwartz, M. A.: Bull. Soc. Nat. Chir., 55:148, 1921.

30. Maxfield, J. E.: Os calcis fractures: treatment of calcaneal fractures by open reduction. J. Bone Joint Surg., 45A:868, 1963.

31. Maxfield, J. E., and McDermott, F. J.: Experience with the Palmer open reduction of fractures of the calcaneus. J. Bone Joint Surg., 37A:99, 1955.

32. Geckeler, E. O.: Comminuted fractures of the os calcis, choice of treatment. Arch. Surg., 61:469, 1950.

33. Von Stockum: Operative Behandlung der Calcaneus und Talus Fractur. Z. Chir., 39:1438, 1912.

34. Wilson, P. D.: Treatment of fractures of the os calcis by arthrodesis of the subastragalar joint. J.A.M.A, 80:1676, 1927.

35. Hall, M. C., and Pennal, G. F.: Primary subtalar arthrodesis in the treatment of severe fractures of the calcaneum. J. Bone Joint Surg., 42B:336, 1960.

36. Schein, A. J.: Paper presented at the Hospital for Joint Disease, New York, May 1978.

37. Deyerle, W. M.: Long term follow-up of fractures of the os calcis — diagnostic peroneal synoviagram. Orthop. Clin. North Am., 4:213, 1973.

38. Crenshaw, A. H. (ed.): Campbell's Operative Orthopaedics, 4th ed., Vol. 1. St. Louis, C. V. Mosby Co., 1963, p. 403.

39. McLaughlin, H. L.: Treatment of late complications after os calcis fractures. Clin. Orthop. Rel. Res., No. 30 (12), 1963, p. 111.

40. Barnard, L.: Non-operative treatment of fractures of the calcaneus. J. Bone Joint Surg., 45A:865, 1963.

41. Lance, E. M., Carey, E. J., Jr., and Wade, P. A.: Fractures of the os calcis: treatment by early mobilization. Clin. Orthop. Rel. Res., 12:79, 1963.

42. Kuhns, J. G.: Changes in elastic adipose tissue. J. Bone Joint Surg., 31A:541, 1949.

43. Sallick, M. A., and Blum, L.: Sensory denervation of the heel for persistent pain following fractures of the calcaneus. J. Bone Joint Surg., 30A:209, 1948.

44. Lea, R. B., and Smith, L.: Non-surgical treatment of tendo Achillis rupture. J. Bone Joint Surg., 54A:1398, 1972.

45. Inglis, A. E., Scott, W. N., Sculco, T. P., and Patterson, A. H.: Ruptures of the tendo Achillis: an objective assessment of surgical and nonsurgical treatment. J. Bone Joint Surg., 58A:990, 1976.

46. Ma, G. W. C., and Griffith, T. G.: Percutaneous repair of acute closed ruptured Achilles tendon—a new technique. Clin. Orthop. Rel. Res., 128:248, 1977.

47. Bosworth, D. M.: Repair of defects in the tendo Achillis. J. Bone Joint Surg., 38A:111, 1956.

48. Hooker, C. H.: Rupture of the tendo Achillis. J. Bone Joint Surg., 45B:360, 1963.

CHAPTER 56

TRAUMA TO THE ANKLE

Joseph J. Conrad, M.D., F.A.C.S.
and Albert H. Tannin, M.D., F.A.C.S.

Injuries in the area of the ankle joint are among the most common injuries to the human body. The volume of the literature concerning fractures of the ankle attests to the fact that these may be extremely difficult injuries to treat. There is still widespread divergence of opinion concerning the treatment of choice. To date, universal agreement has not been reached about whether these injuries should be treated by operative or nonoperative means.

HISTORICAL BACKGROUND

Hippocrates gave a description of lesions about the ankle in about 300 B.C. Cornelius Celsus emphasized the importance of the relationship between the talus and the tibia in the first century A.D. However, it was not until the latter part of the eighteenth century, with the publication of Sir Percivall Pott's detailed description of the pathologic findings of a fracture in the ankle region,[65] that there were attempts to define the pathology and mechanism of ankle fractures. He described a transverse fracture of the fibula 2 to 3 inches above the tip of the fibula, a rupture of the deltoid ligament, and a lateral subluxation of the talus. Pott also discovered that he could achieve a reduction of a fracture-dislocation more easily if the hip and knee were slightly flexed so that the muscles were relaxed.

Dupuytren was the first to try to explain the mechanism of fractures of the ankle by performing experiments on cadavers, describing in detail the findings in experimentally produced fractures.[3] He also described the central dislocation of the talus.[49] In this condition, he recognized the fracture of the fibula with accompanying rupture of the distal tibiofibular ligaments, as well as displacement of the malleoli laterally and proximal dislocation of the talus into the interosseous space between the tibia and fibula. This fracture bears his name. Dupuytren was also the first to describe a method of treatment based on the mechanism of injury that he ascertained from his experiments.

In 1822, Astley Cooper published a treatise on dislocations and fractures of the joints in which he gave a detailed description of many different types of fractures of the ankle.[22] He was probably the first to describe a fracture of the posterior articular margin of the tibia. He also observed that diastasis was necessary to allow upward dislocation of the talus between the tibia and fibula. Maisonneuve was the first to compare the ankle joint to a mortise.[3] In 1840, he noted that it was external rotation that produced the type of ankle fracture with an oblique fracture of the distal fibula and laceration of the deltoid ligament and anterior joint capsule. In experiments on cadavers, he noted differences between the type of fracture seen when the tibiofibular syndesmosis remained intact and that when it was ruptured. His description of a particular fracture-dislocation of the ankle, namely a high fracture of the fibula associated with diastasis of the distal tibiofibular syndesmosis, resulted in the association of his name with this injury complex. In the latter half of the nineteenth century, there continued to be a great deal of work produced based on experiments on cadavers. Huguier supported many of Maisonneuve's ideas.[3] There were also contributions by Honigschmied and Tillaux.[3]

In the beginning of the twentieth century, with the increased use of roentgenography, works were published by Chaput, Destot, and Quenu that correlated the experimental findings of authors of the previous centry with radiographic findings.[3] This included an attempt to determine the mechanism of injury from the appearance of the roentgenogram. During this period, great emphasis was placed on describing fractures of the anterior and posterior lip of the tibia. A landmark was reached in 1922 with the publication of Ashhurst and Bromer's classic study on the classification and mechanics of fractures of the ankle.[1] In 1950, Lauge-Hansen presented a detailed classification of ankle fractures based on the mechanism of injury.[50] This also took into account the ligamentous injuries that accompany fractures about the ankle.

Lane and Lambotte were early advocates of operative treatment of ankle fractures. Since that time, this has been advocated by Danis,[26] who was a pupil of Lambotte. More recently, the principle of open reduction, rigid internal fixation, and early active motion has been advocated by Vasli,[77] the members of the AO Group,[59, 79] and Burwell and Charnley.[10]

ANATOMY OF THE ANKLE

The ankle is a hinge joint. It is formed by the tibia above and medially, the fibula laterally, and the talus below the tibia and between the malleoli. The talus fits into a mortise formed by the tibia and fibula, which is deepened posteriorly by the posterior inferior tibiofibular ligament.

Medially, the distal tibia ends as a short, thick projection, the medial malleolus. This faces anteriorly and laterally and articulates with the medial surface of the trochlea. On the lateral side, the distal end

of the fibula, or lateral malleolus, projects more distally and posteriorly than the medial malleolus. It articulates with the lateral side of the body of the talus. The largest portion of the talus, the body, lies between the medial and lateral malleoli and articulates with the tibia above, the malleoli on either side, and the calcaneus below. Anteriorly, the head of the talus articulates with the navicular. The trochlea, which is the superior articular surface of the talus, is wider anteriorly than it is posteriorly. It is also noted that the inferior articular surface of the tibia is wider anteriorly than it is posteriorly in order for these two articular surfaces to remain congruent. Superiorly, the articular surface of the trochlea is continuous with the articular surfaces on the medial and lateral side of the talus that articulate with the malleoli. The capsule of the ankle joint is reinforced anteriorly and posteriorly by the anterior and posterior capsular ligaments that attach to the edges of the articular cartilage. Despite this, the capsule is thin and weak anteriorly and posteriorly. It is strengthened medially and laterally by strong ligaments.

The medial or deltoid ligament is a very strong triangular band (Fig. 56–1). Its apex is attached to the medial malleolus, and it then broadens distally to attach to the neck of the talus, the navicular, the spring ligament, and the sustentaculum tali. The lateral or fibular collateral ligament is composed of three separate bands (Fig. 56–2): the *posterior talofibular ligament*, which originates at the posterior part of the lateral malleolus and extends backward and downward to attach to the posterior process of the talus; the *calcaneofibular ligament*, which extends downward and slightly posteriorly to insert into the small tubercle on the lateral surface of the calcaneus; and the *anterior talofibular ligament*, which originates from the anterior border of the lateral malleolus and passes forward and somewhat medially to attach to the neck of the talus.

The distal tibiofibular syndesmosis is a very important part of the ankle joint. It is formed by the apposition of the convex medial surface of the fibula to the fibular notch on the lateral aspect of the tibia. Limiting the fibular notch are the prominent anterior and posterior tibial tuber-

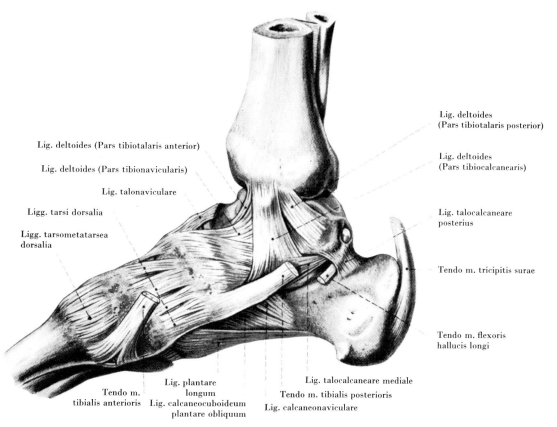

Figure 56–1. *Medial aspect of the ankle. (From Wolf-Heidegger, G.: Atlas der systematischen Anatomie des Menschen. Basel and New York, S. Karger, 1954.)*

Lig. deltoides (Pars tibiotalaris anterior)

Lig. deltoides (Pars tibionavicularis)

Lig. talonaviculare

Ligg. tarsi dorsalia

Ligg. tarsometatarsea dorsalia

Lig. deltoides (Pars tibiotalaris posterior)

Lig. deltoides (Pars tibiocalcanearis)

Lig. talocalcaneare posterius

Tendo m. tricipitis surae

Tendo m. flexoris hallucis longi

Tendo m. tibialis anterioris

Lig. plantare longum

Lig. calcaneocuboideum plantare obliquum

Lig. talocalcaneare mediale

Tendo m. tibialis posterioris

Lig. calcaneonaviculare

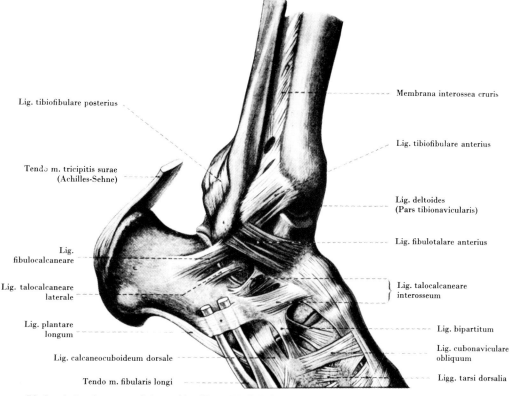

Figure 56–2. *Lateral aspect of the ankle. (From Wolf-Heidegger, G.: Atlas der systematischen Anatomie des Menschen. Basel and New York, S. Karger, 1954.)*

Lig. tibiofibulare posterius

Tendo m. tricipitis surae (Achilles-Sehne)

Lig. fibulocalcaneare

Lig. talocalcaneare laterale

Lig. plantare longum

Lig. calcaneocuboideum dorsale

Tendo m. fibularis longi

Membrana interossea cruris

Lig. tibiofibulare anterius

Lig. deltoides (Pars tibionavicularis)

Lig. fibulotalare anterius

Lig. talocalcaneare interosseum

Lig. bipartitum

Lig. cubonaviculare obliquum

Ligg. tarsi dorsalia

cles. The tibia and fibula are strongly held together in this area by four ligaments: the *interosseous ligament,* which is a distal prolongation of the interosseous membrane; the *anterior inferior tibiofibular ligament,* which extends from the lower end of the tibia laterally and distally to insert on the fibula; the *posterior inferior tibiofibular ligament* (Fig. 56–3), which runs in the same direction as the anterior ligament; and the *transverse ligament,* which is strong and is made up of the deep fibers of the posterior inferior tibiofibular ligament. There is slight fibular motion at the syndesmosis in several planes during normal movement of the ankle joint. Restriction of this motion may result in impaired function of the ankle.

The function of the fibula is not certain. In the past, a weight-bearing function has been attributed to it. It would appear, experimentally, that the fibula is capable of transmitting one sixth of the static load of the leg.[47] Other investigators have replaced this static concept with a dynamic one. Roentgenograms taken while a strong downward thrust was applied through the ball of the foot showed approximation of the fibula to the tibia. It was postulated that this was due to the contraction of the flexor muscles and that the point of greatest stress occurred near the inferior tibiofibular joint.[29] Cineradiographic studies demonstrate a distal migration of the fibula during the stance and push-off phases of gait.[69] During the stance phase of gait, the flexors of the foot cause migration of the fibula distally, deepening the ankle mortise. In addition, this results in tightening of the interosseous membrane, which pulls the fibula medially. The overall effect is to increase the stability of the ankle mortise during activity.

CLASSIFICATION OF ANKLE INJURIES

Dupuytren was the first to suggest a classification of ankle injuries based on the mechanism of injury.[3] However, he recognized only abduction and adduction as forces involved, and therefore, his system was quite limited. Maisonneuve added the concept of the external rotation force.[3] During the remainder of the nineteenth centu-

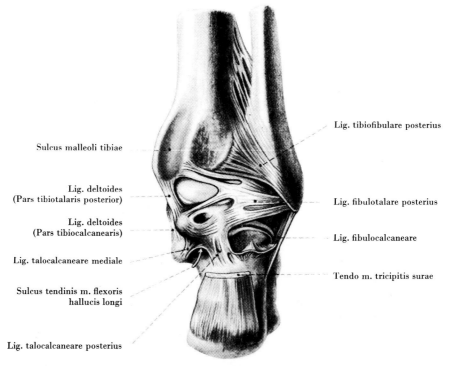

Sulcus malleoli tibiae

Lig. deltoides (Pars tibiotalaris posterior)

Lig. deltoides (Pars tibiocalcanearis)

Lig. talocalcaneare mediale

Sulcus tendinis m. flexoris hallucis longi

Lig. talocalcaneare posterius

Lig. tibiofibulare posterius

Lig. fibulotalare posterius

Lig. fibulocalcaneare

Tendo m. tricipitis surae

Figure 56–3. Posterior aspect of the ankle. (From Wolf-Heidegger, G.: Atlas der systematischen Anatomie des Menschen. Basel and New York, S. Karger, 1954.)

ry, the mechanistic approach was put aside in favor of the anatomic classification. This described ankle fractures as monomalleolar, bimalleolar, or trimalleolar. The anatomic system overemphasized the bony injury and neglected the presence or absence of a ligamentous injury.

At the beginning of this century, interest returned to the use of the mechanism of injury as the basis of classification. By producing fractures in cadaver specimens and doing x-ray studies of the specimens, characteristic images were identified and then classified according to the mechanism of injury and the degree of severity. The first orderly and comprehensive classification of ankle injuries based on the mechanism of injury was presented in a classic paper by Ashhurst and Bromer in 1922.[1] They divided the fractures into three main groups: *external rotation fractures, abduction fractures*, and *adduction fractures*. They further divided each major group into three degrees of injury increasing in severity. The Ashhurst-Bromer classification did not place sufficient emphasis on ligamentous injury, however, and more particularly, did not give enough importance to diastasis of the syndesmosis.

Lauge-Hansen proposed a classification based on experimental, surgical, and roentgenographic studies and used a different terminology.[50] He emphasized the close relationship between ligament injuries and bony lesions about the ankle and classified ankle fractures into four types, according to the manner of production (genesis). These four types of ankle fractures are described by the position of the foot at the moment of the injury and by the direction that the ankle is driven by the injuring force. They are characterized by the localization and form of the fracture of the fibula. The stages in each individual type of fracture are determined according to the combination of the fibular fracture with one or more additional injuries involving other parts of the ankle. Together with the use of "genetic roentgen diagnosis," Lauge-Hansen proposed the use of "genetic reduction." The type of reduction performed in each instance is based on reversing the direction of the injuring force.

A *supination-eversion (SE) fracture* is produced by the application of an external rotation force to the foot, which is fixed in supination. The deltoid ligament is relaxed, and outward rotation of the talus puts pressure on the lateral malleolus, resulting in rupture of the anterior inferior tibiofibular ligament (Stage 1). Continuing pressure produces a spiral fracture of the distal fibula (Stage 2). Further outward rotation of the talus will cause a pull on the posterior inferior tibiofibular ligament, as well as pressure on the posterolateral edge of the tibia. This produces a fracture of the posterolateral border of the tibia (Stage 3). If the force continues, the medial malleolus will be avulsed or there will be a rupture of the deltoid ligament (Stage 4). (See Figure 56–4). Characteristic of the SE fracture is a spiral fracture of the supramalleolar portion of the fibula.

The *supination-adduction (SA) fracture* results when the supinated foot is subjected to a medially directed force. The cal-

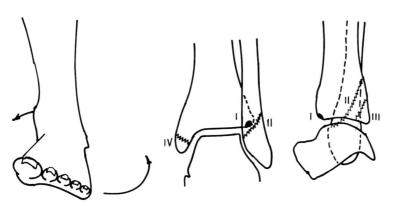

Figure 56–4. *Supination-eversion (SE) fracture. (Modified from Vasli, S.: Acta Chir. Scand. (Suppl.), 226:1, 1957 and Klossner, O.: Acta Chir. Scand. (Suppl.), 293:1, 1962.)*

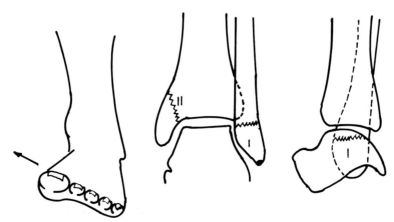

Figure 56–5. *Supination-adduction (SA) fracture. (Modified from Vasli, S.: Acta Chir. Scand. (Suppl.), 226:1, 1957 and Klossner, O.: Acta Chir. Scand. (Suppl.), 293:1, 1962.)*

caneofibular ligament is tightened so that there is either a rupture of the fibular collateral ligament or a transverse fracture of the lateral malleolus (Stage 1). This may be followed by a vertical fracture of the medial malleolus (Stage 2). (See Figure 56–5.) The characteristic feature of the SA fracture is a transverse fracture of the lateral malleolus.

A *pronation-abduction (PA) fracture* is produced by a laterally directed force on the foot fixed in pronation. Since this tightens the deltoid ligament, it will result in either a fracture of the medial malleolus or a rupture of the deltoid ligament (Stage 1). If the force is continued, the anterior and posterior tibiofibular ligaments will rupture, frequently avulsing a small fragment of bone from the anterior tibial tubercle

and a larger fragment of bone from the posterior margin of the tibia (Stage 2). Finally, there will be a short, oblique fracture of the fibula just above the ankle (Stage 3), which is the characteristic feature of this fracture. (See Figure 56–6.)

A *pronation-eversion (PE) fracture* results from an outward rotation of the fixed, pronated foot. The deltoid ligament is tightened, and there is either a fracture of the medial malleolus or a rupture of the deltoid ligament (Stage 1). Progression of the externally rotating force will then cause a tear of the anterior inferior tibiofibular and interosseous ligaments, as well as of the interosseous membrane (Stage 2). As the force continues, there will be a spiral fracture of the shaft of the fibula at a level proximal to the syndesmosis and

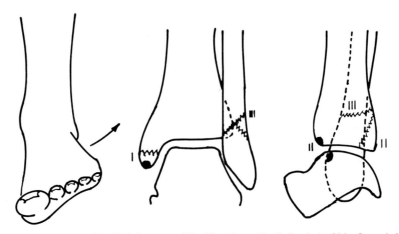

Figure 56–6. *Pronation-abduction (PA) fracture. (Modified from Vasli, S.: Acta Chir. Scand. (Suppl.), 226:1, 1957 and Klossner, O.: Acta Chir. Scand. (Suppl.), 293:1, 1962.)*

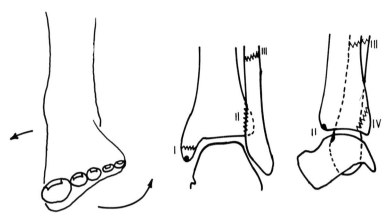

Figure 56–7. *Pronation-eversion (PE) fracture. (Modified from Vasli, S.: Acta Chir. Scand. (Suppl.), 226:1, 1957 and Klossner, O.: Acta Chir. Scand. (Suppl.), 293:1, 1962.)*

even sometimes as high as the neck of the fibula (Stage 3). Finally, there will be a fracture of the posterolateral margin of the tibia (Stage 4). (See Figure 56–7.) Characteristic of the PE injury is a spiral fracture of the fibula at a variable distance above the syndesmosis.

Subsequently, Lauge-Hansen described a fifth type of fracture of the ankle, the *pronation-dorsiflexion fracture*.[53] This type of fracture is produced by a fall on the foot from a considerable height, which drives the talus into the articular surface of the distal tibia. It may occur in four stages: Stage 1 is represented by a fracture of the medial malleolus; Stage 2 is characterized by an avulsion of a large fragment from the anterior lip of the tibia; Stage 3 is demonstrated by a fracture of the fibula just above the level of the malleoli; and Stage 4 is represented by a transverse fracture of the posterior aspect of the tibia level with the proximal margin of the large tibial fragment. Thus, if Stage 4 is reached, the fracture consists of a comminuted intra-articular fracture of the distal end of the tibia and a fracture of the fibula.

The Lauge-Hansen classification has been valuable because of its emphasis on the recognition of ligamentous injuries accompanying ankle fractures, and it has some practical use in the treatment of certain fractures. Its value in treatment is somewhat diminished, however, by its complexity. In actual practice, it is just too difficult to remember and too cumbersome to use.

In practice, a more useful method of classification is that advocated by Weber.[79] This classification is a modification of one proposed earlier by Danis. Weber's classification places significance on the presence or absence of injury to the syndesmosis. The likelihood of injury to the syndesmosis can be inferred from the nature and level of the fibular fracture. (The more proximal on the shaft the fracture of the fibula is, the greater the likelihood of damage to the syndesmosis.)

There are three basic types of injury in this classification (Fig. 56–8). *Type A* is a fracture of the fibula at the level of the ankle joint or distal to it. This may or may not be accompanied by a fracture of the medial malleolus. An equivalent injury would be a rupture of the lateral collateral ligament. Injuries to the syndesmosis, interosseous membrane, or deltoid ligament are never present in this type of fracture. *Type B* is a fracture of the fibula at the level of the syndesmosis, with or without a fracture of the medial malleolus. An equivalent injury would be a rupture of the deltoid ligament if the medial malleolus remains intact. This type of fracture may or may not be associated with an injury to the syndesmosis. *Type C* is a fracture of the fibula above the level of the syndesmosis. This injury is associated with either a rupture of the deltoid ligament or a fracture of the medial malleolus. There is always a rupture of the syndesmosis, with varying degrees of damage to the interosseous membrane.

All three types of injury may be associated with a fracture of the posterior portion

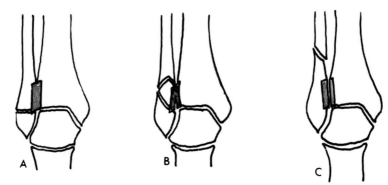

Figure 56–8. *Weber classification — Types A, B, and C ankle fractures. (From Weber, B.G.: Die Verletzungen des oberen Sprunggelenkes. Bern, Stuttgart, and Wien, Verlag Hans Huber, 1972.)*

of the tibia. In Type A fractures, the posterior fragment is medial and adjacent to the medial malleolus. The posterior syndesmosis remains intact. In Types B and C, the posterior fragment is lateral, adjacent to the lateral malleolus, and remains attached to the lower fibular fragment by the posterior tibiofibular ligament. It is apparent that the extent of damage to the syndesmosis progresses in severity from Type A to Type C. In all fractures in which the talus is displaced, there may be accompanying ligamentous injuries or fractures that do not show on roentgenograms. In addition, there is frequently damage to the articular cartilage of the distal tibia and of the talus.

We find that this method of classification has been especially valuable when treating displaced fractures of the ankle joint with rigid internal fixation and early joint motion.

EMERGENCY TREATMENT OF ANKLE FRACTURES

It is important to evaluate the general condition of the patient prior to treatment.[35] The recognition and treatment of emergency conditions, such as airway obstruction, intrathoracic injuries, abdominal injuries, coma, and hemorrhage, take precedence over the ankle injury. As soon as these life-threatening problems are treated and the patient's condition is stabilized, the ankle is examined. Following this, in the evaluation of the injured ankle, one looks for deformity, areas of swelling and tenderness, and loss of function, as well as

for the presence or absence of neurovascular compromise. Examination of the proximal fibula on the injured side is mandatory in the evaluation of ankle injuries.

If there is marked distortion of ankle anatomy with imminent circulatory embarrassment of the skin, an immediate manipulation should be done in the emergency room prior to x-ray studies. This diminishes tension on the skin, thus avoiding the possible complication of converting a closed fracture to an open fracture prior to treatment, and relieves neurovascular embarrassment. The limb is then splinted. There are various methods of accomplishing this, including the use of an air splint, a rigid splint or a pillow splint (Fig. 56–9).

ROENTGENOGRAPHIC EVALUATION

Roentgenographic evaluation of the ankle injury should include anteroposterior and lateral views, as well as an oblique view with the extremity in 20 to 30 degrees of medial rotation (mortise view). It is also helpful to obtain roentgenograms of the entire tibia and fibula, since in some cases there may be a fibular fracture proximal to the ankle joint level. If there is any question about the nature of the ankle injury, comparison views of the opposite ankle are mandatory. Ordinarily, stress films of the ankle are not required. However, if rupture of the ligaments is suspected, stress films can be extremely helpful.

In the presence of a fibular fracture with a possible lesion of the deltoid ligament, the proper stress roentgenogram is one in which the foot and ankle joint are placed

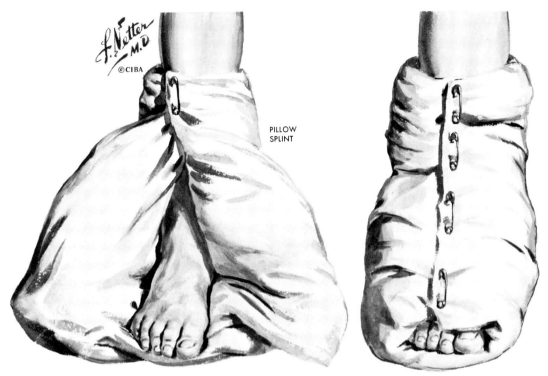

Figure 56–9. *Pillow splint. (© Copyright 1955 CIBA Pharmaceutical Company, Division of CIBA-GEIGY Corporation. Reprinted with permission from Clinical Symposia, illustrated by Frank H. Netter, M.D. All rights reserved.)*

in marked external rotation in relation to the leg. Ordinarily, the space between the superior dome of the talus and the inferior articular surface of the tibia is equal in width to the space between the lateral articular surface of the medial malleolus and the medial articular surface of the talus. A separation of 2 to 4 mm between the medial malleolus and the medial border of the talus is suggestive of joint widening. When the widening is borderline, it is more probable that the patient has a Grade II sprain of the deltoid ligament, rather than a Grade III sprain. If there is complete disruption of the deltoid ligament (Grade III sprain), the distance between the talus and the medial malleolus is sufficient to be characteristic. (See Figure 56–14B.)

In cases of suspected complete rupture of the fibular collateral ligament, roentgenograms should be taken with the ankle placed in a position of forced inversion. This will be discussed in more detail in the section on ruptures of the fibular collateral ligament. Sometimes the use of

arthrography may be helpful in evaluating obscure traumatic lesions.[74]

TREATMENT

Traditionally, the treatment of fractures of the ankle has been nonoperative. However, long-term follow-up studies of fractures treated by closed methods show a disappointingly high proportion of poor results.[56] These poor results are directly related to the inability to obtain and maintain anatomic reduction of the fracture fragments,[77] which predisposes to an increased incidence of osteoarthrosis.[80] In order to avoid this complication, an increasing number of surgeons began to treat displaced ankle fractures by open reduction and internal fixation. Initially the results were only slightly better than those achieved by closed reduction. However, when open reduction and internal fixation were combined with early active motion, the results began to improve.[77] More rigid fixation combined with early active motion, as advocated by other investigators, including the AO Group, resulted in marked improvement in functional results.[5, 10, 27]

The advantages of closed reduction are that a prolonged operative procedure may be avoided and, except in the case of treatment of open fractures, infection does not become a serious consideration. The disadvantages of closed reduction are that anatomic reduction of all the components of the fracture complex is frequently impossible; maintenance of the reduction frequently requires that the foot be placed in an abnormal position; and a period of prolonged plaster immobilization is required, often resulting in "fracture disease," with subsequent swelling, edema, and stiffness of the involved joint.

Open reduction provides an opportunity to adequately visualize all injuries, both bony and ligamentous. It permits anatomic reduction and fixation of the bony fragments, as well as operative repair of the soft-tissue injuries. With rigid fixation, early functional aftertreatment is possible, diminishing the incidence of "fracture disease." The main disadvantages of surgery are the presence of incisional scars, the need for a prolonged operative procedure under anesthesia, and the possibility of postoperative wound infection.

Generalized medical problems, such as diabetic acidosis, congestive heart failure, and cardiac arrhythmia, are temporary contraindications to operative stabilization of the fracture. However, medical consultation and prompt, aggressive treatment will usually correct these problems within 24 hours. If the local skin condition is satisfactory at that time, surgery may be performed.

Some of the local contraindications to surgery include eczematous skin lesions, excessive swelling of the injured foot and ankle, and the presence of fracture blisters. Frequently, the rapid and massive swelling that is seen in severely displaced ankle injuries is surprising. If surgery is not performed promptly, swelling may become so severe that surgery is contraindicated. We have found that elevation of the limb and the administration of furosemide (Lasix), 20 mg by mouth twice a day for two to three days, will help control the local edema. Modified Quigley traction[63] is

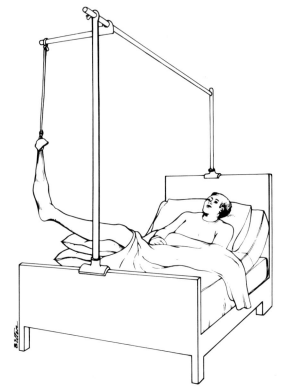

Figure 56–10. *Modified Quigley traction.*

a convenient method of insuring continued elevation of the limb (Fig. 56–10).

Age per se is no contraindication to open reduction of these fractures. In fact, it is our opinion that in the elderly patient, open reduction and early mobilization cause less strain on the cardiovascular system of the patient than does closed reduction followed by subsequent attempts at ambulation in a long leg cast using a walker without bearing weight on the involved extremity.

Closed Reduction

To treat fractures of the ankle by closed reduction, an understanding of the mechanism of ankle injury is required. Reversal of this mechanism facilitates reduction of the fracture. As mentioned previously, there are several methods of classification. A simple practical method for the closed treatment of fractures of the ankle is the classification of Dupuytren, which also was subsequently used by McLaughlin.[55] This classification divides ankle fractures into two groups according to the mechanism of injury — abduction and adduction.

In the *abduction injury*, the foot is forced out into abduction by the deforming force. This will result in an avulsion type of injury medially, so that either the deltoid ligament is torn or there is a transverse fracture of the medial malleolus. The key to the diagnosis of an abduction injury is the presence of a torn deltoid ligament or a transverse fracture of the medial malleolus.

With an *adduction injury*, the foot is brought into adduction and varus. As a result, the talus is driven into the medial malleolus like a chisel. This causes a shearing fracture of the medial malleolus, starting at the junction of the medial malleolus with the tibial plafond. The fracture line proceeds proximally and medially into the tibia. Here again, the location and direction of the fracture line in the medial malleolus are the key to identifying the mechanism of injury.

The classification of Lauge-Hansen certainly gives more specific information about the nature of the deforming forces. In addition, it aids in identifying accompanying ligamentous injuries. However, it is complicated and becomes cumbersome to recall and to use at the time of actual closed reduction. Nevertheless, it does provide a better means for securing more exact repositioning of the fracture fragments with closed reduction.[44]

Technique of Closed Reduction

Adequate closed reduction usually requires general anesthesia. After administration of anesthesia, the involved extremity is permitted to hang over the edge of the fracture table. Flexion of the knee relaxes the gastrocnemius and permits better manipulation of the ankle. It has been noted that "the astragalus, the medial malleolus, the third malleolus, and the lateral malleolus all move as one piece, since their ligamentous connections have remained intact."[13] In view of this, reduction is secured by concentrating on replacing the astragalus anatomically in the ankle mortise. As the astragalus is replaced, the other fragments move along with it and assume a more or less normal position. With an abduction injury, a small segment of the superior portion of the medial malleolus usually remains attached to the main tibial fragment. As the astragalus is reduced, it can be stabilized against the intact segment of the medial malleolus, which acts as a buttress. In an adduction injury, the buttress is usually lacking, and therefore, these reductions are unstable. "Overreduction" should be avoided. Following reduction, an above-the-knee cast is applied and "re-check" roentgenograms are taken.

Several errors have been found to occur commonly in reducing a fracture-dislocation of the ankle.[13] If there is a posterior malleolar fragment of significant size, attempts to keep the foot at a right angle to the leg frequently result in subluxation of the fragment. Satisfactory reduction is often obtained only by placing the talus and the foot in plantar flexion in order to prevent this subluxation.

In closing the mortise, when pressure is applied equally to both sides of the ankle, the talus cannot move. The talus will move and the ankle mortise will "close" only when there is a differential application of pressure. To accomplish this, pressure is applied over the lateral malleolus and also over the lower end of the tibia medially, just above the medial malleolus.

Most ankle injuries result from an external rotation force. To insure proper reduction of the fragments under closed treatment, an internal rotation force is included in the reduction maneuver. If this is not done, the fracture of the lateral malleolus will most likely remain unreduced. Sometimes, the medial malleolar fragment also is difficult to reduce. On the anteroposterior roentgenogram, the reduction appears satisfactory, whereas on the lateral view, there is inferior angulation of the anterior portion of the medial malleolus. Placement of a felt pad under the tip of the medial malleolus can occasionally help to maintain its position. More frequently, however, the malleolus persists in tilting inferiorly despite all attempts at maintaining the position of the reduction, thus resulting in malunion of the medial malleolar fragment.

In bimalleolar fractures, the reduction can usually be held only by some combination of varus and internal rotation of the ankle.[83] This stress causes the talus to move back into position. At some point, the talus stops moving, usually because of the impingement of the lateral malleolus on the proximal fibular fragment. Further forceful internal rotation will accomplish reduction of the talus, provided there is stability medially. This reduction, however, is obtained by stretching of the fibular collateral ligaments. Once the internal rotation stress is discontinued, the talus will return to its displaced position.

It would appear, then, that the lateral malleolus is the key to anatomic reduction of displaced malleolar fragments. Stability of the ankle is restored only when the integrity of the lateral malleolus is reestablished. It represents an important, if not the most important, element in securing anatomic reduction of these injuries.[83]

Roentgenographic Criteria for Closed Reduction

The question of what constitutes an adequate reduction of a fracture-dislocation of the ankle is still undecided. The following roentgenographic criteria have been suggested as evidence of satisfactory reduction: (1) no malposition of the talus; (2) no lateral and/or medial displacement of the malleolar fragments; (3) less than 2 mm of backward displacement of the lateral malleolar fragment; (4) less than 2 mm of proximal displacement of the posterior tibial fragment; and (5) less than 2 mm of backward, forward, or longitudinal displacement of the medial malleolar fragment.[77] In this connection, some experimental work that has been done is helpful.[64] These investigators have found that a 1-mm lateral displacement of the talus would result in the loss of approximately 42 per cent of the contact surface between the tibia and the superior dome of the talus. If the weight that is placed on the ankle joint during the stance phase of gait is taken into account, minimal lateral displacement of the talus results in considerable increase in stress concentration at the joint surface. In order to diminish the possibility of future disability from osteoarthrosis, anatomic reduction of the talus in the mortise is mandatory.

When displacement of the posterior malleolar fragment is evident on the roentgenogram, a "step" is created in the articular surface. If the fragment is larger than 25 per cent of the articular surface, there is loss of congruity between the tibia and the talus. This may result in posterior subluxation of the talus and early disabling osteoarthrosis. Therefore, when the posterior malleolar fragment is greater than 25 per cent of the articular surface, internal fixation is necessary to maintain an anatomic reduction of the fracture fragments.[55]

With closed reduction, the width between the medial border of the talus and the medial malleolus should be approximately equal to that of the space between the superior dome of the talus and the inferior articular surface of the tibia on the anteroposterior view. Any widening of this space is suggestive of incomplete restoration of the ankle mortise. This may be due to interposition of the deltoid ligament medially or incomplete reduction of the lateral malleolar fragment.

Evaluation of the injuries to the syndesmosis is difficult. in these cases, it is mandatory that roentgenograms provide clear visualization of the distal end of the fibula, as well as of the lateral portion of the distal tibia. Sophisticated guidelines are available for the diagnosis of these injuries and for evaluation of the reduction.[3, 54]

If postreduction roentgenograms are satisfactory, the cast is extended above the flexed knee to the upper thigh.

Postreduction Treatment

When swelling subsides, the patient is permitted to ambulate with crutches or a walker with no weight bearing on the involved extremity. Roentgenograms are taken at intervals of one week, two weeks, and four weeks, since displacement of the fracture fragments may occur up to four weeks after reduction. Any loss of position as shown on the roentgenograms may be an indication for either remanipulation or open reduction. Six weeks after reduction, the above-the-knee cast is removed, and a below-the-knee cast is applied under roentgenographic control. Two weeks later, the patient is permitted to bear weight in plaster. The cast can usually be removed at the end of 10 weeks. Active exercises of the ankle as well as increased weight bearing on the involved extremity are emphasized. In general, most patients do not require formal physical therapy after closed reduction. If the patient is unable to cooperate with a program of active exercises at home or is anxious, exercising under the direction of a skilled physiotherapist may be helpful. There is no substitute, however, for active use of the injured extremity by the patient.

Open Reduction

In the open treatment of fracture-dislocations of the ankle, we have found Weber's method of classification[79] to be extremely useful. Therefore, in the following discussion of open reduction, this classification will be used as a guide.

Type A Fracture-Dislocations. In this injury, by definition, the fibular fracture is located below the level of the syndesmosis (see Figure 56–8). The syndesmosis is not involved in the injury. Clinically, the objective findings are confined mainly to the lateral aspect of the joint, at or below the level of the lateral malleolus. At times, additional pathology can also be identified on the medial side of the joint. Roentgenograms show an avulsion fracture of the tip of the lateral malleolus or a transverse fracture of the lateral malleolus below the level of the syndesmosis (Fig. 56–11). When the injury is confined solely to the region of the lateral malleolus, it is preferable to treat the patient nonoperatively. A below-the-knee cast is applied with the ankle in neutral position. Weight bearing is permitted, and the cast may be removed after six weeks.

In elderly patients, the use of a plaster cast creates additional difficulties. An acceptable alternate method of treatment for them is the use of an Unna boot. The Unna boot is changed at approximately two-week intervals for a total of six weeks. At the end of that time, the immobilization is discontinued, and the patient wears an outer heel wedge on his shoe. The weakened peroneal muscles are protected in this manner, thus diminishing the risk of "turning over" on the ankle. With this technique, few problems are found both during and after the immobilization period.

The patient with an avulsion fracture of the tip of the lateral malleolus deserves

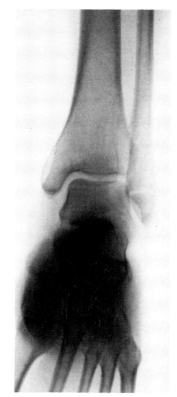

Figure 56–11. *Type A ankle fracture.*

special attention. This usually represents an incomplete avulsion of the attachment of the fibular collateral ligament. However, it could possibly represent a rupture of the fibular collateral ligament, and this must be ruled out.

The *fibular collateral ligament* has an important role in providing stability for the ankle joint. In experimental studies, division of the fibular collateral ligament resulted in approximately 30 degrees of external rotatory instability, as well as marked talar instability.[83] Therefore, after this injury, significant disability would be expected to occur in the ankle. The diagnosis is suspected by a history of severe injury, marked swelling below the tip of the lateral malleolus, tenderness over the fibular collateral ligament, a positive drawer test, and the presence of a talar tilt on the standard anteroposterior roentgenogram. The drawer test is performed as follows: "With the knee flexed and the foot held in 20 degrees of plantar flexion, one hand is applied to the anterior aspect of the tibia, exerting pressure posteriorly,

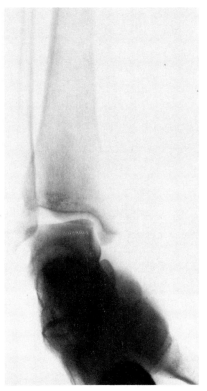

Figure 56–12. *Abnormal inversion stress roentgenogram.*

while the other grasps the calcaneus, exerting pressure anteriorly."[30] At this point, when the test is positive, the talus can be felt to sublux anteriorly. In cases of suspected rupture of the fibular collateral ligament, inversion stress roentgenograms of both ankles in plantar flexion and neutral position are taken. Comparsion views of the uninjured ankle should also be taken. When the stress roentgenogram in neutral position is normal and the stress roentgenogram in plantar flexion shows a talar tilt, usually only the anterior talofibular ligament is ruptured. This should be treated with plaster immobilization for a period of four to six weeks. The patient may then bear weight in the cast. If, however, the roentgenograms show a significant tilt when the ankle is stressed both in plantar flexion and in the neutral position, there is a rupture of both the anterior talofibular and calcaneofibular ligaments (Fig. 56–12).

In the elderly individual, simultaneous ruptures of the anterior talofibular and calcaneofibular ligaments are treated by

immobilization in a below-the-knee weight-bearing cast for six weeks. After the cast is removed, the patient should wear an outer heel wedge for six to eight weeks.

In the younger individual, more strenuous measures are required to secure the optimal result. There has been a recent trend, especially in young athletic individuals, toward immediate operative repair of complete ruptures of the fibular collateral ligament. This has resulted in a definite improvement in functional results.[33, 68, 75]

Type B Fracture-Dislocation. In Type B injuries, the fracture of the fibula is located at the level of the syndesmosis (see Figure 56–8). In this case, there may or may not be involvement of the syndesmosis, depending on the location and direction of the fracture line. The most common ankle fracture, the "external rotation" fracture of the lateral malleolus, is in this group (Fig. 56–13). It can be identified by its unique appearance on the lateral roentgenogram; the fracture line starts anteriorly at the level of the ankle joint and pro-

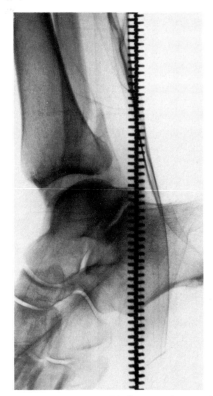

Figure 56–13. *Type B ankle fracture (external rotation fracture).*

ceeds in an oblique manner superiorly into the posterior portion of the fibula. The syndesmosis may or may not be involved in this injury. However, experience has shown that with this particular injury, consistently good results can be obtained by plaster immobilization alone. Therefore, the patient is treated with a below-the-knee cast for four to six weeks. Weight bearing is permitted in the cast. When the cast is removed, the patient wears a shoe with an outer heel wedge for an additional six weeks.

At times, the external rotation fracture of the lateral malleolus may be accompanied by a *complete rupture of the deltoid ligament medially.* This situation can be a trap for the unwary surgeon, as the initial roentgenograms show only the fracture of the lateral malleolus. However, alerted by the abnormal swelling below the medial malleolus, tenderness, and pain below the tip of the medial malleolus, the surgeon should order external rotation stress roentgenograms. These reveal that in addition to the fibular fracture, there is now evidence of widening of the ankle mortise, indicative of loss of stability both medially and laterally (Fig. 56–14).

In a *combined injury*, i.e., a *fracture of the lateral malleolus with a complete rupture of the deltoid ligament,* both closed reduction[17, 38, 42] and open reduction[3, 4, 43, 63] have been proposed. The advocates of each method have claimed good results with their suggested form of treatment. In deciding which method to use, consideration should be given to the fact that the combined medial and lateral joint injuries create a situation in which there is little remaining inherent stability in the ankle mortise. If this injury is treated by closed reduction, the patient is immobilized in an above-the-knee cast with the leg in a position of medial rotation. Roentgenograms are taken at two-week intervals during the first four weeks to insure early detection of loss of reduction. No weight bearing is permitted on the fractured ankle during this period. At the end of six weeks, the cast is removed, roentgenograms are taken, and if the reduction has been maintained, a below-the-knee cast is applied. Weight bearing is permitted in this new cast, which is worn for an additional four weeks.

Recently, there has been a trend toward the operative treatment of this injury.

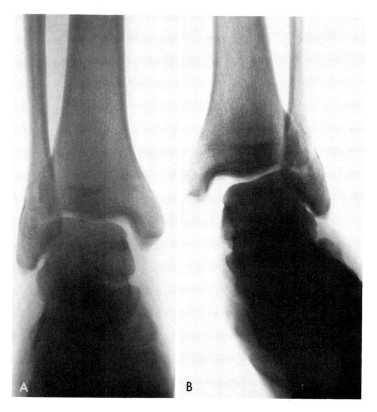

Figure 56–14. *(A) Anteroposterior roentgenogram of an injured ankle. (B) External rotation stress roentgenogram of the same ankle.*

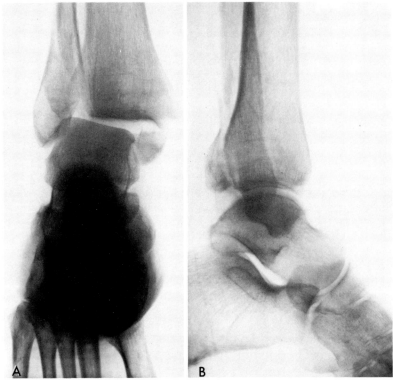

Figure 56–15. *(A) Anteroposterior view of a Type B fracture-dislocation. (B) Lateral view of a Type B fracture-dislocation.*

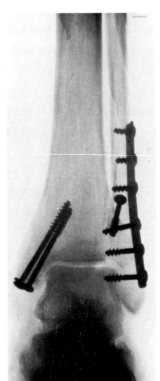

Figure 56–16. *Postoperative roentgenogram of a Type B fracture-dislocation after open reduction and internal fixation.*

Open reduction permits diagnosis and treatment of entrapment of the deltoid ligament between the talus and medial malleolus;[4] interposition of the posterior tibial tendon can be discovered and treated;[21] and primary suturing of the ruptured deltoid ligament can be performed.[16]

Type B ankle fractures may present as fractures of the lateral and medial malleoli. Sometimes, in addition, the posterolateral border of the distal articular surface of the tibia (the so-called "posterior malleolus") is fractured (Fig. 56–15). It is our preference to treat displaced fracture-dislocations of the ankle by open reduction and internal fixation. Both the medial and lateral malleoli should be fixed (Fig. 56–16), and if there is a fracture of the posterior malleolus involving more than 25 per cent of the articular surface, this should also be treated with internal fixation.

Type C Fracture-Dislocation. The Type C injury is identified by the presence of a fracture of the fibula proximal to the syndesmosis (see Figure 56–8). The fracture itself may occur at any level from just

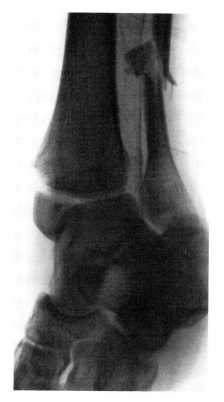

Figure 56–17. *Type C fracture-dislocation with fibular fracture just proximal to the syndesmosis.*

proximal to the syndesmosis (Fig. 56–17) up to the level of the neck of the fibula (Fig. 56–18A,B). Medially, the injury may be either a fracture of the medial malleolus or a rupture of the deltoid ligament. There may also be an accompanying fracture of the posterior malleolus. Closed reduction of this fracture-dislocation usually is not difficult. However, this is an extremely unstable injury, and frequently plaster immobilization alone is not sufficient to maintain the reduction. Therefore, we advise open reduction and rigid internal fixation of these injuries.

At surgery, a tranfixion screw is often required to protect the repair of the syndesmosis (Fig. 56–18C). It has been recommended that the fixation screw be removed at the end of six to eight weeks postoperatively and prior to the onset of weight bearing. There have been reports of patients complaining of a "wooden feeling" in the ankle joint during walking when the screw has not been removed. In addition, there have been reports of breaking of the screw from motion of the fibula during gait. If a 3.5-mm cortex screw is used for fixation of the distal tibiofibular syndesmosis, it is frequently permitted to remain in place even after the onset of weight bearing. Our patients have not reported any complications from this procedure, and although evidence of motion of the screw in the tibia is visible roentgenographically, there does not appear to be any untoward effect. In this injury complex, the cast remains on for 10 to 12 weeks in order to insure complete healing of the ligamentous injuries.

When open treatment is selected for any of these injuries, attention should be paid not only to the bony injuries, but also the ligamentous injuries. The surgical repair of these accompanying ligamentous injuries is as important to a good result as the repair of the bony injuries visualized on roentgenograms.[2, 12, 70, 79]

Fractures of the Distal End of the Tibia Involving the Ankle Joint. These fractures are of three main types: *anterior marginal fractures, posterior marginal fractures,* and *"explosion" (Pilon) fractures* of the distal tibia. The position of the talus at the time of impact will determine the type of fracture. When the talus is in a position of plantar flexion at the time of

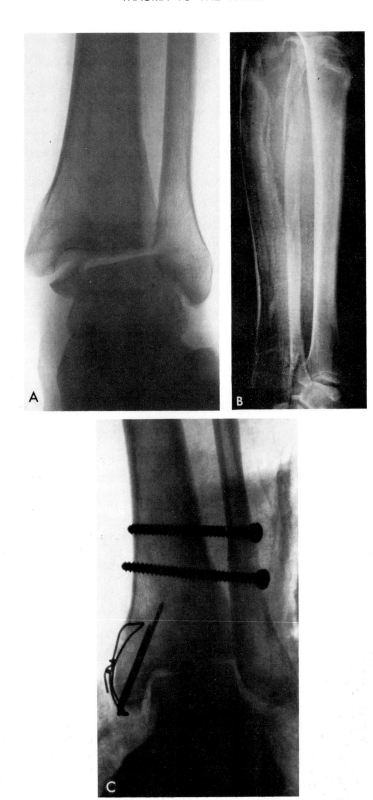

Figure 56–18. *(A) Type C fracture-dislocation (proximal fibular fracture not visualized on ankle roentgenogram). (B) Roentgenogram of the same patient showing the proximal fibular fracture. (C) Postoperative roentgenogram.*

impact, a posterior marginal fracture will be produced. If, however, the talus is in a position of dorsiflexion, an anterior marginal fracture will result. When the talus is in a neutral position, the "explosion" type of fracture occurs. All three fracture types involve the distal articular surface of the tibia. Therefore, in addition to the bony injury that is seen on roentgenograms, there may be injuries of the articular cartilage of the distal tibia and of the talus. These fractures may be treated by open or closed methods. However, as with most intra-articular fractures, the principles of anatomic restoration of the fracture fragments surgically, combined with early active motion, can be expected to produce functional results that are superior to those obtained with nonoperative treatment.

Since fractures of the anterior and posterior margin of the distal tibia are usually of significant size, internal fixation is preferred. This prevents loss of position in plaster with resulting joint incongruity and subluxation leading to subsequent painful osteoarthrosis.

Pilon fractures of the distal tibia present an entirely different problem (Fig. 56–19A). In this injury, the joint is usually totally disrupted by the presence of multiple displaced fracture fragments. Treatment with plaster immobilization is not satisfactory, since anatomic repositioning of the fragments is not possible with this method. In addition, a long period of immobilization in plaster is required. This will usually result in a stiff joint, and frequently painful osteoarthrosis ensues.[23] An alternative is the use of skeletal traction. The technique described by Shelton and Anderson is preferred.[71] Traction is obtained by means of a Steinmann pin inserted into the os calcis. Active motion of the ankle in traction is encouraged for five to six weeks. A cast incorporating a pin in the tibia above the fracture and in the os calcis below the fracture is then applied. The cast and pins are left in place for a total of about 12 weeks. After removal of the cast and pins, a cast brace may be required for an additional three to six months. With this technique, it is essential to maintain the talus centered in the mortise. Hopefully the early active motion of the talus will mold the fracture fragments into a shape congruent with the superior dome of the talus. At the same time, early motion ensures a satisfactory range of motion in the ankle.

In the hands of the experienced surgeon, open reduction of some of these injuries may be considered. It should be pointed out, however, that the operation is frequently long in duration and technically difficult and requires a thorough knowledge of the principles of internal fixation. Open reduction should not be undertaken by the surgeon who treats these injuries infrequently. The principles of operative treatment of this injury have been well presented by members of the AO Group[66] and are outlined below.

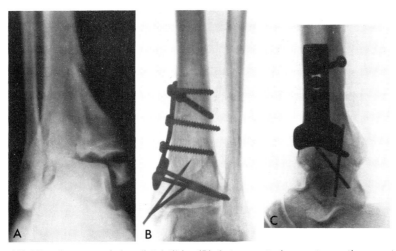

Figure 56–19. *(A) Pilon fracture of the distal tibia. (B) Anteroposterior postoperative roentgenogram. (C) Lateral postoperative roentgenogram.*

RESTORATION OF FIBULAR LENGTH.
This includes not only restoration of the
full length of the fibula, but also correction of any axis deviation, which
must be the first step in the operative
procedure. As a result, the tibia will be
restored to its normal length. After anatomic reduction of the fibula has been accomplished, internal fixation of the fibula
must be performed to prevent displacement during the remaining portion of the
operative procedure.

RECONSTRUCTION OF THE LOWER AR-
TICULAR SURFACE OF THE TIBIA. Depending on the number of fragments, this
stage of the procedure can become quite
complicated. It has been suggested that
the talus be used as a template upon which
the articular surface of the tibia may be
reconstructed. After the fragments have
been repositioned, temporary internal fixation of the fragments with Kirschner
wires is performed. At this point, the extent of the bony defect in the distal tibia
can be properly evaluated.

INTERNAL FIXATION OF THE TIBIA. In
"explosion" fractures of the distal tibia,
there is a tendency for the development of
varus deformities. These deformities may
be prevented by applying a medial buttress plate to the distal tibia (Fig. 56–
19B,C).

CANCELLOUS BONE GRAFTS. After the
articular surface has been restored, a metaphyseal defect is frequently observed.
This defect must be filled in with cancellous bone in order to provide support for
the reconstructed joint surface. At the time
of surgery, lesions of the articular cartilage
of the talus are often noted. These may
consist of bruising and fissuring of the
cartilage, as well as flaking and fractures of
the articular cartilage. Excision of the
loose pieces of cartilage is required. Injury
to the articular cartilage may prejudice the
functional result despite a satisfactory operative procedure.

With this technique, good functional results have been reported in more than 73
per cent of patients followed for a minimal
period of 50 months.[67] After the operative
procedure, it has been noted that if the
patient is going to develop a post-
traumatic arthrosis of the ankle joint, the
clinical symptoms become manifest within
one to two years of the accident. If the
patient has a good result at the end of one
year, the chances are excellent that he will
maintain this good result for an indefinite
time.

Postoperative Treatment

Postoperatively, patients who have undergone open reduction of an ankle fracture are placed in a below-the-knee cast.
Forty-eight hours later, the anterior portion of the lower half of the cast is removed. The patient is then encouraged to
engage in active dorsiflexion exercises of
the ankle (Fig. 56–20). There is no urgency
in performing plantar flexion exercises,
since the restoration of plantar flexion
postoperatively rarely presents a problem.

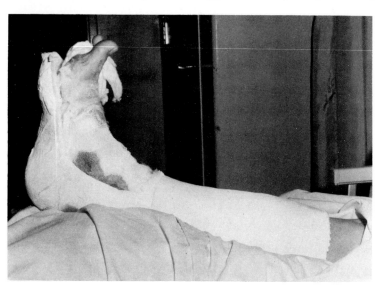

Figure 56–20. Patient performing early active exercises
after open reduction of an ankle
fracture.

When the patient has recovered a satisfactory range of dorsiflexion, the cast is closed. He is then permitted to ambulate using crutches or a walker. The cast is changed at the time of suture removal. Ordinarily, no weight bearing has been permitted on the operated extremity for six to eight weeks. However, recently in some elderly patients who have not required internal fixation of a fracture of the posterior malleolus, weight bearing in a short leg cast has been permitted two to four weeks postoperatively. The cast is left on for a total of 8 to 10 weeks; most recently, this has been shortened to a total of 4 to 6 weeks. If there has been internal fixation of a fractured posterior malleolus, weight bearing is not permitted until 10 weeks postoperatively, and the cast is removed 12 weeks postoperatively. After removal of the cast, treatment is the same as for patients who have had a closed reduction of an ankle fracture.

TREATMENT OF OPEN FRACTURES

An open fracture-dislocation of the ankle is the result of severe trauma with marked displacement of the fractured fragments. Careful examination for injuries to other body systems is made. After the patient's condition has been stabilized, the ankle is examined for the presence of neurovascular embarrassment. If this is present, manipulation is performed immediately in order to relieve circulatory distress. The wound is then dressed and the extremity is splinted. No further examination of the wound is performed until the patient is in the operating room. A broad-spectrum bactericidal antibiotic is administered intravenously as soon as possible in the emergency room prior to roentgenographic evaluation. Tetanus toxoid and tetanus antitoxin are administered as indicated. When the patient's condition permits, roentgenograms are taken and he is brought to the operating room. After the patient has been anesthetized, the dressings are removed and the wound is inspected. No cultures of the wound are taken at this time because it is our opinion that the results of these tests do not provide helpful information if a postoperative

wound infection should develop. Several problems present themselves for consideration, namely, the treatment of accompanying injuries, treatment of the soft-tissue wound, and treatment of the bony and ligamentous injuries. In evaluating the wound, a satisfactory and convenient method of classification is that of the AO Group[57]:

Grade I. A spike of bone protrudes through the skin, causing a laceration, the so-called compounding "from within out." The size of the lesion may vary, but the site of the trauma is localized to a well-defined area of the skin.

Grade II. The trauma occurs from the "outside" to the skin and underlying muscles.

Grade III. The degree of injury to the skin and underlying muscles is very severe. Frequently nerves and blood vessels are also involved. The end result of severe Grade III injuries may be amputation of the limb.

After the wound has been evaluated, a wide area of skin is shaved around the open wound and possible areas of operative intervention are shaved as well. They are then scrubbed with soap and sterile water, and the skin is prepared and draped in the usual manner, as for the standard operative treatment of a fractured ankle.

The wound is debrided. Any areas of impaired or suspected viability are excised. An excellent description of the principles involved in debridement is contained in this paraphrase of an old surgical verse:

From the skin take a piece quite thin;
The tighter the fascia, the more you slash 'er;
Of the muscle much more, till you see fresh gore;
Leave the bone, unless quite alone.

Statements concerning the use of a fixed quantity of irrigation material are misleading. The use of excessive quantities of irrigation solutions, e.g., 15 to 20 liters of saline, is unnecessary and time-consuming. It is preferable to use the quantity of fluid necessary to perform the function of irrigation. Irrigation is used to flush foreign bodies, clots, debris, and possibly some surface bacteria from the wound. It does not, however, eliminate the bacteria from the depths of the wound.[76] We have found the use of Surgi-Lav most helpful in the treatment of open fractures. All damaged tissues are excised by sharp dissection.

Following debridement, the method of stabilization of the fracture is considered. If one accepts the premise that rest of an area is required to aid nature's defenses in fighting infection, internal fixation seems a logical approach. A cast is not bone-tight, and even with a skintight cast, it is difficult to prevent motion of the fracture fragments. This motion further traumatizes the soft tissues and interferes with healing. The use of nonoperative treatment hinders functional aftertreatment of these injuries, and for this reason, internal fixation of Grade I and Grade II open fractures has been recommended by some as a preferred method of treatment.[15, 40, 57] However, the use of internal fixation in this situation should only be considered by the surgeon who can be certain from experience that his debridement has been sufficient and adequate.[40] An interesting technique has been described as being used at the Mayo Clinic in these situations. Cabanela recommends that initially a careful debridement of the wounds of compounding be performed, followed by closed reduction of the fractures.[11] The wounds are packed open, and the limb is immobilized in a compression dressing. Two to five days later, if no signs of infection are present and the wound appears to be granulating satisfactorily, a definitive open reduction and internal fixation are performed. Again, we would advocate that this technique be used only by the experienced surgeon.

In Grade III injuries, survival of the limb is the primary consideration. There are several available techniques that may be of help in achieving this. The use of a transarticular Steinmann pin fixation, as advocated by Childress,[14] should be considered. In this technique, a Steinmann pin (or multiple Kirschner wires) may be inserted through the inferior aspect of the os calcis, at the junction of the middle and anterior thirds. The ankle is held in a position of plantar flexion, and the Steinmann pin is drilled up through the talus, across the tibiotalar joint, and into the lower portion of the tibia (Fig. 56–21). This serves the function of rigidly holding the position of the foot and talus in relation to

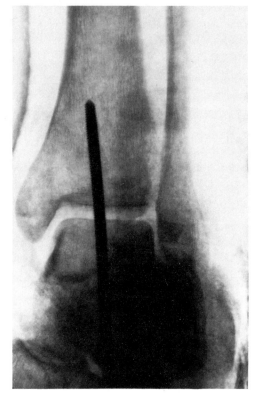

Figure 56–21. *Transarticular fixation of the ankle joint with a Steinmann pin.*

the tibia. Care of the wound is facilitated considerably with this simple procedure.

Another technique is the use of pins above and below the fracture, with incorporation of the pins in the cast. However, the local treatment of the wound is made extremely difficult by the presence of the cast. In some cases of Grade II or Grade III compounding, the use of an external fixation device may facilitate wound care while maintaining partial immobilization of bony fragments at the same time.

Brown has condemned the practice of primary closure of the wound of compounding in open fractures.[6] Premature closure of the wound may result in a sequence of infection, pyarthrosis, osteomyelitis, and perhaps even eventual amputation of the limb. Any surgical extensions of the original wound of compounding and elective incisions made for the purpose of introducing internal fixation may be closed. The original wound of compounding is left open and dressed. Four to five days later, the wound is reexamined in the operating room. Further wound care is based on the concept of bacterial contamination, as outlined by Krizek and Robson, "that the tissue level is more important than the surface contamination."[46] In order for contaminating bacteria to infect a wound, they must be present at a critical level, namely in excess of 10^5 per gram of tissue. (Coincidentally, this is also the same tissue level of bacteria that is required to demonstrate bacteria on a Gram stain slide.) Accordingly, the surface of the wound is cleaned with 70 per cent alcohol, and a biopsy of the wound is taken and sent to the laboratory. This tissue is prepared and examined by the method outlined by Krizek and Robson.[46] The presence of even a few bacteria on the slide is evidence of a tissue level of bacteria in excess of 10^5 per gram of tissue. This contraindicates closure of the wound. Additional specimens are sent to the laboratory for culture and antibiotic sensitivity tests. The wound is then packed and evaluated daily for signs of a developing infection. When no bacteria are observed on the Gram stain slide, the tissue level of bacteria is assumed to be below 10^5 per gram of tissue, and delayed primary closure of the wound may be performed. Aftercare follows the same principles as outlined under the treatment of open reduction of fractures of the ankle.

Antibiotics

There are some areas of controversy about the use of antibiotics in the treatment of open fractures. It has been shown that when antibiotics are administered three or more hours after the introduction of bacteria into a skin lesion in animals, the resultant skin lesion is equal in size to that developing in animals similarly traumatized but who had received no antibiotics.[8] Therefore, as soon as the presence of an open fracture is recognized in the emergency room, a broad-spectrum bactericidal antibiotic is administered intravenously. This route is selected because of the certainty and speed of absorption. It is preferable to give antibiotics as a "bolus" injection.

The administration of systemic antibiotics more than three hours after injury does not affect the presence of bacteria in the wound.[45] In view of these findings, it has been recommended that antibiotics be given for three days after injury,[15] as compared with previous recommendations that they be administered for five days after injury.[62]

Certain investigators have reported no advantage in using systemic prophylactic antibiotics in Grade I and II injuries.[57] They did, however, find a definite decrease in deep soft-tissue infections in those Grade III injuries treated with prophylactic antibiotics.

It is our practice to treat Grade I and Grade II open fractures with broad-spectrum bactericidal systemic antibiotics for 12 to 36 hours after injury. In Grade III open fractures, the antibiotics are continued until the danger of infection has passed.

In summary, the following measures are of proven value in helping to prevent infection following open fracture-dislocations of the ankle: administration of a broad-spectrum bactericidal antibiotic intravenously as soon as possible after the injury of compounding, preferably within less than three hours of the injury; continuation of the antibiotics for no longer than 72 hours, especially since with prolonged use, the possibility of complications such as toxicity, sensitivity, allergy, development of resistant organisms, and superinfection developing from the antibiotics is increased; adequate and meticulous surgical debridement of the wound; consideration of the use of internal fixation by the experienced surgeon, as indicated in Grade I and Grade II open fractures, and consideration of an external fixation mechanism in fractures of Grade III severity; and finally, the use of delayed primary and secondary wound closure.

OPERATIVE TECHNIQUE FOR OPEN REDUCTION

Open reductions are performed as soon as feasible in order to obviate the difficulties presented by swelling of the soft tissues. However, it is our opinion that these procedures are best done in an unhurried and relaxed atmosphere. A difficult ankle reconstruction performed at the end of the day by a tired surgeon assisted by a skeleton crew in the operating room is not designed to give the patient the best possible result. We therefore prefer to perform the open reduction as soon as possible and yet at a time when a full operating team is available, together with complete facilities in the operating room. In general, our patients are operated on within 24 to 48 hours of admission to the hospital.

Many surgeons prefer to prepare the leg the day before surgery. However, the studies by Cruse and Ford[24] show a correlation between postoperative infection and the time interval between skin preparation and surgery. Therefore, our patients are prepared under anesthesia in the operating room immediately prior to surgery.

In the operating room, after the anesthesia has been administered, a tourniquet is applied to the involved extremity. The foot is then hung by the first two toes from an IV stand using a 4- × 4-inch bandage and a Kocher clamp. Routinely, we scrub the foot, ankle, and leg with Betadine solution and sterile water. Following this, several layers of Betadine are applied to the skin. After appropriate draping, the tourniquet is inflated. An incision is made over the lateral aspect of the ankle, beginning over the lower end of the fibula and proceeding distally, curving anteriorly at the level of the malleolus and extending distally and parallel to the peroneus brevis tendon. The incision is continued to the periosteum, providing excellent visualization of the fracture site. With undermining in a medial direction, exposure of the anterior inferior tibiofibular ligament can be obtained. Attention is then directed to the medial side of the ankle and an incision is made centering over the medial malleolus. The incision extends along the posteromedial border of the lower tibia and proceeds distally, curving at the level of the medial malleolus and extending distally and parallel to the posterior tibial tendon. After both fracture sites have been identified and examined, the tourniquet is released, and the bleeding points are cauterized. Usually the tourniquet is not reinflated during the remaining portion of the procedure.

Type A Fracture. When the fibular collateral ligament alone is ruptured, one can proceed with repair of the ligament as described by Ruth.[68] If the insertion of the fibular collateral ligament has been avulsed with a fragment of bone, a decision must be made about this piece of bone. If there is a small chip of bone, it is preferable to excise the fragment and treat the lesion as an isolated rupture of the fibular collateral ligament. It may be necessary in this case to make drill holes in the distal fibula in order to suture the ligaments to the tip of the fibula.

A significant bony fragment accompanying this injury requires internal fixation. The fragment is reduced and fixed with two Kirschner wires (2.0 mm) and a figure-of-eight tension band wire. These lesions may also be accompanied by a fracture of the medial malleolus. In this case, the fracture of the medial malleolus is of significant size and usually starts at the level of the tibial plafond and extends proximally and medially. We have found that excellent fixation can be obtained by the use of two 4.0-mm cancellous screws. (These are introduced according to the technique of the AO Group.) The fracture is temporarily held in place by means of two Kirschner wires, and a 2.0-mm drill hole is then made through the distal fracture fragment across the fracture line into the tibial metaphysis. The drill hole is tapped with a 3.5-mm tap, and a 4.0-mm cancellous screw is then inserted. This is

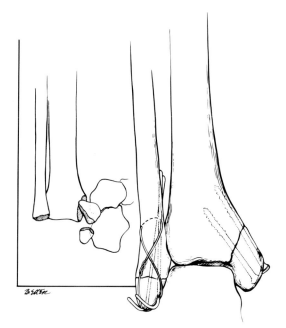

Figure 56–22. *Internal fixation of a Type A fracture.*

followed by removal of one of the Kirschner wires, tapping of the empty hole and insertion of the second cancellous screw. The remaining Kirschner wire can then be removed (Fig. 56–22). At this point, the fracture is tested for stability. If stable, active motion of the ankle is permitted in the immediate postoperative period. If stability is in question, active motion is deferred.

In the Type A group of fracture-dislocations, there is a variant in which a fracture of the posteromedial border of the tibia is present. This may be part of the medial malleolar fragment or may be separate. In any case, additional fixation with a cancellous screw introduced in an anteroposterior direction is frequently required. Even though, by definition, the syndesmosis is not involved in this type of fracture-dislocation, it is always inspected at this point, and the ankle is tested again for stability. Prior to closure, a suction drain may be inserted. Standard wound closure then follows and a short leg cast is applied.

Type B Fracture. The initial approach to the Type B fracture is identical to that for a Type A fracture, that is, both medial and lateral aspects of the ankle are exposed prior to any attempts at surgical repair. After identification of the lesions, one proceeds to the medial side of the joint. If the deltoid ligament is entrapped in the joint, it is removed, and the distal end is held fixed with an Allis clamp to keep it out of the joint during subsequent repair. If there has been a fracture, the ankle is dislocated and any bony debris is removed from the medial joint compartment by irrigation. The ankle dislocation is then reduced and the medial lesion is left unrepaired for the present. Attention is then directed laterally, and the fracture of the lateral malleolus is reduced. If there is a long oblique fracture, it may be safely fixed by means of two 4.0-mm cancellous screws or two 3.5-mm cortex screws (Fig. 56–23). With a short oblique fracture, there are two methods of treatment. The first method is fixation of the fracture site by means of a screw introduced across the fracture site so as to provide interfragmentary compression. This is accomplished by using either a 3.5-mm cortex screw introduced as a "lag" screw or a single 4.0-

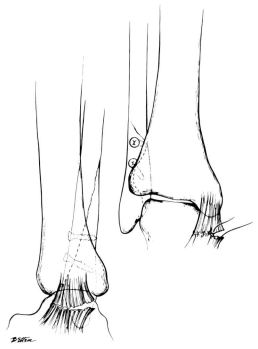

Figure 56–23. *Open reduction of a Type B fracture with a long, oblique fracture of the fibula.*

mm cancellous screw. If the 3.5-mm cortex screw is to be used, a "gliding hole" is drilled in the proximal cortex with a 3.5-mm drill bit. The drill guide is inserted, and the thread hole is drilled in the distal cortex with a 2.0-mm drill bit. After removal of the drill guide, a thread is cut in the distal cortex using a 3.5-mm tap. When the cortex screw is inserted, it is thus capable of exerting compression between the two fragments. After interfragmentary compression has been obtained, a one-third tubular plate is applied to the lateral border of the fibula. The plate must be shaped to fit the contour of the distal end of the fibula prior to its application. This is necessary in order to ensure the maintenance of the normal valgus angle of the distal end of the fibula.

An alternative method in the case of a Type B short oblique fracture is the use of four Kirschner wires introduced according to the method of Willenegger.[37, 80] Two Kirschner wires are introduced from the tip of the lateral malleolus longitudinally up the shaft of the fibula across the fracture site to engage in the medial cortex of the fibula proximal to the fracture. Two addi-

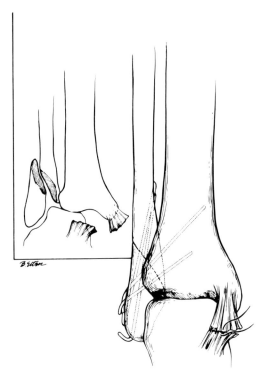

Figure 56–24. *Type B fracture. Fibula fixed with multiple Kirschner wires.*

tional Kirschner wires are then introduced distal to the fracture site, but more proximal than the first two. These wires diverge and cross the fracture site at different angles, penetrating the medial fibular cortex and entering into the tibial shaft (Fig. 56–24). The fracture is tested for stability at this point. Attention is then directed to the medial side of the ankle. To secure adequate visualization of the ligamentous lesion, it is necessary to open the tendon sheath of the posterior tibial tendon, since part of the deltoid ligament extends posteriorly behind the posterior tibial tendon. The ruptured ligament is approximated with interrupted sutures of either 2-0 nylon or 2-0 Vicryl. If possible, the ruptured deltoid ligament should be repaired in two layers as advocated by Close.[17] At this time, the anterior capsule of the ankle joint is repaired.

When a fracture of the medial malleolus is present, it is fixed as described previously. A small fragment is fixed with two Kirschner wires and a figure-of-eight wire suture according to the tension band technique; a large fragment is fixed with two

4.0-mm cancellous screws. Again, at this point the fracture is tested for stability. If the subcutaneous tissues along the medial border of the lateral wound are undermined in a medial direction, the syndesmosis is easily examined. Frequently, the anterior inferior tibiofibular ligament is ruptured. When it is avulsed from its tibial attachment, a fragment of bone may be carried along with it. The fragment is reduced and fixed by means of a 4.0-mm cancellous screw (Fig. 56–25). If the ligament is ruptured in its substance, it can be repaired with a continuous over-and-over suture of 2-0 Dexon or 2-0 Vicryl. When the ligament is avulsed from its fibular insertion, drill holes are made in the fibula for reattachment of the ligament. At times there may be an accompanying fracture of the posterior malleolus. When the fracture fragment consists of less than 25 per cent of the distal articular surface of the tibia, it is not fixed internally. However, if the posterior malleolar fragment is larger than

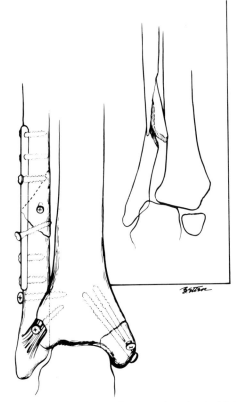

Figure 56–25. *Internal fixation of avulsed tibial attachment of the anterior tibiofibular ligament.*

25 per cent of the distal articular surface of the tibia, internal fixation of the fragment is mandatory. Internal fixation of the posterior malleolus is performed after the fixation of the lateral malleolus and before repair of the medial lesion.

Type C Fracture. By definition, there is involvement of the syndesmosis in the Type C fracture-dislocation of the ankle. Fractures of the posterior malleolus occur more frequently in this group. Incisions are made on the medial and lateral aspects of the ankle. Both injuries are examined before reduction and fixation are performed. Fixation of the fibular fracture is performed first. Since the fibular fracture may occur at any level proximal to the syndesmosis, various options may be exercised. When the fracture is in the lower portion of the fibula, fixation is obtained by means of a tension band plate or a neutralization plate in conjunction with one or more 3.5-mm cortex screws, which provide interfragmentary compression at the fracture site. The rupture of the syndesmosis is repaired using 2-0 Vicryl or 2-0 Dexon. In order to protect the repair of the syndes-

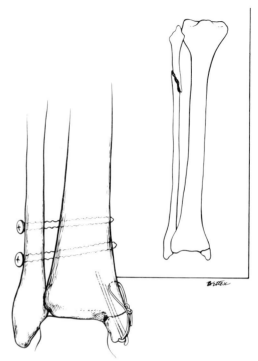

Figure 56–27. *Protection of the syndesmosis repair with screws in treatment of a Type C fracture of proximal fibula.*

mosis, a transfixion screw (3.5-mm cortex screw) may be inserted from the fibula into the tibia, just above the level of the fibular notch. The screw penetrates both cortices of the fibula and only the lateral cortex of the tibia. It should be inserted with the ankle in dorsiflexion. All three cortices are tapped prior to insertion of the screws so as to avoid compression between the tibia and the fibula. Depending on the site of the fibular fracture, the transfixion screw is inserted through a hole in the plate, or it is inserted distal to the plate. It is important to remember also that normally, the fibula lies posterior to the tibia, so that the screw must be introduced in a posteroanterior direction in order to adequately grip the tibia (Fig. 56–26).

When the fracture occurs in the proximal third of the fibula, a different technique involving indirect fixation of the fracture is used. The distal fibula is reduced into the fibular notch of the tibia and provisionally fixed with Kirschner wires. Two 4.5-mm cortex screws are then inserted through the fibula into the tibia, just proximal to the fibular notch of the tibia. In this case,

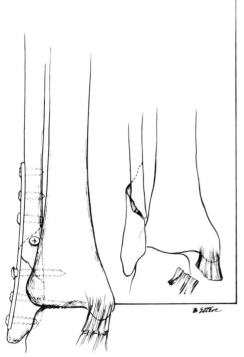

Figure 56–26. *Use of a syndesmosis screw for a Type C fracture of the distal fibula.*

the screws go through both cortices of the fibula and both cortices of the tibia. The entire length of the screw hole is tapped so that no compression occurs when the screw is inserted (Fig. 56–27). The 4.5-mm cortex screws should be removed prior to weight bearing. The 3.5-mm cortex screw may stay in place during ambulation.

If there is a large posterior malleolar fragment, it is now fixed. Weber's technique[79] is recommended. The posterior malleolus is approached with an incision made in the periosteum at the posteromedial border of the tibia. With subperiosteal dissection both proximally and distally, the exposure is extended to the lateral border of the tibia. Prior internal fixation of the fibula has restored the fibula to its normal length, and concomittantly, the intact posterior tibiofibular ligament has repositioned the posterior malleolar fragment. With minimal manipulation, an anatomic reduction can be obtained. A stab wound is made anteriorly, and two 4.0-mm cancellous screws are inserted in an anteroposterior direction (Fig. 56–28 and 56–29). Attention is then directed to

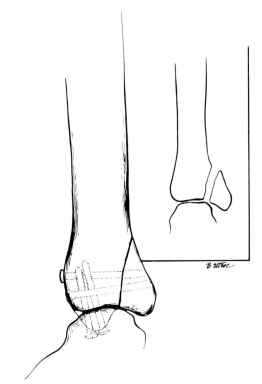

Figure 56–29. *Internal fixation of the posterior malleolus in a Type B fracture.*

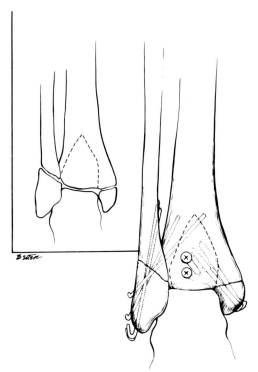

Figure 56–28. *Internal fixation of the posterior malleolus in a Type B fracture (anteroposterior view).*

the medial side of the ankle, and the fractured medial malleolar fragment is fixed as described previously, or if there is a ruptured deltoid ligament, this is repaired. Stability of the ankle is tested again at this point. Roentgenograms are taken of the ankle prior to wound closure to insure that the internal fixation material does not enter the ankle joint itself and to confirm the accuracy of reduction. If required, a suction wound drain is inserted. The wounds are closed, and a short leg cast is applied with the ankle in neutral position. Postoperative care has been described previously. However, in the case of the patient who has had a complete rupture of the syndesmosis, we delay active exercises of the ankle until the cast is removed.

REFERENCES

1. Ashhurst, P. C., and Bromer, R. S.: Classification and mechanism of fractures of the leg bone involving the ankle. Arch. Surg., 4:51, 1922.
2. Bezes, H., Bochio, J. J., Autones, M., et al.: De la réparation des lésions ligamentaires au cours des fractures bimalléolaires. Lyon Chir., 70:248, 1974.

3. Bonnin, J. G.: Injuries to the Ankle. Darien, Connecticut, Hafner Publishing Co., 1970.
4. Braunstein, P. W., and Wade, P. A.: Treatment of unstable fractures of the ankle. Ann. Surg., 149:217, 1959.
5. Brodie, I. A. O. D., and Denham, R. A.: Treatment of unstable ankle fractures. J. Bone Joint Surg., 56B:256, 1974.
6. Brown, P. W.: The prevention of infection in open wounds. Clin. Orthop., 96:42, 1973.
7. Burgess, E.: Fractures of the ankle. J. Bone Joint Surg., 26:721, 1944.
8. Burke, J. F.: The effective period of preventive antibiotic action in experimental incisions and dermal lesions. Surgery, 50:161, 1961.
9. Burke, J. F.: Symposium on antibiotic prophylaxis and therapy. Cont. Surg., 10:38, 1977.
10. Burwell, H. N., and Charnley, A. D.: The treatment of displaced fractures at the ankle by rigid internal fixation and early joint movement. J. Bone Joint Surg., 47B:634, 1965.
11. Cabanela, M. E.: Fractures and dislocations in adults. In Coventry, M. B. (ed.): Year Book of Orthopedics and Traumatic Surgery. Chicago, Year Book Medical Publishers, 1978.
12. Cedell, C. A., and Wiberg, G.: Treatment of eversion-supination fracture of the ankle (2nd degree). Acta Chir. Scand., 124:41, 1962.
13. Charnley, J.: Closed treatment of common fractures, 3rd ed. Baltimore, Williams and Wilkins Co., 1961.
14. Childress, H. M.: Vertical transarticular pin fixation of unstable ankle fractures. Impressions after fifteen years of experience. Presentation of the 43rd annual meeting of the American Academy of Orthopaedic Surgeons, New Orleans, 1976.
15. Clancy, G. J., and Hansen, S. G., Jr.: Open fractures of the tibia. A review of 102 cases. J. Bone Joint Surg., 60A:118, 1978.
16. Clayton, M. L., and Weir, G. J.: Experimental investigations of ligamentous healing. Am. J. Surg., 98:373, 1959.
17. Close, J. R.: Some applications of the functional anatomy of the ankle joint. J. Bone Joint Surg., 38A:761, 1956.
18. Colton, C. L.: Fracture-diastasis of the inferior tibiofibular joint. J. Bone Joint Surg., 50B:830, 1968.
19. Colton, C. L.: The treatment of Dupuytren's fracture-dislocation of the ankle. J. Bone Joint Surg., 53B:63, 1971.
20. Coonrad, R. W.: Fracture-dislocations of the ankle joint with impaction injury of the lateral weight bearing surface of the tibia. J. Bone Joint Surg., 52A:1337, 1970.
21. Coonrad, R. W., and Bugg, E. I., Jr.: Trapping of the posterior tibial tendon and interposition of soft tissue in severe fractures about the ankle joint. J. Bone Joint Surg., 36A:744, 1954.
22. Cooper, A. P.: On dislocations of the ankle joint. On fractures of the tibia and fibula near the ankle joint. Reprinted in Clin. Orthop., 42:3, 1965.
23. Cox, F. J.: Fractures of the ankle involving the lower articular surface of the tibia. Clin. Orthop., 42:51, 1965.
24. Cruse, P. J. E., and Ford, R.: Five year prospective study of 23,649 surgical wounds. Arch. Surg., 107:206, 1973.
25. Daniel, W. J., and Wilson, F. C.: Trimalleolar fractures of the ankle. Clin. Orthop., 122:37, 1977.
26. Danis, R.: Le vrai but et les dangers de l'ostéosynthèse. Lyon Chir., 51:740, 1956.
27. Denham, R. A.: Internal fixation for unstable ankle fractures. J. Bone Joint Surg., 46B:206, 1964.
28. Devas, M.: Geriatric Orthopaedics. New York, Academic Press, 1977.
29. Devas, M.: Stress fractures of the fibula. J. Bone Joint Surg., 38B:818, 1956.
30. Fowler, P. J.: Ligamentous anatomy and physical examination. Am. J. Sports Med., 5:229, 1977.
31. Freeman, M. A. R.: Treatment of ruptures of the lateral ligaments of the ankle. J. Bone Joint Surg., 47B:661, 1965.
32. Gherlinzoni, G., Fiore, T., and Commessatti, P.: Le Fratture del Collo del Piede. Bologna, Aulo Gaggi Editore, 1968.
33. Gordon, S. L., Dunn, E. J., and Malin, T. H.: Lateral collateral ligament ankle injuries in young athletic individuals. J. Trauma, 16:225, 1976.
34. Grath, G. B.: Widening of the ankle mortise. Acta Chir. Scand. (Suppl.), 263:1, 1960.
35. Hartman, J. T.: Fracture Management: A Practical Approach. Philadelphia, Lea and Febiger, 1978.
36. Harvey, J. P., Jr.: Fractures of the ankle. Clin. Orthop., 42:57, 1965.
37. Heim, U., and Pfeiffer, K. M.: Small Fragments Set Manual. New York, Springer-Verlag, 1974.
38. Jergesen, F.: Open reduction of fractures and dislocations of the ankle. Am. J. Surg., 98:136, 1959.
39. Joy, G., Patzakis, M. J., and Harvey, J. P., Jr.: Precise evaluation of the reduction of severe ankle fractures. J. Bone Joint Surg., 56A:979, 1974.
40. Ketenjian, A. Y., and Shelton, M. L.: Primary internal fixation of open fractures: a retrospective study of the use of metallic internal fixation in fresh open fractures. J. Trauma, 12:756, 1972.
41. Kleiger, B.: The mechanism of ankle injuries. J. Bone Joint Surg., 38A:59, 1956.
42. Kleiger, B.: The treatment of oblique fractures of the fibula. J. Bone Joint Surg., 43A:969, 1961.
43. Klossner, O.: Late results of operative and nonoperative treatment of severe ankle fractures. Acta Chir. Scand. (Suppl.), 293:1, 1962.
44. Kristensen, T. B.: Treatment of malleolar fractures according to Lauge-Hansen's method. Acta Chir. Scand., 97:363, 1949.
45. Krizek, T.: Symposium on antibiotic prophylaxis and therapy. Cont. Surg., 10:45, 1977.
46. Krizek, T. J., and Robson, M. C.: Biology of surgical infection. Surg. Clin. North Am., 55:1261, 1975.
47. Lambert, K.: The weight-bearing function of the fibula. J. Bone Joint Surg., 53A:507, 1971.
48. Laskin, R. S.: Steinmann pin fixation in the treatment of unstable fractures of the ankle. J. Bone Joint Surg., 56A:549, 1974.
49. Lauge, N.: Fractures of the ankle: analytical historical survey as the basis of new experimental, roentgenologic and clinical investigations. Arch. Surg., 56:259, 1948.
50. Lauge-Hansen, N.: Fractures of the ankle. II: Combined experimental-surgical and experimental-roentgenologic investigations. Arch. Surg., 60:957, 1950.
51. Lauge-Hansen, N.: Fractures of the ankle: clinical use of genetic roentgen diagnosis and genetic reduction. Arch. Surg., 64:488, 1952.
52. Lauge-Hansen, N.: Fractures of the ankle: genetic roentgenologic diagnosis of fractures of the ankle. Am. J. Roentgenol., 71:456, 1954.
53. Lauge-Hansen, N.: Fractures of the ankle. V: pronation-dorsiflexion fracture. Arch. Surg., 67:813, 1953.
54. McDade, W. C.: Diagnosis and treatment of ankle injuries. Acad. Orthop. Surg., Instructional Course Lectures, 24:251, 1975.
55. McLaughlin, H. L.: Trauma. Philadelphia, W. B. Saunders Company, 1959.
56. Magnusson, R.: Late results in non-operated cases of malleolar fracture. Acta Chir. Scand. (Suppl.), 84:1, 1944.
57. Matter, P., and Rittmann, W. W.: The Open Fracture. Bern, Stuttgart, and Vienna, Verlag Hans Huber, 1978.
58. Monk, E. J. E.: Injuries of the tibiofubular ligaments. J. Bone Joint Surg., 51B:330, 1969.
59. Müller, M. E., Allgower, M., and Willenegger, H.: Manu-

al of Internal Fixation. New York, Springer-Verlag, 1970.

60. Pankovich, A. M.: Fractures of the fibula proximal to the distal tibiofibular syndesmosis. J. Bone Joint Surg., 60A:221, 1978.

61. Patrick, J.: Direct approach to trimalleolar fractures. J. Bone Joint Surg., 47B:236, 1965.

62. Patzakis, M. J., Harvey, J. P., Jr., and Ivler, D.: The role of antibiotics in the management of open fractures. J. Bone Joint Surg., 56A:532, 1974.

63. Quigley, T. B.: Fractures and ligament injuries of the ankle. Am. J. Surg., 98:477, 1959.

64. Ramsey, P. L., and Hamilton, W.: Changes in tibiotalar area of contact caused by lateral talar shift. J. Bone Joint Surg., 58A:356, 1976.

65. Rang, M.: Anthology of Orthopaedics. Edinburgh and London, E. and S. Livingstone, Ltd., 1966.

66. Rüedi, T., and Allgower, M.: Fractures of the lower end of the tibia into the ankle joint. Injury, 1:92, 1969.

67. Rüedi, T.: Fractures of the lower end of the tibia into the ankle joint: results of nine years after open operation and internal fixation. Injury, 5:130, 1973.

68. Ruth, C. J.: The surgical treatment of injuries of the fibular collateral ligaments of the ankle. J. Bone Joint Surg., 43A:229, 1961.

69. Scranton, P. E., Jr., McMaster, J. H., and Kelly, E.: Dynamic fibular function: a new concept. Clin. Orthop., 118:76, 1976.

70. Shelton, M. L.: Diagnosis and treatment of acute injuries to the ankle joint. Graduate course presented at the 62nd meeting of American College of Surgeons, Chicago, 1976.

71. Shelton, M. L., and Anderson, R. L., Jr.: Complications of fractures and dislocations of the ankle. In Epps, C. H., Jr. (ed.): Complications in Orthopedic Surgery. Philadelphia, J. B. Lippincott, 1978.

72. Sneppen, O.: Long term course in 119 cases of pseudarthrosis of the medial malleolus. Acta Orthop. Scand., 40:807, 1970.

73. Solonen, K. A., and Luattamus, L.: Operative treatment of ankle fractures. Acta Orthop. Scand., 39:223, 1968.

74. Spiegel, P. K., and Staples, O. S.: Arthrography of the ankle joint: problems in diagnosis of acute lateral ligament injuries. Radiology, 114:587, 1975.

75. Staples, O. S.: Rupture of fibular collateral ligaments of the ankle: result study of immediate surgical treatment. J. Bone Joint Surg., 57A:101, 1975.

76. Taylor, F. W.: An experimental evaluation of operative wound irrigation. Surg. Gynecol. Obstet., 113:465, 1961.

77. Vasli, S.: Operative treatment of ankle fractures. Acta Chir. Scand. (Suppl.), 226:1, 1957.

78. Wade, P. A., and Lance, E. M.: The operative treatment of fracture-dislocation of the ankle joint. Clin. Orthop., 42:37, 1965.

79. Weber, B. G.: Die Verletzungen des oberen Sprunggelenkes. Bern, Stuttgart, and Wien, Verlag Hans Huber, 1972.

80. Willenegger, H.: Die Behandlung der Luxionsfracturen des oberen Sprunggelenkes nach biomechanische Gesichtspunkten. Helv. Chir. Acta, 28:225, 1961.

81. Wilson, F. C., and Skilbred, L. A.: Long-term results of the treatment of displaced bimalleolar fractures. J. Bone Joint Surg., 48A:1065, 1966.

82. Wolf-Heidegger, G.: Atlas der systematischen Anatomie des Menschen. Basel and New York, S. Karger, 1954.

83. Yablon, I. G., Heller, F. G., and Shouse, L.: The key role of the lateral malleolus in displaced fractures of the ankle. J. Bone Joint Surg., 59A:169, 1977.

CHAPTER 57

SPORTS INJURIES TO THE FOOT AND ANKLE

Tom P. Coker, Jr., M.D.,
and James A. Arnold, M.D.

After years of indolence and inactivity, the 1960's ushered in a great wave of awareness of the need for regular exercise in order to maintain the human body in a reasonably healthy condition. Armed with this new knowledge, people of all ages and sizes rushed out with great vigor to participate in some sport or other, with the result that the foot and ankle were, and still are, being subjected to a new variety of stresses.

The patient who sees his physician volunteers, "I hurt my . . .," and names an anatomic region. Often this area is detectable by inspection, and nearly always so by palpation. Therefore, this chapter is arranged by anatomic sections under the injury headings of (1) fractures, (2) dislocations, (3) sprains, (4) tendon problems, (5) impingement syndrome, (6) static problems, (7) bursitis, and (8) leg pain. Concluding sections consider the particular problems of the runner and jogger. The type of problem that is likely to be seen will vary greatly from sport to sport and from one region or country to another. The most common injuries related to specific sports are as follows:

1. *Ballet:* Fractured sesamoids, stress fractures, ankle fractures and sprains, tendon ruptures, tendinitis, peritendinitis, tenosynovitis, bunions, blisters, clavi, and calluses. (See Chapter 59.)

2. *Baseball:* Ankle fractures, avulsion fractures of the dorsal navicular (talonavicular joint), enlargement and fractures of Stieda's process, ankle sprains, and impingement exostoses (anterior talotibial).

3. *Basketball:* Fractures of the base of the fifth metatarsal, ankle fractures and sprains, rupture and peritendinitis of the Achilles tendon, and blisters.

4. *Bicycling:* Toe fractures, sprains, and spoke injuries (e.g., abrasions, lacerations, and skin slough).

5. *Football:* Fractured sesamoids, fractures of the fifth metatarsal, ankle fractures and sprains, sprains of the first metatarsophalangeal joint, rupture and peritendinitis of the Achilles tendon, impingement exostoses (anterior talotibial), periarticular bony ridges, ossifying hematomas, and compartment syndromes.

6. *Gymnastics:* Toe fractures and dislocations, fractures of the base of the fifth metatarsal, ankle sprains, anterior ankle capsular sprains, and posterior talotibial impingements (Stieda's process).

7. *Skiing:* Ankle fractures and sprains, avulsion fractures of the os calcis, subtalar dislocations, and dislocations of the peroneal tendons.

8. *Soccer:* Forefoot fractures, especially fifth metatarsal stress fractures, ankle fractures and sprains, rupture and peritendinitis of the Achilles tendon, shin splints, and compartment syndromes.

9. *Track and Jogging:* Stress fractures, ankle sprains, rupture and peritendinitis of the Achilles tendon, fasciitis, bursitis, heel pain, blisters, shin splints, and compartment syndromes.

10. *Tennis:* Ankle sprains, tendo-Achillis rupture and peritendinitis, including the medial head of the gastrocnemius ("tennis leg"), heel pain, and blisters.

11. *Wrestling:* Fractures of the base of the fifth metatarsal, ankle sprains, and peritendinitis of the Achilles tendon (a result of training).

In addition, it is often helpful to try to group the activity according to what it requires of an athlete. We know that some sports put emphasis on maneuverability and "cutting," others on endurance, and still others on collisions. This is extremely helpful in differential diagnosis. For example, those sports that put a premium on maneuverability produce strains, avulsion fractures, and blisters. Endurance activities predictably cause tenosynovitis, shin splints, compartment syndromes, fasciitis, and stress fractures. Collisions typically induce fractures and contusions.

HISTORY

The physician must listen to the patient explain his particular position and his sport and what is troubling him. He should specifically inquire about the type of surface the athlete is running or playing on and discuss his shoes. With the patient's help, the practitioner should be able to arrive at a conclusion regarding the acuteness of onset (the exact mechanism) and whether or not the patient's condition is becoming better or worse. The patient may also be asked about changes in training methods, distance times, and equipment. It should be determined whether or not this problem has occurred before, and if so and relief was sought, what treatment modalities were tried. It is judicious to know the success or failure of various remedies.

PHYSICAL EXAMINATION

Inspection. Examination shorts can easily be provided for the patient in the clinical setting. The physician can then observe the patient's natural gait and heel and toe walking. In certain instances, either in a long hallway or outdoors, one can watch the patient jog and observe the stance he assumes. Abnormalities of gait are recorded. Areas of callus distribution, trophic skin changes, swelling, and discoloration are noted. Footwear, orthoses, and other equipment should be thoroughly examined for distribution of gait patterns and excessive wear.

Palpation. Probably the single most important part of the examination is knowing where the patient hurts, how specific the area of tenderness is, and whether or not it is aggravated by position changes in the foot or activation of underlying tendons and joints. The examining physician can determine whether or not the tenderness is aggravated by either passive stretching or active use of a tendon. This portion of the examination should include a search for the appropriate pulses and reflexes. Joint stability and range of motion are observed from the ankle distally to the toes. Hip and knee abnormalities are quickly noted.

Auscultation. This can be helpful in determining the presence of tenosynovitis and occasionally in the search for pulses.

Percussion. Percussion is used primarily in the testing of reflexes. It is also occasionally helpful to determine if the foot is tender to firm fist percussion or to light tapping over involved areas of inflammation.

ROENTGENOGRAMS

The reader is referred to Chapters 4 and 6 for a detailed explanation of roentgenograms and methods of obtaining the specific views desired. Roentgenograms should not be used sparingly, as, for example, in the search for a stress fracture. It may be necessary to obtain repeat views at reasonable intervals. Special techniques such as stress films, arthrograms, tenograms, and tomograms should be utilized where indicated. The examining physician should be familiar with what is likely to be seen on anteroposterior and true lateral views of the foot as well as on oblique views. Anteroposterior and lateral roentgenograms should be taken with the patient bearing weight. The true architecture of the foot as it is used is thus revealed.

TREATMENT

Treatment will vary markedly with the diagnosis; however, certain generalities apply. Ice therapy, compression, and elevation are useful in virtually all acute injuries (remember I-C-E). Rest is an important adjunct to these modalities, and in fact, if ice therapy, compression, and elevation are used to the fullest, they will necessitate rest. Usually, rest from heavy activity does not preclude early, gentle motion.

In the participating athlete, a cast should be avoided unless mandatory.[1] It has been our experience that immobilization of a part in a cast will delay rehabilitation. Muscle atrophy and joint stiffness will occur, and the athlete will sustain a loss of coordination that will affect his performance. At the same time, the use of the cast is disadvantageous to the athlete psychologically and to his body image.

Acute Phase

Ice Therapy. Ice may be useful in several forms.[2] It has been shown scientifically that the best way to cool a part is still with ordinary crushed ice. Whenever ice is used, the skin should be protected, and one advantage of a chemical ice pack is that the time of its duration precludes frostbite. Cold may also be applied by means of immersion, but this virtually always requires dependency, which, in itself, may be harmful. Ice massage is a convenient way for the athlete to treat himself, holding the cube by a tongue-blade handle moving the ice slowly over the affected area for 20 minutes.

Compression. A satisfactory way of obtaining cooling and compression at the same time is to use a wet elastic bandage. The wetness allows the cold to penetrate,

but at the same time the layer of Ace bandage protects the skin from direct contact with the ice. This is useful on the sidelines during an athletic contest for immediate treatment of an acute injury. Later, in order to maintain some compression and allow the patient to be ambulatory at the same time, application of tape, Elastoplast, or an Unna boot may be more practical. In the athletic setting and in the training room, positive-pressure stockings can be applied intermittently. The more frequently that this is done during a 24-hour period, the more beneficial it is likely to be. Intermittent Jobst compression is used at 15 to 25 mm Hg, depending on the patient's tolerance. It is employed in a cycle of 90 seconds on and 120 seconds off for a total treatment period of 90 minutes.

Elevation. Elevation of the foot above the level of the heart is useful to prevent swelling, especially in the first 24 to 48 hours after injury. It has been our observation that prevention of swelling during this time will subtract days from the recovery and rehabilitation period, allowing much earlier return to athletic endeavors.

Rest. Rest in bed will generally accompany the use of ice therapy, compression, and elevation. However, after this initial period has passed, the patient will want to be more active. The use of a cane, crutches, taping, and, in rare instances, a cast will allow the athlete to pursue his studies or occupation.

Early, Gentle Motion. In cases of trauma that are amenable to it, motion can be provided by exercise, either active or passive, or by deep massage.[3] Motion decreases edema, aids circulation, and helps the cells in healing tissue to "line up" in relation to the ligaments and tendons. This produces a stronger scar with less undesirable adherence to bone and capsule.[4] Movement is least likely to cause pain if it is begun before abnormal attachments are formed to adjacent structures. Restoration of proprioceptive reflexes is assisted by motion. Ice massage will aid this early, gentle motion.

Recovery Phase

Whirlpool. During the recovery phase, it may be advantageous to continue with compression and intermittent periods of rest. At this stage, however, the use of a whirlpool can be added for 20 minutes, four times a day. It should be remembered, however, that dependency is unfortunately a part of this treatment if tank-type whirlpools are used. Adjacent hot and cold machines can be used with a whirlpool so that contrast baths can be taken. The temperatures of these baths are in the range of 106°F and 50°F. The patient starts in the 106° bath for four minutes, and then spends two minutes in the 50° bath; this is repeated four times.

Ultrasound. The indiscriminate use of ultrasound is to be deplored; however, in certain conditions, such as tenosynovitis, its proper use can speed recovery. Ultrasound should be used only when the examining physician has a particular objective in mind. The patient's condition should be assessed frequently. The usual treatment is for five minutes, under water, at 1 to 1.5 watts/cm².

Rehabilitation Phase

Initial Stage. Athletics include running and cutting maneuvers, and the patient should understand that if he cannot perform these maneuvers, he is not yet ready to resume his sport. Therefore, he should begin with walking and progress to jogging, running and cutting—in that order. It is of no use for him to try to omit a stage in rehabilitation. The patient should begin with walking until he can walk normally without limping. He then jogs, gradually increasing his jogging speed and stride until he can run. The patient is advised to run straight without sudden stops or starts until he has reached his maximum controlled speed. He can then begin starts and stops and subsequently utilize cutting maneuvers. These are most easily accomplished by running figures-of-eight around pylons, which are originally set out over 20 yards for a complete figure-of-eight loop and are then placed closer together, over 15, 10, and finally 5 yards. Obviously this can easily be done by the recreational athlete in his own backyard. When he is able to make a sharp figure-of-eight within 5 yards, he is allowed to resume his athletic activities.

Proprioceptive Exercises. The aforementioned rehabilitation efforts are easily

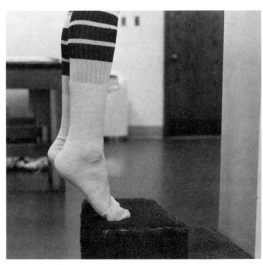

Figure 57–1. *Active toe-raises strengthen the heel cords and aid in rehabilitation.*

carried out. They can be aided by specific exercises, such as proprioceptive exercises, which can be performed on a tilt-board.[5] The board can initially be placed on a cylinder, which gives a two-dimensional effect and then eventually placed on half of a croquet ball, which will give a three-dimensional tilt.

Strengthening Exercises. Strengthening exercises can be performed isometrically. For example, if the patient is a student, in the classroom he can place the heel of the foot on the floor and invert, evert, dorsiflex or plantar flex it against a

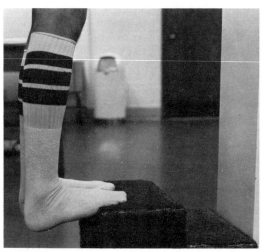

Figure 57–2. *Heel-cord stretching is a preventive measure against ankle sprains. This box is the same type that is used for lateral leg strengthening in rehabilitation of the knee.*

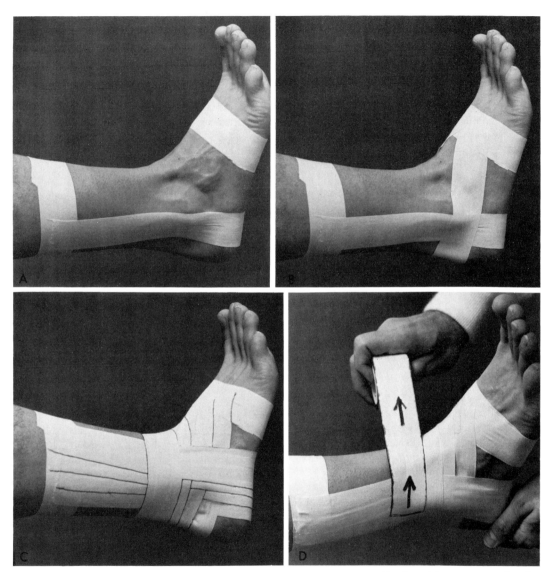

Figure 57–3. *The method of prophylactic ankle taping found to be most effective. This same type of taping, applied directly to the skin after applications of a protective layer of tincture of benzoin, is used therapeutically. For prophylaxis, a single layer of J-wrap is applied first next to the skin. This is highly satisfactory to the athlete who must have his ankle taped every day. (A) Circumferential bands of 1.5-inch-wide tape are applied for adhesion and the first stirrup is in place. (B) The middle of a strip of tape is placed posteriorly on the heel and brought forward along each side of the foot. (C) Similar strips are then alternated to complete the basket-weave stirrup. (D) Heel-lock started. (Note the medial-to-lateral relations in E–J.)*

Illustration continued on following page

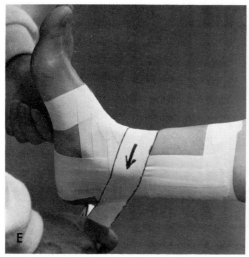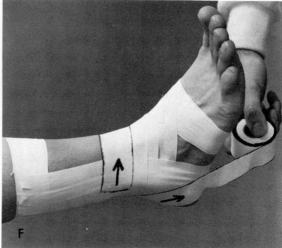

Figure 57–3 *Continued.   (E) Medial view. The ankle turn begun in B is continued onto the medial side and sloped toward the heel. (F) Lateral view. The medial ankle turn becomes the lateral heel-lock and is continued on the sole of the foot.*

Illustration continued on following page

fixed object in front of him, such as another student's desk.

Stretching Exercises. Stretching exercises are an integral part not only of rehabilitation but of prevention. Heel-cord stretching has been shown to be vital in the prevention of ankle sprains by McClusky and associates.[6] and can be carried out by doing toe-raises on the edge of a box or standing against an inclined plane (Figs. 57–1 and 57–2). Single-legged toe-raises utilize the peroneal muscles more actively than dual-legged toe-raises. This aids rehabilitation of proper lateral balance.

Protection. Protection can be offered by the judicious use of braces, splints, and. of course, casts. For more practical purposes in athletics, support is often offered by various means of taping. Taping is important in the treatment of athletic injuries, and the basic methods of taping are illustrated in Figures 57–3 to 57–5. We believe in prophylactic ankle taping, and there is scientific evidence to support this time-honored practice,[7, 8] although some authors do not use it.[9] In a study of intramural athletics, the incidence rate of ankle sprains per 1000 participant games in subjects wearing high-top shoes was 6.5 per cent in those whose ankles were taped compared with 30.4 per cent in those with untaped ankles.[10] In low-top shoes, the incidence rate was 17.6 per cent in those

with taped ankles and 33.4 per cent in those with untaped ankles.

FRACTURES

Injuries to the Great Toe

Injuries to the great toe–first metatarsal area are common in football today, especially in football played in soccer-style shoes on artificial turf.[11, 12] By means of questionnaires sent to a random sampling of athletic trainers throughout the United States, Coker, Arnold, and Weber ascertained that injuries to first metatarsophalangeal joint were significant in football and were seen more frequently with the advent of non–leather-soled shoes and artificial turf.[12] They compared their experience with injuries to the first metatarsophalangeal joint in football players at the University of Arkansas with a study of ankle sprains. Although there were more ankle sprains than toe injuries during the period of the comparison, the latter were more disabling to the players in terms of missed practices and games. Playing on artificial surfaces is also a factor in injuries incurred in other sports, as demonstrated by Bowers and Martin at the University of West Virginia in 1974; they determined that the parameters of stopping time and average acceleration

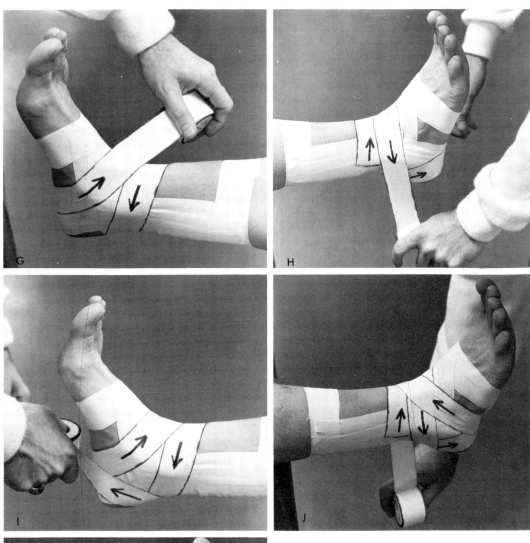

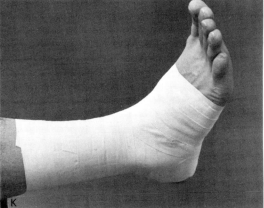

Figure 57–3 *Continued. (G) Medial view. From the sole, the tape is drawn over the arch of the foot. (H) Lateral view. From the arch, the tape is angled toward the heel. (I) Medial view. The tape is then wrapped around the posterior aspect of the heel and becomes the medial heel-lock. (J) Lateral view. The tape is directed under the arch, back over the instep laterally to medially, and then around the ankle to the starting point. (K) Open skin areas and the basket-weave stirrup are covered by additional circumferential strips of tape to complete the bandage.*

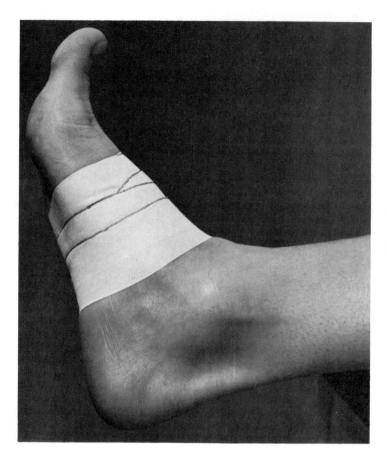

Figure 57–4. Taping for arch strain. In more severe cases, this is combined with longitudinal strips of tape along the course of the posterior tibial tendon.

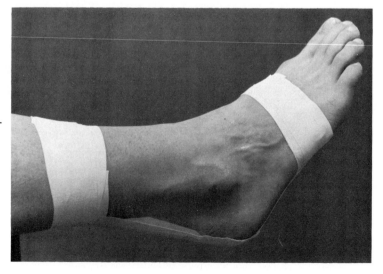

Figure 57–5. Protection is provided for the Achilles tendon.

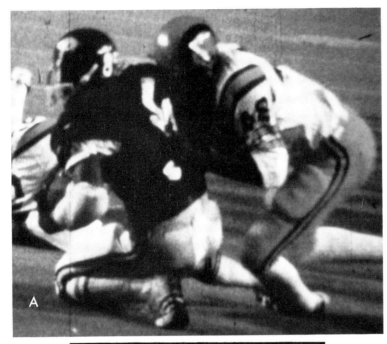

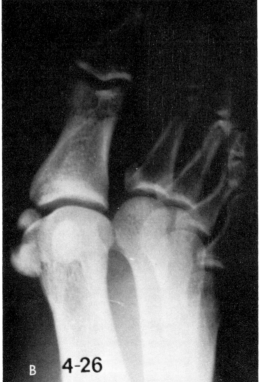

Figure 57–6. (A) "Turf-toe" in the making. This specific injury resulted in a fractured sesamoid. The athlete's own body weight was transmitted through his buttock onto his heel, producing acute hyperextension. (B) Fractured sesamoid in a football player, a hyperextension injury.

and deceleration all approached those on asphalt as the artificial turf aged.[13] The emphasis that coaches place on speed and traction has resulted in a deterioration of the support given by footwear. In addition, nearly all popular brands of football shoes are fitted primarily by length and are available only in a standard width.

A prospective study conducted in 1976 failed to reveal a relationship between injury and pre-season range of motion of the metatarsophalangeal joint. The mechanism of injury seen most frequently involved a player lying in the prone position with the toes on the playing surface and the heel in the air. A subsequent pile-up, with other players falling across the back of the player's leg, hyperextended the metatarsophalangeal joint (Fig. 57–6). Other injuries to the toes and metatarsals as well as Lisfranc fracture or dislocation of the foot may also occur with this same mechanism (Figs. 57–7 and 57–8).

An occurrence of more gradual onset involved a basic valgus type of injury,

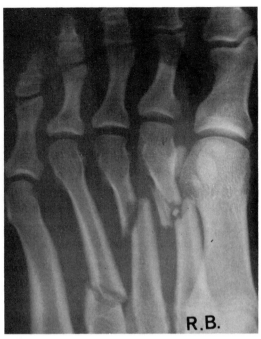

Figure 57–8. *These metatarsal injuries occurred in a patient wearing tennis shoes and playing on grass, but with the same mechanism of forces as in "turf-toe" injuries.*

particularly seen in offensive linemen or backs assuming their stance. In this position, the great toe is pushed, through the soft shoes, into a position of hallux valgus, causing a swollen, painful metatarsophalangeal joint that becomes more severe with time (Fig. 57–9).

Treatment of the acute injury is primarily nonoperative, with the primary component being joint rest. Depending on the severity of the injury, this may include plaster immobilization, walking with crutches or simply walking on the heels to avoid painful motion of the toe. Ice therapy, compression, and elevation are used early. Later, ultrasound, contrast baths or paraffin baths offer some benefit. The player is asked to walk at a speed and in a weight-bearing configuration that is within his range of comfort; under no circumstances should this produce a painful gait. Typically, this therapy will progress from flatfooted walking to a normal gait, and then the player is permitted to jog at increasing speeds with a normal stride until he can run straight ahead at full speed. He is then encouraged to start running from a stance position until he can do so without

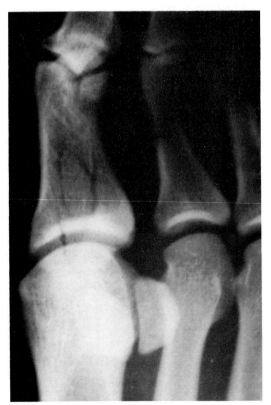

Figure 57–7. *Fracture of the proximal phalanx of the great toe in a "turf-toe" injury.*

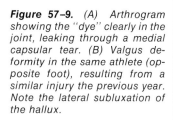
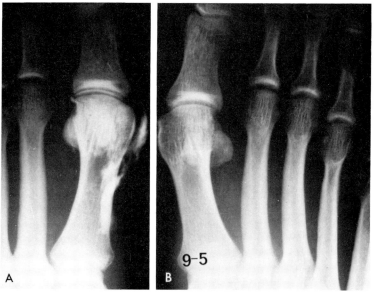

Figure 57–9. (A) Arthrogram showing the "dye" clearly in the joint, leaking through a medial capsular tear. (B) Valgus deformity in the same athlete (opposite foot), resulting from a similar injury the previous year. Note the lateral subluxation of the hallux.

discomfort. Finally, he performs cutting maneuvers. Throughout this period of jogging, the patient is to wear shoes that are modified to produce increased stability of the distal forefoot and toe areas. A 0.51-mm spring-steel splint extending from the forward edge of the heel to the forward edge of the inner sole of the shoe has been utilized routinely (Fig. 57–10). In addition, taping of the toe to prevent it from assuming the configuration of the original injury, as suggested by Weber, head trainer at the University of Arkansas, has been of considerable benefit in most cases (Fig. 57–11). In the opinion of Coker, Arnold, and Weber, steroid injections were of absolutely no benefit and could be detrimental if they masked symptoms that would have prevented a premature return to activity.

Even with the nonoperative therapy as outlined, there have been failures that have led to the necessity of surgery. It was difficult to determine from the initial examination or studies just which injuries would fail to respond to nonoperative therapy. For example, some capsular tears responded to three weeks of conservative therapy, whereas others did not improve even after several months. However, later operative repair was beneficial in such cases. In one patient, a fractured sesamoid resulted in a permanent impairment, whereas in another patient, the same injury caused only two missed practices.

Operative intervention was performed when roentgenograms indicated serious disruption (Figs. 57–6B and 57–12) or when specific symptoms persisted (Fig. 57–13). The operative procedure was

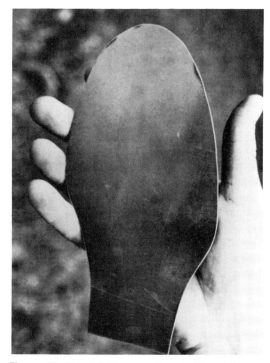

Figure 57–10. A 0.51-mm spring-steel insert that reinforces the forefoot area of athletic shoes. It is placed within the sole.

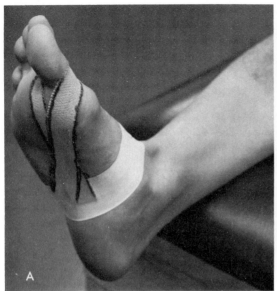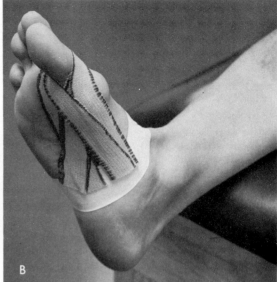

Figure 57–11. *(A) Toe strapping utilizing elastic adherent strips. (B) Completed strapping used in hyperextension injuries to help prevent further dorsiflexion. The ends of the elastic strips are covered with a zinc oxide band.*

directed toward the defect demonstrated, which to date has always been unique to the turf toe series. In the patient in Figure 57–12, a medial incision was made, and the plantar capsule of the first metatarsophalangeal joint was found to be avulsed from the base of the proximal phalanx, accompanied by a fragment of bone less than one millimeter in its largest diameter. The plantar capsule was reattached with sutures through small drill holes in the proximal phalanx. The soft-tissue calcifica-

tion which was located dorsally, beneath avulsed periosteum, resolved. The player was a college senior and did not engage in competitive athletics postoperatively. However, nine years later, he was still active in recreational sports, but experienced occasional mild pain.

The individual in Figure 57–13 and another athlete with negative roentgenograms had persistent point tenderness medially. They were found to have, respectively, (1) an old capsular tear with firm adherence of the capsule to the articular cartilage of the metatarsal head, and (2) three small, loose, cartilaginous bodies within the metatarsophalangeal joint. In the latter case, the loose bodies were removed and the joint was irrigated. A thickened area of the capsule medially was thought to represent spontaneous healing. This was excised, and the capsule was tightened and repaired. Four years later, the patient was still playing basketball without discomfort. He had resumed this sport two and a half months postoperatively. Whereas, four and a half months of preoperative conservative treatment had left him with point tenderness and pain with activity.

The patient with capsular adherence underwent correction through a direct medial approach five months after the injury occurred. The capsule was skived off the

Figure 57–12. *Disruption of the first metatarsophalangeal joint. Arrow points to the area of soft-tissue calcification.*

1-22-69

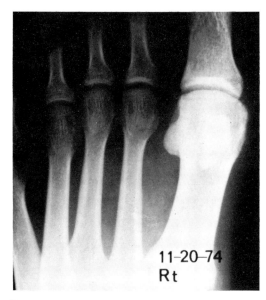

Figure 57–13. *In this patient with persistent point tenderness on the medial aspect of the great toe, the mildest change seen roentgenographically was a minimal narrowing of the medial aspect of the metatarsophalangeal joint and some flattening of the first metatarsal head.*

articular cartilage, and the capsular rent was sutured. The athlete returned to playing football and played through his senior year, three years later.

Based on their clinical experience and responses from major college athletic trainers to their questionnaire, Coker, Arnold, and Weber drew the following conclusions:

1. Injury to the first metatarsophalangeal joint complex was significant and appeared to be on the increase. This was probably related to shoe construction and types of playing surfaces (Fig. 57–14).

2. The mechanism of injury may be hyperextension, hyperflexion, or valgus, depending on the applied stress.

3. The specific structures involved vary greatly.

4. Initial treatment of choice includes rest, ice therapy, compression, and elevation. Attempts to force the cure with injection of steroids, and particularly with injection of local anesthetic agents, are contraindicated.

5. Shoe modification and taping may allow earlier return to athletic activities.

6. Surgery may be required in the event of joint capsular tears and in fractures of the sesamoids. Those athletes not able to jog without a good, painless range of motion three weeks after injury may require surgical repair.

7. When surgery was required, even late repair appeared to be effective, particularly when the primary pathology had been a capsular tear.

8. Proper shoe fitting and sole reinforcement may reduce the instance of this injury.

Fractures of the Sesamoids

Fractures of the sesamoids are typically produced by a fall from a height (as in ballet) or by forced dorsiflexion of the great toe (as in football). The diagnosis is made by findings of local tenderness and pain on dorsiflexion and by roentgenograms. Tangential sesamoid views made in a plane from toe to heel with the toe dorsiflexed may be helpful. This view silhouettes the sesamoids. The treatment of a fractured sesamoid consists of cast immobilization for three weeks. If symptoms persist after eight weeks, the fractured sesamoid may be treated like a fractured patella, with removal of the least significant fragment and repair of the flexor brevis mechanism. In cases of fracture of the medial sesamoid, a medial incision is made. The lateral sesamoid is best approached dorsally. A small lamina spreader is used to open the space between the first two metatarsals. O'Donoghue recommends division of the plantar fascia in cases involving a cavus foot to

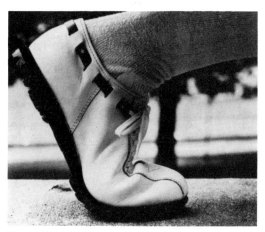

Figure 57–14. *Hyperextension forces are easily applied to the foot at the metatarsophalangeal joint. Inadequate support may play a role.*

relieve pressure on the sesamoid.[14] The first metatarsophalangeal joint may also be the site of valgus deformity (hallus valgus), avulsion fractures, and tenosynovitis, all of which are commonly seen in ballet dancers (see Chapter 59).

Injuries of the Small Toes

Injuries of the lateral four toes are not specific for sports. We have seen such injuries particularly in football players, and they are treated as they are when not sports-related, with ice therapy, elevation, and rest. A cast should be avoided, and the athlete may return to competition as soon as he can run and cut.

Fractures of the Metatarsals

The most common injuries of the metatarsals related to sports are fractures. Stress fractures are particularly common and are usually associated with a sudden increase in distance traveled either by running or hiking.[15] They are unrelated to age, height, or weight.[16] When suspected, stress fractures are diagnosed by local, very specific tenderness over the metatarsal, not in the interspace. Roentgenograms are usually positive in three to six weeks, and the stress fracture may appear either as a reactive callus or as a small fracture line. Stress fractures are best treated with Elastoplast strapping, a stiff-soled shoe, and a properly placed metatarsal pad.[17] The shoe should contain a steel shank. Casts are to be avoided. The prognosis is good for return to competition in approximately six weeks.

Fractures of the base of the fifth metatarsal are a result of either eversion or inversion injury and pull of the peroneus brevis tendon. They are very frequently seen in basketball when the player involved is coming down from a rebound and lands on another player's foot that is already solidly planted. Dameron emphasizes the recognition of two separate basilar fractures.[18] The first is of the tuberosity (Fig. 57–15) and heals quickly, as demonstrated both clinically (in three weeks) and roentgenographically (in eight weeks). Symptomatic treatment suffices, and plaster immobilization is usually not required. The second of the fractures of the fifth metatarsal occurs

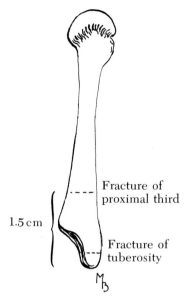

Figure 57–15. *Fractures of the tuberosity of the fifth metatarsal and of the proximal shaft of the fifth metatarsal differ widely in treatment and prognosis.*

more infrequently but is much more significant. This is a transverse fracture near the diaphyseal-metaphyseal juncture, just distal to the flare of the metatarsal base (Fig. 57–15). Delayed union and nonunion are common. Symptoms interfering with competitive athletics are not unusual. Initial treatment, whether symptomatic or with a plaster cast, did not influence the result in 20 patients reported by Dameron.[18] Those requiring bone grafting did well, leading to the suggestion that early bone grafting can be considered in the serious athlete. Bone may be obtained locally from the malleolus, and fixation may be added in the form of a wire loop or metatarsal screw.

Fractures of the Midfoot

Midfoot injuries usually involve avulsion fractures that are not specific for any sport but that are associated with those in which maneuverability and cutting are at a premium. As a rule, they are diagnosed by local tenderness and roentgenograms and are treated conservatively. On rare occasions, the avulsed fragment will need to be removed. A specific avulsion fracture is that of the navicular tuberosity. This is treated by immobilization in an inversion cast for three weeks, followed by inversion strapping for three weeks. If the patient remains symptomatic after conservative treatment, this fragment can be removed and the posterior tibial tendon repositioned on the plantar surface of the remaining navicular.[14]

Fractures of the Hindfoot

Fractures of the beak of the os calcis[19] are frequently produced by adduction of the forefoot, usually with the foot in equinus, and therefore, they occur in sports that require maneuverability. They are caused by the pull of the bifurcate ligament (Fig. 57–16). The patient complains of pain and has local point tenderness in an area halfway between the lateral malleolus and the base of the fifth metatarsal and one finger's breadth anterior to that point. Convalescence is usually slow, requiring six to eight weeks, but there is a good eventual prognosis. Treatment during the acute stage is by strapping and, occasionally, a short leg cast. A noteworthy piece of advice about this fracture is to suspect that it has occurred, since it frequently causes foot pain that persists for weeks following acute injury before being diagnosed. Heel fractures in sports also include avulsion of the Achilles tendon attachment, a fracture that often requires screw fixation and a short leg cast.

The dome of the talus may be fractured. This is diagnosed by the presence of chronic, persistent ankle pain and instability and is frequently confirmed by tomograms. The fractured fragment may turn over.[20] Removal of the loose body is usually required. Postoperatively the patient is rapidly mobilized, thereby remolding the articular surfaces. The prognosis for this fracture is good if it is recognized and treated before significant arthritic changes in the ankle joint become apparent.

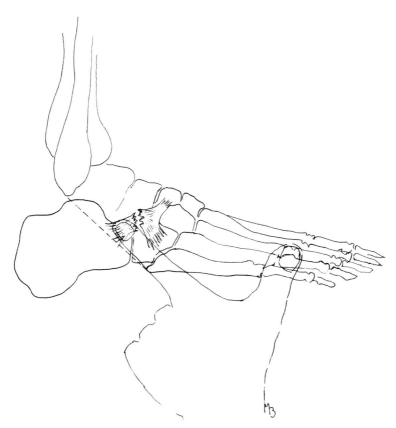

Figure 57–16. *In a fracture of the beak of the os calcis, the tender point is one finger's breadth anterior to the midpoint of a line connecting the lateral malleolus to the base of the fifth metatarsal.*

DISLOCATIONS

Most dislocations are not sport-specific, for example, interphalangeal and metatarsophalangeal dislocations. One that is frequently seen in athletics, however, is a dislocation between the base of the first and second metatarsals.[14, 21] This dislocation extends proximally between the first and second cuboids and then laterally across the foot. In addition to the history and physical examination, the diagnosis is made by roentgenographic evidence of widening between the bases of the first and second metatarsals. A fracture of the base of the second metatarsal or the cuboid or a loss of the normal few degrees of varus of the first metatarsal are clues that this dislocation has occurred (Fig. 57–17). This injury, like turf toe, often occurs with the

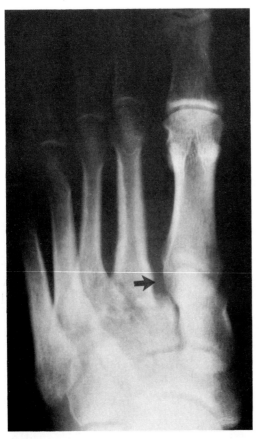

Figure 57–17. *Note the widening between the first and second metatarsal bases (arrow) and the loss of the normal metatarsus primus varus. On the original roentgenograms, avulsion fractures of the second metatarsal base and the cuboid were seen.*

victim in the prone position and in a pile-up. His heel or calf is fallen upon, forcing his forefoot into the turf. Treatment is best accomplished by open reduction and internal fixation to reapproximate this area of separation. Persistent symptoms in a patient seen late are best treated by first metatarsal–cuneiform fusion.

Of perhaps more concern because of the normal-appearing roentgenograms are sprains of the first metatarsal–cuneiform joint, with or without minimal widening between the first and second metatarsal bases. Six weeks of immobilization in plaster with a molded arch will prevent the change of pronation and the collapse of the first metatarsal–cuneiform joint seen in untreated individuals.

Tarsometatarsal dislocations may also occur. We have seen these on a few occasions in football players. Treatment is again best accomplished by open reduction and fixation of the first and fifth tarsometatarsal joints with Kirschner wires,[22] the distal ends of which are left palpable beneath the skin. The foot is immobilized in plaster for six weeks, and the wires are removed at that time under local anesthesia. Gradual rehabilitation is begun with the expectation of active participation in sports in six to nine months. The prognosis is surprisingly good for a satisfactorily functioning foot, despite some changes remaining on roentgenograms. However, the athlete is likely to lose some of his quickness and power.

SPRAINS

Sprains of the foot are most often seen in the first metatarsophalangeal joint and over the laterodorsal surface of the foot. One of the most disabling injuries to an athlete is an acute arch sprain in which the foot is actively dorsiflexed. The complaints and pain in this case are localized to the medial longitudinal arch, and this area of the foot is often swollen. Within a few days the player is able to walk flatfooted perfectly well, but is unable to rise on his toes and has no strength in push-off for three to six weeks. His coach must be apprised of the seriousness of his injury. When a coach sees this apparently healthy player on the sidelines or even jogging or running around the track, he does not understand the athlete's lack of playing effectiveness, which is due to the loss of power in push-off and speed of acceleration. This combination of apparent health and ineffectiveness is common in foot injuries.

Ankle Sprains

Ankle sprains are discussed in Chapters 28 and 56. We would like to suggest that when the time interval between injury and return to play is critical, the athlete has significant advantages. Ice therapy can be used in combination with intermittent Jobst compression.[23] This treatment is repeated three or four times daily, which is often impractical outside of the training room.

The aspiration-injection technique[24] is used for ankle sprains with significant swelling and tenderness laterally and anterolaterally still present after 48 to 72 hours. Ankle stability should be established by stress films and/or arthrograms and/or peroneal tenograms. The ankle joint is then aspirated, and 5 to 10 ml of bloody fluid is usually obtained from sites at the anterolateral and anteromedial cornices of the joint. A mixture of 3 ml of hyaluronidase and 3 ml of lidocaine is then injected into the areas of the anterior talofibular and anterior tibiofibular ligaments.

The sprained ankle is strapped with adhesive plaster as rehabilitation is begun, with emphasis on proprioceptive reflexes, running stride, and coordination and strengthening.

Surgery for Chronic Lateral Ankle Instability

Chronic lateral ankle instability is a major problem in the competing or recreational athlete. Lateral ligamentous instability of the ankle may involve the anterior talofibular ligament and calcaneofibular ligament either separately or in combination. One of the difficulties in reconstruction of these ligaments has been the requirement of substitution by fascial repair or utilization of adjacent musculotendinous units with the inherent problems of fascial elongation and sacrifice of normal functional units. One of our associates,

John Park, has devised an operation that has proved beneficial. It utilizes a Dacron graft.[25] The use of Dacron as an augmentation graft has been reported for the patellar tendon, coracoclavicular ligament, Achilles tendon, and other sites. We have used the double velour woven Dacron graft in coracoclavicular ligaments as a coracoclavicular ligament substitution, based on work in animals showing marked fibrous ingrowth with maturing and organization of collagen throughout the graft, incorporating the Dacron fibrils into the newly forming ligament. Fibrous ingrowth is associated with an increase in strength in the Dacron template. The advantages of Dacron augmentation for lateral ligamentous reconstruction in the ankle include preservation of important musculotendinous units about the ankle, no risk of fascial elongation, and no unnecessary restriction of subtalar motion, unless the graft is placed specifically to assist the calcaneofibular ligament complex. It should be stressed that the maximum follow-up on this new procedure has been two years. The results to date are promising. There have not been any adverse reactions.

Operative Procedure. The technique is a modification of that described by Sefton and associates[26] (Fig. 57–18). A transverse skin incision is made 1.5 cm above the tip of the fibula, originating 1 cm posterior to the fibula and extending to the talar neck. The peroneal tendon sheath is dissected subperiosteally from the posterior aspect of the fibula in its inferior 2 cm, and the peroneal tendons are retracted and protected posteriorly. A 9/64-inch drill hole is made transversely 1.5 cm from the tip of the fibula from anterior to posterior, and a second 9/64-inch drill hole is made angling inferiorly on the anterior surface of the fibula, approximately 1 cm above the tip of the fibula. After elevation of the extensor brevis musculature and sinus tarsi structures, a third 9/64-inch drill hole is made through the lateral margin of the talar neck. A 0.25-inch buttress of cortical bone is preserved. A fourth 9/64-inch drill hole is then made in the talar body anterior to its lateral articulation with the fibula. A prestretched 6-mm Dacron graft is passed from anterior to posterior through the inferior fibular drill hole and then from posterior to anterior through the superior fibu-

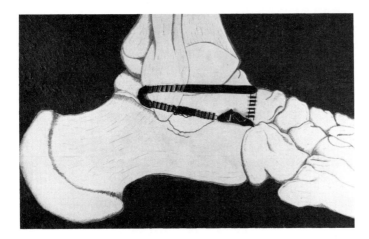

Figure 57–18. Reconstruction of the anterior talofibular ligament.

lar drill hole. The superior limb of the graft is passed from superior to inferior through the talar neck, and the inferior limb is passed from posterior to anterior through the talar body. With the ankle held at 90 degrees and the foot in mild eversion, the graft is tied securely in the sinus tarsi region with a figure-of-eight knot. The ends are cut short. Sutures of nonabsorbable Dacron are utilized to secure the free ends.

Care must be taken during passage of the graft to tighten each portion of the graft as it is passed, as excessive pressures can fracture the thin cortical bridge of the talar neck. If this occurs, the graft should be secured with a staple. If the calcaneofibular ligament is also insufficient, dissection is carried down to the calcaneus directly beneath the fibula, and two drill holes are placed obliquely, approximately 1 cm apart (Fig. 57–19). The Dacron graft is first passed through these drill holes, with both limbs of the graft then entering the posteri-

or aspect of the fibular drill holes, and the remainder of the Dacron graft passage is carried out as previously described. Passage of the graft is made easier if the graft is soaked in a saline or similar solution. The peroneals are replaced and the retinacula are sutured. The soft tissues are reapproximated with interrupted absorbable sutures, and the skin is closed with a running subcuticular nonabsorbable suture.

Postoperative Care. The limb is initially maintained in a well-padded posterior splint with the ankle held in neutral position and slight eversion. After one week to 10 days, the splint and sutures are removed. A short leg walking cast is then applied with the ankle in neutral and the foot in comfortable eversion. This is maintained for a period of four weeks. At the end of four weeks, the cast is removed, and a rehabilitation program is initiated, including active range of motion to the ankle in all planes and gastrocnemius and

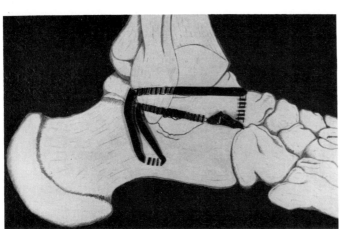

Figure 57–19. Reconstruction of the anterior talofibular ligament and the calcaneofibular ligament.

peroneal-strengthtening exercises. The patient gradually progresses to more vigorous activities, such as jogging on level ground and full-speed running, by three months postoperatively. Taping or strapping of the ankle is recommended during the first six weeks after cast removal until range of motion and muscle strength have returned.

TENDON PROBLEMS

Tendon problems may be divided into tendinitis, peritendinitis, tenosynovitis, acute rupture, stenosis of the tendon sheath, and dislocation. Injuries of the Achilles tendon, including tendinitis, peritendinitis, and rupture, are discussed in Chapters 27, 28, 29, and 55.

Tenosynovitis is a product of repetitive overuse. It is frequently seen in the anterior and posterior tibial tendons, the peroneal tendons, and the tendons of the extensors and flexors, particularly those of the great toe. The diagnosis of tenosynovitis is made easier when the athlete discloses that he participates in an endurance sport. He will have tenderness along the involved tendon, very frequently with redness and crepitation. Passive stretching of the tendon or active use of it against resistance will cause discomfort. It is well at this point to remember that an increased uric acid level can cause the symptoms of either an acute tenosynovitis or an acute joint sprain. The essential component of treatment is rest, which is very difficult to accomplish in a confirmed amateur jogger or professional runner. However, three weeks of rest at this point, accompanied by immobilization, will often effectively relieve the need for more serious measures later. A reduction in the amount of running and relative rest of the Achilles tendon by elevation of the heel are often sufficient. Proper footwear (see Chapter 64) cannot be overemphasized, since only minimal alterations in heel height may cause profound symptom changes in a competitive long-distance runner. Anti-inflammatory medications may be beneficial. This is one lesion that often responds quickly to a single steroid injection.

Stenosis of the tendon sheath may occur in activities that require persistent performance, such as ballet and track. It may involve diverse tendons, including the flexor hallucis longus peroneal, and Achilles tendons. The peroneal tendons are frequently involved by either ankle sprains or os calcis fractures. A peroneal tenogram is made by injecting 6 to 15 ml of sodium iothalamate or meglumine iothalamate directly into the sheath 5 cm proximal to the tip of the fibula. This will indicate stenosis, and leakage of radiopaque material into the joint is indicative of rupture of the calcaneofibular ligament. By the time that stenosis has occurred a direct surgical approach is often necessary to release the tendon sheath. An injection of steroid into the sheath should be tried before resorting to surgery, however. It is of benefit only in a small number of cases, but in those it may give complete relief. The stenosis is usually preceded by tenosynovitis or, in the case of the Achilles tendon, peritendinitis.

Peritendinitis is a frequent complication of distance running. If seen within the first few days of complaint, two weeks of rest will suffice as treatment. If seen after two weeks of persistent symptoms, a prolonged period of rest of as much as six weeks is often required. After six weeks of persistent symptoms, direct operative intervention in the area of the peritendinitis is necessary. The peritenon is opened and debrided of all adhesions, and the sheath is left open. No immobilization is required, and running is permitted as soon as it can be tolerated by the athlete.[28]

Acute rupture of the tendons may occur, and in addition to the Achilles tendon, these are seen most frequently in the anterior tibial tendon. A direct surgical approach to the involved tendon and repair as necessary, usually by means of a Bunnell pull-out wire, are indicated.

Dislocations of the tendons of the foot and ankle usually involve the peroneal tendons. The history is one of eversion and dorsiflexion, although the foot may have been in plantar flexion. The tendons usually reduce spontaneously, and the area remains tender and swollen posterior to the lateral malleolus. It may often be confused with an acute sprain. This problem used to be seen particularly in individuals skiing with the older shoes and bindings, and it now is an occasional product of football, wrestling, soccer, and ballet. The damage inflicted strips the superior peritoneal retinaculum from the fibula, and in approximately 50 per cent of the cases, a fleck of bone is associated with it. This may be visible on the roentgenogram.[29] Although the tendons often reduce spontaneously, chronic dislocation is a problem. The acute cases in the participating athlete are best treated surgically, approaching the lateral malleolus directly through the peroneal sheath and reattaching the retinaculum. If necessary, the groove can be deepened with a gouge. The retinaculum is reattached by means of a drill hole through the bone and small sutures. A short leg cast is worn for four to six weeks.

Chronic cases are often confused with recurrent ankle sprain. Tenderness and swelling along the course of the peroneal tendons may be present. The diagnosis is easier in those cases characterized by a repetitive snapping with dislocation of the peroneal tendons or by a persistent peroneal dislocation.

This injury, when recurrent, may be repaired by a modified Kelly procedure[30, 31] (Fig. 57–20). The skin incision overlies the peroneal tendons posterior and distal to the lateral malleolus. The outer portion of the distal 3 cm of the lateral malleolus is osteotomized in the sagittal plane and swung posteriorly 4 to 5 mm. Kelly originally fixed this with short leg screws. His later modification utilized dovetailing to avoid use of the screws. Watson-Jones fixed the posteriorly displaced graft with sutures and stressed that it should be left attached proximally with its soft tissue and periosteum and in order to preserve its blood supply.[32] His graft was thinner, being an "osteoperiosteal flap." The graft is superficial to the lateral ligaments. Plaster protection for three weeks is sufficient if screws are used. Otherwise six weeks of plaster protection are preferred.

DuVries modified this bone graft by using only the central 1 cm of the Kelly graft, displacing it posteriorly and fixing it with a screw.[33] This avoids the area of ligamentous origin.

A soft-tissue procedure, the Jones

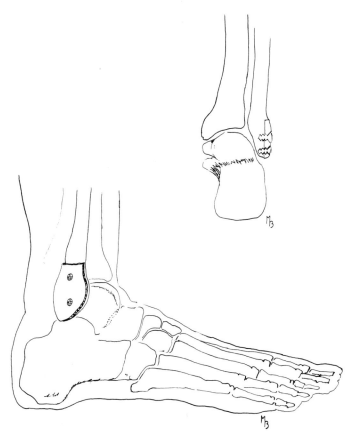

Figure 57–20. *The Kelly procedure for treatment of dislocation of the peroneal tendons deepens the peroneal groove by displacing the outer cortex of the lateral malleolus posteriorly.*

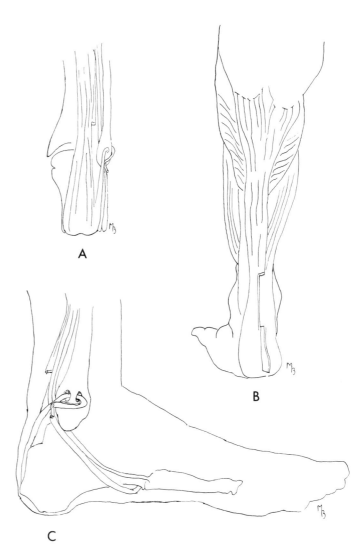

Figure 57–21. *(A–C) The Jones sling operation for imprisoning the peroneal tendons beneath a strip of the Achilles tendon that is looped through the fibular malleolus.*

sling, utilizes a lateral strip of Achilles tendon based distally[34, 35] (Fig. 57–21). The approach is posterior to the distal 5 cm of the fibula. A strip 5 cm long by 0.5 cm wide is dissected from the lateral border of the tendo Achillis, leaving it attached distally to the calcaneus. An anteroposterior drill hole is made in the outer fibular cortex superficial to the peroneal tendon. The free end of the strip is drawn through this hole and sutured back onto itself, holding the peroneal tendons deep to it.

IMPINGEMENT SYNDROME

The anterior impingement syndrome[14] is a result of impingement of the anterior aspect of the tibia against the superior portion of the neck of the talus. This particular syndrome is not a result of traction. It is very common in people who are or were active in athletics during high school and college. For example, 50 per cent of professional major league baseball players have been shown to have this impingement syndrome.[36] It is perhaps most bothersome in a football player, although it does occur in individuals who participate in all running sports. A football player will give a history of a loss of drive or pushoff, a diminution of top speed, and vague anterior ankle pain. Once more, the effect on the athlete may be more devastating than appreciated by casual observation. The impairment of his ability may be noted only in efforts of peak demand. Examination shows pain on forced dorsiflexion and

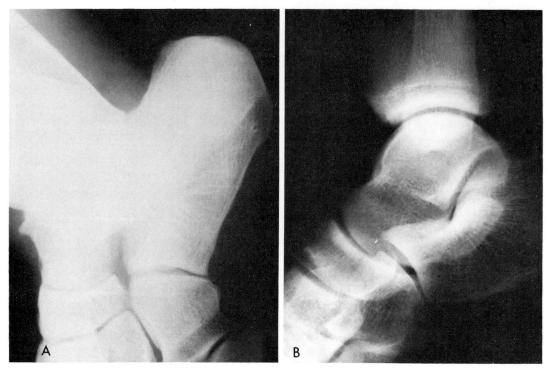

Figure 57–22. *Anterior spur formation on the neck of the talus may be more obvious on the oblique view (A) than on the true lateral roentgenogram (B).*

point tenderness at the area of impingement. Roentgenograms will reveal a spur on the superior aspect of the talus or on the anterior aspect of the tibia, or both (Fig. 57–22). With the foot in a neutral position, the angle between the bevel of the anterior tibia and the neck of the talus should be 60 degrees (Fig. 57–23). This impingement produces a ridge on the anterior tibia and the bevel is lost. With the typical impingement exostosis, other degenerative signs such as narrowing of the joint space are not seen. In the majority of these lesions, treatment is careful neglect. However, if they become symptomatic, particularly in the football player who complains of loss of speed and drive, excision of the exostosis and the anterior lip of the tibia is necessary.

The loss of motion and associated decreased excursion of tendons and muscles produce a shorter stride in the runner. This causes a loss of thigh power, speed, and agility, with force transfer to the big toe and knee.[37] Pain is often found in these areas, as well as in the tibiofibular and calcaneocuboid joints.

The operation is performed through an

anterolateral approach, and the ankle capsule is opened. The tibial exostosis is removed, restoring the normal bevel to the anterior surface. By firm retraction, the

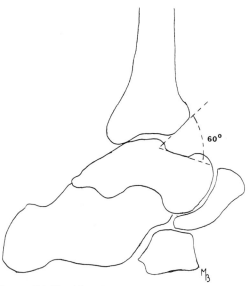

Figure 57–23. *The 60-degree angle between the bevel of the anterior tibia and the neck of the talus with the ankle in neutral position.*

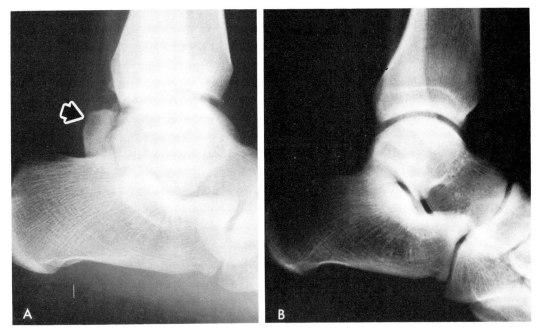

Figure 57–24. *(A) Old fracture of an overdeveloped os trigonum (arrow). This was symptomatic, with pain produced by vigorous running, and allowed limited plantar flexion. (B) After excision of the fragment. The patient is now a professional baseball player without symptoms.*

neck of the talus is visualized and its normal anatomic appearance is restored. If necessary, further removal medially may be done through a separate anteromedial approach. The patient's leg is immobilized in a cast for three weeks, with weight bearing being permitted after the initial pain and swelling subside. On removal of the cast, active rehabilitation is started. In addition to the exostosis of impingement, a calcification may be seen in the anterior aspect of the ankle. This has been described by McMurray as a "footballer's ankle."[38] He saw this in soccer players and related it to kicking the ball with the foot in equinus.

Another area of impingement, but one that is infrequently seen, is the os trigonum. This exostosis may be so large as to prevent plantar flexion and be quite symptomatic after an injury, which may include fracture. If conservative measures fail, operative excision is indicated. The fragment is removed from a medial approach posterior to the malleolus (Fig. 57–24). The neurovascular bundle is retracted anteriorly, and the bony fragment is shelled from the flexor hallucis longus. Postoperative treatment is similar to that for anterior impingement syndrome.

STATIC PROBLEMS

Tight heel cords are one such problem. Normal dorsiflexion is 20 degrees. Athletes average only five to ten degrees.[6] When the ankle is forced into dorsiflexion against a tight heel cord, the subtalar joint supinates[39] because of the normal buffering aspect of the medial malleolus and the taut deltoid ligament. This supination increases the stress on the lateral collateral ligament and produces a tendency toward sprain. The prevention of a tight heel cord has been discussed previously. This is particularly important as prophylaxis for ankle sprains in those sports in which it is common, such as football, basketball, and baseball.

Forefoot varus, pronated feet, heel pain, and plantar fasciitis are discussed in the last sections of this chapter on running and jogging.

BURSITIS

Tendo-Achillis bursitis may be located superficially between the tendon and the skin or deep between the bone and the tendon. It is very often inflammatory and

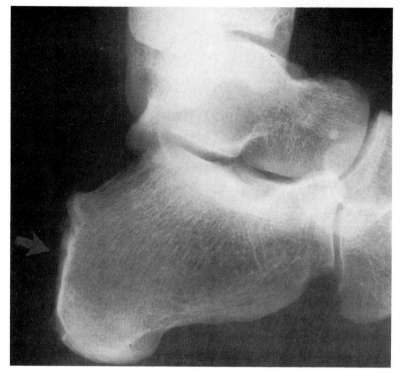

Figure 57–25.   *Amount of bone excised for chronic tendo-Achillis bursitis (arrow).*

quite discernible. The patient has a specific area of tenderness, and treatment includes rest, ice therapy, or hot soaks, proper shoes without a counter and with an elevated heel, injection of steroids, and oral anti-inflammatory drugs. For chronic cases that have been unresponsive to these measures, operative intervention may be required. This includes removal of a large portion of the posterior beak of the os calcis along with the inflamed bursa (Fig. 57–25).

LEG PAIN SYNDROMES

Although leg pain syndromes occur most often in the runner, they will be discussed here to emphasize that they occur in individuals who participate in any sport that requires repetitive foot and ankle activity, for example, ballet, football, basketball, and soccer, not just in track endeavors. The divisions used here are arbitrary, but they serve as aids in diagnosis, differential diagnosis, treatment and prognosis. When the patient presents in the examining room, the distinct divisions tend to blur, as

in the transition from stress fracture to tibial stress syndrome[40] to shin splints. Nearly every reported series of one diagnosis has one or two cases that seem to represent a different entity. Nevertheless, in the following section we make a distinction and, we hope, give sufficient reasons for doing so.

Leg pain syndromes are divided into (1) shin splints, (2) tibial stress syndrome,[40] (3) stress fractures, (4) compartment syndromes (acute and chronic), (5) posttraumatic ossifying hematoma of the interosseous tibiofibular ligament, (6) muscle (fascial) hernias, and (7) tenosynovitis.

Shin Splints

In 1966, "The Standard Nomenclature of Athletic Injuries" was prepared by a subcommittee of the Committee on the Medical Aspects of Sports of the American Medical Association.[41] The term "shin splints" was reserved for those cases presenting as "pain and discomfort in the leg from repetitive running on a hard surface or forcible excessive use of foot flexors; diagnosis should be limited to musculotendinous inflammation, excluding fracture or ischemic disorder."[41] Slocum subsequently stated that "the term can no longer be used as a catch-all for any condition causing pain in the lower part of the leg after exertion, but must be applied to a specific syndrome with a distinct anatomic location and typical clinical course."[42]

The diagnosis is primarily one of exclusion. Direct trauma is excluded by history. Tenderness distal to the ankle, along the tendons, with inflammation and crepitation, is likely to be tenosynovitis. Muscle hernias are usually visible and are palpable at the sites of pain and tenderness. Stress fractures may be visible on roentgenograms, have a more specific point tenderness, and usually have palpable periosteal thickening. However, in early cases, the patient's history with regard to stress fractures, tibial stress syndrome, chronic compartment syndromes, and shin splints may be similar. Tibial stress syndromes occasionally show roentgenographic changes of periostitis or a single cortex fracture, have been localized to the lower third of the tibia posteromedially, and demonstrate localized periosteal induration and thickening. Acute compartment syndromes are much more devastating by history, usually with more acute onset of severe pain, firmness over the involved compartment, glossy skin over the area, and possibly neurologic changes and exquisite pain on muscle stretching. Chronic compartment syndromes are notably resistant to conservative treatment in that they will recur with activity even after months of rest. At the initial visit, however, the history may be similar to that indicating shin splints. The story of pain with activity relieved by a few minutes of rest is more likely to be a compartment syndrome. Walking is painless. The entire anterior compartment is tender. The distinctive feature is increased interstitial fluid pressure, which is present in compartment syndrome[43] but not in shin splint syndrome.[44] The pressure may be determined as suggested by these authors and others,[45] or it may be clinically palpable. Post-traumatic ossifying hematomas are visible on roentgenogram and, as the name suggests, are associated with a history of trauma.

Thus the patient who presents is an athlete engaged in running, jumping, or dancing who has usually increased or changed his training program recently. He may notice that the leg pain is made worse by running on a hard surface and in one direction along a road or around a track and that it is related to the amount of activity, becoming worse if he persists in his efforts. It may be relieved by a few days of rest, only to recur when running is resumed. Tenderness is usually in the middle third of the leg, where the tibialis posterior originates from the tibia. The lower one fourth to one fifth of the posterior tibia is *bare* of any muscle origin. If the anterior muscle group is involved, tenderness is present along the lateral surface of the tibia, usually in the middle third.

The pathophysiology of shin splint syndrome is still debated. A derangement of muscle attachment to bone is the usual explanation. It follows that this lesion is differentiated from fractures and vascular conditions and would be expected to respond to conservative measures.

The sine qua non of treatment is rest. This may vary from complete abstinence from running to simply reducing distance and running on a softer surface. Depending on the muscle involved, changes can be made in heel and/or sole height, and the shoe should be one that provides a cushioning effect. Adhesive strapping for muscle support may be beneficial. Interestingly, the results that were hoped for were not obtained with the prophylactic use of heel padding, heel-cord stretching, or graduated running prior to the normal physical education routine in a group of midshipmen.[46]

Tibial Stress Syndrome

In 1958, Devas published an article in which he described "shin soreness" or "shin splints" as being "caused by a particular type of stress fracture involving only one cortex of the bone and not apparent in the radiographs until a later stage."[47] This description is apt. However, we prefer to differentiate this condition from shin splints and from the typical stress fracture. We therefore prefer the term "tibial stress syndrome" used by Clement[40] and reported subsequently by others.[48]

Tibial stress syndrome differs from shin

splints in that bone is involved, specifically the posteromedial border of the tibia at the junction of the proximal two thirds and distal one third (or proximal three fourths and distal one fourth). Tenderness is increased by direct pressure over the bone at that point and is not aggravated by muscle or tendon palpation. Tendon motion, either active use against resistance or passive stretching, does not elicit the pain. It is magnified by weight-bearing activity and relieved by rest, especially early in the course of the condition. The pain does become longer-lasting.

In addition to the pain and tenderness, the athlete may have local periosteal induration. Roentgenographic signs are late and irregular. It is believed that early recognition and rest decrease the incidence of positive changes. When such

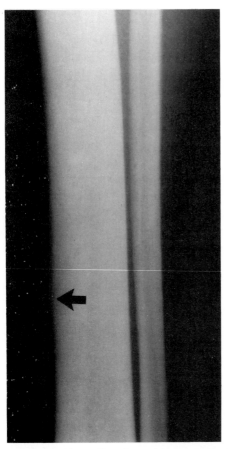

Figure 57–26. *A small periosteal bulge (arrow) is sometimes seen in tibial stress syndrome. A fracture line through one cortex may be seen in some cases.*

changes are present, they are usually along the posterior cortex and begin as well-localized new periosteal bone, as seen in Figure 57–26. A cortical fracture involving only one cortex may appear later. This is obliqued anteroproximally. Jackson and Baily found tibial stress syndrome responsible for the condition of 26 of 40 young athletes seen for "shin splints" (other diagnoses were four typical stress fractures, seven musculotendinous inflammations, or true shin splints, one chronic anterior compartment syndrome, one fascial hernia, and one periosteal reaction, proximo-anterolateral on the tibia).[48] In their series, seven of the 26 athletes demonstrated roentgenographic changes (four with a periosteal reaction, two with cortical hypertrophy, and one with oblique cortical disruption). These roentgenographic changes are differentiated from the usual stress fractures that involve both cortices and show new endosteal as well as new periosteal bone. These fractures are typically transverse.

Treatment consists of rest. This means forbearance from running, jumping, dancing, and any painful activity. This restriction may last from two to six weeks. Local and systemic steroids and other anti-inflammatory agents have been of no benefit. After relief of pain is initially obtained with rest, which is usually within a week, isometric exercises, consisting of dorsiflexion and plantar flexion are started, as recommended by Clement. After two weeks, progressive, resistance, isotonic exercises are instituted.

Stress Fractures

Although these occur in many different sites, fractures of the fibula and tibia present in the leg pain syndromes. Pain usually appears gradually, but may be sudden, following strenuous, repetitive activity. It becomes worse with activity and improves with rest. Does this sound familiar? It should, because the same may be said of the early stages of shin splints, tibial stress syndrome, and chronic compartment syndromes. However, differentiation is relatively unimportant *at this stage*, because the treatment for all of these conditions is rest.

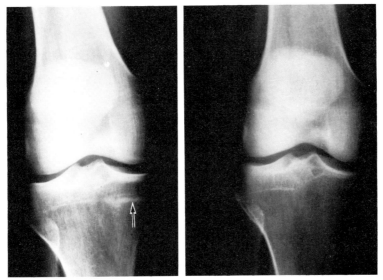

Figure 57–27. *The stress fracture in the proximal tibia (arrow) in the roentgenogram on the left appeared six weeks after the roentgenogram on the right was taken.*

Examination may reveal tenderness, local heat, induration, and swelling. As stated above, the eventual appearance of a stress fracture on roentgenogram is one of new periosteal and endosteal bone and transverse fracture through both cortices. There are exceptions, such as the typical fracture of the middle third of the tibia in ballet dancers, which may involve only the anterior cortex. We have seen many months elapse between onset of symptoms and positive roentgenograms. Unfortunately, recurrence in the same or opposite extremity in subsequent seasons is all too common. Typical sites are the proximal tibia in military recruits, the anterior mid-tibia in ballet dancers, and the distal tibial metaphysis in the middle-aged. In the fibula, stress fractures are typically in the metaphysis in the middle-aged, approximately 3.5 cm from the distal tip.[39] In young athletes, the fracture is usually in the distal third of the diaphysis, 5 cm or more from the distal tip. A "typical" atypical stress fracture is seen in Figure 57–27.

Treatment consists of rest in the case of stress fractures of the fibula. We have found that the only way to provide rest and protection in the young athlete who has a stress fracture of the tibia is by plaster immobilization for six weeks. Sarmineto-type fixation with a movable ankle joint is ideal.

Compartment Syndromes

Compartment syndromes are discussed in Chapter 43. They are mentioned here only as an important factor in differential diagnosis.

Acute Compartment Syndromes. An acute compartment syndrome is an emergency, and time is of the essence.[50] Certainly results begin to deteriorate after four hours.

Symptoms: Severe pain, beginning with or shortly following activity. This may be over a period of many minutes or acutely, within a few steps (we are concerned here only with the compartment syndrome of overuse). The pain is severe, out of the ordinary, and described as "burning," "tearing," or "cramping." Paresthesias may be present.

Signs: Tenseness over the involved compartment (anterior, lateral, posterior), sensory loss, motor loss, pain or tendon activation, tenderness, and particularly the glossy, tight appearance of the skin over the involved compartment.

Treatment is fasciotomy without delay.

The open method allows inspection and excision of necrotic muscle and is preferred for acute compartment syndromes.

Chronic Compartment Syndromes. These are more applicable to this section because they may be diagnosed as shin splints, especially cases seen early. The usual pain on exertion and relief at rest are seen. However, with a chronic compartment syndrome, even several months of rest will not suffice, and any attempt to resume training will result in the reappearance of symptoms. The compartment is tense, which can usually be detected clinically and certainly by pressure determination. Neurologic signs are rare.

This chronic form of compartment syndrome is relieved by fasciotomy. The closed type of fasciotomy utilizing a 1-cm incision and meniscotome is applicable to the anterior compartment, the presence of the peroneal nerve makes this a risky procedure in the lateral compartment. It is interesting to note that the first description of this entity[51] included fasciotomy, with the opening repaired by a fascia lata graft. We do not believe this repair is indicated. Muscle necrosis is rare.[52]

Post-Traumatic Ossifying Hematoma

In this condition, the history of previous injury and the roentgenographic appearance of ossification are diagnostic. At the time of the original injury, varus stress pries the fibula from the tibia, tearing the interosseous membrane and the anterior and posterior tibiofibular ligaments.[53] For some reason, bone forms, which may give rise to the subsequent symptom of aching pain with activity. This is probably due to incomplete cross-ossification and the loss of elasticity of normal tissues.

If indicated, treatment consists of removal of *mature* bone and stabilization of the tibiofibular ligament. We have used the peroneus brevis for this stabilization, weaving it from the fibula to the tibia and back again. Chronic tibiofibular instability is treated in the same manner. The skin incision overlies the course of the peroneal tendons in the distal third of the leg and beyond the fibular malleolus. The peroneus brevis tendon is freed proximally from the muscle mass, and the fascia of this muscle is affixed to the peroneus longus. A strip of tendon approximately 15 cm long, as measured from its insertion, is needed. A drill hole large enough for passage of the tendon is made from distoanteriorly to proximoposteriorly, as in the Evans procedure for repair of chronic ankle sprains. The tendon should emerge from the fibula 1 cm proximal to the joint line. A posteroanterior drill hole is then placed in the lateral margin of the tibia, and the tendon is routed through it and back to the anterior margin of the fibula. The area of the anterior and posterior tibiofibular ligaments is freshened, and a transfixon screw is placed from the fibula through the tibia and is tightened with the ankle in dorsiflexion. The tendon placement reinforces the area of the anterior and posterior tibiofibular ligaments. Fixation of its end to periosteum suffices, since the fixation screw provides the strength necessary for adequate coaptation of the fibula to the tibia. A short leg cast is worn for six weeks, and the screw is removed in three months. This procedure has allowed resumption of competitive athletics by those who would otherwise be incapacitated.

Muscle Hernias

Muscle hernias are diagnosed by the usually visible and nearly always palpable defects at the site of complaint. However, it should be understood that for each symptomatic case there are many asymptomatic ones. A muscle hernia may be an important clue in chronic compartment syndromes, the theory being that chronically increased compartment pressure produces the hernias. This brings us to a word of caution in treatment. In the leg, if surgical treatment is necessary, the defect should not be repaired by direct suturing. Compartment syndromes have been seen following this type of repair. The defect can simply be enlarged by fasciotomy. The buttonhole effect of muscle herniating through a small defect is relieved by converting it to a large defect. If repair is indicated for some reason, a fascia lata graft should be used to close the defect *without tension*.

Tenosynovitis

This pain is usually at or distal to the ankle following the course of the involved tendon. Activity aggravates the pain. It is accompanied by inflammation, heat, redness, and induration. Crepitation may be present. Treatment is discussed in the preceding section on "Tendon Problems."

FOOT PROBLEMS IN DISTANCE RUNNERS

Runners account for an increasing number of patients being seen, because a very large number of otherwise healthy athletes are attempting to log extremely high mileage. This group of patients generally has unique common syndromes due to overuse, as each foot may be subjected to 5000 or more strikes hourly. Many of these people are highly motivated and dedicated athletes who experience the symptoms of a syndrome only with running, whereas other recreational athletic activities do not cause symptoms. Minor alterations of mechanics, form, or training routine may cause pain anywhere from the big toe to the buttock. Subtle alterations in the foot mechanics may be incapacitating to the distance runner if untreated.

Probably in no other type of patient is a complete history more important, since most of the runner's problems are related to errors in training and therefore are easiest to treat. A careful history of training trends should be made, as excessive or rather sudden changes in the runner's routine or track surface, a change from running on a flat surface to running on hills, or an alteration of shoes are very common causes of these overuse syndromes. Indoor track running frequently stresses the left leg (that on the inner part of the track), whereas outdoor running stresses the right leg (that uppermost on the crest of the road).

James and associates have studied the etiology of running problems and found the causes of the disorders to fall into three categories: (1) training errors, (2) anatomic factors, and (3) shoes and surfaces.[54]

Training Errors. Training errors were associated with 60 per cent of the injuries, with excessive distances being the prima-ry mistake. In addition, unusually tense workouts on a hard-surface track and with spiked shoes and rapid changes in the training routine or surface contour were also common.

Anatomic Factors. In the study by James and associates the weight-bearing configuration of the foot in symptomatic runners was studied. Fifty-eight per cent were found to be pronated; 20 per cent had a cavus configuration; and 22 per cent were neutral. Secondary pronation seemed to follow tibia vara, functional equinus with a tight gastrocnemius, subtalar varus, and/or forefoot supination. Individuals with cavus feet generally do not tolerate distance running well, and they seem to be the most intractable and difficult cases to manage. This is apparently because of the relative rigidity of the cavus foot, which is not truly adapted to the loading characteristics of a distance runner.

Shoes. The running shoe market has been a rather lucrative one with varieties of styles and colors, but most are poorly designed; frequently they come only in one width and are improperly fitted. Most feet cannot function on man-made surfaces without support within the shoe, and unfortunately, the universally adequate shoe with proper designs still does not exist. For example, the standard spiked track shoe is made for a runner with metatarsus adductus, with an adducted last, even though only a small percentage of the population has a foot with such a shape. This frequently causes pain over the fifth toe and fifth metatarsal head. The training shoe appears to be designed for an athlete whose third toe is the longest, which presents a problem to the athlete with a long hallux or second toe. The standard training shoe is for a pronated foot. Short spikes are not allowed on track shoes, although they are effective to increase the interface between the surface and shoe, allowing a little torque between the shoe and the ground and subsequently absorbing transverse torque. One of the major problems with training shoes is the lack of support on the medial longitudinal arch, although the wide–toe-box shoes are becoming more popular with public acceptance of comfort for relief of forefoot symptoms.

The last on these shoes is basically no different from that on the earlier shoes, however. The heel counter should be firm to control the hindfoot. A well-molded Achilles pad and tongue protect the Achilles tendon and instep, respectively. The last should be straight, as this has been found to be more comfortable for runners than the standard adductus last. The sole should have moderate cushioning but be flexible under the metatarsal heads to allow adequate dorsiflexion at the metatarsophalangeal joints. A cushioned heel elevated 12 to 15 mm higher than the sole gives additional shock absorption. The "waffle sole" with small rubber studs produces additional cushioning, but some runners have experienced knee, calf, and tendon problems after shifting to the widest heel style. This may be due to too much stability, and occasionally it is necessary to trim the flange. The beveled heel provides stability and also allows the foot to be more easily plantar flexed following heel-strike. A long and adequately high toe-box prevents crowding of the toes. An interesting consumer input to marketing has been carried out in recent issues of "Runner's World," in which large numbers of runners have tested various prototypes of training shoes with subjective scoring. It is hoped that this impetus for an adequately designed shoe will help diminish the number of problems resulting from long-distance running, excluding training errors and the more severe anatomic disorders.

Recent shoe modifications consist of changing the contour of the heel to fit an individual heel configuration, allowing selection of widths in the training shoe, changing the midsole cushion under the forefoot and heel, adding a varus wedge, and the use of closed cellular neoprene insoles, which have been shown to absorb shearing forces acting on the feet and therefore diminish the frequency of blisters, calluses, and trophic ulcers. A closed insole (Spenco insole) has been developed that will absorb 1 cm of shear force in the fore, aft, and lateral motions with 25 degrees of rotary shear. A tape has also been developed for absorption of similar shear forces on the sides or top of the foot.[55] An advancement in replacement of worn outer heel edges prolongs life of the heel and diminishes the subsequent imbalance at heel-strike.

Running Surfaces. Many areas have excellent soft grass fields, but most people ignore these and are found running on concrete surfaces. A soft yet nonyielding surface is good. Too soft a surface allows pronation and results in subsequent overuse syndrome. Hilly areas cause difficulty as the descent of the hills may cause significant patellofemoral compression. Many foot injuries occur with running on the beach owing to the canted surface and pronating through the softer sand. A wood-chip running surface is ideal, yet natural grass causes fewer chronic overuse injuries than synthetic surfaces for daily training.

Orthotic Appliances. Orthoses prescribed in the review of James and associates gave 78 per cent beneficial results.[54] Softer, flexible appliances can be made of a flexible material by an orthotist, but the longevity of soft orthoses is limited, and they provide less precise control. Rigid orthoses are more durable and provide better foot control, and they appear to be better tolerated by long-distance runners. They are particularly effective in compensatory foot pronation, and although they are not a "cure-all," they are useful when properly prescribed and utilized.

In general, it is our preference to begin the use of orthoses in jogging with soft appliances made in the office. Felt is used primarily because it can be easily carved and cut; it provides impact absorption; it lasts for several weeks; and importantly, the patient can remodel it at home by shaving it down where necessary. Heel pads, arch supports, metatarsal pads, and heel and forefoot wedges can be made in this manner. The ideal weight-bearing alignment is seen in Figure 57–28. Those who do not have this ideal alignment are given support in such a way as to approach this configuration. One unusual means of attaining this that is often used in runners is to leave the foot as it is and bring the ground to the foot, for example, by utilizing a medial wedge for a supinated forefoot. A lateral wedge would be the first consideration, but for the participant, correction of deformity may produce strain and therefore is secondary to comfort.

The next stage is a soft but more perma-

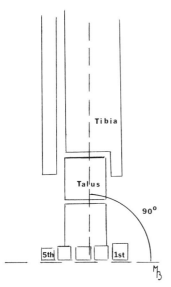

Figure 57–28. *Schematic drawing of the correct leg-heel-forefoot relation. The os calcis is parallel to the tibia, and both are perpendicular to the metatarsal heads.*

nent appliance. For this we use Dow-Corning Silastic 385 Elastomer fashioned by the orthotist. It is lasting, impact-resistant, comfortable, and moisture-proof (perspiration).

When rigid appliances are considered, the concern is usually heel pain or a pronated foot. For heel pain, the polyethylene heel seats* that are pre-formed according to size are used. They should fit so as to be snug to the heel, neither pinching (too tight) or falling off the dependent heel easily (too loose).

For the pronated foot in need of support on a permanent basis, a multitude of products are available. Most are time-consuming and require a positive mold of the foot in corrected posture in order to produce them. High temperatures are required in the manufacturing process. Acrylic, polypropylene, or polyethylene are materials that are strong but workable under high temperatures. A UCB type of foot support that lifts the arch and molds the heel is used.

In the office setting, Orthoplast is useful since it is malleable at temperatures attainable by hot water. Its major drawback is the thickness required to hold the heel.

An interesting, comfortable padding and arch support can be provided by a cork-latex mixture† that is poured into the shoe and allowed to harden to the contours of the foot in about four hours. This does not mold the heel, and it obviously molds to the uncorrected contours of the foot, but it provides impact absorption and is useful in preventing pressure areas and calluses.

DISORDERS IN DISTANCE RUNNERS AND JOGGERS

Posterior Tibial Syndrome

The most common condition noted in distance runners is "posterior tibial syndrome," with tenderness along the course of the posterior tibial muscle. Sheehan feels that this disorder results from a combination of structural and postural problems compounded by the type of shoes worn, the nature of the running surface, and the presence of a short, powerful gastrocnemius and weak anterior compartment groups.[56] He feels that running on hard surfaces and wearing shoes that provide little shock absorption along with fast starts exacerbate the condition. He suggests the following: (1) add a 0.25- to 0.50-inch felt heel lift, (2) stretch the calf muscles with wall push-ups (10 push-ups twice daily), (3) strengthen the muscle groups around the ankle, and (4) ice therapy after competition.

Knee Pain

Knee pain is a frequent complaint in distance runners and may in fact be chondromalacia, but more often it is parapatellar pain due to abnormal transverse rotation. Frequently, the parapatellar pain is associated with a cavus foot that does not handle shock well or tight calf muscles that diminish shock absorption. In addition, shoes with an inadequate amount of rubber at the front or at the heel have poor impact absorption characteristics. In winter weather, a runner may run on a

---

*These may be obtained from Apex Foot Products, 118 W. 22nd Street, New York, New York 10011.

†Contour-A-Mold—available from Professional Products Company, 612 Bayshore Drive, Tarpon Springs, Florida.

tight, curved indoor track in a counter-clockwise direction. This involves internal rotation of the left leg, and subsequent push-off may cause pain in the left calf, whereas the externally rotated right foot may cause some lateral-riding patellar problems. The converse may occur in running outdoors, with the leg uppermost on the road being stressed.

Stress Fractures

Stress fractures have been discussed previously but must be watched for, as toe running has become more common, even in long-distance runners. Orthoses have been particularly beneficial, allowing these athletes to continue to run. The fifth metatarsal stress fracture is particularly common in runners who use an indoor track with banked turns and a hard-packed surface. Stress fractures are often treated differently in distance runners, as rest is unacceptable to the competitive runner.

Achilles Tendinitis

Achilles tendinitis has been a significant problem in the track athlete.[27] In the treatment of this overuse syndrome at the University of Arkansas, only very minimal changes were made in footwear, orthoses, or training methods. Major changes were not tolerated well by the competitive athlete. Clancy and associates pointed out that tenosynovitis of the Achilles tendon may become intractable and require paratenon release.[27]

Plantar Fasciitis

Plantar fasciitis presents as a painful heel with an insidious onset of pain in the area of the plantar fascia. This pain is usually worse on arising and on running increased distances. There is tenderness directly over the medial insertion of the plantar fascia on the calcaneus. It is very difficult to differentiate plantar fasciitis from a medial arch strain, but most runners, whether they run heel-toe or flatfooted, roll to the outside of the foot with the foot in a supinated position, followed by foot-flat, and roll into pronation and subsequently back into supination.[54] This rel-ative supination of the forefoot is a more stable condition and an ideal mechanism, but in individuals with abnormal pronation or other anatomic disorders, unusual stresses are placed on the medial side of the longitudinal arch and plantar fascia. Therefore, orthoses may be beneficial in this regard. Playing shoes with very thick soles under the metatarsophalangeal joints absorb stresses, but the lack of flexibility causes strain on the Achilles tendon. Frequently, the sole of the shoe can be cut with a hacksaw so that the shoe can flex more readily, relieving this problem. Anterior heels shorten the lever arm from the ankle to the forefoot so that the Achilles tendon can lift the heel off, but most importantly a stretching program to strengthen and stretch the gastrocnemius-soleus musculotendinous unit is essential.

Leach and associates have called attention to the entity of rupture of the plantar fascia.[57] This had not previously been reported, although it has occasionally been seen. Five of their six patients had been long-distance runners and their sixth, as well as a patient whom we treated recently, were basketball players. The athlete presents with sudden, marked onset of pain, tenderness, and swelling. There may have been an audible or palpable pop in the plantar aspect of the foot. Often the swelling causes the medial longitudinal arch to take on a convex, rather than concave, appearance. Later, as the swelling recedes, a palpable defect may present in the plantar fascia, or the area may fill with a firm, painful nodule. Five of the six patients of Leach and associates had received multiple steroid injections,[57] but the relationship of steroids to rupture of the fascia can only be conjectured.

Treatment consists of phenylbutazone, 100 mg three times a day for a week, ice applied locally for 15 minutes three times a day, and the sine qua non of relative rest. Crutches are used until the patient can walk painlessly, usually for about two or three weeks. Running and jumping are permitted when the patient can stand on tiptoes without pain. Taping and soft arch pads are helpful supports for the arch. Most athletes can run effectively in six weeks.

If a painful nodule appears, it may require surgical excision. Transection of the plantar fascia does not adversely affect the runner.

Heel Pain

Typical heel pain is located on the plantar surface of the os calcis and is often said to be caused by "heel spurs." This is frequently seen in joggers, as they strike the heel first, and in fact, it is called "jogger's heel" in those athletes.[38] A history of pain on first arising in the morning or after sitting for a long period of time, with relief after taking several steps, but worsening again after prolonged activity, such as standing on hard floors or jogging, should suggest this diagnosis. The tenderness is quite specific and is located further posteriorly than the attachment of the plantar fascia. Roentgenograms may be perfectly normal, or they may demonstrate an os calcis spur that is a "red herring." Several modes of treatment are beneficial and will almost always work without surgical intervention being required. Since the pathology involved is a disruption of the fibrofatty hydraulic system of the heel, anything that increases padding, such as sponge or felt, will be helpful. Heat or cold will often give temporary relief. Anti-inflammatory agents and local anesthetics with steroids are occasionally useful. Of perhaps the most significant benefit is the well-fitted heel cup, which will alter the strike pattern and can be worn inside the jogging shoe. The runner should also confine his activity to softer surfaces. As an individual preference to complete rest from running, the athlete may switch from distance running or jogging (heel-strike) to sprinting (forefoot-strike).

Jogger's Toe

Jogger's toe is very similar to tennis toe, being caused by repeated traumatization of the nail of the hallux by sudden deceleration against the toe-box of the training shoe. There are two forms of jogger's toe. The first is a subungual hematoma that is frequently experienced by distance runners who wear a tight-fitting shoe that provides such good traction that the runner's foot is forced into the toe-box of the

shoe during deceleration or downhill running, traumatizing the nail of the hallux.[58] The patient frequently presents some three to four weeks after the incident with an asymptomatic bluish discoloration of the nail. This disorder has responded extremely well to treatment consisting of a properly fitting shoe, soft toe padding, and neoprene shoe liners. A second form of jogger's toe may involve any of the toes and is frequently bilateral, involving the toe that is most forward in the toe-box. It is interesting as a stigma particular to joggers, with a highly characteristic traumatic petechial eruption of the fat pad of the toe tip. The etiology is similar to the subungual hemorrhage of the runner wearing a tight-fitting shoe. It is seen in training as a result of a forefoot-strike, often combined with much hill work. There is no real clinical significance in this discoloration, although it has been mistaken by the untrained eye for plantar verrucae and even for malignant melanoma. Most long-distance runners eventually show damage to the toenails, with the small nails often being lost or becoming thickened secondary to the petechial eruption and repeated trauma.

Conclusions

The foot is often neglected, unless it is your own; it then becomes the pedestal on which the rest of you stands.

REFERENCES

1. Quigley, T. B.: Management of ankle injuries sustained in sports. J. A. M. A., 169:1451, 1959.
2. McMaster, W. D.: A literary review of ice therapy in injuries. J. Sports Med., 5:124, 1977.
3. Cyriax, J.: Textbook of Orthopaedic Medicine, 6th ed. London, Baillière Tindall, 1975, Vol. 1, p. 19.
4. Stearns, M. L.: Studies of development of connective tissue in transparent chambers in the rabbit's ear. Am. J. Anat., 67:55, 1940.
5. Freeman, M. A. R., Dean, M. R. E., and Hanhan, I. W. F.: The etiology and prevention of functional instability of the foot. J. Bone Joint Surg., 47B:678, 1965.
6. McCluskey, G. M., Blackburn, T. A., and Lewis, T.: Prevention of ankle sprains. Am. J. Sports Med., 4:151, 1976.
7. Darick, G. L., Bigley, G., Karst, R., and Malina, R. M.: The measurable support of the ankle joint by conventional methods of taping. J. Bone Joint Surg., 44A:1183, 1962.
8. Ryan, A. J.: In support of ankles. Clin. Pediatr., 8:618, 1969.

9. Ferguson, A. B.: The case against ankle taping. J. Sports Med., *1*:46, 1973.

10. Glick, J. G., and Requa, R. K.: Role of external support in the prevention of ankle sprains. Med. Sci. Sports, 5:200, 1973.

11. Bowers, K. D., Jr., and Martin, R. B.: Turf-toe, a shoe-surface related football injury. Med. Sci. Sports, 8:81, 1976.

12. Coker, T. P., Arnold, J. A., and Weber, D. L.: Traumatic lesions of the metatarsophalangeal joint of the great toe in athletes. J. Arkansas Med. Soc., 74:309, 1978.

13. Bowers, K. D., Jr., and Martin, R. B.: Impact absorption, new and old Astroturf at West Virginia University. Med. Sci. Sports, 6:217, 1974.

14. O'Donoghue, D. H.: Treatment of Injuries to Athletes, 3rd ed. Philadelphia, W. B. Saunders Co., 1976, Vol. I.

15. Clancy, W. G., Jr.: Lower extremity injuries in the jogger and distance runner. Phys. Sports Med., 2:47, 1974.

16. Bernstein, A., and Stone, J. R.: March fracture: a report of three hundred and seven cases, and a new method of treatment. J. Bone Joint Surg., 26:743, 1944.

17. Rockwood, C. A., and Green, D. P.: Fractures, 1st ed. Philadelphia, J. B. Lippincott Co., 1975, Vol. 2, p. 1400.

18. Dameron, T. B.: Fractures and anatomical variations of the fifth metatarsal. J. Bone Joint Surg., 57A:788, 1975.

19. Gellmen, M.: Fractures of the anterior process of the calcaneus. J. Bone Joint Surg., 33B:382, 1951.

20. Nisbet, M. W.: Dome fractures of the talus. J. Bone Joint Surg., 36B:244, 1954.

21. Funk, F. J.: Tarsometatarsal dislocations. Presented at the Internal Meeting of the American Orthopaedic Society for Sports Medicine, Dallas, February, 1978.

22. Aitken, A. P., and Poulson, D.: Dislocations of the tarsometatarsal joint. J. Bone Joint. Surg., 45A:246, 1963.

23. Starkey, J. A.: Treatment of ankle sprains by simultaneous use of intermittent compression and ice pack. Sports Med., 4:142, 1976.

24. Brady, T. A., and Arnold, A.: Aspiration injection treatment for varus sprain of the ankle. J. Bone Joint Surg., 54A:1257, 1972.

25. Park, J.: Personal communication.

26. Sefton, G. K., George, J., Fitton, J. M., et al.: Reconstruction of the anterior talofibular ligament for the treatment of the unstable ankle. J. Bone Joint Surg. 61B:352, 1979.

27. Clancy, W. G., Neidhart, D., and Brand, R. L.: Achilles tendinitis in runners: a report of five cases. Am. J. Sports Med., 4:46, 1976.

28. Snook, O. A.: Achilles tendon tenosynovitis in long-distance runners. Med. Sci. Sports, 4:155, 1972.

29. Earle, A. A., Mortiz, J. E., and Tapper, E. H.: Dislocation of the peroneal tendons at the ankle: an analysis of 25 ski injuries. Northwest. Med., 71:108, 1972.

30. Marti, R.: Dislocation of the peroneal tendons. Am. J. Sports Med., 5:19, 1977.

31. Kelly, R. E.: An operation for chronic dislocation of peroneal tendons. Br. J. Surg., 7:502, 1920.

32. Watson-Jones, R.: Fractures and Joint Injuries, 4th ed. Baltimore, Williams and Wilkins, 1955, Vol. 2, p. 830.

33. Crenshaw, A. H. (ed.): Campbell's Operative Orthopaedics, 5th ed. St. Louis, C. V. Mosby Co., 1971, Vol. 2, p. 1495.

34. Jones, E.: Operative treatment of chronic dislocation of the peroneal tendons. J. Bone Joint Surg., 14:547, 1932.

35. Savastano, A. A. : The treatment of recurrent dislocations of the common peroneal tendons. Presented at the Eighth Annual Meeting of the American Orthopaedic Foot Society, Inc., Dallas, February 1978.

36. King, J. W., Tullos, H., Stanley, R., et al.: Lesions of the feet in athletes. South. Med. J., 64:45, 1971.

37. Nicholas, J. A.: Ankle injuries in athletes. Orthop. Clin. North Am., 5:153, 1974.

38. McMurray, T. P.: Footballer's ankle. J. Bone Joint Surg., 32B:68, 1950.

39. Cahill, B. R.: Chronic orthopaedic problems in the young athlete. J. Sports Med., 3:35, 1973.

40. Clement, D. B.: Tibial stress syndrome in athletes. J. Sports Med., 2:81, 1974.

41. Rachun, A., et al.: Standard Nomenclature of Athletic Injuries. Chicago, American Medical Association, 1966, p. 126.

42. Slocum, D. B.: The shin splint syndrome. Am. J. Surg., 114:875, 1967.

43. Reneman, R. S.: The anterior and the lateral compartmental syndrome of the leg due to intensive use of muscles. Clin. Orthop., 113:69, 1975.

44. D'Ambrosia, R. D., Zelic, R. F., Chuinard, R. G., and Wilmore, J.: Interstitial pressure measurements in the anterior and posterior compartments in athletes with shin splints. J. Sports Med., 5:127, 1977.

45. Whitesides, T. E., Haney, T. C., Morimoto, K., and Harada, H.: Tissue pressure measurements as a determinant for the need for fasciotomy. Clin. Orthop., 113:43, 1975.

46. Andrish, J. T., Bergfeld, J. A., and Walheim, J.: A prospective study of the management of shin splints. J. Bone Joint Surg., 56A:1697, 1974.

47. Devas, M. B.: Stress fractures of the tibia in athletes, or "shin soreness." J. Bone Joint Surg., 40B:227, 1958.

48. Jackson, D. W., and Bailey, D.: Shin splints in the young athlete: a nonspecific diagnosis. Phys. Sports Med., 3:45, 1975.

49. Burrows, H. J.: Fatigue fractures of the fibula. J. Bone Joint Surg., 30B:266, 1948.

50. Wiggins, H. E.: The anterior tibial compartmental syndrome. Clin. Orthop., 113:9, 1975.

51. Mavor, G. E.: The anterior tibial syndrome. J. Bone Joint Surg., 38B:513, 1956.

52. Puranen, J.: The medial tibial syndrome. J. Bone Joint Surg., 56B:712, 1974.

53. Levinthal, D. H., and Kaplan, L.: Post-traumatic ossifying hematoma of the interosseous tibiofibular ligament in the lower leg. Clin. Orthop., 23:171, 1962.

54. James, S. L., Bates, B. T., and Osternig, L. R.: Injuries to runners. Am. J. Sports Med., 6:40, 1978.

55. Spence, W. R., and Shields, M. N.: Prevention of blisters, callosities and ulcers by absorption of shear forces. J. Am. Podiatry Assoc., 58:428, 1968.

56. Sheehan, G.: Personal communication.

57. Leach, R., Jones, R., and Silva, T.: Rupture of the plantar fascia in athletes. J. Bone Joint Surg., 60A:537, 1978.

58. Schuster, D. P. M., and Richard, O.: Podiatry in the foot of the athlete. J. Am. Podiatry Assoc., 62:465, 1972.

CHAPTER 58

INDUSTRIAL INJURIES TO THE FOOT AND ANKLE AND THEIR PREVENTION

Hamilton Hall, M.D., F.R.C.S.(C.)

THE PROBLEM

In 1975, the Department of Environmental Health at the University of Washington instituted a national occupational hazard survey.[1] One of the questions asked was "Do weak or painful feet make your life miserable?" Of the workers responding to the questionnaire, 7.4 per cent said yes. Of this group, 72 per cent related their foot problem to their occupation. No other symptom questioned carried a higher job-related incidence. Kleiger, basing his opinion on 1971 National Safety Council figures, estimated that 16.5 per cent of work accidents involved the foot and ankle.[2] A report prepared in 1973 by the Construction Safety Association of Ontario (CSAO) estimated that 10.6 per cent of the 17,500 work injuries that occurred that year in the province of Ontario involved the foot.[3] In describing occupational injuries in Australia in 1975, Wigglesworth estimated that trauma to the foot constituted 9 per cent of the total.[4]

Accidents involving the foot and ankle remain a major economic concern. The National Safety Council estimated that in the United States during 1971 almost 600 million dollars were paid in compensation for work-related injuries to the ankle and foot.[5] In 1960, a Canadian estimate placed the cost of each foot accident at about one thousand dollars. The estimated direct cost to Canadian industry was about three million dollars.[6] In preparation for the Canadian Conference on Personal Protective Equipment in 1978, the Construction Safety Association of Ontario carried out a new survey on industrial injury in Canada.[7] They estimated that the direct cost of foot injuries in Canada had risen from three million to almost 50 million dollars. The indirect costs, including lost productivity, approaches 200 million dollars a year. On an even larger scale, an increase in compensation costs continues in the United States. The economic significance of injuries to the foot and ankle cannot be ignored.

The results of a survey submitted by the Construction Safety Association of Ontario to the American National Standards Institute in 1975 stated that 48.6 per cent of the foot and ankle injuries reviewed occurred in men doing heavy labor.[8] Sixty-seven per cent of these laborers were employed in construction. The next largest single group were carpenters, who constituted only 9.6 per cent of the total. Although foot and

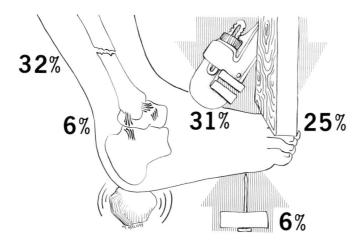

32%

6%   31%   25%

6%

Figure 58–1. Crushing produces most of the trauma to the midfoot and toes. Ankle injuries result from both direct blows and inversion or eversion strains. Puncture wounds and trauma to the heel each account for 6 per cent of the total.

ankle injuries may occur in any industrial setting, it is obvious that heavy construction, particularly the building trades, carries the greatest risk.

This same survey found that 30 per cent of the injuries to the foot occurred on the sole, 23 per cent involved the midfoot, and 22 per cent affected the toes. Punctures were the most common injury, accounting for 31 per cent of the total. About 25 per cent of the injuries involved fractures.

The 1977 Canadian Injury Survey of foot and ankle injuries produced a comprehensive look at the industrial accident pattern in North America.[7] In this survey, 32 per cent of the injuries involved the ankle; 31 per cent involved the metatarsal area of the foot; toe injuries accounted for 25 per cent; and heel and sole injuries constituted 6 per cent each (Fig. 58–1). The reasons for the significant reduction in the incidence of puncture wounds is discussed later in the chapter.

Most industrial accidents occur to young, inexperienced workmen. According to the Australian figures, men are injured six times more often than women, but the type and site of injury are the same for both sexes.[4] Fifty-five per cent of the accidents reported in the Canadian study occurred to workmen under 30 years of age; 65 per cent of the accidents involved workmen with less than five years experience in their occupation. The vulnerability of this group can be illustrated in a different way. Using the figures from Statistics Canada for 1976, it is found that the probability of a worker under 24 years old being injured on the job is 65 per cent. The probability of injury for those over 24 years

old is only 35 per cent. This government statistic applies to all industrial injuries. The CSAO survey, however, confirmed a parallel frequency in injuries confined to the foot and ankle.

Part of this preponderance of industrial injuries among the younger age group may be explained by the fact that they are the largest single group of workers. However, their percentage of injuries is higher than their proportion to the total work force. Moreover, as already noted, 65 per cent of industrial accidents to the foot and ankle involved workers with less than five years experience in their occupation, regardless of their age. Inexperience is a major cause of accidents.

The Australian study[4] adds several interesting facts. Injuries were most common on Mondays, and the frequency decreased during the rest of the week. Each day the frequency of accidents increased just before lunch and again late in the afternoon. Friday morning was the most accident-free period of the week. Over 25 per cent of the injuries to the foot and ankle were caused by slips or falls, often while the workman was hurrying. Almost one third of the injuries involved contact with the floor or ground.

Although personal protective equipment is important, it is obviously not enough. A safe work site and personal safety habits are necessary if the frequency of foot and ankle injuries is to be reduced, but the overall statistic remains constant. Surveys from the mid 1960's to the present continue to show an incidence of industrial foot and ankle injury of about 10 per cent. For every 300 men working in heavy industry, 15 working days per month continue to be lost as a result of foot problems.[9]

Once a compensable injury has occurred, the recovery period may be prolonged. The patient suffering chronic pain from an old ankle injury is a typical example of the problem that confounds rehabilitation workers. Four factors can be recognized as acting to prevent the patient from returning to work. The prolonged absence of a regular work routine makes resumption of the daily schedule difficult. This fact, often imbued with deep psychiatric significance, may in reality be little different than the natural reluctance most people feel on being forced to return to work after a prolonged holiday. The injured workman's absence has been no holiday, however, and his return to work may physically increase his pain. His natural reluctance is reinforced by the fact that he experiences, perhaps for the first time in several weeks, a return of his ankle symptoms. The third factor working against successful rehabilitation is lack of patient understanding. The workman justifiably equates his increase in pain with increasing damage and the possibility of permanent injury. He is afraid to return to work for fear of causing further harm. The last factor influencing the situation is obviously the compensation payments. When the first three components are combined with the fact that the workman may be receiving as much or more after-tax income from his injury benefits as he did from his regular employment, it is little wonder that patients receiving compensation perform more poorly than those recovering from noncompensable injuries.

THE AREAS OF INJURY

The Toes

Most toe injuries are caused by objects falling on the foot. Trauma ranges from frequent minor soft-tissue contusions to fortunately uncommon severe crush injuries of the phalanges. In reviewing the injury records of a manufacturing plant in Massachusetts, Johnson showed that 50 per cent of the fractures occurring in the forefoot were in the great toe and first metatarsal, with the distal phalanx of the large toe being the most common single site of injury.[10] Twenty-five per cent of the fractures involved the fifth ray, and the remaining 25 per cent involved the middle three rays combined.

As will be discussed later in the chapter, adequate toe protection is available, yet toe injuries continue to account for 25 per cent of the trauma in this area. The hazard has been underestimated.

Treatment depends on the severity of the injury and ranges from simple protection and methods of external or internal fixation to amputation of the injured digit.[11] I agree with Johnson that most toe injuries have been overtreated in the past. The majority of closed phalangeal fractures require only protective splinting to the adjacent digit, simple analgesia, and early ambulation in the protective shoe. Walking casts are generally not required. A moderate amount of angulation or rotation is acceptable and will not produce functional disability. In Johnson's series, only 8 per cent of workers suffering isolated phalangeal fractures lost time from work.[10]

The Metatarsal Region

Like toe injuries, most trauma to the metatarsal area of the foot is caused by a direct blow (Fig. 58–2). Occasional crushing injuries may result from a foot being trapped beneath heavy equipment or under a wheel. A forced plantar-flexion inversion injury, similar to that producing lateral ligament disruption in the ankle, may also damage the midfoot. The frequency of industrial injury to this area is second only to that involving the ankle.

Fortunately, severe injuries are rare, but minor injuries from direct trauma, including soft-tissue bruising, traumatic synovitis of the dorsal tendon sheaths, and hemorrhage into the extensor digitorum brevis, are common. Small avulsion fractures of the tarsal bones from inversion strain are also typical. Fracture-dislocation at the tarsometatarsal joint (Lisfranc's fracture) and fracture-dislocation through the midtarsal joints (Chopart's fracture) are rare and are usually associated with both direct and indirect violence.

The severity of a soft-tissue crush injury of the midfoot may be difficult to deter-

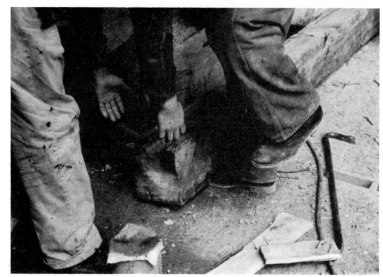

Figure 58–2. *This crush injury involved the entire forefoot. A steel toecap in the work boot reduced the severity of the trauma to the toes. All the metatarsals were fractured.*

mine. A careful history to elicit the exact mechanism of injury along with an assessment of the magnitude and duration of the crushing force is essential. Radiographic evidence of multiple fractures or fracture-dislocations may indicate an unsuspected severity. The application of a snug below-the-knee cast for the treatment of apparently minor metatarsal fractures can lead to serious problems with skin slough, vascular insufficiency, and muscle necrosis due to severe edema. The devastating effects of the soft-tissue damage must not be overlooked.

The treatment of metatarsal injuries is similar to that for trauma to the toes. Simple metatarsal fractures without soft-tissue crushing can be well treated with careful padding, a metatarsal support, elastic bandaging, and an oversized work shoe with a rigid shank. Because the first and fifth metatarsals are major weight-bearing components of the foot, midshaft fractures of these bones may produce prolonged disability. Their treatment requires a longer period of immobilization than that necessary for fractures of the internal rays. Multiple fractures, fracture-dislocations, or extensive crush injuries may require hospitalization for careful observation and possible fasciotomy or open reduction with internal fixation.

Time off from work because of metatarsal injuries is substantially greater than that associated with trauma to the toes. In general, as the point of injury moves proximally from the tips of the digits, the consequences become more serious. MacFarlane cited the case of a 23-year-old welder injured when a metal truss fell on his right foot.[12] He sustained fractures of the first and second metatarsals, which were treated by immobilization in a below-the-knee cast. The patient continued to complain of severe pain in the region of the first metatarsophalangeal joint, but the physical examination revealed only restricted movement and local tenderness. Because the workman's pain was sufficient to keep him from work, a first metatarsophalangeal fusion was performed 10 months after the primary injury. The fusion failed to relieve his pain, and a repeat operation was done eight months later. The third attempt at surgery took place six months after that. Four months after his last operation, the workman was still in pain and out of work. The total cost of the claim was in excess of $29,000. In compensable industrial injuries, the role of surgery, particularly repeat surgery, must be critically assessed.

The Ankle

According to the Canadian survey,[7] the ankle joint is the most common site of industrial trauma in this region. Soft-tissue ankle injuries occurred frequently, and in

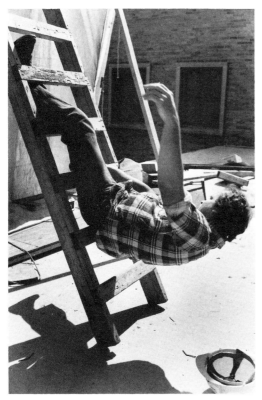

Figure 58–3. *Not all ankle injuries are this dramatic. However, over 50 per cent of trauma to the ankle is produced by slips or falls causing inversion or eversion strains.*

this group, "sprains and strains" were the most common diagnoses. Most of these injuries occurred as the result of contact with a surface or a "trip over" or a "slip on" something (Fig. 58–3). This mechanism alone accounted for more than 50 per cent of ankle injuries. The second most common source of soft-tissue damage was blunt trauma to the ankle from a moving object. Because of the exposed position of the ankle outside the shoe, cuts and burns were more frequent about the ankle than on the rest of the foot. Fractures were uncommon, accounting for only 3 per cent of the total.

Treatment depends on the nature and severity of the injury. Minor soft-tissue injuries can be supported with simple adhesive strapping inside the firm, high-cut work boot. With return to work, however, the possibility of re-injury must be taken into account. According to Wilson, one third of patients suffering adduction in-

juries of the ankle will remember a previous sprain of the same ankle.[13] An extended period of pain occasionally follows ankle injury and may significantly interfere with the rehabilitation effort. Therapy may be further hampered by the unsatisfactory response of the patient receiving compensation.[14]

The Heel

Trauma to the heel is uncommon compared with the other industrial injuries of the foot and ankle. The heel pad is a uniquely structured cushion consisting of small cells of fat held within a honeycomb of elastic connective tissue. It may be damaged by a direct blow, such as a fall on the heel, or by repetitive minor trauma, such as prolonged walking on hard surfaces. Scarring of the heel pad may be a source of chronic pain. Symptoms of heel-pad damage must be differentiated from the pain arising at the anterior border of the calcaneal tuberosity with plantar fasciitis. Fasciitis itself may also be the result of industrial injury. More often, the chronic inflammation is aggravated by poorly fitting work boots and extended periods of time on the feet.

It is fortunate that bony injuries to the heel are rare. Fractures of the os calcis have always had a poor prognosis. In 1908, Cotton and Wilson stated that "ordinarily speaking, the man who breaks his heel bone is 'done,' so far as his industrial future is concerned."[15] Treatment has ranged from use of Böhler's clamp to open reduction to studied neglect, but no one form of treatment has been universally accepted. Although they may be a little too pessimistic, Giannestras and Sammarco have considerable support when they state, "In spite of the extensive experience with this injury through the ages, its major economic impact from the standpoint of the amount of time lost, and the attention given it in recent years throughout the world, there is still no method of treatment that yields good — or even predictable — results."[11]

The Sole

With the use of safety boots on the job, lacerations of the sole of the foot are unusual. Deep plantar lacerations do occur, however, and are usually associated with crush injuries to the rest of the foot. Treatment of the laceration itself is generally conservative. Yancey reports that the majority of surgeons he surveyed preferred not to repair isolated tendon lacerations other than those of the flexor hallucis longus.[16] The functional result, even after extensive laceration in this area, is surprisingly good.

Most industrial injuries to the sole of the foot are puncture wounds (Fig. 58–4). Because the injury seems so innocuous, patients may receive inadequate management or may decide not to seek treatment at all. Puncture wounds can have serious complications, however; the incidence of established infection following punctures in the sole has been reported to be as high as 10 per cent. To minimize the problem, the treatment of puncture wounds should include a careful history, tetanus prophy-

laxis, cleansing, probing, and debridement of the wound. Antibiotics are not routinely required but should be reserved for an established infection.[17]

A review of the Canadian industrial accident statistics between 1967 and 1977 revealed a dramatic drop in the incidence of puncture wounds of the foot. In 1967, 36 per cent of all injuries occurring in construction laborers were puncture wounds. By 1977, the incidence of puncture wounds in this group had fallen to 6 per cent, an outstanding demonstration of the influence that industrial safety can exert. This tremendous reduction in incidence was the result of three factors. The lumber formwork and shoring used in the pouring of concrete were largely replaced with prefabricated metal ones. The Construction Safety Association of Ontario estimated that the elimination of an enormous number of nail-studded scraps of lumber reduced the potential for puncture wounds from 36 per cent to 15 per cent. The further reduction to 6 per cent was the result of both an intensive safety program and the compulsory use of safety shoes with steel insoles on all construction sites.

SPECIFIC JOB-RELATED INJURIES

Few foot or ankle injuries have been so elegantly related to a specific occupation as "aviator's astragalus."[18] The use of a rudder bar rather than foot pedals in British aircraft during World War II created a unique injury situation. The localized pressure of the bar beneath the forefoot in a head-on crash caused forced dorsiflexion of the foot and a fracture of the neck of the talus against the anterior margin of the tibia. Although similar fractures of the talar neck have occurred in many other ways, the particular circumstances and high incidence of the injury in pilots led to the classic designation.

Fractures of the os calcis have also had many designations. "Lover's heel," for example, denotes a fracture that occurs after a hasty exit from a second-story window. This mechanism has little to do with the average industrial setting. The injury, however, is more common in occupations such as structural steel construction and firefighting, which require work at a

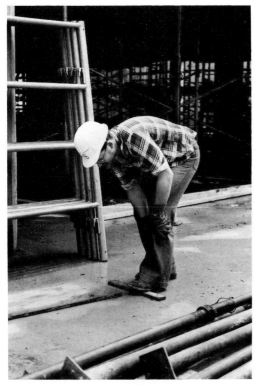

Figure 58–4. *Until recently, a puncture wound in the sole was the most common industrial foot injury. Although initially painful, the injury can be underestimated and inadequately treated. The use of steel insoles has greatly reduced the incidence.*

height. During World War II, fractures of the calcaneus were well documented in the armed forces.[19] Unfortunately, in many cases the very occupation leading to a fracture of the heel bone is the type in which the residual disability proves the greatest handicap. This is one reason that fractures of the os calcis have such a poor prognosis.

As reflected in all the available statistics, individuals who do heavy labor in the building trades are at the highest risk for ankle and foot injury. Most are nonspecific injuries resulting mainly from falls or crush injuries of the foot. The incidence of puncture wounds, in the Canadian work force at least, has been greatly reduced.

Burns and Thermal Injuries

Burns involving the foot and ankle are not unique to industry. They are a particular hazard, however, when combined with the misuse of personal protective equipment. High-cut work boots may be required in an industry in which the risk of ankle injury is significant, but wearing the boots open at the top provides access to the foot and can actually increase the possibility of a serious accident. Welders, for example, have been severely burned by metal fragments falling inside the boot. Cases of severe second-degree burns have occurred when cleaners accidentally hosed scalding water inside their boots and were then unable to remove them quickly enough to prevent serious injury (Fig. 58–5). Some companies now require that trouser legs be worn outside the boots to prevent such accidents.

Not all burns to the foot and ankle are so obvious. Because work boots are usually worn with heavy socks, which absorb toxic material, burns may occur gradually without the workman being aware of the injury. Figure 58–6 shows the result of rock salt burns. The patient was unaware that any salt had gotten inside his boot, and because of the insidious onset, he did not appreciate the severity of the burn.

Injuries due to cold are not common in industry. With the exception of a few special circumstances, such as pipeline workers in the far north, most workmen are not exposed to dangerous extremes of temperature. Although cold feet rarely harm the

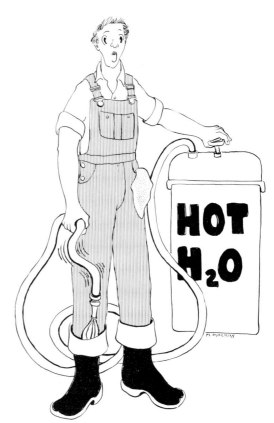

Figure 58–5. *Severe second-degree burns may be caused by the accidental hosing of hot water inside the boot. The depth of the burn is increased because the sock and boot hold the water in contact with the skin.*

workman, they are a common excuse for failure to wear safety shoes during the winter months, and this lack of protection can lead to serious injury. It is a widely held belief that the steel toecap of the safety boot causes excessive loss of heat from the foot. In fact, this is not true. Research has shown that the only difference in the rate of heat loss between safety and nonsafety boots occurs over the toecap but has demonstrated that nonsafety, uninsulated boots tend to lose heat faster.[20] The use of protective footwear should not be abandoned during the winter months.

Electrical Injuries

Contact with high-voltage electrical equipment is an occupational hazard in several industries. Electrical injuries are not isolated to the feet, but since the lower

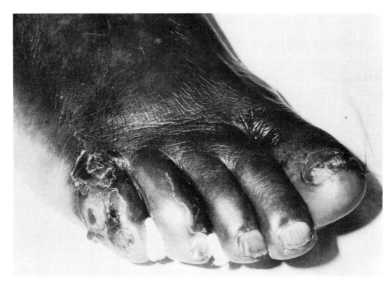

Figure 58–6. *This chemical burn (from rock salt) produced edema and maceration of the tissue between the toes. A superficial ulcer is present on the lateral aspect of the fifth toe. Treatment includes rest, warm water soaks, and exposure to the air. (Courtesy of Melvin H. Jahss, M.D.)*

limbs usually conduct the current to ground, the workman's feet and footwear are almost always involved (Fig. 58–7).

PROTECTION

Thirty-two per cent of industrial foot injuries are caused by falling objects, either equipment or working materials. Most of these accidents result in trauma to the toes or metatarsal area. It is to be anticipated that an object falling on the foot would have an equal chance of landing on either the midfoot or the toes. This assumption was supported in the CSAO survey that reviewed the frequency of injuries to these two areas in workmen wearing ordinary

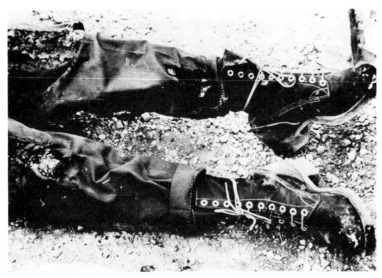

Figure 58–7. *Eight thousand volts passed through this workman's body, killing him instantly. Extensive leg burns are obvious. The charred toes of his safety boots illustrate the conductivity of the steel toecaps. (Photo courtesy of Ontario Hydro.)*

shoes. Toe injuries accounted for 28 per cent of the total number of injuries, whereas metatarsal injuries accounted for 29 per cent. The statistic for workmen wearing safety boots with steel toecaps was 24 per cent toe injuries compared with 31 per cent metatarsal injuries. From these figures, it appears that toe protection in the modern safety boot reduces the expected incidence of injury by only 7 per cent. A further increase in protection is obviously required, but even the 7 per cent improvement represents a saving of over three million dollars to the economy.

Typical of legislation enacted to promote foot protection is section 115 of the Ontario Industrial Safety Act, which states that "where a person is exposed to the hazard of foot injury from (a) falling or crushing objects; (b) hot, corrosive, or poisonous substances; (c) sharp objects; or (d) wet locations, he shall wear foot protection appropriate in the circumstances."

"Foot protection appropriate in the circumstances" can hardly be considered confining legislation. For many years, independent safety organizations such as the National Safety Council, the American National Standards Institute, and the Canadian Standards Association have attempted to provide specifications, specific performance requirements, and methods of testing for safety footwear. In 1940, at the urging of the War Production Board, a project on safety shoes was organized under the specialized procedures for American War Standards. This resulted in the development of nine safety standards under the general classification Z41,

which were approved in 1944. In 1963, the American National Standards Committee on Performance Requirements for Protective Occupational Footwear Z41 was established, with special subcommittees designed to update the Z41 war standards. Several revisions have been done; the most recent was published in 1976 by the American National Standards Institute.[21] Specifications have been developed for protection of the toes and metatarsal region and protection against penetration of the sole, electrical conductivity, and electrical hazards. The testing procedures and minimum requirements for each category are well summarized by Gould[22] and are discussed in Chapter 64.

The average life of a safety shoe is about six months. Continuous use and exposure to a destructive environment make frequent replacement necessary. Worn safety boots offer little protection. Loss of the tread or insulating capacity of the sole, corrosion of the toecap, or defects in the upper part of the shoe all expose the foot to potential hazards. Fortunately, the cost to the workman of regular replacement is low. Most companies in heavy industry and a growing number of others provide a replacement subsidy, and the retail price of safety shoes is generally about half the price of their nonsafety counterparts.

By current definition, a safety shoe implies merely the inclusion of a steel toecap. Using information obtained from the 1977 Canadian Injury Survey, the Construction Safety Association of Ontario has calculated typical energy levels produced by falling objects landing on the toe for

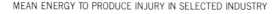

MEAN ENERGY TO PRODUCE INJURY IN SELECTED INDUSTRY

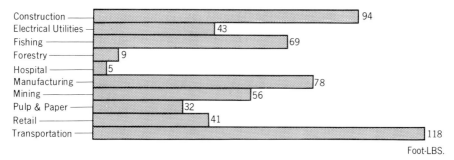

Foot-LBS.

Figure 58–8. *Workers in the transportation, construction, and manufacturing industries are more likely to receive high-energy trauma to their feet. The calculation in foot-pounds is based on the average weight of the falling object and the height from which it falls.*

ENERGY EXCHANGE PRODUCING INJURY

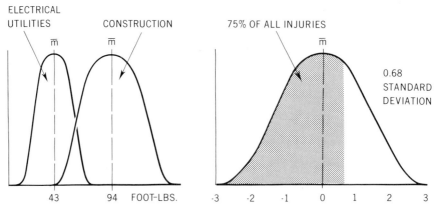

Figure 58–9. *The same values displayed in Figure 58–8 are shown here as bell curves. Notice the higher energy involved in injuries to construction workers compared with that in injuries to electrical workers. Calculation of the standard deviations for each curve leads to a determination of the energy required to produce 75 per cent of all crushing foot injuries in each industry.*

several industries. The results, calculated in foot-pounds, are shown in Figure 58–8. Figure 58–9 shows typical values obtained for electrical utilities and the construction industry. By plotting the values on a bell curve and calculating the standard deviation, it is possible to determine the energy level producing 75 per cent of the crush injuries of the foot in each industry. Obviously, the level of energy absorption required in a steel toecap to prevent 75 per cent of these injuries must be the same as that required to produce them. The amounts calculated for 75 per cent protection in the various industries are shown in Figure 58–10. The current maximum

(Class I) Z41 requirement with regard to energy absorption for toe protection is 75 foot-pounds.

Despite the apparent discrepancy in these figures, the issue of increased toe protection in standard safety boots is not clear-cut. Test methods must be improved and standardized to verify the energy levels reported in the Canadian survey. The German D.I.N. Standard for toecap impact resistance is 200 ft-lbs. The British Standard is 150 ft-lbs. Both of these standards are far higher than the maximum Z41 requirement of 75 ft-lbs, but test methods differ from country to country. When samples of both British and American safety

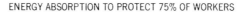
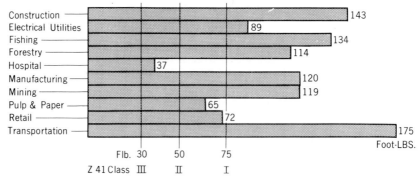

Figure 58–10. *The Z41 Class I requirement of 75 ft-lbs. offers 75 per cent protection to retail, pulp and paper, and hospital workers only. Based on the energy absorption estimates alone, it appears that the current level of toe protection available in North America is inadequate for most of the work force.*

shoes were tested, it was found that they easily passed their own country's test and failed when examined using the foreign testing method.[23] The apparent discrepancy in impact strength may not be as great as the present values indicate. If agreement can be reached on acceptable impact levels, there is still a need to develop a reliable nondestructive test method that can be used for quality control during shoe manufacture.

The issue is further clouded by the question of style. An increase in protection may require a change in appearance that the worker will not accept. Without user acceptance, the value of any protective footwear is lost.

The Sole

Slips and falls are major factors in the production of ankle injuries in industry. A slip results from insufficient friction between the soles or heels of the worker's shoes and the surface on which he is walking. Obviously, both the surface and the sole must be considered.

According to the Ontario Hospital Association, 63 per cent of the falls among their employees resulted from foreign matter spilled on the floor.[24] The floor surface must be kept as clean and as dry as possible. The floor may be modified with a number of nonslip products, such as abrasive paints, abrasive strips, rubber matting, or even racks in areas where water gathers. Where it can be used, modern commercial carpeting virtually eliminates slipping.

"Slip-resistant" soles abound, but no one knows for sure which sole material slips least on what.[25] The basic elements of sole design that relate to slip resistance can be simply outlined:
1. Abrasive (friction) qualities
   a. Of the basic sole material
   b. Of "additives"
2. Tread design
   a. For squeegee action
   b. For suction
   c. For traction on soft substrata

The slip resistance of the basic material is at least partially related to softness. Hard soles of leather and the old synthetic rubbers are rated less slip-resistant than soles of the soft rubbers and crepes. The abrasive quality can be further enhanced by the addition of abrasive ingredients or "grits." Of prime importance to the continued slip resistance of soles is their ability to resist absorption of the slippery substances commonly found on plant floors. Soles impregnated with grease or oils or turned mushy by solvents are about as slip-resistant as wet, bare feet.

There are almost as many tread designs on safety shoe soles as there are on automobile tires. Because no tread is suitable for all conditions, compromises are required. Cleats, ribs, suction cups, and squeegee designs are all combined in a fascinating array of patterns. Performance data are lacking, however. The gains that have already been made have not yet been established, and the search for a perfect combination of tread and sole material continues.

Protection against penetration through the sole is gradually being accepted as an integral part of the safety shoe. In Ontario, safety boots with steel insoles are mandatory in the construction trades. In 1977, the incidence of puncture wounds in the province was less than half the national average and six times less than the incidence prior to the general use of sole protection. In an effort to reduce weight and improve flexibility, various materials have been substituted for the steel insoles. To date no satisfactory "puncture-proof" replacement has been found.

Nonconductive soles are required in industries in which workmen handle high-voltage equipment. Electrical hazard shoes employ outsoles and heels of a highly electrically resistant composition. No metal parts extend into either the sole or the heel. Nonconductive footwear, however, does not always have to be specially designed.

Figure 58–11 shows the result of a fatal contact between the boom of an auger and an 8000-volt rural feeder line. The workman was electrocuted by a current that passed through the nails in the soles of his boots. Within a week of this accident, a second case was reported involving a father and son erecting a television antenna that also came in contact with an 8000-volt line. Both suffered only minor injuries; the father was wearing rubber boots and the son had on dry sneakers.[26]

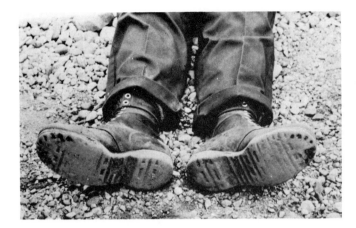

Figure 58–11. *This workman was killed by an 8000-volt current. The small burns around the front of each foot represent the points through which the current was conducted to the ground by the nails in the soles of his boots. (Photo courtesy of Ontario Hydro.)*

The Toecap

The principal role of the safety shoe is toe protection. Crush injuries, fractures, and lacerations of the toes continue to account for 25 per cent of all industrial foot injuries. Although the incidence of trauma to the digits remains high, the nature of the trauma would undoubtedly be far more serious without the current level of protection.

A few case histories illustrate the type of forefoot injury that can occur.

A steel plant employee had his foot caught under a load of angle irons when an end support collapsed and tipped the load onto his forefoot. The estimated total weight of the angle irons was 15 tons. The workman's safety boot is shown in Figure 58–12. His only injury was a laceration of the fifth toe. There was no crush injury and no fracture.

A worker in a plant producing sheet metal had an eight-ton cylinder of steel plating roll across his forefoot. His only injury was moderate soft-tissue bruising. He sustained no fractures and no significant neurovascular damage. Recovery from the soft-tissue injury was complete. His work boot is shown in Figure 58–13.

A steel crossbeam weighing about 1700 pounds tipped onto the toe of a construction laborer's work boot. The effect of impact on the steel toecap is shown in Figure 58–14. The laborer's foot was not injured.

An employee in a canning factory slipped and caught his foot in a below-the-floor con-

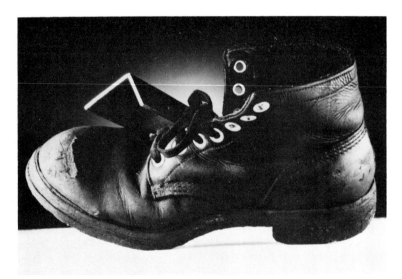

Figure 58–12. *Notice the indentation that marks the proximal edge of the toecap of this safety boot. Although the weight applied to the workman's foot was certainly less than the total weight of the load that fell, it would have easily produced a severe crush injury without the protection of this safety boot.*

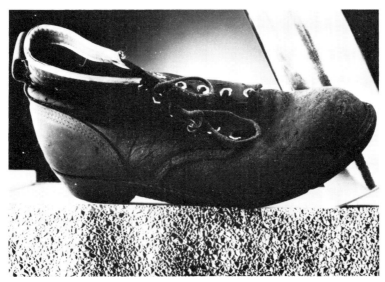

Figure 58–13. *This boot shows little evidence of having been compressed by an eight-ton steel cylinder. The toecap maintained its height and offered sufficient protection to allow only a minor soft-tissue injury.*

veyor belt. The result of the accident on his work boot is shown in Figure 58–15. His foot was not injured.

A railroad boxcar ran over the front of a yard worker's foot. Figure 58–16 shows the result of the accident. The workman sustained only a severe soft-tissue injury to the medial side of his foot and a fractured proximal phalanx of his fifth toe.

In each of these cases, the accident described would have produced at least a severe crush injury to the toes or perhaps even a complete traumatic amputation if the workman had been wearing shoes without steel toecaps. However, the presence of a steel toecap converted the injury into a relatively minor one or prevented injury altogether.

The Metatarsal Area

Z41 performance requirements for metatarsal protection are incorporated into safety shoes manufactured in North America. Despite the protection in this area, however, almost one third of foot injuries involve the midfoot.

Additional metatarsal protection in the form of a metatarsal shield is available. This additional protection is not widely used and is found mainly in the shoes of steel and foundry workers or in those of loggers in the pulp and paper industry. The metatarsal shield, like the rest of the safety shoe, must meet rigid specifications. To gain the approval of the Canadian Standards Association, for example, a metatarsal shield must be an integral part of the shoe; it must overlap or rest on the

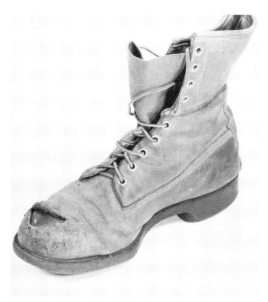

Figure 58–14. *The leather on the toe of this boot was torn by the impact of a 1700-lb steel crossbeam. The steel toecap was hardly marked. Without this protection, the accident would probably have produced traumatic amputation of the toes, but because he was wearing safety boots, the worker escaped injury.*

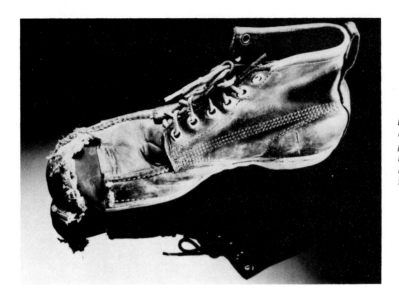

Figure 58–15. Movement of a conveyor belt tore the toe and part of the sole off this work boot. The steel toecap remained in place, and the employee's foot was not injured.

Figure 58–16. Although the official accident report described the boxcar as "running over" the foot, it is likely that the workman's boot was caught and pushed ahead of the wheel. The force was sufficient, however, to crush the steel toecap to less than half its normal height. Despite this severe trauma, the foot was saved and recovery was complete.

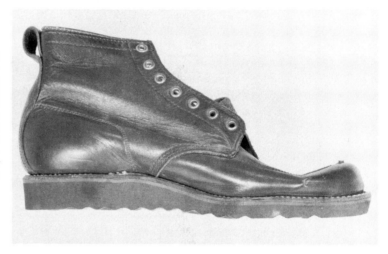

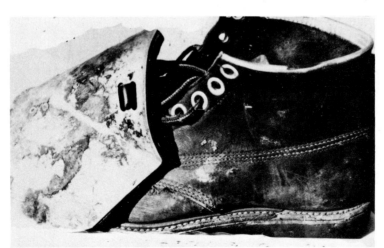

Figure 58–17. A 5- by 7-ft steel plate fell 10 feet and struck the employee on top of the foot. Without metatarsal protection, his forefoot would have been traumatically amputated. The line of impact can be seen running across the metatarsal shield.

toecap; and it must be of sufficient height and width to completely cover the dorsum of the foot. Figure 58–17 graphically demonstrates the value of additional metatarsal protection.

The Ankle

Most ankle injuries, both industrial and nonindustrial, are the result of indirect violence that produces tears of the lateral ligaments. High-cut safety boots do not appear to decrease the frequency of this type of ankle injury.

The other common ankle injury results from direct trauma. Blunt trauma from wheels or the edges of heavy equipment is reduced by the ankle protection afforded by high boots. In the glass industry, for example, the use of protective leather or canvas gaiters about the ankle and lower leg has significantly lowered the incidence of lacerations.

As mentioned previously, wearing boots incorrectly open at the top allows access to the foot and may be a factor in the production of thermal or chemical burns.

PREVENTION

The major limiting factor in the implementation of any safety shoe program is consumer acceptance. Style is critical, particularly in North America. The recorded higher impact strength of the German steel toecap is due in large measure to its bulky, square shape. Although this appearance may be acceptable in a conventional work boot, it has proved to be highly unpopular with the North American worker in all other types of safety shoe. The term "safety shoe" is properly used only to denote the presence of a steel toecap, but to many workers it implies heavy, box-like, poorly styled footwear. This is far from the truth. Lack of style is no longer a valid excuse for failure to wear safety shoes (Fig. 58–18).

On moral grounds, it is hard to challenge the statement that regardless of cost, better protective equipment is required. "It is impossible to put a price tag on suffering." Yet if the price of research, engineering, education and enforcement exceeds the savings that result, it is economically questionable whether the work should proceed. In the case of foot and ankle protection, however, improvements are currently available at no additional cost. The design of the protective steel toecap is constantly being improved to add strength from altered design characteristics and not from increased thickness. The components that provide protection do not significantly increase the cost. In the past, safety shoe manufacturers have had difficulty in complying with the required Z41 standards while supplying the styles demanded by

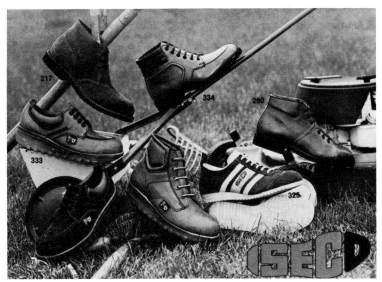

Figure 58–18. *Pictured here are a few styles of "safety shoe." Each, including the low-cut sneaker, contains a steel toecap that meets current safety requirements.*

the public. These problems have largely been overcome, and the steel toecaps currently available exceed the required specifications.[27] Whether the specifications themselves should now be increased is a matter of continuing debate.

For a shoe to be safe in addition to a safety shoe, the design should include accommodation to the work surface, a good, comfortable fit, and additional protection, such as a nonconductive sole for electrical hazards. Finally, to be acceptable to the workman, the design must conform to the current styles of nonsafety footwear.

Safety Programs

Prevention of industrial injuries to the foot and ankle obviously requires more than the use of safety shoes. The Ontario Hospital Association provided its members with the following list of considerations for formulating policy on safe footwear[24]:

1. *Surface:* The type of floor or surface on which the employees work for the major portion of the day is an important consideration. One sole may be quite acceptable on one type of floor surface but not on another.

2. *Time Spent on the Feet:* The amount of time the average employee spends on his feet either standing or walking is another consideration. Comfort and good shoe fit are of prime importance. Well-fitting shoes ease fatigue and prevent backache and painful calluses, all of which could lead to accidents.

3. *Condition of the Floor:* Exposure to situations in which the floor is often wet is another concern. Those employees working outdoors must be considered.

4. *The Noise Factor:* If an employee works in patient areas, soft-soled shoes should be considered to keep noise to a minimum. Studies have shown that the accumulation of many small noises can cause actual discomfort to the patient.

5. *Hazards in the Work Areas:* Each department will have potential hazards unique to the area. The Dietary Department must consider the possibility of spills of hot fluids, and porters may require additional heel and ankle protecton to prevent injury from the carts they transport.

6. *Accident Record:* Previous accidents in the department that could have been caused by improper footwear or that could have been prevented by a change in footwear should be reviewed.

Creating policy is generally the responsibility of management; putting the policy into practice requires the cooperation of all the employees. The concerns listed by the Ontario Hospital Association are a commendable guide to management but have no immediate effect on the prevention of foot and ankle injuries. In describing the Australian experience in the area of eye protection, Wigglesworth stated that the use of passive protection such as shielding attached directly to a machine proved far more effective than active protection such as the use of safety glasses, which required the conscious cooperation of the worker.[4] Unfortunately, there is no reason to doubt that the same difference exists between the value of passive and active foot and ankle protection.

Simply having the protective equipment available is not enough. Employees must be educated to use it. Westinghouse Canada Limited in Hamilton, Ontario, produced a dramatic decline in the incidence of toe injuries through a program of "positive reinforcement" that encouraged the use of safety shoes.[28] Workers were given ample explanation of the program and a reasonable period for adjustment without penalty. They received financial assistance in purchasing their safety shoes, and purchases could be made from a local supplier right at the plant. This approach resulted in all but two of 4000 employees willingly accepting the use of toe protection. Twenty-eight toe injuries were reported in the six months prior to the safety campaign; only two injuries were reported in the six months immediately afterward, and both of these involved the foot above the toes.

Another positive approach to the acceptance of foot safety is the Ten-on-Two Club organized in the Province of Ontario by the Industrial Accident Prevention Association (IAPA). Membership in the club is extended to anyone whose protective foot equipment prevented the loss of toes or other serious foot injury on or off the job. A detailed description of the accident as well as a photograph of the safety shoe is forwarded to the IAPA by the company to allow verification. Since its inception in

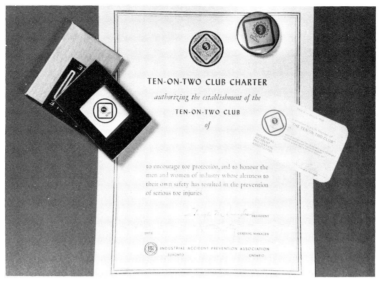

Figure 58–19. *More than 550 companies have received Ten-on-Two Club charters. Individual members receive a button, card, and tape measure bearing the club insignia.*

1957, the Ten-on-Two Club has accepted over 2200 members (Fig. 58–19).

It is not surprising that the majority of foot and ankle injuries occurred in heavy industry and the construction trades, but it is significant that almost three fourths of the injuries occurred where workers had no access to a safety program.[7] Half of the injured workers reported wearing protective equipment at the time of their accident. Of the "protected" group, however, almost half were using equipment that could not be certified to meet the minimum safety requirements. These figures suggest that nearly three fourths of the foot and ankle injuries occurred in workmen who were not wearing adequate foot protection.

The alternative to the institution of safety programs is legislation to require the compulsory use of protective footwear. In Ontario, Ministry of Labor inspectors are presently empowered to fine workers found on the job site without protective equipment. Instead of reporting the infraction to a supervisor or management representative, the inspector issues a "ticket" directly to the worker in the manner of those given for a speeding violation. Through this program, the incidence of industrial foot and ankle injuries is being reduced.

Home Injuries

The pattern of injury has changed slightly in the past decade. Puncture wounds, which formerly accounted for 30 per cent of the industrial foot injuries in Ontario, are now uncommon following a program of education and the enactment of legislation requiring the wearing of puncture-resistant soles. Most injuries continue to occur in young, inexperienced workers. Fortunately, the majority of the injuries are not severe; 40 per cent are only sprains and bruises. The current distribution of traumatic injuries — 30 per cent to the ankle, 30 per cent to the metatarsal area, and 25 per cent to the toes — indicates the regions that require additional protection.

With this increased awareness, a new problem has arisen. Most safety organizations now recognize that injuries to the foot and ankle occurring at home are a major cause of time off from work. Too often the use of safety equipment ends with the end of the shift. Before the magnitude of the home-injury problem was recognized, one company even painted the toes of all its safety boots orange so that the workers would not accidentally wear them home.

The greatest single cause of serious foot injuries away from work is the power lawn

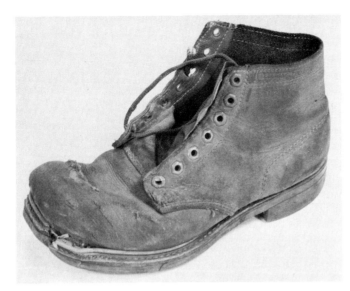

Figure 58–20. Lawn mower blades grazed the top and side of this work boot and split the front of the sole. The force of their impact was dissipated against the steel toecap, and the workman escaped serious injury.

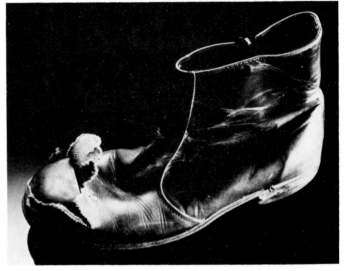

Figure 58–21. A lawn mower blade sliced cleanly through the leather toe of this safety boot. The steel toecap resisted the blow. Without this protection, the supervisor would have lost most of his toes.

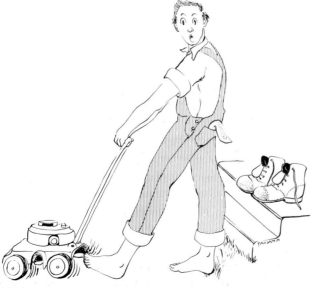

Figure 58–22. A workman who would refuse to stay on the job without adequate foot protection often ignores comparable safety standards around his own home.

mower. Several years ago, the National Safety council recorded an annual incidence in the United States of 10,000 power lawn mower injuries to the foot. The number continues to rise. "In fact, it is rare for an orthopaedic surgeon to go through a summer without seeing at least one mutilated forefoot injury."[29] Without protective footwear, the effects can be devastating.

While trimming grass on a cloverleaf the operator of a large riding mower lost control of his machine and allowed it to run over his foot. Figure 58–20 shows the safety shoe he was wearing. The workman sustained a laceration to the side of his foot but had no fractures or major neurovascular injury.

While helping to cut the grass outside a small factory, a member of a supervisory staff got his foot caught under the lawn mower. His dress-type safety shoe was badly damaged as shown in Figure 58–21, but his foot was not injured.

Unfortunately, this type of lawn mower injury frequently happens around the house when the home gardener does not have or has neglected to wear his safety boots (Fig. 58–22). The application of safety standards and the education of the worker must extend beyond the limits of his place of employment. Regardless of how or where a toe is lost, nobody wants to join the Nine-on-Two Club.

Acknowledgements

I gratefully acknowledge the assistance of the following people in the preparation of this chapter: Mr. Robert Litster, Construction Safety Association of Ontario; Mrs. Denes Corless, Mr. Peter Cheng, Mr. Milton Norris, and Mr. George Anderson, Industrial Accident Prevention Association; and Mr. Gary Munnings, Industrial Safety Equipment Company, Limited (ISECO).

REFERENCES

1. Discher, D. P., Kleinman, G. D., and Foster, F. J.: Pilot Study for Development of an Occupational Disease Surveillance Method. Washington, D.C., Department of Health, Education and Welfare, May 1975 (NIOSH 75–162).
2. Kleigher, B.: Work-related injuries of the foot and ankle. *In* Bateman, J. E. (ed.): Foot Science. Philadelphia, W. B. Saunders Company, 1976, pp. 254–256.
3. Construction Safety Association of Ontario: Foot Protection. Toronto, Construction Safety Association of Ontario, Research and Development Department, Publication No. 2, 1973.
4. Wigglesworth, E. C.: Occupational injuries: an explor-

5. National Safety Council: Accident Facts. 1972, pp. 23–39.
6. Dennis, R.: Better safety boots are needed — but who will buy? Shoe and Leather Journal, June 1969, p. 24.
7. Litster, R.: Review of 1977 Canadian Injury Survey. Proceedings Paper, Canadian Conference on Personal Protective Equipment. Toronto, January, 1978.
8. Construction Safety Association of Ontario: Summary of a Foot Injury Study. Toronto, Construction Safety Association of Ontario, 1975.
9. Hillegass, R. C.: Injuries to the mid-foot: a major cause of industrial morbidity. *In* Bateman, J. E. (ed.): Foot Science. Philadelphia, W. B. Saunders Company, 1976, pp. 266–271.
10. Johnson, V. S.: Treatment of fractures of the forefoot in industry. *In* Bateman, J. E. (ed.): Foot Science. Philadelphia, W. B. Saunders Company, 1976, pp. 257–265.
11. Giannestras, N. J., and Sammarco, G. J.: Fractures and dislocations in the foot. *In* Rockwood, C. A., and Green, D. P. (eds.): Fractures. Philadelphia, J. B. Lippincott Co., 1975, pp. 1400–1490.
12. MacFarlane, E. J.: Foot Injuries. Proceedings Paper, Canadian Conference on Personal Protective Equipment. Toronto, January 1978.
13. Wilson, F. C.: Fractures and dislocations of the ankle. *In* Rockwood, C. A., and Green, D. P. (eds.): Fractures. Philadelphia, J. B. Lippincott Co., 1975, p. 1384.
14. Beals, R. K., and Hickman, N. W.: Industrial injuries of the back and extremities. J. Bone Joint Surg., 54A:1593, 1972.
15. Cotton, F. J., and Wilson, L. T.: Fractures of the os calcis. Boston Med. Surg. J., 159:559, 1908.
16. Yancey, H. A.: Lacerations of the plantar aspect of the foot. Clin. Orthop., 122:46, 1977.
17. Fitzgerald, R. H., and Cowan, J. D. E.: Puncture wounds of the foot. Orthop. Clin. North Am., 6:965, 1975.
18. Coltart, W. D.: Aviator's astragalus. J. Bone Joint Surg., 34B:545, 1952.
19. Watson-Jones, R.: Fractures and Joint Injuries, 4th ed. Baltimore, Williams and Wilkins, 1956, Vol. 2, p. 862.
20. Popplewell, D.: Thermal Aspects of Foot Protection. Proceedings Paper, Canadian Conference on Personal Protective Equipment. Toronto, January 1978.
21. American National Standards Institute: American National Standards for Safety — Toe Footwear, Z41. New York, American National Standards Institute, 1976.
22. Gould, N.: Safety shoes for industry. *In* Bateman, J. E. (ed.): Foot Science. Philadelphia, W. B. Saunders Company, 1976, pp. 272–283.
23. Gray, B. E.: Performance Standards for Safety Footwear in the U.S.A. Proceedings Paper, Canadian Conference on Personal Protective Equipment. Toronto, January 1978.
24. Ontario Hospital Association: Safe Footwear. Hospital Accident Prevention Department, Ontario Hospital Association, October 1976.
25. Hopkins, S. K.: Elusive factor in falls: the shoe sole. National Safety News, November 1966.
26. Greenway, P.: Non-Conductive Footwear, the Second Line of Defense. Proceedings Paper, Canadian Conference on Personal Protective Equipment. Toronto, January 1978.
27. Carlson, E. J.: The Protective Steel Toecap for Safety Footwear. Proceedings Paper, Canadian Conference on Personal Protective Equipment. Toronto, January 1978.
28. Praise, rather than blame, improves safety record. Industrial Accident Prevention Association Magazine, October 1973, p. 6.
29. Anderson, L. D.: Injuries of the forefoot. Clin. Orthop., 122:18, 1977.

atory analysis of successful Australian strategies. Med. J. Aust., 1:335, 1976.

CHAPTER 59

THE FOOT AND ANKLE IN CLASSICAL BALLET AND MODERN DANCE

G. James Sammarco, M.D., F.A.C.S.

They love dancing well that dance barefoot upon thorns.

THOMAS FULLER
Gnomologia No. 4966

TRAINING FOR DANCE

The bones of the foot and ankle are formed in the first trimester of gestation (see Chapter 1), and active contraction of embryonic muscles insures the development of proper joint motion.[1,2] True joint laxity, which is uncommon, and diseases of the muscles that require bracing or reconstructive surgery preclude dance as a career. Dance requires all three functional joint requisites: stability, a full range of motion, which is often the upper limits of normal, and freedom from pain.[3,4] The last may be debated at length by both dancers and physicians.

Children dance and jump in a burst of joy, but their motions are only instinctive manifestations of joy. To elevate this motion to the height of art and style, it must be given a definite form. The process begins with the study of the rapid steps and turns that constitutes a ballet class[5] (Fig. 59–1). Children develop at different rates, depending on hereditary, ethnic background, and nutrition. The dance training they receive must therefore be individualized. Over the centuries, ballet

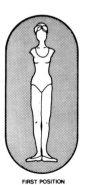 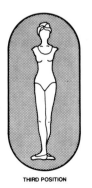 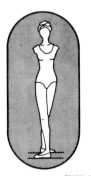 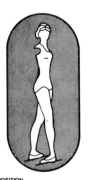 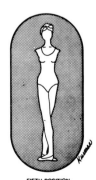

FIRST POSITION　　SECOND POSITION　　THIRD POSITION　　FOURTH POSITION　　FIFTH POSITION

Figure 59–1. *The five basic positions of the feet in classical ballet.*

masters have developed their own rules through experience. In northern European countries, children are allowed to begin ballet at ages nine to twelve, and in southern European countries, at ages eight to ten. Pointe dancing before the age of 11 is not permitted because of the lack of intellectual ability to understand body control and because of the lack of muscle strength to control the body.[6, 7] Modern rationale dictates that the decision to allow a child to dance *en pointe* be based on several factors. The girl should have had at least three to three and a half years of ballet training and should have mastered the basic steps at the *barre*. Other requisites include: all exercises on the *demi-pointe* (half pointe) must be mastered with the supporting knee straight; the feet must be free from sickling in or out; and the toes must be used correctly in soft shoes. She should be at least 12 years old[5, 8-10] and must have developed good ankle "extension" (i.e., plantar flexion or flexion). The arch of the foot must be well developed, a

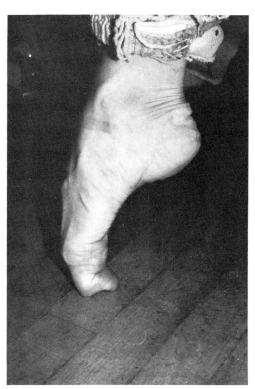

Figure 59–3. *"Clutching," "curling," or "knuckling over." The dancer is bearing full weight, demonstrating what happens within the ballet pointe shoe when a dancer is permitted to dance "en pointe" prior to being physically able to do so.*

process that takes several months. The purpose of early training is to make the dancer aware of her body by developing balance, strength, and coordination while permitting normal body and ligamentous growth at the same time.

The three "balance points" of the foot are: (1) ¼ pointe — the weight is not over the metatarsal arch. This is used by males in staging many poses. (2) ½ pointe — the weight is over the metatarsal arch. This is used in pirouettes and rises for females when a full pointe is not being utilized, and it is used extensively by males. (3) ¾ pointe — the body rises as high as possible on the foot. This is desirable for all quick footwork because it lends lightness and speed rarely attained or made in pirouettes or in a holding pose. Dancing *sur les pointes* (on the tips of the toes) requires good coordination of the whole body, with each part holding its place and moving to new positions correctly and without strain.[5, 7, 8] Pointe dancing (Fig. 59–2) before the dancer is ready results in several

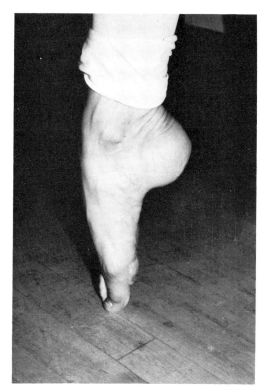

Figure 59–2. *The foot and ankle bearing weight "sur la pointe." This dancer is unusual in that she is able to support herself without a ballet pointe shoe.*

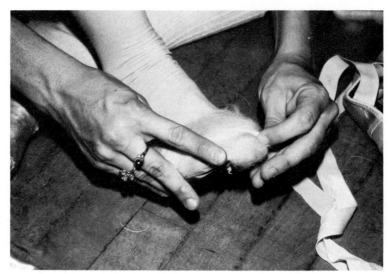

Figure 59–4. *A ballet dancer molding lamb's wool around her toes prior to putting on the ballet pointe shoe.*

problems. If the ankle has not attained full "extension" (plantar-flexion) and the foot is stiff, this predisposes the ankle to lateral strains. Balance must then be controlled by the calf muscles, with the hips and knees flexed. The lumbar spine compensates by hyperextending rather than being erect. This lack of posture causes an unaesthetic style, overdevelopment and fatigue of calf muscles, and in later years symptomatic arthritis of the spine.[5, 7, 8] The arch of the foot is not developed, and thus the toes tend to "clutch," "curl," or "knuckle-over" (hyperflex) in the pointe shoe (Fig. 59–3). No amount of lamb's wool padding in the pointe shoe (Fig. 59–4) will substitute for a well-developed arch and adequate ankle motion. The enthusiasm of the young dancer masks pain until symptoms are obvious. Treatment consists of discontinuing dancing *sur la pointe* until such time as the child has been adequately prepared.

Developing the Arch

A high arch, long considered desirable for the dancer, gives an aesthetic appearance of the entire leg. Suppleness of the foot combines with the arch, enabling the dancer to perform quick and difficult steps in a graceful manner. Nijinsky had so high

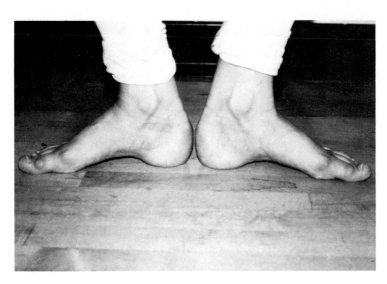

Figure 59–5. *The well-formed arches of a ballet dancer.*

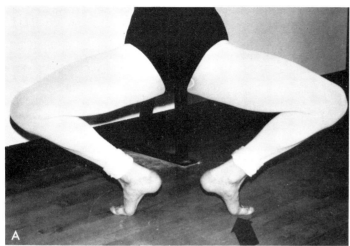

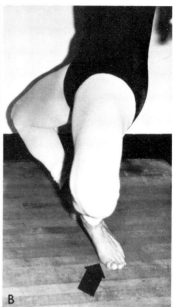

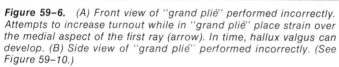

Figure 59–6. *(A) Front view of "grand plié" performed incorrectly. Attempts to increase turnout while in "grand plié" place strain over the medial aspect of the first ray (arrow). In time, hallux valgus can develop. (B) Side view of "grand plié" performed incorrectly. (See Figure 59–10.)*

and supple an arch that he was able to clasp the back of the ankle of his other leg as though it were a hand, a position called *sur le cou de pied*.[11] An important goal of early training is the development of both the intrinsic and extrinsic foot muscles in order to raise the arch (Fig. 59–5). It is necessary that all dancers develop this control, because the long-standing strain caused by training tends to stretch the medial foot ligaments. A student with flexible pes planus can develop this actively supported arch within six months to one year. If it is not developed sufficiently, dancing may become quite painful, and the student will discontinue her studies. Males usually begin dance training later than females. Their tarsal bones and ligaments tend to be less supple, and this can cause "rolling in" as the dancer attempts to increase his turnout. A result of such chronic strain is hallux valgus (see Figure 59–6.)

Congenital Abnormalities

Children with rigid flatfoot from whatever cause are quickly eliminated from dance class. The discipline of dance requires a high, supple arch for rapid, difficult steps. The etiology of this condition is therefore unimportant.

Polydactyly has usually been surgically corrected prior to beginning dance class. A slightly broadened foot should not prevent the fitting of a ballet or pointe shoe. The foot of the child with complete ray duplication will not fit into a ballet shoe. The foot of a student who has undergone ray resection will be stiff, preventing arch development. This leads to pain, fatigue, and eventual discontinuance of class. Partial limb deficiencies[12] that permit dancing as therapy or recreation differ from those that would allow a career of dance. Terminal and intercalary hemimelias, which shorten or distort the extremity, compromise the graceful line and symmetry of the leg. Terminal partial forefoot hemimelias do not permit control of push-off at the three "balance points" of the foot.[13] In addition to the lack of bony support and muscular control in the foot and ankle, associated congenital fusions of the tarsal bones are common. This stiffens the foot even more. Paraxial hemimelias that do not shorten the foot may still cause stiffness and prevent arch development.

However, it must be remembered that the desire for achievement in art often overcomes a physical handicap. In modern dance, in which asymmetric positions are common, steps may be developed by a dancer to cover a physical deformity. The

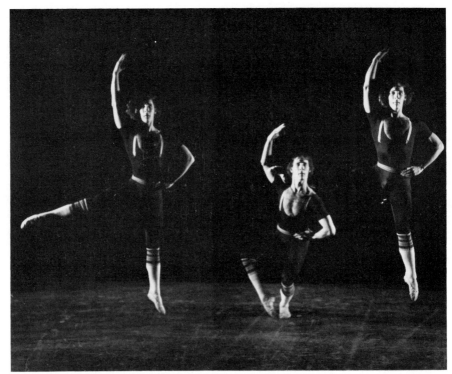

Figure 59–7. "Ballon." A strobiscopic photograph that shows the dancer in midair (right), then landing on his left foot and flexing his knee (center), and immediately springing into the next step (left). "Ballon" is the smooth transition of landing from one step and immediately beginning another.

great seventeenth-century dancer Bournonville perfected *ballon* to hide his own foot deformity (Fig. 59–7). Children with pes planus or a congenital or acquired foot deformity should not be discouraged from dance. If they are discouraged, they will feel as though they have been cheated, and they must therefore find out for themselves if they are able to dance. For minor deformities, cotton or wool padding in the ballet and pointe shoe is recommended. A forefoot prosthesis, however, causes loss of the proprioceptive feedback needed from foot contact with the floor and is not recommended.

THE DANCER'S NORMAL FOOT

The ideal foot for dancing *sur la pointe* might be considered to be that which has a second toe that is equal in length to the hallux. This would allow weight to be evenly distributed across these two medial toes (Fig. 59–8). However, this is not necessarily the case. If the second toe is

longer than the hallux, flexion of the distal interphalangeal joint occurs (Fig. 59–9). There is floor contact across these two toes but through the hallux and the flexed distal interphalangeal joint of the second toe. This causes no difficulty, and surgery to "correct the second toe" is condemned. The foot with toes in a "falling away" shape, that is, with each of the lateral four toes shorter than its medially adjacent neighbor, is not commonly found in toe dancers. In such a foot, all floor contact occurs through the tip of the hallux while dancing *sur la pointe.* Load concentration is too high and thus painful. The dancer with this type of foot does not commonly dance *sur la pointe* because of discomfort. The average area of contact between the floor and the shoe is about four square centimeters.

Bunions

Bunions are common in both male and female dancers.[10] The etiology of the acquired condition in non-dancers has been

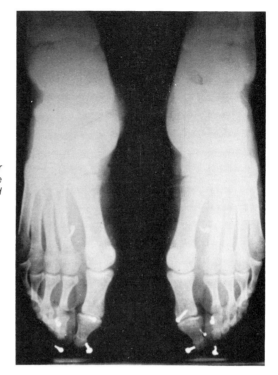

Figure 59–8. *A roentgenogram of a ballet dancer standing "sur les pointes." The second toe is the same length as the first toe. The weight is evenly distributed between the two.*

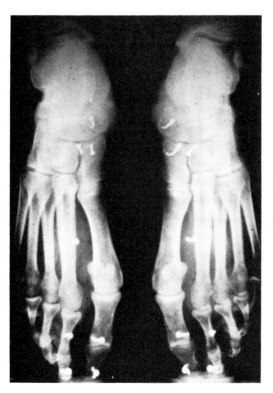

Figure 59–9. *A roentgenogram of a ballet dancer standing "sur les pointes." The second toe is longer than the first toe, and consequently, the distal interphalangeal joint of the second toe is flexed, allowing the weight to be borne across that joint rather than on the tuft.*

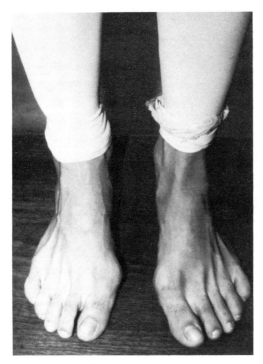

Figure 59–10. *A 19-year-old dancer with asymptomatic bunions already developing.*

Figure 59–11. *A dancer standing at the barre in the first position displaying the naturally externally rotated hips of a dancer. This dancer has developed excellent turn-out.*

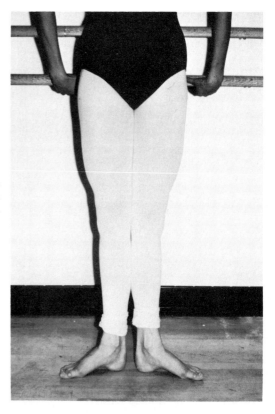

documented.[14-16] One important cause of bunion formation in female dancers is the static deforming forces within the pointe shoe holding the metatarsal heads together and forcing the great toe into adduction. At the same time, the lateral toes are forced into adduction, with the weight line passing through the first and second toes. The deforming forces of body weight plus the force of the constraining shape of the pointe shoe contribute to the development of hallux valgus (Fig. 59–10). Associated mallet deformity of the second toe or a hammer toe may accompany the deformity. Such deformities may be seen by the age of 18 years if the dancer has been dancing *sur la pointe* since the age of 11. Symptoms of pain over the medial portion of the first metatarsal usually occur after rehearsing *en pointe* and abate within a few hours. This pain is common and may be associated with an acute bursitis. Pain in the second toe at the medial aspect of the proximal interphalangeal joint is also caused by hallux pressure.

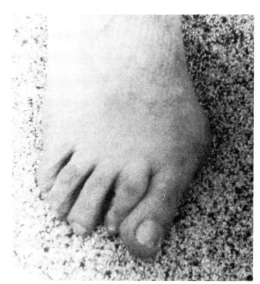

Figure 59–13. *The foot of a dancer in his sixth decade. In attempting to improve his turnout as a youth, he forced the weight of his body across his forefoot while in "grand plié"; he had severe pain daily. (See Figure 59–6.) He subsequently developed hallux valgus, associated with fixed hammer-toe deformities.*

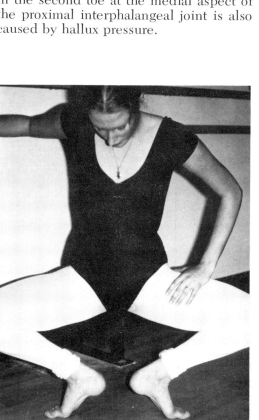

Figure 59–12. *A dancer performing a "grand plié," that is, bending deeply at the knees while holding the second position.*

Males may develop hallux valgus by improper training to improve turnout through performance of a forced *grand plié*. During a *grand plié* (bending the knees deeply in the first or second position), the dancer rolls forward, putting stress on the medial aspect of the first metatarsophalangeal joint (Figs. 59–11 and 59–12). (See also Figure 59–6A.) This stretches the medial ligaments and is painful. If not corrected, severe hallux valgus may develop (Fig. 59–13).

Treatment of minor foot pains consists of elevation after class for a period of two hours, with the feet elevated above the knees, which are slightly bent, and in turn elevated above the level of the hips. Active motion and elevation provide "milking action" to the foot. Classes need not be interrupted, but a longer "warm-up" period with stretching exercises of the toes for a minimum of five minutes is helpful.

Hammer Toe

The mechanics of hammer toes are also known.[14, 17] The closed space of the pointe shoe contributes to their development in dancers by forcibly shortening the toes. The dancers spend much of their time on the "balance points" of the foot with the metatarsophalangeal joints extended and the proximal interphalangeal joints flexed. Flexible hammer-toe deformity develops at a rapid rate and may become fixed in the older dancer (Fig. 59–13). Associated soft-tissue changes include callus and blister formation over the dorsum of the proximal interphalangeal joint. Callosities at the terminal tuft and beneath the metatarsal head of the respective toe are usually not symptomatic.

Splayfoot

Long hours of practice each day are spent on the forefoot. The ballet shoe is made of soft, lightweight leather and cannot restrict metatarsal spread. The intermetatarsal ligaments stretch with time. The long flexor tendons may slip between the metatarsal heads during weight bearing, and the dancer thus bears weight directly on the metatarsal heads without the benefit of the flexor tendons for cushioning. The foot may have a narrow appearance when no weight is being borne; however, the forefoot spreads when weight is applied. In younger dancers, both male and female, the feet are asymptomatic. However, older dancers, particularly males in their fourth and fifth decades, develop painful forefeet when standing for long periods of time. The medial longitudinal arch is retained, but bunion and hammertoes can develop in spite of the splaying.

The best treatment for the symptomatic splayfoot consists of properly fitting ballet and pointe shoes. In the older dancer, a full-insole, molded, leather arch support with an elevated medial longitudinal arch and a metatarsal pad 0.25 inch high is prescribed. This is worn when during class and in street shoes. Dancers do not wear such orthoses during performances because they decrease the sensitivity of the foot.

Hallux Rigidus

While dancing *en pointe*, increased loads crossing the non–weight-bearing portion of the hallucal metatarsophalangeal joint

can hasten the onset of arthritis. Acute flexion injury to the hallucal metatarsophalangeal joint can produce a dorsal tear of the joint capsule and also lead to the formation of osteophytes. The result of these unusual stresses can be the uncommon finding of hallux rigidus, which can be difficult to treat in dancers. Since full dorsiflexion of the hallucal metatarsophalangeal joint is most important in dancing in the *demi pointe* position, the position in which a dancer spends most of his performing time, limitation of this motion, particularly if it is painful, causes dramatic alteration in dancing style and technique.

Osteophytes form on all sides of the joint. The joint space decreases, and painful motion makes it difficult to dance. Going from the *demi pointe* position to *pointe* position becomes uncomfortable, and this may predispose to further injury. The dancer attempts to dance until stiffness and pain have significantly changed her style. At this point, she will discontinue dancing and seek medical advice. Treatment is based on the amount of pain and limitation of motion. Even the occurrence of osteophytes at the joint will not preclude fitting a pointe shoe. Appropriate padding can be made if this is painful, but most of the pain occurs with motion of the toe, not with pressure over osteophytes.

Surgical debridement of the metatarsophalangeal joint through a medial curvilinear incision should be performed only after appropriate counseling of the dancer as to alternatives, including cessation of her career or performing dances that do not require such forced dorsiflexion. If surgical debridement is performed, a full range of dorsiflexion, approaching 90 degrees, should be obtained at the operating table. Silastic prosthetic replacement of the proximal hallucal phalanx has been performed rarely, and the results in classical ballet dancers are unpredictable. Arthrodesis of the joint precludes motion and, therefore, is not recommended.

Indications for Surgery

Severely symptomatic bunions or splayfoot in the dancer is uncommon during a dancing career, and therefore surgery is seldom indicated. Since dancers tend to be self-sacrificing, goal-oriented individuals, they usually tolerate a considerable amount of discomfort. A full range of motion in the hallux is required for the dancer — from 90 degrees of extension to 25 degrees of plantar flexion. Since most procedures for bunion correction require six to twelve months for recovery, time lost from the *barre*, with loss of muscle tone and coordination, may result in the termination of a theatrical dance career. No procedure for splayfoot correction has yet been devised that will allow a consistently good result in a dancer without the risk of disaster. If surgery is to be considered it should be discussed in detail with the dancer and with full recognition of the potential necessity to choose alternative career goals, e.g., teaching or choreography.

A hammer toe tends to be flexible and minimally symptomatic during the period of a professional dancer's career. Procedures that shorten or stiffen toes in order to "align" them often lead to permanent loss of coordination and painful adjacent joints. There is no indication for correction of the mallet deformity of the second toe in the pointe dancer since this is the weight-bearing characteristic of a commonly shaped forefoot, i.e., the second toe is longer than the first.

ROENTGENOGRAPHIC CHARACTERISTICS

The Ankle

Roentgenographic studies of the dancer's ankle may show osteophytes on the anterior lip of the tibia and the superior portion of the talar neck (Fig. 59–14). This is to be expected, since it is seen in individuals in other professions that require forced dorsiflexion of the ankle (e.g., professional baseball catchers). Calcification within the medial and lateral ankle ligaments is not common without a history of previous ankle injury. Diastasis of the tibiofibular syndesmosis has not been observed in dancers without a history of injury. Osteochondritis dissecans can be confused with an osteochondral fracture but is usually asymptomatic (Fig. 59–15).

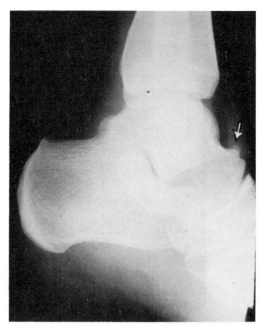

Figure 59–14. *A lateral view of the ankle joint showing an osteophyte over the talar neck (arrow). The dancer was unable to "plié" in a symmetric manner because the osteophyte prevented complete dorsiflexion of the ankle. Following the excision of the osteophyte, the ability to perform a symmetric "grand plié" returned. (Courtesy of E.H. Miller, M.D.)*

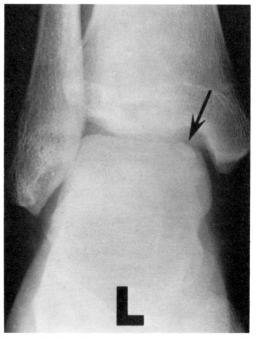

Figure 59–15. *An anteroposterior view of the ankle showing osteochondritis dissecans (arrow). This should not be confused with an osteochondral fracture.*

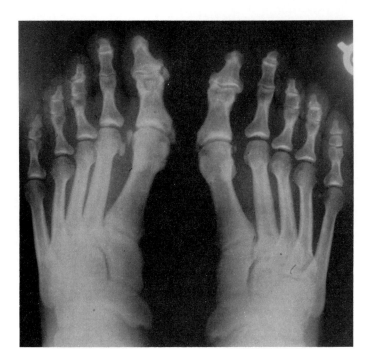

Figure 59–16. An anteroposterior view of the feet of a ballet dancer in his fourth decade showing extensive ligament calcification and osteophyte formation. (Courtesy of E.H. Miller, M.D.)

The Foot

Characteristics of the tarsal bones in dancers can be divided into two categories, those in dancers who began ballet training before cessation of bone growth and those in dancers who began training when or after growth of the foot was completed. Nikolic and Zimmerman examined 60 feet in dancers and compared them with normal tarsal bones.[18, 19] They found that in those who began training at a younger age, the grooves for tendons and areas of attachment of intrinsic foot muscles were prominent, whereas arthritic changes characterized by osteophyte formation and ossification within ligaments occurred in those who began training at an older age (Fig. 59–16). The arch of the ballet dancer, particularly that of a female is elevated. However, pes planus, although not common, does occur in dancers. Bony changes associated with pes planus, including a flattened longitudinal arch, may be seen in roentgenograms. This is usually not due to a plantar flexed talus.

The diaphysis of the second and occasionally the third metatarsal has an ir-

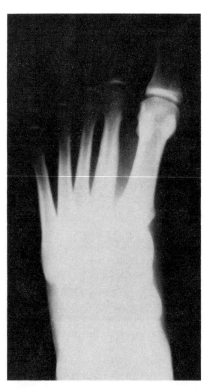

Figure 59–17. A thickened second metatarsal shaft secondary to increased loading on the forefoot.

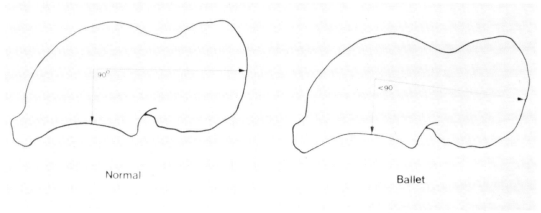

Normal   Ballet

Figure 59–18. *The angle of inclination of the talar neck in ballet dancers (right) is slightly less than the 90-degree angle of inclination in non-dancers.*

regularly thickened cortex (Figs. 59–9 and 59–17). Although this may occur in females as a result of dancing *sur la pointe* or as a sequela to a healing fatigue fracture,[20, 21] it is also quite common in asymptomatic females and males who dance both ballet and modern dance. The etiology is most likely that of diaphyseal cortical hypertrophy secondary to chronic stress on the forefoot through the most rigid portion of the foot.[22]

An increased sclerosis can also be seen in the subchondral bone of the metatarsophalangeal and interphalangeal joints of the hallux and occasionally along the lateral cortex of the first metatarsal.

The tarsal navicular is somewhat flatter and shorter than normal in dancers. The dorsoplantar angle of inclination of the talar neck is slightly less than 90 degrees when compared with that in non-dancers[18] (Fig. 59–18).

FATIGUE FRACTURES

In dance, the foot and ankle are commonly stressed beyond their limits of repair. Some floor surfaces on which dancers are forced to perform may be of concrete or of linoleum on concrete or wood. The recommended floor is one of hard wood that rests on springs or hard wood on wood rafters anchored directly to the walls without support beneath the center, the so-called floating floor. These wood floors absorb the energy of foot-floor reaction forces more than other more rigid surfaces, which require the foot and body to absorb almost all of the force.

When the microfractures that occur with everyday dancing do not have time to heal before the next day's class, a fatigue fracture begins to develop. Symptoms may precede roentgenographic findings by several months. An area of tenderness about the fracture is noted. As time goes on, the pain may become pinpointed over the fracture or remain diffuse, causing confusion of the diagnosis with chronic muscle fatigue, ligament strain, or periostitis. A sudden sharp pain is felt after several weeks of "ache" about the particular site. Roentgenographic evidence of a fracture may be lacking even at this stage. Radioactive bone scanning has been used to localize such fractures.

A common fibular fatigue fracture occurs in the distal third of the shaft, 10 cm above the lateral malleolus[20] (Fig. 59–19). A second common area is the proximal fibular shaft. The fracture may recur in the same area within several months of complete healing if training is accelerated at too rapid a pace. Fractures of the tibia occur in all portions of the bone and may be multiple but are more common in the diaphysis. They are not within the scope of this chapter. Fatigue fractures of the distal tibial metaphysis and plafond are uncommon. Recommended treatment is limited weight bearing on crutches for four weeks.

The load-bearing characteristics within the foot and the load distribution at the foot-floor interface suggest that normal or increased loads are transmitted through the second metatarsal.[22] A fatigue fracture may occur in any portion of the second metatarsal, including the neck, shaft, and

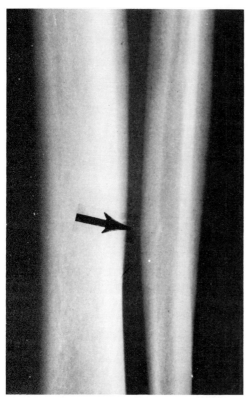

Figure 59–19. *An anteroposterior roentgenogram of the tibia and fibula showing a stress fracture of the fibula (arrow). This occurs 10 cm above the lateral malleolus. (Courtesy of E.H. Miller, M.D.)*

bony union. Although roentgenographic evidence of remodeling at the fracture site or periosteal reaction may remain for some time, this alone should not prevent return to a full dance routine. The ability of the dancer to suffer pain for the sake of her art is not to be underestimated, and the desire to remain a principal dancer often outweighs the symptoms of several fatigue fractures.[20] The dancer may even deny symptoms or refuse treatment. The art of medicine must be weighed against the science of therapy. The loss of a principal dancer in a small company may mean financial disaster.

Fatigue fractures of the phalanges occur but are uncommon. If such occurs, taping of the fractured toe to the adjacent toe with placement of a cotton pad in the web space for three weeks will suffice. The tape is changed daily, and dancing *sur la pointe* is restricted until symptoms abate. The toe of

base (Fig. 59–20). The diagnosis may be difficult and may elude the examiner for several months, even in the presence of marked symptoms. Close scrutiny of anteroposterior and oblique roentgenograms and comparison with views of the opposite foot may be necessary to determine if a suspected fracture enters Lisfranc's joint.

Application of a short leg, weight-bearing cast is indicated for four weeks. The use of an elastic adhesive dressing and crutches is offered as an alternative, but a cast broadens the area of weight bearing to include the entire plantar surface of the foot, whereas the elastic dressing permits weight bearing through the fracture site. After cast removal, a rehabilitation period of six to eight weeks is required. During this time, the patient may complain of symptoms similar to those noted earlier. She is not to be permitted to return to an unrestricted routine until there is roentgenographic evidence of

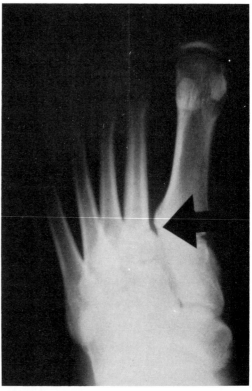

Figure 59–20. *An anteroposterior roentgenogram of a dancer's foot showing a fatigue fracture through the base of the second metatarsal (arrow). The patient had symptoms for six months prior to developing roentgenographic changes.*

the ballet or pointe shoe should be padded with lambs' wool to relieve pressure.

ABNORMAL FOOT POSITIONS

Generations of ballet masters have defined the correct ballet form. Modern dance changed or discarded many of these rigid rules to suit its own needs. However, those who study modern dance still require a foundation in classical ballet for control of balance, technique, and style.

Sickling

The position of the pointing foot is described in several standard texts.[5, 6, 23] Normally, when the foot is raised *en pointe*, the ankle is flexed (plantar flexed), the instep is forced forward, and the "pointe" is forced downward so that the heel is forward (Fig. 59–21A). Sickling develops from early faulty training. The foot is raised *en pointe* and the ankle is plantar flexed, but the instep is held inward, forcing the pointe downward and inward

and the heel outward (Fig. 59–21B). Females who sickle *en pointe* bear weight on the third and fourth toes rather than on the hallux and second toe. This not only causes the toes to become painful but also predisposes the ankle to inversion injuries.

Males are also commonly affected. As a rule, as noted previously, male dancers begin dancing at a later age, and the foot is more mature and consequently stiffer, particularly over the lateral aspect. This may result in severe inversion-type injuries when quick steps with the pointed foot are performed, for example, *emboîté* (Fig. 59–22). The injury occurs from a "bad landing," and often takes place at the end of the day, when the dancer is tired.

Lesser injuries include chronic ankle and foot strain and peroneal tendinitis. Sickling must be corrected early in training, or a compromised style as well as predisposition to injuries will result.

Rolling In

The turnout is a basic principle of classical ballet form and should come from the

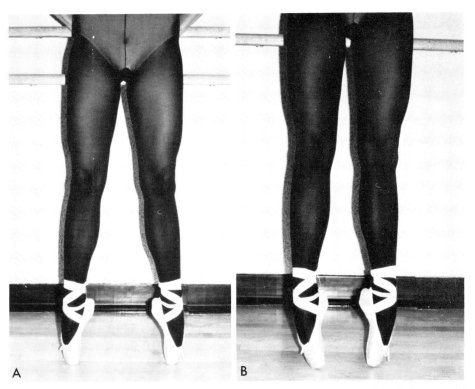

Figure 59–21. *(A) A dancer "sur les pointes." (B) A dancer standing "sur les pointes" demonstrating sickling.*

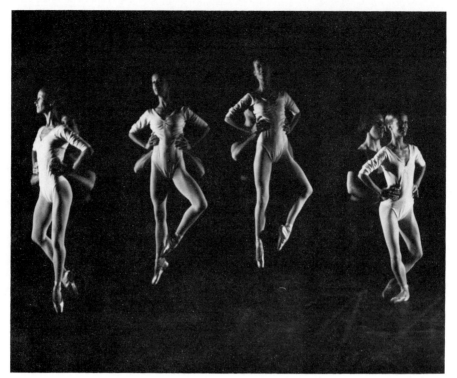

Figure 59–22. A stroboscopic photo of "emboîté." "Emboîté" is performed beginning (from right to left) in fifth position, followed by "demi plié" and a jumping up with the left leg bent 45 degrees. The dancer then lands on the left foot into "demi plié." While in the air, the dancer moves the left leg forward, bending it. Jumping up again, the dancer will move the right leg forward.

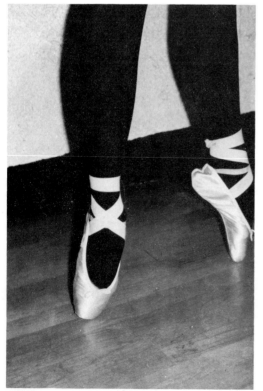

Figure 59–23. A dancer standing "sur les pointes" demonstrating "rolling in." The weight of the body is borne over the medial aspect of the foot. This fault is bad form.

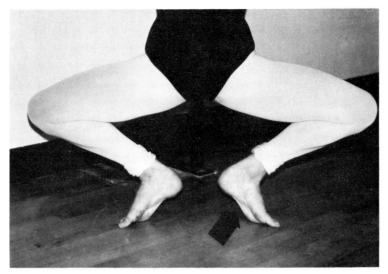

Figure 59–24. A dancer performing a "grand plié" and demonstrating "rolling out" of the feet (arrow).

hip (see Figure 59–11). To achieve this, the foot is firmly placed flat on the floor and external rotation is forced at the hip. Several years are required to achieve this by stretching the hip capsule. However, if this movement is not developed correctly, the medial ligaments of the knee and foot are also stretched. Weight is borne over the medial part of the foot, and the foot will abduct, allowing the medial longitudinal arch to flatten or "roll in" (Fig. 59–23). This "fault" represents bad form. It also leads to medial foot strain. Treatment consists of correcting the fault by turning out less. Rest, elevation, and anti-inflammatory drugs, the most effective of which is aspirin, are recommended. When *grand plié* is attempted with "rolling in," great pressure is applied medially to the hallux. This causes pain at the medial aspect of the first metatarsophalangeal joint and may lead to severe hallux valgus over many years (see Figure 59–13).

Rolling Out

In order to increase *plié* by increasing dorsiflexion of the ankle, there is a tendency to bring the foot into varus (Fig. 59–24). *Plié* is increased in an effort to stretch the

Figure 59–25. "Clawing" of the toes.

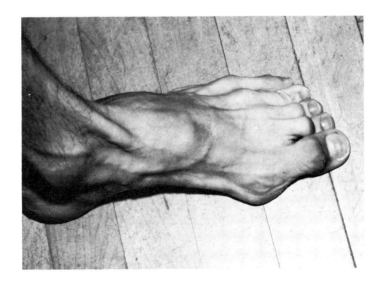

Achilles tendon, which is desirable in classical ballet. Nijinsky, one of the greatest ballet dancers, had an excess of ankle dorsiflexion and a long Achilles tendon, both of which contributed to his ability to perform great leaps. "Rolling out," however, is not only bad form but may predispose the dancer to inversion injuries.

Clawing of the Toes

In an effort to hold a position, the dancer tenses the muscles of the foot and leg, giving the toes the appearance of gripping the floor (Fig. 59–25). In addition to the "fault" in technique, this produces muscle spasm in the intrinsic muscles of the foot. Treatment consists of correcting the fault and gently stretching the toes with the hands. Slow, active, non–weight-bearing flexion and extension of the toes for three to five minutes during warm-up are followed by exercises to gently stretch the intrinsic muscles, such as squatting on the ball of the foot. This is followed by passive hyperextension of the hallux and small toes with the knee extended for three minutes.[24] A diet with an adequate intake of carbohydrates and supplemented with potassium and sodium is also important for the prevention of associated muscle cramps.

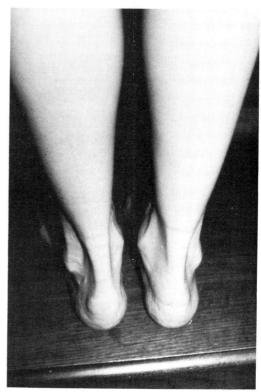

Figure 59–26. *View of the ankles from behind showing ribbon marks. These should not be confused or associated with Achilles tendinitis.*

TENDON PROBLEMS ABOUT THE ANKLE

Tendo Achillis

Dancers are particularly prone to develop tendinitis and tears of the tendo Achillis. The more common of these is tendinitis, which occurs 3 cm above the insertion of the Achilles tendon into the calcaneus. It is common when beginning a new or different exercise or when returning to dancing after vacation. It occurs in both males and females, but it is not associated with the ribbons of the ballet toe shoes, which are wrapped about the ankle (Fig. 59–26).

Pain is noted on landing owing to deceleration activity of the triceps surae. Tenderness occurs over a 5-cm area of the tendon, which may be associated with swelling and redness. A "leather bottle" crepitation may be noted on palpation. Often, however, pain and tenderness are the only symptoms. Treatment consists of elevation and the application of heat over the affected area. Anti-inflammatory drugs such as aspirin, indomethacin, or phenylbutazone (Butazolidin) are also recommended. A 1-inch heel lift should be worn in street shoes. A prolonged warm-up period of active and passive stretching of the tendons for 10 minutes is necessary. Since tendinitis represents microruptures of the tendon, one should be aware of a possible impending tendo-Achillis rupture. The dancer should refrain from high leaps until the pain has subsided.

Pain at the insertion of the tendo Achillis occurs more commonly in dancers who have not yet completed their growth. The pain occurs during *plié* and on landing following a leap. It probably represents a form of partial avulsion of the tendo Achillis from the calcaneus. Equivalent injuries about the knee are jumper's knee and Osgood-Schlatter disease. Roentgenograms are negative since the tendon inserts into the cartilaginous calcaneal apophysis. Tenderness on palpation at the Achilles insertion confirms the diagnosis. Treatment with analgesics, a 1-inch heel lift in street shoes, and a prolonged warm-up of active and passive ankle flexion (dorsiflexion) for 10 minutes are indicated.

Partial rupture at the musculotendinous junction of the gastrocnemius muscle occurs in the skeletally mature dancer. Symptoms are a sharp pain in the mid-posterior calf following a leap without a palpable defect on palpation of the muscle. An antalgic gait is noted. Dancing should cease for seven to ten days. Elevation of the legs, analgesics, and a 1-inch heel lift are prescribed. When dancing is resumed, calf-stretching exercises should be performed for 10 to 15 minutes as part of warm-up.[25] Calf-stretching is performed as follows: The dancer faces the wall, and places his hands against the wall. His feet are 1 meter away from the wall. He then leans forward without allowing his heels to leave the floor. The body is kept in a straight line. The dancer then returns to the initial position again. To increase stretching, he takes a 6-inch step backward from his previous position so that he is able to stretch (dorsiflex) the tendon more before his body reaches the wall. Successive steps away from the wall increase the limit that the ankle may be stretched.

Complete rupture of the tendo Achillis is a catastrophic event. It may signal the end of the dancer's career as a professional performer. The diagnosis is obvious, with a palpable defect about 10 cm above the tendon insertion. Signs include loss of plantar flexion, acute severe pain, and inability to walk. Treatment consists of surgical repair by one of several methods.[26, 27] Immobilization in a cast for six weeks is required postoperatively, followed by slow mobilization. Prognosis is guarded for return of a principal dancer to the roles danced prior to this injury. I know of only two cases of return to major roles following complete rupture of the Achilles tendon.[28]

Posteromedial Compartment Tendons

Tendinitis of the Tibialis Posterior, Flexor Digitorum Longus, and Flexor Hallucis Longus

Tendinitis of the long flexor tendons at the medial aspect of the ankle is common. It occurs with equal frequency in the tibialis posterior and flexor hallucis longus tendons. The primary symptom is posteromedial pain while *en pointe*, which may be exacerbated by attempts to arch the foot. One technique of dancing *sur la pointe* that attempted to increase muscle pull of the deep calf muscles while using the gastrocnemius muscle less resulted in an epidemic of flexor hallucis longus tendinitis among students. Diagnosis of acute tendinitis of the tibialis posterior is made by palpating the tendon just behind the medial malleolus of the ankle and following the tibialis posterior tendon proximally while the dancer plantar flexes the ankle and inverts the foot. Tenderness is noted in a 5-cm area of tendon adjacent to the ankle. Treatment is symptomatic, with elevation, application of heat, and anti-inflammatory drugs.

Tendinitis of the flexor digitorum longus is less common. Tenderness is noted on palpation behind the tibialis posterior tendon. It may be treated in the same manner as tibialis posterior tendinitis. Traumatic neuritis of the tibial nerve and traumatic posterior tibial arteritis are uncommon in dancers.

The diagnosis of flexor hallucis longus tendinitis is made by palpating deeply 2 cm posterior to the lateral malleolus just proximal to the tendo Achillis.[29] As the dancer moves the ankle and hallux through a range of motion, pain is noted as the tendon slides beneath the palpating finger. Crepitation is not uncommon. Symptoms may be present for several weeks, gradually increasing. Treatment consists of elevation and application of hot packs during periods of acute symptoms. This may require loss of a day of rehearsal time. On return to the *barre*, warm-up periods of 10 to 20 minutes may be required to prevent further injury. Anti-inflammatory medications are also quite helpful.

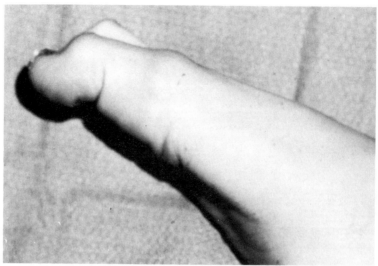

Figure 59–27. *Lateral view of the forefoot showing the great toe locked in the triggered position. Note the flexion at the interphalangeal joint.*

Partial Rupture of the Flexor Hallucis Longus Tendon (Trigger Toe)

When a dancer begins to show triggering of the hallux, partial rupture of the flexor hallucis longus tendon should be suspected.[30] It is characterized by the following: When the foot is in neutral position, the hallux can be flexed with ease. As the foot is brought into plantar flexion (extension), the ability to flex the hallux is lost. In this position, the toe can be flexed passively, but not with a forcible, active contraction of the flexor hallucis longus; a snap or pop is noted in the posteromedial region of the ankle and the toe flexes acutely. The dancer is then unable to extend the interphalangeal and metatarsophalangeal joints of the hallux. When the ankle is then passively brought back into neutral position, clawing of the hallux is apparent, with extension of the metatarsophalangeal joint and flexion of the interphalangeal joint caused by the

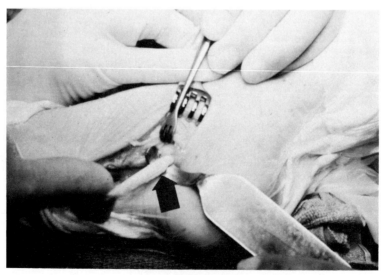

Figure 59–28. *The tendon of the flexor hallucis longus is exposed, and the anterior retractor beneath the tendon shows the fusiform swelling in the tendon (arrow). The toes are to the right.*

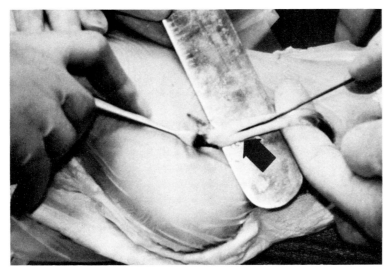

Figure 59–29. *The flexor hallucis longus is exposed in another dancer with a trigger toe. (The toes are to the left.) A probe has been passed into the longitudinal rent in the tendon (arrow), which may measure as long as 3 cm.*

tenodesis effect of the tethered flexor hallucis longus tendon (Fig. 59–27). Passive extension of the interphalangeal joint of the hallux produces a painless pop in the posteromedial region of the ankle, with subsequent freeing of motion in the great toe.

If the tendon is palpated in the posteromedial compartment of the ankle 2 cm posterior to the lateral malleolus and 1 cm above the calcaneus during the periods of flexion and extension of the hallux, a popping sensation is felt at a point 2 cm posterior to the lateral malleolus and 1 cm above the superior border of the calcaneus.

At surgery, through a posteromedial curvilinear incision 7 cm in length, the neurocirculatory structures of the posteromedial compartment of the ankle are retracted anteriorly. The flexor hallucis longus tendon is identified by its muscle fibers lying posteriorly in the compartment anterior to the tendo Achillis. On opening its retracular tunnel, a fusiform thickening in the tendon is observed in the portion distal to the retinaculum beneath the calcaneus (Fig. 59–28). The peripheral fibers appear intact. The longitudinal rent is found in the tendon (Fig. 59–29). The central fibers of the tendon rupture and contract, thus causing a thickening in the region of the contracted fibers and a narrowing just proximal to this fusiform enlargement. A

general closure is made, and a light compression dressing is applied after division of the retinaculum, with the tendon moving freely in its bony groove.

Active range of motion is begun three days postoperatively. Exercises at the *barre*, using the good leg and with active motion of the hallux, are started in 10 days. The dancer is permitted to return to dancing *en pointe* three months postoperatively.

Complete Rupture of the Flexor Hallucis Longus Tendon

Complete rupture of the flexor hallucis longus tendon occurs rarely. Diagnosis is made when there is complete and sudden loss of interphalangeal flexion of the great toe.[28] The rupture lies just beneath the calcaneus, distal to the tendon tunnel at the posteromedial compartment of the ankle. Direct repair of the tendon with six weeks of immobilization in plaster is required before dancing is resumed. One full year is to be expected for recovery.

Lateral Compartment Tendons

Tendinitis of the Peroneus Brevis and Peroneus Longus

Peroneal tendinitis is common to all dancers. An area of tenderness is noted just behind the lateral malleolus and may

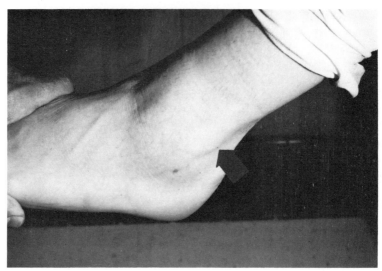

Figure 59–30. *Swelling along the course of the peroneal tendon, just posterior to the lateral malleolus (arrow). This is a common finding in peroneal tendinitis in dancers.*

extend several centimeters proximally into the lateral compartment. Occasionally, swelling is noted behind the lateral malleolus (Fig. 59–30). Steps such as *relevé* (rising up on the toes) cause aching, which increases as the dancer tires. Abnormal postures, such as "rolling in" the foot during attempts to improve turnout, may contribute to the condition. Treatment includes elevation of the feet at the end of the day for two hours as well as anti-inflammatory drugs and application of hot packs. There should be a warm-up period

of 10 to 20 minutes before class during which slow, active motion is performed. A device used for warming up the calf muscles to increase control at the ankle is the "exercise board" (Fig. 59–31). This is a circular platform made of 0.5-inch-thick wood with a 2-inch-long post with a rounded tip on the center of the underside of the board. The platform is placed post down on the floor, and the dancer stands at the barre. The foot of the affected side is placed in the center of the circular platform, and the dancer slowly rotates the

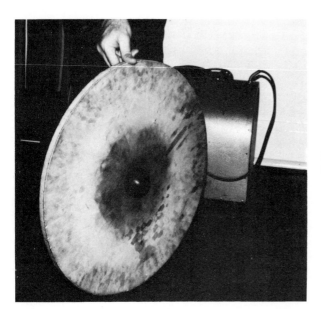

Figure 59–31. *The foot exercise board. (Courtesy of The Royal Ballet.)*

foot from side to side and fore and aft, causing the platform to rise and fall in the desired direction. The exercise is performed slowly before each class for 10 minutes.

Tendinitis of the peroneus longus can also occur at the point where the tendon turns beneath the cuboid bone. Pain may be exacerbated by a *ronde de jambe* (Fig. 59–32). There is tenderness on palpation at the lateral plantar border of the cuboid. Roentgenograms are of no help in diagnosing this condition and in fact may cause confusion with a fracture if the sesamoid bone is present in the peroneus longus tendon, which is a common finding. The differential diagnosis includes partial avulsion of the peroneus brevis tendon at its insertion and Jones fracture, both of which cause tenderness over the styloid process of the fifth metatarsal. A fracture of the cuboid has an associated history of trauma, with positive roentgenographic findings. Treatment of peroneus longus tendinitis is similar to that of peroneus brevis tendinitis. Injection of corticosteroid preparations is mentioned only to be condemned.

Dislocation of the peroneal tendons at the lateral malleolus occurs during *relevé sur la pointe* (rising to the pointe) and less commonly during *demi plié* or *grand plié*, and deep bending with flexion (dorsiflexion) of the ankle. Symptoms consist of a snap along with a feeling of giving way at the lateral malleolus. Palpation during *relevé* confirms the diagnosis. Roentgenograms may reveal a small chip fracture at the peroneal groove of the fibula if the injury is acute. Periosteal reaction may occur in the area where the peroneal retinaculum has been pulled from the fibula. Treatment of the acute dislocation is plaster immobilization for six weeks in a short leg, weight-bearing cast.

Chronic recurrent dislocation requires surgical repair. The recommended procedure is through a posterolateral curved incision, avoiding the prominence of the lateral malleolus. The sural nerve is protected, because injury to this nerve causes numbness over the lateral forefoot. The superior peroneal retinaculum will have been pulled from its attachment to the posterior fibula. If the groove for the peroneal tendon is shallow, it may be deepened. The retinaculum is then reattached to the bones, snugly across the tendons through drill holes in the bone, with 3–0 synthetic nonabsorbable suture material or by a check ligament formed from the tendo Achillis.[31] A general clo-

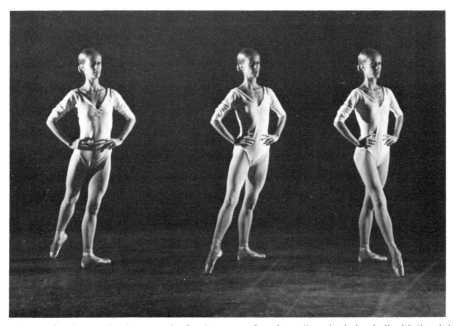

Figure 59–32. *Stroboscopic photograph of a dancer performing a "ronde de jambe" with the right foot.*

sure is made, and immobilization for six weeks in a non–weight-bearing cast with the foot in a neutral position is necessary. The prognosis in such cases is guarded, and discussion of the risks and problems of surgery with the dancer is mandatory. Stiffness in the ankle requires six to eight months to resolve. Any bony procedure, including deepening of the peroneal groove, bone block, or periosteal flap (the last two procedures are not recommended), may permanently stiffen the ankle.

Anterior Tendons

Tendinitis of the Tibialis Anterior and Extensor Digitorum Longus

Tibialis anterior and extensor digitorum longus tendinitis is easily diagnosed by palpation over the respective tendons at the ankle joint. They may be treated as is tendinitis of other tendons, with rest, elevation after classes, and anti-inflammatory drugs. Occasionally, dancing must cease for several days until symptoms subside.

THE ANKLE JOINT

Synovitis and Anterior Tibiofibular Ligament Strain

The most common symptom of synovitis is pain at the anterolateral and anteromedial tibiotalar joint line. Continued motion of the ankle joint at its extremes may contribute to the chronic irritation by alternating stretching and impingement of the synovium between the tibia and talar neck. Pain after dance class at the joint line increases over a period of weeks, and the dancer may become anxious about the possible necessity of terminating her career. The diagnosis is made by palpating between the medial malleolus and the tibialis anterior tendon or between the lateral malleolus and extensor digitorum longus tendon. A visible or palpable ankle effusion is usually not present. Anterolateral pain may be confused with anterior tibiofibular ligament strain. However, anterior tibiofibular ligament strain extends 2 cm proximally, whereas synovitis causes tenderness at the talar neck. This differential diagnosis may also be made by injecting 3 ml of 1 per cent lidocaine into

the ankle joint. The pain of synovitis should disappear, but pain from chronic ligament strain will remain. Osteophyte formation may be seen on the anterior tibial joint line and talar neck in the third and fourth decades and occurs independently of synovitis. Treatment of such osteophytes is usually nonsurgical unless it prevents ankle flexion (dorsiflexion) (see Figure 59–14). Treatment of synovitis consists of prolonged warm-up periods with slow stretching and use of the exercise board (see Figure 59–31) and analgesics and anti-inflammatory drugs (i.e., aspirin, indomethacin, Motrin), along with wrapping of the ankle prior to dance class. Adhesive taping about the ankle and foot is applied with the skin dry. If pointe dancing is to be performed, the ankle is plantar-flexed 10 degrees prior to application of the wrap. The wrap consists of an elastic adhesive bandage applied about the foot and ankle in a figure-of-eight manner.

Chronic synovitis may lead to loss of several months of dancing and may even end the career of a dancer. Steroid injections into the ankle joint in a professional dancer may cause destruction of the articular cartilage. Therefore, the future of the dancer must be considered before any such injection is administered. Synovectomy of the ankle is recommended only as a last resort. Postoperative recovery time is at least one year. Interruption of dance training for one year is an alternative to surgery. The prognosis for chronic synovitis is guarded for returning to a career of ballet or modern dance.

IMPINGEMENT OF THE OS TRIGONUM (OS TRIGONUM SYNDROME)

Impingement of the os trigonum is not uncommon. The os trigonum is a common accessory bone that occurs behind the posterior tip of the talus, where the talar dome and the posterior facet of the talus meet as the dancer stands *sur les pointes*. The posterior border of the flexed tibia impinges this accessory bone between itself and the calcaneus. This can become quite painful, and arthritis may develop from repeated trauma while dancing *sur les pointes*. If the osteophytes on this bone grow and the activity remains unchanged, the resultant irritation causes pain above the calcaneus at the posterior ankle joint. On palpation, tenderness is noted medial and deep to the peroneal tendons at the joint line.[32]

The differential diagnosis of this condition includes tendinitis of the flexor hallucis longus tendon, trigger toe, peroneal tendinitis at the lateral malleolus, and synovitis of the ankle. A lateral roentgenogram of the ankle joint reveals the presence of an os trigonum with or without osteophyte formation, fragmentation of the bone, or a rotated position of the bone (Fig. 59–33).

The condition is treated by prolonged warm-ups of the ankle joint and the application of an elastic adhesive dressing to the ankle, especially during class and rehearsals, for a period of two weeks, along with anti-inflammatory medication. In cases that persist for several months, with progressive fragmentation of the bone or the development of osteophytes, a steadily

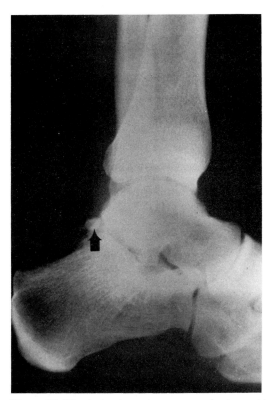

Figure 59–33. *Lateral roentgenogram of a dancer's ankle showing the os trigonum (arrow). Relief of symptoms may require surgical excision.*

decreasing activity in dance may occur. The dancer should then be counseled for posterior arthrotomy of the ankle with excision of the bone. The incision is made in the posterolateral aspect of the ankle behind the lateral malleolus and peroneal tendons. Care is taken to retract the subcutaneous sural nerve anteriorly to prevent its injury. Since the joint is quite deep, an incision 5 cm in length is necessary. A posterior ankle arthrotomy is performed, and the bone is excised.

Postoperative healing and rehabilitation may take as long as four to six months. The classical ballet dancer should be cautioned, because the period of time before she is able to dance *sur les pointes* without difficulty may be close to a year.

LIGAMENT INJURIES

Strains

There are five ligaments that control lateral stability of the ankle. Strain of the anterior tibiofibular ligament was discussed previously. The most common lateral ligament strain in dancers occurs in the anterior talofibular ligament. This may happen after changing a dance routine or intensifying rehearsals prior to a performance. Pain is noted in the specific anatomic area anterior to the fibula. Less commonly, the fibulocalcaneal ligament is also tender. Instability is not associated with these strains. Strapping, elevation, analgesics, and a prolonged warm-up period for the calf muscles with use of the foot exercise board are prescribed. If symptoms are severe, restriction of dancing *en pointe* is necessary for one week, but exercise at the *barre* should continue.

Inversion Injuries

Inversion injuries resulting from a "bad landing," sickling, or rolling out are accompanied by acute lateral swelling and tenderness, restriction of motion, and lateral pain. If instability and an anterior drawer sign are present, a complete tear of the anterior talofibular and fibulocalcaneal ligaments, a serious dance injury, is indicated. Roentgenograms may reveal a chip fracture of the fibula adjacent to the talus. Application of a short leg walking cast for six weeks is necessary, followed by a program of rehabilitation for at least six weeks. The dancer may not be able to return to dancing *en pointe* for a period of at least two months. The prognosis is good, however, for in six months the dancer should return to a full routine. Chronic lateral instability requires a direct repair of the ligaments and at least one year for recovery, and the younger the dancer, the less guarded the prognosis.

Eversion Injuries

Strain from eversion forces causes injury to the anterior portion of the deltoid ligament and may be associated with injury to the anterior tibiofibular ligament (see previous discussion of synovitis). Rapid turns *sur la pointe* or at 3/4 pointe, as in *fouetté*, are a common cause. In modern dance, rising from the floor while pushing off from the medial side of the foot can also cause this injury. Symptoms may also occur from chronic forced flexion (dorsiflexion) of the ankle. Proper warm-up along with multiple rest periods to recover

from fatigue is stressed. An elastic anklet gives some support, but strapping the ankle during rehearsal is recommended if vigorous dance steps are necessary. Elevation of the feet at the end of the day, analgesics and anti-inflammatory drugs, and an elastic bandage are all helpful.

Isolated complete tear of the deltoid ligament is rare. It requires cast immobilization for six weeks.

Pain from ligament strain persists for several months. Most dancers learn to live with such pain. However, the occasional dancer may require two to three months off from dancing in order to fully heal his injury. If instability dictates surgical repair, recovery will require at least one year. The prognosis is guarded, because ankle motion will be decreased. Thus, the dancer must be counseled with respect to his or her career.

FRACTURES

Many factors contribute to the etiology of ankle fractures, including the hardness

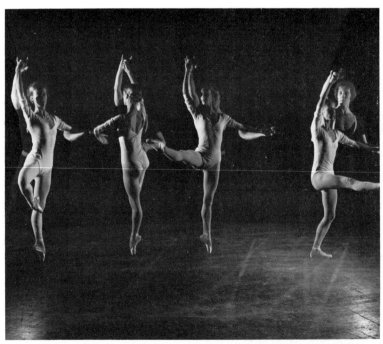

Figure 59–34. *"Fouetté" performed with assistance to demonstrate the particular movement from left to right. The body quickly turns away from the ankle of support from a "demi plié" on the left leg (foot of support). The right leg at the same time opens to second position and turns "en dehors" (with turnout) on the left leg. During the turn, the right leg swings behind the left calf and is then placed in front of the calf. The stop is made again in "demi plié."*

of the floor and the size, weight, age, and fatigue of the dancer. When a dancer is tired, timing is off and balance is poor. This is the time when fractures occur.

Eversion Fracture (*Fouetté* Type)

This fracture is caused by poor balance and fatigue when initiating a turn. It occurs in the "ankle of support," i.e., that of the weight-bearing leg (Fig. 59–34).

Fracture of the fibula with tearing of the deltoid ligament and diastasis of the syndesmosis occurs (Fig. 59–35). Treatment of the fracture is anatomic reduction under general anesthesia; an image intensifier is helpful. If closed reduction is impossible, open reduction is indicated. Postoperatively, the ankle must be placed in a cast in neutral position for five weeks, followed by active range of motion and passive stretching. The prognosis is guarded for

returning to professional dancing *en pointe*. The female dancer may return to dancing *sur la pointe*, but this may take as long as two years.

An epiphyseal fracture of the distal fibula may occur in the dancer who is skeletally immature. Closed reduction in a short leg, non–weight-bearing cast for six weeks is the treatment of choice. Because this injury occurs in younger dancers, prognosis is ultimately good, but return to full motion (equal to that of the opposite ankle) may be restricted for at least two years.

Inversion Fractures (*Emboîté* Type)

When the dancer inverts the foot and plantar flexes the ankle from fatigue or poor form, he is at risk of incurring an inversion fracture (Fig. 59–36). The abnormal posture of sickling predisposes the ankle to such an injury. Dance steps such as *emboîté* (see Figure 59–22) or *saut de basque* for which quick steps are required

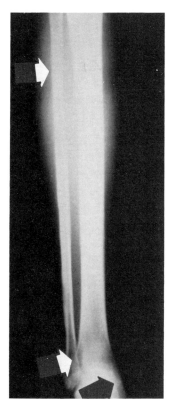

Figure 59–35. *A dancer with an injury due to a fracture caused during the performance of a "fouetté." A tear of the deltoid ligament, disruption of the tibiofibular syndesmosis, and a fracture of the proximal shaft of the fibula are noted (arrows).*

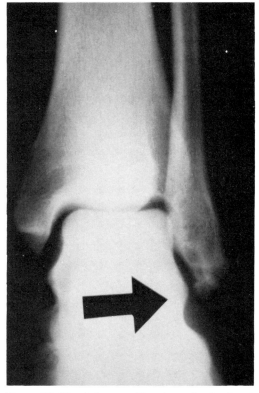

Figure 59–36. *A dancer with an inversion fracture (a fracture of the lateral malleolus [arrow] that occurred during an "emboîté" step.*

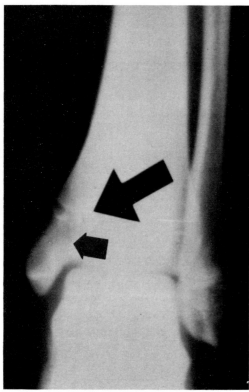

Figure 59–37. *Fracture of the medial malleolus through the epiphyseal line (arrows) secondary to an inversion injury.*

the dancer trips. This injury is more common in males.

Treatment is closed anatomic reduction with plaster immobilization for six weeks, followed by a gradual increase in active and passive motion. Dancing is begun after two months. Prognosis is guarded for recovery of a full range of motion before two years.

Fracture of the medial malleolus may also occur. If the dancer is skeletally immature, an epiphyseal fracture may result (Fig. 59–37). Such injuries carry a guarded prognosis because of the possibility of early epiphyseal closure. However, since it occurs in very young dancers, the chance of complete recovery with only a slightly limited range of motion may be expected.

Fractures of the Talar Dome

Fractures of the talus are uncommon, but they do occur.[33] Fracture of the posterior dome of the talus occurs from acute plantar flexion of the ankle (Fig. 59–38). The central portion of the talar dome is not involved, and the posterior blood supply of the talar dome insures healing without avascular necrosis.[34] The synovial attachments of the posterior fragment prevent loose body formation. However, even with minor displacement, several months of rehabilitation are required before return of a full range of motion can be expected.

Osteochondritis dissecans of the talar dome may cause symptoms of pain with a

also predispose the dancer to such an injury. The fatigue of long rehearsals contributes to loss of timing. Body weight falls on the lateral side of the forefoot, and

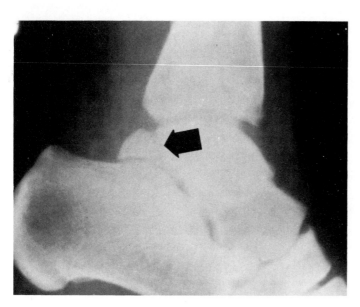

Figure 59–38. *Fracture of the talar dome (arrow) secondary to forcing the foot into plantar flexion while landing from a jump.*

limited range of motion (see Figure 59–15). Confusion with synovitis of the ankle is eliminated by finding the characteristic lesion on the roentgenogram. If a free fragment is present and causes locking, this should be removed. The use of roentgenograms to localize the fragment is important at the time of surgery. Postoperative care includes the application of a posterior splint for 10 days, followed by removal of sutures and initiation of active range of motion with weight bearing as tolerated. Recovery time may be as long as one year.

THE FOOT

Trauma to the Fifth Metatarsal

Soft-tissue trauma to the base of the fifth metatarsal may occur by direct force applied to the lateral aspect of the bare foot in modern dance. Such an injury is minor, requiring symptomatic pain medication or a thin felt pad wrapped about the midfoot to provide appropriate relief in the area of tenderness.

The Jones Fracture

The Jones fracture is the avulsion of the peroneus brevis tendon with a bony frag-ment from its insertion at the styloid process of the fifth metatarsal when the foot is abruptly inverted.[35] Pain and swelling are present over the styloid process of the fifth metatarsal. Passive inversion is quite painful. Roentgenograms reveal the characteristic Jones fracture, which includes the styloid process and occasionally a portion of the tarsometatarsal joint surface (Fig. 59–39). A fracture through the base of the fifth metatarsal is uncommon in dancers. Treatment is application of an elastic adhesive dressing for three weeks, followed by a slow return to active exercises at the *barre*. Recovery of full range of motion and strength may be expected in three months.

In skeletally immature dancers, partial avulsion of the peroneus brevis tendon may present the same symptoms. In these patients, there is usually no roentgenographic evidence of a fracture. Confusion with an ossifying styloid apophysis is eliminated by comparison views of the opposite foot. Treatment is application of an elastic adhesive dressing for two weeks, followed by *barre* and warm-up exercises on the exercise board (see Figure 59–31).

Fracture of the Fifth Metatarsal Neck and Shaft

Fracture of the fifth metatarsal also occurs in the distal shaft or neck regions

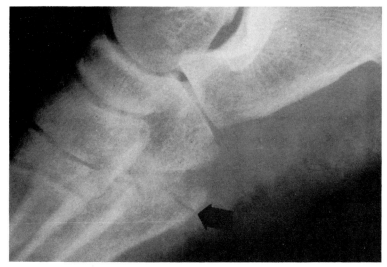

Figure 59–39. *Jones fracture. A fracture of the styloid process of the fifth metatarsal (arrow) caused by landing off balance and attempting to compensate by forceful contracture of the peroneus brevis muscle.*

of the bone. This injury usually occurs through inversion as a result of fatigue or "horseplay." The will to dance is such that dancers have been known to complete an entire act of a full-length ballet before recognizing that an injury has occurred. Tired lateral calf muscles may predispose to the injury. Loss of fine coordination through muscle fatigue or unusual or strange steps has also been known to cause it. Significant displacement or angulation of the distal fragment is not uncommon. Such a fracture may take five months to heal with simple immobilization. If alignment is not anatomic, an open reduction may be necessary. Experience has shown that the fracture requires no longer to heal with open reduction and internal fixation than if treated by the closed method with cast immobilization. The patient may require cast immobilization for two months following surgery. Then active rehabilitation is required for an additional two months. Full use of the foot should not be permitted until there is roentgenographic evidence of bony union.

Ligament and Muscle Sprains

Stressing the midfoot may cause acute ligament strain at the intertarsal joints. Tenderness is usually localized over the particular area of strain. Holding the heel firmly and gently manipulating the forefoot with the other hand will also help to locate the area. Roentgenograms may reveal evidence of a chip fracture. Treatment consists of elevation, analgesics, and elastic taping of the foot while dancing. There are periods of exacerbation and remissions. Muscle spasm may be quite disabling and can cause loss of rehearsal time. Clawing of the toes is common in beginning dancers (see previous discussion and Figure 59–25). It is caused by spasm of the intrinsic muscles of the foot.

Spasm of the abductor hallucis muscle is characterized by medial longitudinal arch pain associated with stiffness of the hallux. Such acute problems respond to massage and gentle passive stretching of the toes.[24] In the summer or in subtropical climates, electrolyte balance is of great importance. Rehearsals and classes must be balanced with periods of rest. Since lumbar spine disease is common among dancers, unilateral cramping of the foot may mask a herniated disc syndrome.

Dorsal Cutaneous Neuritis

The medial terminal branch of the deep peroneal nerve may be chronically traumatized as it crosses the tarsometatarsal joint dorsally. Direct trauma is caused by repetitive sitting on the inverted dorsum of the bare foot, as is required within certain modern dance steps. Stretching while dancing *en pointe* can also cause this. Chronic irritation from the elastic strap that crosses the dorsum of the foot and holds the ballet shoe on is rarely the cause because of its more proximal position at the ankle. Neither have the ribbons on pointe shoes been the cause. A positive Tinel's sign confirms the diagnosis, with characteristics of radicular paresthesia noted in the first web space. Treatment consists of application of paper adhesive tape across the tender area to decrease skin friction or use of a thin, foam-rubber pad over the dorsal midfoot. Moving the elastic strap of the ballet shoe away from the involved area may also correct the problem.

Aneurysm of the Dorsalis Pedis Artery

An aneurysm of the dorsalis pedis artery can occur as a result of trauma to the artery as it passes from beneath the extensor retinaculum on the anterior ankle across the cuneiforms to the first intermetatarsal space[36] (Fig. 59–40). The main symptom is pain, which may be accompanied by a pulsatile mass at the tarsometatarsal joint. An arteriogram is diagnostic and necessary, but a Doppler study is also helpful and is noninvasive. Treatment consists of ligation and section of the aneurysm. One must be sure that the posterior tibial artery is present prior to surgery. Counseling the dancer before surgery is important. Recovery time is six months, and the prognosis is good.

Plantar Fasciitis

Plantar fasciitis causes plantar pain on passive extension of the hallux and direct

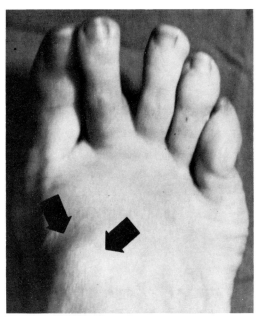

Figure 59–40. *Aneurysm of the dorsalis pedis artery (arrows). (Courtesy of Garrett Pipkin, M.D.)*

tenderness over the plantar fascia. No nodules are palpable. The dancer is restricted from rehearsal for two to three days until acute symptoms subside. A stiff-soled (wooden) shoe is recommended along with elevation of the foot and analgesics. Forefoot exercises[37] are performed before class for five to ten minutes during warm-up. This condition may progress to a chronic fasciitis but is not related to the nodular variety.

Arch Supports

The use of arch supports in treating dancers is important. The older dancer with the chronic deformities previously noted (see Splayfoot) finds classes painful and fatiguing. A full-insole, leather arch support is recommended, with longitudinal medial arch elevation and a metatarsal pad of rubber or Silastic. Appropriate relief is obtained if these arch supports and pads are placed around painful areas such as the metatarsal heads or the hallux tuft. These appliances are not recommended for theatrical professional dancers during rehearsal or performance. The use of arch supports while dancing stiffens the shoe and compromises foot flexibility, allowing the foot to slide within the shoe itself. In addition, the proprioceptive feedback mechanism between the foot-floor interface is lost owing to the thickness of the orthosis.

FOREFOOT INJURIES

Injuries to the Hallux

Fracture

Fracture of the proximal phalanx is uncommon in ballet. Certain movements of folk dance, such as the Spanish flamenco, in which the toe is forcibly and rapidly driven against the floor have caused such fractures, particularly in the student. The hallux is normally not subjected to such trauma, and study must proceed at a prudent rate to allow the bone to hypertrophy. Treatment consists of taping the hallux to the second toe und wearing a stiff-soled shoe for three weeks. Recovery may require three months and is associated with metatarsophalangeal stiffness that remains for several months.

Injury to the Sesamoids

Sesamoiditis may occur in dancers whose routine requires rapid slapping of the forefoot. Certain folk dances, for example, Javanese dance, require such slapping steps. The ball of the foot becomes tender shortly after the routine is begun. Within one month, it is quite painful beneath the medial sesamoid. Extension of the hallux allows the area of tenderness to advance owing to the phalangeal insertion of the flexor hallucis brevis tendon. The sesamoid view on roentgenogram reveals a compression fracture of the tibial sesamoid (Fig. 59–41). Treatment consists of shaping a 3/8-inch felt pad beneath the tender area of the sesamoid for relief. Since symptoms require as much as six months to subside, a leather arch support placed beneath the first metatarsal head may be necessary to provide relief. Prognosis is ultimately good.

Fracture of the sesamoid occurs from landing after a leap. It also occurs more commonly in the tibial sesamoid (Fig. 59–42). Treatment consists of placing a 1-cm-thick felt pad shaped to relieve the area of the sesamoids about the first metatarsal

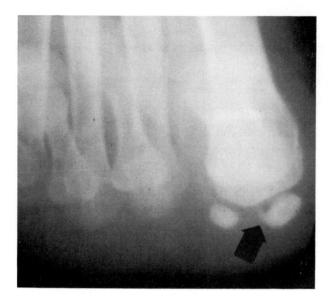

Figure 59–41. *Compression fracture of the tibial sesamoid (arrow). This occurs as a result of slapping steps that are performed in modern dance and ethnic dance.*

head. Dancing is restricted until the pain subsides.

Flexion Injury

A common injury among dancers, more frequently of males, is acute hyperflexion injury of the metatarsophalangeal joint of the hallux. The injury is caused by "falling over" the foot during quick steps. The hallux is forcibly flexed as the tip of the toe is caught. The body weight falls on the flexed joint, causing the dorsal portion of the capsule to tear. Pain is immediate and disabling, and motion is lost. Tenderness over the dorsal aspect of the joint and pain on active flexion of the toe are present. Stability, however, is not lost. Roentgenograms are helpful only in excluding fracture. Treatment consists of elastic adhesive strapping of the great toe and forefoot. Splints are not required, but a stiff-soled shoe and crutches are helpful. After 10 days, gentle, active and passive motion is begun. Full motion should return within six weeks.

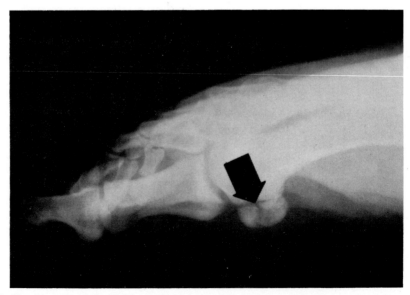

Figure 59–42. *Fracture of the tibial sesamoid (arrow) caused by landing from a jump ("tour en l'air").*

Injury to the Interphalangeal Joint

Acute strain of the interphalangeal joint of the hallux has been seen in the ballet student using pointe shoes that no longer have sufficient stiffness in the toe-box. The student may not have the strength to support herself (see Training for Dance). *En pointe* pain and swelling accompanied by inability to dance *sur la pointe* follow. Diagnosis is made by gently rotating the distal phalanx of the hallux while holding the metatarsophalangeal joint. This elicits pain over the dorsum and sides of the joint. No instability is noted. Dancing *sur la pointe* is restricted for several days. Obtaining new, properly fitted pointe shoes and knowing when to change shoes are important in preventing recurrence.

Chronic hyperflexion of the interphalangeal joint of the hallux in children may result from allowing the student to dance *en pointe* prior to what her ability, training, balance, and maturity dictate (see Knuckling Over). The distal phalanx bears weight over the dorsum and nail in the pointe shoes. The result of such overzealous advancement by teachers or parents may result in termination of the ballet training.

Hyperextension of the interphalangeal joint of the hallux is not uncommon. It develops in toe dancers and is seldom symptomatic. If symptoms occur, padding with lamb's wool is helpful, but surgery, especially arthrodesis to permanently stiffen the joint, is contraindicated (see Bunions).

Dislocation of the Toes

Strain of the metatarsophalangeal joints of the lateral toes is common. However, accidents such as striking the forefoot against scenery, can cause dislocation of a metatarsophalangeal joint (Fig. 59–43). This is immediately incapacitating. Dorsal displacement of the proximal phalanx causes an obvious deformity. Treatment is closed reduction by hyperextending the toe, followed by application of traction distally and, finally, flexing of the toe. The affected toe is then taped to the adjacent uninjured toe for three weeks. *Barre* exercises are begun following this, but it may require several months for full motion to return.

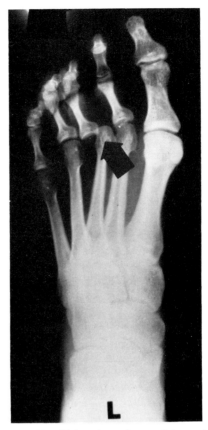

Figure 59–43. *Dislocation of a metatarsophalangeal joint (arrow) in a male dancer. (Courtesy of E.H. Miller, M.D.)*

Calluses and Soft Corns

The pointe shoe is designed to distribute the weight of the dancer across the entire forefoot, gradually concentrating it on the hallux and second toe. It is then transmitted through the pointe shoe to the floor.

Callus formation over the medial interphalangeal joint of the hallux and the dorsal portions of the proximal interphalangeal joints is normal in the toe dancer, as is callus formation over the lateral aspects of the fourth and fifth toes (Fig. 59–44). These are usually asymptomatic when toughened by daily classes *en pointe*. When tender or painful, porous paper adhesive tape is wrapped about the toe to decrease friction. This is usually enough to decrease the pain.

The design of the ballet and pointe shoes results in medial compression of the forefoot. The areas between the toes, par-

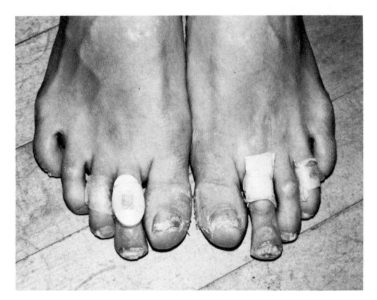

Figure 59–44. *The normal feet of a dancer showing areas of callus formation, padding over areas of tenderness, onycholysis, and, in particular, heavy callus formation over the second toe, which is longer than the first and used to bear weight on the flexed distal interphalangeal joint when in the pointe shoe. Notice that the circular pad over the second toe of the right foot has a hole in it large enough to permit the tender corn to fit into it.*

ticularly the skin medial and lateral to the proximal interphalangeal joints of the second, third, and fourth toes, as well as that of the medial aspect of the fifth toe, may macerate if not allowed to dry. A small ulcer forms, which may become infected. Chronic extrinsic pressure on the sides of the interphalangeal joints leads to osteophyte formation and contributes to the localized pain and ulcer formation. Maceration of skin due to web-space pressure may also lead to abscess formation. The abscess is located deep within the web space. This may develop over a period of months and may be accompanied by intermittent drainage. Plain forefoot roentgenograms are not helpful. A sinogram, however, often demonstrates the sinus tract and abscess.

Painful soft corns are best treated with a felt or foam-rubber U-shaped pad made from material that is 0.25 inch thick. These must be individually fashioned so that the base of the U-shaped pad lies distally in the web space and the legs extend dorsal and plantar to the painful area. The pad is then attached between the toes using 0.25-inch paper adhesive tape applied to dry skin. Squeezing the toes together should elicit no pain if the pad is properly applied.

Treatment of abscess formation is surgical incision and drainage through the dorsal web space, with excision of the sinus tract. Sutures are removed after 10 days, and this may be followed by weight bear-

ing and *barre* exercises 20 days postoperatively. Cultures are taken preoperatively and intraoperatively, and appropriate antibiotics are administered. Surgical excision of osteophytes is not recommended unless all conservative measures have been tried. If this is necessary, however, a short longitudinal incision is made through the corn without excision of skin, the osteophyte is removed with a thin-nosed rongeur. Since the basic cause of ulcerations remains, that is, the design of the ballet and pointe shoes, the use of U-shaped pads or "donut" pads is mandatory after dancing is resumed to prevent recurrence.

Problems of the Nails

Common complaints from dancers almost always include the nails. Paronychia is common in the hallux on either side of the nail. Treatment of the mild condition includes soaking, elevation of the foot after class or rehearsal, and appropriate antibiotics. Padding the pointe shoe with lamb's wool is helpful. The lamb's wool must be adjusted by each dancer so that it is in the most comfortable position. Surgical incision and drainage may require partial removal of a 0.25-inch portion of nail adjacent to the abscess, leaving the remaining 0.75 inch of the nail to protect the hallux. Under no circumstances should the entire nail be removed, since it is needed for protection of the hallux and may require one year to regrow. Destruction of the germinal area of the nail is likewise condemned, since the empty nail bed remains tender. After total removal of the nails, the dancer is not able to dance *en pointe* without considerable discomfort.

Onycholysis occurs transversely. The body weight is placed axially on the tuft of the hallux in the pointe shoe, bending the distal portion of the nail upward. This also causes the nail to delaminate (see Figure 59–44). Ballet dancers commonly lose portions of all their nails, with occasional subungual hematoma. Although this is not anesthetic in appearance, it is usually painless. If the dancer stops dancing *sur la pointe*, the nail grows in a natural manner. Protection of the nail with several applications of clear nail polish will help contain cracking. The application of a single layer of adhesive tape will protect a loosened portion of the nail; the dancer should be cautioned against removing it.

Onychomycosis is best treated with oral griseofulvin and controlled locally with Tinactin. Although this condition is annoying, it should not affect dancing.

REFERENCES

1. Drachman, D. B., and Coulombre, A. J.: Experimental clubfoot and arthrogryposis multiplex congenital. Lancet, 2:523, 1962.
2. Swinyard, C. A.: Limb Development and Deformity: Problems of Evaluation and Rehabilitation. Springfield, Illinois, Charles C Thomas, 1969, Chapters 2–23.
3. Steindler, A.: Kinesiology. Springfield, Illinois, Charles C Thomas, 1961.
4. Sammarco, G. J., Burstein, A. H., and Frankel, V. H.: Biomechanics of the ankle; a kinematic study. Orthop. Clin. North Am., 4:75, 1973.
5. Vaganova, A.: Basic Principles of Classical Ballet. New York, Dover Publications, Inc., 1969.
6. Beaumont, C. W., and Idzikowski, S.: A Manual of the Theory and Practice of Classical Theatrical Dancing. New York, Dover Publications, Inc., 1970.
7. Martin, A.: (Dancer): Personal communication.
8. McLain, D. (Artistic Director, Cincinnati Ballet Company): Personal communication.
9. Seblette, S. (Chairwoman, Chautauqua Institution, Dance Department): Personal communication, 1978.
10. Sparger, C.: Anatomy and Ballet, 5th ed. London, Adam and Charles Black, 1970.
11. Rambert, M.: Quicksilver. London, Macmillan Press, 1972.
12. Frantz, C.., and O'Rahilly, R.: Congenital skeletal limb deficiencies. J. Bone Joint Surg., 43A:1202, 1964.
13. Lawson, J.: Classical Ballet, Its Style and Technique. New York, Macmillan, 1960, Chapter 4.
14. Sim-Fook, L., and Hodgson, A. R.: Comparison of foot forms among the non-shoe and the shoe wearing Chinese population. J. Bone Joint Surg., 40A:1058, 1958.
15. Hewitt, D., Stewart, A. M., and Webb, J. W.: The prevalence of foot defects among wartime recruits. Br. Med. J., 2:745, 1953.
16. Hardy, R. H., and Clapham, J. C.: Observations on hallux valgus. J. Bone Joint Surg., 33B:376, 1951.
17. Inman, V. (ed.): DuVries' Surgery of the Foot, 3rd ed. St. Louis, C. V. Mosby Co., 1973, pp. 248–249.
18. Nikolic, V., and Zimmermann, B.: Functional changes of tarsal bones of ballet dancers. Rad. Med. Fak. Zagrebu, 16:131, 1968.
19. Zimmermann, B.: Adaptation, function and injuries of the upper and lower foot joint in ballet dancers. Arh. Hig. Rada. Toksikol., 21, 1970.
20. Miller, E. H., Schneider, H. J., Bronson, J. L., and McLain, D.: A new consideration in athletic injuries— the classical ballet dancer. Clin. Orthop., 111:181, 1975.
21. Burrows, H. J.: Fatigue infraction (incomplete fracture) of the middle of the tibia in ballet dancers. J. Bone Joint Surg., 38B:83, 1956.
22. Collis, W. J. M., and Jayson, M. I. V.: Measurement of pedal pressures. Ann. Rheum. Dis., 31:217, 1972.
23. Messerer, A.: Classes in Classical Ballet. Garden City, New York, Doubleday and Co., Inc., 1975, pp. 29–51.
24. Como, W.: Raoul Gelabert's Anatomy for the Dancer with Exercises to Improve Technique and Prevent Injuries. New York, Danad Publishing Co., Inc., 1964, pp. 51–57.
25. University of Cincinnati, Department of Orthopaedics: Flexibility Program, Calf Stretching.
26. Lynn, T..: Repair of the torn achilles tendon, using the plantaris tendon as a reinforcing membrane. J. Bone Joint Surg., 48A:268, 1966.
27. Lindholm, A.: A new method of operation in the subcutaneous rupture of the Achilles tendon. Acta Chir. Scand., 117:261, 1959.
28. Karlholm, S.: Personal communications on the Swedish Ballet.
29. Hamilton, W. G.: Tendinitis about the ankle joint in classical ballet dancers. J. Sports Med., 5:84, 1977.
30. Sammarco, G. J., and Miller, E. H.: Partial rupture of the flexor hallucis longus tendon in classical ballet dancers. J. Bone Joint Surg., 61:149, 1979.
31. Jones, E.: Operative treatment of chronic dislocations of the peroneal tendons. J. Bone Joint Surg., 14:574, 1932.
32. Quirk, R.: Personal communication, 1980.
33. Stojanovie, S., Marenie, S., and Ukropina, D.: Diseases in ballet dancers. Srpski Arh. Celok. Lek., 91:903, 1963.
34. Mulfinger, G. L., and Trueta, J.: The blood supply of the talus. J. Bone Joint Surg., 52B:160, 1970.
35. Jones, R.: Fractures of the fifth metatarsal bone. Liverpool Med. Surg. J., 42:103, 1902.
36. Pipkin, G.: Personal communication.
37. O'Donoghue, D. H.: Treatment of Injuries to Athletes, 3rd ed. Philadelphia, W. B. Saunders Company, 1976, p. 755.
38. Kleiger, B.: Personal communication, 1981.

CHAPTER 60

TRAUMA TO THE CHILD'S FOOT AND ANKLE, INCLUDING GROWTH PLATE AND EPIPHYSEAL INJURIES

Robert S. Siffert, M.D.,
and David J. Feldman, M.D.

In addition to the bone and soft-tissue injuries that may be sustained by an adult, children present special problems relating to the effect of trauma on growing bone and the potential for future deformities. This chapter will correlate basic principles concerning growth and development of the child's foot with management of trauma. An understanding of the pathologic anatomy of an injured part at each year of age and the capacity for repair, coupled with considerations of the amount of growth remaining, the projected natural history that may lead to deformity, and the risks of intervention, allow the orthopaedic surgeon the opportunity to consider all alternatives in making the wisest treatment choice.

INCIDENCE OF TRAUMA IN CHILDHOOD

It has been reported that death due to accident leads all other causes of death in children under 14 years of age.[26, 118] In their evaluation of nonfatal injuries in childhood in a small geographic area of approximately 500,000 people, Izant and Hubay found that 49 per cent of all those admitted to the emergency facilities of the hospitals were children.[52] The most common injuries were lacerations (32 per cent), contusions and abrasions (22 per cent), and fractures and dislocations (8.7 per cent). Falls accounted for 45 per cent of the injuries, 71 per cent of which occurred in the home or yard. Forty-three per cent resulted from sports, with football being involved most frequently. In a one-year review of pediatric hospital admissions from the emergency ward, those requiring orthopaedic care made up 17 per cent of the total. Manheimer and associates reported the expected yearly injury rate for children to be 246 per thousand.[67] In a review of 330 growth-plate injuries from the Mayo Clinic, Peterson and Peterson observed that the rate of injury of the proximal to distal physis of the lower extremity was 1.6:1.[79] Boys sustained injuries more than twice as often as girls. An analysis of the incidence of growth plates injured revealed that the distal tibial was involved in 17.8 per cent of the cases, the distal fibula in 63 per cent, the phalanges in 3.3 per cent, and the metatarsals in 1.8 per cent. The male-female ratio of the rate of injuries to the distal tibia was 2.7:1, with the maximum incidence in boys of 13 to 14 years of age and in girls of 11 to 12 years of age. With regard to injuries to the distal fibula, the male-female ratio was 1.3:1, with a maximum incidence in 12-year-old boys and 8-year-old girls. The age range for both tibial and fibular fractures was from ages 2 to 16 years. Metatarsal and phalangeal fractures occurred with equal frequency, with the maximum incidence both in girls and boys occurring at about 11 to 12 years of age, with a range from ages 6 to 15.

The foot links the body to its environment in its every standing, walking, and running motion, and it is one of the areas most commonly injured. It has been estimated that 12 per cent of all injuries are of the ankle,[8] with a higher incidence occurring in violent sports and ballet[94] and motor vehicle accidents.[51]

With the growing emphasis on sports and physical activities, the incidence of injuries to the extremities in children and adolescents is increasing, being greater in nonorganized than planned activities.[56] Since prevention is wiser than treatment, proper supervision, conditioning and training, selection of the appropriate sport for a youngster's age, height, weight, agility, and motivation, as well as appropriate selection of equipment, protective gear, and playing fields are factors that minimize athletic injuries in children.

GROWTH

The most important consideration in evaluating the effect of trauma to a child's foot and ankle is its potential effect on future growth. An apparently benign injury may result in a severe deformity several years later. Understanding normal and abnormal growth patterns of the foot and ankle will aid in planning appropriate treatment, and parental education and guidance may stimulate early recognition of a problem that is developing to permit more effective management.

Growth of the foot starts during the embryonic period, four weeks postovulation, and continues to the age of 16 in boys and 14 in girls, when the foot reaches its mature length.[8] The tibia attains its mature length at age 17 in boys and 15 in girls.[1] Approximately 20 per cent of the length of the entire lower extremity is derived from the distal tibia.[29] The tibia itself grows approximately 1.6 cm per year (from age 4 through maturity), with approximately 40 per cent of the growth occurring at the distal tibial growth plate.[1, 29, 42] After an initial sharp increase from infancy to age 5, the foot increases in length at an average of 0.9 cm per year from ages 5 to 12 in girls and from ages 5 to 14 in boys. Thus, since the foot matures earlier than the tibia,[106] factors that inhibit growth below the leg of a child (e.g., vascular conditions, muscle weakness) would ultimately affect the length of the foot proportionately less than the length of the tibia.

Throughout the period of growth in the child, except for the membranous ossification that occurs directly from the fibrous periosteal mesenchyme in the skull and clavicle, the growth potential of bone is invested in the growth cartilage through the process of endochondral ossification. Within the lower limb bud, which forms by the fourth postovulatory week, slightly later than the upper limb bud, are genetically directed cartilage models, containing all the skeletal elements of the foot arising from condensation of mesenchyme (Fig. 60–1). Congenital deformities of the foot, therefore, occur prior to the seventh postovulatory week of intrauterine life, when the structural and skeletal components are determined. At the seventh week, the end of the embryonic period, ossification of the foot begins and progresses through postnatal life.[25, 39, 77] The general sequence of ossification of the foot is as follows: The distal phalanges are the first to ossify at approximately the seventh postovulatory week. At birth, the ossification centers of the calcaneus, talus, and cuboid are usually present. The calcaneus begins to ossify by the third fetal month, followed by the talus and then the cuboid. The average age of the appearance of the primary ossification centers of the foot and ankle and the average age for fusion of the centers are available in detail.[9, 106] The original cartilage model of the foot proliferates

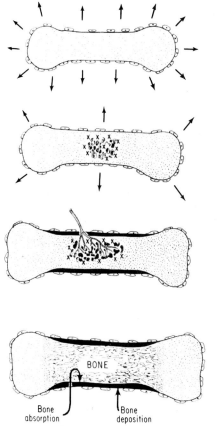

Figure 60–1. *Mechanism of bone replacement of fetal cartilage model.*

throughout growth until it is totally replaced by bone by two mechanisms, endochondral and periosteal ossification.

The cartilage model of a long bone is invaded by blood vessels, and osteogenesis occurs. As bone replaces the model, surface periosteum forms, adding width to the enlarging bone (Fig. 60–1). Future growth in width consists of periosteal (membrane) apposition and endosteal absorption, maintaining a relatively constant cortical thickness. As cartilage is replaced by bone proximally and distally, the diaphysis becomes tubulated until a genetically determined point when bone replacement slows to keep pace with the rate of cartilage formation in the epiphysis. In a manner similar to ossification of the long bone model, a bony centrum appears in the epiphysis and enlarges to form a bony end plate, and a definable longitudinal growth plate is established (Fig. 60–2). Surface epiphyseal cartilage proliferation keeps pace with bony centrum replacement to maintain a relatively constant but decreasing mass of epiphyseal growth cartilage throughout adolescence.

Since a post-traumatic deformity may be the result of alterations in this growth mechanism, the functions of the growth plate will be discussed briefly.

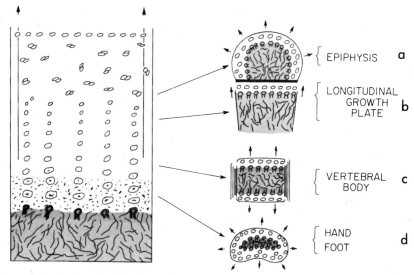

Figure 60–2. *Model of enchondral (endochondral) growth indicating that the mechanism is similar regardless of its location or shape. (a) Dome-shaped epiphysis and dome-shaped growth plate. (b) Longitudinal end plate delineating epiphysis and metaphysis. (c) Horizontal growth plate. (d) Circumferential growth plate.*

Endochondral Ossification

Growth occurs by enlargement of a cartilage model by multiplication of cells and elaboration of an intercellular matrix.[95-97] The cells undergo changes that prepare the matrix for calcification, and finally the calcified cartilage is replaced by bone. At the growth plate of long bones (physis), the proliferating cells are separated from the epiphyseal bony end plate by a thin layer of reserve cells through which vessels penetrate. In the hemispheric growing epiphysis and in the intra-articular epiphysoid bones of the hand and foot, the growth cartilage mechanism is spherical in shape, and the proliferating cells are located as a layer at the periphery (Fig. 60–2).

Nutrition to growth cartilage cells is obtained by diffusion through the matrix. Nutrients derived from joint fluid as a result of pressure diffusion accomplished by the movement of opposing joint surfaces penetrate to an undetermined extent in the epiphysis and epiphysoid bones, with the deeper layers being supplied from the bony centrum itself. At the longitudinal growth plate, blood vessels that enter the epiphysis penetrate the bony end plate and terminate as capillaries in the subjacent growth cartilage matrix.[111, 112]

Blood vessels that enter the epiphysis are involved in both osteogenesis and chondrogenesis (Fig. 60–3). In osteogenesis, they are involved in diffusion of nutrients to the deeper layers of the growth cartilage of the epiphysis (and epiphysoid bones) (Fig. 60–3A). In chondrogenesis, they play a part in new bone formation within the epiphysis (and epiphysoid bones) (Fig. 60–3B); maintaining the health of mature bone within the epiphysis (and epiphysoid bones) (Fig. 60–3C); and penetrating the bony end plate to nourish proliferation cartilage of the longitudinal growth plate (Fig. 60–3D). Interruption of these vessels produces predictable deformities in the growing bony epiphysis and long bone.

Division of the longitudinal growth plate (physis) into (1) the *zone of growth,* (2) the *zone of cartilage transformation* and (3) the *zone of ossification* forms a basis and fundamental anatomic and physiologic model that is useful in understanding the effect of trauma on the growth plate (Fig. 60–4).

The Zone of Growth. Multiplication and growth of the relatively glycogen-free cells of the germinal layer and production of a hyaline intercellular matrix containing few collagen fibers[15, 32] provide the mechanism for the expansion of the growth plate and the steady increase in the distance between the epiphysis and the metaphysis. The perichondral ring contributes to the widening of the plate.[91] Nutrition to the proliferating cells is derived from blood vessels that course through the epiphysis and penetrate the bony end plate.[47, 111, 114] Irreparable injury to the proliferating cells profoundly affects longitudinal bone growth.

The Zone of Cartilage Transformation. The zone of cartilage transformation is concerned with preparing cartilage formed in the zone of growth for ossification. Details of this complex physiologic mechanism, which accompanies cell enlargement and eventual destruction, are beyond the scope of this summary.[13, 15] Calcification is essential before orderly osteogenesis can occur. The enzymatic and biochemical changes in the zone of cartilage transformation and their roles in the preparation of the cartilage for calcification are complex and are still being studied.[16] Injuries to the zone of transformation do not generally affect cell prolifer-

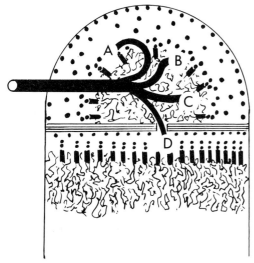

Figure 60–3. *Blood vessels of the epiphysis. (See text.) (From Siffert, R. S.: Skeletal Radiol., 2:21, 1977.)*

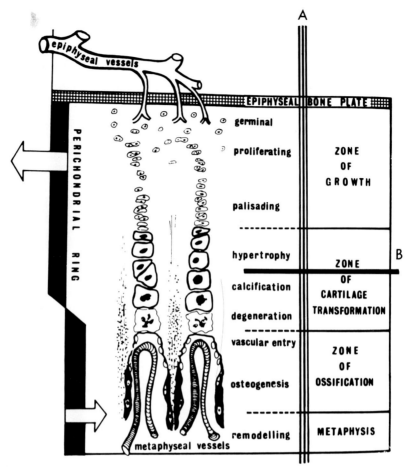

Figure 60–4. *Model of longitudinal growth plate indicating major zones of growth and vascularity. The effect of trauma on the plate depends basically on injury to germinal cells or their blood supply or whether epiphysiodesis occurs as a result of bone growing between the epiphysis and metaphysis. (A) Longitudinal injury through all zones. (B) Horizontal injury through zone of transformation, sparing germinal cells and their vascularity. (From Siffert, R. S.: Skeletal Radiol., 2:21, 1977.)*

ation and growth. Fractures or physiologic alterations (rickets) temporarily widen the plate as growth cartilage accumulates until repair occurs and the normal plate is restored.

The Zone of Ossification. In the zone of ossification, the removal of cellular and calcified remnants of the growth cartilage matrix and the elaboration of new bone take place. Terminal branches of metaphyseal vessels invade the calcified cartilage as vascular loops and penetrate the degenerating cells. Osteoblasts arise from the multipotential perivascular or endosteal cells and form osteoid on intercellular cartilage remnants (primary spongiosa). The new bone is subsequently remodeled in the maturing metaphysis and diaphysis.

Growth continues, and maturing cartilage calcifies undisturbed when bone formation is inhibited as a result of injury to the zone of ossification. The widened plate rapidly returns to normal when metaphyseal vascularity is restored.

ENVIRONMENTAL EFFECTS (TRAUMA) ON THE GROWTH PLATE AND EPIPHYSIS

For reasons still unclear, fractures of the metaphysis or diaphysis of long bones, not involving the epiphysis, may result in the temporary stimulation of longitudinal growth. Chronic inflammation producing hyperemia has a similar effect, whereas

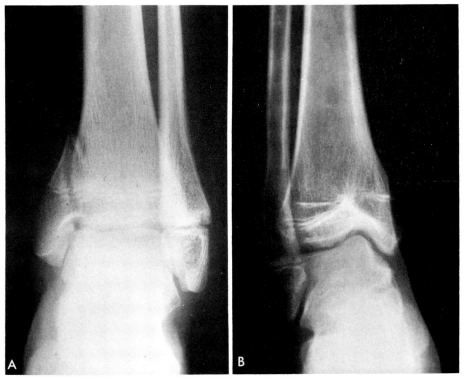

Figure 60-5. *(A) Transepiphyseal injury with growth arrest potential (Salter-Harris Type IV). (B) Eccentric epiphysiodesis and angulation that results from a bony bridge from epiphysis to metaphysis.*

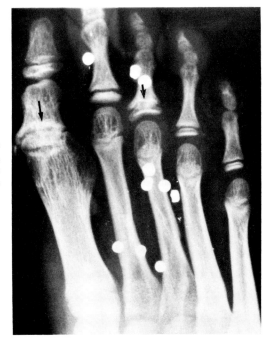

Figure 60-6. *Old shotgun injury. Note the epiphyseal damage with shortening of the proximal phalanx of the hallux (arrow) as well as the damage to the epiphysis of the proximal phalanx of the third toe (arrow). (Courtesy of Melvin H. Jahss, M.D.)*

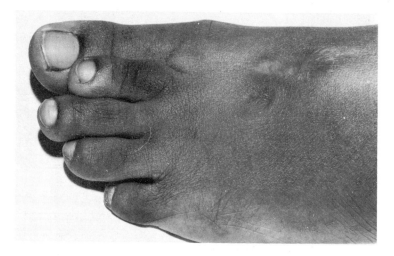

Figure 60–7. *Osteomyelitis of the second metatarsal with shortening of the metatarsal. A mild callus under the third metatarsal head was due to decreased weight bearing under the second metatarsal head. Treatment was syndactylization of the second toe to the third toe. (Courtesy of Melvin H. Jahss, M.D.)*

atrophy, disuse, and malnutrition may be associated with decreased growth rates.[5, 10, 83] When a portion of the growth plate is damaged eccentrically by acute trauma and the unaffected segment continues to grow, the predictable deformity is in direct relationship to the tethering effect of the epiphysiodesis and the growth potential of the uninvolved segment. Angular deformities may also result from chronic pressure effects, which slow growth eccentrically (Fig. 60–5).

Direct damage to an epiphysis or epiphyseal plate may occur, as in gunshot wounds (Fig. 60–6). Similarly, osteomyelitis may cause damage to the epiphyseal plate, with resulting ray shortening (Fig. 60–7) or tarsal bone irregularity leading to osteoarthritis in adulthood.

MECHANISMS OF TRAUMA

The cartilaginous epiphyseal plate is weaker than the bone[82, 86] and is certainly weaker than the ligamentous structures, although it does have a higher elastic modulus than the fibrous periosteum.[13] Because only shearing and avulsion forces can separate the epiphysis, fractures through bone are much more common in childhood than epiphyseal separations. When axially loaded in compression, the viscoelastic properties of cartilage, aided by its containment by the perichondral ring, and the ossification groove and periosteum may protect the growth plate. However, the porous nature of a child's

bone[82] allows failure not only in tension but in compression as well, resulting in the characteristic complete or incomplete fractures that occur.

Trauma to the longitudinal growth plate may be one of four types: avulsion, shearing, splitting, or crushing. Experimentally, Bright, Burstein, and Ellmore found that epiphyseal displacement depended on the age of the animal and the direction in which the force was applied — the older the animal, the more force required.[13, 14] The plate was least resistant to torsion and most resistant to traction force, with approximately 0.5 mm of displacement before separation occurred. Salter and Harris attributed the growth plate's resistance to shearing force to the longitudinally oriented collagen fibers in the amorphous matrix, which function much like the steel rods used to reinforce concrete.[86]

The weakest segment of the growth plate appears to be the layer of hypertrophic cells where the matrix has thinned and collagen fibers have not yet thickened and become longitudinally oriented, as in the subsequent zone of calcification.[46, 105] Depending on the nature and magnitude of the forces applied and the age and species of animal, failures may occur at almost any level and are often associated with tears and clefts across the entire plate,[13] accounting for the unpredictable prognosis of this type of injury.

Regardless of the exact biomechanical events, it is apparent that normal growth should continue unless the proliferating cells or their nutrition is damaged or a transepiphyseal injury occurs and the fracture extending across the plate opens a channel for the formation of a bony bridge between the epiphysis and metaphysis, which would act as a restraint to growth.

Injection studies by Trueta and associates have demonstrated two sources of blood vessels to the longitudinal growth plate: (1) the epiphyseal system, arising from vessels in the epiphysis that penetrate the bony end plate of the epiphysis and terminate as capillary loops among the proliferating cells in the zone of growth; and (2) the metaphyseal system, terminating in vascular loops in the zone of ossification.[112, 113]

Acute trauma that results in eccentric epiphysiodesis and chronic pressure that retards multiplication of proliferating cells have similar effects, namely progressive angular deformity. Angulation of a long bone, asymmetric pressures as the result of asymmetric muscle pull or joint laxity, or the application of corrective braces or casts may produce angular forces sufficient to result in deformity by slowing growth on the side of compression.[2, 96] Foot and ankle deformity secondary to paralysis, imbalance of the foot, and the flat-topped talus are examples that growth cartilage of the longitudinal growth plate and epiphysoid bones is sensitive to the effects of pressure regardless of its anatomic location. Rapidly applied excessive pressures, as with compression devices,[117] may produce irreversible intraphyseal damage. Mild or chronic pressures due to malposition (Blount's disease) of braces and staples slow cartilage cell proliferation and may be reversible when the pressure is relieved, but they may cause epiphysiodesis if sustained for long periods of time.[97]

If epiphysiodesis does occur, its recognition may present diagnostic problems. The normal growth plate as it appears on roentgenogram consists of a lucent line bordered by bone density. The lucency represents the cartilage of the plate, and the adjacent dense lines represent the bony end plate and the metaphyseal new bone, respectively.[93] Roentgenograms of good quality and positioning that permit the central x-ray beam to parallel these structures produce this classic image. The major normal bone roentgenographic markers of the epiphyseal and metaphyse-

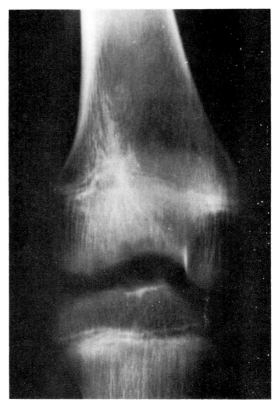

Figure 60–8. *Tomogram demonstrating central epiphysiodesis.*

al sides of the growth plate are the cortical and subcortical densities. Intramedullary central epiphysiodesis may be obscured by these normal peripheral projections, and tomography may be required for its detection (Fig. 60–8). Prompt attention to the extent and nature of a progressing deformity by serial scanograms permits early planning of management (including nonsurgical therapy, epiphysiodesis, shortening, lengthening, or resection of an epiphysiodesis.[11, 49, 60-62] The potential for progressive deformity is related in large part to the future growth of the undamaged segment of the growth cartilage. The younger the patient, the longer the period of growth and, consequently, the greater the potential for deformity. Once a deformity has become established and angulation of the bone has occurred, abnormal mechanical forces may produce further progression of a deformity that has been initiated by an acute or chronic injury to the growth plate.

INJURIES TO THE EPIPHYSIS

Injuries to an epiphysis may affect the articular growth cartilage, the bony epiphysis, or both. Pyarthrosis, synovial disease, synovectomy, the injection of intra-articular steroids, penetrating and surgical injuries, and other direct insults to the joint surface have been implicated in the production of articular, cartilage cell, and matrix degeneration. Direct laceration other than that which occurs at the time of surgery is a rare clinical entity. Experimentally, lacerations of articular cartilage are associated with an apparent initial short-lived increase in cartilage cell metabolism in an attempt at repair, but a degenerative matrix changes generally result in a local articular defect.[108] Lacerations extending deeper into subjacent bone have a greater capacity to heal, as granulation tissue and vessels from the underlying bony epiphysis invade the laceration gap, eventually producing a fibrocartilaginous repair. Although there is little information as to the long-term character and the degree of the mechanical integrity of this type of healing, it is apparent that results can be expected to be more satisfactory if the articular surface is restored by an anatomic reduction and the

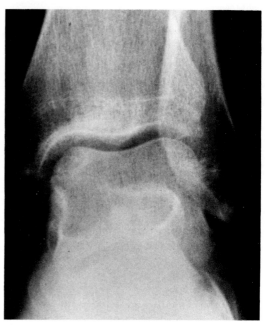

Figure 60–9. *An osteochondral fracture at the medial border of the talus. There was no displacement, and this injury healed without complications.*

integrity of the joint surface is re-established. Clinically, if osteochondral fractures, in which the fragment contains both bone and cartilage, are replaced by

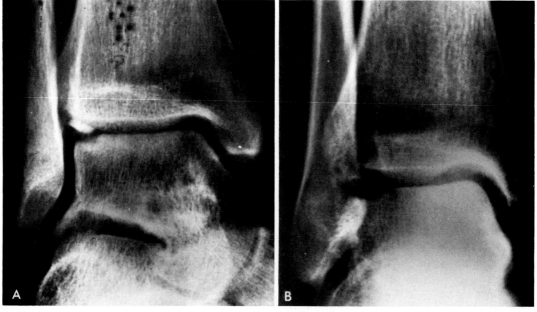

Figure 60–10. *(A) An osteochondral fracture at the lateral talar border that did not heal, produced symptoms, and required surgical excision (B).*

accurate closed or open reduction, bone may heal, permitting the thin cartilage laceration to fill with fibrocartilage (Fig. 60–9). If the bony fragment does not heal properly, it may be unstable, and degenerative articular changes may occur as a result of normal interference with joint forces required for diffusion of nutrients. A loose body may form if both bone and cartilage become necrotic. Osteochondritis dissecans is probably the result of a sharp impact of one joint surface against another in a rotatory or angular fashion. A fragment of subchondral bone may be fractured, as on the talar border of the ankle. The fracture may heal promptly without abnormality; however, lack of immobilization of the fragment may result in nonunion, bone necrosis, and often partial absorption. The lower overlying cartilage may degenerate because of loss of its firm base, which is necessary to maintain diffusional forces, and fragments of cartilage and bone may separate into the joint (Fig. 60–10). In addition to osteochondral injuries, avulsion fractures at the site of ligamentous or tendon attachment (base of the phalanx or tibial spine), which should be reduced open or closed to prevent joint instability, or compression fractures may occur.

Injuries to the Bony Epiphysis

Injuries to the bony epiphysis[95] may be the result of causes that are (1) extraosseous, (2) intraosseous, or (3) idiopathic. *Extraosseous conditions* are most notably fractures, which interfere with vascular supply to the epiphysis, laceration due to injury or surgery, or thrombosis, which may lead to avascular necrosis. *Intraosseous conditions* are characterized by nutritional deprivation of the trabeculae within the epiphysis. Sickle cell crisis may be induced by trauma, as, theoretically, may traumatic avascular necrosis. The pressure of intraosseous diseases (Gaucher's disease, systemic steroids) may predispose an epiphysis to injury. *Idiopathic avascular necrosis* of the epiphysis, including Perthes' disease of the hip and Köhler's disease of the tarsal navicular, is another source of injury to the bony epiphysis.

INJURIES TO THE GROWTH PLATE

Classifications of growth-plate trauma provide terminology for accurate description of an injury and serve as excellent guides for management and prognosis. In 1895, Poland proposed a simple classification, including epiphyseal slip, vertical fracture of the epiphysis not extending through the growth plate, and vertical fracture through the epiphysis and metaphysis that crosses the growth plate.[81] Salter and Harris elaborated on this classification based on the pathomechanics of different patterns of injury.[86, 87] Basically, there are five categories (Fig. 60–11):

The *Type I injury* is essentially a slip of the epiphyseal plate. If the periosteum is not torn, there is no displacement. If the periosteum is torn on one side, displace-

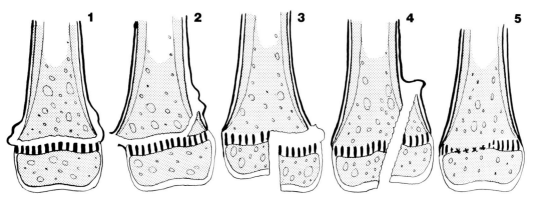

Figure 60–11. *Salter-Harris classification of epiphyseal injuries. (See text.) (From Siffert, R. S.: Skeletal Radiol., 2:21, 1977.)*

ment is usually easily reduced and stabilized by the intact periosteum on the other side acting as a hinge. These injuries are usually the results of shearing forces, torsion, or avulsion. Metabolic diseases such as scurvy, rickets, osteomyelitis, and hormone imbalance are associated with Type I injury.

In a *Type II injury*, a fracture is produced by a lateral displacement force that passes partially through the plate before it fractures through the metaphysis (Thurston-Holland fragment) on the side of the intact periosteum. It has been suggested that weight bearing in addition to a lateral force produces a Type II rather than a Type I injury. This fracture is also easily reduced and held in place by the intact periosteal hinge.

A *Type III injury* is a fracture of the epiphysis associated with separation of the growth plate along with the epiphyseal fragment. If displaced, this intra-articular fracture requires accurate reduction to prevent malarticulation.

A *Type III fracture* generally occurs during adolescence as the growth plate begins its closure from one side to the other.[57] A force that begins as a Type I fracture can extend across the plate only to the point of closure and then fractures through the epiphysis at that junction, or it may represent an avulsion of the epiphysis

through the unclosed segment of the plate.

In a *Type IV injury*, a fracture crosses the joint surface, the growth plate, and the metaphysis. The intra-articular deformity should not be left unreduced (Fig. 60–12).

A *Type V injury*, a crushing of the growth plate, may involve all or part of the plate.

In general, a Type I injury, except for that of the distal femur, usually does not result in growth arrest. However, with Type II injuries, growth arrest may occur, presumably because of the force of weight bearing and impingement of the metaphyseal fragment on the growth plate or passage of the undulating fracture line into the epiphysis and metaphysis. Type III and Type IV injuries frequently result in epiphysiodesis as bone grows across the epiphysis to the metaphysis, producing a tether. Thin Kirschner wires may be used to fix unstable fractures and epiphyseal displacements and generally produce no harmful effects if centrally placed, small, and unthreaded.[4] Although central transepiphyseal bridging results, not unlike a Type IV fracture, its volume is small relative to the overall size of the plate so that it soon atrophies and is replaced by normal growth cartilage. If the bridge is large and asymmetric, as in a separated fracture of

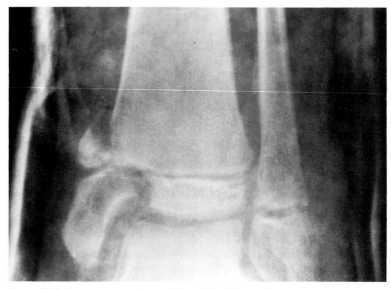

Figure 60–12. *Type IV Salter-Harris fracture of the distal tibia with potential epiphysiodesis and articular surface deformity. This injury requires accurate reduction.*

the plate, attenuation will occur locally. Increasing deformity will be related to continued growth at a distance from the tether and the age of the patient. If the bridge is large and centrally located, it may halt growth completely, whereas small bridges will have relatively little effect. Angular deformities may also occur as a result of injuries to the perichondral ring, most commonly observed in lawn mower scalping injuries of the medial side of the ankle (Type VI — Rang classification).[82] Epiphyseal and metaphyseal bone join across the plate, producing progressive angular deformity.

A Type V (crush) injury is not evident on the roentgenogram at the time of initial examination, and the diagnosis is usually made in retrospect, as shortening or angulation deformity develops later.

The prognosis of injuries to the extremity during growth is not always predictable. Severe soft-tissue trauma without fracture or fracture of a long bone distant from the plate may result in growth deformity, and parents should be made aware of this possibility at the time of trauma.

FRACTURES ABOUT THE ANKLE

Classification of Injury. In 1898, in his study of epiphyseal injuries, Poland stated his belief that those injuries involving the distal tibial and fibular epiphyses could not be classified on the basis of mechanism of injury.[81] However, Ashhurst and Bromer,[3] Bishop,[7] Carothers and Crenshaw,[17] and Crenshaw[22] found similar patterns of injury based on the mechanism of injury. Five major groups were used: (1) abduction injuries, (2) external rotation injuries, (3) plantar flexion injuries, (4) axial compression injuries (and those caused by direct violence), and (5) adduction injuries. Kleiger defined the mechanism of injury as the direction in which the joint is moved, which is determined by the position of the foot, the direction and intensity of the applied force, and the resistance of the structures making up the joint.[58] Since exact information may be difficult to obtain from the child,[89] there is, as Rang emphasized,[82] a conjectural nature to this type of classification. Thus, classification based on

the specific anatomic nature of the damage that is produced provides the best information regarding prognosis.

Fracture Types

Fibular Fractures

Type I epiphyseal injuries are quite common at the distal end of the fibula. The fracture is generally caused by an adduction or inversion strain, resulting in avulsion of the distal fibular epiphysis from the metaphysis. The displacement usually reduces to its normal position spontaneously as a result of the elastic recoil of the soft tissues.

Although the injury may not be apparent on the roentgenogram, it can be recognized clinically by swelling and tenderness over the growth plate of the fibula. Stress films taken with the patient under anesthesia will demonstrate the injury, but they are rarely necessary. Diagnosis can be confirmed two weeks after injury by the presence of distal fibular metaphyseal periosteal new bone formation. Recommended treatment is immobilization in a plaster walking cast for three weeks. The average age for this injury is reported as 12 years and three months, and none of the cases reported required surgical treatment.[100] Premature closure of the growth plate with shortening was observed, but no angular deformity of the ankle joint was noted.

Type II fractures of the distal fibula generally heal uneventfully with immobilization without deformity or complications.[100]

Tibial Fractures

Type I Tibial Fractures. Speigel and associates reported the average age of the patients in their study with this injury to be 10 years and six months, and 25 per cent had associated fractures of the shaft of the fibula.[100] Of the 28 patients who were followed adequately, there was one closure of the distal tibial epiphyseal plate (1.3 cm of shortening) and occasional stimulation of growth (not exceeding 1.5 cm). Slight postreduction residual angular deformity corrected spontaneously, and none of the patients required surgery.

Type II Tibial Fractures. Rang described plantar flexion and inversion injuries that produced displacement of the distal tibial epiphysis and that may be accompanied by a greenstick fracture of the fibula.[82] Reduction is easily accomplished by closed manipulation, and the ankle joint is rarely disrupted in children. The talotibial relationship is maintained by the three major groups of ligaments. Rang accepts up to 20 degrees of valgus, with the expectation that remodeling will correct this deformity, and suggests the application of a long leg cast with a walking heel for a period of six weeks. However, in their report of 91 patients, Spiegel and associates noted that if angular displacement was not reduced, it often remained as a permanent deformity.[100] In both series, an acceptable amount of shortening was noted occasionally. In this type of fracture, as in all fractures of an extremity, any sign of interference with the vascular supply calls for at least immediate partial reduction of the fracture without anesthesia as a first-aid measure. Posttraumatic aseptic necrosis of the distal tibial epiphysis has been reported in one patient who had a displaced Type II fracture, a fibular fracture, and presumably a crush element and who sustained multiple severe trauma in a motor vehicle accident.[92]

Type III Tibial Fractures. Two types of Type III tibial fractures have been reported, depending on the age of the patient and, therefore, the stage of closure of the epiphyseal plate of the distal tibia. Kleiger and Mankin determined that the distal tibial epiphyseal plate closes over a period of one and a half years in an asymmetric manner, first centrally, then on the medial side, and finally laterally at varying ages from 14 to 18.[57] The same external rotation force may therefore produce two different patterns of injury, depending on the stage of plate closure.

TYPE III TIBIAL FRACTURES WITH AN OPEN GROWTH PLATE. Fractures through the base of the medial malleolus are difficult to differentiate (whether type III, Type IV, Type V) on the roentgenogram because the x-ray beam cannot clearly delineate the inner margin of the growth plate and comminution is common. Posttraumatic epiphysiodesis is a frequent re-

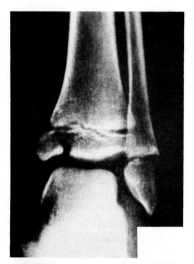

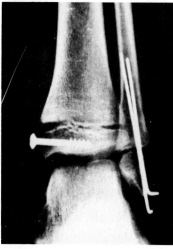

Figure 60–13. *A Type III distal tibial fracture and a Type I fibular fracture which required open reduction. The compression screw provides excellent alignment of articular cartilage without risk to the germinal cells of the plate. The small, smooth pins will not affect longitudinal growth of the fibula.*

sidual, leading to varus deformity of the ankle, accompanied by overgrowth of the fibula. Anatomically, reduction of a separated fragment is essential to close the gap in the growth plate and to restore the articular surface, and transepiphyseal pins can be used to maintain the reduction. Reduction of an epiphyseal fracture can be accomplished by use of a compression screw placed parallel to the growth plate in the center of the epiphysis (Fig. 60–13).

Type III Tibial Fractures with a Closing Growth Plate. A fracture of the lateral portion of the distal end of the tibia was originally described in adults as the fracture of Tillaux.[57, 119] At the age of 13 to 14 years, the medial half of the distal tibial growth plate is closing; the lateral half remains open. An external rotation force applied to the anterior tibiofibular ligament (connecting the tibial epiphysis with the fibula metaphysis) avulses the anterior lateral corner of the distal tibial epiphysis. Rang suggested that this injury is the equivalent of a traumatic diastasis in the adult.[82] If the fragments are small and cannot be reduced by closed reduction, open reduction to restore articular integrity is indicated.[30, 73]

Type IV Tibial Fractures. Although transepiphyseal fractures may occur medially, laterally, or centrally, they are most common at the base of the medial malleolus. Undisplaced comminuted and crush injuries of the plate are treated by above-the-knee plaster immobilization and have a high incidence of epiphyseal closure.[87, 100]

Type V Injuries. Type V injuries usually occur on the medial side of the distal tibial epiphysis.[87] This injury occurs as a result of a severe varus angulation and crushing force applied to the ankle. The injury is difficult to recognize initially both clinically and radiographically, and only a careful history of the mechanism of injury may lead to suspicion of a Type V injury. It is generally a diagnosis made in retrospect when deformity occurs. Repeated tibial osteotomies in order to control a progressive angular deformity or attempted resection of the epiphysiodesis may be indicated.[11, 61, 62]

Type VI Injuries. Rang described an ablation of the perichondral ring, generally secondary to lawn mower and degloving injuries that incise the perichondral ring at the time of trauma.[82] A callus bridge forms between the epiphysis and the metaphysis, resulting in a tethering action and a varus deformity. Langenskiöld[61, 62] and Bright[11, 12] confirmed this injury experimentally and found it possible to prevent the ingrowth of callus by inserting fat or silicone, respectively, after excision of the bridged growth plate.

Triplane Fractures

Approximately 6 per cent of distal epiphyseal fractures are triplane,[20] a combination of Salter-Harris Type III and Type II fractures. The fracture lines are in three planes, extending from the articular surface of the growth plate, along the growth plate, and into the metaphysis. The goal of treatment is restoration of normal anatomy. If closed reduction in internal rotation fails to obliterate the gap to less than 2 mm, open reduction and internal fixation[20, 66, 68, 109] are necessary to reconstitute the joint articulation and reduce the growth plate fracture. Tomograms can be helpful in determining the degree of displacement and the size and location of the fracture fragments.

Miscellaneous Injuries

Rang described the avulsion of both malleoli,[82] which, depending on the size of the fragment, may require open reduction and internal fixation. An ossicle may form, with enlargement of the entire epiphysis and no interference with function. An unusual injury is external rotation at the distal tibial growth plate, with or without displacement of the distal fibular epiphysis. Unless the knee and ankle are included on the same roentgenogram, an oblique view of the ankle may have the appearance of a normal anteroposterior projection.

COMPLICATIONS OF EPIPHYSEAL FRACTURES OF THE ANKLE

Since any type of epiphyseal fracture may result in epiphysiodesis, parents should be informed of this possibility at the time of injury. They should be instructed to observe the ankle for changes in shape, as may occur with angular deformity, and limp caused by shortening. Follow-up examination and roentgenograms at 6 and 12 months is advisable. If a growth arrest line occurs, it can be a valuable indication of symmetric growth or asymmetric growth arrest due to partial epiphysiodesis (Fig. 60–14).

In general, Type I and Type II fibular fractures have a low incidence of epiphy-

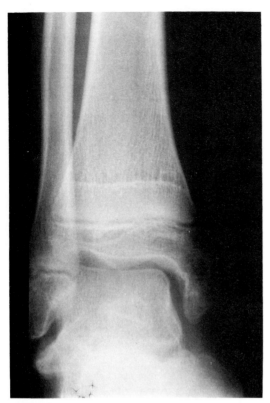

Figure 60–14. *Growth arrest line on the distal tibia. The symmetric line indicates equal growth from the plate and no potential angular deformity.*

siodesis,[100] and if closure should occur, resulting in a short fibula, there is usually no disturbance in the tibiotalar joint or ankle joint dysfunction. Type I tibial fractures are also considered to have a low risk for epiphysiodesis. A Type II distal tibial fracture generally occurs when there is a partially closed plate, near the end of growth, so that even if epiphysiodesis does occur, there is little or no deformity or shortening. Type IV distal tibial fractures with minimal displacement (less than 2 mm) may not be associated with epiphysiodesis, but it is difficult to evaluate the degree of separation in a transepiphyseal fracture, and this criterion is unreliable. All Type IV fractures, therefore, must be considered to have a potentially high risk for epiphysiodesis. Similarly, other fractures that cross the plate resulting in a diastasis into which bone may grow from epiphysis and metaphysis in the formation of an epiphysiodesis must be considered

high-risk. These include displaced Type III and Type IV, juvenile Tillaux, and triplane fractures, any comminuted tibial epiphyseal trauma, and Type V crush injuries.

Open reduction is indicated in high-risk displaced fractures primarily to restore joint alignment and to prevent later articular deformity, with the recognition that if epiphysiodesis does occur, it can be managed by equalizing procedures during growth.

INJURIES TO THE CHILD'S FOOT

Blount,[9] Tachdjian,[106] and Rang[82] noted the relatively low incidence of injury to the child's foot compared with that of the adult in which problems are generally much more complex. The child's foot is flexible and resilient, and the force of trauma is generally transmitted proximally to the ankle and leg, frequently producing ligamentous, bony, or epiphyseal injury. Blount stressed the recuperative powers of the child's foot and emphasized that closed attempts at acceptable rather than anatomic alignment, coupled with immobilization, elevation, and when possible, compression, generally yield satisfactory results.[9] Although traumatized growing bone and soft tissues tend toward remodeling and repair with restoration of normal architecture, there are certain situations that require special attention and that should be emphasized on the general discussion of injuries to the child's foot.

Fractures of the Talus

Fractures of the talus are relatively uncommon in children[82] and, in contrast to those in adults, heal satisfactorily without serious residuals.[9] Avascular necrosis has been described as an unusual complication[9] but has been reported in children as well as in adults.[99]

The gross anatomy of the talus in children is essentially similar to that in adults, with strong ligaments but no muscular attachments and with seven articular facets. The bony centrum of the talus is completely enveloped in growth cartilage in early infancy, but through childhood and adolescence the nonarticular surfaces develop periosteal coverings, until adult life, when two fifths of the surface is bone.

The relatively small surface that is covered with periosteum is the site of entrance of blood vessels arising from the three main arteries of the leg — the posterior tibial, peroneal, and dorsalis pedis arteries.[45] The major vascular supply is from the discrete vessels of the artery of the sinus tarsi and the artery of the tarsal canal, usually found as a branch of the dorsalis pedis artery, entering the talus at the lateral part of its capsular attachment.[45, 98] In general, vascularity is extremely variable, through inconstant anastamosis and vessels penetrating directly and at ligamentous attachments.[70] Dislocation, which disrupts the capsule and ligaments, and fractures through the neck at the site of richest vascularity represent a risk of subsequent avascular necrosis.

The majority of fractures of the talus occur through the neck, which is the weakest segment of the bone.[99] In dorsiflexion injuries, such as those that occur in a forward fall, the lower anterior margin of the tibia is driven into the talus like a chisel. The fracture may be simple without dislocation, with dislocation, or with partial dislocation. The majority of simple fractures heal without subsequent avascular necrosis after six weeks of immobilization and early weight bearing. Fractures of the neck with dislocation and partial dislocation, which have higher risk of avascular necrosis, can be reduced and fixed in full plantar flexion and eversion and maintained in this position for approximately eight weeks without risk to the function of the foot. At eight weeks, the foot may be brought into neutral position, and it is kept in plaster for another two weeks. Concomitant compression fracture of the head of the talus may occur.[99] Displaced fractures of the body of the talus may require open reduction with Kirschner-wire fixation. During the wide exposure required to allow visualization of fracture surfaces, there is a risk of damage to vascularity, and care should be taken to avoid removing soft-tissue attachments to the bony fragments. The degree of joint stiffness appears to be proportional to the involvement and disruption of the joint surfaces, notably those of the subtalar joint.

Fracture of the lateral process of the talus, which may involve the talofibular articulation of the ankle joint and the posterior talocalcaneal articulation of the subtalar joint, may be an avulsion in nature[99] or may be due to a compression force that is produced when the inverted foot is severely dorsiflexed.[48] This injury is difficult to recognize initially. Pain and joint tenderness in front of the lateral malleolus may persist, and oblique roentgenograms or tomograms may demonstrate loose bodies, which when excised, generally provide relief.

Osteochondritis Dissecans

The most common site of osteochondritis dissecans is the medial corner of the superior surface of the talus[106] (see Figure 60–7). The lesion is observed most frequently in adolescents and generally heals with rest. Despite roentgenographic changes of bony fragmentation and partial absorption, exploration may disclose normal overlying articular cartilage, which derives nutrition from the joint fluid. In later adolescence, the subchondral bony fragment may fail to unite, leading to cartilage fragmentation, articular irregularity, and occasionally, extrusion of the fragment into the joint.

An arthrogram may visualize clefts or partial separation of the overlying cartilage that may not be apparent on a plain roentgenogram.[6] Severe involvement with degeneration of articular cartilage is generally treated by excision of the fragment and drilling of the eburnated base into bleeding bone to allow the defect to be filled with fibrous tissue, which matures into fibrocartilage.

Fracture-Dislocation of the Talus

Fracture-dislocation of the talus is very rare in children and is generally followed by avascular necrosis of the talus and degenerative joint disease. Open reduction has been necessary in the cases reported.[27, 104]

Fractures of the Calcaneus

All authors agree that fractures of the calcaneus should be treated nonsurgically during childhood because of the great deal of restoration of form and function that occurs despite involvement of the subtalar joint.[9, 69, 83, 106, 107] Treatment consists of elevation and compression until swelling and pain subside, followed by early mobilization and avoidance of weight bearing until the fracture has healed (approximately six weeks). There has been a question as to whether avascular necrosis occurs, but it is of no apparent clinical significance since it does not appear to be associated with deformity or late sequelae.[107]

Osteochondrosis of the calcaneus (Sever's disease) is a clinical diagnosis based on the syndrome of tenderness and pain in the heel.[90] Avascular necrosis of the apophysis, Achilles tendinitis, traumatic periostitis, and other theoretical etiologies have been implicated to explain the pain and roentgenographic irregularity of the apophysis, which is generally viewed as a normal developmental finding. Therefore, the syndrome may have many causes. Density and fragmentation of the apophysis, which are also present in children with no pain, are probably normal findings.

Midtarsal Injuries

Midtarsal injuries are usually caused by direct crushing (Fig. 60–15). In view of the marked amount of soft-tissue trauma that accompanies deeper bone and joint injury, there is a risk of massive edema, vascular impairment, and delayed skin loss. Un-

less it is urgent to attend to an open fracture or dangerously displaced fragments, treatment of the soft-tissue injury by hospitalization, elevation, compression, application of cold, and occasionally decompression, when necessary, takes priority. Closed reduction using Kirschner wires is preferable, followed later by plaster immobilization when the swelling and the effects of soft-tissue trauma have decreased.

Acute crush injuries of the navicular are rare and should not be confused with Köhler's disease (Fig. 60–16), which is an osteochondrosis.[59] Although it has been suggested that osteochondritis may be related to repetitive trauma in a susceptible growing epiphysis and may perhaps be associated with constitutional predisposition (to account for familial incidence[24] and bilaterality), there is no evidence of this with respect to the foot. Aseptic necrosis may be seen in the adult navicular and in metatarsal heads whose growth plates have been closed for a long time. In either case, Köhler's disease is self-limited and heals with normal or near-normal reconstitution.

Metatarsal Fractures

Metatarsal fractures may be either single or multiple. Blount emphasizes that the metatarsals in young children have excellent remodeling potential and that following healing of a fracture, a nearly normal roentgenographic appearance can be

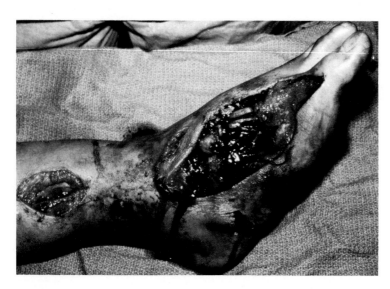

Figure 60–15. *A direct crush injury of the midfoot with marked soft-tissue injury that required open reduction, internal fixation, and a split-thickness skin graft.*

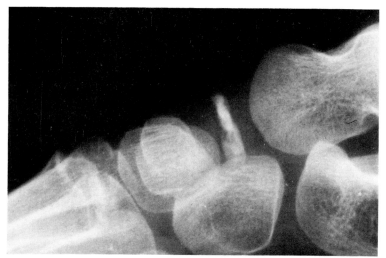

Figure 60–16. *Köhler's disease. A roentgenogram demonstrating the necrotic bony centrum of the navicular and the continued normal growth of the circumferential growth plate as indicated by the maintenance of the normal space between the talus and the cuneiform. When the centrum is revascularized, a near-normal navicular reconstitutes and may be demonstrated roentgenographically. (From Siffert, R. S.: Skeletal Radiol., 2:21, 1977.)*

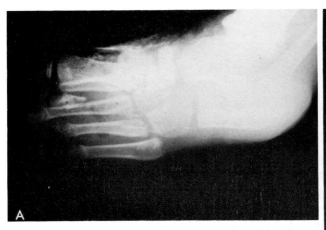

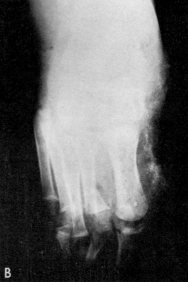

Figure 60–17. *(A and B) Direct trauma produced metatarsal fractures, tarsometatarsal dislocations, and metatarsophalangeal dislocation with severe soft-tissue injury. (C and D) Satisfactory alignment achieved wtih open reduction and multiple pin fixation.*

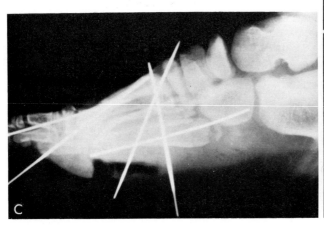

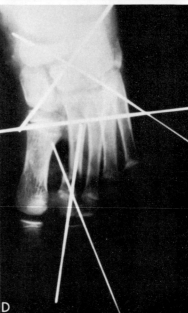

expected within one or two years, with excellent functional results.[9] When stability cannot be obtained by manipulation, alignment may be accomplished by temporary skin traction applied to the toes. Skeletal traction is rarely necessary. The focus of treatment should be directed toward maintaining the arch and preventing depression of the metatarsal heads and metatarsal shortening. Intramedullary fixation with Kirschner wires may be employed for unstable fractures.

Jones Fracture. A Jones fracture occurs through the tuberosity at the base of the fifth metatarsal. In a child, a fracture of the tuberosity can be differentiated from the normal appearance of the apophysis since fractures are usually oriented at a right angle to the shaft and usually extend to the articulations between the fifth metatarsal and the cuboid and between the fourth and fifth metatarsals, whereas the apophyseal line traverses the tubercle in a direction almost parallel to the long axis of the shaft and does not extend proximally into the metatarsocuboid joint or medially into the joint between the fourth and fifth metatarsals.[23] Healing generally occurs without residuals, and treatment is symptomatic, consisting of elastic support, a compression dressing, and partial weight bearing with support or with a walking cast if symptoms are severe.

Trauma to the Metatarsal Heads. In 1914, Freiberg described painful distortions in the metatarsal heads of six patients, four of whom had a preceding history of trauma.[38] He believed that the previous injury caused the deformity and produced pain, and he used the term "infraction" to describe this condition. Steindler explained the high frequency of involvement of the second metatarsal as being due to the fact that it is the metatarsal most vulnerable to trauma since it is the longest and most rigidly fixed at its base.[103] Unrecognized acute trauma or the effect of repeated trauma producing stress consequences, or both, have been implicated as the etiologic factors. These painful distortions may be associated with stress (march) fracture of the metatarsal diaphysis in the same or opposite foot.[24]

Transverse Fractures of the Metatarsals. Crushing blows and direct trauma may result in transverse fractures of the

metatarsals[19] (Fig. 60–17). Fractures of the diaphysis that heal with angluation may leave local bony prominences that become sources of pain owing to shoe pressure, prominence of a metatarsal head and plantar hyperkeratosis, and hammer toes. Fractures of the proximal third of a metatarsal, comminuted transverse fractures of the diaphysis, or oblique and spiral fractures of the neck may be treated by a short leg, walking cast or a modified shoe, depending on the severity of the injury and the patient's symptoms. Displaced metatarsal shaft fractures that result in dorsal or plantar angulation should be reduced. Medial and lateral displacement does not usually present a problem with alignment of the toes and generally is more acceptable. If closed reduction is not adequate or is unstable, internal fixation can be attained by use of an intramedullary wire or crossed Kirschner wires. The wire is removed after three weeks without weight bearing, and this is followed by immobilization in a

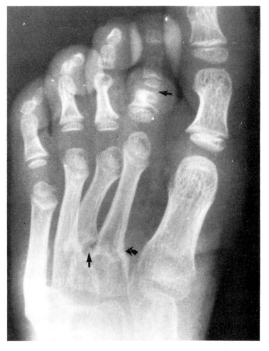

Figure 60–18. *Roentgenogram taken one and a half years after an automobile crush injury. Note the delayed union of the base of the second metatarsal, nonunion of the base of the third metatarsal, and nonunion of the proximal phalanx of the second toe (arrows). (Courtesy of Melvin H. Jahss, M.D.)*

short leg, walking cast until the fracture is fully healed.

Occasionally in multiple trauma, fractures associated with a crush injury to the foot may be overlooked even on roentgenograms, such as that of a toe or metatarsal, which may progress to nonunion (Fig. 60–18). Similarly, an undisplaced fracture of the talus may be missed and may result in aseptic necrosis, occasionally leading to significant deformity.

Metatarsophalangeal Joint Dislocation

The great toe is the most common site of metatarsophalangeal dislocation as the proximal phalanx displaces dorsally, medially, or laterally. Closed reduction can generally be accomplished, with good stability obtained by splinting or cast immobilization. Irreducible dislocation because of buttonholing of the metatarsal head through the volar capsule requiring open reduction has been reported.[41] Percutaneous pinning may be employed when there is instability.[40]

Fractures of the Phalanx

A fracture of the large toe that has displaced and required reduction should be immobilized. Open reduction of displaced intra-articular fractures of the large toe may be necessary to avoid growth arrest, particularly joint incongruity and later degenerative changes. Rang reported such growth arrest, presumably as a result of Type V fracture after stubbing of the great toe.[82]

The little toe is the most commonly fractured phalanx. Fracture of a phalanx in a child is generally characterized by an epiphyseal separation, which can be easily reduced under local anesthesia and immobilized by splinting the toe to the adjacent toe. Gross angulation and rotation should be avoided. If multiple digits are fractured, closed reduction and a padded walking cast with a toe plate extending beyond the toes usually enable the patient to walk comfortably. Comfort can be improved by placing small pieces of absorbent cotton between the digits.

Lisfranc Joint Dislocation (Tarsometatarsal Fracture-Dislocation)

The lateral four metatarsals are jointed by a transverse ligament. The medial cuneiform and the second metatarsal are united by a ligament, and the base of the second metatarsal is locked and recessed between the medial and lateral cuneiforms.[120] A Lisfranc joint dislocation therefore disrupts this interval, creating a fracture of the second metatarsal and extending laterally through the cuboid. A stable, closed reduction generally heals after six weeks of plaster immobilization. Percutaneous pinning may be necessary if instability exists. Open reduction is occasionally required. Short-term results are good, but later degenerative joint disease can be anticipated.[106]

Midfoot Fractures and Dislocations

Midfoot fractures and dislocations in childhood are rare, and the general approach and management are similar for a navicular, cuneiform, or cuboid fracture and for dislocation of the talonavicular joint or cuneiform and cuboid bones. Priority is given to soft-tissue and potential vascular injury by elevation, compression, and ice therapy. Dislocated and displaced fractures can generally be reduced closed and maintained in plaster with or without Kirschner wires. Open reduction is rarely required. Diagnosis may be difficult, and all suspected injuries demand careful roentgenographic examination, including at least four views: (1) dorsoplantar view to include the metatarsal heads, (2) lateral view to include the ankle and metatarsals, including the metatarsal heads, (3) anteroposterior view of the ankle, and (4) oblique view of the foot.

Accessory Bones

Accessory ossicles and sesamoid bones may cause confusion in differential diagnosis from chip fractures in the region of the midfoot. Knowledge of the normal location of accessory ossicles may be helpful, as are detailed roentgenograms that are clear enough to allow differentiation of a smooth cortical border from an irregular fractured edge. Chip fractures are rarely displaced enough to result in ligamentous problems or to be bothersome as loose bodies. Elastic support or a walking cast is usually sufficient treatment, and parents should be informed of the possibility of failure of the fracture to heal, which will not be associated with functional abnormality.

Stress Fractures

Stress or fatigue fractures, which are the result of repetitive injury focused on a particular segment of bone, are not associated with a history of acute trauma but may occur as a result of overuse (e.g., dancing, jumping, or running). The child presents with a painful gait pattern, and initial roentgenograms may be normal or may suggest a faint area of lucency. The clinical diagnosis is made on the basis of knowledge of the most common sites of stress fractures coupled with a careful history.[28, 33] Pain, which may be associated with tenderness and swelling occurs on activity and is relieved by rest. Roentgenograms taken at 10 to 14 days begin to show periosteal reaction of reparative osteogenesis, with or without the appearance of a fracture line. At this stage, the roentgenographic appearance and biopsy specimens may mimic inflammatory or malignant disease. Finally, the callus is absorbed as remodeling takes place. Treatment consists solely of rest and support to relieve the symptoms and a change of activity or orthotic supports to help prevent recurrence.

In infants, the most frequent site of stress fractures is the lower half of the fibula, although the callus may extend higher. Other sites of stress fractures in children are the second and third metatarsals, the sesamoids,[43] the fifth metatarsal in a partially corrected clubfoot,[82] the calcaneus,[63, 102] and the tarsal navicular.[110]

Athletic Injuries to the Ankle and Foot

As a result of the increased interest in athletics and more organized sports, chil-dren are exposed to an environment that may produce injury to the foot and ankle. Turco presented a review of these injuries.[116] Certain principles should be emphasized. The same etiologic, diagnostic, and therapeutic considerations pertain to nonathletic as well as athletic injuries, with the differences being related to the mechanism of trauma as determined by a careful history. Although the young athlete is often pressured to return to participation in his sport by team and personal motivation pressures, as well as by his parents, injured parts should be allowed to heal fully and to be completely rehabilitated before subjected again to damaging trauma. Analysis of the cause of an injury may be helpful in prevention.

Direct Injuries

A direct blow will cause contusion of skin, subcutaneous tissues, deeper muscles, nerves, tendons, and ligaments and traumatic periostitis, with swelling and discoloration. Initial treatment should be elevation, application of cold, and compression. Disabling periostitis, as occurs frequently in the heel, is common in running sports and may delay return to activity. The peroneal tendons may sublux as a result of a direct blow or twisting trauma to the ankle. The torn or stretched tethering retinaculum generally heals with rest, but if there is chronic disability, surgical correction, as described by O'Donoghue[75] and Savastano,[88] may offer satisfactory results.

Achilles Tendinitis

Achilles tendinitis is generally the result of excessive stretching of a tight heel cord. Rest, local application of heat, and a heel lift generally relieve this problem, and when relief has been obtained, gentle stretching is begun to avoid recurrence. Rupture of the Achilles tendon is uncommon during childhood.

Ankle Sprains

Lateral Ligament Sprain. Ankle sprains occur frequently during sports, most commonly to the anterior talofibular component of a lateral ankle ligament. In a young athlete, there may be an avulsion fracture of the tip of the lateral malleolus, at the point of ligament attachment. In addition, an unchecked inverting force of the ankle often results in a secondary fracture of the medial malleolus. The program of treatment, which depends on the severity of the injury, begins with a period of rest, ice therapy, elevation, and compression, followed by active motion as tolerated. When weight bearing is permitted, strapping or external support is employed. Any suspicion of ligament tear should be treated by immobilization in a plaster cast for several weeks. Immediate surgical repair of a documented torn ligament has been recommended in the older adolescent.[44, 101]

Medial Ligament Sprain. Isolated injury to the deltoid ligament is rare and is usually accompanied by fracture of the fibula, lateral displacement of the talus, or separation of the tibiofibular syndesmosis. Oblique postreduction roentgenograms are essential to insure that there is reduction of the fibula and no widening of the space between the medial malleolus and the talus. The injury should be immobilized in plaster for approximately eight weeks.

Tibiofibular Ligament Sprain. A sudden "pop" at the ankle noted as the foot is sharply hyperdorsiflexed suggests a tibiofibular sprain, as may occur in running or jumping sports or in hockey when the skate strikes the board. Usually, there is little swelling, with point tenderness localized over the anterior and posterior tibiofibular ligaments. Compression of both malleoli may produce pain over the syndesmosis. The patient may prefer to walk on his toes to avoid stretching of the ligament in dorsiflexion. Mild injuries are treated symptomatically, and plaster immobilization in equinus is recommended for more severe injuries. Even without separation, there may be persistent pain over the syndesmosis anteriorly and posteriorly for months, and displaced injuries may be associated with prolonged symptoms, with aggravation during push-off activities. If it is initially unrecognized, roentgenograms may demonstrate later calcification in the interosseous space between the tibia and the fibula. Surgery is reserved for irreducible or unstable separations.

Severe Ankle Injuries

In addition to the separation of the tibiofibular syndesmosis and rupture of the tibiofibular ligaments, fracture of the lateral malleolus above the level of the ankle and tearing of the deltoid ligament may be the result of violent injuries. The foot and fibula are displaced laterally. If closed reduction is not stable, open reduction of the fibula and transfixion of the fibula to the tibia, followed by repair of the deltoid ligament, may be indicated.

Traumatic Separation of the First and Second Metatarsals

Traumatic separation of the first and second metatarsals is known as sagittal diastasis. This common injury may occur in any of the jumping and running sports, usually resulting from concentration of the body weight on the ball of the foot. The patient presents with immediate severe pain and inability to bear weight. Swelling develops over the forefoot and may eventually spread to between the first and second toes. An avulsion fracture at the base of the first metatarsal or medial cuneiform is practically pathognomonic of this injury, which may be accompanied by slight widening between the first and second metatarsals, as compared with the normal side. Initial treatment is application of a compression dressing with elevation, followed by plaster immobilization for approximately five to six weeks. Symptoms may persist for many months, and protective supports may be required.

Puncture Wounds of the Foot

Puncture wounds of the foot and their complications are not uncommon during childhood and adolescence.[55, 72, 80] The majority of 887 children reviewed by Fitzgerald and Cowan sustained their wounds between May and October, with the largest number occurring during the month of July.[37] Most of the children were 15 years of age or younger; approximately 70 per cent were boys and 30 per cent were girls. Puncture by a nail accounted for 98 per cent of the injuries. An accurate history is important and should include the type of puncture wound, the geographic location and time of injury, the estimated depth of penetration, and the status of tetanus immunization. The wound should be cleansed in a detergent solution of iodophor, since Pseudomonas contamination has been noted in hexachlorophene detergents that have been opened. Local debridement and probing under strict sterile conditions may be effective in removing the foreign-body remnant. Fitzgerald and Cowan treated the wounds with dry, sterile dressings, elevation, and rest without prophylactic antibiotics, since only two of the 467 patients treated on the first day of injury required later incision and drainage. Antibiotics were reserved for untreated patients who presented with late cellulitis or an established infection. Staphylococcus was the most common organism, and patients were treated with a semisynthetic penicillinase-resistant penicillin until results of culture studies were known. Pseudomonas has also been described as an occasional offender, often associated with osteomyelitis or joint involvement.[36, 55, 72]

Power Mower Injuries

Power mower injuries in children can produce devastating damage to the foot. The energy a typical motor blade approximately 66 cm long can produce rotating at 3000 rpm is about 2100 foot-pounds.[78] The type of injuries encountered have been described as complete or partial amputation of the foot or leg, major lacerations of skin and tendons, and fractures and fracture-dislocations.[64] Self-propelled mowers were involved in collision injuries, including open tibial fractures and fractures of the upper extremity. Missile injuries are the direct result of pieces of metal parts or objects on the ground thrown at high speed by the power mower. The initial wound may be small and belie the presence of a deep injury or foreign body, which may result in infection. All injuries associated with a lawn mower must be assumed to be contaminated with anaerobic organisms and should not be closed primarily, for fear of complications, including skin slough, gangrene, wound dehiscence, and infection. Patients with lawn mower wounds should receive human antitetanus globulin,[21] since the wounds must be assumed to have Clostridium contamination, and should receive prophylactic broad-spectrum antibiotics.

Thorough debridement should be done with exploration under general anesthesia, because the depth of the wound may be deceptive, and tissue planes may fall together after the blade has passed through. Degloved skin should be cleansed, defatted, and reapplied. Finally, skin grafting on clean, granulated tissue may be performed after about 7 to 10 days.

Rang described a perichondral ring injury (Salter Type VI) resulting in peripheral epiphysiodesis and progressive angular deformity because the blade sliced the surface of the growth plate. Most lawn mower injuries are the result of operator error and carelessness and may be prevented by better education and better design of the equipment.

Bicycle Spoke Injuries

Bicycle spoke injuries present problems in management, primarily because they initially appear to be minor injuries. Izant and associates reviewed 60 cases of this injury in children under the age of 14 and found a striking similarity between bicycle spoke injuries and ringer injuries of the arm; they felt that the initial examination did not reveal the true extent of the injury.[53] In almost every instance, the injury occurred while two children were on a bicycle built for one with a passenger riding on the handlebar, the cross frame, or the rear fender. The foot became impinged between the areas of the spokes of the wheel and the frame of the bicycle. The kinetic energy of stopping the bike is transmitted to the trapped foot, resulting in laceration of the tissues from the knife-like action of the spoke, crushing from the impingement between the wheel and frame of the bicycle, and/or shearing injury. Laceration was usually at the malleoli, the Achilles tendon area of the heel, or the dorsum of the foot, and most often occurred in children from ages two to eight. Tendon and bone and skin sloughs, particularly of the heel pad, may become necrotic since the extent of devitalization may not be apparent at the initial examination. Compression necrosis due to injured blood vessels that have thrombosed and soft tissue that has been sheared from underlying fixed points might not be apparent for three or four days. Therefore, the decision to graft skin must either await delineation of necrosis or follow wide debridement. After fracture has been ruled out and areas of abrasion or tissue loss have been treated by dressing and mild fluff compression, the extremity is elevated and the circulation observed, and the extremity is often immobilized in a simple splint. Debridement of devitalized tissue is performed as necessary at frequent dressing changes, and early skin grafting of the dorsum of the foot or malleoli is recommended. Primary closure of lacerations should be performed only after careful debridement.

Burns

The degree and character of a residual deformity depend on the extent and severity of a burn and the adequacy and effectiveness of treatment.[34, 35] The potentially severe systemic effect of burns should not be neglected while attention is being paid to the affected skin. The bone and joint changes complicating burns have been well described[34,35] and are beyond the scope of this discussion. (See Chapter 61.) Evans and associates noted that contractures of joints are major complications of severe burns and are often the result of the contraction tendency of the burn wound or its covering graft. Contractures of joints may be minimized by proper positioning, use of supportive splints, judicious use of skeletal traction and suspension, and maintenance of joint mobility. The ideal treatment for the burn patient is that provided by the burn team, which includes plastic, general, and orthopaedic surgeons, pediatricians, occupational and physical therapists, and nursing personnel. Burns may result in either growth stimulation or retardation or epiphysiodesis.

Freezing Injuries

Freezing produces local effects similar to those of burns. However, the duration and severity of exposure make the response to this type of trauma unpredictable. Hermann and coworkers classified freezing injuries into two types — frostbite and wet immersion foot.[50] The effect of freezing is a profound reduction of blood flow, followed by rupture of small blood vessels and edema. When the injured tissues begin to thaw, an intense vasoconstriction occurs at the junction of the uninvolved and the involved tissues. Treatment generally consists of rapid rewarming of the foot and local care. Frozen parts should be placed in a warming bath for rapid rewarming, at a temperature of no more than 42°C.[31, 71]

Traumatic Skin Loss

Except for slight differences, the principles of skin coverage are similar for both the child and the adult. Skin replacement in children below the age of 10[85] can generally be by a split graft in the lower extremity. Heel injuries in children as the result of avulsion in relatively slow-moving vehicle accidents should be debrided promptly.[65] The defatted skin is sutured back into position. If a defect remains, a posterior thigh flap may be prepared simultaneously to facilitate early grafting.

Amputations

The techniques for management of traumatic and elective amputations in children and the use of prostheses have been well established, and new methods have been considered.[18] Patellar-tendon–bearing prostheses and the Syme amputation prosthesis with a solid ankle, cushioned heel, and spacers that move as the level of amputation moves distally with growth are well known. Generally, the amputation of single toes may lead to deformities of the foot as a whole unless the space previously occupied is filled. Loss of the great toe may impair rapid gait or running and can create excessive pressures·in the lateral metatarsal heads. New techniques of microsurgery that have been employed successfully in the hand are now being attempted in the foot. Onizuka and associates repaired an amputated great toe in two cases in young children and repaired brachydactyly of the great toe in a nine-month-old boy with a congenital defect, using a plantar flap with the pedicle on the root of the amputated great toe.[76] Experimental attempts are being made to transplant epiphyses with their vascular supply intact to permit replacement of essential damaged growth plates. Bone lengthening for cosmetic and functional purposes has been successful, mainly in metatarsal defects and congenital problems.[54, 117]

Major Limb Replantation

Most efforts in major limb replantation have been directed toward the upper extremity, which has no prosthetic equal. Highly trained teams are directing expertise toward lower limb replantation as well.[74] The value of this procedure and its attendant morbidity, risks, and costs with limited gain if sensation and function are not maintained must be weighed against the advantages of early, highly effective, lower-extremity prosthetic fitting.

Iatrogenic Trauma

In the previous sections, it is apparent that the child's foot is particularly vulnerable to a number of harmful environmental influences. In planning intervention, the values of all possible surgical and nonsurgical alternatives must be weighed against the possible complications, including the high risk of morbidity, infection, damage to the epiphyses, necrosis, and gangrene. Iatrogenic deformities due to abnormal forces applied to growing bones of a child's foot, which ordinarily might be tolerated by an adult, may include flat-topped talus, rocker-bottom foot, pes planovalgus, and rotational and angular deformities of bone. For example, the compressive forces inherent in persistent, forceful plaster corrections for clubfeet may result in flattening of the talar dome or, rarely, damage to the lower tibial epiphysis (Fig. 60–19). X-ray therapy, once advocated for plantar warts in children, may result in metatarsal epiphyseal plate damage, with secondary ray shortening.

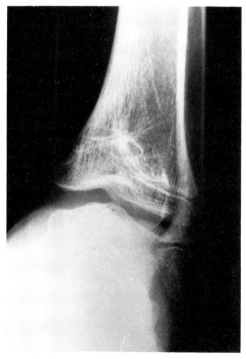

Figure 60–19. *Clubfoot. Note the epiphyseal damage, with premature closure of half of the lower tibial epiphysis and the irregular talar dome. (Courtesy of Melvin H. Jahss, M.D.)*

REFERENCES

1. Anderson, M., and Green, W. T.: Lengths of the femur and the tibia: norms derived from orthoroentgenograms of children from five years of age until epiphysial closure. Am. J. Dis. Child., 75:279, 1948.
2. Arkin, A. M., and Katz, J. F.: The effects of pressure on epiphyseal growth. The mechanism of plasticity of growing bone. J. Bone Joint Surg., 38A:1056, 1956.
3. Ashhurst, A. P. C., and Bromer, R. S.: Classification and mechanism of fractures of the leg bones involving the ankle. Arch. Surg., 4:51, 1922.
4. Barash, E. S., and Siffert, R. S.: The potential for growth of experimentally produced hemi-epiphyses. In Proceedings of the Orthopaedic Research Society. J. Bone Joint Surg., 47A:1100, 1965.
5. Barnicot, N. A., and Datta, S. P.: Vitamin A and bone. In Bourne, G. H. (ed.): The Biochemistry and Physiology of Bone, 2nd ed. New York and London, Academic Press, 1972, Vol. 2, Chapter 5.
6. Berndt, A. L., and Harty, M.: Transchondral fractures (osteochondritis dissecans) of the talus. J. Bone Joint Surg., 41A:988, 1959.
7. Bishop, P. A.: Fractures and epiphyseal separation fractures of the ankle — a classification of 332 cases according to the mechanism of their production. Am. J. Roentgenol., 28:49, 1932.
8. Blais, M. M., Green, W. T., and Anderson, M.: Lengths of the growing foot. J. Bone Joint Surg., 38A:998, 1956.
9. Blount, W. P.: Fractures in Children. Baltimore, Williams and Wilkins, 1955.
10. Bourne, G. H.: Vitamin C and bone. In Bourne, G. H. (ed.): The Biochemistry and Physiology of Bone, 2nd ed. New York and London, Academic Press, 1972, Vol. 2, Chapter 5.
11. Bright, R. W.: Operative correction of partial epiphyseal plate closure by osseous-bridge resection and silicone-rubber implant. J. Bone Joint Surg., 56A:655, 1974.

12. Bright, R. W.: Surgical correction of partial epiphyseal plate closure in dogs by bone bridge resection and use of silicone rubber implants. In Proceedings of the Orthopaedic Research Society. J. Bone Joint Surg., 54A:1133, 1972.

13. Bright, R. W., Burstein, A. H., and Elmore, S. M.: Epiphyseal-plate cartilage. A biomechanical and histological analysis of failure modes. J. Bone Joint Surg., 56A:688, 1974.

14. Bright, R. W., and Elmore, S. M.: Physical properties of epiphyseal plate cartilage. Surg. Forum, 19:463, 1968.

15. Brighton, C. T.: Clinical problems in epiphyseal plate growth and development. AAOS Instructional Course Lectures, St. Louis, C. V. Mosby Co., 1974, Vol. 23, pp. 105–122.

16. Brighton, C. T., and Hunt, R. M.: The Role of Mitochondria in growth plate calcification as demonstrated in a rachitic model. J. Bone Joint Surg., 60A:630, 1978.

17. Carothers, C. O., and Crenshaw, A. H.: Clinical significance of a classification of epiphyseal injuries at the ankle. Am. J. Surg., 89:879, 1955.

18. Cary, J. M., and Norton, C. W. M.: Tibial Diaphyseal Amputations in Children — A Problem in Growth Dysfunction. Paper presented at the Newington Children's Hospital Sixteenth Annual Orthopaedic Clinical Meeting and Alumni Reunion. October 1978.

19. Colville, J.: Drain-cover injuries in children. Br. Med. J., 1:564, 1977.

20. Cooperman, D. R., Spiegel, P. G., and Laros, G. S.: Tibial fractures involving the ankle in children. The so-called triplane epiphyseal fracture. J. Bone Joint Surg., 60A:1040, 1978.

21. Cooperman, E. M.: Anaerobes in clinical practice: frequently forgotten. Can. Med. Assoc. J., 115:298, 1976.

22. Crenshaw, A. H.: Injuries of the distal tibial epiphysis. Clin. Orthop., 41:98, 1965.

23. Dameron, T. B., Jr.: Fractures and anatomical variations of the proximal portion of the fifth metatarsal. J. Bone Joint Surg., 57A:788, 1975.

24. Davidson, J. K.: Aseptic Necrosis of Bone. New York, Elsevier, 1976.

25. Davies, D. A., and Parsons, F. G.: The age order of the appearance and union of the normal epiphyses as seen by x-rays. J. Anat., 62:57, 1927.

26. Department of Health, Education, and Welfare: Health Statistics. Washington, D.C., U.S. Government Printing Office, 1963.

27. Detenbeck, L. C., and Kelly, P. J.: Total dislocation of the talus. J. Bone Joint Surg., 51A:283, 1969.

28. Devas, M. B.: Stress fractures in children. J. Bone Joint Surg., 45B:528, 1963.

29. Digby, K. H.: The measurement of diaphysial growth in proximal and distal directions. J. Anat. Physiol., 1:187, 1915–1916.

30. Dingeman, R. D., and Shaver, G. B., Jr.: Operative treatment of displaced Salter-Harris III distal tibial fractures. Clin. Orthop., 135:101, 1978.

31. DuVries, H. L.: In Inman, V. T. (ed.): DuVries' Surgery of The Foot, 3rd ed. St. Louis, C. V. Mosby Co., 1973.

32. Ehrlich, M. G., Mankin, H. J., and Treadwell, B. V.: Biochemical and physiological events during closure of the stapled distal femoral epiphyseal plate in rats. J. Bone Joint Surg., 54A:309, 1972.

33. Engh, C. A., Robinson, R. A., and Milgram, J.: Stress fractures in children. J. Trauma, 10:532, 1970.

34. Evans, E. B.: Current practices in the prevention and correction of deformity in the severely burned. J. Bone Joint Surg., 52B:782, 1970.

35. Evans, E. B.: Orthopaedic measures in the treatment of severe burns. J. Bone Joint Surg., 48A:643, 1966.

36. Feigin, R. D., Mc Alister, W. H., San Joaquin, V. H., and Middlekamp, J. N.: Osteomyelitis of the calcaneus. Report of eight cases. Am. J. Dis. Child., 119:61, 1970.

37. Fitzgerald, R. N., and Cowan, J. D.: Puncture wounds of the foot. Orthop. Clin. North Am., 6:965, 1975.

38. Freiberg, A. H.: Infraction of the second metatarsal bone, a typical injury. Surg. Gynecol. Obstet., 19:191, 1914.

39. Gardner, E., Gray, D. J., and O'Rahilly, R.: The prenatal development of the skeleton and joints of the human foot. J. Bone Joint Surg., 41A:847, 1959.

40. Giannestras, N. J.: Foot Disorders: Medical and Surgical Management, 2nd ed. Philadelphia, Lea and Febiger, 1973.

41. Giannestras, N. J.: Fractures and dislocations in the foot. In Rockwood, C. A., Jr., and Green, D. P. (eds.): Fractures. Philadelphia, J. B. Lippincott Co., 1975, Vol. 2, pp. 1400–1495.

42. Gill, G. G., and Abbott, L. C.: Practical method of predicting growth of the femur and tibia in the child. Arch. Surg., 45:286, 1942.

43. Golding, C.: Museum pages, V. The sesamoids of the hallux. J. Bone Joint Surg., 42B:840, 1960.

44. Good, C. J., Jones, M. A., and Livingstone, B. N.: Reconstruction of the lateral ligament of the ankle. Injury, 7:63, 1975–1976.

45. Haliburton, R. A., Sullivan, C. R., Kelly, P. J., and Peterson, L. F. A.: The extraosseous and intraosseous blood supply of the talus. J. Bone Joint Surg., 40A:1115, 1956.

46. Harris, W. R.: The endocrine basis for slipping of the upper femoral epiphysis — an experimental study. J. Bone Joint Surg., 32B:5, 1950.

47. Harris, W. R., Martin, R., and Tile, M.: Transplantation of epiphyseal plates — an experimental study. J. Bone Joint Surg., 47A:897, 1965.

48. Hawkins, L. G.: Fracture of the lateral process of the talus. J. Bone Joint Surg., 47A:1170, 1965.

49. Heikel, H. V. A.: Experimental epiphyseal transplantation. Part III. Histological observations. Acta Orthop. Scand., 30:1, 1960–1961.

50. Hermann, G., Schechter, D. C., Owens, J. C., and Starzl, T. E.: The problem of frostbite in civilian medical practice. Surg. Clin. North Am., 43:519, 1963.

51. Huelke, D. F.: Extremity injuries produced in motor vehicle collisions. J. Trauma, 10:189, 1970.

52. Izant, R. J., Jr., and Hubay, C. A.: The annual injury of 15,000,000 children: a limited study of childhood accidental injury and death. J. Trauma, 6:65, 1966.

53. Izant, R. J., Jr., Rothman, B. F., and Frankel, V. H.: Bicycle spoke injuries of the foot and ankle in children: an underestimated "minor" injury. J. Pediatr. Surg., 4:654, 1969.

54. Jinnaka, S.: Jinnaka's Orthopaedics, 20th ed. (revised and edited by T. Ohako). Tokyo, Nan Zando, 1972, pp. 1278–1279.

55. Johanson, P. N.: Pseudomonas infections of the foot following puncture wounds. J.A.M.A., 204:170, 1968.

56. Keddy, J. A.: Accidents in childhood: a report on 17,141 accidents. Can. Med. Assoc. J., 91:675, 1964.

57. Kleiger, B., and Mankin, H. J.: Fracture of the lateral portion of the distal tibial epiphysis. J. Bone Joint Surg., 46A:25, 1964.

58. Kleiger, B.: Mechanisms of ankle injury. Orthop. Clin. North Am., 5:127, 1974.

59. Köhler, A.: Ueber Eine Haufige Bisher Anscheinend' Unbekannte Erkrankung Eizelner Kindlicher Knochen. Munch. Med. Wochenschr., 45:1923, 1908.

60. Langenskiöld, A., and Edgren, W.: Imitation of chondrodysplasia by localized roentgen ray injury — an experimental study of bone growth. Acta Chir. Scand., 99:353, 1950.

61. Langenskiöld, A.: The possibilities of eliminating pre-

mature partial closure of an epiphyseal plate caused by trauma or disease. Acta Orthop. Scand., 38:267, 1967.

62. Langenskiöld, A.: Partial closure of the epiphyseal plate: principles of treatment. International Orthopaedics (SICOT), 2:95, 1978.

63. Leabhart, J. W.: Stress fractures of the calcaneus. J. Bone Joint Surg., 41A:1285, 1959.

64. Letts, R. M., and Mardirosian, A.: Lawnmower injuries in children. Can. Med. Assoc. J., 116:1151, 1977.

65. Lodha, S. C., Mehta, M. C., and Bapna, P. L.: Automobile accidents in children and surface covering of heel defect by thigh graft: a new method. Br. J. Surg., 57:538, 1970.

66. Lynn, M. D.: The triplane distal tibial epiphyseal fracture. Clin. Orthop., 86:187, 1972.

67. Manheimer, D. I., Dewey, J., Mellinger, G. D., et al.: 50,000 child-years of accidental injuries. Public Health Rep., 81:519, 1966.

68. Marmor, L.: An unusual fracture of the tibial epiphysis. Clin. Orthop., 73:132, 1970.

69. Matteri, R. E., and Frymoyer, J. W.: Fracture of the calcaneus in young children, report of three cases. J. Bone Joint Surg., 55A:1091, 1973.

70. McKeever, F. M.: Fracture of the neck of the astragalus. Arch. Surg., 46:720, 1943.

71. Mills, W. J., Jr., Fis, W., and Whiley, R.: Frostbite — experience with rapid rewarming and ultrasonic therapy. Alaska Med., 3:28, 1961.

72. Minnefor, A. B., Olson, M. I., and Carver, D. H.: Pseudomonas osteomyelitis following puncture wounds of the foot. Pediatrics, 47:598, 1971.

73. Milster, A., Sreide, O., Solhaug, J. H., and Raugstad, T. S.: Fractures of the lateral part of the distal tibial epiphysis (Tillaux or Kleiger fracture). Injury, 8:260, 1976–1977.

74. Morrison, W. A., O'Brien, B. M., and MacLeod, A. M.: Major limb replantation. Orthop. Clin. North Am., 8:343, 1977.

75. O'Donoghue, D. H.: Treatment of Injuries to Athletes, 3rd ed. Philadelphia, W. B. Saunders Company, 1976.

76. Onizuka, T., Noda, H., and Sumiya N.: Repair of the amputated great toe. J. Trauma, 16:836, 1976.

77. O'Rahilly, R., Gardner, E., and Gray, D. J.: The skeletal development of the foot. Clin. Orthop., 16:7, 1960.

78. Park, W. H., and DeMuth, W. E., Jr.: Wounding capacity of rotary lawn mowers. J. Trauma, 15:36, 1975.

79. Peterson, C. A., and Peterson, H. A.: Analysis of the incidence of injuries to the epiphyseal growth plate. J. Trauma, 12:275, 1972.

80. Peterson, H. A., Tressler, H. A., Lang, A. G., et al.: Fracture conference. Puncture wounds of the foot. Minn. Med., 56:787, 1973.

81. Poland, J.: Traumatic Separation of the Epiphyses. London, Smith Elder, 1898.

82. Rang, M.: Children's Fractures. Philadelphia, J. B. Lippincott Co., 1974.

83. Ray, R. D., Asling, C. W., Walker, D. G., et al.: Growth and differentiation of the skeleton in thyroidectomized-hypophysectomized rats treated with thyroxin, growth hormone and the combination. J. Bone Joint Surg., 36A:94, 1954.

84. Roser, L. A., and Clawson, D. K.: Football injuries in the very young athlete. Clin. Orthop., 69:219, 1970.

85. Saad, M. N.: The problems of traumatic skin loss of the lower limbs, especially when associated with skeletal injury. Br. J. Surg., 57:601, 1970.

86. Salter, R. B., and Harris, W. R.: Injuries involving the epiphyseal plate. J. Bone Joint Surg., 45A:587, 1963.

87. Salter, R. B.: Injuries of the ankle in children. Orthop. Clin. North Am., 5:147, 1974.

88. Savastano, A. A.: Surgical Treatment of Recurrent Dis-

89. Schweitzer, G.: Injuries to the distal tibial epiphysis. S. Afr. Med. J., 43:1258, 1969.

90. Sever, J. W.: Apophysitis of the os calcis. N.Y. Med. J., 95:1025, 1912.

91. Shapiro, F., Holtrop, M. E., and Glimcher, M. J.: Organization and cellular biology of the perichondral ossification groove of Ranvier: a morphological study in rabbits. J. Bone Joint Surg., 59A:703, 1977.

92. Siffert, R. S.: The effect of trauma to the epiphysis and growth plate. Skeletal Radiol., 2:21, 1977.

93. Siffert, R. S., and Arkin, A. M.: Post-traumatic aseptic necrosis of the distal tibial epiphysis: report of a case. J. Bone Joint Surg., 32A:691, 1950.

94. Siffert, R. S., and Levy, R. N.: Athletic injuries in children. Pediatr. Clin. North Am., 12:1027, 1965.

95. Siffert, R. S.: Osteochondrosis of the proximal femoral epiphysis. AAOS Instructional Course Lectures. St. Louis, C. V. Mosby Co., 1973, Vol. 22, p. 270.

96. Siffert, R. S.: The effect of staples and longitudinal wires on epiphyseal growth, an experimental study. J. Bone Joint Surg., 38A:1077, 1956.

97. Siffert, R. S.: The growth plate and its affections. J. Bone Joint Surg., 48A:546, 1966.

98. Sneed, W. L.: The astragalus; a case of dislocation, excision and replacement; an attempt to demonstrate the circulation in this bone. J. Bone Joint Surg., 7:384, 1925.

99. Spak, I.: Fractures of the talus in children. Acta Chir. Scand., 107:553, 1954.

100. Spiegel, P. G., Cooperman, D. R., and Laros, G. S.: Epiphyseal fractures of the distal ends of the tibia and fibula. A retrospective study of two hundred and thirty-seven cases in children. J. Bone Joint Surg., 60A:1046, 1978.

101. Staples, O. S.: Ruptures of the fibular collateral ligaments of the ankle: result study of immediate surgical treatment. J. Bone Joint Surg., 57A:101, 1975.

102. Stein, R. E., and Stelling, F. H.: Stress fracture of the calcaneus in a child with cerebral palsy. J. Bone Joint Surg., 59A:131, 1977.

103. Steindler, A.: Kinesiology of the Human Body Under Normal and Pathological Conditions. Springfield, Illinois, Charles C Thomas, 1955.

104. Stephens, N. A.: Fracture-dislocation of the talus in childhood: a report of two cases. Br. J. Surg., 43:600, 1956.

105. Sutro, C. J.: Slipping of the capital epiphysis of the femur in adolescence. Arch. Surg., 31:345, 1935.

106. Tachdjian, M. O.: Pediatric Orthopaedics. Philadelphia, W. B. Saunders Company, 1972.

107. Thomas, H. M.: Calcaneal fracture in childhood. Br. J. Surg., 56:664, 1969.

108. Tonna, E. A., and Cronkite, E. P.: Cellular response to fracture studied with tritiated thymidine. J. Bone Joint Surg., 43A:352, 1961.

109. Torg, J. S., and Ruggiero, R. A.: Comminuted epiphyseal fracture of the distal tibia. A case report and review of the literature. Clin. Orthop., 110:215, 1975.

110. Towne, L. C., Blazina, M. E., and Cozen, L. N.: Fatigue fracture of the tarsal navicular. J. Bone Joint Surg., 52A:376, 1970.

111. Trueta, J.: The role of the vessels in osteogenesis. J. Bone Joint Surg., 45B:402, 1963.

112. Trueta, J., and Amato, V. P.: The vascular contribution to osteogenesis. III. Changes in the growth cartilage caused by experimentally induced ischaemia. J. Bone Joint Surg., 42B:571, 1960.

113. Trueta, J., and Little, K.: The vascular contribution to osteogenesis. II. Studies with the electron microscope. J. Bone Joint Surg., 42B:367, 1960.

114. Trueta, J., and Morgan, J. D.: The vascular contribution

location Peroneal Tendons. American Academy of Orthopaedic Surgeons, Film Library.

to osteogenesis. I. Studies by the injection method. J. Bone Joint Surg., *42B*:97, 1960.

115. Trueta, J., and Trias, A.: The vascular contribution to osteogenesis. IV. The effect of pressure upon the epiphyseal cartilage of the rabbit. J. Bone Joint Surg., *43B*:800, 1961.

116. Turco, V. J.: Injuries to the ankle and foot in athletics. Orthop. Clin. North Am., 8:669, 1977.

117. Urano, Y., and Kobayashi, A.: Bone-lengthening for shortness of the fourth toe. J. Bone Joint Surg., *60A*:91, 1978.

118. U.S. Bureau of the Census: U.S. Census of Population and Housing 1960, Census Tracts Final Report: PHC (1)-28. Washington, D.C., U.S. Government Printing Office, 1962.

119. Watson-Jones, R.: Fractures and Joint Injuries, 4th ed. Baltimore, Williams and Wilkins, 4th ed. 1957.

120. Wiley, J. J.: The mechanism of tarso-metatarsal joint injuries. J. Bone Joint Surg., *53B*:474, 1971.

CHAPTER 61

BURNS OF THE FOOT

James E. C. Norris, M.D.

A burn of the foot can be an exceedingly disabling injury. Unless prompt healing of the burned extremity is achieved and stringent rehabilitative measures are undertaken, the patient may be consigned to a degree of disability and discomfort far out of proportion to the extent of his injury. The economic costs due to lost wages and medical care can be staggering — a reality that is compounded when treatment is delayed or inappropriate.

It is therefore incumbent on all concerned with the management of the patient with burns of the feet that four principles of care be rigorously followed: (1) accurate diagnosis of the extent of the injury, (2) immediate institution of measures to lessen the effects of the injuring agent, (3) early closure of the wound, and (4) prompt initiation of rehabilitative measures.

Burn injury may occur from thermal agents, chemicals, electricity, or radiation. As diverse as the agents are, there are many facets that they have in common. The severity of the burn is determined by the intensity of the injuring agent and the duration of contact. Additional factors that influence the severity of burns are the age of the patient and the presence of associated diseases, such as diabetes and arteriosclerosis.

The overall principles of treatment are not affected by the cause of the injury, but the basic treatment plan will have to be modified depending on the injuring agent. Management of thermal burns will be presented in detail. Salient points in the management of electrical, chemical, and radiation burns will be discussed.

THERMAL BURNS

Thermal burns may occur from fire, scalding, or contact with hot objects. Flame burns of the feet are uncommon and are usually seen in the more severely burned patients.[1]

Scalding is a common cause of burns of the feet. It is frequently seen in young children. Symmetric scalding of a child's feet should be viewed with suspicion, as child abuse is an important factor in childhood injury. No cause of injury demands a more thorough history and explanation of the circumstances of the injury than a scald burn in a child.

Contact burns may result from such diverse causes as an elderly person falling asleep with a hot water bag on his foot or molten metal injuries in industry.

Pathophysiology

Although it is common to think of burns in terms of first-, second-, and third-degree injury, it is more accurate to express the depth of injury as partial-thickness and full-thickness. Partial-thickness injury extends through the epidermis and part of the dermis. Full-thickness injury results from destruction of the epidermis, the entire thickness of the dermis, and the skin appendages.

Burn depth is difficult to discern in the

early stages of the injury because the burned area is viewed two-dimensionally, whereas the depth of injury involves the third dimension. There is no simple, accurate method to detect the depth of a burn. Dyes such as Evans' Blue[2] and fluorescein,[3] thermography,[4] and ultrasound[5] have been proposed to measure burn depth, but none has proved to be both simple and accurate.

Another reason burn depth is difficult to discern is that the burn injury is progressive.[6] Progression of the burn injury occurs from the prolonged heat of the tissues and from the tissue injury per se. The graphs shown in Figure 61–1 summarize three facts about the heating and cooling of tissues[7]: (1) The duration of overheating of tissues is considerably longer than contact with the external burning agent; (2) after removal of the heat source, heat continues to penetrate into the depths of the tissues; and (3) cooling of the burned area will result in shortening of the overheating time.

The fact that the severity of the burn injury may progress beyond the moment that the heat source is removed from the tissues has great import clinically. Experimental studies in animals have shown conclusively that cooling will prevent injury

to deeper tissue levels, reduce edema in the burn wound, and reduce mortality.[8-13] Even initiation of cooling three hours after injury is effective in ameliorating the effects of thermal injuries on animals. There is not a great body of experimental data on the cooling of burn wounds in humans because of the obvious difficulties encountered in human experimentation.

Progression of the burn injury unrelated to thermal factors has been documented repeatedly. In his experiments, Hinshaw showed that progression of the injury continued over a 48-hour period following the initial insult.[6] Stasis with sludging of red blood cells in the capillaries and subsequent thrombosis have been observed. Jackson was among the first to outline the histopathology.[14, 15] He described three zones of injury in the burn wound — the zone of hyperemia, the zone of stasis, and the zone of coagulation (Fig. 61–2):

The zone of hyperemia (1) is red and blanches on pressure until it is epithelialized by about 7 days. The zone of stasis (2) is also red to start with and blanches on pressure immediately after burning; but the capillary blood flow stops after some minutes or hours, being complete by the end of 24 hours. After stasis of the capillary circulation, this zone, though still red, no longer blanches on pres-

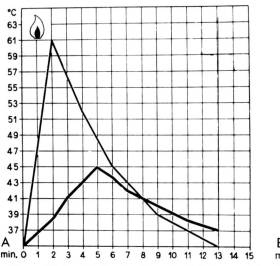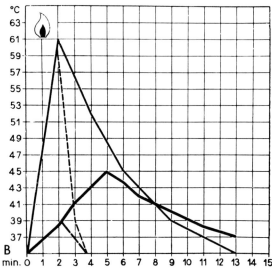

Figure 61–1. *(A) Overheating of rabbit tissues following burning with a flame for two minutes. Light line represents measurements under the skin and heavy line represents measurements at depth of 1 cm. (B) Broken line shows effects of cooling tissues with water at 8° C. (From Rudowski, W.: Burn Therapy and Research. Baltimore, The Johns Hopkins University Press, 1976, pp. 16–17.)*

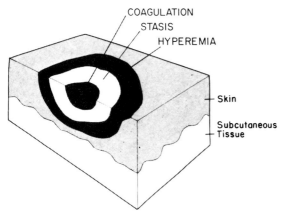

COAGULATION
STASIS
HYPEREMIA

Skin

Subcutaneous
Tissue

Figure 61–2. *The three zones of injury in the burn wound. (Modified from Jackson, D. M.: Br. J. Surg., 40:588, 1953.)*

sure. At this stage histologic examination shows the capillaries dilated and stuffed with red cells. During the next 4 days or so the zone of stasis becomes mottled red and white; it may develop petechial hemorrhages and some pink staining due to hemolysis, and then it becomes white and indistinguishable from the central zone.

The central zone of coagulation (3) is white from the start, and histologically the capillaries are contracted and empty of red cells, as if they had been coagulated in a state of spasm. After about 4 days, zones (1) and (2) are both white and indistinguishable from each other.[14]

The zone of stasis is where progressive dermal ischemia occurs during the first 24 hours after injury.

Robson and associates have postulated that prostaglandins might be responsible for the progressive dermal ischemia.[16, 17] In 1978, Robson and coworkers reported their findings in burned rats in which they demonstrated that leukocytes adhered to the endothelium of vessels of the mesentery, resulting in increased capillary pressure and partial occlusion.[16] That these changes in the microcirculation might be caused by prostaglandins is suggested by the fact that thromboxane A_2 synthesis is increased by injury and/or ischemia. Thromboxane A_2 is produced by platelets and functions as a platelet aggregator and vasoconstrictor. Robson and associates hypothesized that specific antiprostaglandins might neutralize the effects of the prostaglandins and thereby prevent the progression of dermal ischemia. In an experiment

with thermally injured guinea pigs, they demonstrated that the dermal ischemia could be prevented and even reversed by the administration of pharmacologic agents with antiprostaglandin properties.[17] The agents used were indomethacin, acetylsalicylic acid, and 1 per cent topical methylprednisolone.

Zawacki feels that the primary cause of necrosis in the zone of stasis is neither heat nor vascular occlusion, but wound dehydration.[18] He presented evidence demonstrating that through the appropriate prevention of wound dehydration, capillary stasis may be reversed and necrosis may be prevented. In guinea pigs on which he inflicted 5 per cent BSA (body surface area) burns at 75 degrees for 10 seconds, he could reverse capillary stasis through the immediate application of homografts to the burned areas.

Although there is indisputable evidence that immediately following burning there is a progression of dermal ischemia that leads to a deepening necrosis of the burn wound, the causes of this phenomenon are unclear. The solution to the problem will provide the surgeon with an effective weapon to lessen the effects of the injury.

Management of the Acute Burn

Assessment

The first step in managing the acute burn is a careful assessment of the problem. An accurate history of how the burn occurred, the agent that caused the injury, and the time of injury is recorded. The patient is evaluated thoroughly, with special emphasis on the extent and location of the burn injuries, the surface area of the body burned, and the presence of associated injuries. As previously discussed, the depth of the burn is difficult to assess immediately following injury, but the examiner should attempt to assess the depth as accurately as possible. Inspection of the wound and testing for sensation by pinprick will provide most of the information needed to assess the depth of injury.

Armed with a history of the injury and a careful assessment of the wound, intelligent decisions can be made with respect to fluid administration, antibiotic therapy, wound care, and the need for an escharotomy. Unless the burn is definitely superficial (first-degree) or quite small, patients with burns of the foot are best managed in a hospital.

Fluid administration in burn injury is beyond the scope of this chapter.

Circulatory Status

It is essential to perform a baseline evaluation of the circulatory status of the foot at the first examination. Evidence of pre-injury circulatory impairment should be noted. Pre-injury arterial insufficiency, venous insufficiency, or lymphatic obstruction will affect the prognosis in every case.

The lower extremity that has been burned circumferentially must be observed closely. If the burn is full-thickness, the eschar may become a virtual constricting band. Edema from injury will result in occlusion of the blood vessels and gangrene of the distal extremity unless relieved. A cool, cyanotic, painful, pulseless foot is in extreme danger and probably will not be salvable unless an escharotomy and, if necessary, a fasciotomy are performed immediately. It must be kept in mind, however, that clinical assessment of the extremity to determine the need for an escharotomy or fasciotomy may be misleading. Monitoring of the circulatory status with Doppler ultrasound has been advocated as a more objective means of assessment, but tissue ischemia may be present despite evidence of perfusion utilizing Doppler ultrasound.[19]

The measurement of tissue pressure as described by Kingsley and associates[20] and Whitesides and coworkers[21] provides the most accurate assessment of the circulatory status. In any event, if there is doubt as to the circulatory status of the foot, it is best to perform a release.

The technique of escharotomy consists of incising the burned skin through midlateral incisions. The incisions should be started at the margin of unburned skin and burned skin and carried through the eschar until unburned skin is reached. No anesthesia is necessary, as the eschar is anesthetic. Division of the fascia is indicated if the escharotomy fails to result in circulatory improvement of the foot.

Edema of the foot predisposes it to infection, circulatory compromise, and poor healing. It should be counteracted vigorously. The simplest and most expedient measure to counteract edema is strict bed rest with elevation of the foot.

Antibiotic Therapy

Antibiotic therapy may be administered systemically or topically. Systemic antibiotic therapy in burn wound management is not obligatory. Antibiotics should be prescribed intelligently, taking into consideration the mode of injury, the degree of contamination, the past medical history of the patient, and the state of the wound. It is obligatory, however, to do culture studies of the wound before initiating antibiotic therapy.

Topical antibiotic therapy is not obligatory and should be administered with the same considerations as systemic antibiotics.

There is no dearth of agents or substances to apply to burn wounds. There are, however, few substances that meet the criteria for optimal topical therapy for a burn wound. Agents should be low in toxicity, have minimal metabolic effects, should be easy to apply, easy to remove, and effective against the bacterial population of the burn wound, and should penetrate the eschar effectively in order to reduce subescharic infection. Wound healing should not be affected.

Currently, there are three agents used in burn treatment that meet most of these criteria. Delay in eschar separation has been listed as a disadvantage of all three of these agents. Actually, delay of eschar separation is an indication of the effectiveness of the agents against bacterial invasion (see discussion of debridement under Care of the Burn Wound). All three agents listed in Table 61–1 have broad antibacterial spectra, but it is prudent to monitor the wound bacteria by serial cultures and sensitivity studies to ensure that strains resistant to the topical antibiotic are not present.[22]

Care of the Burn Wound

The objectives in care of the burn wound are:
1. To prevent progression of the injury.
2. To prevent infection.

TABLE 61–1. Topical Antimicrobial Agents Employed in Burn Wound Treatment

	SILVER NITRATE	MAFENIDE ACETATE (SULFAMYALON)	SILVER SULFADIAZINE (SILVERDENE)
Bacteriostatic	+	+	+
Hypersensitivity	0	+ 7%	+
Neutropenia	0	0	+
Electrolyte effects	+	0	0
Metabolic effects	0	+	0
Methemoglobinemia	+	0	0
Penetrates eschar	0	+ + + +	+
Painful	0	+ + + +	+
Ease of application	dressing	yes	yes
Stains	+ + + +	0	0

0 = negligible
+ = graded effect, with one + representing the least effect and four + representing the maximal effect

3. To provide an environment in which healing will proceed as rapidly as possible.

Progression of the injury may be retarded by cooling the burned area. No standards have been established for cooling the burn wound in humans,[23] but on the basis of animal studies, the following suggestions are made. Extremely cold water or ice should not be applied. Water cooled to a temperature of about 25° C (77° F) applied for 30 to 45 minutes is probably the safest cooling method. Systemic hypothermia should be avoided.[24]

Progression of the injury may also be retarded by the prevention of drying of the wound.[18, 25] Blisters are left intact. If the blister is tense, aspiration may be performed, but the epidermis should be left on the wound.

In superficial partial-thickness injury, simply covering the wound with gauze impregnated with petrolatum or an antiseptic in a petrolatum base (Xeroform, scarlet red) will provide a protective covering. Application of a biologic dressing such as a xenograft or homograft may effectively impede the progression of the dermal ischemia and provide protection for a wound surface and an optimal environment for healing of the burn wound.[26]

If necrosis has resulted from the burn injury, the wound will not only have to be protected from bacterial contamination, but an environment inimical to bacterial proliferation must be maintained. Necrosis of the burn wound indicates a deep partial-thickness burn or a full-thickness injury.

There are presently no simple, reliable methods to accurately determine the depth of injury. Therefore, the surgeon's judgment is crucial in deciding how the deep partial-thickness or full-thickness burn will be managed. Depending on the condition of the patient, the extent of the burns, and the overall therapeutic objectives, the surgeon may elect to excise the eschar and perform an immediate graft, or he may delay the grafting. He may also treat the wound expectantly, applying topical antibiotics and evaluating the wound daily for evidence of healing. Figure 61–3 indicates an outline of an approach to the deep dermal or full-thickness burn.

Even small burns of the foot that do not show evidence of healing within 8 to 10 days should be debrided and grafted. The wound that heals over a prolonged period by contraction and epithelialization leaves an unstable scar that is subject to repeated breakdown; rehabilitation is delayed, and permanent deformities may develop.

The technique of grafting is as follows: The wound is prepared with topical antibi-

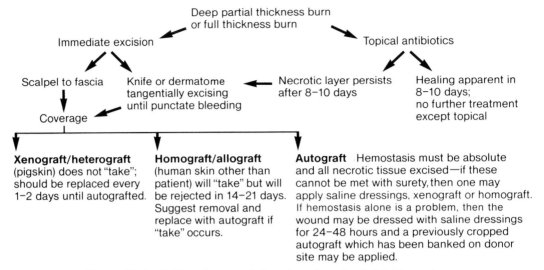

Figure 61–3. *Outline of approach to a deep dermal or full-thickness burn.*

otics until the day before surgery; saline dressings are then applied every three to four hours to reduce the debris and bacterial count of the wound. A wound culture is taken 48 hours before surgery. If laboratory facilities are available, a quantitative culture is taken before the grafting procedure is performed.[27]

The debridement is done surgically, and a xenograft, homograft, or autograft is applied. One should not hesitate to withhold application of the autograft if conditions for its "take" are not favorable. The conditions for "take" are absolute hemostasis, adequate debridement, and a quantitative bacterial count of the wound of less than 10^5 bacteria per gram of tissue. If the autograft is not applied, the freshly debrided wound must be protected from desiccation or a neoeschar will develop, and there will be a new layer of necrosis on the wound. A biologic dressing provides the best protection for the freshly debrided wound.

The skin graft is best taken with a mechanical dermatome, such as the Brown dermatome. The lateral thigh is an excellent donor area, but in a young female, it is better to utilize the buttocks areas (areas beneath the bathing suit) if sufficient skin can be obtained. The skin can be applied as a sheet or passed through the Tanner mesh graft machine.[28] The Tanner mesh graft machine was devised so that numerous slits are cut into the graft to permit expansion of the graft. There are four expansion ratios of mesh grafts available: 1:1.5, 1:3, 1:6, and 1:9. It should rarely be necessary to go beyond the 1:3 expansion ratio. The 1:1.5 expansion ratio is sufficient in nearly all cases. Expanded mesh grafts do cause unsightly scars, so only in situations in which donor skin is not adequate should the skin be expanded. A very acceptable cosmetic result can be obtained by using unexpanded meshed skin grafts, and at the same time, the advantage of drainage is gained. The graft can be covered with a layer of Xeroform or scarlet red dressing and nonfilled gauze and wrapped with a Kling bandage, and if the graft extends over a joint, a well-padded, carefully molded plaster of Paris posterior splint is applied to protect the grafted site from shearing forces. The grafted area is inspected on the fifth postoperative day. Ambulation may be started on the tenth to twelfth postoperative day, but only after the application of an elastic bandage as support for the grafted area.

BURN DEFORMITIES

The management of the burned foot does not end with a healed wound. Should the surgeon terminate management of the injury without making provisions for preventing contracture formation, it may prove costly for the patient. Despite the fact that no open wound exists, the wound bed will contract unless it meets an opposing force.[29] Therefore, forces must be exerted to oppose the burn scar contraction and the eventual contracture formation.

It is helpful to examine the burn deformity in a foot in which no therapeutic program has been carried out.[30-32] Obviously the deformity will depend on where the burn injury occurs. Most burns occur on the dorsal aspect of the foot. The dorsal burn wound contracture usually results in dorsiflexion and hyperextension at the metatarsophalangeal joints. The toes are pulled toward the midaxial line (Fig. 61–4). The deformities result from deep partial-thickness burns, full-thickness burns, or full-thickness burns to which autografts have been applied. Deformities on the plantar surface of the foot consist of flexion of the foot and toes and an equinus deformity.

Prevention of these deformities begins

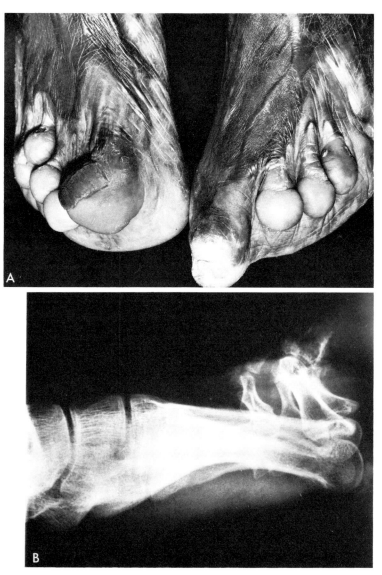

Figure 61–4. (A) Contracture of the dorsal aspect of foot. The toes are pulled toward the midaxial line and hyperextension of the metatarsophalangeal joints exists. (B) Radiograph demonstrating marked hyperextension of metatarsophalangeal joints in a dorsal burn wound contracture. (Courtesy of Melvin H. Jahss, M.D.)

with the initial care of the burn wound. Properly constructed splints will help prevent the equinus deformity.[33] Expeditious closure of the wound will permit the physiatrist to devise an effective plan of physiotherapy. The sooner a molded shoe with padding to oppose the contractile forces of the burn wound is constructed, the greater the chances of preventing the burn scar deformity.[34] The advanced deformity may even respond to a vigorous program of therapy and serial adjustments of a molded shoe. If the deformity cannot be corrected by these measures, a surgical release should be performed.

Surgery for Burn Deformities

The key to successful reconstructive surgery is planning. The technical aspects of the surgery are straightforward and can be mastered with ease, provided one pays attention to every detail. Planning the reconstruction is more demanding. It requires an understanding of the pathophysiology of the deformity, judgment, and the ability to anticipate problems. Regardless of the technical superiority of the surgeon, a poorly planned procedure will fail or at least fall short of the objectives of reconstruction.

Numerous questions must be answered in the planning stage: When is the most propitious time to operate? Is the patient capable of cooperating? Are the conditions of the foot favorable for reconstructive surgery? Is there irreparable bony deformity? Is there tendon shortening? Has rehabilitation medicine personnel been apprised of the planned surgery? What is the most feasible reconstructive plan for the deformity? The only one of these questions in which the answer may be controversial is the first question — When is the most propitious time to operate? The best answer to this question is when all wounds are well healed, the scar is matured, and the patient has achieved maximum benefit from his physical therapy.

The reconstructive surgical procedures have been covered in other chapters, but for most burn scar deformities, release of the contracture and split-thickness skin grafting will suffice. Figure 61–5 illustrates the steps in a release and skin graft of a dorsal foot contracture. It is best to perform the releases under tourniquet. Dorsal foot contractures are released by incising transversely to uninvolved skin or to the midaxial line. Placing the incision in the area of maximum tension assures the greatest release. In extensively contracted wounds, two transverse incisions — one placed proximally and one placed distally — may give a better release. Darting of the incision will give greater release laterally and medially. All contracted bands must be divided to normal tissue. Incisions over tendons should be done with care to avoid dividing the peritenon or even the tendon. It is rarely necessary to excise scar tissue.

Tenotomies need not be done in the reconstruction of the contracted, burned foot. In nearly all cases, the contractures can be overcome by skeletal traction.[33] The recalcitrant equinus deformity may be corrected by the technique of Pannier and associates, in which lengthening of the Achilles tendon is performed.[32]

Absolute hemostasis of the wound is mandatory. A split-thickness skin graft 16 to 18/1000 inch or 0.40 to 0.45 mm thick should be applied. The graft is best taken with a manual dermatome, such as the Reese-Padgett dermatome. A single sheet of skin provides the best coverage. If a single sheet is not available, more than one sheet may be applied, but they should be joined transversely. Sutures (4-0 silk) tied over a cotton bolster will hold the graft in intimate contact with the wound bed. A plaster cast or posterior and anterior plaster splints will provide further immobilization. The stent or bolster dressing may be removed on the third to fifth postoperative day. Splinting of the foot may continue for another five days. By this time, beginning contracture formation can be discerned, and the foot should be placed in a molded splint. Weight bearing or wearing a shoe may not be permitted for another 10 days.

ELECTRICAL BURNS

An electrical burn of the foot may be either low-tension or high-tension and may occur from one of two mechanisms — passage of current through the limb or arcing. The burn does not occur from the

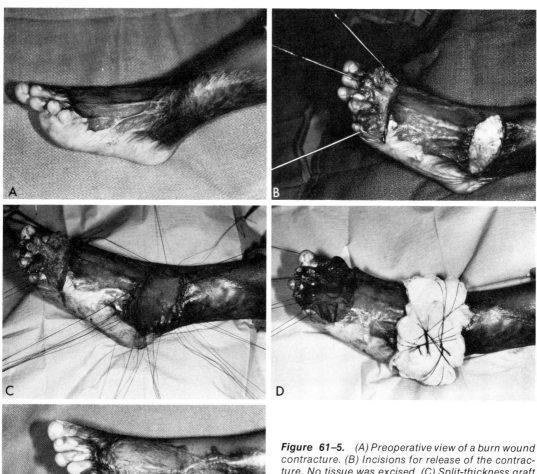

Figure 61–5. *(A) Preoperative view of a burn wound contracture. (B) Incisions for release of the contracture. No tissue was excised. (C) Split-thickness graft sutured in place in the proximal defect. (D) Sutures have been tied over a cotton bolster or stent. The distal defect is covered with a graft. (E) Postoperative view of the deformity six months after the patient was released from the hospital.*

electricity per se, but results when the electrical energy is converted to thermal energy on meeting resistance. The type of current (alternating or direct), amperage of the current, voltage, area of the body through which the current passes, duration of exposure to the current, and the resistance of the body structures all influence the magnitude of injury.

Alternating current is more destructive than direct current because tetanic muscle contractions result, and the victim may be held to the source of the current. Amperage, which in essence is the amount of electricity, or the intensity and voltage, which make up the force behind the pas-

sage of the current, are extremely important in influencing the degree of injury. A low-tension injury occurs when the voltage is not in excess of 1000 volts. In Sweden, 380 volts is the borderline.[35] The low-tension injury is characteristically seen in household situations. High-tension injury is caused when the voltage exceeds 1000 volts. This type of injury is seen in situations such as contact with a power line.

The electricity may enter at a distant point in the body, pass through the limb, and exit from the extremity or vice versa. The wound of entry characteristically has a central area of charring, which is surrounded by a grey-white zone of necrosis. This zone is surrounded by an outer zone of partially necrotic and hyperemic tissue. The wound of exit will have the appearance as though the tissues exploded. Between these wounds, the skin may appear normal, yet underlying the apparently normal skin, there may be extensive soft-tissue injury. The blood vessels may be damaged, and thrombosis or rupture may be imminent.

In the arc-type injury, the current leaps from one conductor to the other. The usual situation is between a source of electricity and part of the body that acts as a conductor. The arc results from ionization of the air between the conductors. Intense heat is generated, reaching a magnitude of 4000° F.

The resistance of the body is at two levels. The first level is that of the skin, which varies according to the thickness; the greater the thickness and the dryer the skin, the greater the resistance. The second level of resistance is afforded by the various tissues below the skin. Bone offers the greatest resistance and nerve the least. The structures in diminishing order of resistance between bone and nerve are fat, tendon, muscle, and blood vessels.[36]

Salvage of the extremity will depend on the extent of the injury, the integrity of the blood vessels, and prevention of ischemic necrosis. The single factor over which the surgeon has greatest control in the emergency care of the electrically injured foot is ischemia. In high-tension injuries, immediate escharotomy and a decompression fasciotomy are imperative.[37] As soon as the patient's condition is stable, debridement of all necrotic tissue should be done. Caution should be exercised, however, in the debridement of nerves. Several operations may be required before debridement is complete.

It is tempting to autograft the wound following initial debridement, but one should be sure of the viability of the tissues in the wound. The best test for viability of the tissues in the wound is by grafting with an allograft. If the allograft "takes," one may safely proceed with reconstruction utilizing an autograft or flap coverage. The selection of the form of coverage (skin graft versus skin flap) will

depend on the location of the wound and whether vital structures are exposed.

CHEMICAL BURNS

Chemical burns of the skin might be more appropriately labeled chemical injuries to the skin. Jelenko stresses that chemical agents coagulate protein by oxidation, reduction, salt formation, corrosion, protoplasmic poisoning, metabolic competitive inhibition, desiccation, and vesicant activity.[38] Injury by thermal activity may occur during the heat of reaction, but this does not occur with all chemical agents.

Factors that influence the severity of a chemical injury are the concentration or pH of the solution, the mode of action of the agent, the vehicle, the volume, and the duration of contact.

Emergency treatment of a chemical injury hinges on knowing what agent caused the injury and the application of the proper antidote. In all chemical injuries, clothing, shoes, and socks should be removed, and all particulate matter should be cleaned away. In nearly all chemical injuries, the most effective expedient is water — immediately and copiously applied. A continuous stream of water (tap water is best; it is readily available and abundant) dilutes and washes away the chemical, reduces the rate of reaction, mitigates the hygroscopic action of the chemical, and restores the pH of the wound to normal.[39]

Chemical injury due to hydrofluoric acid and phosphorus require special treatment beyond irrigation with water. Jelenko feels that water should not be used following injury by these agents.[38] He advocates a boric acid or sodium bicarbonate ($NaHCO_3$) wash for injuries due to hydrofluoric acid and a 2 per cent copper sulfate ($CuSO_4$) solution for injuries due to white phosphorus. In these injuries, the copper sulfate solution should be used only to identify the phosphorus particles; immediate removal of the phosphorus particles is mandatory.[41] (The references at the end of the chapter should be consulted for more details of treatment for specific chemicals.) Tables 61–2 and 61–3 provide

TABLE 61–2. The Pathophysiology and Treatment of Acid Chemical Injury to the Skin*

THE PATHOPHYSIOLOGY OF ACID CHEMICAL INJURY			
Agent (acid)	*Mechanism of action*	*Appearance*	*Texture*
Sulfuric Nitric Hydrochloric Trichloroacetic Phenol	Exothermic reaction, cellular dehydration, and protein precipitation	Gray, yellow, brown, or black	Soft to leathery
Hydrofluoric	Same as other acids + liquefaction and decalcification	Erythema + central necrosis	Painful, leathery eschar

TREATMENT OF ACID INJURY			
Agent (acid)	*Cleansing*	*Neutralization*	*Debridement*
Sulfuric Nitric Hydrochloric Trichloroacetic	Water	Sodium bicarbonate solution, if available (not necessary)	Loose, nonviable tissue and blebs
Phenol	Ethyl alcohol Water	Sodium bicarbonate solution, if available (not necessary)	Debride loose, nonviable tissue and blebs
Hydrofluoric	Water	Zephiran or Hyamine chloride soaks	Debride nonviable tissue and blebs
(Consider primary excision of full-thickness injuries)			

*From Salisbury, R. E., and Pruitt, B. A.: Burns of the Upper Extremity. Vol. XIX in the series Major Problems in Clinical Surgery. Philadelphia, W. B. Saunders Company, 1976.

TABLE 61–3. The Pathophysiology and Treatment of Alkali Chemical Injury to the Skin*

PATHOPHYSIOLOGY OF ALKALI CHEMICAL INJURY			
Agent	*Mechanism of action*	*Appearance*	*Treatment*
Potassium hydroxide Sodium hydroxide Lime	Exothermic reaction; hygroscopic cellular dehydration with saponification of fat and protein precipitation	Erythema with bullae	Painful; "soapy" or slick eschar
Ammonia	Same as other bases; laryngeal and pulmonary edema	Gray, yellow, brown or black often very deep	Soft to leathery
PATHOPHYSIOLOGY OF OTHER CHEMICAL INJURIES			
Phosphorus	Thermal effect, melts at body temperature, runs, ignites at 34°C, acid effect of H_2PO_4	Gray or blue green Glows in dark	Depressed leathery eschar
Mustard gas	Vesicant, alkalization effect	Marked erythema with vesicles and bullae	Painful, soft vesicles and bullae
Tear gas	Weak acid effect	Similar to mild second-degree flame burn	Soft and wet
TREATMENT OF ALKALI INJURY			
Agent	*Cleansing*	*Neutralization*	*Debridement*
Potassium hydroxide Sodium hydroxide Ammonia	Water	0.5–5.0% acetic acid, if available (not necessary)	Debride loose, nonviable tissue
Lime	Brush off powder, then wash with water	0.5%–5.0% acetic acid, if available (not necessary)	Debride loose, nonviable tissue
TREATMENT OF OTHER CHEMICAL INJURIES			
Phosphorus	Water	1% copper sulfate, rinse	Debride and remove particles; keep particles moist
Mustard gas	Water	M-5 ointment	Aspirate; then excise blebs during flushing with water
Tear gas	Water	Sodium bicarbonate solution	Debride loose tissue

*From Salisbury, R. E., and Pruitt, B. A.: Burns of the Upper Extremity. Vol. XIX in the series Major Problems in Clinical Surgery. Philadelphia, W. B. Saunders Company, 1976.

a guide for initial care of the patient with a chemical injury.[42]

Once the emergency treatment of the chemical injury is terminated, the wound is managed just as that of a thermal burn (see Care of the Burn Wound).

RADIATION BURNS

Radiation burns result from damage to cells by exposure to ionizing radiation. There are several types of radiation that may result in injury, but the most common types are alpha particles, beta particles, and gamma particles. The extent of the damage will therefore be determined by the type of irradiation, the amount of irradiation, and the period of exposure. The radiation burn may be described as acute or chronic.

The acute changes may subside completely, and there may be a period of years or months before the late effects are witnessed. The late effects, which are of greatest concern to the surgeon, are radiodermatitis and radionecrosis. These changes are caused by three distinct characteristics of radiation injury: (1) an endarteritis obliterans, (2) excessive fibrosis of the tissue, and (3) cellular changes that occur at the chromosomal level and adversely affect cellular replication.[43] Owing to the propensity of radiation-damaged tissue to develop neoplasia, tissue biopsies should be thoroughly studied before any reconstructive procedures are undertaken.[44]

Chronic ulceration due to radionecrosis affecting the foot may be managed by a number of techniques. Skin grafts will be perfectly adequate in situations in which radiodermatitis has taken place and radionecrosis is superficial. A well-vascularized wound is a prerequisite for grafting.

For the deeper lesions involving tendon, muscle, and even bone, flap coverage should be considered. In the foot that has sustained radiation damage, local flap op-

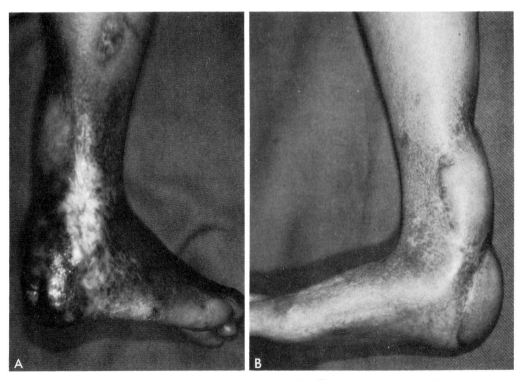

Figure 61–6. *(A) Radiation ulcer of heel of eight years' duration. The patient received radiation to the area 31 years prior to the appearance of the ulcer. Malignancy was suspected, but multiple biopsies were negative. The ulcer and the posterior calcaneus were excised. The defect was covered wtih a cross-leg flap. (B) Postoperative appearance of the heel one year after surgery.*

tions are limited. Distant flaps are among the more prudent alternatives, but radiation injury to the vasculature may preclude the usage of two types of distant flaps — the island flap and the free flap. Figure 61–6 demonstrates a radiation ulcer of the heel that was closed with a pedicle flap.

REFERENCES

1. Artz, C. P., and Moncrief, J. A.: The Treatment of Burns, 2nd ed. Philadelphia, W. B. Saunders Company, 1969.
2. Goulian, D., Jr.: Early differentiation between necrotic and viable tissue in burns. Review of the problem and development of a new clinical approach. Plast. Reconstr. Surg., 27:359, 1961.
3. Bechtold, F., and Lipin, R. J.: Differentiation of full thickness and partial thickness burn with the aid of fluorescein. Am. J. Surg., 109:436, 1965.
4. Mladick, R., Georgiade, H., and Thorne, F.: Clinical evaluation of thermography in determining degree of injury. Plast. Reconstr. Surg., 38:512, 1966.
5. Goans, R. E.: Ultrasonic pulse-echo determination of thermal injury in deep dermal burns. Med. Phys., 4:259, 1977.
6. Hinshaw, R. J.: Early changes in the depth of burns. Ann. N.Y. Acad. Sci., 150:548, 1968.
7. Rudowski, W.: Burn Therapy and Research. Baltimore, The Johns Hopkins University Press, 1976, Chapter 3, pp. 16–17.
8. Ofeigsson, O. J., Mitchell, R., and Patrick, R. S.: Observations on the cold water treatment of cutaneous burns. J. Pathol., 108:145, 1972.
9. Wiedeman, M. P., and Brigham, M. P.: The effects of cooling on the microvasculature after thermal injury. Microvasc. Res., 3:154, 1971.
10. Shulman, A. G., and Wagner, K.: Effect of cold water immersion on burn edema in rabbits. Surg. Gynecol. Obstet., 115:557, 1962.
11. Ofeigsson, O. J.: Water cooling; first aid treatment for burns. Surgery, 57:391, 1965.
12. Ferrer, J. M., Crikelair, G. F., and Armstrong, D.: Some effects of cooling on scald burns in the rat. Surg. Forum, 13:486, 1962.
13. King, T. C., Zimmerman, J. M., and Price, P. B.: Effect of immediate short-term cooling on extensive burns. Surg. Forum. 13:487, 1962.
14. Jackson, D. M.: The diagnosis of depth of burning. Br. J. Surg., 40:588, 1953.
15. Jackson, D. M.: Second thoughts on the burn wound. J. Trauma, 9:839, 1969.
16. Robson, M., C., Kucan, J. O., Paik, K. I., and Ericksson, E.: Prevention of dermal ischemia after thermal trauma. Arch. Surg., 113:621, 1978.
17. Robson, M. C., Del Beccaro, E. J., and Heggars, J. P.: The effect of prostaglandins on the dermal microcirculation after burning, and the inhibition of the effect by specific pharmacological agents. Plast. Reconstr. Surg., 63:781, 1979.
18. Zawacki, B. E.: Reversal of capillary stasis and prevention of necrosis in burns. Ann. Surg., 180:98, 1974.
19. Salisbury, R. E., McKeel, D. W., and Manson, A. D.: Ischemic necrosis of intrinsic muscles of the hand after thermal injuries. J. Bone Joint Surg., 56A:1701, 1974.
20. Kingsley, N. W., Stein, J. M., and Levenson, S. M.: Measuring tissue pressure to assess the severity of burn-induced ischemia. Plast. Reconstr. Surg., 63:404, 1979.
21. Whitesides, T. E., Haney, T. C., Morimoto, K., and Harada, H.: Tissue pressure measurements as a determinant for the need of fasciotomy. Clin. Orthop., 113:43, 1975.
22. Nathan, P., Law, E. J., Murphy, D. F., and MacMillan, B. G.: Laboratory method for selection of topical antimicrobial agents to treat infected burn wounds. Burns, 4:177, 1977–78.
23. Clark, W. R.: Personal communication.
24. Epstein, M. F., and Crawford, J. D.: Cooling in the emergency treatment of burns. Pediatrics, 52:430, 1973.
25. Forage, A. V.: The effects of removing the epidermis from burnt skin. Lancet, 2:690, 1962.
26. Miller, T. A., Switzer, W. E., Foley, F. D., and Moncrief, J. A.: Early homografting of second degree burns. Plast. Reconstr. Surg., 40:117, 1967.
27. Robson, M. C., Krizek, T. J., and Heggers, J. P.: Biology of surgical infection. Curr. Probl. Surg., 10:3, 1973.
28. Tanner, J. C., Jr., Vandeput, J., and Olley, J. F.: The mesh skin graft. Plast. Reconstr. Surg., 34:287, 1964.
29. Larson, D. L., Abston, S., Evans, E. B., et al.: Techniques for decreasing scar formation and contractures in the burned patient. J. Trauma, 11:807, 1971.
30. Heimburger, R. A., Marten, E., Larson, D. L., et al.: Burned feet in children. Am. J. Surg., 125:575, 1973.
31. Achaner, B. M., Bartlett, R. H., and Wilson, L. F.: Burns of the feet. J. Foot Surg., 15:43, 1976.
32. Pannier, M., Visset, J., and Mousseau, P. A.: Surgical treatment of equinus deformities of the ankle following burns. Ann. Chir. Plast., 21:289, 1976.
33. Evans, E. B., Larson, D. L., Abston, S., and Willis, B.: Prevention and correction of deformity after severe burns. Surg. Clin. North Am., 50:1361, 1970.
34. Holley, D., and Harris, C. N.: Hyperextension deformity of burned toes. Burns, 3:215, 1977.
35. Skoog, T.: Electrical injuries. J. Trauma, 10:816, 1970.
36. Robinson, D. W., Masters, F. W., and Forrest, W. J.: Electrical burns. A review and analysis of 33 cases. Surgery, 57:385, 1965.
37. Mann, R. J., and Wallquist, J. M.: Early decompression fasciotomy in the treatment of high voltage electrical burns of the extremities. South. Med. J., 68:1103, 1975.
38. Jelenko, C., III: Chemicals that "burn." J. Trauma, 14:65, 1974.
39. Bromberg, B. E., Song, I. C., and Walden, R. H.: Hydrotherapy of chemical burns. Plast. Reconstr. Surg., 35:85, 1965.
40. Walfort, F. G., DeMeester, T., Knorr, N., and Edgerton, M.: Surgical management of cutaneous lye burns. Surg. Gynecol. Obstet., 131:873, 1970.
41. Orcutt, T. J., and Pruitt, B. A.: Chemical injuries of the upper extremity. In Salisbury, R. E., and Pruitt, B. A. (eds.): Burns of the Upper Extremity (Volume XIX in the series: Major Problems in Clinical Surgery). Philadelphia, W. B. Saunders Company, 1976.
42. Salisbury, R. E., and Pruitt, B. A.: Burns of the Upper Extremity. Vol. XIX in the series Major Problems in Clinical Surgery. Philadelphia, W. B. Saunders Company, 1976.
43. Robinson, D. W.: Surgical problems in the excision and repair of radiated tissue. Plast. Reconstr. Surg., 55:41, 1975.
44. Hartwell, S. W., Huger, W., Jr., and Pickrell, K.: Radiation dermatitis and radiogenic neoplasms of the hands. Ann. Surg., 160:828, 1964.

Part VII

ORTHOTIC FOOT MANAGEMENT

CHAPTER 62

PADDING AND DEVICES TO RELIEVE THE PAINFUL FOOT

Joseph E. Milgram, M.D.

An astonishing number of people annually seek relief from temporary and prolonged attacks of foot pain. If a fifth of the population of the United States complained, 100 million feet would become centers of attention each year. Usually, the vast bulk of complaints reach the shoe salesman first. The suppliers and fitters of footwear are currently increasingly aware of the need for information.

Some of the office measures that may be used to relieve patients suffering from pain acute enough to direct them to medical services are simple and often mechanical in nature. Some are of temporary value, useful as adjuncts to other forms of therapy; still others are of a more lasting character.

The patient's history, including the complaint, past and present, is essential to diagnosis. Judicious questions will help to indicate whether the lesion is dermatologic, single or multiple, of central or peripheral origin, or associated with vascular patterns of appearance and relief, with neurologic defects, or other diseases.

Although the physician's initial examination of the foot is general, it is critical to his evaluation and plans for further diagnostic laboratory and roentgenographic measures. It must be a functional examination that takes into account sensory, peripheral vascular, and motor kinesiologic details. The physician must be acutely attentive to findings that might serve to indicate that the foot is but a peripheral clue to another condition, such as tabes, diabetes, peripheral vascular disease, a discal or foramenal spinal encroachment, an unsuspected meningomyelocele, a blood dyscrasia, an epiphyseal dysplasia, an inherited blood abnormality, a neoplasm, a metabolic defect such as gout, or just unusual environmental, habitual, or athletic propensities. The patient's shoes must also be examined. Finally, after the physician has studied the roentgenograms for common and uncommon lesions, including early stress fracture, and has requested blood and urine tests for the next visit, he makes a probable diagnosis. He again seeks evidence from the patient that the pain could reasonably arise from the presumed cause and then determines the form of treatment that is most likely to provide relief.

This chapter considers briefly some aspects of the use of pads as protectors and stress shifters and their continued comfortable presence on insoles and in appropriate shoes. Padding for relief of the pain of Morton's neuroma will be mentioned in some detail. The utilization of pads to relieve the discomfort of hallux rigidus will exemplify their use to shift and change the point of application of weight-bearing stresses. Padding for the hammer toe and short heel cord will also be mentioned. Sole alterations in stiff ankles will be suggested as more simple means of relieving foot pain. Pads and strapping are also beneficial for painful ligaments and lesions causing heel pain.

PADS

Pads are applied for the following reasons:

1. To transfer weight-bearing stresses from painful areas to selected painless zones (as for joint ligament or metatarsal pain, Freiberg's osteochondritis of the metatarsal head, a fractured sesamoid, or a calcaneal spur area).

2. To shield skin lesions, such as boils, those associated with gout, calluses, corns, warts, and areas to which medication has been applied, from weight-bearing stress or shoe contact.

3. To guard against pressure breakdown of hypesthetic, sensitive, marginally vascular areas of skin and fascia during use of the foot and to bypass dangerous zones (areas of excessive skin pressure) and shield skin nerves from pressure.

4. To shield painful areas (e.g., bunion bursae, corns, exostoses ["Überbeins"], hammer toes).

5. To separate structures that are compressing or in contact with a tender structure (e.g., the metatarsals adjacent to a Morton's neuroma, toes with soft corns and exostoses on their adjacent surfaces, for which both metatarsal spreading and toe spreading are sought).

6. To maintain, by passive support, painless alignment of bones during gait, which otherwise can be maintained only by active and fatiguing muscle activity (e.g., in hallux rigidus).

7. To diminish weight-bearing stresses on operatively realigned structures until shoes or supports of permanently protective nature can be provided or until healing has been completed (as after metatarsophalangeal joint resections in arthritic feet).

8. To facilitate function of shortened, cocked-up toes (with hammer toes, for example, a toe crest pad "brings the ground up to the toes" and permits them to function during gait and takes some stress off the metatarsal heads).

9. To tilt the foot to relieve pain (e.g., a heel raise for a calcaneal spur or a longitudinal arch support for painful, relaxed flatfoot with tender talonavicular ligaments).

Pads may be made of felt or rubber, but long ago I learned that pads made of prepared ¼-inch, adhesive-backed, medium-density sponge rubber are much easier to prepare and apply. The sponge (not foam) rubber does not collapse on use, for it contains encysted air bubbles without communication, in contrast to those in soft foam rubber. Such special sponge rubber is furnished in yard-long rolls that are 8 inches wide and with the adhesive surface covered with a removable protective layer of corrugated plastic or paper. The pad is easily cut into the desired shape with bandage scissors. During this process, the plastic protective layer should remain in place to prevent the adhesive backing from sticking to the scissors. To facilitate removal of the plastic, one edge should project beyond the rubber. If this is not done, separating the plastic from the completed rubber pad may be difficult. The pad is cut into its final shape with its edges beveled with the scissors. If necessary, the pad may be built up in areas by adding an additional layer or a trimmed half layer of rubber. When completed, the adhesive surface of the pad is applied to the skin of the foot in the appropriate area, usually proximal to the tender area, over a protective adhesive that has been applied previously and has dried.

Skin Preparation and Care for Pad Application

The skin is first protected with a skin glue or varnish. The formula of Leo Roth, recently marketed as B-D Adherent, has been most satisfactory in preventing local allergic reactions to the rubber pad. I have encountered only two instances of sensitivity, neither of which was severe. Compound tincture of benzoin (aerosol packed) is almost equally good, but it dries more slowly.

For relief of pain "beneath the metatarsals," the pad is placed in the desired location not beneath but directly proximal to the palpable and often tender bony prominences. It is finally covered with a layer of adhesive tape. I prefer to use Dermicel, a nylon adhesive tape that is 1 inch wide and packed in rolls. The first strip of tape is tucked in against the back edge of the pad, where it is fastened to the skin with pressure from a finger to prevent the tape from migrating toward the heel under the repeated impact of weight bearing, especially in women who wear high heels.

It may not be amiss at this point to remark that in removing adhesive tape and a pad glued anywhere to the plantar surface, the distal edge should first be elevated from the skin. After the adhesive strapping has been carefully split with bandage scissors, both it and the pad can be peeled off safely, always working toward the heel. The "grain" of the skin of the foot appears to be such that if an adherent callus or tape is peeled off toward the toes instead of toward the heel, there is a tendency to pull off the skin and tear deeper into skin layers, often causing bleeding.

When patients who are wearing such pads are bathing, they are advised to cover the foot with a plastic bag held in place with rubber bands. The foot, toes, and nails may be carefully washed separately to avoid maceration of the skin beneath the pad and tape.

If strapping has to be applied to the foot and ankle, the wearing of boots is liable to markedly increase and spread a silent infection from the nails. Knee-high boots are even worse.

Metatarsal Pads

Pads are designed for the individual foot and problem; they should not be applied empirically, but on the basis of the specific kinesiologic problem of the foot. They are the means of relieving one portion of a foot from painful pressure by transferring weight-bearing stresses and function to other precisely outlined areas, usually adjacent areas, where weight bearing can be tolerated painlessly.

In the metatarsal area, the painful weight-bearing zones are commonly situated over bony prominences such as the metatarsal heads, especially if they are depressed and exposed by hammer-toe dorsiflexion of the proximal phalanges, an equinus position of the foot, shortening of the first metatarsal shaft, distal migration of subcutaneous pads, or rotation (pronation or supination) of the fore part of the foot. Pads are therefore designed to transfer and distribute the body weight to the commonly painless necks and shafts of specific metatarsals.

The triangular or pear-shaped pads of sponge rubber of different sizes that are usually stocked by shoe and drug stores are occasionally grossly useful and partially adequate if the lesion involves mainly the third and fourth metatarsals. These pads are less efficient for lesions of the second metatarsal head. They are poorly shaped and almost useless if the metatarsophalangeal joint of the hallux is the site of stress and distress, unless they are very thick, in which case they may afford partial relief initially, but they subsequently initiate new complaints. Pads must be made accurately to fit the individual patient's needs. Stock pads should not be relied on.

The most useful pad for decompressing painful areas beneath the second, third, and fourth metatarsal heads is one that precisely transfers stresses to the neck and distal portion of the shaft of the first metatarsal, which is by far the sturdiest metatarsal and tolerates weight-bearing burdens with apparent ease. A pear-shaped pad will not transfer the stress in this way. A special right-angle pad (Fig. 62–1) is most often found to be necessary. The longitudinal portion of this pad, which is parallel to the long axis of the foot, is located under the shafts and necks of the second, third, and often the fourth metatarsals, proximal to their heads. The other arm of the right angle, which is parallel to the transverse axis of the foot, is located beneath the neck and shaft of the first meta-

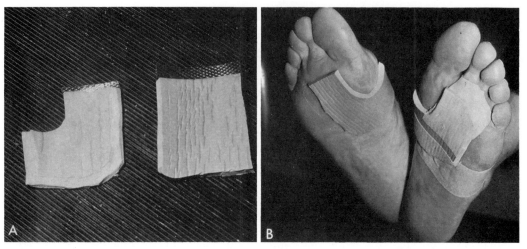

Figure 62–1. *(A) Right-angle pad edges are beveled. (B) Pads applied to transfer stress off the first metatarsal heads.*

tarsal, just behind the head and sesamoids. This arm should extend and wrap well around the shaft medially and along the shaft proximally for 1.0 to 1.5 inches to provide an adequate area of support for the body weight by the first metatarsal shaft.

For contact pain limited to the big toe or the sesamoids, the longitudinal arm is extended forward, with its terminal ½ inch thinned a bit, under the heads of the second, third, and fourth metatarsals, not just under the shafts, and the broad, transverse arm of the pad is adjusted to fit snugly behind the metatarsal head and sesamoids of the big toe (Fig. 62–2). This arm can be built up with an additional full or half layer of sponge rubber (or felt). When the second metatarsal head area is painful, as occurs when the first metatarsal is congenitally short, the longitudinal arm of the pad should end just behind the second metatarsal head, and the transverse arm should

extend under the first metatarsal to just behind its head.

Extensions of pads directly beneath the second, third, and fourth metatarsal heads when they are painless permit these structures to bear part of the weight of a painful first metatarsophalangeal joint, provided the neck of the first metatarsal is made to bear the major portion through use of a pad shaped in this way (see Figures 61–1B and 61–11B, C).

It may be noted that no use has been made of the area of the fifth metatarsal shaft in designing most pads for weight bearing. In the majority of patients, the shaft of the fifth metatarsal should not be supported. The pad should be accurately trimmed and thinned laterally, so that when applied, it will not raise the fifth metatarsal shaft off the sole of the shoe or the insole surface.

This rule should be disregarded, howev-

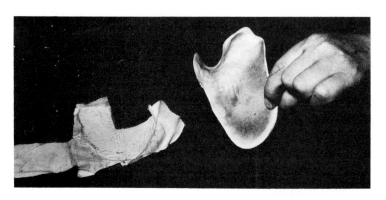

Figure 62–2. *Right-angle pad replaced by a short insole for a shoe for a patient with a sesamoid injury.*

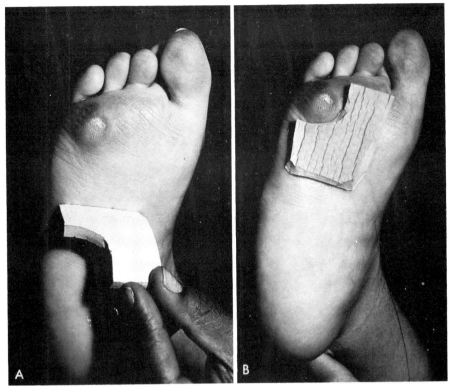

Figure 62–3. *(A) Painful prominence of the fifth metatarsal head. (B) Pad applied to relieve the area of stress on weight bearing.*

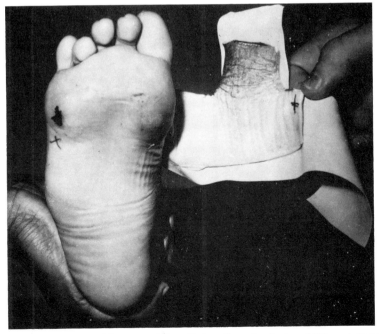

Figure 62–4. *T-shaped pad used in cavus deformity to relieve the first and fifth metatarsal head areas.*

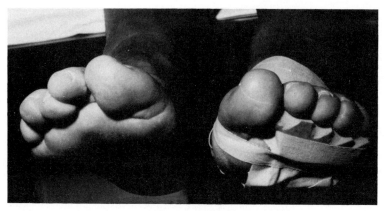

Figure 62–5. *End view of a scalloped toe crest pad.*

er, when the fifth metatarsal head area is the site of a painful callus or a plantar wart, when the fifth metatarsal is in an equinus position relative to the rest of the foot, when the heel cord is tight and the patient must wear high heels, or when the fifth metatarsal is shortened as the result of trauma or growth disturbance. In such cases, the weight-supporting transverse arm of the pad must be extended laterally and must be carefully shaped to be thickest proximal to the palpably prominent fifth metatarsal head (Fig. 62–3). If lateral shielding from the shoe is needed, a separate curved shield is cut from stock and applied temporarily.

For a cavus foot, a T-shaped pad with both a lateral and a medial transverse arm may be used (Fig. 62–4).

Toe Crest Pad

In cases of excessive tenderness in the metatarsal area, it is at times useful to apply an adherent rubber toe crest pad. It consists of a slightly curved, ½-inch-wide strip of sponge rubber that is convex distally and sometimes scalloped to fit behind the second through fourth toes and possibly the fifth toe. It fills the space under each proximal phalanx and gives each toe an additional fulcrum on which to press. Thereby some stress is taken off the tender metatarsophalangeal joint area. The toe

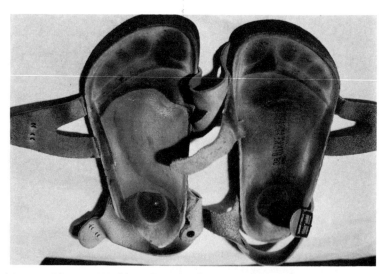

Figure 62–6. *A toe crest incorporated into the sole of a sandal (seen best on the right). The left sandal is modified by inserting a pad shaped to transfer stress to the neck and shaft of the first metatarsal.*

crest pad is shaped to each foot individually; usually the hallux and the fifth toe are excluded. If it is properly cut, the pad is found to be comfortable at once. Scalloping is easily and rapidly accomplished with bandage scissors (Fig. 62–5). The toe crest pad is held in place by a cross strip of nylon adhesive tape.

Such pads are very frequently incorporated on an insole or the strap or sole of the shoe (Fig. 62–6). Separate commercial toe crest "sausages" that are held in place with elastic are available.

MORTON'S NEUROMA

On further study, the adult patient, usually female, with paroxysms of forefoot pain radiating into two toes is often found to be suffering from the lesion described by Durlacher in 1845[2] and Morton in 1876[8] and attributed by Betts in 1940[1] to a neuroma of the digital nerve. Reed and Bliss directed attention to fibrinoid deposition if fibroadipose tissue adjacent to the so-called neuroma and interpreted the findings as regressive and productive intermetatarsal elastofibrositis. In 1976, Lassmann and associates described the Morton lesion as perineural thickening with endoneural edema, nerve fiber degeneration, and vascular wall thickening and hyalinization. Adjacent tissues, such as the intermetatarsal bursa, are also involved. In any case, excision of the lesion has given most patients complete relief. Recurrence is seldom experienced and seldom reported. New York City colleagues estimated their failure rate to be between 3 per cent and 7 per cent. Several patients experienced very disturbing causalgic pain with recurrence.

I have treated many patients with Morton's neuroma with a "spread pad." The first such patient was pregnant, and the second had a cardiac condition; both had been refused surgery for excision of the neuroma. They both obtained prompt relief from treatment with a spread pad.

I have also treated with a spread pad 22 patients who had recurrence after having undergone surgery for excision of the neuroma. Of these 22 patients, three left to seek relief elsewhere and 19, four of whom experienced causalgia after recurrence, achieved comfort and ability to walk freely, provided they continued to use their corrective footwear.

In the past 19 years, 25 patients with classic nonoperated Morton's neuroma have also been so treated. In 21 of the 25 individuals, complaints of foot pain ceased after treatment. Consequently, I continue to use spread pads, applying this very simple principle: "One seeks to spread the metatarsals at the affected interspace and keep them spread on weight bearing."

With the foot supported comfortably at the level of the physician's eye, the patient is requested to relax and look elsewhere. The physician uses the tip of his index finger to explore just behind the palpable involved metatarsal heads. Pressure is applied with the finger tip, seeking a precise, small area where pressure will cause the two affected toes to visibly separate. This spot is outlined with a pen for application of a spread pad.

The pad, which is approximately ¼ inch thick, ⅜ to ½ inch wide, and ¾ inch long, is cut in advance from adhesive-backed, rubber stock. Glue is applied to the skin, and when it has dried, the pad is applied to the pressure site (Fig. 62–7A). Pressure on the pad at this site must demonstrably cause the toes to separate, or it is shifted to where it will do so (Fig. 62–7B). The pad is covered with strips of 1-inch-wide, thin, nylon Dermicel tape.

It is my current practice to provide an additional L-shaped pad that supports the first metatarsal shaft up to its head as well as the neck and shaft of the second metatarsal (Fig. 62–8). This pad is separate from the spread pad. The vertical limb is ½ to ¾ inch wide and about 1¼ inches long. The horizontal limb under the first metatarsal is about 1¼ to 1½ inches wide. I also supply the patient with several small, ¼-inch, square rubber pads, one of which is to be worn between the affected toes to reinforce toe spreading.

In several severe cases, the padding, which must be worn constantly, was renewed at 7- to 12-day intervals for several months before encircling thin leather straps were applied or permanent insoles were made (with the removed straps being used as models by the insole maker).

If leather straps are used, a 1-inch square of adhesive, half on the skin of the

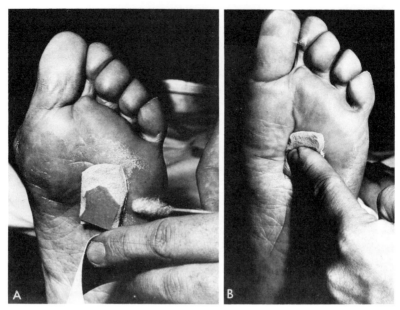

Figure 62–7. *(A) Small spread pad for Morton's neuroma. (B) Test for correct placement. Pressure on this spread pad visibly separates the third and fourth toes.*

sole and half on the leather, spread-pad metatarsal strap, is applied by the patient until shrinkage holds the strap in place. The stocking is worn over the strap. Usually, a replica insole replaces the strap at a later date and is worn in all types of footwear indefinitely.

At the initial visit, the patient is usually able to judge instantly if the pads will relieve the pain on standing and walking.

Shoes with an adequate width are essential. Since changes are painstaking, sufficient office time must be provided initially for often prolonged trials.

After relief has been obtained with the spread pad, the choice of surgical excision of the neuroma with a relatively small percentage of failure or of continued painstaking insole and shoe attention is presented to the patient. Of the previously

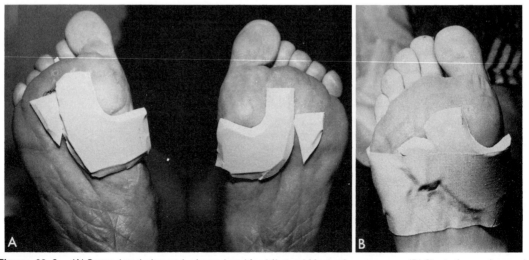

Figure 62–8. *(A) Spread pad plus an L-shaped pad for bilateral Morton's neuromas. (B) Start of securing pads in place.*

mentioned 18 patients with Morton's neuroma who obtained relief with a spread pad, none chose to undergo surgery. Nevertheless, in my opinion, surgical excision is still the best method of providing prompt and usually lasting relief to patients suffering from the most severe forms of this disturbing pathologic lesion. However, I am obliged to offer the alternative of prolonged and troublesome conservative care by letting the patient actually experience treatment and relief with a spread pad. Such a conservative program amplifies the statistical information that the patient must consider to grant adequately informed consent for surgical excision of the involved area of nerve.

HALLUX RIGIDUS GAIT

Consideration of the gait in hallux rigidus (hallux flexus) suggests therapeutic measures that usually permit the orthopaedist to provide prompt relief in his office to patients suffering from what may often be severe pain and disability of the big toe. As the foot is placed on the ground in normal gait, body weight is borne first on the heel and then progressively along the outer border of the foot until the weight is on the metatarsal area. The metatarsophalangeal joints then dorsiflex, and as the foot leaves the ground, the toes, especially the big toe, plantar flex and push away from the ground. If the metatarsophalangeal joint of the hallux is incapable of even passive dorsiflexion because of rigidity, body weight forcibly dorsiflexes the big toe, producing instant and usually severe metatarsophalangeal joint pain. It is for this complaint that the patient with hallux rigidus most commonly seeks relief.

If patients with severe hallux rigidus are observed walking barefoot, it is evident that weight is borne on the outer border of the foot, until the weight is on the region of the fifth metatarsal head (Fig. 62–9A). The patient then actively plantar flexes the big toe and the lesser toes and inverts and adducts the fore part of the foot, with the result that the foot leaves the ground from the tip of the terminal phalanx of the big toe without motion of the metatarsophalangeal joint. In this way, the painful metatarsophalangeal joint is bypassed. To walk

in this way, the patient must contract the strong flexor muscles of the hallux and transfer the body weight from the tip of the big toe through the first metatarsal shaft, with the first metatarsal head and metatarsophalangeal joint held off the ground. Such active effort is very tiring (Fig. 62–9B). As time passes, the skin under the terminal phalanx thickens, whereas that under the first metatarsophalangeal joint appears thin or even abnormally delicate (Fig. 62–9C).

Evidence of this type of gait can be seen in the patient's shoe: (1) the crease at the break of the shoe is oblique instead of transverse; (2) the sole shows most wear along the back of the outer side of the heel and under the fifth metatarsal base, whereas medially the sole is worn just proximal to the point where the end of the oblique crease intersects the medial border of the shoe (area of pivoting on the great toe); (3) the area of the sole under the metatarsophalangeal joint of the big toe shows no wear; and (4) a well or depression appears in the sole where the terminal phalanx of the big toe pivots actively in equinus as the fore part of the foot leaves the ground.

To provide relief conservatively:

1. Choose a shoe last that permits the fore part of the foot to adduct and provides enough room for the big toe to plantar flex freely, particularly for the metatarsal and metatarsophalangeal joint to rise without the dorsum of the metatarsophalangeal joint being abraded by the lining of the shoe. In other words, the adducted forefoot last shoe must provide increased space above the metatarsophalangeal joint of the big toe (Fig. 62–10). An upper made of flexible leather is also helpful.

2. Under the shaft of the first metatarsal, insert an adequate (considerable) raise that does not extend under the metatarsophalangeal joint. The shaft should be passively supported, thus relieving the plantar flexors of the great toe of an otherwise almost intolerable burden (Fig. 62–11). The raise is made high enough (double) to permit the big toe to be flexed and extends laterally, diminishing in thickness under the second and third metatarsals. Such a doubly thick, right-angle rubber pad is shaped with scissors and is applied in the office initially. Later, an insole is

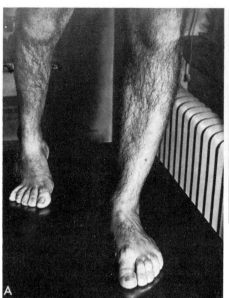

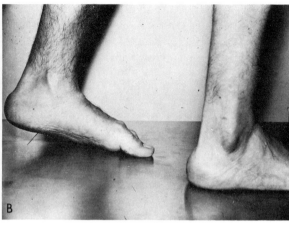

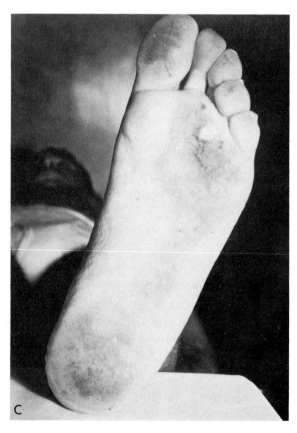

Figure 62–9. *(A) Hallux rigidus gait. Compensation for inability to dorsiflex the big toe. The metatarsophalangeal joint of the big toe supports weight and stress by plantar flexing. (B) Tiring flexor support. (C) Characteristic soiling pattern of the sole in hallux rigidus. The phalanx of the big toe, the other toes, and the outer border of the foot are soiled. The skin over the first metatarsophalangeal joint is soft and clean (untouched in gait).*

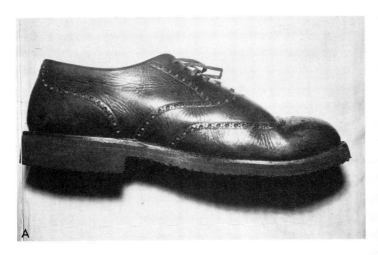

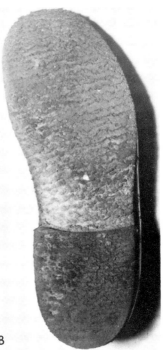

Figure 62–10. *(A) Shoe for hallux rigidus provides room for big toe motion. (B) Adducted forefoot last. Latex sole.*

made incorporating this raise, or the raise can be built into the molded inner sole of the shoe.

3. A genuine latex sole (not merely rubber) on the shoe tends to compensate automatically for any error in shoe correction provided.

In practice, the patient who limps into the office with acutely painful hallux rigidus can usually be relieved promptly by two measures: (1) application of a right-angle pad with adequate (often double-layer) thickening extending distally to just behind the first, second, and third metatarsal heads and (2) stretching the shoe in the "bunion area" with a shoemaker's "swan" (Fig. 62–12) or, with the patient's permission, splitting the shoe (often a blucher in men) to create adequate room over the big toe for plantar flexion during walking.

A new shoe with its fore part adducted (adducted last) is then ordered for the promptest possible delivery. This new shoe is stretched locally over the area of the hallux with a wooden screw shoe stretcher to which a dorsal hump has been attached to the last in the area to be stretched. Moistening the leather locally helps fix the correction. The proprietor of the orthopaedic shoe store or the insole

maker will usually make this adjustment, following the instructions of the orthopaedist. Latex-soled shoes with adducted lasts are commercially available. Custom-made shoes are rarely needed. Molded space shoes are usually beneficial if design is supervised.

After the patient has been relieved of acute pain, surgical correction by a permanent type of joint resection procedure should be considered. A hallux rigidus is often gouty and is more common in men, and blood tests are regularly ordered. I have found that after they have obtained relief of pain, most men will elect to continue conservative treatment indefinitely. Women, however, are much more likely to request surgical treatment because it will enable them to wear regular shoes with higher heels. They are informed that the resected joint will be weaker but relatively painless and that metatarsal padding will be of value in the future.

Patients with hallux rigidus should trim their nails long and, of course, transversely. Because it pivots in plantar flexion, the big toe especially may develop an ingrown toenail if the nail is cut short.

In long-standing unoperated cases, the interphalangeal joint of the big toe usually

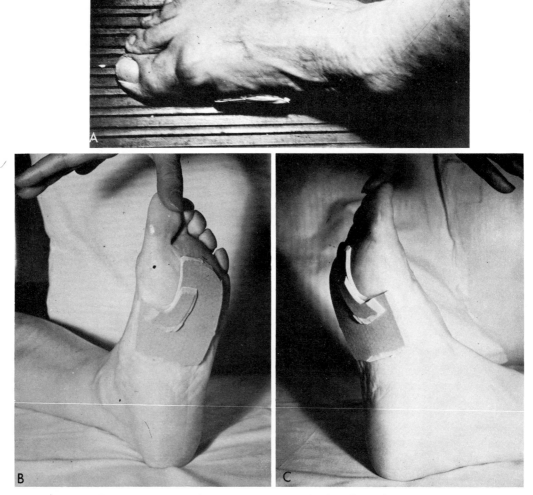

Figure 62–11. *(A) Support beneath the first metatarsal on application of pad gives prompt relief. (B and C) Pad applied. There is a raise of double thickness beneath the second and third metatarsal shafts, providing support to the neck and shaft of the first metatarsal.*

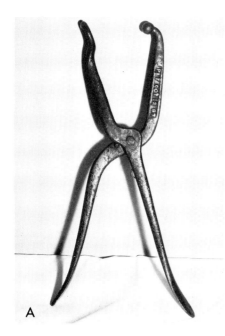

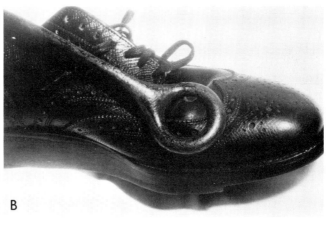

Figure 62–12. *(A) Shoemaker's "swan" for stretching a local area of a shoe. (B) "Swan" in use. The leather should be moistened before swan is used.*

acquires an increased range of dorsiflexion in addition to its normal plantar flexion, providing a partial substitute for some lost metatarsophalangeal joint plantar flexion.

PAINFUL HAMMER TOES

Hammer toes, even those with metatarsophalangeal subluxation or dislocation, may be made comfortable temporarily by local shields of various materials. A supply of commercial polyurethane tubing of assorted diameters can be cheaply stocked in the office and cut to shape, with one end cut transversely and the proximal end cut obliquely. The patient can be taught to cut the tubing himself. The proximal thickness of the shield, which is glued to skin, will serve to give immediate comfort. Under-and-over application of an adhesive strip can be used to hold a flexible hammer toe back in place between the two toes adjacent to it. There are also commercially available plantar rubber plates with rubber tubes to retain the toe if the contracture is not too severe, but they are not easy for the patient to apply.

A shoemaker's "swan" enables the patient's shoe to be stretched in the office (see Figure 62–12).

Daily manipulation by stretching the dorsal metatarsophalangeal joint capsule and elongating the deformed toe with gentle but firm tension has materially improved moderate or early cases of hammer toe, somewhat to my surprise.

After patients with severely contracted hammer toes have been provided with immediate relief in the office, if possible, they are advised as to the degree of the relief of pain and of deformity and the alternate state of function that can be expected from any operation proposed. They are informed about what they can reasonably expect from operative correction of the toes and about the metatarsophalangeal subluxation or dislocation if either is present.

If hallux surgery is contemplated simultaneously after relief of pain has been attained in the initial office visit, such discussions are outlined and noted on the patient's chart. Informative notes may assist the patient's judgment later if recriminations are made concerning treatment.

SHORT HEEL CORD

A common clinical syndrome seen in young children and adolescents with relatively normal-appearing gaits is characterized by foot fatigue. In these cases, the arch is more often elevated than depressed, and slight ankle valgus becomes manifest in the standing position. There is splaying of the fore part of the foot, but more often, there is a tendency for dorsal callosities to develop over the toes, no matter how roomy the shoes appear to be. Later, slight clawing of the toes appears, and with it prominence of the metatarsal heads on the plantar surface, and there is a tendency to develop hammer toes. In severe cases, clawing and hammer toes may progress to the point where function of the toes in weight bearing becomes negligible. Hammer-toe correction in such equinus feet is difficult when the patient is at an age when heel-cord lengthening is unwise.

Shaffer[11] and Hibbs[3] suggested that this syndrome in the foot was due to shortening of the heel cord. There has been some debate as to how short a heel cord must be to be considered short. It has also been debated whether a foot that does not dorsiflex to a right angle when it is held in the position of peritalar inversion is really abnormal. I believe it is functionally inadequate if the foot in inversion, with the knee extended, fails to passively attain right-angle flexion in relationship to the leg.

In my experience, it is relatively easy to recognize this type of foot when the patient first walks across the examination room barefoot. The toes dorsiflex convulsively at times before the foot as a whole begins to dorsiflex (Fig. 62–13). Just as the platysma and other accessory muscles of respiration function when the asthmatic patient tries to elevate the thoracic cage, so

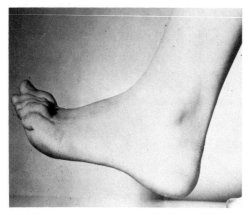

Figure 62–13. *Toe dorsiflexion gait in a foot with a short heel cord.*

do the toe extensor muscles stand out as efforts are made involuntarily to assist the tibialis anterior to dorsiflex the foot against the abnormal resistance of short calf structures. If dorsiflexion is tested with the foot inverted, the outer border of the foot may stop 15 to 20 degrees short of a right angle with the leg. Equally significant is the observation that if the knee is then flexed, the inverted foot can now be dorsiflexed well past the right angle (Fig. 62–14). In these feet the last needed degrees of dorsiflexion are achieved not in the ankle joint but in the subtalar and midtarsal joints by everting the foot maximally. It is this constant eversion demand that tires these feet. Furthermore, abnormal toe dorsiflexion causes stress on the metatarsal heads. This type of fatigue is difficult to relieve. For cock-up deformities, an insole with a good toe-crest "brings the ground up to the toes" and enables these retracted toes to regain push-off function (Fig. 62–15). The crest also takes part of the body weight off the "exposed" metatarsal heads (Fig. 62–16). Latex soles are particularly restful for these feet. The heels of the shoes cannot be lowered in the presence of short heel cords, although, strangely enough, these patients can often walk comfortably barefoot on grass. Many women are able to walk best and most comfortably in high-heeled shoes in later years.

For many years, for children, I have advised classic heel-cord stretching exercises, which are started as soon as the short heel cords are discovered and are performed in accordance with the following instructions:

1. Face the wall, emphasizing toeing-in, with the toes initially 8 inches from wall and the heels 7 to 8 inches apart. Touch the abdomen to wall, keeping the heels on the ground. This is performed 30 times morning, noon, and night, and the distance from the wall is gradually increased as calf tension becomes tolerated (Fig. 62–17).

2. Advance one foot, keeping the rear foot toeing in. Charge! This exercise, which stretches the heel cord of the rear foot, is performed 30 times, with the position of the feet being alternated.

Just how useful these exercises are may be somewhat doubtful, but it is possible that they may effect some change in childhood, when the lesion is often first en-

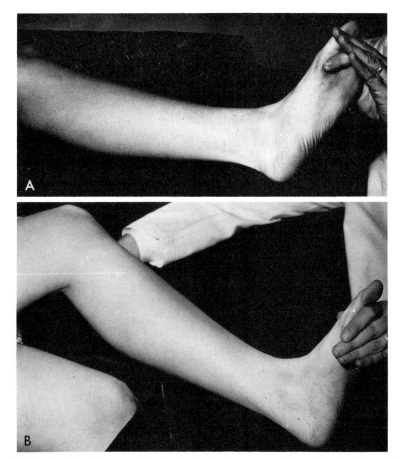

Figure 62–14. *(A) Limited dorsiflexion of the foot with the knee extended and the foot tested in inversion. (B) With the knee flexed, foot dorsiflexes past a right angle. Permitting the foot to evert adds materially to the range of dorsiflexion.*

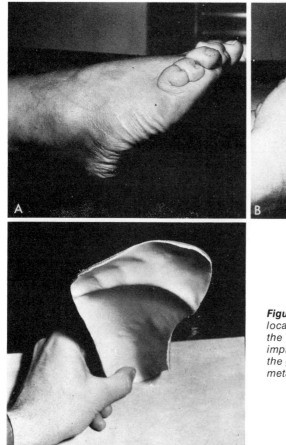
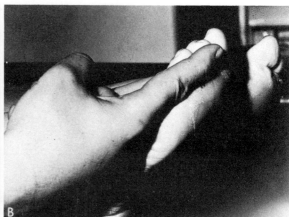

Figure 62–15. *(A) Contracted, cocked-up toes increase local metatarsal head stresses. (B) Finger demonstrates the position of the toe crest to provide a fulcrum for improved toe action. (C) A toe crest on an insole "brings the ground up to the toes." However, this insole lacks a metatarsal elevation.*

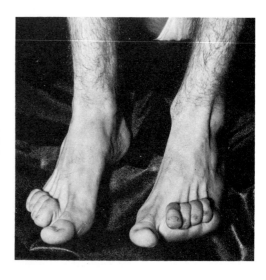

Figure 62–16. *Patient with short heel cords at age 15. "Exposed" metatarsal heads have appeared. When the patient was seen at age 7.5, there were minimal toe deformities.*

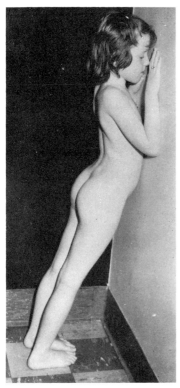

Figure 62–17. Heel-cord stretching exercises performed toeing-in.

countered. Hibbs used to advise such patients to go mountain climbing, which would have the same stretching effect on the heel cords.

It is essential to recognize this very common foot handicap and to understand why relatively normal-looking feet are painful and why toe-crested, long insoles such as those in molded "space" shoes often help patients who have a closet full of ordinary shoes and short insoles but obtain no relief from them. Such molded insoles of adequate length can be fabricated for shoes of reasonably acceptable appearance. The patient had best be informed in advance, however, that the initial pair of costly molded "space" shoes may have to be replaced by a longer pair as the hammer toes spontaneously straighten and the shoes become too short.

So-called "space" shoes gained popularity for a number of reasons. They provided molded insoles for relatively normal feet and for feet with shortened heel cords and retracted toes. However, since the molds are usually made in the trade with the patient standing, they often permit the foot to splay. In particular, they supply toe crests under the retracted phalanges of the second to fifth toes and, by their shortness, a fulcrum for toe function, so that the often cocked-up toes with their limited plantar flexion can help to decompress the overstressed metatarsal areas (see Figure 62–16). This is a valuable feature. As mentioned previously, as the toes are mobilized, they tend to elongate, and the shoes often become too short for the feet. Because of this, we urged long ago that there should be separate and replaceable insoles for "space" shoes, which can be modified as the need arises. It is the molded insole,

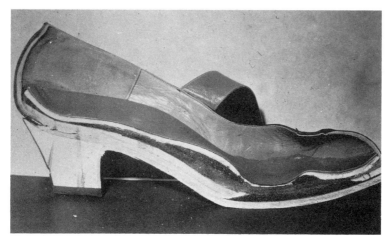

Figure 62–18. Hemisection of a shoe containing an insole with a toe crest made on a mold of the foot.

not primarily the shoe, that provides most of the relief (Fig. 62–18).

The thick, latex sole of the "space" shoe is also a desirable feature. This sole has a somewhat bizarre appearance, emphasized at times by bright colors and vein-like modeling of the shoe uppers, but the relief frequently afforded by these shoes is considerable and compensates for their appearance. Such features seem to have made these shoes a status symbol and, hence, to have given them trade value. However, the stock shoes that incorporate the external features of the custom-made shoes without the molded toe crest or other corrections and that often have foam-rubber rather than latex soles have no special therapeutic value.

Another advantage of a custom-made shoe fabricated on a good mold of the foot is the provision of a snug, medial counter and a properly cupped heel of the shoe that grips the foot when needed.

Sandals

Today, many women wear open-toed, sandal-like footwear. Some of these shoes control only toe spread. Others, extending more proximally, encircle the metatarsal shafts. Some are built on a straight medial line last. Others are pointed, and the sides converge from the metatarsophalangeal joints to the tip in the line of the third metatarsal. The latter conformation encourages development or worsening of hallux valgus and nail deformities.

The heel height of modern sandal-like shoes varies from very low heels to wedged heels that are frequently three inches high. In such shoes, the heel is usually free, and when the ankle joint is dorsiflexed, the dorsum of the foot strikes the anterior dorsal retaining strap, which tenses the attachments anchoring the sole on each side just anterior to the heel of the shoe in gait. The equinus position of the foot is frequently relieved momentarily during periods of standing at rest. At such times, the wearer stands mainly on one foot, but while doing so, she everts the other at the peritalar joint. This foot then comes into dorsiflexion on the leg, and the shoe visibly tips into eversion. The ankle equinus is for a moment overcome. When equinus is not unremitting or constant, equinus contracture will neither develop nor increase. From my observations, high heels in sandals do not aggravate heel-cord shortening.

INSOLES AND MOLDS

Insoles properly planned and accurately fabricated of varied new materials, cork compounds, thermoplastic and plastic compounds, and various metals provide a practical means of providing foot support and comfort for many patients who have areas of contact discomfort (Fig. 62–18). Although an orthopaedist or an expert insole maker can often modify a stock insole to fit, in more difficult cases insoles made directly by the physician or made on his molds of the patient's feet will be much more likely to provide successful decompression. Molds are best made by the orthopaedist, who imposes the desired corrections on them as he makes them.

Molds should be made with the foot in the corrected position, not in the deformed position, as is commonly done by some insole makers, who are later obliged to impose guessed corrections on the completed positive. To make a plaster mold for a corrective insole that will control splaying of the foot, the mold is preferably made with the patient lying relaxed, either prone or supine. If the mold is made with the patient sitting on an ordinary chair, it is difficult to manually control the foot for corrections to be imposed on it. Weight bearing is avoided. If the heel cords are short, the molds are made with the knees flexed 90 degrees and the patient in the prone position, so that a replica of the foot with the ankle at a right angle can be made.

A complicated apparatus to record weight-bearing correction produced by ingenious adjustable contour pegs for making insoles without molds was tried experimentally in the early days of World War II, but it proved to be too impractical for regular use.

Manually made molds of plaster of Paris are practical (Fig. 62–19). Some orthopaedists use roller bandages that are 6 inches wide, but I prefer to use 6-inch-wide, plaster of Paris, edge-contacting reverses, five layers thick, applied to the talcum-

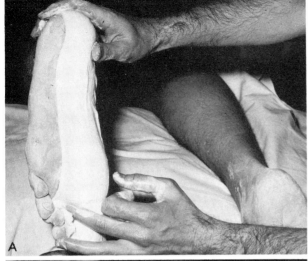
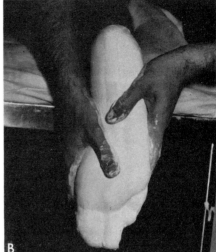
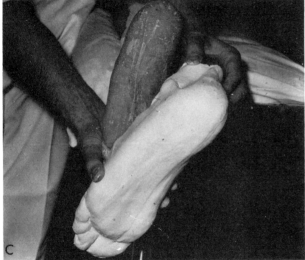

Figure 62–19. (A) Making a plaster mold with the patient supine. The toes are modeled with care. (B) Modeling the longitudinal arch and metatarsals. (C) Removal of the completed ankle-height mold.

powdered foot. The thin mold should extend to well above the malleoli, so that the insole maker can see the foot in erect alignment. As the plaster sets, it is rapidly and snugly modeled to compress the soft tissues where weight will be borne in the following areas:

1. Behind each metatarsal head and particularly along the shaft and snugly behind the head of the first metatarsal, where special care is exercised.

2. Distal to the metatarsal areas, with the plaster being carefully modeled into the spaces beneath and between the phalanges of the toes so that a toe crest can be made on the completed insole. Alignment of metatarsal heads and the degree of forefoot spread or compression are monitored.

3. About the heel, with the plaster mold being cupped firmly on both sides of the os calcis and flattened or hollowed on the plantar surface to compress or relieve the soft tissues against the calcaneus as tenderness may dictate.

4. Along the medial and lateral borders of the foot, with the plaster being stroked firmly along the longitudinal arch and along the lateral border of the foot. Navicular and cuboid areas are modeled.

As the foot is being aligned, the orthopaedist should remember that when the

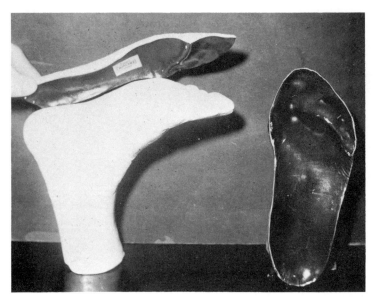

Figure 62-20. *Positive model and insole.*

patient is standing, the foot will be on a relatively flat, horizontal surface. Hence, there must be no inversion or eversion of the foot on the leg or of the forefoot on the hindfoot, nor should the fore part of the foot be plantar flexed on the hind part as the mold is completed. Peritalar function must also be considered.

The medial and lateral contiguous margins of the reverses need not quite meet on the dorsum of the foot if insoles (not shoes) are planned. With this narrow gap anteriorly, the mold can be spread without cutting, and it will tend to spring back into shape after it has been removed from the foot. A few transverse lines penciled across the gap before the mold is removed make it easier to realign the mold after removal. The insole maker will later fill the powdered mold and make a positive plaster last on which he can fabricate the insole without trimming or making corrections (Fig. 62-20). The chances are good that a leather-cork-steel insole made on such a model will fit and serve well. However, it must be used in a shoe with a counter strong enough to prevent sagging of the insole and with a heel that fits accurately and snugly, preventing the calcaneus from tilting in the peritalar joint. Only long insoles stay in place; short insoles may shift. In most cases, toe crests need to be attached to the insole, which must be full length, extending under the toes.

SHOES

Since the Egyptian sandal with a leather thong between the first and second toes and the rawhide shoes worn in early Britain, which were akin to the American Indian's moccasin, few basic changes or improvements have appeared in the sole in footwear design. The medieval dandy wore shoes with such long, pointed toes that they were actually tied to his belt; the men portrayed by Dürer and contemporaries of Henry VIII wore shoes almost as broad as they were long; Chinese women had their feet bound; and in the twentieth century shoes with pointed toes have periodically sacrificed female feet on the altar of local fashion; today feet have not fared too badly, however, for it usually proves unprofitable to design a shoe that generates more curiosity than customers.

At present, good shoes do exist, but selection and fitting are not always informed or available everywhere. Joggers are one segment of the population who tend to take care in choosing their footwear.

Since there is such variation in foot shape that no ideal shoe could conceivably

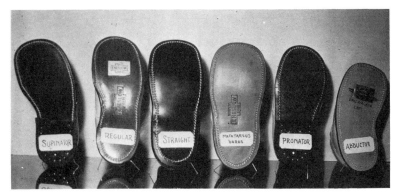

Figure 62–21. *Different children's shoe lasts with neutral, adducted, and abducted forefeet.*

be made on one last, many lasts are need-ed. On the American market, there are many well-designed and sturdily con-structed shoes. Orthopaedists training res-idents would be well advised to request the managers and shoe fitters of the stores they recommend to bring sample shoes with neutral, adducted, markedly adduct-ed, abducted, and bunion lasts (Figs. 62–21 and 62–22), and with different heel heights and heel widths and cupped heel seatings to the hospital for staff discus-sion. Shoes with counters of different de-grees of rigidity and with well-shanked soles of various types should be stocked locally. A craftsman capable of modifying

shoes of adults and children according to the specific prescription of the ortho-paedist is very desirable and worthy of support.

The normal foot can tolerate almost any bad shoe at least for a while. For centuries, the feet of rich and poor alike have been forced for short periods into abnormally shaped shoes. Even though right and left shoes were made in antiquity, there have been many periods in history when shoes were made the same for both feet. Even Dr. Johnson seemed to believe that shoes were interchangeable. He criticized Shake-speare's line, "Had falsely thrust (his slip-pers) upon contrary feet," remarking that

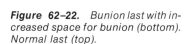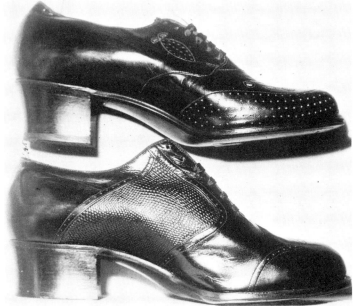

Figure 62–22. *Bunion last with in-creased space for bunion (bottom). Normal last (top).*

the Bard was confusing shoes with gloves, since either shoe would equally admit either foot. As late as the American Civil War, soldiers were initially issued "two shoes for two feet."

Fitting Shoes

An experienced shoe fitter can fit feet with heels and fore parts of different widths, sizes, and proportions, and feet with unusual heel-to-ball-to-toe ratios, unusual toes, abnormal flexibility, and many other deviations from the so-called normal with shoes in stock. An adequate stock, particularly for small and growing children, is the sine qua non of a satisfactory shoe store. The foot must never be fitted into shoes that merely happen to be available, as regrettably occurs at times in inadequately stocked stores. Toe deformities and deviations, hammer toes, ingrown toenails, and hard as well as soft corns are often caused by shoe-fitting errors committed during childhood or later.

To be able to fit children from infancy to age 12 years, one responsible shoe merchant of my acquaintance currently stocks all 30 sizes in half sizes, with each in four widths (when manufactured) in each of four varieties of last. These lasts are (1) the so-called straight last (ordinary last, which is in slight forefoot adduction), (2) the neutral or medius last (nonadducted forefoot), (3) the adducted forefoot last, and (4) the abducted forefoot last. He provides these 480 different pairs of shoes as the basic fitting stock. In addition, he has other shoes with different types of heels, and special degrees of correction — for example, for clubfeet — as may be indicated by the attending orthopaedist. One to four of the 480 pairs of shoes are stocked and replenished daily. It is then possible to fit infants and children precisely when accurate fitting is needed. He finds that the variety is essential and not a luxury. Several other local merchants are completing and enlarging their own inventories to be able to provide comparable satisfactory fitting service.

SOLE ALTERATIONS

Properly placed leather or rubber blocks and patches attached to the anterior portion of the sole of the shoe behind the metatarsal heads will transmit weight-bearing stresses to areas proximal to the metatarsal heads, provided the sole of the shoe is yielding, according to Jones and Steindler. If the sole is rigid and unyielding, however, there is no corrective or local selective supportive effect since stresses are transmitted through the sole to the whole foot. Sole alterations are therefore more often useful for a thin-soled woman's shoe than for the relatively rigid sole of a man's leather shoe. Although properly designed insoles or pads in the shoe of an adult are generally more dependable than "anterior heels" as a means of changing the transmission of stress, "anterior heels" carefully located and shaped (Fig. 62–23) are still of value. Straight, oblique, curved, or comma-shaped, they are applied to the shoes for local support as desired. They should be covered with a thin layer of cemented rubber to ensure that the correction does not wear down rapidly and to diminish the sometimes objectionable clatter that they make.

Unless the shoe is very sturdily constructed, sole or heel wedges are of only temporary value, since the shoe counter breaks down under the stress exerted by the hind part of the foot.

A Thomas-type medially elongated heel provides little better insurance that the shoe counter will remain supportive than does an ordinary heel with a well-built modern shoe counter and a strong shank. When counters become deformed, they should be replaced.

A good insole has the advantage that it can be shifted from shoe to shoe of the same type without requiring modification of each new pair of shoes, which, for children, is often a nuisance and a not inconsiderable expense to the parent. A child can also benefit from properly designed insoles when shoes that are available are inadequate for his particular needs.

Rocker Sole

Special modifications of the shoe may be beneficial in the presence of a fused ankle joint. In such instances, a shoe with a rocker-bottom sole provides a substitute "ankle joint on the ground" (Fig. 62–24). The length of the curved surface of the

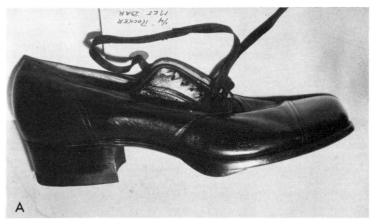

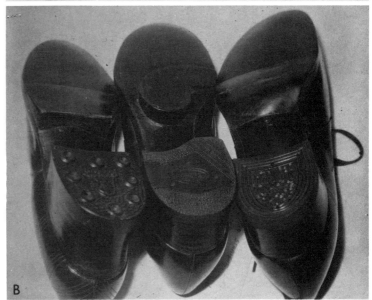

Figure 62–23. (A) Placement of an anterior heel on a thin sole. (B) Various anterior heels and a Thomas heel.

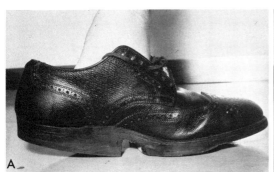

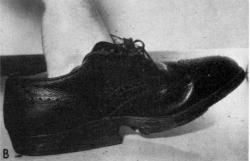

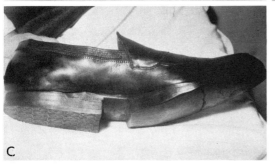

Figure 62–24. (A) A rocker sole on the forefoot. (B) A rocker sole on the heel. (C) Plantar view of another rocker sole.

rocker tends to determine the length of the step. The strain on the fused ankle is markedly diminished by the rocker.

The tibial axis is extended in a vertical line to the ground, passing a bit in front of the midpoint (on the lateral roentgenogram) of the tibiotalar joint. This line marks the apex of the curve of the rocker sole attached to the shoe. To complete the rocker, the heel is shaved down posteriorly. It need not be too high. The heel on the normal foot should be elevated or a heel lift should be supplied inside the shoe to keep standing posture symmetric. A commercial shoe popular for a while featured an analogous curved sole for relatively normal feet. The orthopaedist must personally instruct the craftsman in the design of the rocker, otherwise the apex of the curve may be located too far anteriorly, where it will only cause increased dorsiflexion stress on the ankle joint instead of reducing it.

It is unfortunate that custom-made shoes for relatively normal feet, which are often of definite therapeutic value, can seldom be obtained in the United States at reasonable cost.

STRAPPING

Ankle Strapping

Strapping of the ankle region has long been employed for many conditions. In acute static foot strain, it often affords temporary relief. Local arthritic involvement may be partially helped, but gout is seldom benefited. Strapping is beneficial as an adjunctive measure for local tenosynovitis treated by Novocain infiltration. As mentioned previously, the wearing of high boots encourages the spread of tinea under strappings.

Inversional "Sprained Ankle" — Diagnostic Difficulties and Treatment, Including Strapping

Strapping is perhaps most frequently employed in connection with "sprain of the ankle." As this term implies, it was long believed that this injury was limited to the anterolateral and lateral ligaments of the ankle joint. Hughes, however, has convincingly demonstrated the surprising frequency of osteochondral damage of the contiguous joint surfaces of the tibiotalar

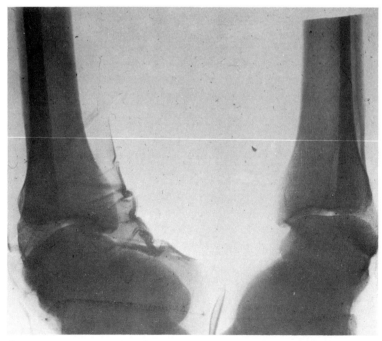

Figure 62–25. *Stress roentgenogram showing subluxation of the talus occurring under a 10-day-old loosened strapping.*

joint caused by the subluxation that occurs during injury.[4] Osteochondral injuries of the lateral malleolus are also often demonstrable.

In my experience, osteochondral avulsions, reduced and checked on stress and other appropriate roentgenograms, are best treated by cast immobilization and no weight bearing on crutches until union is attained. The sprained ankle must therefore be carefully assessed before eversion strapping and ambulation, as prescribed for the common anterolateral ligamentous injury, are chosen for treatment (Fig. 62–25).

It is important to be aware that the subtalar joint can also be "sprained" and may sustain ligamentous injury and avulsion fractures of the margins of the articular surfaces, with production of lateral pedicled osteochondral bodies.

Fissure fractures of adjacent bones stressed by the inversion accident are not uncommon. These include fractures of the anterior beak of the calcaneus in the subtalar joint and of the margins of the calcaneocuboid joint, with infraction of the cuboid or avulsion of the margin of the navicular in the region of the attachment of the anterior tibial tendon. Traumatic persistent subluxations of the tarsometatarsal joints have resulted from forced inversion. They are not easy to recognize on roentgenograms.

The effect of an inversion injury on the peroneus brevis muscle may be demonstrated by avulsion of the epiphysis at the base of the fifth metatarsal or by an avulsion fracture in this region if the epiphysis has fused. The peroneus longus tendon may be damaged and may become calcified near its sesamoid bone opposite to the cuboid; it may rupture and retract posteriorly along with its sesamoid; it may shred and create a stenosing tenosynovitis where it angulates around the "pulley" of the peroneal tubercle on the anterolateral aspect of the calcaneus; or it may create a crepitating synovitis behind the malleolus. This tendon may jump out of its confining groove behind the lateral malleolus and sublux onto the outer surface of the fibula. This subluxation may be encountered in the extremely active adolescent, in the adult as the result of injury, and in the newborn infant with calcaneovalgus deformities. In each, inversion strapping may be helpful.

These and other sequelae of inversional sprains emphasize the necessity for study and accurate diagnosis before a definitive program of treatment is formulated and prognosis is hazarded. Initially, in the office, however, strapping often provides useful support and relief of pain on motion, if not on weight bearing.

Nighttime barefoot stub fractures of the phalanges of the fifth toe are readily immobilized by strapping the fifth toe to the fourth toe, with a layer of cotton interposed between them for aeration.

Suggestions for Strapping

Strapping should be simple and be able to be applied quickly. With the improved adherence of modern adhesive tape, complicated woven or basket-weave strappings last no longer than simpler types. Seven or eight parallel strips of 2-inch-wide adhesive tape of adequate length, lapped one over the other and applied after preparation of the skin with B-D Adherent, hold securely. Tincture of benzoin will do, but it is not quite as satisfactory. In the rare patient with known adhesive sensitivity, a protective layer of thin, cotton flannel is applied free or glued to the skin painted with narrow strips of B-D Adherent before the adhesive strapping is applied.

Nonwaterproof, nonperforated adhesive tape is preferred, as the waterproof tape wrinkles and the porous tape stretches. Depending on the diagnosis, strappings are planned to evert or invert the foot or to maintain it in a relatively neutral position; they are best applied with the foot dorsiflexed and in the desired (usually everted) position, with a $1/2$- by $1^1/2$-inch strip of $1/8$-inch felt protecting the tendons anterior to the ankle. When the foot comes down from dorsiflexion, the adhesive will be smooth and stretched, and thus dorsal creasing and subsequent local irritation over the moving tendons will be minimized. Strappings not renewed and permitted to loosen may not control subluxation (Fig. 62–25).

If the foot is strapped in the everted and dorsiflexed position for control of the common ligamentous ankle sprain, two additional long, circumferential, horizontally placed strips of 2-inch-wide tape, one below and one above the malleoli, reinforce and tighten the oblique strapping considerably. Although this procedure is quite harmless, it is advisable to mark these strips with a pencil to indicate where the patient should cut them in the event that they become too tight for any reason.

Tape is best stored in the refrigerator and dispensed from a central spindle through its core to avoid manual compression of the roll during use.

Examples of Special Strappings

Strapping for Incomplete Rupture of the Calf Muscles or Heel Cord

Incomplete rupture of the calf muscles or of the heel cord is a diagnosis that should be made with circumspection, considering the ease with which the more frequent complete rupture may be mis-

judged as incomplete (Fig. 62–26). Incomplete rupture is well treated by six weeks of strapping in equinus position, aided and enforced with a raise of at least ¾ inch under each heel (Fig. 62–27).

The strips of 2-inch-wide adhesive may extend back from the toes along the sole of the foot, over the heel, and up the back of the calf to below the knee. A triple thickness of superimposed layers of adhesive is employed. The ankle is maintained in equinus position while the tape is applied to the previously shaved and Adherent-coated skin of the ankle and leg. Circumferential turns of adhesive avoided in the leg and calf areas secure the adhesive strips firmly only to the fore part of the foot. A small felt pad is then placed over the anterior aspect of the ankle and foot, and finally, the ankle, leg, and adhesive strips are smoothly covered with an elastic adherent casing such as Elastoplast or Tensoplast. A ½-inch-thick tapered pad of

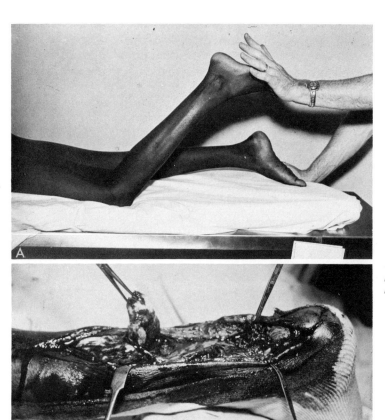

Figure 62–26. *(A) Complete rupture of the tendo Achillis is deceptive. Note the retained equinus power owing to the lateral and big toe muscles. (B) Marked separation of many inches is present at operation performed the morning after the photograph shown in A was taken.*

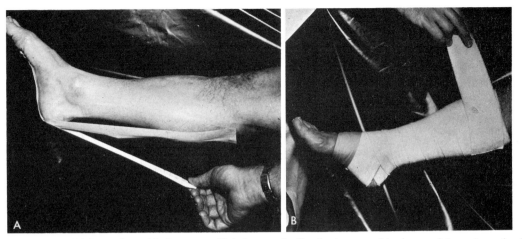

Figure 62–27. *(A) Strapping with deeper multiple layers of adhesive tape used for incomplete rupture of calf muscle tendon apparatus. (B) Final layer of Elastoplast and a ¾-inch heel raise is used in the shoe worn.*

firm felt is taped into the heel of each shoe as a raise, and the patient is referred to a shoemaker for a more permanent type of tapered heel raise for both heels, tapered from ½ inch in front to ¾ inch behind. Elevation and strapping should be continued for six weeks, with the strapping being reinforced at intervals of seven to ten days and being changed if it becomes loose. Longer fixation may seem necessary in some cases.

Strapping for Hammer Toes

Strapping of hammer toes with or without a protective pad on top of the toe and with "over-and-under" application of a strip of adhesive tape, depending on whether the toe is rigid or flexible, helps temporarily to keep toes aligned before surgery (Figs. 62–28 and 62–29). This procedure also provides prompt comfort at the initial visit. Often, such realignment of a second toe dorsally misplaced by a hallux valgus deformity helps diminish the associated bunion before surgical correction. As a temporary measure stretching the shoe with a "swan" or even (rarely) making a crescentic transverse incision through the dorsum of the shoe can provide prompt relief from intolerable pain caused by toe-shoe contact.

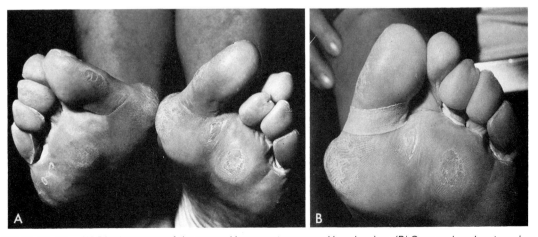

Figure 62–28. *(A) Displacement of the second hammer toe caused by a bunion. (B) Over-and-under strapping provides retention of alignment prior to surgical correction.*

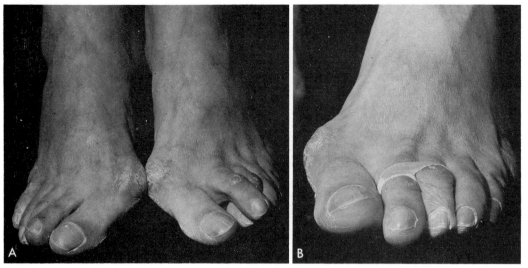

Figure 62–29. *(A) Another hammer toe. (B) Retentive over-and-under strapping.*

Strapping for Painful Flatfeet

Painful flatfeet can frequently be temporarily relieved by supportive strappings of the foot and ankle. In general, pain in relaxed feet is associated with eversion strain of the subtalar joint. This type of strain can be manifested by eversion spasm or localized ligamentous tenderness. Strapping applied at the first office visit and maintained for several weeks helps to temporarily invert the calcaneus under the talus. A supportive pad also is of value. This procedure is followed by provision of insoles and shoes that grip the heel, diminishing eversion. Good insoles help support the region of the talonavicular joint and the so-called medial pillar of the foot.

Some children with untreated relaxed flatfeet have pain (Fig. 62–30), and a trial of strapping in such cases is often followed by striking clinical improvement, which may then be continued by the use of properly designed supports and shoes. Properly fitted heel cups are of value in diminishing heel eversion in some children.

Rigid, painful flatfeet in children with radiologically demonstrable congenital bone anomalies can also be temporarily partially relieved of pain by strapping the feet to control their fixed eversion. The possibility of restoring subtalar joint motion when feasible, as indicated roentgenographically, can be proposed to the parent. Mechanical support should be provided pending surgical treatment to obtain more permanent relief if possible.

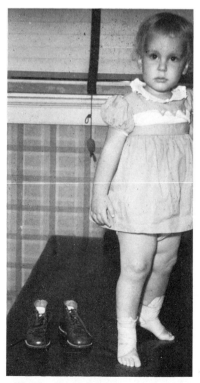

Figure 62–30. *Strapping gave prompt relief from pain in this child with flatfeet. Insoles and shoes subsequently fitted continued relief.*

BURSITIS, TENDINITIS, AND TENOSYNOVITIS

Pads and strapping are also useful in connection with the injection treatment of tendon and bursal inflammatory lesions. Once suspected, these common and very painful lesions are diagnosed mainly by the presence of point tenderness at the site of the lesion or by pain on resisted function of the involved tendon. Calcific tendinitis in lumbrical areas or near the os peroneum can be demonstrated roentgenographically. Weight-transferring pads or strapping may be valuable supplements to local injection therapy, using Novocain and puncturing the calcium deposit areas of inflammation in the tendon and tendon sheath. Vascularization injections of this type are frequently helpful in tendinitis, bursitis, and particularly tenosynovitis. Often these injections give prompt temporary and, not infrequently, permanent relief. In obscure plantar foot pain, lesions of this type should be systematically searched for by palpation and resisted muscle-contraction tests. Such tendons as the tibialis posterior and the long flexors in the sole of the foot, particularly at points of tendon crossing, are common sites of these lesions. Areas of tendon angulation, such as that of the peroneus longus in its "pulley" at the peroneal tubercle, or at the cuboid, are occasional sites.

The injection of steroid preparations into tendons and even about tendons is certainly not without its hazards. We no longer employ it for such purposes, for we have observed ruptures of tendons following its brief local employment. Both the tendo Achillis and the tibialis posterior have separated in continuity during its use. In the case of the tibialis posterior, a unilateral flatfoot appeared as a consequence of its degeneration and rupture.

HEEL PAIN

Pain and local tenderness in the region of the anterior tubercle of the calcaneus with or without a spur visible on roentgenogram are usually promptly improved by heel elevation and the use of a plantar horseshoe heel pad open anteriorly. It is fashioned from two or three skived and shaped layers of ¼-inch sponge rubber, with the top layer being the longest. The pad is usually placed in the shoe so that it causes weight bearing to take place on the periphery of the heel area instead of centrally and simultaneously raises the heel, thereby shifting more weight onto the fore part of the foot. Both shoes should be similarly treated. A ring pad is not as satisfactory. The heels of both shoes should be elevated ½ to ¾ inch by the shoemaker. In severe cases, the horseshoe pad may be glued to the skin to ensure retention in position for one or two weeks.

For a painful subcutaneous bursa over the attachment of the tendo Achillis on the heel, local aspiration coupled with protection of the heel from contact with the back of the shoe will be helpful (Fig. 62–31). A pad of rubber glued on either side of the bursa will enable the patient to wait until a gusset of soft material can be provided to replace the back of the shoe, which produced the lesion. High-heeled shoes are not the only offenders; flat shoes may also have badly contoured backs. In some resistant cases, excision may ultimately be required if conservative measures fail.

Lesions of the deeper tendo Achillis bursa (Albert's bursitis, motorman's heel, retrocalcaneal bursa), extending between the anterior surface of the tendo Achillis and the posterior surface of the calcaneus, are much more troublesome. Local infiltration with Novocain alone coupled with strapping with the foot in equinus and a considerable bilateral heel raise has sometimes been successful. Rest with the foot held in equinus is also important. A search for systemic disease, such as gout, should be carried out next. If there is still no relief after these measures, resection of the portion of the calcaneus in contact with the tendon sheath above its insertion has been advised. I have not used this procedure, except in cases involving severe traumatic lesions of the calcaneus.

Chronic tenosynovitis of the pseudosheath of the tendo Achillis often benefits from dissection and sheath excision. It may be partially relieved by inserting a considerable rubber heel raise inside the shoe at the patient's initial visit.

Involvement of the sheath, and even of the tendon, by an obscure pathologic proc-

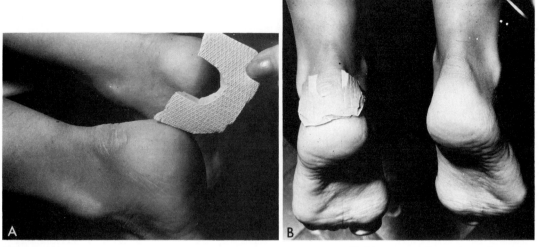

Figure 62–31. (A) Protection for a painful subcutaneous heel bursa. (B) Placement of a pad to relieve shoe pressure.

ess is not infrequently found at operation. A needle biopsy of the sheath performed in the office may provide early definitive information. Xanthoma and leukemic infiltration were diagnosed by this means in two instances.

As mentioned previously, local injection of steroid into the tendon is inadvisable, as it may serve to precipitate rupture of the tendon.

REFERENCES

1. Betts, L. O.: Morton's metatarsalgia: neuritis of the fourth digital nerve. Med. J. Aust., *1*:514, 1940.
2. Durlacher, L.: Treatise on Corns, Bunions, the Diseases of Nails and the General Management of the Feet. London, Simpkin, Marshall, 1845, p. 52.
3. Hibbs, R. A.: Muscle bound feet. N.Y. Med. J., *100*:797, 1914.
4. Hughes, J. R.: The articular damage in complete ruptures of the lateral ligaments of the ankle. *In* Proceedings of the British Orthopaedic Association. J. Bone Joint Surg., *37B*:723, 1955.
5. Jones, R.: "Plantar Neuralgia." Liverpool Medico-Chirurgical Journal, January 1897.
6. Lassmann, G., Lassmann, H., and Stockinger, L.: Morton's metatarsalgia. Light and electron microscopic observations and their relation to entrapment neuropathies. Virchows Arch. [Pathol. Anat.], *370*:307, 1976.
7. Milgram, J. E.: Office measures for relief of the painful foot. J. Bone Joint Surg., *46A*:1095, 1964.
8. Morton, J. G.: A peculiar and painful affection of the fourth metatarsophalangeal articulation. Am. J. Med. Sci., *71*:37, 1876.
9. Omer, G., and Spinner, M.: Management of Peripheral Nerve Problems. Philadelphia, W. B. Saunders Company, 1980.
10. Reed, R. J., and Bliss, B. O.: Morton's neuroma. Regressive and productive intermetatarsal elastofibrosis. Arch. Pathol., *95*:123, 1973.
11. Shaffer, N. M.: Non-deforming clubfoot with remarks on its pathology. Med. Rec., *27*:561, 1885.
12. Silverman, L. G.: Morton's toe or Morton's neuralgia: its recognition and treatment. J. Am. Podiatry Assoc., *66*:749, 1976.

CHAPTER 63

ARCH SUPPORTS AND MISCELLANEOUS DEVICES

Melvin H. Jahss, M.D.

An orthosis is a mechanical device made for the foot or toes that is used to either stabilize the foot or hold it in optimum position, increase function, limit motion of a painful joint, decrease the weight bearing on painful areas, or protect the foot or toes from pressure or excess friction against each other or the shoe. The protective devices are called shields and are usually used for toe deformities or any foot prominences that unduly press against the shoe. The shields, as with arch supports, are preferably custom-made, although some are available commercially. They may be adhered to the foot in the office for temporary relief of discomfort or made into permanent removable devices. Arch supports are one group of these orthoses. Most frequently, they are not used as a support for the arch but to relieve painful, keratotic, or ulcerated areas on the plantar aspect of the foot.

INTERRELATIONSHIPS OF SHOES AND FOOT ORTHOSES[1, 5, 9, 20]

An orthosis, especially an arch support, must be held securely in the shoe to be effective. Ideally, it should be held in place by sturdy orthopaedic oxfords with long medial counters, especially if it is one of the more flexible appliances. Otherwise, the foot will simply bulge out the medial longitudinal arch flange of the appliance as well as the shoe over the longitudinal arch. The problem of supporting orthoses in athletes wearing sneakers may be partially offset by the use of better supportive leather high-top sneakers. A well-made shoe has a snug heel counter to grip the heel plus a steel shank, which prevents any tendency for pronation.[16] A shoe with a heel over 2 inches high, especially if poorly constructed, results in a decrease of heel-to-toe length by deformation of the tarsus.[17] In addition, the patient tends to slide down any incorporated arch support. Accurately placed corrections will no longer line up with the foot deformities, especially toe crests. High heels will not only render metatarsal support inneffectual but will thrust further weight bearing under the metatarsal heads. Usually the patient requires a shoe with a width one size larger than he customarily wears because of the added bulk of the arch support. With thicker arch supports over 3/16 inch thick, patients will require extra-depth shoes, which are commercially available. Supports that are thicker than ¼ inch require a custom-made shoe.

Shoes may supplement the effect of an orthosis. A rubber-soled wedgie will give added support in the shank as well as provide further resiliency on weight bearing. A metatarsal bar will supplement the effect of a metatarsal pad or a metatarsal raise in an arch support. However, a patient with hypersensitive feet may only be able to tolerate a weak correction, such as a low metatarsal pad or just a Denver heel. In general, arch supports or inside shoe corrections (e.g., a metatarsal or sesamoid pad) are more effective than outer sole corrections such as Denver heels.

A high toe-box will give the necessary room for hammer toes and hammer-toe shields, and a bunion last oxford will accommodate a bunion or a bunion shield. It should always be kept in mind that the more bulk added inside the shoe, the tighter the shoe may become, defeating the purpose of the shields. A wider shoe will be too loose, especially about the heel.

In formulating the conservative treatment of any ankle, foot, or toe pathology or deformity all the possibilities of orthoses, shielding, appropriate shoes, and shoe modifications must be considered. If the treating physician is not able to provide such corrections in his office, he is obliged to prescribe in written detail to his orthotist or pedorthist (member of Prescription Footwear Association) the exact shoes and corrections needed. The orthopaedist must then evaluate the correction after about three weeks of use to determine if any adjustments are necessary.

ARCH SUPPORTS[1, 5, 7, 9, 15]

One of the advantages of arch supports, compared with fixed, cemented in-shoe inserts, is that they can be transferred from one shoe into another. Commercial "shelf" supports are relatively useless compared with custom-made ones modeled from casts of the patient's feet since every foot is different and the casts may reveal a different pathology.

Arch supports have had a recent resurgence of use with the increasing popularity of jogging and especially long-distance running. Although many of these patients have a generalized aching of their feet, they often complain more bitterly of medial or lateral knee pain. The soft rubber

support in runners' shoes may be insufficient in providing significant knee relief. The mechanism of relief with arch supports may be that the more even distribution of weight bearing in the foot in turn transmits these repeated impact forces, more equally dispersed, into the knee. In patients with pes planovalgus, the plaster mold is usually taken to minimize the valgus strain. It has been advised that the optimum supportive position is at that point at which the foot suddenly "gives" while gently swinging it from inversion to eversion. By stabilizing the subtalar joint in optimum position, the arch support probably also decreases rotatory forces among the foot, ankle, and knee.

Rigid Supports

Arch supports were originally conceived to function as an external method of supporting the foot and of actively correcting physiologic deformities. Thus, it was felt that in a "weak" foot, such as a flatfoot, the arch support could not only relieve ligamentous strain but, if worn at an early enough age, would also assist in the development of a normal longitudinal arch. Such supports, therefore, were necessarily rigid, initially being made of steel and later Duralumin, and included a medial flange to support the arch. To give some flexibility, spring steel was later used. The steel was occasionally covered with leather. The supports were made from casts of the patient's feet, and minor corrections could be obtained by hammering the steel over heavy lead blocks.

One of the most popular supports was the Whitman arch support[19] made for mobile pes planus in children. The plaster mold is taken as follows: Freshly mixed plaster of Paris is placed over a slanted board. The foot is placed in slight inversion into the plaster, which is then molded partly up the entire foot and heel and allowed to set. The exposed portion of the foot and the adjacent plaster are powdered, and the remaining plaster is applied to cover the rest of the foot. The negative mold therefore comes apart, and after shellacking the insides, more plaster is poured into it to make the positive mold. A small amount of plaster is then added to the lateral aspect to compensate for the soft-tissue compression that occurs when

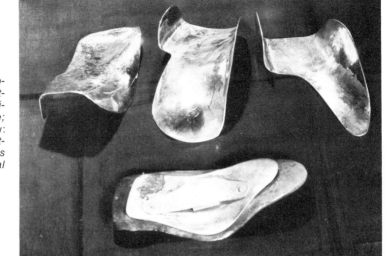

Figure 63–1. *Steel arch supports.* Top row (left to right): *bottom and top surfaces of a combination Whitman-style plate; Whitman plate.* Bottom row: *Spring steel Shaffer plate, bottom surface. Most steel supports end proximal to the metatarsal heads.*

the foot is in inversion. While walking with the Whitman plate, there is an active, inversion, rocking "corrective" force on the heel. The Whitman plate extends up on either side of the heel (Fig. 63–1). This heel control principle is similar to that of the presently used UCBL insert (Fig. 63–2), which is also being used for pes planovalgus, although with questionable results.[12]

Other steel supports (Fig. 63–1) besides supporting the longitudinal arch often included a metatarsal raise for anterior metatarsalgia and metatarsal calluses. The metatarsal raise was the first attempt to relieve symptoms rather than correct a deformity. This was a step forward, as attempting to correct a genetically predetermined deformity by external support is wishful thinking. The rigid supports were heavy, uncomfortable (considering one was walking on steel), and could not be sufficiently molded to relieve small areas of weight-bearing discomfort.

An improved type of rigid support is that made of heat-molded plastics and thermoplastics[7] (Fig. 63–3). They are slightly more flexible and weigh less than metal, but, again, they cannot be accurately molded or adjusted, although softer materials can usually be cemented onto them (with polyadhesive glue) for added com-

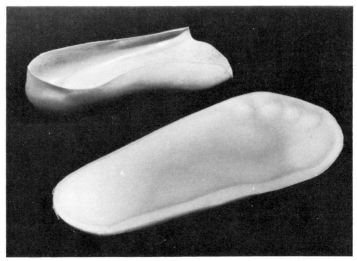

Figure 63–2. Top: *UCBL laminated plastic insert.* Bottom: *Polyethylene foam arch support.*

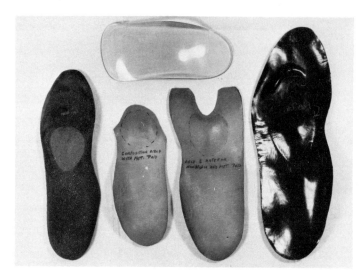

Figure 63–3. Semi-rigid arch supports. Top: *Moderately rigid acrylic support.* Bottom: *Cork-rubber supports (left to right) — plantar view illustrating addition of moderately firm metatarsal pad; metatarsal arch support ending proximal to the metatarsal heads; horseshoe arch support with metatarsal raise; soft arch support with metatarsal raise and toe crest.*

fort and corrections. The four most frequently used rigid plastics are: polypropylene, laminated plastics, acrylics, and polyethylene. Polypropylene, a thermoplastic, is softened and made pliable by heating it to 400°F for eight to ten minutes. It is then vacuum-formed over the custom-made foot mold. It is opaque white in color. The laminated plastics consist of a polyester with a matrix of nylon and fiber glass. They come in a liquid form to which is added a catalyst plus a "promotor." The endothermic reaction of the promotor solidifies the liquid. UCBL inserts are either custom-made from laminated plastics (Fig. 63–2) or made for stock with polypropylene. Polyethylene is also thermoplastic and rigid, but it is slightly softer than polypropylene. Acrylic nylon, which is also rigid, was originally made clear amber in color, but more recently is deep red. It is also thermoplastic, requiring heating to 284° F to soften, and is similarly molded. Thermoplastics can be spot corrected by using a heat gun with a nozzle.

Although an experienced orthotist or arch support technician is capable of taking an accurate mold of the foot, the orthopaedist may wish to do this himself. Merely tracing an outline about the patient's feet is totally inadequate. The simplest method of making an accurate mold is as follows: the patient lies in the supine position, and the feet are powdered. A roll of 4- or 5-inch-wide plaster is loosely rolled up and down the patient's foot, being carefully molded to the arch and conformities.

Before the plaster sets, the hollow behind the metatarsal heads is compressed, thereby providing an accurate corrective support behind the heads. This hollow will vary in depth from patient to patient. If a toe crest is to be incorporated into the arch support, the plaster must extend to the ends of the toes and be molded into the hollows under the bases of the toes. The plaster is quickly removed from the foot and, just before it sets, is placed on a hard, flat surface, on which the metatarsal head area is flattened out straight across to give a plantigrade foot rather than any rocking motion. If desired, a positive mold may be made by pouring in plain plaster of Paris after the negative mold is shellacked. The positive is then removed, and adjustments may be made by adding some plaster over pressure points. This will create a depression or "well" in the arch support. If added height is desired in the arch support, then that area is scooped out on the positive mold. Final minor corrections may be made on the arch support itself by spot heating with a heat gun.

Semi-Rigid and Soft Arch Supports[3-5, 7, 9, 18]

The semi-rigid and soft supports heralded a new era of comfort and function (Figs. 63–2 to 63–5). These consist essentially of rubber, cork-rubber, cork compositions, and polyethylene foam, quite frequently in combination (i.e., layers). Soft arch supports provide resiliency, to compensate for

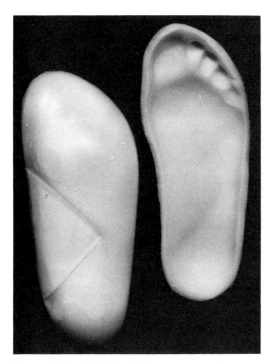

Figure 63–4. *Unfinished Plastazote arch support reinforced in the longitudinal arch.*

any atrophy that occurs in plantar foot pads. They lessen the force of hard interfaces against the weight-bearing portions of the foot, such as the heel and metatarsal heads. They are also used to protect areas of excessive weight bearing of deformed feet. Because soft arch supports are pliable, they can usually be molded to conform to even minor deformities. They permit very accurate correction, essentially by means of "raises" under areas of too little weight

bearing and "wells" or depressions under areas of excessive weight bearing, which are clinically demonstrated by calluses. Soft arch supports are used to conform to the following principles for obtaining foot relief where there are fixed deformities, as are usually present in the adult:

1. Never attempt to correct a fixed deformity by adding a raise under the calloused prominent area. It will only increase the pain under the callus and, in patients with neurologic sensory and/or vascular deficiency, may cause local sloughing from the excess pressure.

2. The floor must be brought up to the foot, thereby obtaining a plantigrade foot by distributing the weight bearing over the entire foot. This is also the principle of the total contact cast.

3. Pressure must be taken away from areas of excess weight bearing. This is determined by the presence of calluses and also by means of inking devices, such as the Harris mat, Brand's slipper, forceplates, and thermograms[2, 6] (see Chapter 46). Too little weight bearing is indicated by soft, baby-like skin.

4. Weight bearing should be added to areas of too little weight bearing as well as non–weight-bearing areas, such as the longitudinal arch and the sole of the foot behind the metatarsal heads.

Thus, if the forefoot is in fixed varus, the non–weight-bearing *medial* portion of the forefoot requires a raise to shift the weight bearing away from the calloused lateral aspect of the plantar aspect of the foot, as in an old clubfoot deformity. A similar, more common example is the support

Figure 63–5. Top: *One-inch-thick, cork-rubber, adjustable Levy mold made in conjunction with custom-made shoes. Support consists of a top layer of medium-soft rubber, a middle layer of firmer cork-rubber, and a bottom layer of firm cork.* Bottom: *Support with a top layer of moderately firm rubber, a middle layer of softer rubber, and a bottom layer of cork. The firm top layer has been ground down under the tender area of the heel, permitting the heel to rest in softer rubber.*

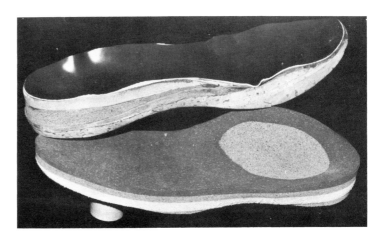

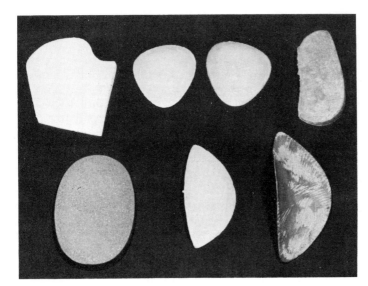

Figure 63–6. Commercial pads that may be glued with rubber cement over the insole or incorporated into arch supports. Top row (left to right): sesamoid (dancer's) pad; left and right metatarsal pads; ⅛-inch rubber wedge. Bottom row (left to right): ³/₁₆-inch rubber tapered heel lift; rubber and leather scaphoids.

modifications made for metatarsal calluses secondary to pes cavus or forefoot equinus. By raising the support in the normally non–weight-bearing areas of the longitudinal arch and behind the metatarsal heads, the excess weight bearing is redistributed away from the metatarsal heads. This is best achieved, as previously noted, by pressing and molding the still-wet plaster cast behind the metatarsal heads. As mentioned earlier, a "well' is a depression made in the support under areas of painful calluses. For accuracy, the callus may be marked out on the foot with lipstick, which is then transferred to the support by pressing the support against the marked foot. Both the raises and the wells should have smooth, rounded edges. The wells should have a relatively soft base. Foam-rubber or polyethylene supports may be supplemented with firmer rubber or cork-rubber composition beneath them (Fig. 63–6). Cork-rubber, rubber, and polyethylene may be accurately ground down with sanding discs. Rubber cement and plastic cements are used to bind the various materials of the support together.

Foam-rubber arch supports consist of two types, an open-celled type, which is more porous, providing better aeration, and a closed-cell form (microcellular), which provides better resiliency. The latter is preferable. The foam is produced by blowing nitrogen bubbles through the material, which can also be adjusted to produce various densities, usually designated as soft, medium, or firm. However, intermediate grades of consistency can be made. Foam polyethylene is usually closed cell and is made similarly. Both the rubber and polyethylene are made in sheets. The rubber is usually manufactured in thicknesses of ⅛ to 3/16 inch and can be adhesive-backed or non–adhesive-backed. The adhesive-backed 3/16-inch closed-cell variety (Milgram's adhesive-backed rubber latex) is ideal for plantar padding and shielding.[13] Polyethylene is not adhesive-backed and is manufactured in sheets of thicknesses up to ½ inch. It is known under different trade names such as Plastazote, Pelite, and Aliplast.

It is not advisable to use the soft variety, except as a thin lining under "wells," since excess softness causes undue pistoning in the shoe, resulting in friction and blister formation, especially about the heel. In addition, any significant weight put on too soft a material causes compression, with loss of resiliency. The medium-firm materials are much more ideal but must be at least 3/16 inch thick to be effective. Thicker arch supports of up to 1 inch are even more desirable in more severe plantar deformities, such as prominent tender metatarsal heads underlying atrophied metatarsal fat pads, as seen in rheumatoid arthritis and long-standing pes cavus or in peripheral neuropathies with trophic ulcers. Such arch supports require custom-made shoes.

Rubber and polyethylene arch supports

should be covered with a thin, porous, durable, smooth, soft layer of material, preferably leather, permitting aeration, longer wear, and less shearing force than if the plantar skin were in direct contact with the foam.

Closed-cell polyethylene is currently the most popular material used for soft insoles[6, 8] and has the advantage of being able to be readily molded in the office. It becomes pliable when heated at relatively low temperatures permitting molding to the foot. Owing to the closed cells and the excellent insulating capacity, the surface rapidly cools, allowing comfort of application while the deeper, hotter layers still remain pliable. The heated Plastazote may also be molded onto a plaster mold of the foot. Once cool, which takes but a few seconds, the polyethylene maintains its shape ("memory"). While still hot, polyethylene becomes tacky, permitting autoadhesion of additional pieces. However, it is usually simpler to add supplementary pieces (especially in the longitudinal arch) or other materials with special plastic cements. Most soft as well as hard plastics that are heat pliable are made "stress relieved," which prevents shrinkage with heating. However, excess temperature does result in progressive shrinkage. At 200°F, Plastazote is moderately pliable, does not shrink, and is only slightly tacky. At 225°F, it is more pliable, permitting better contouring, with accurate "wells" forming under prominent plantar bony prominences with weight bearing before it cools. However, at this temperature, it is tackier, and there is approximately 10 per cent shrinkage, for which allowance must be made when originally outlining the foot on the Plastazote. Thin Plastazote requires about two to three minutes of heating, whereas thicker pieces (3/16 inch) require five minutes.

The one problem with polyethylene foam is that it tends to "bottom out" or pack down with use. An unsupported polyethylene insole will bottom out in about two months. This problem is partially obviated by adding support, such as cork-rubber, under the polyethylene, which extends its usefulness to about six months.

Polyethylene foam arch supports may be readily made in the office. The patient stands on a piece of Plastazote (preferably 3/16 inch thick), and his feet are outlined on it in pencil. The supports are then easily cut out with bandage scissors. The supports are placed in a small oven at 200°F for two to three minutes, first putting a small amount of talcum on the inside of the oven or on the support to avoid a tendency for sticking. When the support becomes slightly soft and limp, it is removed from the oven, flipped a few times in the hands to cool it off, slightly and then molded up against the patient's sole and behind the metatarsals. It rapidly cools and sets. Additional support of polyethylene, cork-rubber, and finally lining may be added to the support. Before the lining is added, the perimeter is skived (beveled). The polyethylene support is quite lightweight and comfortable. Polyethylene slipper shoes that incorporate custom-made polyethylene insoles and have uppers that may be partially molded are commercially available. They are useful as temporary footwear in patients with draining ulcers and sinuses. The polyethylene may be readily washed and cleansed.

Arch Supports of Miscellaneous Materials

Cork and cork-rubber compositions are used more frequently for arch supports by pedorthists. These materials are also layered under soft rubber or polyethylene arch supports (see Figure 63–5) and are used as "build-ups" for leg length discrepancy. Thermocork is heat pliable at 120° to 150°C, at which point it is also autoadhesive. It does not bottom out. It comes in sheets of ¼-inch thickness. Rubber "butter" is a cork compound that is applied with a spatula to small areas over cork supports to provide build-ups.

Celastic is occasionally used for arch supports. It is manufactured in thin, hard sheets that become pliable with an activator.

Molo is a rubber compound manufactured as pre-formed 1/16-inch-thick insoles. These insoles are soft and compressible with weight bearing, molding to any deformities. They may be superimposed over each other and glued together with rubber cement. They remain compressed, having no "memory."

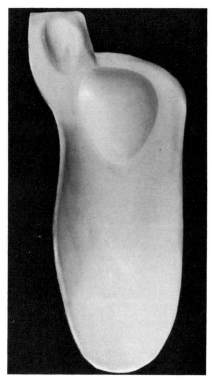

Figure 63–7. *Cork-rubber arch support with a Morton's extension and a "well" under the interphalangeal joint of hallux plus a metatarsal pad.*

Specific Supports and Corrections

Special types of arch supports may be constructed in accordance with the patient's pathology and based on the same principles as listed previously. When

there is too little weight bearing under the first and fifth metatarsal heads associated with calluses under the middle metatarsal heads, a standard metatarsal raise may not be sufficient. The arch support should be horseshoe-shaped, with the lateral raised flanges extending beyond the first and fifth metatarsal heads in addition to the metatarsal raise behind the three middle metatarsal heads; this is known as a horseshoe correction (see Figure 63–3). In cases of sesamoiditis or when there is an isolated callus under the head of the first metatarsal, a sesamoid pad or dancer's pad is incorporated into the arch support. This is done by extending the metatarsal raise medially to behind the first metatarsal head (see Figure 63–6). In patients with Morton's syndrome, a raised medial flange extending past the head of the first metatarsal is used. If there is an associated callus under the first interphalangeal joint, the flange is further extended to include a well under the callus (Fig. 63–7).

An arch support may be made with the heel cupped for an associated heel spur syndrome. Alernatives are commercially made plastic heel cups or the addition of a calcaneal heel[5] to the outer sole. The calcaneal heel is a heel extension added medially just distal to the breast of the heel. The most satisfactory correction, however, is the Steindler heel spur correction[9] (see Chapter 33).

In patients who have advanced deformities, such as rheumatoid arthritis and severe splayfeet, and in diabetics with neu-

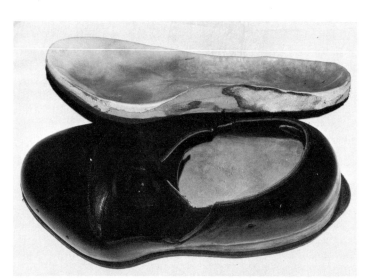

Figure 63–8. *Custom-made shoe, a thick, rubber-soled wedgie with a 1-inch-thick, custom-made, adjustable, cork-rubber Levy mold.*

rovascular foot pathology, the best type of footwear is a custom-made shoe with thick, rubber, wedgie outsoles. These shoes are made with removable, 1-inch-thick, custom-made, rubber and cork-rubber arch supports (adjustable Levy molds) (Fig. 63–8). Wells are made under calluses, ulcers, and bony prominences, and non–weight-bearing areas are given extra support. The support consists of the following from top to bottom: leather covering, medium-soft rubber, firmer cork-rubber, and finally plain cork, the firmest and least resilient layer. Since the uppers are made from casts of the patient's feet, the shoe will conform to any toe deformities such as bunions or hammer toes. If the foot or ankle is somewhat stiff, the wedgie outsole may be supplemented with a wedged (SACH-type) rubber heel combined with a long sole rocker.

Arch supports are occasionally used in conjunction with braces. Such supports are usually made of steel, a characteristic perhaps carried over from earlier concepts that stressed the desirability of stability and rigidity to control the instability associated with muscle weakness, such as that due to poliomyelitis. Such foot plates should preferably be covered with soft material for added comfort (Fig. 63–9). When associated foot support and relief are required in conjunction with a brace or rigid leg orthosis, especially when there is sensory deficit, the brace should preferably be attached to heel calipers, and the feet should be provided with custom-made soft supports. In cases of neuropathic feet and trophic ulcers, the most effective method of unloading the metatarsal heads is by means of a PTB orthosis attached to heel calipers. It may also be used for Charcot feet and ankles. The support should consist of the previously mentioned 1-inch-thick, cork-rubber, adjustable Levy molds in conjunction with custom-made shoes with rubber, wedgie outsoles.

TOE ORTHOSES

Toe orthoses are small mechanical devices and shields that are applied to the toes.[18] They protect deformed toes from painful pressure against each other, as is seen with interdigital soft corns. They also protect the toe from rubbing against the toe-box, as happens with hammer toes (Fig. 63–10) or a hard corn over the lateral aspect of the fifth toe. Toe orthoses also protect toes from painful contact against the insole, as occurs with end corns and the paraungual corn of a rotated fifth toe. They may be used to assist in toe function, as does the toe crest under dorsally subluxed hammer toes. Finally, they may be used as corrective devices to hold a hammer toe that has been operated on in corrected position, as does the Budin splint (see Chapter 33).

Permanent, custom-made, removable shields are the most satisfactory toe orthoses (Fig. 63–11). Toe shields are readily available commercially, but unfortunately, they are of poor quality, usually being made of too soft and too thin a rubber or polyurethane (Fig. 63–12).

With the advent of commercial and orthopaedic shoes with high, wide toe-boxes, extra-depth shoes, and custom-made

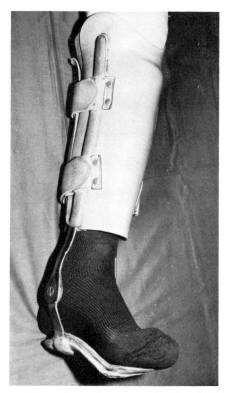

Figure 63–9. *A patellar-tendon–bearing (PTB) orthosis with the foot plate covered with rubber and leather for a diabetic Charcot ankle.*

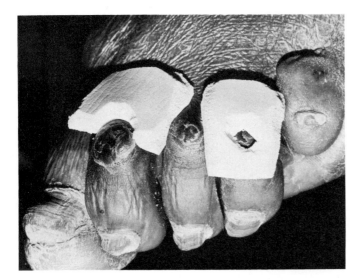

Figure 63–10. Office-made dorsal hammer-toe shields of ³/₁₆-inch closed-cell rubber latex. Note the skiving (beveling) of the edges.

Figure 63–11. Removable, custom-made latex shield for a bunion. Note the build-up proximal to the bunion. The shield was made from a cast of the first ray.

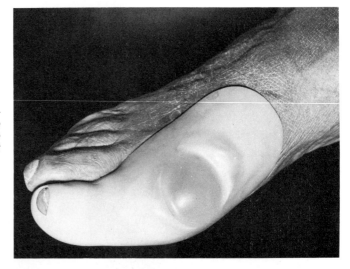

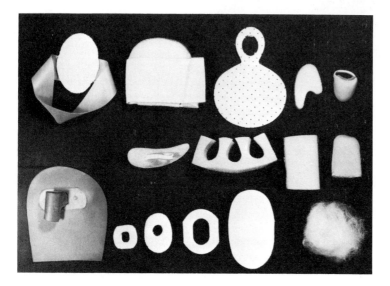

Figure 63–12. Commercial shields and materials. Top row (left to right): bunion shield; two types of metatarsal pads; interdigital soft-corn shield; and hard-corn shield for the fifth toe. Middle row (left to right): toe crest; toe separator; toe sleeve, and toe cap. Bottom row (left to right): Budin splint; four adhesive-backed corn and callus shields; and lamb's wool.

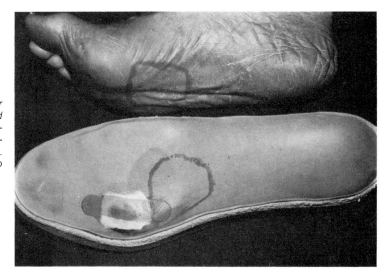

Figure 63–13. Trophic ulcer under the first metatarsal head from diabetic peripheral neuropathy. Lipstick on the foot indicates the area to be built up. Note the lipstick transference to the arch support.

shoes, the need for toe shielding has been minimized.

CORNS AND CALLUSES

It must be remembered that before any shield or metatarsal support is applied, calluses should be pared. This is done by means of a scalpel, using repeated light strokes and shaving off very thin layers one at a time. A thin layer of callus should be preserved to avoid bleeding or any undue tenderness on weight bearing. The one exception to this rule is when the callus is unduly tender, especially when associated with any underlying hemorrhage or inflammatory reaction. In such cases, further paring often reveals underlying slough, most frequently due to an early trophic ulcer secondary to diabetes or a peripheral neuropathy. Any overhanging keratotic or necrotic edges should be removed with a convex cuticle nipper to permit adequate drainage.

FOLLOW-UP

It is relatively simple to evaluate the effect of an arch support by relief of symptoms and decrease in the rate of pressure keratosis formation. How is the efficiency of an arch support evaluated in patients with sensory loss (e.g., peripheral neuropathy), considering that the patient is probably being treated for painless plan-

tar ulcerations? Aside from biomechanical studies with pressure-sensitive devices[2] (see Chapter 46) or thermograms, the most practical method is to apply lipstick on the patient's foot in the areas needing wells or elevations. The arch support is simply pressed up against the patient's foot, there-

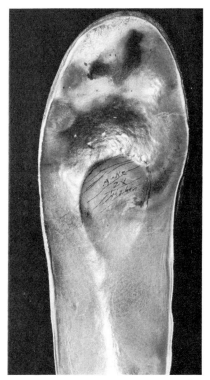

Figure 63–14. Flexible arch support showing wear of the leather, indicating poor distribution of weight bearing. The metatarsal pad should be doubled in height.

by accurately transferring the lipstick markings to the support (Fig. 63–13). In about six weeks, the arch support should reveal evidence of even wear (weight distribution) by brown staining of the normally beige leather covering of the arch support (Fig. 63–14).

Long-term check-up of arch supports is also necessary, as soft supports may compress, metal may become deformed, foot pathology may change or advance, splayfeet may become wider, and unsuspected diagnoses may become evident. What was originally surmised to be a simple mechanical plantar heel spur syndrome or hallux valgus may demonstrate evidence of collagen disease or psoriasis as the underlying etiology.

REFERENCES

1. Anderson, A. D.: The Shoe and Leather Lexicon, 15th ed. New York, 1952.
2. Brand, P. W., and Ebner, J. D.: Pressure sensitive devices for denervated hands and feet. J. Bone Joint Surg., *51A*:109, 1969.
3. Carleton, F. J.: Shoes and Feet. West Chester, PA, Charles H. Andress, 1940.
4. Dickson, F. D., and Diveley, R. L.: Functional Disorders of the Foot, 2nd ed. Philadelphia, J. B. Lippincott Co., 1944.
5. Diveley, R. L.: Foot appliances and shoe alterations. *In* American Academy of Orthopaedic Surgeons: Orthopaedic Appliances Atlas, Vol. I. Ann Arbor, Michigan, J. W. Edwards, 1952, pp. 439–478.
6. Enna, C. D., Brand, P. W., Reed, J. K., Jr., and Welch, D.: The orthotic care of the denervated foot in Hansen's disease. Orthot. Prosth., *30*:33, 1976.
7. Gibbard, L. C. (ed.): Charlesworth's Chiropodial Orthopaedics, 2nd ed. London, Baillière, Tindall and Cassell, 1968.
8. Hertzman, C. A.: Use of Plastazote in foot disabilities. Am. J. Phys. Med., *52*:289, 1973.
9. Jahss, M. H.: Shoes and shoe modifications. *In* American Academy of Orthopaedic Surgeons: Atlas of Orthotics. Biomechanical Principles and Application. St. Louis, C. V. Mosby Co., 1975, pp. 267–279,
10. Jahss, M. H.: Geriatric aspects of the foot and ankle. *In* Rossmann, I. (ed.): Clinical Geriatrics, 2nd ed. Philadelphia, J. B. Lippincott Co., 1979, pp. 638–650.
11. Jordan, H. H.: Orthopaedic Appliances, 2nd ed. Springfield, Illinois, Charles C Thomas, 1963.
12. Mereday, C., Dolan, C. M. E., and Lusskin, R.: Evaluation of the University of California Biomechanics Laboratory shoe insert in "flexible" pes planus. Clin. Orthop., *82*:45, 1972.
13. Milgram, J. E.: Office measures for relief of the painful foot. J. Bone Joint Surg., *46A*:1095, 1964.
14. Morton, D. J.: The Human Foot. Its Evolution, Physiology and Functional Disorders. Morningside Heights, New York, Columbia University Press, 1935, pp. 220–221.
15. Schuster, O. N.: Foot Orthopaedics, 2nd ed. Albany, New York, J. B. Lyon Co., 1939.
16. Schwartz, R. P., Heath, A. L., and Misiek, W.: The influence of the shoe on gait. J. Bone Joint Surg., *17*:406, 1935.
17. Schwartz, R. P., and Heath, A. L.: Preliminary findings from a roentgenographic study of the influence of heel height and empirical shank curvature on osteoarticular relationships in the normal female. J. Bone Joint Surg., *41A*:1065, 1959.
18. Sonderling, H.: *In* Lewi, M. J. (ed.): Modern Foot Therapy. Long Island, New York, Modern Foot Therapy Publishing Co., 1948, pp. 518–626.
19. Whitman, R.: A Treatise on Orthopaedic Surgery, 8th ed. Philadelphia, Lea and Febiger, 1927, pp. 736–926, 933.
20. Wickstrom, J., and Williams, R. A.: Shoe corrections and orthopaedic foot supports. Clin. Orthop., *70*:30, 1970.

CHAPTER 64

SHOES AND SHOE MODIFICATIONS

Nathaniel Gould, M.D.

HISTORY

For thousands of years, man has worn shoes. Even the early cave man recognized the possibility of injury to his foot by sharp rocks, sticks, the bite of a snake, or the sting of a scorpion or insect, and he attempted to provide protection by covering the foot with the hide of an animal he had slain. Repeated references to feet and shoes are noted throughout the Bible, and flexible sandals were the order of the day in those times. Early Egyptians wove sandals from plaited papyrus leaves. Today, sandals continue to be the most generally worn form of footwear in most very warm countries. During the past decade, sandals have come into vogue in the United States and have, to some extent, supplanted sneakers and loafers for summer footwear. The thickness and flexibility of the platform sole seem to be quite standard, but numerous variations are noted in the method of binding the sandal to the foot. Even in early times, some styling of sandals was important, but the texture of materials denoted the social status and degree of wealth of the individual. The Japanese, in particular, have continued to make distinctive sandals for the imperial household and for people in varying professions and vocations. The Greeks, always the lovers of beauty, attempted to depict this love even in their classic designs on sandals. The Romans employed a standard design for the military, but the sandals of their ruling class were bedecked with gold and precious stones.

People in cold countries turn to the moccasin for foot protection. This is bound and molded to the foot by the "puckering string." The North American Indians, the Eskimos, the Laplanders did make and continue to make their own foot coverings from the skins of animals.

In medieval and Renaissance times, boredom and the fopperies of the Court, whether in England, France, Italy, Spain, or the Teutonic countries, brought a most consistent early evidence of styling. Pointed toes assumed a position of prominence. This extravagance of style was exemplified by the peak shoe, or crackow, with the toe so long that it sometimes made walking almost impossible. In Oriental countries, long tails were attached to these points and were tied about the waist. Femininity in male apparel had "its day" and with it came harmful shoe styling. Some styles portrayed the wildest stretches of human imagination, and foot comfort was disregarded.

Until the middle of the nineteenth century, most shoes were made with absolutely straight lasts, and there was no difference in the appearance of the right and left shoes. At first, there were only two widths to a size, and the basic last used was what was known as the "slim shoe." In order to make the "fat" or "stout" shoe, a pad of leather was placed over the last to create whatever additional foot room was necessary.

Until the nineteenth century, tools for making shoes were practically the same as what had been utilized in early Biblical times. Basic implements consisted of the curved awl, which is a light knife and scraper, a form of pincers, the lapstone, a hammer, and a variety of rubbing sticks for finishing edges and heels. The average shoemaker, who did all work by hand, managed to make only one pair of shoes per day. In the days of the early American settlers, the traveling shoemaker would "live in" with a family and proceed to make enough shoes to supply the entire family for a year. He would then move on to the next family.

It was not until 1854 that the first machine came into use in the shoe industry. This was the Rolling machine,[26] which replaced the lapstone and hammer that had been used by the hand shoemaker to pound leather to compact its fibers. In 1854, the Davey pegging machine was patented. This allowed the sole to be fastened to the upper with small wooden pegs, and with this machine, the average operator could peg 600 pairs of shoes per day. From that time on, a rapid succession of various types of machinery was improvised. Gordon McKay purchased the patterns of Lyman R. Lake, a shoemaker, who had invented a machine for sewing the soles of shoes to the uppers. He found it difficult to sell these machines or to interest people in employing them because of their high cost. He therefore came up with the idea of issuing "royalty stamps." The shoe manufacturer could "rent the use of this machine" and paid for this rental by "royalty payment" for each pair of shoes made. This system is still popular, and today, in most shoe manufacturing plants, machines are rented or leased, thereby allowing the small manufacturer to survive the changes in lasting and styling that have continued through the years without increasing his overhead.

In 1875, the first Goodyear welt sewing machine, the forerunner of the various welting and auxiliary machinery of today, was developed. Huge sums of money have been expended in perfecting the modern

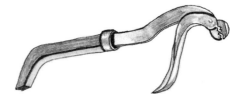

Figure 64–1. *Lasting pincer.*

shoemaking machinery. This progress may be illustrated by the developments that have taken place with regard to the lasting pincer (Fig. 64–1), a simple combination of a gripper and a lever, which for centuries was the shoemaker's only tool in shaping the leather of the shoe around the form on which it was made. This was supplemented by the pull of the thumbs and the use of tacks. Today, the automatic toe laster for Goodyear welt shoes can last 1200 pairs of shoes in eight hours.

THE MANUFACTURE OF SHOES[1, 5, 26]

Principal Parts of the Shoe

The basic major parts of the shoe are the *upper*, the *insole*, the *outsole*, and the *heel* (Fig. 64–2). The insole has been referred to by shoemakers as the "backbone" of the

THE WELT SHOE

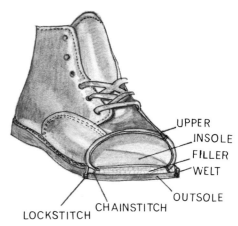

UPPER

INSOLE

FILLER

WELT

OUTSOLE

LOCKSTITCH   CHAINSTITCH

Figure 64–2. *The basic parts of the shoe.*

shoe with shank

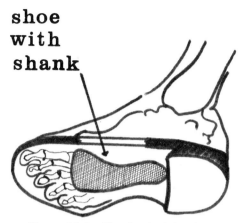

Figure 64–3. *The shank of the shoe.*

foundation of the shoe; the upper is what is seen on the top of the shoe; and the outsole and heel need no explanation. The *ball* of the shoe refers to the area of the metatarsal heads. The *shank* is the area between the heel and the ball of the shoe (Fig. 64–3). It reinforces the arch and is usually made of carefully shaped steel, steel and leather board, or wood strip positioned between the insole and outsole to conform to the arch, strengthening this part of the shoe and, therefore, supporting the foot. The forepart of the shoe is the part extending from the ball to the toe. The extreme forepart of the shoe is called the *tip*, and the vertical height of the shoe in this area is the *toe-box*. This part of the

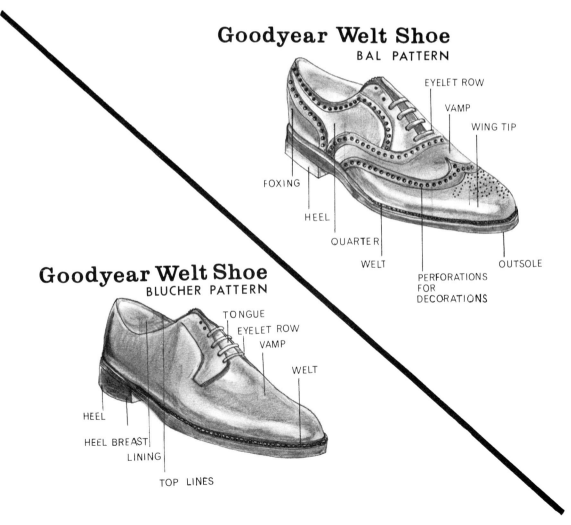

Figure 64–4. *The Bal and blucher styles of men's shoe.*

shoe is usually put through a stiffening process to maintain the contour. Behind the tip is the area called the *vamp* (see Figure 64–4), which extends backward over the ball and instep and then joins to the back part and sides of the upper of the shoe, an area commonly called the *quarters*. The quarters are joined in back by the *back seam*. In high boots, the quarter may be referred to as the *top*. The forepart of the heel is known as the *heel breast*. The margin of the upper of the shoe through which the foot enters the shoe is referred to as the *top line*.

Men's shoes are made in two basic styles (Fig. 64–4): (1) the Bal last, which is a front-laced shoe in which the quarters meet and the vamp is stitched over the quarters at the front of the "throat" of the shoe. The name of this shoe is an abbreviation of Balmoral, a Scottish castle, where such shoes were first worn. (2) The blucher, named after the Prussian general von Blücher, is a shoe patterned after a half boot. The quarters are left loose at the inner edge and made to lace across the tongue. The "throat" of the shoe is the central part of the shoe vamp opening, where it is seamed to the front of the quarter.

Common Shoe Terminology [8]

Boot: Any closed shoe with an upper rising above the ankle.

Bootee: A knitted foot-covering used largely for infants.

Box toe: A stiffener used to maintain the shape of the toe of the shoe, thus preserving the toe room within the shoe and protecting the wearer's foot to some extent.

Brogue: A heavy, low-cut, laced shoe, usually having a long wing tip trimmed with pinking, perforations, and unusual stitching.

Brushed leather: Side leather that is "sueded" on the flesh side, for example, a pigskin.

Buck: Leather that is "sueded" on the grain with a short nap.

Casual: A shoe designed for informal wear, usually soft, unlined, and roomy.

Cordovan: Genuine horsehide leather with a smooth, highly polished finish.

Cushioning sole: An insole padded with felt, cork, sponge, or foam-rubber cushioning material.

Dull calf or kid: Leather having a smooth but dull, unglazed finish.

Dutchman: A thick wedge of leather, fiberboard, or plastic inserted between the insole and outsole or between the lifts of the heel and designed to throw the foot inward or outward.

Flat: A shoe having no heel or an extremely low heel.

Foxing: A design feature of a shoe in which a portion of the shoe comes over the counter, where it is overlaid, seamed, or tacked.

Ghillie: A tie shoe with scalloped eye stays, usually open from the vamp throat to the instep.

Jodhpur boot: A short riding boot with a top just above the ankle and held in place by a strap around the back of the ankle. It is worn with or without leggings.

Kiltie: A fringed tongue adapted from Scottish shoes.

Last: A three-dimensional wooden or plastic form shaped in the general outline of the foot over which a shoe is fashioned.[1]

Loafer: A type of slip-on shoe.

Mule: A woman's shoe with a low back.

Open shank shoe: A woman's dress shoe in which cutouts are made at the shank of the shoe.

Orthopaedic shoe: A shoe that usually has a ⅛-inch heel wedge, a long counter, a solid shank, and a Thomas heel; in the larger sense, a shoe that has been specially designed for a particular patient with particular disabilities or requirements.

Outsole: The bottom of the shoe, the full outer surface of which is exposed to wear.

Oxford: Any low-cut shoe held to the foot by means of lacing, straps, or other adjustments.

Pac: Moccasin-type shoe with the top extending up to or above the ankle.

Patent leather: A leather with a finish produced by covering the leather with coats of varnish.

Perforations: Punched holes used to decorate the shoe.

Pinking: A method of fringing leather that is used purely for decorative purposes.

Platform: A thick midsole.

Plug: A separate piece of leather inserted in the shoe upper, usually for "stiffening" purposes.

Pump: Any shoe not built above the vamp and quarter lines and held to the foot without any fastenings.

Romeo: A man's slipper with a high back and front and low-cut sides.

Sabot strap: A single, wide instep strap usually used on children's footwear and women's so-called "comfort" shoes.

Saddle shoe: An oxford-type shoe having an overlay, usually of leather, that extends across the instep and is fastened on both sides of the sole. The overlap may be in one or two parts and is located between the vamp and the quarter. "Saddle" refers to the overlay.

Sandal: Open-designed lightweight footwear featuring straps and thong arrangements attached to a sole.

Scotch grain: Heavily textured side leather, derived from classic heavy British brogue.

Suede: An upper with a velvety finish.

Sling strap: The strap that encircles the heel in an open-heel patterned shoe.

Stacked heel: A thick, short heel now seen on women's high-fashion footwear, formerly found only on "old women's shoes."

Swivel strap: A movable strap that can be worn across the instep or pushed back to fit around the heel of the shoe.

Synthetics: Manmade materials, as opposed to leather, rubber, and wood. Synthetics and shoe upper materials come in three basic types: poromeric, expanded vinyls, and nonexpanded vinyls.

Welt: A narrow strip of leather or plastic stitched to a sole between the upper and the sole.

Shoe Sizes

The measurement of shoes by sizes was established in 1324 by King Edward II. He decreed that three barley corns taken from the center of the ear of corn, placed end to end, equaled 1 inch. It was found that 39 barley corns so placed equaled the length of the longest normal foot. At that time, because 39 was divisible by three, the longest normal foot was found to be size 13, and sizing since then has been graded down or up by one barley corn or $\frac{1}{3}$ inch to a size. Width sizing usually consists of 12 widths, ranging from 5A to 4E. Only four to six widths — that is, A to D or AA or E — are normally made in adult shoes for street and dress wear. Widths increase circumferentially at the ball by $\frac{1}{4}$ inch.

This arithmetical form of shoe sizing came into vogue with the advent of shoe-making machinery about the time of the American Civil War, and thereafter, shoes were mass produced rather than made for a particular individual. American shoes are made in more than 300 sizes, with widths to fit every foot. Length ranges in half sizes by groups from an infant's size 0 to a man's size 16. Two hundred and thirty-nine shoe sizes and widths were required for the U.S. Army during World War II, since the average foot at that time was approximately a size 8. With the improvement in nutrition, resulting in larger feet, even more sizing may be necessary in the future, unless changes with regard to sizing are made.

It is obvious that to combine the present arithmetical sizing of shoes with the style of shoe requires an enormous economic output, both in the manufacture of the shoe and in the stocking of the shoes by the retail outlets. Attempts have been made to determine methods of sizing that would diminish the enormous expenditure and that would function satisfactorily in the fitting of the shoes. One proposal was the Dynametric One sizing, which would maintain the present length sizes but would do away with the multiple widths from the present 12 to a maximum of six, leaving out every other width. Dynametric Two would maintain the present width but would change the arithmetical half size lengths to three-quarter size lengths. It is estimated that a combination of both Dynametric types could conceivably save the industry at least 30 per cent of its outlay in product and economics for each style of shoe. The most recently adopted proportional grade sizing by a large part of the shoe industry has already resulted in the saving of millions of dollars. Adoption of the metric system of measurement, which is probably soon to come, would require expenditures of many millions of dollars and a drastic change-over in the industry.

The Last

Figure 64–5 shows a reproduction of the approximate shape of the human foot, and over this form, a shoe is shaped. Before 1820, all lasts were made entirely by hand, and no distinction was made between right and left feet; one shape of wood served for both feet. In 1850, Thomas Blanchard invented a duplicating lathe for turning gunstocks, and this was later used to "turn shoe lasts." Within five years, a "grading" machine was developed with which larger or smaller sizes could be turned from the same model on the principle of the pantograph, an instrument for copying an object on any desired scale.

Children's feet differ considerably in shape and size from those of an adult. They have not been molded by activity and time, so shoe sizing for them must be worked out on a different scale, depending on the age of the individual. In growth, feet increase in length faster than they do in width. This growth occurs in spurts in varying characteristics. Because of these varying characteristics, lasts have been grouped under standard classifications (Fig. 64–6): Infant's sizes 1 to 5, children's sizes 8 to 12, little gents' sizes 8½ to 13½, misses' sizes 8½ to 13½, youths' sizes 1 to 3, boys' sizes 1½ to 6, growing girls' sizes 2½ to 9, women's sizes 3 to 10, and men's sizes 6 to 12. Actually, each grouping has been extended beyond the size quoted to cover any extreme, particularly in "king-size" individuals, and the groups do overlap in general size but not in character. Infant's soft shoes are normally made without using lasts.

In 1888, the Retail Boot and Shoe Dealers' National Association set up what became known as "The Standard Measurement of Lasts," and it is still the norm from which last makers work. This sets up exact schedules, giving the length, width, or girth, waist, and instep girth measurements for each last group (see Figure 64–5). Lasts increase ⅓ inch in length and ¼ inch in girth between sizes. The lathes used are pantographic in principle, and the fixed ⅓-inch and ¼-inch mount for each increases with each last size increase. This, of course, is not rigidly adhered to, since this principle would result in lasts having rather ludicrously higher heels in the large sizes as compared with the small sizes of the same style. The arch of the last

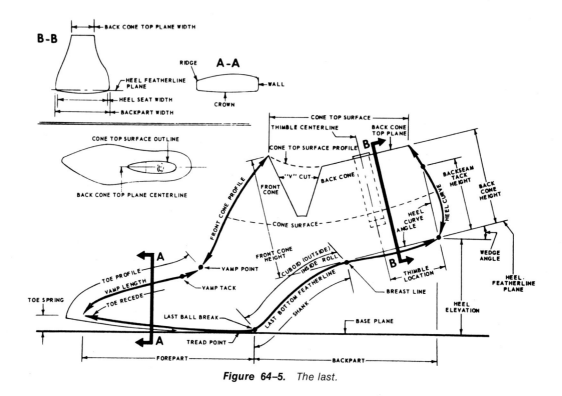

Figure 64–5. *The last.*

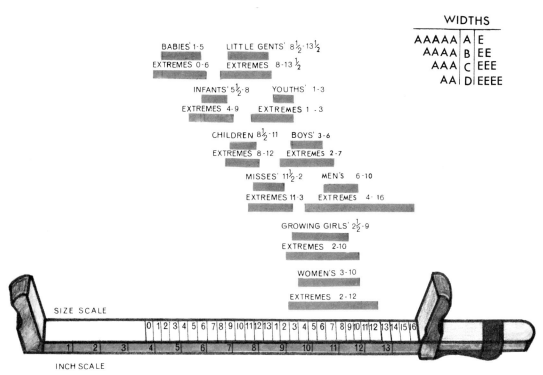

Figure 64–6. *Shoe size classifications.*

would also be seriously and adversely affected. Therefore, the measurement of a last is with the specific measurements listed in "The Standard Measurement of Lasts."

Different styles of footwear would call for "different distribution of the wood" about a last, but this was still within the basic volumetric total of the standard last measurements. The girth measurement is identical in each case illustrated in figure 64–7; however, the distribution of the area enclosed is different. In last making, the problem of holding a woman's pump on the foot differs from that of holding on a riding boot or an Oxford. The human foot seems to be adaptable in certain areas and "distributes itself within the shoe." In the area where the foot is not adaptable, the last makers carefully avoid any attempted distribution. Variations in style can usually be achieved by changing the shape of the toe, and since shoes are normally supposedly fitted several sizes longer than the actual foot, these changes do little to affect the comfort and fit of the shoe. The variations in the last with regard to the toe are confined to the fully mature adult foot, and

fitting in the retail outlet is carefully adhered to. It is hoped that compression of the foot within is minimal and is usually not deforming. However, this is the area of shoemaking that can cause manmade foot deformities and that prompted the American Academy of Orthopaedic Surgeons Resolution of 1965 with regard to "stylizing of children's shoes."

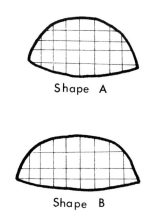

Figure 64–7. *The girth of the last at the ball of the foot.*

During the past several years, there has appeared in the shoe market an ever-increasing tendency toward "stylizing" children's and teenager's shoes, an apparent attempt by the manufacturers at duplication of the adult female's pointed toe styles. In many parts of the country, only these "styled" shoes are available for purchase.

Since it is the aim of the orthopaedic surgeon to "maintain and preserve" the musculoskeletal system, then it is his moral responsibility to guide the proper development of the growing child. With this principle in mind, and knowing that this improper footwear can result in various foot deformities, be it here resolved that the American Academy of Orthopaedic Surgeons decry the influx of these "stylized shoes" and urge the shoe industry to carefully review this problem and to redesign this footwear to allow the unencumbered development of the growing foot.[12a]

Because of the tremendous number of variables, last makers usually create individual models for each "group" of lasts by hand. The surfaces of the lasts, which are curved in several directions, must be carefully smoothed. The last is then turned from the model on the duplicating lathe. Shoe patterns are made from this, and the shoes are made and tried on selected feet for fit and appearance. Often, many changes must be made, and a number of lasts are discarded before a shoe manufacturer feels warranted in approving such a last and adding a given shoe to his line of manufacture.

Last making[1] is a custom business, and lasts are made to order to the shoe manufacturer's requirements. Many large shoe manufacturers have 30 to 60 active last styles with 80 to 90 sizes and widths in each style, representing a total of 2400 to 5400 different lasts, and to produce shoes in volume, many pairs of lasts are needed in each style, size, and width. It is readily understood that long-range planning is necessary to prepare for new styles. Months and even years go by between the preparation of a proposed last and the actual finished shoe.

Foreign imported shoes, which are frequently made in only average widths and with less adherence to the careful American methods of sizing, can be produced in a far less costly fashion and accordingly are "successful" in an American market. At last count, foreign imports constituted about 40 per cent of the retail shoe sales in this country. Many American manufacturers have adopted this plan of producing shoes for the average foot and thereby reduce their cost of manufacture.

The footwear industry of America has taken pride in its accomplishments in supplying good materials and precise shaping and sizing of shoes by adhering to the aforementioned principles, but with the rising cost of labor, many of the outstanding "name" shoe manufacturers have been forced into bankruptcy or have sold their patterns to other manufacturers. There has also been a shifting of the site of manufacture from what was once the dominant northeast sector of the country to a more dispersed production throughout the South and West.

Upper Patterns

Since the shoe upper parts are cut from flat materials, it is necessary to translate the three-dimensional shape of the last into the two dimensions of a piece of leather that is a flat plane. The pattern maker is a highly skilled, knowledgeable individual who must cut his leather patterns in such a way that the tip of the finished shoe appears straight. Dies are employed to cut these patterns on other materials. In the art of shoemaking, the method of attaching the upper to the sole has resulted in a number of constructions and combinations of construction, each of which particularly fills a specific footwear need. In women's shoes, these constructions (Fig. 64–8) are usually cement, Littleways, slip lasted, and turns. Goodyear welting is chiefly employed in men's and boys' shoes, "stitch downs" and "prewelts" in children's shoes, and "McKays" and "nailed" or molding in work shoes. The cement sole-attaching process is the most popular method and is also about the least expensive. Basically, depending on the method used to attach the upper to the outsole, shoes may be described as cemented shoes, nailed shoes, sewed shoes, and direct molded shoes. Various combinations may occur in one type of shoe. The attachments vary with the economics of luxury styling and also with the variety of activities in which men, women, and children participate and for which the footwear is intended.

The Shoemaking Process

The modern shoe factory is usually divided into eight production departments called "rooms": (1) upper cutting room, (2) upper fitting room or stitching room, (3) stocking fitting, or sole leather room, (4) lasting room, (5) bottoming room, (6) making room, (7) finishing room, and (8) treeing and packing room. For details as to what transpires in each of these areas, the reader is referred to the United Shoe Machinery Booklet, *How American Shoes are Made.*[26] For the sake of brevity and for

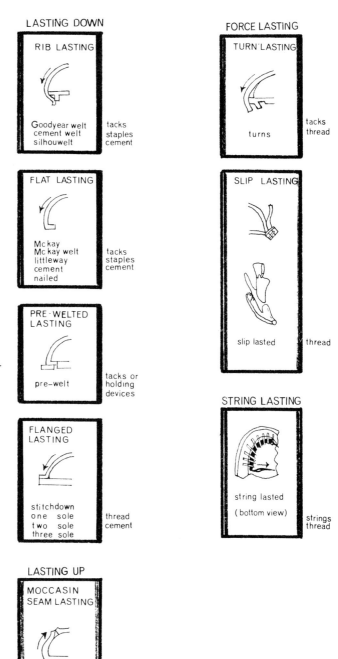

Figure 64–8. *Methods of lasting.*

comprehension, the intricacies of design and manufacture of shoes have been omitted here, but this short review will serve to acquaint the reader with the massive economics and the enormous number of highly trained individuals involved in the shoemaking industry.

About 15 years ago, when shoe production was at its highest, the total number of shoes produced annually was about 630 million pairs. There were approximately 1000 shoe manufacturing firms employing 213,000 men and women, with a total payroll of over 750 million dollars. The skill of those workers added over a billion dollars a year to the value of the materials that made up the shoes.

A satisfactory shoe begins with the hide of the animal and is then worked on by tanners, welters, lasters, and shoe manufacturers and is distributed to wholesalers, retail outlets, and shoe fitters. The improper fitting of shoes by unknowledgeable shoe salesmen nullifies all this work and the complexities of production.

At one time, an individual owned just one pair of shoes because of the difficulty in manufacture and procurement. With the machine age, owning two or more pairs of shoes became common. With today's luxuries and styling, most adults, particularly women, own many pairs of shoes to complement clothing and activities. In recent years, even the growing child possesses several pairs of shoes of various styles and colors, which could lead to problems. The unpredictability of growth coupled with the styling and poor fitting of shoes may create deformities in the foot of the growing child.

BASIC REQUISITES FOR THE PROPER SHOE

In July 1965, the original shoe committee for the American Academy of Orthopaedic Surgeons forwarded a letter to the then National Footwear Manufacturers Association, stating that proper shoes "cover the foot, conform to the foot, complement the foot, but never compress the foot." If these essentials are kept in mind, the necessary requisites for the designing of the proper shoe can readily be developed.

Fitting of the Shoes. Proper fitting of the shoes is a primary requisite. For example, the short, broad foot, the long, narrow foot, the wide splayed foot, the foot with a narrow heel, the foot with a wide forefoot, the high-arch or the low-arch foot all require different shoe configurations. Although the custom making, configuration, and fitting of shoes would be extremely valuable, it is as yet completely impractical economically. The day may not be too far away, however, when an individual can walk into an establishment, step into a particular mold and return some hours later to pick up his own individualized pair of shoes.

At present, a large retail outlet with a well-trained shoe fitter provides a better opportunity for correct selection of the proper shoe. However, the individual himself should be knowledgeable about his foot and should know what type of shoe is correct for him. He should also know about his own foot deformities and should not be satisfied with what only one store can provide but, if necessary should determine if other shops may be able to provide shoes that fill his needs more completely. The shoe should feel "right" from the start and should require little or no "breaking in." The child manifests his dissatisfaction with the fitting of his shoes by their frequent removal or, if the shoes remain on, possible limping and signs of skin irritation. The adult recognizes within a very short period that a certain style or type of shoe is not right for him because of local foot discomfort, irritation, redness, corns, blisters, burning, or more dispersed complaints such as leg aches, unusual tiredness, or even backaches.

Conformity and Attachment of the Shoe to the Foot. It is not sufficient to manufacture shoes that conform to the foot; attention must also be paid to how this conforming shoe is attached to the foot. No improvement has yet been made in satisfactory lacing of shoes. Lacing allows for the expanding volume of the foot from morning to night and holds the conforming upper snugly about the foot. Attempts have been made to employ zippers, snaps, side lacings, and clasps on shoes, but these devices do not hold the shoe snugly to the foot and so handicap and fail to complement the foot. For good lacing, four or five pairs of eyelets are necessary, so that the entire length of the throat of the vamp of the shoe is fitted snugly to the foot. A proper tongue that is smoothly stitched and adequately padded prevents irritation underneath the lacing. The average adult foot may increase approximately 4 per cent in volume from morning to night and expands two sizes in width from non-weight-bearing to weight-bearing status. The individual should know his own expansion status and make appropriate determinations as to the proper size of the shoes based on this measurement. It has also been found that the average foot lengthens only half a size with weight bearing, that is, $\frac{1}{6}$ inch, and this must also be taken into consideration in determining the proper type and size shoe.

In summary, the shoe should conform to the shape of the individual's foot. Theoretically, it should be shaped to the width of the heel and the width of the forefoot. This may require, in women particularly, a sling-back type of arrangement for the heel and/or an open toe for the forefoot. Lacing is advisable to allow for the expanding characteristics of the foot from morning to night that occur with prolonged occupational or recreational weight bearing.

The Shoe Must "Complement" the Foot. This third quality of a proper shoe is intertwined with the first two requisites to some degree. For a shoe to conform to and "complement" the foot, the longitudinal arch must be well protected by a satisfactory shank that is flexible, and the general alignment of the arch must be such that the high-arch foot is not placed in a low-arch shoe. With increased activity, support in this longitudinal arch area maintains the strength of the foot, prevents fatigue, and increases the individual's productiveness throughout the day. Therefore, conformity and "complementation" are interrelated.

Flexibility of the sole of the shoe allows the metatarsophalangeal joints to function properly, and proper contouring in this area maintains the proper contour of the forefoot.

A proper heel, which is preferably made of rubber and has an adequate diameter, provides cushioning stability during heel-strike. Heel height should not be greater than 1 to $1\frac{1}{2}$ inches and aids in balance and take-off and complements posture.

When shoes with negative heels were tested with dynamic granule staining slipper socks, unusual gripping of the toes and imbalance were demonstrated in the normally plantigrade foot.

Flexibility and lightness of the material in the upper allow unhampered and complementary flexibility of the foot. A straight inside last and a wide outflare for the toes provide the foot with the roominess and mobility required for dynamic expression of a proper gait.

The application of a proper water-repellent material to both the upper and sole is a further protective measure.

To date, leather has proved to be the only "breathing" material, preventing burning and unusual perspiration and fatigue of the foot. Socks made of 100 per cent cotton or wool also allow the foot to "breathe" and are a tremendous asset to the good health of the individual.

In summary, "complementation" of the shoe to the foot allows the foot to carry on its dynamic properties in gait by the use of "breathing," lightweight, protective materials that conform to the foot, complemented by a shank that is "springy," and a slight elevation in the heel. Cushioning of the heel with rubber and a sole made of non-slippery, flexible leather also provide "complementation."

The warning to *never compress the foot* (Fig. 64–9) is entirely one of common sense. Many foot problems and deformities are man-made, with the greatest single factor in creating them being a shoe that is improperly manufactured or fitted or both. Blisters, bunions, calluses, corns, ingrown toenails, heel spurs, and painful bursae are common examples of conditions that result from wearing improper shoes. To be sure, some are the result of contracture of the leg muscles during the growth period; some may be due to congenital or inherited characteristics; and some may be caused by the fetal position in utero, but in general, the shoe is most often responsible.

When all of the preceding factors were recognized at the time of World War II, there was an attempt to develop a uniform shoe design that would be most satisfactory for all military personnel. M. B. Howorth, an orthopaedic surgeon, was a pioneer of proper footwear,[14] and the prop-

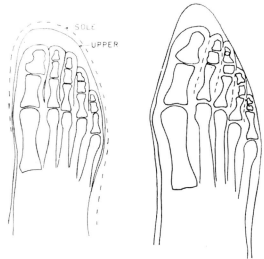

Figure 64–9. *Compression of the foot by the shoe. (From Howorth, M. B.: Consumers' Research Bulletin, May 1943.)*

er shoe that he designed is depicted in Figure 64–10.

FOOTWEAR FOR CHILDREN

An infant whose feet are essentially in neutral position does not need shoes or requires only a pair of bootees for warmth. Footwear is really not necessary until he begins to ambulate. In the pre-walking stage, soft leather "nothing" shoes are available, which have some shape but are usually not made on the last. These consist of one piece of leather that was die-cut on

a flat plane and stitched around, giving the general shape of a pair of shoes, although the right and left shoes are sometimes interchangeable.

There is a controversy among orthopaedic surgeons as to whether the outsole of the shoe should be a hard platform or flexible and soft in nature in the early walking phase of development. A semisoft, flexible outsole seems to allow better take-off and balance and greater toe control. It also seems to allow the child to be warned by trial and error of the perils beneath his feet, such as obstructions, moving objects, and ground or floor irregularities.

The upper should be soft and flexible to allow mobility of the foot and to prevent irritation of the child's delicate skin. A straight inside last, a wide toe outflare, and a good toe-box provide sufficient roominess for all the toes in the weight-bearing position. The upper should be of the high boot variety, rising above the ankle to supply stability there; the lacings should have multiple eyelets; and the tongue should be soft. The last characteristic prevents skin irritation, and the multiple-eyelet lacing supplies further stability to the foot and ankle until good balance and control have been achieved. Care must be taken in fitting, since children are often quite stoic and frequently curl the toes down, and shoes can inadvertently be put on with the toes flexed or with the foot inadequately placed in the shoe. Furthermore, care must be taken to avoid wrinkling of socks or of the leather at the

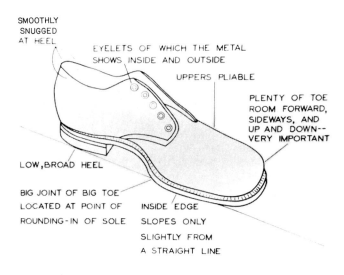

SMOOTHLY SNUGGED AT HEEL

EYELETS OF WHICH THE METAL SHOWS INSIDE AND OUTSIDE

UPPERS PLIABLE

PLENTY OF TOE ROOM FORWARD, SIDEWAYS, AND UP AND DOWN-- VERY IMPORTANT

LOW, BROAD HEEL

BIG JOINT OF BIG TOE LOCATED AT POINT OF ROUNDING-IN OF SOLE

INSIDE EDGE SLOPES ONLY SLIGHTLY FROM A STRAIGHT LINE

Figure 64–10. *Howorth's proper shoe. (From Howorth, M. B.: Consumers' Research Bulletin, May 1943.)*

tongue. Lacings should be tight at the bottom of the eyelet scale and looser with progression toward the top.

Parents can check to determine whether or not the shoes still fit satisfactorily in a number of ways. Taking off the shoe and sock rather rapidly and searching the toes for signs of redness and irritation is one method. Unlacing the shoe widely and studying the sweat pattern of the toes within the shoe gives a clue as to whether or not it is time to visit the shoe store again. Abnormal creasing of the flexible shoes at the line of the ball of the foot is further evidence that new shoes are required. By palpation, tightness and compression may be determined, particularly with regard to the width of the shoes, and signs of these may even be visible. In the growing child, footwear usually needs to be changed about every three months. Shoes should not be handed down in a large family unless they are fitted and approved by the orthopaedic surgeon.

The softness of the leather may be preserved by the use of saddle soap or other similar substances, and the shape of the shoes should be maintained by stuffing them each night either with the discarded dirty socks, paper, or rags. A badly fitted or outgrown shoe should be discarded immediately, because irritations of the skin of the foot in a child at this age are particularly difficult to heal and because there is also an adverse effect on the child's attitude about the further wearing of shoes.

All shoe corrections should be scrupulously avoided until the child is walking with satisfactory balance, which usually occurs by the time the child has been walking for about four months. The outsole may be made firmer with succeeding pairs of shoes. The heel is continuous with the sole ("cack") to prevent catching of the breast of the heel.

At first, a high shoe should be employed to aid in stabilizing the ankle. A child this young is very top-heavy, with short legs with musculature that is soft and not completely developed. In addition, the knee and ankle and foot joints are rather unstable and wobbly, and the youngster has difficulty maintaining his balance. Therefore, the easiest way to handle the problem is to stabilize the ankle joint to a large degree with a high shoe and lacings. As

the activity of the youngster increases and the musculature becomes stronger, the need to provide stability at the ankle diminishes, and the shoes may be low-cut. For many years, some orthopaedic surgeons felt that this transfer into low-cut shoes should be postponed until the child was about four years old. However, shoe manufacturers have disagreed, and it is rather difficult to obtain high-cut shoes for these youngsters in the larger sizes. Therefore, a compromise should be reached. The usual age of transfer is when the child is 20 to 30 months old.

Some have labeled the time from ages two to six as "the years of disregard," during which shoes take a terrible beating. It is during this period, from an economic standpoint, that it is important to reinforce the toe-box. Growth during this period is exceptionally slow, and shoes must be more durable, since size changes need to be observed about once every four months. The youngster is difficult to control, scuffs his shoes, walks through puddles, and goes about with complete nonchalance and disregard. This is probably the only period during the growing years of a child when it may be necessary to visit the cobbler to have shoes repaired rather than to discard them because they have been outgrown. In addition, heels are present on the shoes of children at this age, and they wear down and need repair. Further care of the shoes such as rubbing saddle soap into the leather prior to the first wearing of the shoe by the child, may be necessary and is probably advisable. This protects the leather from the snow and water. Polishing the shoes at least once a week also serves to repel water. Protecting the shoes in this way will maintain the integrity of the leather and keep it from hardening in spots and from discoloration.

When a child reaches school age, several factors create problems: (1) From ages six to nine, the child is entering into the second fastest growth period of his life, and shoes may sometimes be rapidly outgrown. (2) Because the child is now associating with other children, he begins to become somewhat style-conscious and wants shoes like those he sees others wearing. If the child is being followed on an annual basis by an orthopaedic surgeon or a pediatrician, one or the other will make the problem less difficult to manage by utilizing his position of authority to insure that proper footwear is chosen. The shoes of the school-age child should be durable but flexible, satisfactorily roomy and the oxford type of shoe with long lacings and should maintain the straight inside last with a wide outflare for the toes.

This is the age when a second pair of shoes is in order, and the ability of the child to wear a stylish shoe for a few hours a day supplies a satisfactory compromise among the doctor, the parents, and the child. Mary Janes, cowboy boots, Ghillies, loafers, or sneakers may be worn for just a short period of time, such as for play, to go to Sunday school, or for a social gathering. However, the basic shoes should be worn for the greatest part of the day, and there should be no wavering in this regard. Functional shoes for a particular interest or avocation, are in order, of course, such as ballet slippers, sneakers for play, boots for riding, and special shoes for sports.

From the ages of 10 to 14 years, styling becomes all important to the preteen and teenager. Resistance to the wearing of the basic oxford shoe has mounted. The rapidity of growth during this age of puberty until the feet have reached approximate maturity at 14 years of age, when the epiphyses are closed, requires a number of pairs of shoes each year. However, the basic shoes are most essential at this time, since they lessen the possibility of cramping of the toes and irritations of the feet. The wearing of loafers, loafer-like shoes, sandals, and sneakers, none of which support the arch, tire the feet and may even cause leg cramps and backache. This is a difficult time, when proper education of the child with regard to footwear must be insisted upon. One suggestion offered for how this would be done is the adoption of standard uniforms by all schools, private, public, and parochial. This would probably solve the problem most completely, since the education would then be confined to the governing bodies in their respective schools. If conformity is the rule at school, the wearing of proper footwear would ensue during the major part of the day. Once that habit is begun, it can be carried through the vacation months by parents or counselors.

The following recommendations were made to Her Majesty's Government through the Council of the British Medical Association in this regard:

1. A school footcare service should be established; this service is to include regular inspection of children's feet and footwear.
2. There should be control of footwear worn for school; this footwear to be of approved design.
3. All footwear approved as above to be free of purchase tax.
4. The Government will be requested to increase its efforts of health education in this connection.[28]

The adoption of school uniforms would be the most democratic as well as the most practical way to approach the problem. This would also probably reduce the budget in most families by eliminating individuality of dress and the competition for style by the children.

Once the feet have reached full growth, aberration of styling may still, of course, create deformities and problems with the feet and legs; however, it is felt that the formation of good habits in the years of development with regard to proper footwear will be carried over into the adult years. This part of the populace will continue to be conscious of shoe comfort and, in most instances, will wear shoes with the basic designs throughout most of the day.

FOOTWEAR FOR ADULTS

People do not purchase footwear based solely on its styling. Many individuals do not have feet that can be covered by just any shoe, despite the multiple sizing and shaping so carefully fabricated by most American shoe manufacturers. As noted previously, for proper "shoeing," an individual must know his own feet and their peculiarities. Nearly 100 per cent of the adult population have two feet that are not alike, and this factor must also be considered.

Shoe Requirements in Foot Deformities and Problems

Position-in-Utero Deformities

1. *Windblown Hips* (Fig. 64–11). In this deformity, at birth one foot is usually neutral in alignment and muscle balance (oc-

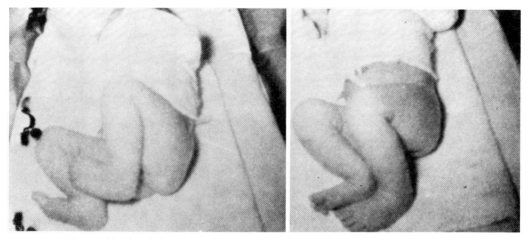

Figure 64–11. "Windblown hips." (From Gould, N.: Am. J. Orthop., 4:46, 1962.)

casionally in cavovarus), whereas the other is calcaneovalgus. If the deformity is greater than mild and these feet are not treated soon after birth, muscle imbalance can remain, and the adult feet will differ. The calcaneovalgus foot will be longer, probably wider, and pes planus may ensue. The shoe shank requirements and shoe sizing for each foot will differ.

2. *Calcaneovalgus Feet.* If untreated, shortly after birth, pronation and/or pes planus of varying degree may result, and shoe shank requirements will vary from the average neutral foot.

3. *Metatarsus Adductus.* This deformity, treated or incompletely treated, will require variations in the forepart of the shoe.

Developmental Deformities. The foot is not to be considered as a separate entity. It is attached to the rest of the body, and any variables in static alignment of the legs and the trunk do affect the dynamics of the foot in weight bearing and balance.

1. *Leg Length Discrepancies.* Whether due to trauma, disease, or heredity, leg length discrepancies place variable weight-bearing requirements on the two feet, and shoes must be correspondingly chosen.

2. *Genu Valgum and Genu Varum.* In a neutral line of weight bearing, a plumb line dropped from the anterosuperior spine of the ilium and bisecting the patella should then align itself between the first and second rays of the foot. If the static line is medial to this reference point, spe-

cial shoe shank requirements will be necessary.

3. *Tight Heel Cords.* If at all possible, contracted calf muscles, no matter what the cause, should be treated by exercise or surgery, so that heel heights may be evenly maintained at 1 to 1½ inches as the most desirable for the two shoes. However, owing to uncorrectable circumstances, a variable may ensue. A shoe heel height of 1 to 1½ inches does not seem to affect body balance and actually appears to complement forward propulsion in gait. Maintenance of contracture of the calf musculature does not allow the normal first heel-strike to take place and places an undue amount of stress on the forepart of the foot and shoe, mainly on the metatarsal head region.

4. *Contracted Plantar Structures.* Whether the condition is due to disease, heredity, or trauma, shank requirements of the shoe must be more carefully screened in the cavus foot. Blucher-style shoes and boots with looser lacing, preferably with four or five eyelets, and a smooth tongue are also essential.

5. *Bunions.* The vertical height of the toe-box must be carefully measured. An increase in the vertical height at the toe and at the first metatarsophalangeal joint may require a bunion last (Fig. 64–12) or an extra-depth shoe. After measurement of more than 1000 feet, I have determined that the vertical height of the average adult great toe measures ⅞ inch (2.2 cm). The average height of the adult foot at the first metatarsal head is 1¾ inches (4.5 cm).

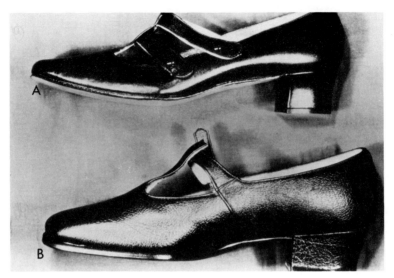

Figure 64–12. *(A) Regular last. (B) Bunion last.*

6. *Short First Metatarsal and Long Lesser Toes.* The straight inside last shoe with the wide outflare for the toes will probably be essential to prevent hammer toes with attendant callosities and metatarsalgia.

7. *Narrow Heel and Wide Forefoot.* Combination-last shoes have largely been discontinued from manufacture for reasons of economy. Compromising the feet by wearing a shoe that is a "little loose" at the heel and a "little tight at the ball" is not advisable. Women can still obtain satisfactory "walking shoes," the so-called "nurse's shoes," which retain the combination last. Sling backs, open-toed shoes, and sandals also solve the problem.

Genetic Deformities. Wide variations in sizing and configuration are common in bilateral genetic foot deformities (e.g., clubfeet, cavus feet). Frequently, there is only unilateral involvement (e.g., clubfoot, Charcot-Marie-Tooth disease).

Disease. Feet with neuropathies and rheumatoid arthritis, which necessitate special insole requirements with total-contact support at the sole, call for the extra-depth shoe, which can provide the space required for the special insole. Footwear must be carefully cushion lined, with an upper of "breathing" leather.

Trauma. Commonly, one foot suffers the insult and requires a special shoe or shoe corrections.

SIZING AND THE SHOE

The angle between the first and second metatarsals with weight bearing should measure less than 10 degrees on the roentgenogram. The rather rigid angle between the second and fourth metatarsals should measure about 6 degrees. The flexible outer intermetatarsal angle, between the fourth and fifth metatarsals, should also measure about 6 degrees. Any appreciably greater measurements probably indicate a splayfoot.

In my experience, as mentioned previously, with weight bearing, the average adult foot increases in girth at the area of the metatarsal head ½ inch, or two width sizes. The average adult foot also lengthens ⅙ inch, or one half a shoe size with weight bearing. It is important to measure the feet with and without weight bearing, so that the "larger" foot can be determined (as noted previously nearly 100 per cent of adults have different size feet), which should determine the shoe sizing necessary.

MATERIALS IN THE DAILY SHOE

Rubber Heels. Rubber heels help cushion heel-strike.

Leather Uppers and Leather Soles. To date, no material has been discovered to supplant leather for "breathing." With the rise in cost of petroleum products, however, synthetics now rival and in some instances even surpass leather in economic outlay. Soft calf leather creates the most flexible upper, constricts the least, and contours best to the variable configurations of the foot. Steer leather is somewhat firmer and is what is usually employed. The best "belly" leather is utilized for the showy part of the shoe — that is, at the toe and vamp — and the "back" leather is reserved for the back and sides of the shoe. Pig leather tends to form hard and soft spots with perspiration and other wetness. Horse leather is not usually as soft or as flexible as cow leather.

Rubber soles are heavy and do not "breathe." Crepe is also heavy and heightens the interface, making walking a foot-lifting process and thus increasing the work-energy effort expended. When very wet, the crepe surface becomes slippery.

Cork. Cork is used for filler lightness. Even reducing the average weight of each shoe by just a few ounces makes a remarkable difference in the work-energy effort expended and the fatigue of the individual by the end of the day.

Flexible Steel Shank. Supported footwear complements the biomechanics of

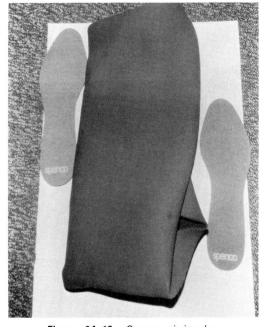

Figure 64–13. *Spenco air insoles.*

walking and reduces the incidence of longitudinal arch strain.

Cushioned Linings and Insoles. Rheumatoid feet, neuropathic feet (as in diabetes), and feet with a tendency toward excessive perspiration are best protected with lined, cushioned footwear. Although cotton and wool are the most "breathing" materials, some nylon is necessary for supportive strength. Air insoles (Fig. 64–13) cushion and protect hypersensitive and insensitive feet.

Vegetable Dyes. Rarely, skin rashes are noted as a result of wearing shoes. If the dermatologist confirms this finding to be the result of an allergic response, special vegetable-dye-treated, nonallergenic footwear is required.

FAULTY FOOTWEAR

Foot Dynamics[7, 15, 17, 21]

Normal weight bearing consists of three phases of gait per foot:

1. *Heel-strike.* The foot strikes the ground in the neutral or slightly rolled-out position, depending on whether the individual has straight or slightly bowed legs or is slightly knock-kneed. At heel-strike, the tibia internally rotates, and the os calcis everts.

2. *Foot-Flat.* The forward progress of the foot renders it flat on the ground, and now with the eversion of the os calcis, the talus rolls inward as much as 14 to 18 degrees and can even slide forward and backward a few millimeters. The foot goes into pronation, with subsequent "unrolling" of the remainder of the bones of the foot depending on the laxity of the ligaments, thus diffusing the shock of weight bearing. The weight bearing moves rapidly medially, from the head of the fifth metatarsal to the head of the first metatarsal.

3. *Toe-Off.* As the center of mass moves forward, weight bearing changes and moves rapidly laterally, from the proximal phalanx of the great toe to the proximal phalanx of the fifth toe. The tibia externally rotates and the foot goes into supination. The bones of the foot "roll back together." As the toes bend, the plantar tissues tighten and shorten the arch, and push-off and

toes-off occur, while heel-strike is occurring on the other foot.

In order for the foot to function as just described, the individual must be walking barefoot or in shoes that (1) are roomy enough not to constrict the toe, (2) have flexible soles, and (3) otherwise do not constrict the dynamics of the foot.

Types of Faulty Footwear

Pointed-Toe Shoe

When one looks carefully at the styling of the shoes of yesteryear, one notes that fashion changed about every 20 to 30 years and that the styling of shoes today is relatively unchanged from that of the past. The pointed-toe shoe dates back to medieval times. Originally, the pointed segment was intended to be a false, styled toe-piece and was not meant to contain the foot. However, adding this type of styling did not add to the aesthetic appearance of the individual, particularly that of women who had long feet. Accordingly, it become common to attempt to squeeze the forepart of the foot into the constricted confines of the tapered toe. This pointed-toe footwear could do nothing but render the foot painful and created corns, calluses, bunions, hammer toes, skin abrasions, ingrown toenails, swollen bursae, and tendinitis.

In the early 1960's, when shoe manufacturers became interested in fabricating a second shoe for the growing child other than the basic footwear that children had worn for many years, it seemed an excellent idea, for little girls, to utilize a pointed-toe styling similar to that of women's shoes. Little girls immediately wished to imitate their mothers, and the basic styled shoes fell into discard. As a result, basic footwear disappeared from the shelves of retail shoe stores. Problems similar to those experienced by women began to appear in the feet of children. This prompted the resolution to be passed by the American Academy of Orthopaedic Surgeons that "decried the influx of stylized footwear which could damage the growing foot." A committee on the foot was established by the American Academy of Orthopaedic Surgeons, and following a number of meetings with nearly 95 per cent of those involved in the children's footwear industry, a virtual promise was obtained that this constricting footwear would gradually be removed from the market, and it was. As rapidly as the pointed-toe shoe disappeared from the children's footwear market, so the pointed-toe shoe disappeared from the adult market. In the past several years, tapered toe footwear for adults has returned to a mild degree, particularly in the so-called "high-styled shoes"; this has been largely in the European markets.

Chisel Last Shoe

In this type of footwear, the vertical height of the toe-box is diminished in the shape of a chisel. The toes are squeezed from above, and as a result, skin abrasions, tendinitis, and other irritations may ensue. If the heel of the shoe is greater than 1 inch or so in height, the necessary room in the toe-box has been removed, and "toe spring"* (dorsiflexion ability of the metatarsophalangeal joints, especially that of the hallux) cannot take place, and further pressure occurs, particularly on the great toe. As stated previously, the average vertical height of the great toe in the adult measures about ⅞ inch, and with this chisel last shoe, the dorsiflexion ability of the great toe is markedly impeded.

High-Heeled Shoes

Styling of the heel of the shoe has been going on for years. When the foot is tipped into a semivertical position, the long foot looks shorter, and actually the longitudinal arch does shorten, as the toes go into dorsiflexion. However, the high-heeled shoe produces an ungainly, mincing gait with a series of fore and aft body curves. The foot cannot carry out its normal dynamic movement and go into pronation but is maintained in supination. Therefore, the shock of weight bearing cannot be dispersed to some degree, as is normal in the foot, but extends vertically upward, not only through the joints of the foot but to

---

*When referring to shoe construction, "toe spring" indicates the usual ½ inch of dorsal curve that the end of the shoe makes with the ground.

the major joints of the leg and even to the back, with possible early traumatic arthritic change. It also increases the work-energy effort. With prolonged wearing, the calf musculature becomes contracted, and weight bearing is unevenly dispersed throughout the anterior tibial musculature of the leg and to the forepart of the foot. Metatarsalgia may ensue, with callosities under the metatarsal heads; this is fostered if the heel seat is not made level by the wedge angle.

In the usual American shoe manufacturing, an attempt is made to level off the heel by the so-called wedge angle, placing the foot in a greater degree of plantar flexion with special flexing through the longitudinal arch, increasing the shank curve of the shoe. However, in the recent styling of a great deal of high-heeled footwear, little or no attention has been paid to the establishment of a wedge angle; the heel is obliquely placed, and the foot simply slides forward in the shoe, placing most of the weight bearing on the metatarsal heads. Such compression of the toes also creates hammer and claw toes, corns, ingrown toenails, and abrasions. This type of shoe corresponds to the detrimental high-heeled footwear of the past.

Negative Heel Footwear

In the 1970's, the "earth shoe" came into being. Originally, this had a negative heel, but with time, changes have been made in manufacture by other companies, and the heel has ranged from negative to zero. It was the impression of the deviser of this shoe that it would cause one to walk and stand straighter. In testing this footwear with the granule slipper sock test, however, it was noted that weight bearing was transmitted to the forepart of the foot and that the toes were constantly digging in, such as when an individual was walking uphill. In addition to complaints of aching calf muscles caused by overstretching, complaints in the forepart of the foot came into being. Symptoms of metatarsalgia became common, and even intermetatarsal neuroma was suspected. All of these complaints could be alleviated and remedied by returning to wearing shoes with proper heels.

Platform Shoes

In the medieval period, the platform shoe, elevated with cork filler, appeared. Originally, such shoes were worn by women to prevent dirtying of the feet in the mud of the streets. Later, it also became the symbol of the hierarchy and suggested elevated social stature.

The wearing of a platform shoe thoroughly destroys the biomechanics of normal gait. It also makes balance difficult, shocks the joints above the foot, and increases the danger of falls, sprains, and fractures. Such a shoe does little else but make the individual feel taller.

Heavy Footwear

With increasing economic strain, short cuts in shoe manufacture were sought. Thus, molded footwear came into being. The heel and the sole were cut with one die and cemented to the upper. Because of gravity and also because of the nonskid interface of the rubber or crepe sole, the work-energy effort expended by the individual because of the heaviness of such a shoe causes fatigue and reduces productivity. The method of molding and cementing may also cause a faulty curling of the sole to the upper.

Footwear Made of "Nonbreathing" Materials

Leather is still the most "breathing" material for shoes. Canvas sneakers, when not wet from perspiration or other means, would be a second choice. Encasing the foot in a shoe made of nonbreathing materials further tires the wearer and makes for discomfort.

Footwear Made of Unyielding Materials

Plastic footwear tends to abrade the foot, fails to conform to the contour of the foot, and makes wearing the shoe, let alone ambulation, a painful effort. Unyielding materials such as plastics are commonly employed in ski boots, skates, and golf shoes. The utilization of an inner boot that is yielding and conforms to the foot in the ski boot and skates overcomes the discomfort to a large extent. Furthermore, because the feet remain in neutral position in the skate and ski boot and forward motion is by sliding rather than ambulation, foot dynamics are not essential.

Slippery Footwear

New shoes with slippery soles can be particularly hazardous to young children. Scuffing the soles prior to wear is helpful. Corrugated rubber circular inserts measuring about 1½ to 2 cm in diameter, one at the heel, one at the first metatarsal head, one at the fifth metatarsal head, and one under the base of the proximal phalanx of the great toe, would probably solve the problem.

"Nonbreathing" Socks

Socks made of 100 per cent wool or cotton are the most comfortable to the foot and the least fatiguing. Multi-size stretch socks made largely of nylon or orlon cause discomfort and promote maceration and abrasion of soft tissues.

SAFETY SHOES FOR INDUSTRY[12, 22, 23]

Including the military forces of the United States, the total national work force is roughly estimated at 85 million people. Because the foot is one of the most vulnerable parts of the body and is liable to be subjected to injury in industry, standards of materials and performance in shoes that protect the foot are required. In 1940, a program for development of safety shoes for all industries was begun, and the committee that evolved to propound these standards was known as the Z41 Committee. Their first meeting was held in 1963. Subcommittees have also been organized, and standards for this Z41 series based on the American war standards have been reviewed, revised, and brought up to date as special requirements for various industries evolved.

National Safety Council. In 1912, a small group "concerned with industrial safety" met in Chicago and discussed the organization of a council that would be a "non-profit, non-governmental, public service organization dedicated to safety education and the development of acci-

dent prevention programs."[23] A charter was granted by Congress, and in 1953, there was a new National Council for Industrial Safety. This was to "arouse and maintain the interest in safety and accident prevention and to encourage the adoption and institution of safety methods by all persons, corporations and other organizations." The headquarters of this self-governing organization remains in Chicago. Its membership is composed of "more than 15,000 individuals and organizations, including manufacturers, transportation organizations, insurance companies, public utilities, hospitals, governmental agencies, associations, schools and all manner of citizen service groups." The Board of Trustees are volunteers from among the members, and there is a "continuous flow of information on safety to and from the membership." Unfortunately, not all industry is associated with the safety movement; only about 30 per cent of the national work force is involved. Finances come from membership dues and from various materials and services performed under contract.

Z41 Committee. Thirty-three organizations were in the original listing of members of the Z41 Committee. About 13 years ago, the American Academy of Orthopaedic Surgeons was added. Standards set forth by the Committee provide specifications, performance requirements, and methods of testing for safety footwear designed primarily to protect the feet of the wearer. No attempt is made by this committee to specify exact materials to be utilized in the manufacture of such shoes, since it is felt that if new materials suddenly appeared on the market that would satisfy the requirements, they could be utilized by the proper manufacturers without necessitating a complete revision of the listed specifications. The armed forces, however, have reserved the right to standardize materials to be used.

It has been estimated that following of the precepts outlined by the Committee has reduced the number of injuries by more than 70 per cent.

Specifications have been instituted for protection of the toes and metatarsals and for protection from penetration of the shoe from below, and from electrical hazards and for electrical conduction.

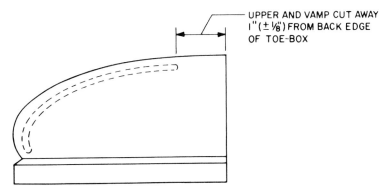

UPPER AND VAMP CUT AWAY
1"($\pm$ 1/8) FROM BACK EDGE
OF TOE-BOX

Figure 64–14. *Toe-box prepared for impact testing. (From Gould, N.: In Bateman, J. E. (ed.): Foot Science. Philadelphia, W. B. Saunders Company, 1976, p. 272.)*

Safety Shoes with Steel Toecaps

A protective toecap, usually made of steel, is incorporated into safety shoes during construction. Its strength is tested by *impact testing* and *compression testing.*

Impact Testing. The specified footwear utilized in impact testing (Fig. 64–14) consists of unworn size 9D men's shoes randomly selected from stock, and three specimens from each style are employed. At least 14 days have had to elapse since the completion of manufacture. The impact testing equipment (Fig. 64–15) is a weight of steel with a plunger 1 inch in diameter and 6 inches long that falls freely from a vertical height. The weight falls from the machine, striking the approximate center of the toe-box (about ½ inch in front of its back edge) of the shoe being tested. The proper class footwear, measured in foot-pounds, is determined by the weight of the material dropped plus the height from which it falls. Therefore, footwear is classified as 75 footwear (tested with a 50-lb weight dropped from a height of 18 inches), 50 footwear (tested with a 50-lb weight dropped from a height of 12 inches), and 30 footwear (tested with a 50-lb weight dropped from a height of 7¼ inches). The owner of the factory or industry where the workers must wear the safety shoes determines just how well the foot of the worker should be protected, judging by the weight of materials that could possibly fall on the foot in that particular environment. The strength of the supporting material at the point of the impact should be such that the inside vertical height of the toe-box of the shoe is not reduced to less than ½ inch.

Compression Testing. The same cut-out specimens of footwear utilized for impact testing are also used for compression testing (Fig. 64–16). Compression tested shoes must pass a loading of 1000 to 5000 lbs plus or minus a 50-lb variable and are so listed in their classification (Fig. 64–17). This type of testing has been given up in

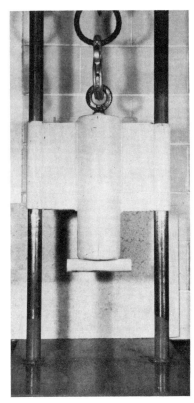

Figure 64–15. *Machine for impact testing. (From Gould, N.: In Bateman, J. E. (ed.): Foot Science. Philadelphia, W. B. Saunders Company, 1976, p. 272.)*

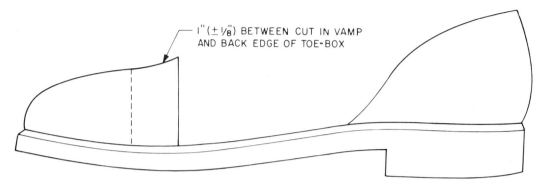

Figure 64–16. Footwear with vamp and upper cut away to facilitate compression testing. (From Gould, N.: In Bateman, J. E. (ed.): Foot Science. Philadelphia, W. B. Saunders Company, 1976, p. 272.)

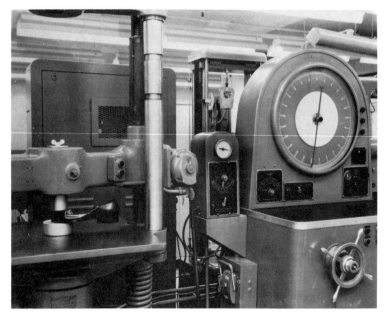

Figure 64–17. Machine for compression testing. (From Gould, N.: In Bateman, J. E. (ed.): Foot Science. Philadelphia, W. B. Saunders Company, 1976, p. 272.)

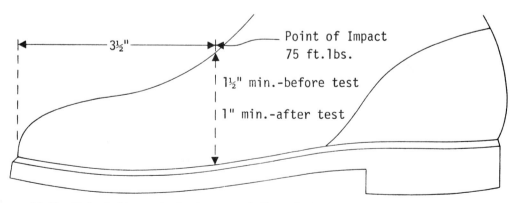

Figure 64–18. Method of impact testing (metatarsal). (From Gould, N.: In Bateman, J. E. (ed.): Foot Science. Philadelphia, W. B. Saunders Company, 1976, p. 272.)

many foreign countries. In the United States, because nearly all injuries arise from impact and because of the uncertainty and variability in compression testing, this type of testing is also expected to be eliminated here in the near future.

Metatarsal Safety Footwear

To test shoes for metatarsal safety, a size 9D shoe with a wax form inserted into it is used. The wax form is prepared in a specific fashion with specific materials, largely paraffin and beeswax in a proportion of 5 to 1, heated and mixed in such a way as to eliminate all bubbles and to obtain a uniformity of material. Testing is done at approximately room temperature. The method of impact testing (Fig. 64–18) is similar to that for safety shoes with steel toecaps, but the point of impact of the test weight is 3⅜ inches back from the tip of the shoe, following a line centered between the heel and toe axis. Metatarsal safety footwear has a clearance of 1½ inches before testing and 1 inch after impact.

Conductive Shoes

These shoes are intended to provide protection from static electricity that may accumulate on personnel and are designed to dissipate this static electricity to the ground and prevent ignition of sensitive explosive mixtures. These are intended for use by individuals operating high-voltage lines when the potential on the person and the energized part must be equal. The footwear intended to dissipate static electricity has been designated as Type 1 and that for high-voltage linesmen as Type 2. All exposed external metal parts must be nonferrous, and zinc is the material commonly used. Type 1 footwear requires a nonmetallic heel. Nail heads are below the tread surface (so-called blind nailing). Type 1 footwear has an electrical resistance in new or unworn shoes ranging from 25,000 to 500,000 ohms. Type 2 footwear has an electrical resistance involving each conductive component in sock lining not exceeding 10,000 ohms when measured.

After the shoe passes the proper testing, it is identified by a three-line stamp: the first line represents the American National Standards Institute (ANSI); the second line indicates the type of shoe; and the third line contains the ANSI standard number and date of approval, with the number following the slash mark indicating the test results for impact and compression as required.

Floor oils, oily cleaning compounds, and some floor waxes cannot be used on floors where conductive shoes are to be worn. In order to function properly, the shoes, particularly the soles and heels, should be clean at all times. Grit, corrosion, and oils damage the effectiveness of the conductivity. Because wool has an insulating property, wool socks cannot be worn with these shoes; slightly dampened cotton, rayon, or nylon socks must be worn. Foot powders tend to insulate and dry and therefore should not be used. Conductive sock linings should not be removed from the shoes nor should they be separated, because this may create excessively high resistance or may show up as a break in the circuit. The shoes are tested periodically. Type 1 shoes are withdrawn from use when the electrical resistance exceeds 1 million ohms, and Type 2 shoes are withdrawn when the electrical resistance exceeds 10,000 ohms.

Electrical Hazards Shoes

Electrical hazards shoes (Fig. 64–19) are intended to provide protection against open circuits of less than 600 volts under dry conditions and are not intended to supplant conductive footwear in conditions when it is required. They also protect the toes from an impact force (a steel toecap must be incorporated into these shoes during their construction). No metal parts may be present in sole or heel of the shoe. The outsole of the shoe is made of a highly electrically resistant composition, not less than 12 irons (1 iron = 1/40 inch) in thickness. The heels are also of electrically resistant composition.

Electrical hazards footwear is used primarily in the aluminum industry. These shoes protect against the high currents operated during the electrolytic production process. Workers in the chlorine or sodium industries also utilize this form of protection.

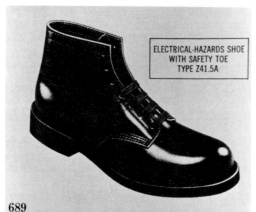

689
Black leather. Oil resistant sole and no-nail
cemented safety heel. Full cushion insole.
Pacifate® vamp lining. Non-conductive shoe
for use where electric hazards are present.
No metal except zinc-coated steel toe.
B 8-13, C 7-13, D, E and EEE 6-13.

Figure 64–19. Electrical hazards shoe.

Problems of leakage have been found in
shoes of welt construction, but other shoe
constructions meet the standards. Three
sample shoes, new, unworn, and about 14
days old, are tested in a dry, nondestructive environment. A blotter soaked in saline solution is inserted into the shoe over
65 per cent or more of the insole (this is a
recently developed test that is utilized
instead of the formerly used wet test). The
shoe is tested immediately for current
leakage with a specific transformer. It may
also be tested utilizing a 5-lb weighted foil

electrode placed within the shoe in contact with at least 60 per cent of the surface
of the insole. If the shoe passes the test, it
is identified as previously stated for conductive shoes, except "electrical hazards
shoe" is listed on the second line. Periodically, worn electrical hazards shoes are
tested to ascertain whether their insulating
properties remain.

Footwear With Puncture-Resistant Soles

In Canada, it has been found that 30 per
cent of injuries to the foot resulted from
puncture. In 1977, the Z41 Committee
proposed the following protective device
and testing to guard against such injury:

The protective device extends from the toe to
the breast of the heel and must withstand a
force of not less than 300 lbs. The device must
show no signs of corrosion after being exposed
to 5% saline solution for twenty-four hours.

Three samples are tested. The test device
(Fig. 64–20) consists of a movable platform
fitted with a fixed 2″ 8D common nail with 1″ of
its pointed end exposed. The platform moves at
a rate of 2″/minute. Each test requires a new
nail with a hardness of Rockwell B 70
plus/minus 8 and a diameter of .132″ plus/minus
.003″.

A 3/4″ (nom) thick female block has a 1/2″
(nom) diameter hole to allow free passage of the
nail as it penetrates through the protective
device during the test.

A minimum of three tests are made on each
protective device being tested. Penetrations
shall be at least 1″ from the edge of the sample

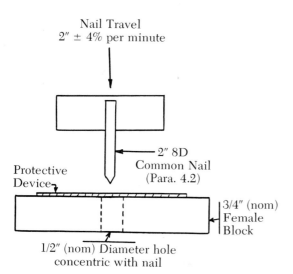

Figure 64–20. Sole puncture-resistance testing device.

and at least 1″ apart. The reading taken shall be at the peak of force when the point of the nail penetrates the sample.

Women's Safety Shoes

Specifications for women's safety shoes have recently been propounded. In general, this footwear is incorporated into the men's standard. The one variation in test requirement for women's sizes is the alteration to a 15/32-inch clearance and a size 8B test shoe. New, somewhat more elegant-appearing safety footwear (Fig. 64–21) has been designed for women and is gradually being accepted.

The military has found that it can fit 95 per cent of its women in the current men's shoes (Fig. 64–22). In general, footwear similar to that worn by men is employed when women are doing work that in the past was delegated to the men.

Summary

Statistics have shown that the foot is a very vulnerable part of the body and is liable to be injured in almost every industry. With these facts in mind and aided by the long-standing know-how of the military, the Z41 Committee of the National Safety Council, with a membership composed of approximately 30 representatives, manufacturers, and utilizers of safety shoes for industry and in the armed forces, has set forth standards for the design and manufacture of safety shoes. The parent National Safety Council is a voluntary effort of American industry to protect its manpower and work force and to eliminate any elements that could impair the industrial economy of the nation.

Unfortunately, people are sometimes careless about self-protection and suffer injury with subsequent loss of income, simply by forgetting to utilize the safeguards that have been provided for them. The emergency rooms of hospitals are beset with injuries that could have been less serious or would not have occurred at all if the injured party had not carelessly omitted to use safety footwear. It is hoped that labor unions, by making definitive demands upon their membership, will require that the work force utilize the safety measures that have been provided for them.

American industry has made rapid strides in these safety endeavors, and more efficient materials are constantly being discovered and used to advantage.

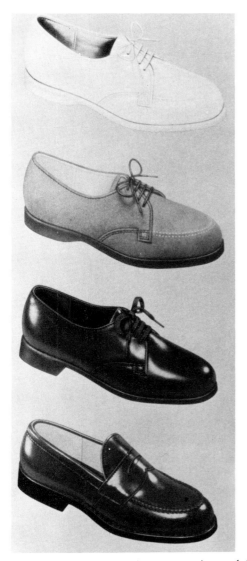

Figure 64–21. *Representative women's safety shoes. (Courtesy of Iron Age Shoe Co., Pittsburgh, Pennsylvania.)*

MILITARY FOOTWEAR[2, 3, 12]

Improper footwear can affect the combat efficiency of any military force, and the careful development of proper materials is constantly in progress and reviewed.

Prior to the establishment of the volun-

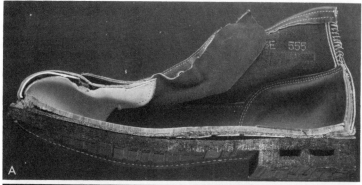

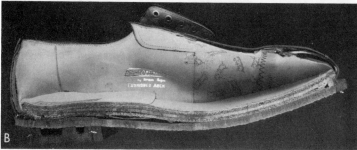

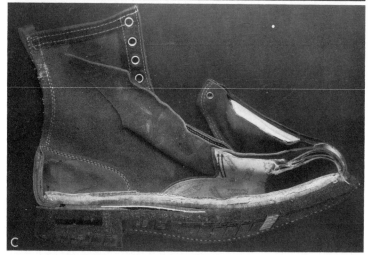

Figure 64–22. *(A) Men's short all-purpose boot made of soft leather and lined for comfort. Other features include steel safety toecap, steel heel protector, and steel shank. The thick neoprene sole and heel are nonskid and difficult to penetrate. (B) Men's dress oxford with cushioned arch, steel safety toecap, steel shank, thick sole, and Goodyear welt. (C) Men's high top, soft leather boot with cushioned arch, steel safety toecap, steel shank, protective reinforced leather tongue, stiffened reinforced leather heel protection, and thick, nonskid, highly impenetrable neoprene sole and heel. (From Gould, N.: In Bateman, J. E. (ed.): Foot Science. Philadelphia, W. B. Saunders Company, 1976, p. 272.)*

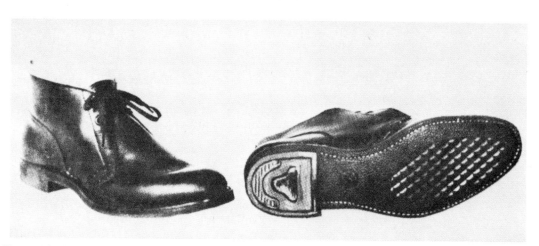

Figure 64–23. *Water-resistant Fleet shoe. (From Bailey, M.: Development of the Navy's New Water Resistant Fleet Shoe. American Shoemaking. June 24, 1959.)*

teer army, consideration was being given to changing the size of military footwear to correspond to Dynametric 1 and 2, as previously described. However, the new military force, in the judgment of the military leaders, justified the maintenance of half sizes in footwear and careful selection of only the best materials.

Navy. The Fleet shoe (Fig. 64–23) is made of water-resistant leather and has nonmarking heels and soles and polyethylene counters. The shoe seams are constructed so that they bar penetration of water through the stitch holes. This has now become the general-purpose shoe, the field shoe, and the flight deck shoe, and it eliminates the need for wearing rubbers with work shoes. The components of the Fleet shoe are sufficiently durable and suitable, so that they may be used on both wet and dry terrain. Proper vulcanization construction would probably reduce their cost.

Army. Booby traps of Panji spikes were prevalent throughout Southeast Asia. Tropical combat boots (Fig. 64–24) were designed with insoles of stainless steel plates 0.012 inch thick and were effective in resisting penetration from these spikes.

Another tropical combat boot (Fig. 64–25) was designed so that it freed itself

fairly readily of mud and maintained a relatively consistent traction capability. The outsole design was developed during the Vietnam conflict.

Special boots are made for use in temperate zones (Fig. 64–26), and other thermal lined boots are available for Arctic and Antarctic areas (Fig. 64–27). For the sake of economy and ease of transport and delivery, research is being carried out for material that will be proper to insert into the combat boot to render it an all-purpose boot suitable to be worn in Arctic areas with temperatures as low as −20°F or in warm climates with temperatures as high as 100°F.

A standardized dress shoe (Fig. 64–28) is now available for all military services. Various measurements were taken of over 20,000 soldiers, and a comfortable shoe was developed, which is quite similar to the old Munson last that was designed during World War I. It has a straight inside last, a wide outflare for the toes, and the toe-box is sufficiently deep to avoid compression of the toes.

FOOTWEAR FOR SPORTS

Physical fitness is the byword of today. The medical profession has encouraged

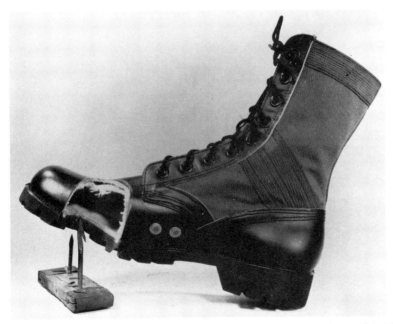

Figure 64–24. *Tropical combat boot. (Courtesy of U.S. Army Natick Laboratories, Natick, Massachusetts.)*

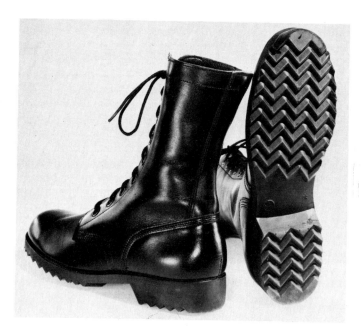

Figure 64–25. *Tropical mud-freeing combat boot. (Courtesy of U.S. Army Natick Laboratories, Natick, Massachusetts.)*

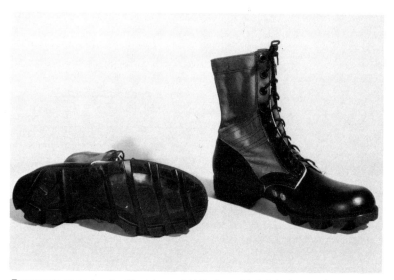

Figure 64–26. *Temperate zone boots. (Courtesy of U.S. Army Natick Laboratories, Natick, Massachusetts.)*

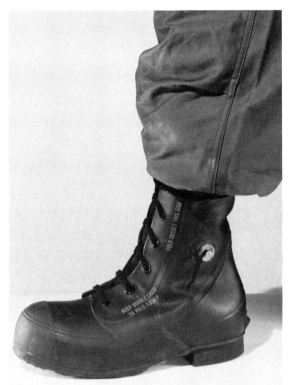

Figure 64–27. *Thermal-lined boots for Arctic and Antarctic areas. (Courtesy of the U.S. Army.)*

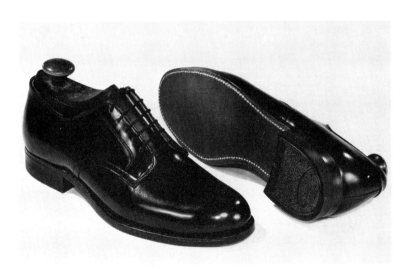

Figure 64–28. *Standardized military dress shoe for all services. (Courtesy of U.S. Army Natick Laboratories, Natick, Massachusetts.)*

daily exercise and a balanced diet for prevention of disease and prolongation of life. The President's Council on Physical Fitness has been formed in Washington. With more participation in sports, more injuries are occurring. Research is being done to prevent such injury. The Academy for Sports Medicine has evolved from the American Academy of Orthopaedic Surgeons, a Sports Medicine Committee has been designated by the American Orthopaedic Foot Society, and other medical organizations have followed suit. With this in-depth study of individual sports, many injuries peculiar to particular sports have been recognized, documented, and reviewed. New equipment has been formulated to prevent such injuries. Of course, in most instances, special footwear designs have been developed.

Running and Jogging. Jogging has swept the country as a leading form of exercise, one which does not require that an individual be a champion but enables him to develop strength in his lower extremities and improve his general body and vital organ tone. Special features to look for in and recommendations about shoes for running and jogging are as follows*:
1. Self-fitting.
2. Sizing varies from manufacturer to manufacturer.
3. Lightweight footwear.
4. Aerated footwear.
5. Use no insoles except for short runs.
6. Take care against sharp inner edges of soles, for they can lacerate the ankle.
7. Padded tongue (also control the tongue by special lacing so that it does not slide down).
8. Contour sole forward and up on the toe and backward and up on the heel to give some rocker effect.

In addition, the recently introduced "varus heel," which reduces excessive pronation, helps to prevent longitudinal arch strain and, for some joggers, offers new comfort.

Tennis. Tennis has had a tremendous resurgence in popularity. Special features to look for in tennis shoes are as follows*:
1. Self-fitting.
2. Well cushioned, providing immediate comfort with weight bearing.
3. Heel slightly higher than the sole.
4. Ridged rubber sole.
5. Aerated insole.
6. Lightweight footwear.
7. Special interface on the toe because of extensive wear on "toe drag."

Football. This is one of today's most popular sports. Special features to look for in and recommendations about shoes for football are as follows†:
1. Self-fitting.
2. For natural turf, seven or eight ½-inch metal cleats on the sole and two to four ½-inch metal cleats on the heel.
3. For artificial turf, the same number of molded rubber ½-inch cleats on the sole and heel.
4. Muslin ankle wrap, but preferably high, above-the-ankle footwear.
5. Lightness and durability.

Skiing. Skiing has increased tremendously in popularity, especially with the growing interest in cross-country skiing, the so-called "safe sport." Footwear for cross-country skiing has a semiflexible upper and sole and should be immediately comfortable. There are no other special requisites.

Special features to look for in and recommendations about boots for downhill skiing are as follows‡:
1. Snug-fitting boots for instant control.
2. Firm heel control.
3. Inner boot and longitudinal arch mold.
4. Allow only forward slide.
5. Use foam and snug-fitting, cushioned inner boot to fill extra space and to promote instant control.

Ice Skating and Ice Hockey. Skates used for ice skating and ice hockey (1) should be snug and self-fitting for instant

---

*Courtesy of Blair Filler, M.D., orthopaedic surgeon and marathon runner.

*Courtesy of Nason Burden, M.D., orthopaedic surgeon and champion tennis player.

†Courtesy of George Snook, M.D., orthopaedic surgeon and college football team physician.

‡Courtesy of Arthur Ellison, M.D., orthopaedic surgeon and Olympic ski team physician.

control and (2) should have firm heel control.

Golf, Baseball, Soccer, Track, and Bowling. Individual self-fitting is required for footwear for all these sports. They should be instantly comfortable and incorporate all the safety features necessary for that individual sport.

Except for skiing and skating, footwear for sports is necessarily lightweight and well-aerated and allows for balance and natural foot dynamics. Ski boots and skates, however, must be snug-fitting for instant control. The heel must be maintained in the neutral position and the inner boot and arch mold fitting utilized for comfort.

Before participating in any sport, an individual should pay careful attention to the selection of proper and well-fitting footwear.

CORRECTION SHOES[16, 19]

The term corrective footwear has been commonly used to denote shoes that have been lasted in a particular shape to suit a particular condition. The nomenclature "corrective" is faulty, however, since a shoe cannot correct. A particular "correction" shoe is utilized simply to maintain a correction that has already been obtained by manipulation, casting, or surgery.

Children's Last Shoes

1. *Conventional last* (Fig. 64–29A). Standard from heel to toe. Rights and lefts. Minor modifications can be made in the shoe for minor corrections.

2. *Straight last* (Fig. 64–29B). Straight, neutral from heel to toe. Rights and lefts, usually interchangeable. Shoes from one company angle slightly, and rights and lefts are recognizable. In the pre-walker type, the toes are open, and the lacing goes to the toes.

3. *Outflare lasts* (Fig. 64–29C). Employed to maintain correction after treatment for metatarsus adductus. The pre-walker shoe laces to the toes and has an instep strap for firmer placement of the foot within the shoe.

4. *Inflare lasts* (Fig. 64–29D). Utilized for maintaining correction after treatment for pronated feet. Pre-walker (with lacing to toes) and walker types.

Adult Shoes

1. *Surgical shoe* (Fig. 64–30A). Usually high-top and laced to the toes. Frequently

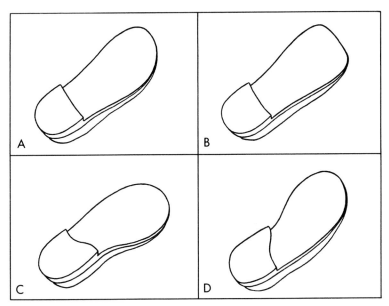

Figure 64–29. *Children's last shoes. (A) Conventional last. (B) Straight last. (C) Outflare last. (D) Inflare last.*

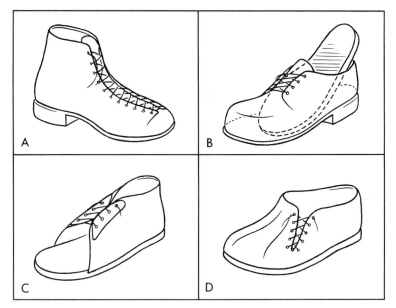

Figure 64–30. *Adult shoes. (A) Surgical shoe. (B) Extra-depth shoe. (C) Postoperative shoe. (D) Custom-molded shoe.*

used in cerebral palsy, peripheral edema or insensitive feet or with prostheses.

2. *Postoperative shoe* (Fig. 64–30C). Similar to a cast boot; however, usually has wooden sole, canvas upper, open toe, and Velcro straps or multiple lacings. Limits foot motion.

3. *Custom molded shoe ("space shoe")* (Fig. 64–30D). Made from a cast of the foot and conforms to all of the deformities of the foot.

4. *Bunion last shoe* (see Figure 64–12B). Extra-depth toe-box in the metatarsal region with soft upper leather to avoid constriction of and to conform to deformities of the toes.

5. *Extra-depth shoe* (Figs. 64–30B and 64–31). The latest in corrective shoes. This shoe measures one size longer (1/3 inch) and two sizes wider (½ inch greater in circumference at the metatarsophalangeal joints) than the individual's usual size and

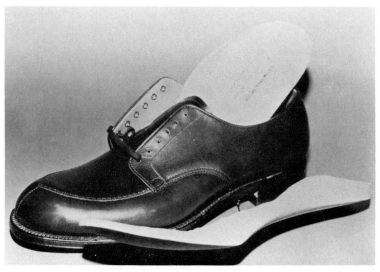

Figure 64–31. *Men's extra-depth shoe.*

allows the insertion of a molded ½-inch insole of Plastazote or a similar material. Most often employed in neuropathic or hypersensitive feet. Excellent in diabetic and rheumatoid conditions.

SHOE CORRECTIONS[13, 16, 19, 24, 27]

Modifications in footwear are made in (1) the last, (2) the heel, (3) the outsole, (4) the insole, or (5) the upper for various problems.

The Last

One of the pioneers in shoe research was Plato Swartz, an orthopaedic surgeon who attempted correction of *pronation* by modifying the last at the heel. He believed the correction should be made as close to the foot as possible, that is, in the last, the form from which the shoe is made.

The Heel

Common types of correction heels are:

1. *Thomas heel* (Fig. 64–32A) — the breast extends medially for ½ inch or so, extending under the sustentaculum tali.

2. *Stone heel* (Fig. 64–32B) — oblique-shaped Thomas heel.

3. *Reverse Thomas heel* (Fig. 64–32C) — the breast extends laterally.

4. *Flare heel* (Fig. 64–32D) — for wider and broader support base.

5. *Offset heel* (Fig. 64–32E) — broader than the flare heel and reinforces the sides of the counter.

6. *Plantar flexion heel* (Fig. 64–32F) — the softer posterior wedge cushions heel-strike; helpful in cases of limited ankle motion and is sometimes combined with a rocker bar.

7. *UCB heel cup* (Fig. 64–33) — a form of heel cup with shank extension to hold the heel in neutral position; sometimes combined with short leg splint or brace; perfected at the University of California at Berkeley.

8. *Heel wedges*

   a. *Medial heel wedge* (Fig. 64–32G) — usually has an elevation of ⅛ to ¼ inch; an attempt to control pronation.

   b. *Lateral heel wedge* (Fig. 64–32H) — has the same elevation as the medial heel wedge.

The Outsole

Various materials are used in the construction of the outsole. Originally, leather, which "breathes" and is flexible, was the material of choice. Later, with advances in technology, composition soles, which are longer wearing and cheaper, were favored. Cushioned crepe and other rubbers gained favor when the more economic molding manufacture was perfected. Rubber is heavy and "non-breathing" but is soft and increases traction. However, as stated previously, the increase in the interface increases the work-energy effort expended. Other rubber modifications include the ribbed and "ripple" soles, which allegedly further increase traction. Modifications of the outsole are:

1. *Lateral sole wedge* (Fig. 64–34A) — ⅛ to ¼ inch elevation, as desired, to attain eversion of the forefoot.

2. *Medial sole wedge* (Fig. 64–34B) — ⅛ to ¼ inch elevation to attain inversion of the forefoot.

3. *Metatarsal bar* — placed across the sole from proximally to the area of the metatarsal heads; ¾ inch wide with 3/16 inch elevation; used to remove pressure from the metatarsal heads. Variations of this are the Mayo bar (Fig. 64–34C), which is curved anteriorly and distally, and the Flush bar (Fig. 64–34D), which is tapered from proximal to distal to prevent tripping on the forward edge.

4. *Denver heel or bar* (Fig. 64–34E) — ¾ inch wide and is placed ¼ inch proximal to the greatest width of the shoe; tapers to a straight anterior distal edge; used for metatarsalgia.

5. *Hauser bar* (Fig. 64–34F) — comma-shaped metatarsal bar — for metatarsalgia; combined with a Thomas heel, it allegedly prevents supination of the fore part of the foot.

6. *Rocker sole* (Fig. 64–34G) — rolled from heel to toe for rigidity of the sole; for use in dynamic treatment for fractures of metatarsals or toes and hallux rigidus and for insensitive feet — to limit weight bearing in the fore part of the foot. Many

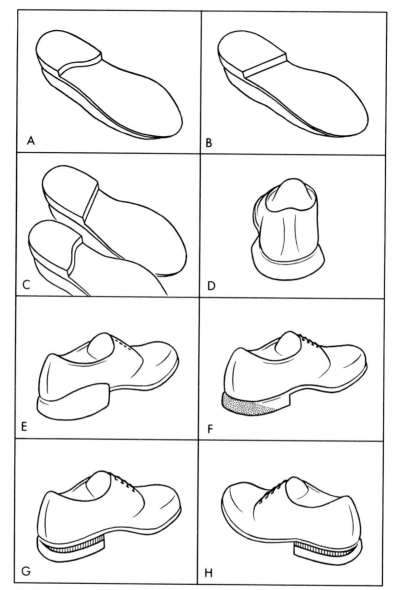

Figure 64–32. Modifications to the heel. (A) Thomas heel. (B) Stone heel. (C) Reverse Thomas and Stone heels. (D) Flare heel. (E) Offset heel. (F) Plantar flexion heel. (G) Medial heel wedge. (H) Lateral heel wedge.

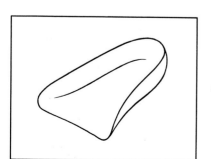

Figure 64–33. UCB heel cup.

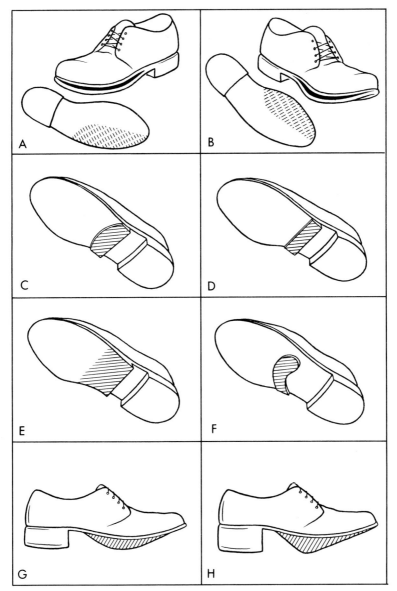

Figure 64–34. *Modifications to the sole. (A) Lateral sole wedge. (B) Medial sole wedge. (C) Mayo metatarsal bar. (D) Flush metatarsal bar. (E) Denver heel or bar. (F) Hauser bar. (G) Rocker sole. (H) Rocker sole (extended and steeper).*

variations of the rocker sole are made (Fig. 64–34H).

The Insole

Insole corrections are discussed in Chapter 63. Briefly, common ones are[16, 20, 27]:

1. *Arch supports* — made of plastic, leather, or steel.

2. *Spenco insoles* (Fig. 64–13) — made of neoprene with nitrogen air cells; for tender soles and heels and to prevent blistering and mild arch strain, especially in athletic footwear.

3. *Longitudinal arch pads* — made of rubber, felt, or other resilient material; for pronation.

4. *Metatarsal pads or bar* — ⅛ to ¼ inch thick, beveled and skived; for metatarsalgia.

5. *Morton pads* — 3/16 inch elevation

between the insole and the outsole to lift a short first metatarsal; used to attempt balanced weight bearing.

6. *Foamed polyethylene* (Plastazote, Pelite, Aliplast) — closed-cell, cross-linked, lightweight materials of variable densities; for total contact support, molds of insensitive and hypersensitive feet, metatarsalgia, and longitudinal arch strain, especially in runners.

The Upper

Some upper corrections are:

1. *Velcro closures* — used when finger disabilities make lacing impossible.

2. *Extended lacing to the toes* — as in a surgical shoe and so that the placement and position of the toes can be observed before lacing, as with insensitive feet.

3. *Balloon patch** — for hammer toe.

4. *Gore elastic piece* — inserted in the upper at the vamp to allow expansion of the foot, such as in peripheral edema.

Summary

There are many variations in the corrections listed (Fig. 64–35). Each pedorthist or highly experienced cobbler has his own technical style. Numerous orthopaedists who have pioneered conservative treatment of feet with footwear also have interesting and well-thought-out modifications.

GENERAL ASPECTS OF THERAPY

Although the conservative treatment of certain conditions with footwear and orthoses has been discussed previously in this chapter, it may be helpful to present the following "specifics" and suggestions for particular conditions with regard to conservative treatment with footwear and footwear corrections.

Bunions and Hallux Valgus
1. Bunion last shoes (Fig. 64–12B).
2. Extra-depth shoes (Figs. 64–30B and 64–31).

---

*Cut-out made in the upper over a hammer toe or any painful prominence and replaced by a loose, ballooned-out patch of soft leather, which is stitched or cemented on.

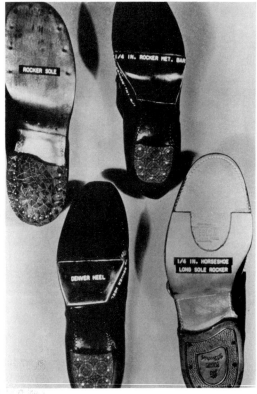

Figure 64–35. *Variations of shoe corrections.*

3. Custom-molded shoe (space shoe) (Fig. 64–30D).

Dorsal Spurs

The most common site of dorsal spurs is at the base of the first metatarsal–medial cuneiform joint, and they reflect developmental stresses during the "growing years" of the foot. Avoid friction to the area by having the patient wear sandals or shoes with soft, smooth, unwrinkled tongues.

Hallux Rigidus
1. For mild cases, low-heeled, "stiff-soled" shoe.
2. Rocker sole (Fig. 64–34G, H).

Longitudinal Arch Strain
1. For the non-athlete: For mild cases, supporting, off-the-shelf footwear that has a resilient shank. For more severe cases, plastic arch supports, which can be transferred from shoe to shoe.
2. For the athlete: Supportive strapping

to arch, longitudinal arch Plastazote mold, or Plastazote mold and varus heel (⅛ inch inside heel wedge) plus re-evaluation of the patient's athletic footwear.

Metatarsalgia
1. Rubber or crepe soles.
2. Cushioned insole.
3. Extra-depth shoe with molded, heat-treated, foamed polyethylene insoles (Figs. 64–30B and 64–31).

Narrow Heel and Wide Forefoot
So-called combination last shoes are not manufactured in any quantity except in "nurse" or "waitress" shoes, and many popular brands are available for women. For dress, suggested footwear is sling-back, open-toed shoes and sandals for summer wear.

Neuropathic Feet (Diabetes, Hyposensitive or Anesthetic Feet)
1. Best treated with molded polyethylene footwear (shoes, sandals, insoles).
2. Milder cases can be treated with Spenco insoles or extra-depth shoes with heat-molded polyethylene insoles.

Pes Cavus with Hammer Toes
1. For mild cases, off-the-shelf shoes with soft leather, nondecorated uppers, a blucher last, four- or five-eyelet lacing with a cushioned tongue, supportive resilient counters and shanks, and roomy toe-box. Conforming plastic arch supports may also be used with such shoes.
2. For moderate cases, extra-depth shoes (one size longer and two sizes wider than the patient's regular shoes), plus a ½-inch Plastazote filler (heat-molded to conform to individual soles).
3. For severe cases, extra-depth shoes with heat-molded Plastazote insoles plus a balloon patch or patches or space shoes (custom-made molded footwear) (Fig. 64–30D).

Plantar Heel Spurs
Plantar heel spurs usually signify longitudinal arch strain, are usually found in individuals with normal or nearly normal longitudinal arches, and require support along the longitudinal arch (e.g., arch supports [best], molded, foamed-polyethylene inserts, UCB insert [Fig. 64–33]). The wearing of supportive footwear (i.e., shoes with a resilient shank having a configuration corresponding to the wearer's feet) will result in gradual subsidence of symptoms in milder cases. The horizontal spur, protruding from the tubercle of the os calcis, simply denotes either long-standing stress or an acute strain with residual calcification.

Pronation
1. In the newborn, the calcaneovalgus foot should be manipulated into the cavoequinovarus position in a plaster of Paris cast, and the cast should be changed weekly for about six weeks.
2. In the early walker, longitudinal arch "cookies" should be used in shoes with flexible semisoft soles. In about four months, when the child walks with reasonable balance, the next pair of shoes may have firmer soles.
3. For the preschooler, in mild cases, longitudinal arch cookies or shoes with resilient supporting shanks should be used. In more severe cases, ⅛-inch inside heel wedges and supportive solid shank shoes with long counters are best.
4. For the preteenager, ⅛-inch inside heel wedges and supportive solid shank shoes with long counters or custom-made plastic arch supports are recommended.
5. For the teenager, custom-made plastic arch supports in four- or five-eyelet laced shoes are suggested.
6. For the adult, custom-made plastic arch supports in four- or five-eyelet laced shoes are recommended.

Rheumatoid Arthritis
Hypersensitive feet are best treated with custom-molded shoes (Fig. 64–30D) or foamed polyethylene footwear (shoes, sandals, insoles).

"Smelly" Feet
Avoid insulating and "nonbreathing" shoe materials, such as all-rubber soles, plastic uppers, all-rubber footwear, as well as prolonged wearing of sneakers and running shoes. Athletic footwear should be cleaned, sun-dried, and well

aerated. Leather is still the best "breathing" material.

Conservative therapy is the skillful combination of the best available footwear with the best orthoses, prostheses, and mechanotherapy to comfort the foot and provide relief to the patient.

Acknowledgments

The author is grateful to the following for their inestimable aid: the American Footwear Industries Association; fellow members of the Z-41 Committee of the National Safety Council; Geri Saks and Gary Nelson, graphic artists; Wing Woon, photographer; and Karen Amidon, secretary.

REFERENCES

1. American Footwear Manufacturers Association: Speaking of Lasts — A Compilation of Last Terms. New York, October 1970.
2. Bailey, M.: Evaluation of New Universal Military Last and Experimental Oxford. Bermuda Project NT001-018, August 31, 1955.
3. Bailey, M.: Development of the Navy's New Water Resistant Fleet Shoe. American Shoemaking. June 24, 1959.
4. Bleck, E. E., and Berzins, U. J.: Conservative management of pes valgus with plantar flexed talus, flexible. Clin. Orthop., *122*:85, 1977.
5. Cucinelli, M.: The Art and Science of Footwear Manufacturing. Arlington, Virginia, America Footwear Industries Association, 1974.
6. Diveley, R. L.: Foot appliances and shoe alterations. *In* American Academy of Orthopaedic Surgeons: Orthopaedic Appliances Atlas, Vol. I, Ann Arbor, Michigan, J. W. Edwards, 1952, pp. 439–478.
7. Elftman, H.: The transverse tarsal joint and its control. Clin. Orthop., *16*:41, 1960.
8. Footwear News: Dictionary of Footwear Terms. New York, March 14, 1965.
9. Giannestras, N. J.: Foot Disorders: Medical and Surgical Management. Philadelphia, Lea and Febiger, 1973.
10. Gould, N.: Positional in-utero deformities. Am. J. Orthop., *4*:46, 1962.
11. Gould, N.: First patterns of gait. Am. J. Orthop., October, 1962.
12. Gould, N.: Safety shoes for industry. *In* Bateman, J. E. (ed.): Foot Science. Philadelphia, W. B. Saunders Company, 1976, pp. 272–283.
12a. Gould, N.: Resolution on Pointed-Toe Shoes in Children's Footwear. AAOS Annual Meeting. Chicago, Illinois, June 1965.
13. Helfet, A. J.: A new way of treating flat feet in children. Lancet, *1*:262, 1956.
14. Howorth, M. B.: Consumer's Research Bulletin, May 1943.
15. Inman, V. T. (ed.): DuVries' Surgery of the Foot. St. Louis, C. V. Mosby Co., 1973.
16. Jahss, M. H.: Shoes and shoe modifications. *In* American Academy of Orthopaedic Surgeons: Atlas of Orthotics. Biomechanical Principles and Application. St. Louis, C. V. Mosby Co., 1975, Chapter 14.
17. Mann, R. A.: Biomechanics of the foot. *In* American Academy of Orthopaedic Surgeons: Atlas of Orthotics. Biomechanical Principles and Application. St. Louis, C. V. Mosby Co., 1975, p. 257.
18. Marshall, H.: Foot Knowledge, 1st ed. Boston, Boot and Shoe Recorder, 1923.
19. McMahan, J., and Schwab, D.: Shoes and Modifications for Pedorthic Practice. Atlanta, Georgia, Rapid Printers, 1975.
20. Milgram, J. E.: Office measures for relief of the painful foot. J. Bone Surg., *46A*:1095, 1964.
21. Morris, J.: Biomechanics of the foot and ankle. Clin. Orthop., *122*:10, 1977.
22. National Safety Council: U.S.A. Standards. Chicago, Z41 Committee, 1977.
23. National Safety Council: Booklet on Development and Aims. Chicago, 1977.
24. Rose, G. K.: Correction of the pronated foot. J. Bone Joint Surg., *44B*:642, 1962.
25. Scholl, W. M.: The Human Foot, 3rd ed. Chicago, Foot Specialist Publishing Co., 1920.
26. United Shoe Machinery: How American Shoes are Made.
27. Wickstrom, J., and Williams, R. A.: Shoe corrections and orthopaedic foot supports. Clin. Orthop., *70*:30, 1970.
28. The Health of Children's Feet. Report of a Conference Held at British Medical Association House, London, November 10, 1964. St. Albans, Fisher Knight and Co., Ltd., Gainsborough Press, 1965, p. 7.

CHAPTER 65

ORTHOTIC AND PROSTHETIC MANAGEMENT OF FOOT DISORDERS

James T. Demopoulos, M.D.

ORTHOTICS

The management of patients with lower-limb pathology, including disorders of the ankle-foot segment, has historically been based on the utilization of one or more treatment methods, including the use of pharmacologic agents to alleviate pain, infection, and other conditions, surgical reconstruction to correct pathomechanics, physical therapy exercises and modalities to improve functional capability, walking aids to assist ambulation and elevation activities, prescription of shoes and shoe corrections, and the fabrication of various orthotic devices.

The last few years have witnessed a rapid evolution in the field of orthotics. Current concepts include the development and use of thermosetting and thermoplastic materials for fabrication, a radically altered technological approach to design and construction of devices, creation of a new functional terminology, introduction of a multidisciplinary team to manage all aspects of the problem, more dependence on engineering principles and instrumentation to precisely develop the orthosis, and an increasing reliance on mathematical and other biomechanical assessment systems to gather and record useful data, develop the prescription, and monitor the outcome.

ORTHOTIC FUNCTIONAL TERMINOLOGY

A lower-limb orthosis is generally defined as a device of varying design and construction that is applied externally to the limb to restrict or facilitate motion, substitute for weakened structures, provide stability of the limb segments to allow locomotion, reduce or redistribute weight-bearing forces, alleviate pain that may be present on motion or ambulation, protect diseased or injured tissues, and enhance total function.

Essentially, the conventional usage of the term brace, particularly the nondescriptive "long leg brace" and "short leg brace," has been abandoned for the more current terminology that considers the anatomic region being corrected by the orthosis. An ankle-foot orthosis (AFO), for example, exerts its influence on the ankle and/or foot, and this term is used in place of the term "short leg brace." Table 65–1 defines the classification of orthoses rec-

TABLE 65–1. Classification of Lower-Limb Orthoses

FOOT ORTHOSES (FO)
  a. Molded shoe insert FO
  b. Bilateral shoe clamp (Denis Browne splint)

ANKLE-FOOT ORTHOSES (AFO)
  a. Metal double-bar AFO
  b. Single-bar AFO
  c. Rigid or solid ankle AFO
  d. Flexible or posterior leaf-spring AFO
  e. Molded spiral AFO
  f. Patellar-tendon–bearing AFO

KNEE ORTHOSES
  a. Molded plastic orthosis
  b. Swedish knee cage (rigid three-point pressure)
  c. Double anterior loop knee orthosis
  d. Hinged knee cage, with plastic, leather, or fabric bands

KNEE-ANKLE-FOOT ORTHOSES (KAFO)
  a. Conventional long leg, double-bar orthosis
  b. Plastic laminated KAFO
  c. Plastic quadrilateral brim, weight-bearing orthosis
  d. Single-bar, knee lock orthosis
  e. Molded supracondylar KAFO, with and without knee joints

HIP ORTHOSES
  a. Hip abduction orthosis
  b. Trilateral socket hip abduction orthosis
  c. Hip control orthosis

HIP-KNEE-ANKLE-FOOT ORTHOSES
  a. Conventional double-bar orthosis, with hip joint and pelvic band
  b. Twister orthosis
  c. Standing orthosis for children
  d. Standing/sitting orthosis for children

ommended by the Committee on Prosthetic-Orthotic Education (CPOE) of the National Academy of Sciences and other national and international groups.

In addition, various terms are used to designate the functional requirement of the orthotic components, since the prescription of orthotic devices is now based more on an analysis and correction of dysfunction rather than on the specific diagnostic criteria. The term "free," implies free joint motion; "assist" indicates the application of an external force to increase the range, velocity, or force of a motion; "resist" indicates the application of an external force to decrease the range, velocity, or force of the motion; "stop" implies the inclusion of a static unit to deter an undesired motion in one direction; "variable" means a unit or component of the orthosis that can be adjusted without making a structural change; "hold" indicates

elimination of all motion in a prescribed plane; and "lock" is a device that will maintain the orthosis in a desired position or attitude.

PLASTICS FOR ORTHOSIS FABRICATION

The choice of materials used in the fabrication of lower-limb orthoses, particularly those for foot disorders, has most recently undergone a considerable change, away from the conventional use of metal alloys and leathers toward an increasing dependence on plastics. Concurrent with the rapidly evolving use of plastics, there has been development of newer technology and significant advances in the training and professionalism of the individual fabricating the orthosis.

Plastics represent a large group of organic, synthetic, or processed materials that can be shaped to the contours of a plaster mold or directly to the lower limb, enabling the fabrication of a multiplicity of orthotic devices. Generally, plastics for orthoses can be categorized as either thermosetting or thermoplastic (Table 65–2).

Thermosetting plastics, which are liquid in their original state, solidify when mixed with a catalytic agent and develop a permanent shape that will not soften when reheated. Polyester laminates are thermosetting and commonly used in orthotics in combinations of a rigid and flexible resin in a matrix that can include nylon, Dacron, or cotton fibers or glass fibers. The polyester laminates are used over inexpensive plaster molds of the limb segment and exhibit excellent weight-strength ratios, are odorless, do not absorb moisture, and can be pigmented, drilled, and sanded. Other materials can be attached to the plastic laminated orthoses. Essentially, the polyester thermosetting laminates provide high tensile, compressive, and flexural strength and impact resistance, making them highly suitable for ischial weight-bearing or patellar-tendon–bearing orthotic sockets, as well as for foot supports.

Thermoplastic materials are available in sheets that become pliable with the application of heat, and in this state, they can be molded over irregular plaster molds by vacuum-forming techniques. On cooling,

TABLE 65-2. Plastics Used in Lower-Limb Orthoses

THERMOPLASTICS

Polyethylene
Characteristics: Tough, waxy material; rigid or flexible; varied colors; odorless; tasteless; well tolerated by skin; available in 1/8-, 3/16-, and 1/4-inch widths.

Fabrication: Heated in an oven for 10 to 15 minutes, material becomes translucent; draped or vacuum-formed over a positive model; easily machined or riveted; may be welded.

Polypropylene
Characteristics: Very rigid material; relatively low cold flow, chemically inert; extremely tough; lightest in weight of this group of materials; unlimited flexibility; resists temperature to 300°F; varied colors; available in widths of 1/8, 3/16, and 1/4 inch; excellent plastic memory.

Fabrication: Heated in an oven at 400°F for 8 to 10 minutes, material becomes extremely tacky; when heated, it must be in a special frame (platen); easily vacuum-formed.

Kydex
Characteristics: Acrylic polyvinyl chloride; outstanding chemical resistance; extremely rigid; easily machined; beige in color.

Fabrication: Heated to 350 to 400°F, material becomes pliable and is easily molded over a positive model.

Plastazote
Characteristics: Closed-cell polyethylene sheet; blown under nitrogen, assuming foam-like characteristics; malleable and autoadhesive in dry heat (284°F); nontoxic; low flammability; easily cut, sanded, and smoothed; available in many densities (most common being soft); used for padding and insoles.

Fabrication: Material is cut to pre-shaped pattern, heated in an oven or with a heat gun, and bonded with contact cement or autobonded to a material that is more resilient.

Ortholene
Characteristics: Extremely high molecular weight polyethylene; superior-notch toughness; resistant to chemical corrosion; not brittle at low temperatures; pink in color; can be sterilized; easily cold-formed; slower return than polypropylene.

Fabrication: Material is cut into a pattern and heated to 350°F for 10 to 15 minutes; conforms to positive mold with Ace bandages.

Pelite
Characteristics: Lightweight foam sheets of polyethylene; used as padding material; white in color; clean; nonallergenic; soft texture; available in different densities.

Fabrication: Material is heated to 180°F for 10 minutes, then pulled over positive mold; may be trimmed or buffed.

Nyloplex
Characteristics: Reddish, clear acrylic base bounded with nylon; tempered for 2 hours at 90°C for maximum strength; available in 2.0-, 2.5-, 3.0-, 3.5-, and 4.0-mm widths; can be sanded and buffed.

Fabrication: Material is cut into a pattern, heated at 284°F for 10 to 15 minutes; pulled over positive mold and formed with Ace bandage to conform to surface irregularities.

Subortholene
Characteristics: Very high molecular weight polyethylene; related to Ortholene, with less toughness and strength, but easier to form under heat; can be machined, welded, and cold-formed; compatible with skin; odorless; resistant to perspiration.

Fabrication: Material is cut into a pattern and heated to 150 to 160°C; excellent deep drawing characteristics; can be vacuum-formed.

THERMOSETTING PLASTICS

Polyester
Characteristics: Liquid in original state; when combined with oxidizing agent, endothermic reaction solidifies the resin; available rigid or flexible; used in matrix of nylon and fiber glass or metal supports; easily machined, buffed, carved, and riveted; slightly moldable with application of heat; many colors available with selection of pigments; may be cut, sanded, and smoothed into proper dimensions.

Fabrication: The liquid resin is mixed with the proper percentage of rigid or flexible resin; catalyst is a benzoperoxide to speed the chemical realignment of polyesters; pigments of various shades are blended into the mix, and a promoter of cobalt or aniline is used to speed the reaction; the resin is poured into a PVA cone pulled over the work; the resin is massaged into the matrix of nylon and fiber glass stockinette; the resin will solidify in one hour.

Acrylic Resin
Characteristics: Available as a liquid in the original state; manufactured on a methylmethacrylate base; two-component resin (flexible and rigid); extremely good weight-strength ratio; will chemically bond to fiber glass and nylon; a selection of pigments of various shades is available; a hardener paste is used to solidify the resin.

Fabrication: Same as for polyester.

the plastic retains the new shape; reheating can again produce contour alterations. Polypropylene sheets are most commonly used, exhibiting extremely high weight-strength ratios, high fatigue resistance, and excellent molding characteristics, and they are lightweight. Furthermore, this material will bond to an interface material in the moldable state and can easily be machined. Polypropylene, together with other thermoplastic materials, is used in orthotics where support is needed together with a spring effect, e.g., to simulate dorsiflexion during the swing phase of an individual gait cycle where weakness of the dorsiflexors exists.

Plastazote is another thermoplastic material available in a foam sheet. The sheet plastic is a polyethylene that is blown under nitrogen to form a sponge or foam-like substance of varying density. Rigid-density Plastazote is commonly used for inserts, and the soft-density type is utilized for padding. A decided advantage is that on heating it becomes pliable and can be applied directly to the patient's skin, avoiding the need for casting of the foot.

Pelite is another closed-cell polyethylene foam that is light in weight and soft in texture. This material is generally used as an interface material between the skin and the internal surface of the orthosis.

Other materials used in the field of orthotics include steel, stainless steel, aluminum alloys, leathers, fabrics, and other metal alloys. However, plastics are quickly replacing the primary use of these materials in the prescription of foot and ankle-foot orthoses.

ADVANTAGES AND INDICATIONS FOR PLASTIC ORTHOSES

Advantages

Normal function during the stance and swing phases of gait demands active and adequate motor units, stable leverage systems, intact sensory reception and interpretation, and central motor control. Conventional braces usually overcompensate for disturbances in muscles, joints, nerves, the spinal cord, or the brain by utilizing rigid and heavy steel and metal alloy com-

TABLE 65–3.   Advantages of Plastic Orthoses

1. Superior cosmesis
2. Lighter weight
3. Favorable weight-strength ratio
4. Biophysiologic motion
5. Improved deformity prevention/correction
6. Minimal or no moving parts
7. Higher degree of comfort
8. Less maintenance
9. Easier and consistent donning
10. Better patient acceptance

ponents that permit motion in only one plane. Plastic orthoses offer lighter weight, favorable weight-strength ratios, improved cosmesis, a higher degree of comfort, more effective prevention and correction of deformities because of their high degree of congruency to the limb contours, less maintenance, consistent and easier donning, better patient acceptance, and more physiologic motion, closely matching that of the normal limb (Table 65–3). A plastic orthosis can be constructed to allow motion in the sagittal plane, ankle dorsiflexion, and plantar flexion, as well as allowing axial rotation of the leg segment and simulating subtalar motion. The conventional double-bar ankle-foot orthosis ("short leg brace") permits only sagittal up-and-down motion of the ankle-foot articulation.

There are disadvantages inherent in plastic orthoses, however, including the higher cost of fabrication and their relative inability to be altered once completed and delivered to the patient. The introduction of newer materials, preformed components, and adjustable orthoses are expected to lessen such disadvantages.

Indications

Plastic lower-limb orthoses, specifically foot and ankle-foot orthoses, are indicated and prescribed for a wide variety of diagnostic categories and disabilities. Table 65–4 delineates conditions that are amenable to orthotic care, particularly when shoes and shoe modifications have failed. A foot orthosis of the molded insert type can be expected to protect ulcerations due

TABLE 65–4.   Foot Disorders Amenable to Orthotic Management

Development disorders
Congenital anomalies
Genetic disturbances
Neurologic disorders
   a. Failure of development
   b. Birth injury (cerebral)
   c. Ataxias
   d. Stroke
   e. Poliomyelitis
   f. Peripheral neuropathies
   g. Charcot foot
   h. Sudeck's atrophy
   i. Insensitive foot
Medical disorders
   a. Gout
   b. Arthritis
   c. Metabolic problems
   d. Blood dyscrasias
Avascular disorders
   a. Diabetes mellitus
   b. Nondiabetic disturbances
Infections
Tumors
Trauma

to infection, diabetes mellitus, burns, and local trauma. The insert is designed so that there is relief of the diseased or injured area; a well-fitted and specifically designed shoe is a vital component of the corrective device. Ankle-foot orthoses usually extend proximally on the below-the-knee limb segment and often to the level of the knee to correct foot disorders. An example is the patellar-tendon–bearing (PTB) orthosis prescribed to unload the ankle in degenerative and other arthritic conditions, reduce painful ankle motion, protect surgical reconstruction until healing has occurred, and prevent pathologic fractures. Plastic orthoses are also indicated when spasticity induced by upper motor neuron disease interferes with gait or when proprioceptive loss requires compensation. Surgical intervention in spinal column disease or injury, as well as total joint replacement surgery of the hip or knee, occasionally produces peripheral nerve injuries that cause motor and sensory loss in the ankle-foot region; various devices are then required to alleviate the problem. A later section of this chapter will detail the different pathologic states and describe the appropriate orthosis.

DEVELOPMENT OF THE ORTHOTIC PRESCRIPTION

The process of orthotically restoring function to a patient with impairment of the ankle-foot segment is a complex endeavor and requires a combined approach by an interdisciplinary group of professionals, with each individual contributing his technical expertise. The process must be designed to meet the total needs of the patient, beyond the simple fabrication and delivery of a device.

Orthotic Service

Experience with patients requiring orthoses to correct varying degrees of pathology indicates that the creation of a well-staffed Orthotic Service is the most effective method to evaluate the total needs of a patient, prescribe the orthosis and training, and provide continuing care (Table 65–5).

Generally, the Orthotic Service is directed by a physician with sound training and experience in the field of orthotics. Furthermore, the physician must possess medical administrative knowledge to assemble and supervise the clinic staff, particularly when the Orthotic Service operates within a large teaching hospital. Sufficient support staff in the secretarial and clerical areas is required to establish and maintain a system of medical records and appointments, schedule and circulate notice of the clinic to all appropriate individuals, maintain relevant statistics, pre-

TABLE 65–5.   Orthotic Service Staffing Pattern

1. Physician — team leader (orthopaedist-physiatrist)
2. Certified orthotist
3. Registered physical therapist
4. Rehabilitation engineer
5. Shoe expert
6. Medical social service worker
7. Psychologist-psychiatrist
8. Vocational rehabilitation counselor
9. Rehabilitation nurse
10. Administrative and secretarial staff
11. House staff (orthopaedic, physiatric, pediatric)
12. Medical students
13. Allied health staff students

pare reports for sponsoring public and private agencies, schedule team conferences, complete and transmit prescription orders, and monitor the patient through the entire process.

Optimally, the Orthotic Service includes a certified orthotist, an expert in shoes and shoe corrections (pedorthist), and a licensed, knowledgeable physical therapist. These individuals should possess evidence of appropriate training, including intensive postgraduate and continuing education in the area of orthotics. The physical therapist, in particular, should devote the major part of his total efforts to orthotics, completing his part of the evaluation, participating in the team decision, and being responsible for the training of the patient. Additionally, as a result of the initial patient evaluation and identification of problem areas, other professionals are consulted to deal with social and economic adjustment, vocational evaluation and guidance, and psychologic difficulties reported by the patient or perceived by the team. The Orthotic Service is also a teaching medium for house staff officers, medical students, allied health students, and others. Depending on available resources, a rehabilitation engineer can assist in the design of a special orthosis, participate in the team decision, and add his competence to the entire operation. Furthermore, various electromechanical systems can be utilized by the team to evaluate certain characteristics, such as gait, before and after prescription of an orthosis. Audiovisual equipment can also be used to document a patient's mobility and locomotion, all in the process of determining the orthotic prescription and detailing the results. Obviously, the scope of the team and available professional input may be limited by many factors, but the concept of total involvement by many different individuals should be pursued.

Orthotic Evaluation

The function of the orthotic team, as just outlined, is to examine and evaluate the patient, jointly prescribe the orthosis and required training, and attend to all other variables that affect the patient's life-style (Table 65–6).

The physician is responsible for devel-

TABLE 65–6.   Orthotic Management Process

1. Diagnosis and functional evaluation by multidisciplinary team
2. Team conference
3. Development of prescription
4. Servicing by all disciplines as indicated
5. Orthotic fabrication
6. Delivery and "check-out"
7. Orthotic training
8. Re-examinations
9. Re-evaluation conferences

oping the relevant medical and surgical history, performing and recording the pertinent aspects of the examination, ordering and reviewing laboratory and radiographic findings, and noting other organ system dysfunctions, such as cardiopulmonary disease. The physician must also determine whether other alternatives to an orthosis are available and feasible, including surgical correction of the problem, use of shoes and shoe modifications plus walking aids to accomplish the same end, or treatment with physical therapy, medication, and other methods. In many instances, all or some of these measures are indicated prior to prescribing an orthosis.

The orthotist and shoe expert participate in the team conference, are given all the available information, including goals and contraindications, and are expected to provide their special expertise, particularly in the area of materials, current technology, and information on the most feasible approach to meet the orthotic restoration criteria. The physical therapist assists in developing and recording the patient's physical status and functional level; training is also rendered by the therapist. It must be stressed that the actual prescription of the specific orthosis is the result of a shared effort by the entire team.

Finally, in establishing the orthotic prescription, it is vital that certain factors be determined and recorded, including trunk and lower-limb muscle strength and endurance, joint motion, joint stability, degree of pain, if present, scope of deformities and contractures, gait and elevation deviations, use and type of walking aids, limb volume fluctuations, sensation, competence of circulation, presence of abnormal reflexes and undesirable movement, other defects, and previous orthotic experience, if any.

Text continued on page 1793

TECHNICAL ANALYSIS FORM   LOWER LIMB

Name _____ No. _____ Age _____ Sex _____

Date of Onset _____ Cause _____

Occupation _____ Present Lower-Limb Equipment _____

Diagnosis _____

_____

Ambulatory ☐   Non-Ambulatory ☐

MAJOR IMPAIRMENTS:

A.   Skeletal
1.   Bone and Joints: Normal ☐   Abnormal _____
2.   Ligaments: Normal ☐   Abnormal ☐   Knee: AC ☐   PC ☐   MC ☐   LC ☐
                                                Ankle: MC ☐   LC ☐

3.   Extremity Shortening: None ☐   Left ☐   Right ☐
     Amount of Discrepancy: A.S.S.-Heel _____   A.S.S.-MTP _____   MTP-Heel _____

B.   Sensation: Normal ☐   Abnormal ☐
1.   Anaesthesia ☐   Hypaesthesia ☐   Location: _____
     Protective Sensation: Retained ☐   Lost ☐
2.   Pain ☐   Location: _____

C.   Skin: Normal ☐   Abnormal: _____

D.   Vascular: Normal ☐   Abnormal ☐   Right ☐   Left ☐

E.   Balance: Normal ☐   Impaired ☐   Support: _____

F.   Gait Deviations: _____

_____

G.   Other Impairments: _____

———————————————————————— LEGEND ————————————————————————

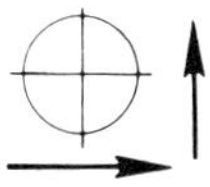

↑ = Direction of Translatory
    Motion

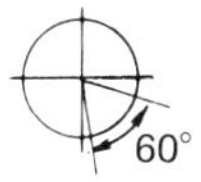

⊕ / 60° = Abnormal Degree of
    Rotary Motion

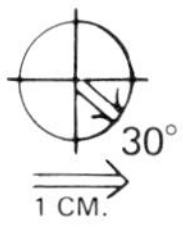

⊕ / 30° = Fixed Position
1 CM. →

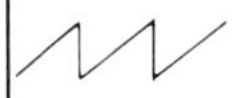

/\/\/ = Fracture

Volitional Force (V)
N   = Normal
G   = Good
F   = Fair
P   = Poor
T   = Trace
Z   = Zero

Hypertonic Muscle (H)
N   = Normal
M   = Mild
Mo = Moderate
S   = Severe

Proprioception (P)
N   = Normal
I   = Impaired
A   = Absent

D   = Local Distension or
      Enlargement

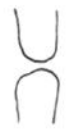

= Pseudarthrosis

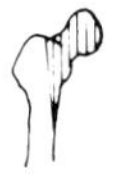

= Absence of Segment

Figure 65–1. *Technical analysis form contains patient information, diagnosis, and notation of major impairments.*

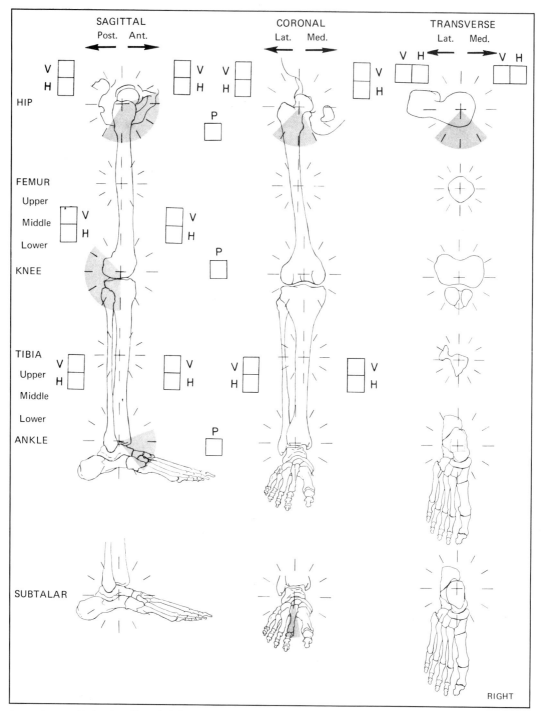

Figure 65–2. *Skeletal outline of right lower limb for recording motion, muscle strength, and degree of hypertonicity.*

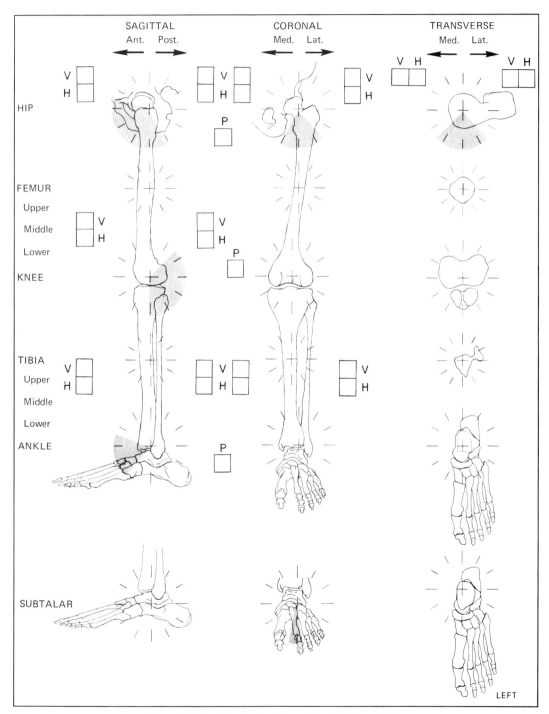

Figure 65–3. *Skeletal outline of the left lower limb.*

Summary of Functional Disability _____

_____

_____

_____

_____

_____

Treatment Objectives:

Prevent/Correct Deformity ☐   Improve Ambulation ☐

Reduce Axial Load ☐   Fracture Treatment ☐

Protect Joint ☐   Other _____

ORTHOTIC RECOMMENDATION

LOWER LIMB		FLEX	EXT	ABD	ADD	ROTATION		AXIAL LOAD
						Int.	Ext.	
HKAO	Hip							
KAO	Thigh							
	Knee							
AFO	Leg							
	Ankle	(Dorsi)	(Plantar)					
	Subtalar					(Inver.)	(Ever.)	
FO Foot	Midtarsal							
	Met.-phal.							

REMARKS:

Signature _____   Date _____

KEY: Use the following symbols to indicate desired control of designated function:

F = FREE — *Free* motion.

A = ASSIST — Application of an external force for the purpose of increasing the range, velocity, or force of a motion.

R = RESIST — Application of an external force for the purpose of decreasing the velocity or force of a motion.

S = STOP — Inclusion of a static unit to deter an undesired motion in one direction.

v = Variable — A unit that can be adjusted without making a structural change.

H = HOLD — Elimination of all motion in prescribed plane (verify position).

L = LOCK — Device includes an optional lock.

Figure 65–4. *Functional disability, treatment objectives, and orthotic recommendations are recorded.*

Following completion of this entire process, the patient is informed about the results of the evaluation, and with his understanding and concurrence, the orthosis is prescribed.

Orthotic Assessment Systems

The creation of an effective Orthotic Service, with active participation by many different professionals, each in turn evaluating and recording his or her specialty findings and submitting recommendations, mandates the use of a technical analysis form and other systems to more logically translate the information into an orthotic prescription. The Committee on Orthotics and Prosthetics of the American Academy of Orthopaedic Surgeons developed a form that utilizes biomechanical analysis of functional impairment of the lower limb to select the appropriate orthotic components; this approach reduces the team's reliance on matching orthoses to specific disease entities, e.g., a "hemiplegic short leg brace" for a stroke patient is no longer the most expeditious manner to prescribe an orthosis. In addition, use of a technical analysis form serves as an educational mechanism as well as a basis for more accurate communication among the members of the orthotic team. Figures 65–1 to 65–4 illustrate the form used to record the location and type of major impairments, diagram motion, indicate fixed positions, note muscle volitional force, hypertonicity, and proprioception, summarize functional disability, outline treatment objectives, and recommend the orthotic prescription. McCollough's chapter in the Atlas of Orthotics fully describes and illustrates the use of this technical analysis form.

FABRICATION OF PLASTIC ORTHOSES

As indicated in the section on Functional Terminology, a patellar-tendon–bearing orthosis relies on the anatomic elements of the knee, notably the patellar tendon and the medial condylar flare to alleviate dysfunction of the ankle and foot, including painful states secondary to arthritis, ulcerations, sequelae of trauma, and other conditions. The design and construction of a PTB orthosis are illustrative of the often complex procedures utilized to produce a plastic lower-limb orthosis (Fig. 65–5).

Fabrication of the all-plastic PTB orthosis involves a two-step casting of the below-the-knee segment with plaster of Paris, cast modifications, two plastic lamination procedures or two-stage vacuum-forming steps, and fitting processes. Prior to the casting procedure, the standard longitudinal, width, and circumferential measurements are recorded.

The patient is seated on a chair with the foot held in 5 degrees of dorsiflexion on the properly selected last. A stockinette is placed on the leg and brought above the knee. An indelible pencil is used to locate the patella, tibial tubercle, crest of the tibia, head of the fibula, lateral flare of the tibia, medial condylar flare, both malleoli, midpoint of the patellar tendon, and the first and fifth metatarsal heads. A cast of the ankle-foot segment to the midcalf level is then made, using an elastic plaster of Paris bandage. After the ankle-foot cast has hardened sufficiently, the knee is placed in 30 degrees of flexion, and the cast is extended above the femoral condyles. The completed cast is removed and filled with plaster of Paris to produce an uncorrected positive mold. This is then modified by removing the plaster in the area of the patellar tendon, under the medial condyle, and along the proximal aspect of the tibia and fibula. In addition, material is added over the head of the fibula, lateral tibial condyle, tibial tubercle, and crest of the tibia. The plantar surface of the mold is modified to form the longitudinal and transverse arches, and finally, relief is provided for the malleoli and base of the fifth metatarsal. The positive mold is then smoothed, covered with special PVA foil, layers of Perlon, and a fiber-glass stockinette. A mixture of 80 per cent Laminar Harz and 20 per cent Degaplast with 4 per cent color and 3 per cent catalyst is laminated under suction, creating the anteroproximal section of the plastic orthosis. The second lamination process also involves PVA foil, Perlon, and fiber-glass stockinette, together with lamination under suction, producing the shank and foot-ankle part. The fitting process consists of application of a stockinette to the patient's

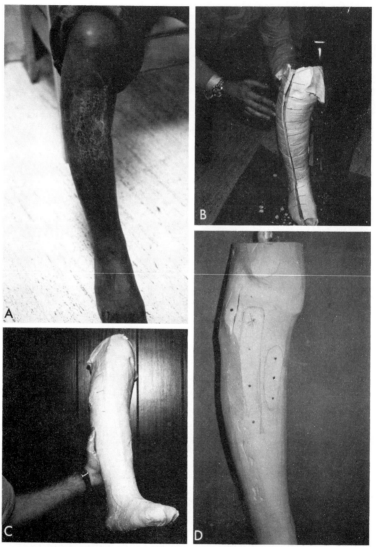

Figure 65–5. *(A) Osteomyelitis, deformity, and delayed union of a fractured tibia prior to fabrication of a PTB orthosis. (B) The negative wrap, with horizontal realignment markings, is removed from the patient. (C) A plaster of Paris splint reseals the negative wrap prior to preparation of the positive mold. (D) Plaster is removed from the positive model to protect sensitive areas, including the fibular head, patella, and other tibial prominences.*

Illustration continued on opposite page

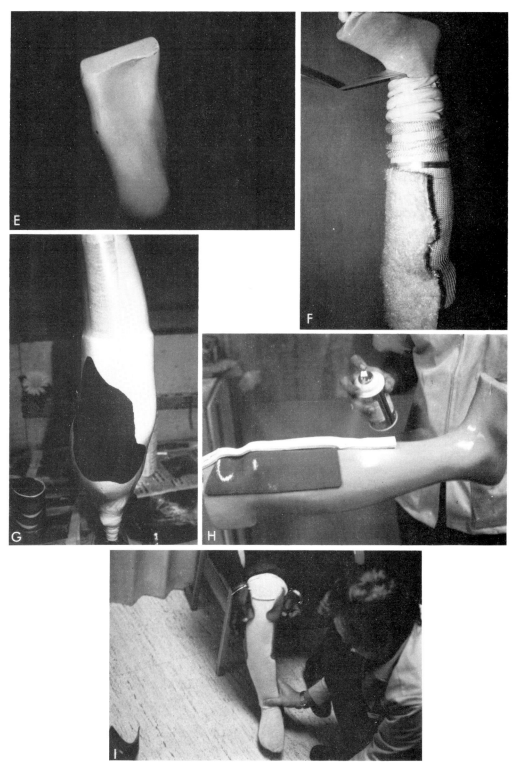

Figure 65–5 Continued (E) Plaster has either been added or removed from the plantar surface of the positive model. (F) Nylon matting, fiber glass, and nylon stockinette have been added in several layers to the positive model prior to lamination. (G) The pretibial shell is laminated by pouring acrylic resin through the filler sleeve. (H) The finished pretibial shell is oriented on the positive model and silicone spray is applied prior to lamination of the lower section of the PTB orthosis. (I) The completed orthosis, without the pretibial shell, is fitted to the patient.

leg and donning of the shank section by spreading apart the patellar-tendon groove and sliding the foot through. The PTB anterior shell is slotted into the shank, with the knee flexed to 90 degrees; Velcro is used to secure the two parts of the orthosis. Normal check-out for a PTB orthosis completes the entire process.

DELIVERY, CHECK-OUT, AND TRAINING

Following completion of the orthosis, a process that requires several visits to the facilities of an orthotist and continuing input by the patient and orthotic team members, the patient is scheduled to re-turn to the Orthotic Service for a procedure that is simply called a "check-out." The team determines adherence to the prescription, patient acceptability, workmanship, correction of the disabling factors, alleviation of pain, if relevant, improved ambulation, cosmesis, ease of donning, and total functional improvement. Generally, various forms are utilized to record the information and to indicate approval (Table 65–7). Once the orthosis has been approved, training is prescribed and then rendered by the physical therapist of the orthotic team. Where available, audiovisual and other instrumentation is used to document the outcome. A final review of the patient's life-style is performed, with appropriate intervention by

TABLE 65–7. Orthotic Check-out — Ankle-Foot Orthosis

IDENTIFYING DATA
  Patient
  Diagnosis
  Disability

—————————— 1. Is the orthosis as prescribed?
  If a recheck, have previous recommendations been accomplished?
—————————— 2. Can the patient don the orthosis without difficulty?

CHECK WITH PATIENT STANDING

Shoe

—————————— 3. Is the shoe satisfactory and does it fit properly?
—————————— 4. Are the sole and heel of the shoe flat on the floor?

Ankle

—————————— 5. Are the mechanical ankle joints aligned so that they coincide approximately with the anatomic ankle?
—————————— 6. Is there satisfactory clearance between the anatomic ankle and the medial and lateral mechanical ankle joints?
—————————— 7. Is sufficient force exerted by the varus or valgus strap or shoe insert to produce the desired support without causing significant discomfort?
—————————— 8. Is there minimal rocking between the shoe insert and the shoe?

Uprights

—————————— 9. Do the uprights conform to the contour of the leg and provide adequate clearance?
—————————— 10. Is each upright at the midline of the leg?
—————————— 11. In a child's orthosis, is there adequate provision for lengthening of the uprights?

Bands and Cuffs

—————————— 12. Is the calf band or cuff of proper width and does it conform to the contours of the leg?
—————————— 13. Is the calf band or cuff comfortable?
—————————— 14. If a patellar-tendon–bearing brim is used, is piston action minimal?
—————————— 15. If a patellar-tendon–bearing brim is used, is there adequate reduction in weight bearing at the heel?
—————————— 16. Is there sufficient clearance between the top of the orthosis and the head of the fibula?
—————————— 17. Is the patient stable?

TABLE 65–7.   Orthotic Check-out—Ankle-Foot Orthosis —*Continued*

CHECK WITH PATIENT WALKING

_____ 18. Is the shoe flat on the floor during the midstance phase of walking?

_____ 19. Is there adequate clearance between the malleoli and the mechanical ankle joints?

_____ 20. Does the varus or valgus strap or shoe insert provide the desired support?

_____ 21. Is the patient's performance in level walking satisfactory?
Indicate below the gait deviations that require attention:

_____ a. Lateral trunk bending		_____ i. Lordosis	
_____ b. Hip hiking		_____ j. Hyperextended knee	
_____ c. Internal (external) hip rotation		_____ k. Knee instability	
_____ d. Circumduction		_____ l. Inadequate dorsiflexion control	
_____ e. Wide walking base		_____ m. Insufficient push-off	
_____ f. Excessive medial (lateral) foot contact		_____ n. Vaulting	
_____ g. Anterior trunk bending		_____ o. Rhythmic abnormalities	
_____ h. Posterior trunk bending		_____ p. Other, including arm motion, noises, etc. (Describe)	

_____ 22. Is the orthosis sufficiently strong and rigid?

_____ 23. Does the orthosis operate quietly?

CHECK WITH PATIENT SITTING

_____ 24. Can the patient sit comfortably with his knees flexed 90 degrees, and can he flex his knee an additional 15 degrees without undue pressure?

_____ 25. Do the mechanical ankle joints provide the prescribed range of motion?

_____ 26. Are the sole and heel of the shoe flat on the floor?

CHECK WITH ORTHOSIS OFF THE PATIENT

_____ 27. Is the leg free from signs of irritation immediately after the orthosis is removed?

Workmanship

_____ 28. Is the shoe firmly attached to the orthosis, and is the shoe shank strong enough for its anticipated use?

_____ 29. Is the heel flat and firmly nailed to the shoe, and are wedges and lifts as neat and as inconspicuous as possible?

_____ 30. Do the ankle joints move without binding?

_____ 31. Do both medial and lateral stops of the ankle joints make simultaneous contact when the joints are fully flexed and extended?

_____ 32. Is the calf band adequately and smoothly lined and padded?

_____ 33. Is there adequate provision for adjustment of the cuff?

_____ 34. Are the metal parts of the orthosis smooth and free from sharp edges and sharp bends?

_____ 35. Is the leather work neat?

_____ 36. Is the general appearance of the orthosis satisfactory?

_____ 37. Does the patient consider the orthosis satisfactory with regard to comfort, function, and appearance?

representatives of the different disciplines. Scheduling of follow-up visits completes the orthotic restoration process.

ORTHOTIC COMPONENTS AND SYSTEMS

The establishment of a multidisciplinary orthotic team, coupled with the introduction of plastic materials and advanced technology, has resulted in an increased capability to design and construct a variety of highly individualized orthoses for virtually any foot disorder. The practitioner is no longer reliant on matching a diagnostic entity with a standard orthosis. Still, there are guidelines and basic orthotic components and systems that can be applied to the majority of foot and ankle-foot impairments.

FOOT ORTHOSES

The molded insert foot orthosis (FO) is fabricated of various high-impact plastic materials and is designed to maintain the foot in a more normal anatomic position, partially correcting abnormal attitudes such as valgus or varus. The plastic foot orthosis possesses many of the characteristics of conventional arch supports that are fabricated with metals, leathers, and other materials, but it closely adheres to the configuration of the foot and is therefore more supportive.

The impaired, malaligned foot is manually corrected to an optimal position and then plaster casted. The plaster model is utilized to fabricate a plastic laminated or vacuum-formed insert that is fairly rigid and will not easily fatigue under continuing application of weight-bearing forces (Fig. 65–6). The upturned lateral and medial walls meet posteriorly and snugly hold the foot in the desired position, minimizing midtarsal and subtalar motion. The plantar surface of the orthosis can be modified to redistribute forces, alleviating pain and preventing ulcerations. A soft heel pad is added to attenuate heel-strike. Often, a cushioned heel and rocker bar must be added to a well-fitted shoe for a normal transition from the terminal stance phase to the early swing phase of gait.

Essentially, the molded insert foot orthosis (Fig. 65–7) is best prescribed to alter minor, passively correctable positional abnormalities of the foot, alleviate pain related to weight bearing or motion of various foot joints, provide relief of ulcerated, in-

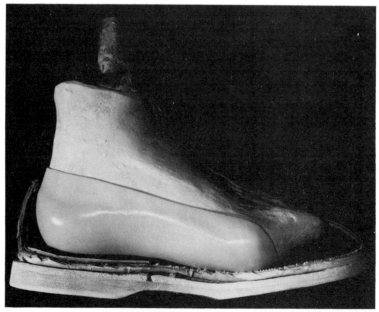

Figure 65–6. *A plaster cast model of the corrected foot position is used to fabricate a plastic laminated foot orthosis.*

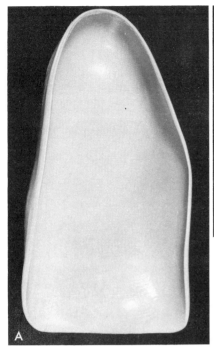
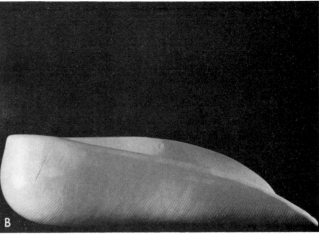

Figure 65–7. (A) Top view of a foot orthosis, demonstrating contouring for the longitudinal arches and metatarsal head area. (B) Side view of a foot orthosis that is used as a shoe insert to correct minor malalignments.

fected, inflamed, or atrophic areas of the sole, and compensate partially for limb length differences, without external modifications of the shoe (Table 65–8). The correction of moderate to severe foot disorders requires consideration of ankle-foot orthoses or orthoses that are dependent on knee contours, the patellar tendon, or the ischial tuberosity–gluteal area for improvement of the problem.

ANKLE-FOOT ORTHOSES

Ankle-foot orthoses (AFOs), as implied by the term, exert their effect primarily on the ankle-foot juncture. Generally, this

TABLE 65–8. Indications for a Molded Shoe Insert

1. Relief of painful, sensitive areas of the sole
2. Avoidance of pressure on atrophic, ulcerated areas
3. Support for longitudinal and transverse arches
4. Relief of metatarsal head discomfort
5. Partial correction of abnormal foot position
6. Ancillary to management of partial foot amputations and major loss of toes
7. Addition to ankle-foot orthoses
8. Reduction of limb length discrepancies
9. Partial restriction of motion of some foot joints

type of orthosis is indicated to prevent deformity, correct existing deformities that are not fixed, assist weakened or totally nonfunctioning muscles, compensate for proprioceptive and other sensory dysfunction, provide ankle joint stability, improve gait and balance, lessen the impact of spasticity, protect the osseous and soft-tissue structures of the ankle-foot articulation, provide immobilization to allow healing following surgical reconstruction or internal fixation of traumatic or pathologic fractures, and lessen pain due to abnormal motion of the ankle and foot joints and, to a much lesser extent, pain resulting from direct weight-bearing forces.

Metal Double-Bar AFO

The double-bar ankle-foot orthosis (Fig. 65–8), known for many years in the orthotic field as a "short leg brace," continues to be used because of its relatively low cost and ease of fabrication. Although the concept of the orthotic team staffed by professionals knowledgeable in and utilizing the most recent developments in materials and technology has not yet been fully diffused throughout the United States, increasingly during the last decade, particularly in larger metropolitan areas where

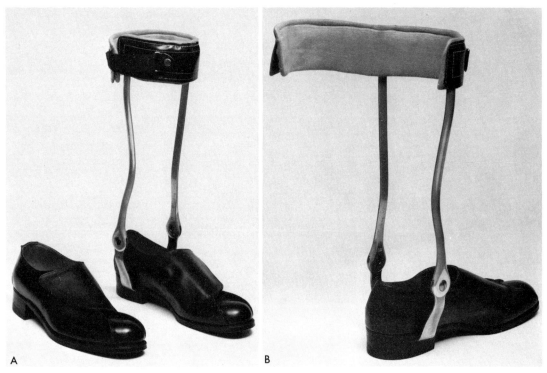

Figure 65–8. (A) Metal and leather double-bar ankle-foot orthosis attached to the shoe with a steel stirrup. (B) Orthotic motion occurs at the junction of the metal uprights and the stirrup; adjustments determine the degree of motion.

such teams are operating, the double-bar AFO is being replaced by various plastic orthoses.

The conventional double-bar AFO consists of two metal alloy uprights, a single metal, leather or plastic-covered calf band, attachment to an appropriately constructed shoe by a steel stirrup, caliper, or shoe plate, and an ankle joint usually placed at the level of the anatomic ankle joint. The ankle joint can include a "posterior or 90-degree ankle stop" that allows unrestricted dorsiflexion but limits plantar flexion below the horizontal plane, an "anterior or reverse stop" that limits dorsiflexion to prevent a patient from walking on his heels, "a limited motion stop" that permits a total of 5 to 10 degrees of ankle motion, or a "free ankle joint" that allows unrestricted motion. Accessory corrective ankle straps or pressure pads, constructed of leather or plastic materials, are attached to the shoe at the junction of the upper segment and the sole and are buckled around the lateral or medial metal upright. To correct a pronated (valgus) foot, the strap is attached to the shoe medially and buckled around the lateral bar. Lateral attachment of the ankle strap to the shoe with buckling around the medial bar corrects supination (varus) of the foot. Furthermore, the metal uprights can be extensible to accommodate for growth in a child (Fig. 65–9).

The double-bar AFO is most often prescribed for those conditions in which an upper motor neuron lesion (e.g., stroke, tumor, or other neurologic central nervous system disorders) or a lower motor neuron disease or injury (e.g., poliomyelitis or surgically or traumatically induced neuropathies) produces weakness of the dorsiflexors, resulting in a "dropped foot" attitude during the swing phase of gait; a "posterior 90-degree ankle stop" or a dorsiflexion spring-assisted mechanism is used in these cases (Table 65–9). In patients with acquired brain damage, such as that due to a cerebral vascular accident, a corrective ankle strap is added to help correct the spastic equinovarus that is usually present. Other conditions aided by

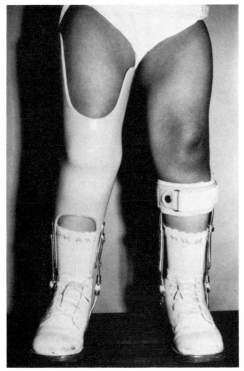

Figure 65–9. *Extensible uprights permit orthotic lengthening as the child grows.*

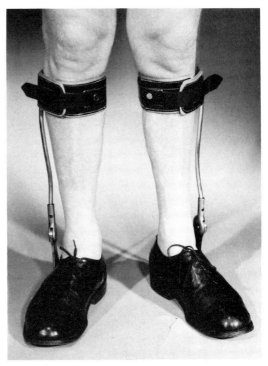

Figure 65–10. *Single-bar ankle-foot orthoses with round bar uprights to permit slight rotation.*

the double-bar AFO include unwanted mediolateral motion secondary to degenerative and other forms of arthritis, foot-ankle injuries, and proprioceptive loss in neuropathic joints. A single-bar ankle-foot orthosis, which has essentially the same components as the double-bar orthosis and is indicated for similar diseases and injuries, is less useful because subtalar motion is poorly controlled (Fig. 65–10).

Other metal ankle-foot orthoses include (1) a double-bar AFO with a molded shoe insert to provide good subtalar stabilization (Fig. 65–11), (2) a double-rod AFO in which the two rods are fabricated of spring steel wire or epoxy–fiber glass, providing reduced weight but very limited mediolateral ankle control (Fig. 65–12), (3) a posterior bar AFO in which there is a spring steel or epoxy–fiber glass posterior bar attached to a calf band and a metal shoe attachment, offering light weight and low cost but little mediolateral ankle stability (Fig. 65–13), and (4) a shoe clasp AFO that combines a metal or plastic calf band, a posterior bar of epoxy–fiber glass and a stainless steel clasp fitted to the heel counter (Fig. 65–14). These lightweight orthoses do biomechanically provide assisted dorsiflexion, but they offer minimal or no mediolateral ankle stabilization, thus severely limiting their usefulness in most clinical situations.

Posterior Leaf-Spring AFO

The posterior leaf-spring AFO, or plastic shell orthosis, is rapidly replacing the metal double-bar orthosis for many ankle-foot disorders, particularly in those condi-

TABLE 65–9. Indications for a Metal Double-Bar AFO

1. Assist ankle dorsiflexion (spring type)
2. Limit dorsiflexion or plantar flexion
3. Restrict all ankle motion
4. Control subtalar motion
5. Correct valgus and varus deformities
6. Reduce ankle-foot spasticity
7. Compensate for proprioceptive sensory loss
8. Relieve painful ankle motion
9. Correct foot imbalance

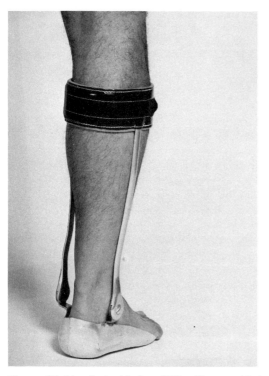

Figure 65–11. A double-bar AFO with a molded shoe insert provides improved subtalar stabilization.

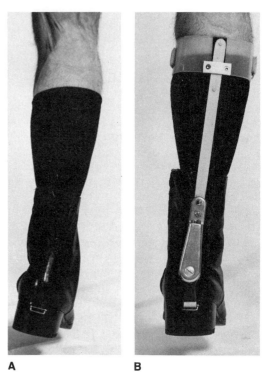

A   **B**

Figure 65–13. Posterior bar AFO. (A) Equinovarus attitude secondary to paralysis. (B) Orthotic correction.

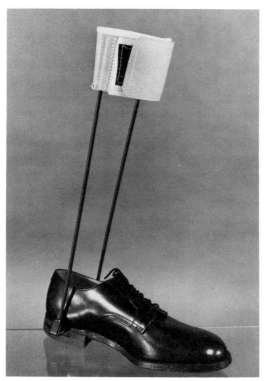

Figure 65–12. Double-rod AFO with lightweight, spring steel wire construction.

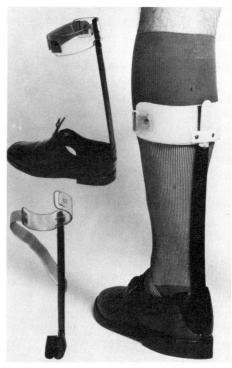

Figure 65–14. Shoe clasp AFO with plastic calf band, posterior bar of epoxy–fiber glass, and a stainless steel clasp fitted to the heel counter.

tions due to disease or injury that require assisted dorsiflexion during the early part of the swing phase. Currently, this orthosis is being fabricated of high-molecular-weight polypropylene, a thermoplastic material that becomes moldable at a temperature of 350° F. In this state, the plastic can be hand-formed, draped, or, more appropriately, vacuum-formed to conform to the irregular surfaces of the ankle-foot plastic mold. Furthermore, in its thermopliable state, the flexible plastic will autobond to itself and to various interfaces such as soft-form Plastazote and Pelite.

In addition to being lightweight, highly fatigue-resistant, cosmetic, and easily donned, the posterior leaf-spring AFO has a high degree of plastic memory, a characteristic of some materials that allows fairly rapid and full return to the original shape following removal of deforming forces. The ankle-foot orthosis is deformed in the direction of plantar flexion following heel-

strike by either active or spastic plantar flexors, with the foot achieving full contact with the floor. Following push-off, the plastic memory returns the orthosis to its previous state, thus simulating dorsiflexion during the swing phase.

The flexible plastic shell orthosis (Fig. 65–15) consists of a molded foot section continuous with a posterior leg segment that terminates 2 to 3 inches below the fibular neck. The foot section is carefully constructed to support the longitudinal and medial arches, correct any abnormal foot position, and provide support in the metatarsal area, if indicated. The posterior trim lines at the ankle level can be varied to permit more or less flexibility, and the medial and lateral trim lines can be heightened to provide mediolateral stabilization. Velcro closure and a slightly larger, well-constructed shoe complete the orthotic system.

The posterior leaf-spring orthosis is pre-

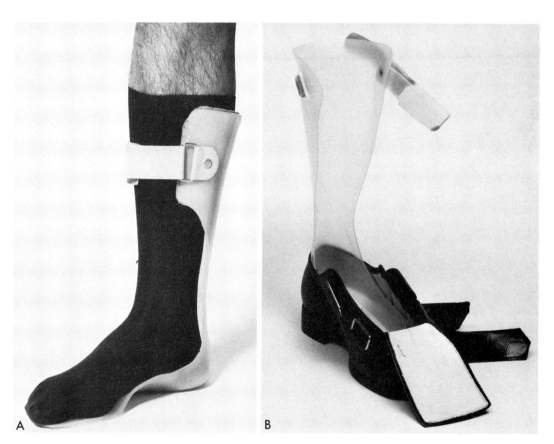

Figure 65–15. *(A) Posterior leaf-spring orthosis to assist dorsiflexion. (B) Polypropylene posterior leaf-spring orthosis with an open flap shoe.*

TABLE 65–10. Indications and Criteria for a Posterior Leaf-Spring AFO

1. Assist absent or weakened dorsiflexors
2. Compensate for loss of ankle proprioception
3. Good foot placement required
4. Functional plantar flexors needed
5. Some valgus or varus acceptable
6. Slight or moderate spasticity not a contraindication
7. Fair to good hip and knee control required
8. Mild to moderate edema acceptable
9. Good mediolateral ankle stability needed

scribed for those conditions in which weakness of the dorsiflexors is the dominant biomechanical deficit, being particularly effective for lower motor neuron disorders that selectively disrupt the anterolateral leg muscles (Table 65–10). As long as spastic deforming forces are not too great, this orthosis can also be used in upper motor neuron disturbances such as stroke. Active or spastic plantar flexors are required to deform the orthosis following heel-strike, and the orthotic memory re-

turns the ankle-foot complex to neutral position during the swing phase. Furthermore, prescription criteria also require good to fair mediolateral ankle stability, passive ankle dorsiflexion, minimal or no abnormal foot deformity (varus or valgus), and adequate knee and hip joint mobility and strength. As noted, deforming forces of a magnitude that creates highly abnormal foot placement are a contraindication for this type of ankle-foot orthosis. In general, this orthosis serves as a lightweight, durable, and more physiologic alternative to the conventional double-bar metal orthosis in those conditions requiring dorsiflexion assistance. However, other plastic orthoses are indicated when significant mediolateral ankle instability and painful motion need correction.

Molded Spiral AFO

The plastic, molded spiral ankle-foot orthosis (Fig. 65–16) is fabricated with vari-

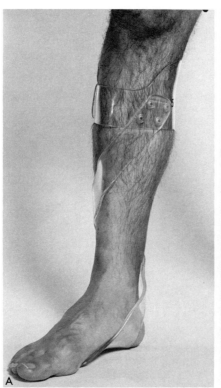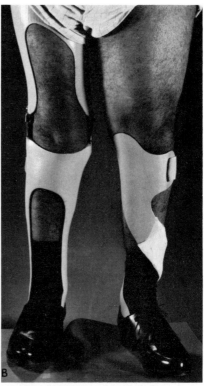

Figure 65–16. (A) A clear plastic, spiral ankle-foot orthosis is worn by a patient with poor ankle control. (B) A plastic laminated, spiral AFO controls the left ankle; an above-the-knee orthosis on the right side stabilizes the knee and ankle joints.

ous materials, including Plexidur, Nyoplex, polypropylene, and plastic laminates. The spiral component of the orthosis originates at the medial aspect of the foot segment, wraps around the leg posteriorly, and ends at the level of the medial tibial condyle; a horizontally placed band provides closure at the calf level. The orthotic foot section is molded to conform to the contours of the plantar surface of the foot, providing medial and longitudinal arch support.

The molded spiral AFO shares the attributes of other lightweight, cosmetic, plastic orthoses. In addition, this orthosis is the one device that most closely matches the normal physiologic motion of the human ankle-foot complex, controlling or simulating motion in the frontal, sagittal, and transverse planes. On weight bearing, shortly following heel-strike, the spiral portion unwinds to permit controlled plantar flexion. Cessation of weight bearing by the limb causes rewinding of the spiral to simulate and cause dorsiflexion of the foot. As the weight-bearing limb moves beyond midstance, the spiral is stressed in the direction of dorsiflexion. Following heel-off, the stressed spiral resists further unwinding and returns to its previous state, thus assisting push-off. In addition, as the spiral winds and unwinds, orthotic transverse rotation occurs, matching the usual subtalar motion that occurs during ambulation. The configuration of the orthotic foot section, its attachment to the spiral, and a three-point pressure system serve to control subtalar motion and provide mediolateral ankle stability. Fabrication of the spiral AFO is thus more complicated, requiring high precision and critical attention to the fitting and check-out procedures.

The spiral AFO is appropriate in those conditions in which there is severe weakness or absence of ankle dorsiflexors and plantar flexors, including stroke, traumatic injury to nerves supplying the leg musculature, lower motor neuron disease, and conditions with proprioceptive loss at the ankle (Table 65–11). The spiral AFO provides more mediolateral stability than the posterior leaf-spring orthosis, assists push-off, and is of use where weakness of the knee muscles exists. The spiral AFO is generally not indicated when there is

TABLE 65–11. Indications and Criteria for a Molded Spiral AFO

1. Weakness or absence of ankle dorsiflexors and plantar flexors
2. Proprioceptive sensory defect at ankle
3. Slight to moderate spasticity acceptable
4. Mediolateral ankle instability not a contraindication
5. Fair to good knee and hip control needed
6. Edema may be a problem

moderate to severe spasticity, poor sensation and circulation, and limb volume fluctuations. Combining these limitations, usually found in disease and injury of the ankle-foot area, with technical fabrication difficulties and a higher-than-usual incidence of breakage, it is not surprising that this very physiologic orthosis has not been widely accepted. Generally, other plastic orthoses can adequately replace this device and allow a choice of flexible or rigid variants.

Solid Ankle-Foot Orthosis

The solid ankle-foot orthosis, or rigid orthosis (Fig. 65–17), is constructed with thermosetting plastic laminates to assure rigidity and minimize material fatigue. As with other orthoses prescribed to control the ankle, the solid AFO is fabricated from an accurate plaster cast, with extension proximally to the medial flare of the tibia. The ankle-foot segment is molded closely to support the arches of the foot, the calcaneus, and the malleoli. The upper medial and lateral trim lines of the orthosis, viewed in the sagittal plane, are carried anterior to the midline to provide more efficient fitting and support; a proximal anterior Velcro strap is utilized for closure. In some instances, an anterior shell is applied to the orthosis to provide increased rigidity where spasticity is severe.

The solid ankle-foot orthosis is primarily prescribed when weakness of the dorsiflexors and plantar flexors is combined with severe spasticity, producing marked equinovarus during the gait cycle (Table 65–12). The orthosis is therefore very useful in stroke and other upper motor neuron disease and injury states in which spasticity distorts foot placement. In addition, a rigid orthosis that totally restricts ankle

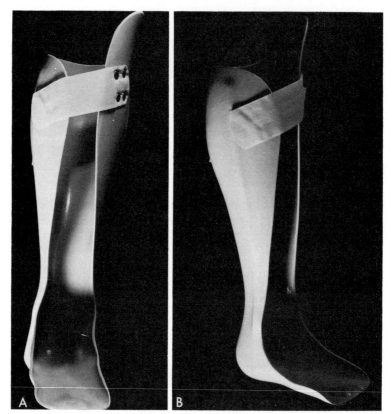

Figure 65–17. *(A) Anterior view of a solid ankle-foot orthosis with proximal Velcro closure. (B) An antero-medial view of a solid ankle-foot orthosis demonstrating the various trim lines.*

and subtalar joint motion is indicated when there is substantial proprioceptive sensory dysfunction secondary to any cause. Painful ankle and subtalar motion due to injury or arthritic destruction is well controlled by this device. Removable immobilization following ankle-foot surgery for reconstruction or fracture reduction is another attribute of the solid AFO. Circulatory and cutaneous sensory disturbances, as well as ankle-foot volume changes, can be contraindications.

TABLE 65–12. Indications and Criteria for a Solid AFO

1. Weakness or absence of dorsiflexors and plantar flexors
2. Moderate to severe proprioceptive loss
3. Painful ankle motion
4. Severe spasticity
5. Postoperative need for stabilization
6. Restriction of ankle motion, any indication
7. Adequate knee and hip control required
8. Edema of significance is a contraindication

The shoe component of this orthotic system requires a compressible rubber heel and rocker bar for a more normal gait pattern since ankle motion is so restricted. As with other orthoses, a larger and wider shoe is required, or a depth inlay shoe with a removable prefabricated inlay removed on the orthotic side and inserted on the sound side may be used.

Patellar-Tendon–Bearing Orthosis

The patellar-tendon–bearing (PTB) orthosis is representative of the close linkage between the fields of prosthetics and orthotics. The concept of utilizing the patellar tendon and the medial condylar area of the tibia for support was initially introduced in prosthetic restoration in below-the-knee amputations. A patient with a hindfoot amputation served as the first model for a PTB orthosis, combining a PTB socket with metal double-bar uprights and a shoe plate (Fig. 65–18). The

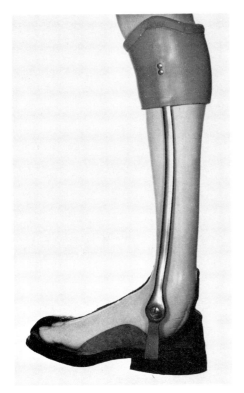

Figure 65–18. *An early model PTB orthosis provides support for a hindfoot amputation site.*

original sketch for the prototype of this orthosis is presented in Figure 65–19.

In the most often used variant of the PTB orthosis, plastic materials are used to develop the PTB socket. Double-bar uprights of lightweight metal alloys are attached proximally to the socket and distally to a shoe plate built of various materials, including well-molded, leather-covered metals (Figs. 65–20 to 65–22). The ankle joint is either fixed or allows limited motion; a cushioned heel assists in the attenuation of heel-strike forces. An all-plastic PTB orthosis (Fig. 65–23) developed by Demopoulos and Eschen utilizes plastic laminates for improved cosmesis and better ankle-foot support; the construction of this type of PTB orthosis was detailed in the preceding section on Fabrication of Plastic Orthoses.

The PTB orthosis finds its widest application in those conditions in which the foot and ankle require partial or complete removal of weight-bearing forces. Previously described ankle-foot devices de-

pend on precise contouring of the foot section to redistribute forces away from painful and ulcerated areas of the plantar surface of the foot. Modifications of orthotic trim lines are also utilized in an attempt to provide more support and thus reduce pain. However, only a PTB orthosis can effectively unload a very painful ankle, particularly pain related to direct weight bearing, and efficiently redistribute forces away from ulcerated areas. Shoe modifications, conventional arch supports, molded inserts, and the other ankle-foot orthoses are only successful with mild to moderate defects.

Biomechanical and other dysfunctional states that respond to prescription of a PTB orthosis include arthritis of the ankle, surgical reduction and fixation of ankle-foot fractures, disease or injury of the sole that produces painful and/or ulcerated lesions, surgical reconstructive procedures that require unloading during the healing process, and neuropathic ankle joints (either acquired or congenital); Table 65–13 details these and other indications.

With regard to most of the prescription criteria for use of a PTB orthosis, studies have demonstrated that effective reduction of weight-bearing forces and other rotational and shear stresses occurs during the heel-strike–to–midstance period. Considerable lessening of the unloading characteristics of this device is observed beyond the midstance interval and at the time of push-off. A rocker-bottom shoe modification and training to avoid push-off significantly obviate the biomechanical deficiency of the PTB orthosis. On some occasions, an ischial weight-bearing orthosis is required to relieve pathology of the ankle-foot region. The conventional ischial weight-bearing "long leg brace" includes a circular proximal band at the ischial tuberosity area, thigh double uprights, knee joints and locks, leg uprights, ankle joints with varying adjustments, knee pads, thigh and calf bands, and a shoe plate (Fig. 65–24). The plastic hip-knee-ankle orthosis includes a quadrilateral socket that is similar to an above-the-knee prosthetic socket, metal or plastic knee joints with a locking capability, and single-unit construction of the leg and molded ankle-foot component (Fig. 65–25). This orthosis is rarely required for

Text continued on page 1812

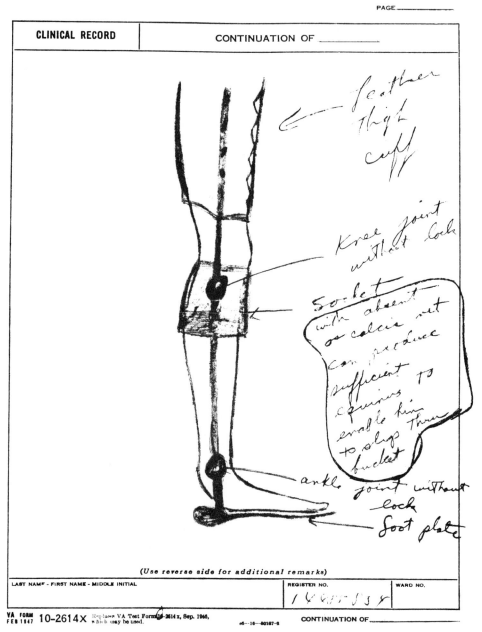

Figure 65–19. *Evolution of the PTB orthosis is shown in a sketch prepared at the V.A. Prosthetic Center.*

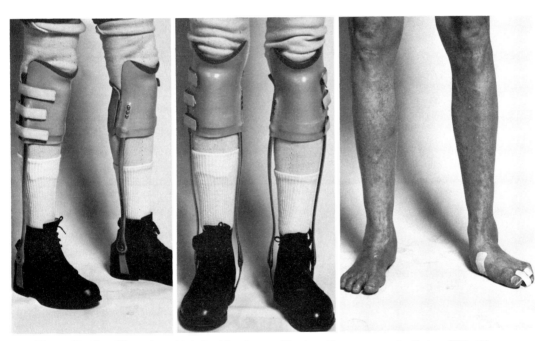

Figure 65-20. *Bilateral, multiple foot fractures with ulcerations managed with two PTB orthoses.*

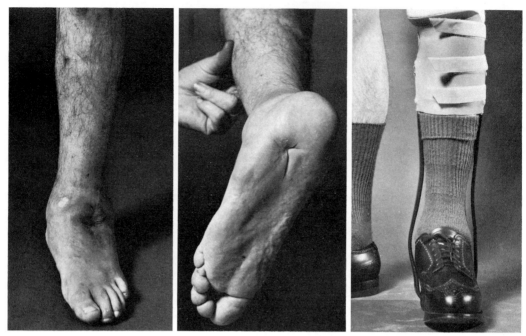

Figure 65–21. *A patient with multiple gunshot wounds fitted with a left PTB orthosis.*

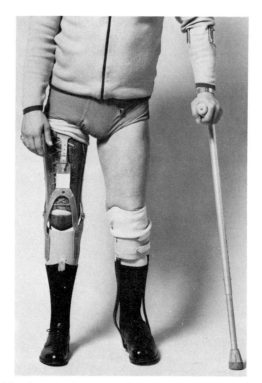

Figure 65–22. *The relationship of prosthetics and orthotics is demonstrated in a patient with a right prosthesis and a left PTB orthosis.*

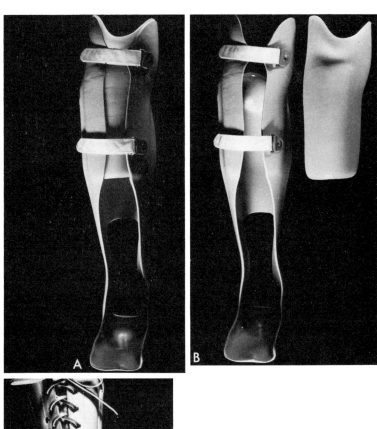

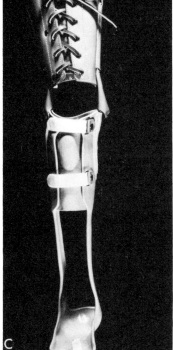

Figure 65–23. (A) An all-plastic PTB orthosis with the pretibial shell in place. (B) The all-plastic PTB orthosis with removal of the pretibial shell. (C) A thigh lacer and knee joints provide knee stability to the all-plastic PTB orthosis.

TABLE 65–13. Indications and Criteria for Patellar-Tendon–Bearing AFO

1. Painful ankle on weight bearing
2. Delayed union or nonunion of the tibia or ankle
3. Failure of arthrodesis of ankle
4. Pathology of sole (e.g., burns, infections, ulcers)
5. Imminent fracture of the tibia (any cause)
6. Acquired or congenital sensory loss at the ankle
7. Unloading of ankle following surgery
8. Good knee and hip control required
9. Edema of slight degree is acceptable

ankle-foot pathology, but it is very effective when prescribed.

PROSTHETICS

Prosthetic restoration, or "the art and science of replacing, by artificial means, body parts that may be missing or defective as a result of surgical intervention, trauma, disease or developmental anomaly," has undergone considerable advancement in the last 37 years, since the end of a World War that inflicted much injury to the lower limbs, particularly the distal seg-

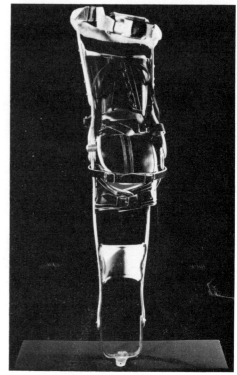

Figure 65–24. *A conventional, ischial, weight-bearing, above-the-knee brace with calf bands, thigh lacer, knee pads, and assorted straps.*

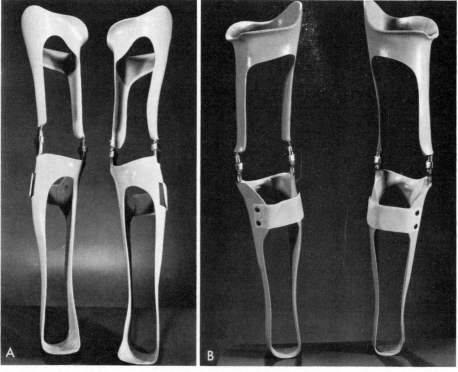

Figure 65–25. *(A) Plastic hip-knee-ankle orthoses stabilize the knees and ankles. (B) Proximal ischial support areas can reduce forces at the feet and ankles.*

ments. A major effort, significantly supported by governmental funds, resulted in the creation of research and development units, evaluation and training units and educational services, all coordinated with the intent of designing and fabricating modern prostheses. Indeed, the use of plastic materials, major technological advances, the introduction of the multidisciplinary team concept, and systematic analysis of pathomechanics, which previously were described, first evolved in the field of prosthetics and were later incorporated into the areas of orthotics.

The management of patients with partial or total amputation of the foot has not, until recently, received adequate allocation of resources and interest, since such amputations were either only minimally disabling (loss of one or two toes) or were temporary measures preceding surgical amputation at a more proximal level. Recognizing that the great majority of lower-limb amputations are performed secondary to progressive disease of the circulatory system, it is understandable that toe and partial foot amputations are often followed by surgical ablation at higher levels. The development of innovative medical care that controls diseases more adequately, coupled with improved surgical techniques, has resulted in the preservation of more limb segments, with a marked shift from standard above-the-knee amputations to procedures at the below-the-knee level. Only 20 years ago, 90 per cent of all lower-limb surgery was performed at a level proximal to the knee, primarily at the midthigh level. Table 65–14 outlines the current ratio of amputations of the lower limb, demonstrating the degree of improved care.

The number, or percentage, of patients with toe and foot amputations is difficult to define since these individuals are not regularly referred to organized Amputee Units. It is known, however, that the total of toe amputations exceeds the combined total of amputations at all the other levels. Further progress is producing even greater preservation of the limb, requiring a review of the prosthetic-orthotic capability to manage this group of patients in a more scientific manner, particularly to intervene and prevent further limb loss. All too often in the past, patient self-care of toe and partial foot amputations produced complications that required higher level amputation. For this reason, a more concentrated effort is required by structured orthotic-prosthetic services.

PROSTHETIC TERMINOLOGY

The Committee on Prosthetic-Orthotic Education (CPOE) of the National Academy of Sciences National Research Council appointed the Task Force on Standardization of Prosthetic-Orthotic Terminology in early 1971. Progress was initially made in the area of orthotics, with creation of a functional nomenclature to describe orthoses. In 1974, the group recommended that the new terminology for classification

TABLE 65–14. Current Ratio of Lower-Limb Amputations

LEVEL	NUMBER
Partial foot and Syme (excludes toe amputations)	325
Below the knee	2300
Knee disarticulation	50
Above the knee	1560
Hip disarticulation or hemipelvectomy	7
Total	4242

TABLE 65–15. Terminology for Lower-Limb Amputation Levels

NEW TERMS	CURRENT TERMS
Pelvic (Pel), complete	Hemicorporectomy
Hip (Hip), complete	Hemipelvectomy
Thigh (Th), complete	Hip disarticulation
Thigh (Th), partial (upper 1/3)	Short (upper-third) AK
Thigh (Th), partial (middle 1/3)	Medium (mid-third) AK
Thigh (Th), partial (lower 1/3)	Long (lower-third) AK
Leg (Leg), complete	Knee disarticulation
Leg (Leg), partial (upper 1/3)	Short (upper-third) BK
Leg (Leg) partial (middle 1/3)	Medium (mid-third) BK
Leg (Leg), partial (lower 1/3)	Long (lower-third) BK
Tarsal (Ta), complete	Ankle disarticulation or Syme amputation
Tarsal (Ta), partial	Known collectively as partial foot amputations, some specifics being:
Metatarsal (MT), complete	
Metatarsal (MT), partial	
Phalangeal (Ph), complete	
Phalangeal (Ph), partial	
	Chopart's amputation
	Forbe's amputation
	Hancock's amputation
	Hey's amputation
	Lisfranc's amputation
	Pirogoff's amputation

of congenital limb deficiencies be adopted, utilizing the transverse deficiencies to describe noncongenital amputations. Table 65–15 details the terminology for amputation levels for the lower limb. In foot disorders, it will be noted that an ankle disarticulation or the slightly more proximal Syme amputation denotes total ablation of the foot, except that the heel pad is preserved in the Syme procedure and in variations of an ankle disarticulation. In the remaining foot amputation levels, partial or total loss of the tarsal bones, metatarsals, or phalanges is considered.

MATERIALS IN ANKLE-FOOT PROSTHETICS

The fabrication of ankle-foot prosthetic devices depends on many of the same materials found useful in orthotics, including fabrics, leathers, metal alloys, rubber variants, and plastics. Following total or partial amputation of the foot, the residual limb is generally more prominent, with thin and often poor skin covering, requiring the use of diverse materials to cushion and protect the area.

The design and construction of prostheses following an ankle disarticulation or Syme amputation rely on thermosetting plastics and polyester or acrylic laminations for rigidity and favorable strength-weight ratios; Dacron, nylon, and fiber-glass cloth or mat are used in a manner similar to that in the fabrication of PTB prostheses or PTB orthoses. Woolen or cotton stump socks of various weights (or "plies") are used to reduce friction, absorb perspiration, and protect the skin. Flexible silicone elastomers are added as a pad or cushion to provide additional protection of the thin tissues at the terminal aspect of the limb.

In developing prosthetic devices for transmetatarsal and toe amputations, liberal utilization of padding material is mandatory. Flexible silicone elastomers are used, as well as leathers (either vegetable or chrome tanned), rubber of the open cell variety, Plastazote of soft density, Pelite, and Silicone gel sheets. Spring steel, a low-carbon steel with "elasticity," is also used in partial foot and toe amputation to assist during push-off.

DEVELOPMENT OF THE ANKLE-FOOT PROSTHETIC PRESCRIPTION

The successful restoration or total rehabilitation of a patient with a partial or total foot amputation generally requires the same multidisciplinary approach proved so valid by the long-established nationwide system of Amputee Clinics.

In the last two or three decades, over 400 Amputee Clinics were established within university-affiliated medical centers in the United States and Canada. The clinics function as a team structure, evaluating and developing a management plan for each amputee. Essentially, the Amputee Clinic is directed by a physician and includes a prosthetist, physical and occupational therapists, and an individual competent in shoe fabrication and modification. Ancillary services available to each Amputee Service vary but most often involve social service, nursing staff, vocational rehabilitation counselors, and psychologists; the larger clinics have access to, or include as a regular member, a rehabilitation engineer. In addition, the administrative and clerical support outlined in the section on orthotics is also critical to the successful operation of an Amputee Service.

The physician who is the team leader develops the medical and surgical history and performs the examination. Again, the patient's secondary medical problems, plus drug management, must be fully considered and documented. Local examination of the amputated area focuses on swelling, discoloration, trophic changes, circulatory status, sensation, joint motion, motor power, tenderness, healing, and other factors. The state of the more proximal segment and the partially amputated limb must also be noted, as must the condition of the other limbs and the trunk. The members of the Amputee Clinic team perform and record their information, with exchange of data taking place in a conference setting. The prescription of a prosthetic device depends on the recommendations of the entire group servicing the amputee. As in orthotics, delivery, checkout, and training follow in an established sequence.

The prescription of foot prostheses is a

less complex process compared with that necessary for more proximal amputation levels and severe disabilities requiring orthotic care. However, it must be done well since vascular disease (responsible for 80 to 85 per cent of lower-limb amputations) is usually progressive. The patient's understanding and cooperation are probably the most important factors in preventing further amputation. The team members need to be available and alert to every minor physical alteration of the residual foot, relying on extremely well-fitting shoes and padding to supplement the prosthetic device. Care and attention to the other limb are also extremely important, for the other limb often requires shoe modifications and foot insert orthoses to prevent damage.

PROSTHETIC COMPONENTS AND SYSTEMS

Prosthetic restoration in patients with partial or total amputation of the foot involves only a minimum of true prosthetic components. The usual combinations of a socket, articulated mechanical joints, suspension units, locking devices, and other components are not required for ankle-foot prostheses. Indeed, many of the appliances prescribed for the patient with an ankle-foot amputation are more recognizable as orthotic devices. Generally, management of this group of patients requires the careful selection and prescription of a molded shoe insert, with padding and contouring materials, a soundly constructed shoe, and shoe modifications to restore balance, support, and ambulation capability.

Toe Amputations

Loss of the small toe often results in a residual bony prominence over the distolateral aspect of the foot. Flexible elastomers, silicone products that are synthetic rubbers, can be contoured and used as padding to avoid tissue injury. Amputation of one or two toes medial to an intact small toe is similarly managed with protective padding. Loss of all the toes or loss of only the large toe requires the construction of a molded shoe insert to maintain foot sup-

port and alignment, affixation of plastic material such as rigid-density Plastazote as a toe filler, addition of a contoured, long, steel spring to the shoe to aid push-off, and a well-developed shoe with a rocker bar; a metal alloy can also be added to maintain the integrity of the toe-box of the shoe. The overriding concern of the Amputee Clinic team is to avoid complications.

Transmetatarsal Amputations

Traumatic or surgical ablation of the metatarsal heads is managed in the same manner as loss of all the toes. More proximal amputations, at the mid-transmetatarsal level, result in muscle imbalance between the dorsiflexors and the plantar flexors, particularly with prolonged walking. A polypropylene posterior leaf-spring orthosis (Figs. 65–26 and 65–27) is prescribed, with the addition of distal, contoured plastic materials serving as padding and as a toe/foot filler. The polypropylene orthosis is modified to permit plantar flexion on heel-strike and toe pick-up during the swing phase. The plantar segment of the orthosis, together with the modified shoe (with long, steel spring and rocker bar), functions as an extension of the residual foot. This partial foot prothesis is also of benefit for total ablation of the metatarsals and for an amputee who has lost most of the toes of one limb and has a more proximal amputation (below or above the knee) of the other limb.

Partial Tarsal Amputations

A partial foot prosthesis, as just described, is useful in instances in which the distal tarsal bones have been amputated or the midtarsal level is the amputation site. A more proximal tarsal amputation such as a Chopart procedure (the talus and calcaneus are retained) results in a shortened residual limb and a plantar-flexion deformity; a plastic laminate "clam-shell" prosthesis is preferred (Fig. 65–28). A hindfoot amputation requires a PTB orthosis for effective management. The PTB orthosis is also indicated in partial foot amputations in which the residual plantar surface is ulcerated or painful and requires unloading. The foot-plate component of the PTB orthosis is modified to include toe-filler

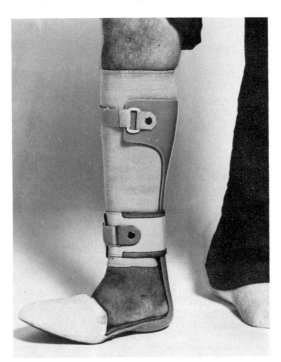

Figure 65–26. *Partial foot prosthesis fitted for a transmetatarsal amputation.*

material, and a shoe rocker bar completes the system (Fig. 65–29).

Total Foot Amputation

As a result of improved medical and surgical care, many patients with vascular disease of the lower limb undergo amputation of only the toes. When this is not possible, the mid-transmetatarsal level is then the preferred amputation site. The next, more proximal site of amputation, if mandated by the patient's condition, should be a Syme amputation, avoiding transtarsal amputations that create contractures and poorly contoured residual limbs.

In the Syme amputation, the entire foot is removed, with the tibia and fibula being sectioned transversely immediately above the ankle joint; the distal ends of the malleoli are excised. The heel pad, with the talus and calcaneus removed, is left attached posteriorly and sutured anteriorly. The heel pad includes the termination of the posterior tibial nerve, the posterior tibial artery, the periosteum of the calcaneus, the specialized adipose tissue, and the plantar aponeurosis. The end-bearing capability of this amputation is very satisfactory, permitting the amputee to walk within his home without any device. Furthermore, there are distinct mechanical advantages in maintaining a long lever arm, and there is less psychologic trauma. The residual limb is 2.5 to 3.25 inches shorter, with a somewhat bulbous distal end; these potential disadvantages can be minimized with careful surgical technique.

The original Syme prosthesis was constructed with a laced leather socket, steel

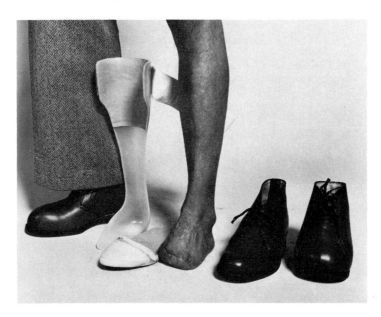

Figure 65–27. *A more flexible, lighter weight posterior leaf-spring orthosis is used with a molded, toe-filler insert and standard size shoe; the previous foreshortened shoe is at the extreme right.*

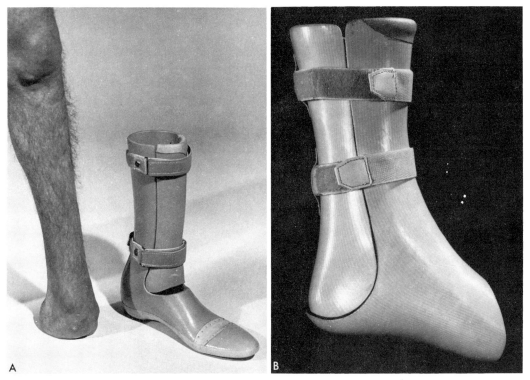

Figure 65–28. *(A) A clam-shell plastic laminated prosthesis provides stability for a Chopart amputation. (B) Posterior opening prosthetic variant for Chopart amputations.*

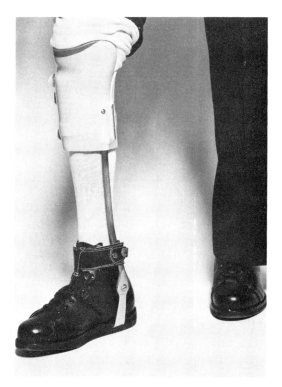

Figure 65–29. *A PTB orthosis can be used with a partial foot prosthesis to unload sensitive, ulcerated areas.*

side straps that terminated distally in an ankle base, and a wooden foot with a terminal toe-break. A Canadian modification of the Syme prosthesis utilized a plastic laminated socket attached to a solid ankle cushioned heel (SACH foot). To allow entry of the residual limb, the socket was split down the medial and lateral sides and hinged together; a strap retained the closure.

The current, modified Syme prosthesis uses a thermosetting plastic laminated socket, carefully contoured to the outlines of the residual limb. In the VAPC variant, the medial window version (Fig. 65–30) the amputee can bypass the narrow waist of the prosthesis with his bulbous stump. The stump (or distal aspect of the residual limb) is passed through the intact brim of the prosthesis to achieve PTB weight-bearing characteristics. The stump is brought out of the window past the narrowest part and reinserted into the socket distally. Replacement of the plastic window achieves suspension. A closed Syme prosthesis, without a window, is used for those individuals who engage in strenuous activity (Fig. 65–31). In this version, the bulbous end is passed through the brim, and passage through the narrow waist is made possible by the fabrication of a flexible inner liner, either removable or attached to the socket. After the bulbous stump has been passed beyond the expandible, flexible waist, the waist regains its previous contour to achieve suspension. In most instances, the medial window variant of the prosthesis is prescribed. Finally, proximal support, at the patellar tendon area, can be added in the early postoperative stage to protect the end of the residual limb; painful or poorly healed areas can thus be alleviated. The modern Syme prosthesis, bolted to a SACH foot, is also used in Pirogoff amputations (retained calcaneus) and true ankle disarticulations. As stated, the Syme amputation is preferred. The decision to perform a

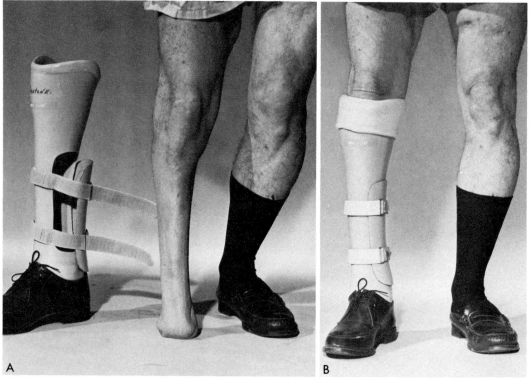

Figure 65–30. *(A) Modified Syme prosthesis with plastic medial closure. (B) Syme prosthesis, fully donned, provides satisfactory function but limited cosmesis.*

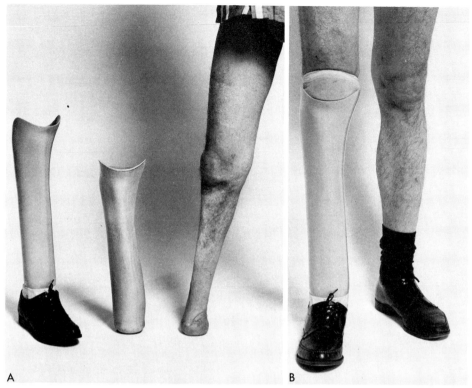

Figure 65–31. *(A) Closed Syme prosthesis with a soft inner liner is preferred for strenuous activity. (B) The closed Syme prosthesis presents poor cosmesis for the female amputee.*

Syme procedure or a more proximal below-the-knee amputation depends on the clinical examination and certain laboratory findings, including the xenon-133 technique, thermography, Doppler studies, angiography, and other measures. The use of immediate postoperative plaster casts and controlled environment methods has increased the percentage of favorable results following Syme and other partial foot amputations.

FUNCTIONAL ELECTRICAL STIMULATION

Electrical stimulators have been used to produce muscle contraction for many years, provided that the stimulus was of adequate strength, duration, and abruptness. It has been confirmed by numerous investigations that a brief stimulus (duration of less than half a millisecond) at a frequency of 40 cycles per second causes an effective tetanic contraction of muscle with minimal pain and discomfort.

The introduction of transistors and other microcircuitry permitted the development of a compact, battery-powered stimulator that evokes contraction of a patient's dorsiflexors and evertors, simulating dorsiflexion of the ankle during swing phase. A shoe switch controls the flow of stimulating current when the involved lower limb is lifted from the floor; the apparatus is illustrated in Figure 65–32.

In general, extensive clinical experience indicates that functional electrical stimulation of the peroneal nerve and the anterior tibial muscle provides acceptable orthotic management of the patient with weakness or absence of the anterolateral compartment musculature of the leg. Prescription of the system requires patient alertness and close monitoring to assure success, since misplaced electrodes, defective wir-

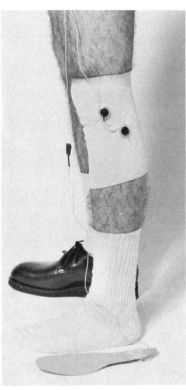
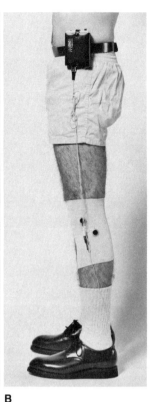

A   **B**

Figure 65-32. *Functional electrical stimulator. (A) Shoe insert with switch controls flow of current to the electrodes at the knee. (B) Compact battery unit provides electrical source for the device.*

ing, or an exhausted power source can cause failure of the device and be a hazard to the patient.

ORTHOTIC-PROSTHETIC CARE OF THE CHILD

The child with a disorder of the ankle-foot area is generally managed with orthotic and prosthetic systems similar to those used in the adult with reliance on a careful biomechanical assessment of functional deficiencies to develop the prescription. A major factor in evaluating disability is growth, particularly when the normal development of a child can aggravate the deformity. Again, a higher probability of successful rehabilitation is assured by assembling a team specialized in the care of handicapped children, a team that will respond not only to the immediate provision of an orthosis or prosthesis, but that will also be sensitive to the child's behavioral reaction and adjustment, social and educational needs, and other aspects of his life that may be affected. The process of evaluation, conference discussions, exami-

nation, patient and parent involvement, development of the prescription, fabrication, delivery, check-out, training, and ongoing re-evaluations follows the standards and criteria developed by adult amputee and orthotic services. However, there is a considerably higher degree of individualization in the devices used in children, the majority of whom will present with diverse congenital or developmental disorders.

In the field of orthotic management of pediatric ankle-foot problems, much reliance is placed on the metal double-bar AFO to correct and prevent deformity, assist weakened or absent muscles, correct abnormal alignment, control or reduce spasticity, and improve other motor and sensory defects. Extensible uprights are utilized to compensate for growth, together with high-top shoes and externally or internally applied shoe modifications. However, plastic orthoses, including all the variants described in preceding sections, are applicable and in most instances offer better prevention of deformity because of the higher degree of orthosis-limb congruency. A major disadvantage of plastic orthoses for the child is the high cost of frequent replacement, since they are not adjustable as the child develops and grows; however, modifications of plastic orthoses are being introduced to lessen this disadvantage. Figure 65–33 demonstrates the combination of a plastic supracondylar section attached to a conventional double-bar AFO; the well-contoured plastic component provides alignment control that is superior to that with the double-bar AFO alone. A solid AFO lined with Pelite, which can be removed later, is one method of anticipating circumferential growth (Fig. 65–34). Figure 65–35 illustrates an experimental solid AFO that is extensible by removing and replacing metal screws. Furthermore, revisions of the spiral section attachment of a plastic spiral AFO can permit lengthening of this device as the child grows; Figure 65–36 displays this concept.

In prosthetics, absence of one or more toes is treated with molded shoe inserts, toe-filler materials, and modified shoes. Traumatic transmetatarsal amputations are managed with partial foot prostheses or a variant that provides more ankle stability, as shown in Figure 65–37. Elective surgical ablation of the congenitally abnormal foot involves the Syme procedure to preserve distal epiphyseal growth centers. The closed Syme prosthesis, or one with a removable posterior section, is most often used. It is beyond the scope of this review to fully detail the many variants of prosthetic appliances; it must be remembered, however, that each child requires an individually designed and constructed unit. For example, Figure 65–38 details the restoration process in a girl with congenital deformities of the right foot, including removal of the toes, wedge resection, and fixation to correct severe pes cavus, and fabrication of a PTB orthosis with cosmetic contouring.

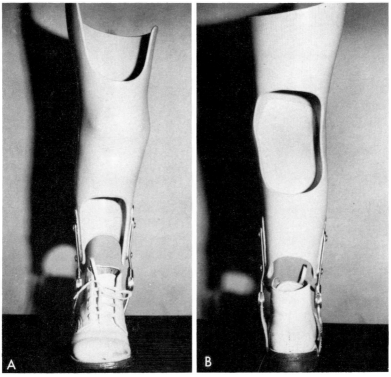

Figure 65–33. (A) Combination of a well-contoured, proximal plastic section and a double-bar AFO result in superior alignment and foot-ankle control. (B) Posterior view of the supracondylar ankle-foot orthosis with extensible double uprights to allow for growth.

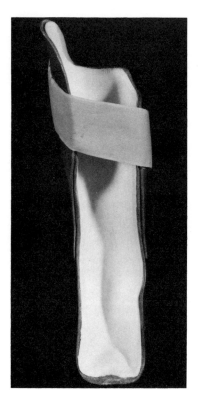

Figure 65–34. *Anterior view of a solid AFO with a Pelite liner that is removable to allow for circumferential growth.*

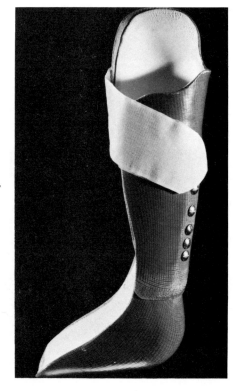

Figure 65–35. *Solid AFO with extensible proximal component, permitting longitudinal growth.*

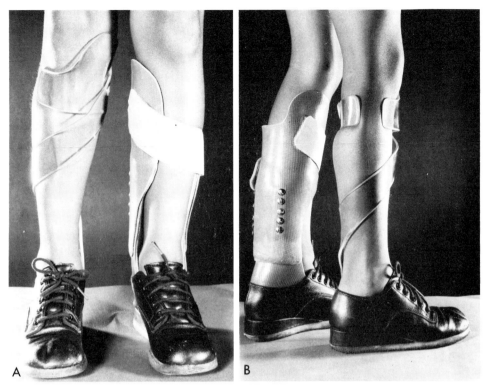

Figure 65–36. (A) Child with a solid AFO on the left and an adjustable spiral AFO on the right. (B) Side view of the solid AFO and the adjustable spiral AFO.

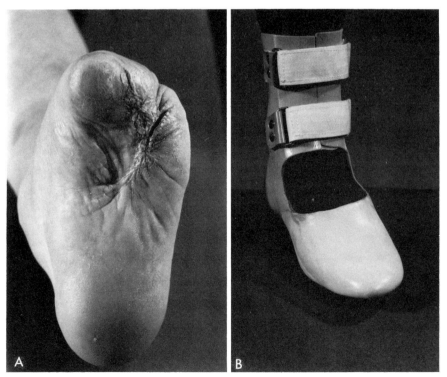

Figure 65–37. (A) Plantar view of a partial foot amputation in a young child, with healing, ulcerated areas secondary to activity. (B) Proximal plastic section with Velcro closure provides added stability to reduce motion between the residual foot and the prosthesis.

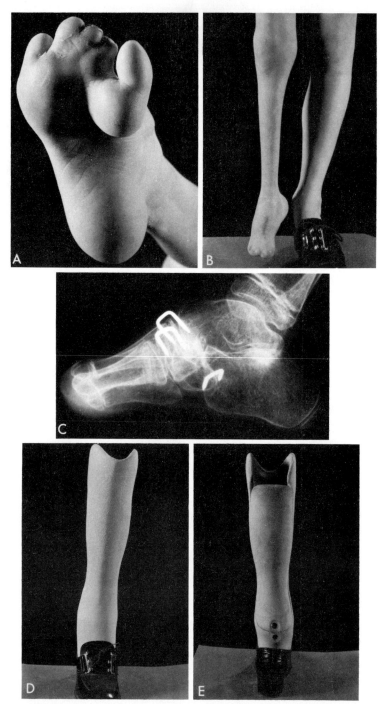

Figure 65–38. (A) Multiple congenital deformities of the right foot prior to surgical and prosthetic restoration. (B) Thin, atrophic right leg with initial ablation of toes. (C) Wedge resection of tarsal bones with staple fixation corrects severe cavus deformity. (D) Anterior view of a PTB prosthesis with cosmetic cover for limb equalization, cosmesis, improved function, and partial unloading of the deformed foot. (E) Posterior view showing hinged panel for donning.

Acknowledgment

I wish to gratefully acknowledge the invaluable assistance of Drs. Gustav Rubin and John E. Eschen; I could not have prepared this chapter without them.

REFERENCES

1. American Academy of Orthopaedic Surgeons: Orthopaedic Appliances Atlas, Vol. 1 (Braces, Splints, Shoe Alterations). Ann Arbor, Michigan, J. E. Edwards, 1952.
2. Artamonov, A.: Vacuum-forming techniques and materials in prosthetics and orthotics. Inter-Clinic Information Bulletin, *11*:10, 1972.
3. Committee on Prosthetics Research and Development, National Academy of Sciences: Report of the Seventh Workshop Panel on Lower Extremity Orthosis of the Subcommittee on Design and Development, National Research Council. Washington, D. C., March 1970.
4. Committee on Prosthetics Research and Development, National Academy of Sciences: A clinical evaluation of four lower-limb orthoses. Report E-5. Washington, D.C., 1972.
5. Committee on Prosthetics Research and Development, National Academy of Sciences: Clinical evaluation of a comprehensive approach to below-knee orthotics. Report E-6. Washington, D.C., 1972.
6. Committee on Prosthetics Research and Development, National Academy of Sciences: Report of eighth workshop. Washington, D.C., October 1972.
7. Committee on Prosthetics Research and Development, National Academy of Sciences: Seventh workshop panel on lower-extremity orthotics. Report of workshop. Washington, D.C., March 1972.
8. Committee on Prosthetics Research and Development, National Academy of Sciences: Clinical evaluation of the Ljubljana functional electrical personal brace. Report E-7. Washington, D.C., 1973.
9. Corcoran, P. J.: Evaluation of plastic short brace (thesis submitted in partial fulfillment of requirements for degree of Master of Science). Seattle, University of Washington, May 24, 1968.
10. Davis, F. J., Fry, L. R., Lippert, F. G., et al.: Patellar tendon-bearing brace: report of 16 patients. J. Trauma, *14*:216, 1974.
11. Demopoulos, J. T., and Cassvan, A.: Experience with plastic orthoses in children: preliminary observations. Bull. Hosp. Joint Dis., *32*:148, 1971.
12. Demopoulos, J. T., Cassvan, A., and Snowden, J. M.: Experience with plastic lower extremity orthoses. Bull. Hosp. Joint Dis., *33*:22, 1972.
13. Demopoulos, J. T., and Eschen, J. E.: Modification of plastic orthoses for children. Bull. Hosp. Joint Dis., *34*:156, 1973.
14. Demopoulos, J. T., and Eschen, J. E.: Experience with a patellar tendon-bearing orthosis. Orthot. Prosthet., *28*:5, 1974.
15. Demopoulos, J. T., and Eschen, J. E.: Variations in plastic orthoses for the developing child. N.Y.U. Inter-Clinic Bulletin, *25*:4, 1976.
16. Eighth Workshop Panel on Lower Limb Orthotics: Report of the Subcommittee on Design and Development, Committee on Prosthetics Research and Development, Division of Medical Sciences, National Research Council, National Academy of Sciences and National Academy of Engineering, Los Angeles, California, October 1972.
17. Engen, T. J.: Research developments of lower extremity orthotic systems for patients with various functional deficits. Houston, Texas Institute for Rehabilitation and Research, 1970.
18. Engen, T. J.: Instructional manual for fabrication and fitting of a below knee corrugated polypropylene orthosis. Houston, Texas Institute for Rehabilitation and Research, 1971.
19. England, C. F., Fannin, R. E., and Skahan, J. E.: *In* Anderson, M. H., et al. (eds.): Manual of Lower Extremities Orthotics. Springfield, Illinois, Charles C Thomas, 1972.
20. Evaluation–VAPC modular single-bar braces. Bull. Prosthet. Res., *10*:152, 1968.
21. Fifth Workshop Panel on Lower Extremity Orthotics: Report of the Subcommittee on Design and Development, Committee on Prosthetics Research and Development, Division of Engineering, National Research Council, National Academy of Sciences and National Academy of Engineering. Atlanta, Georgia, April 1968.
22. Fourth Workshop Panel on Lower Extremity Orthotics: Report of the Subcommittee on Design and Development, Committee on Prosthetics Research and Development, Division of Engineering, National Research Council, National Acdemy of Sciences and National Academy of Engineering. Santa Monica, California, March 1967.
23. Harris, E. E.: A new orthotics terminology—A guide to its use for prescription and fee schedules. Orthot. Prosthet., *27*:6, 1973.
24. Hill, J. T., and Fenwich, A. L.: A contoured, posterior, fiberglass-epoxy drop-foot brace. United States Army Medical Bioengineering Research and Development Laboratory Tech. Rep. 6805. Forest Glen, Maryland, May 1968.
25. Hill, J. T., and Stube, R. W.: The USAMBRL fiberglass dropfoot brace. Prosthet. Int., *3*:9, 1969.
26. Hill, J. T., and Stube, R. W.: An improved manufacturing technique for the USAMBRL fiberglass-epoxy drop-foot brace. United States Army Medical Bioengineering Research and Development Laboratory Tech. Rep. 6910. Forest Glen, Maryland, 1969.
27. Hill, J. T., and Stube, R. W.: Manual for the USAMBRL posterior bar drop-foot brace. United States Army Medical Bioengineering Research and Development Laboratory Tech. Rep. 7003. Forest Glen, Maryland, August 1970.
28. Hill, J. T., and Stube, R. W.: Manual for the USAMBRL lateral rod drop-foot brace. United States Army Medical Bioengineering Research and Development Laboratory Tech. Rep. 7004. Forest Glen, Maryland, August 1970.
29. Isman, R. E., and Inman, V. T.: Anthropometric studies of the human foot and ankle. Bull. Prosthet. Res., *10–11*:97, 1969.
30. Jebsen, R. H., Corcoran, P. J., and Simons, B. C.: Clinical experience with plastic short leg brace. Arch. Phys. Med. Rehabil., *51*:114, 1970.
31. Jebsen, R. H., Simons, B. C., and Corcoran, P. J.: Experimental plastic short leg braces. Arch. Phys. Med. Rehabil., *49*:108, 1968.
32. Kay, H. W.: Clinical applications of the Veterans Administration Prosthetics Center patella-tendon-bearing brace. Artif. Limbs, *15*:46, 1971.
33. Kay, H. W., and Vorchheimer, H.: A Survey of Eight Wearers of the Veterans Administration Prosthetics Center Patellar Tendon-Bearing Brace. School of Engineering and Science, New York University, July 1965.
34. Lehmann, J. F., DeLateur, B. J., Warren, C. G., and Simons, B. C.: Trends in lower extremity bracing. Arch. Phys. Med. Rehabil., *51*:338, 1970.
35. Lehmann, J. F., and Warren, C. G.: Ischial and patellar tendon weight-bearing braces; function, design, adjustment and training. Bull. Prosthet. Res., *19*:6, 1973.
36. Lehmann, J. F., Warren, C. G., and DeLateur, B. J.: Biomechanical evaluation of knee stability in below-knee braces. Arch. Phys. Med. Rehabil., *51*:688, 1970.

37. Lehneis, H. R.: New concepts in lower extremity orthotics. Med. Clin. North Am., 53:585, 1969.
38. Lehneis, H. R.: New developments in lower-limb orthotics through bioengineering. Arch. Phys. Med. Rehabil., 53:303, 1972.
39. Lehneis, H. R.: Final report: Bioengineering design and development of lower extremity orthotic devices. New York, Institute of Rehabilitation Medicine, New York University Medical Center, October 1972.
40. Lehneis, H. R.: Orthotics alignment in the lower limb. Proceedings of the First International Congress on Prosthetics Techniques and Functional Rehabilitation, Paper IV-109, 4:73, 1973.
41. Lehneis, H. R., Frisina, E., Marx, H. W., and Sowell, T.: Bioengineering design and development of lower-extremity orthotic devices. New York, Institute of Rehabilitation Medicine, New York University Medical Center, October 1972.
42. Licht, S. (ed.): Physical Medicine Library, Vol. 9 (Orthotics). Baltimore, Waverly Press, 1966.
43. Lindseth, R. E., and Glancy, J.: Polypropylene lower extremity braces for paraplegia due to myelomeningocele. J. Bone Joint Surg., 56A:556, 1974.
44. Lusskin, R.: The influence of errors in bracing upon deformity of the lower extremity. Arch. Phys. Med. Rehabil., 47:520, 1966.
45. Lyons, C.: Vacuum-formed upper extremity splints. Inter-Clinic Information Bulletin, 11:10, 1972.
46. McCullough, C., III: Introduction to lower extremity orthotics. Instructional course lectures of the American Academy of Orthopaedic Surgeons, 20:116, 1971.
47. McCullough, C., III, Fryer, C. M., and Glancy, J.: A new approach to patient analysis for orthotic prescription. Artif. Limbs, 14:68, 1970.
48. McCullough, C., III, Fryer, C. M., and Glancy, J.: A new approach to patient analysis for orthotic prescription. Part I. The lower extremity. Artif. Limbs, 14:26, 1970.
49. McIlmurray, W. J., and Greenbaum, W.: A below-knee weight-bearing brace. Orthop. Prosthet. Appliance J., 12:81, 1958.
50. McIlmurray, W. J., and Greenbaum, W.: The application of Sach foot principles to orthotics. Orthop. Prosthet. Appliance J., 13:209, 1959.
51. Meyer, P. R., Jr.: Lower limb orthotics. Clin. Orthop., 102:58, 1974.
52. Mooney, V., and Snelson, R.: Fabrication and application of transparent polycarbonate sockets. Orthot. Prosthet., 26:1, 1972.
53. Nitschke, R. O., and Marschall, D.: The PTS knee brace. Orthot. Prosthet., 22:46, 1968.
54. Perry, J., and Hislop, H. J.: Principles of Lower-Extremity Bracing. New York, American Physical Therapy Association, 1967.
55. Rubin, G., and Dixon, M.: The modern ankle-foot orthoses (AFO's). Bull. Prosthet. Res., 19:20, 1973.
56. Sarno, J. E., and Lehneis, H. R.: Prescription and considerations for plastic below-knee orthoses. Arch. Phys. Med. Rehabil., 52:503, 1971.
57. Saunders, J. B. de C. M., Inman, V. T., and Eberhart, H. D.: The major-determinants in normal and pathological gait. J. Bone Joint Surg., 35A:543, 1953.
58. Simons, B. C., Jebsen, R. H., and Wildman, L. E.: Plastic short leg brace fabrication. Orthot. Prosthet., 21:215, 1967.
59. Staros, A.: Joint designs in prosthetics and orthotics. Prosthet. Int., 3:1, 1970.
60. Staros, A.: Nomenclatures and classification of orthotic components. In Murdoch's Prosthetic and Orthotic Practice: A Report of a Conference in Dundee, Scotland, June 1969, London, Edward Arnold Ltd., 1970, pp. 484–488.
61. Staros, A.: Functional analysis of lower-limb orthoses. Proceedings of the First International Congress on Prosthetics Techniques and Functional Rehabilitation, Paper II-75, 2:215, 1973.
62. Staros, A., and Peizer, E.: The clinical engineer. American Society of Mechanical Engineers, Winter Annual Meeting, November 1973.
63. Sutherland, D. H.: An electromyographic study of the plantar flexors of the ankle in normal walking on the level. J. Bone Joint Surg., 48A:66, 1966.
64. Thorndike, A., Murphy, E. F., and Staros, A.: Engineering applied to orthopaedic bracing. Orthop. Prosthet. Appliance J., 10:55, 1956.
65. Wright, D. G., Desai, S. M., and Henderson, W. H.: Action of the subtalar and ankle joint complex during the stance phase of walking. J. Bone Joint Surg., 46A:361, 1964.
66. Yates, G.: A method for the provision of lightweight aesthetic orthopaedic appliances. Orthopaedics, 1:153, 1968.

CHAPTER 66

ORGANIZATION OF A FOOT SERVICE

F. William Wagner, Jr., M.D.

In the past, most adult foot problems have been cared for by Adult Orthopaedic Reconstruction Services. Children's problems have usually been assigned to the Pediatric Orthopaedic Service. Founding of the American Orthopedic Foot Society, continued growth of subspecialization in the orthopaedic field, and continued growth of knowledge in care of the foot have virtually dictated the need for establishment of a Foot Service in each residency program. Many are in operation, although not always distinguished by name. The exact composition of a Foot Service will vary with each institution, depending on the size, the number of departments, the number of residents, and the type of affiliation with a medical school and medical center. The following outlines are intended as general guides only, and variations will be mandated by the wishes of the teaching and attending staff.

OUTPATIENT DIVISION

Patients are divided by age. Adult foot and ankle problems are seen separately. Children's foot problems are treated in a children's foot clinic affiliated with the Pediatric Orthopaedic Service.

A. *Medical Staff*
   1. Attending orthopaedic surgeons: At least two.
   2. Fellows: Postgraduate fellows may be assigned for a six-month to one-year rotation, depending on the size and volume of the Service. This is becoming more attractive, as more orthopaedists are now limiting their practice to the foot.
   3. Residents: Resident assignments should be for at least two months. Some residents may wish to repeat the Service as a senior elective if such is available in their program.
   4. Interns and medical students are assigned for at least one month.
   5. Consultations: Other departments are asked to have representatives available for consultations and conferences as needed.
      a. Vascular Surgery: Diabetic and other dysvascular patients will frequently require revascularization procedures. Noninvasive assessments such as Doppler ultrasound, plethysmography, xenon skin flow tests, and similar studies can be ordered on an outpatient basis in most cases. Angiography is performed when revascularization is indicated. Residents should visit vascular surgery clinics and rounds to gain knowledge of the indications for and the ordering of vascular diagnostic tests.
      b. Dermatology: Skin lesions frequently accompany structural problems in the foot. Systemic

diseases can, on occasion, be manifested in foot eruptions. Hyperhidrosis can be a problem with plastic shoe inserts and orthoses made of other types of material that act as insulators. Consultations with the dermatologist should frequently be on a direct basis for greater learning value to the resident on the Foot Service.

c. Plastic Surgery: Major skin and soft-tissue loss can require more expertise in flap design and transfer techniques than possessed by the orthopaedist. The resident should become familiar with the various techniques for skin grafting. Visits to the plastic surgery clinic and teaching by the plastic surgeon as a consultant in surgical cases aid in learning of basic techniques of plastic surgery.

d. Pediatrician: Medical, genetic, emotional, and similar problems in children can require assistance from the pediatrician.

e. Diabetologist: Good diabetic control is especially important in care of foot problems such as diabetic neuropathy, Charcot joints, and infected ulcers. It is of even more importance during hospitalization for gangrene, infected gangrene, and other severe problems. The best results appear to come from a Service in which diabetic and orthopaedic care are provided by coequal attending and resident staff.

B. *Ancillary Personnel:* Nurses, attendants, social workers, orthopaedic physician's assistant and/or plaster technician, and secretary.

C. *Records:* Records and photographs frequently become an important adjunct to the clinic when results of a particular procedure are being studied. A system should be designed that will allow filing of photographs in the patient's chart for better clinical care and a cross-indexing system to indicate which photographs are available.

D. *Patient Referral:* A registry is maintained, and referrals are made directly to the clinic. Referrals may come from allied clinics such as those for arthritis, diabetes, stroke, spinal surgery, fracture, trauma, and tumor.

E. *Equipment:* Much of the equipment needed for a Foot Service will be that found in any orthopaedic clinic. However, specialized tools for care of the foot and implements for the manufacture of shoe corrections are necessary additions. The following list is not intended to be complete, but it can be supplemented as experience in the clinic shows the need for changes and additions:

Plaster of Paris rolls and splints; new plastic cast material (e.g., Hexcellite, Lite Cast, Cutter-7); cast padding material, cast saws and cutters, cast spreaders, sequestrectomy forceps; different grades of felt, foam rubber, and microcellular rubber; different grades of foamed polyethylene; a small electric oven; moleskin; metatarsal pads, adhesive tape; nail clippers; bone rongeurs (a rongeur makes an excellent nail clipper for ram's horn and other enlarged nails); cuticle nipper; assorted scalpel blades; curettes; Moto-tool with sandpaper discs and burs; Wood's light; tuning fork; percussion hammer; pins; footprint pads; toenail interpositional material; alginate casting material, Doppler ultrasound flowmeter; assorted sphygmomanometer cuffs for thigh-to-toe blood pressure measurements; and commercially available inserts such as cord pads, toe crests, felt and plastic metatarsal supports, night bunion splints, and similar pressure-relieving appliances.

F. *Radiology:* Roentgenograms are essential in the complete examination of the foot and ankle. The history and physical examination should determine the area to be studied and the particular views to be requested. In assessing injuries near joints and epiphyseal lines in children, the contralateral normal side should be studied for comparison. Arthrography, xerography, image intensification, computerized axial tomography, and cineradiography may be used for special problems in consultation with the radiologist.

Not infrequently, the "standard

views" do not provide all of the necessary information. Members of the radiologic and orthopaedic departments should consult and agree on which views constitute a minimal examination. Additional views may then be ordered if further information is necessary.

G. *Electrodiagnosis:* Foot deformities can result from disorders of the neuromuscular system. Electrical tests are correlated with clinical and roentgenographic findings. Nerve conduction tests, electromyography, and tests of neuromuscular excitability are the most common tests performed.

H. *Ancillary Services:* The services of prescription shoe fitters, orthotists, and prosthetists should be readily available. It will depend on each institution whether these are full-time in-house personnel or the services are contracted from local private businesses.

INPATIENT DIVISION

Adequate beds should be assigned and operating time allocated so that unnecessary waiting does not occur between the decision for surgery and its actual performance. The resident or fellow who has seen the patient in the clinic should perform the in-hospital work-up and follow through surgery, convalescence, and outpatient rehabilitation. Residents are allowed to perform surgery in accordance with their proficiency and experience.

Surgical equipment will include standard orthopaedic instruments. In addition, small osteotomes, chisels, curettes, bone clamps, and periosteal elevators will be necessary. They should be supplemented with electric or gas-driven saws, drills, and pin drivers. Small plates, screws, wires, pins, and fixation devices, similar to those used in hand surgery, are frequently required.

RESEARCH AND TRAINING

Series of foot cases lend themselves well to clinical research. Each resident and fellow should be required to study a foot problem during his rotation on the service and to prepare a paper on the results. The use of the walking electromyograph and other gait analysis equipment is beginning to point the way toward laboratory aid in the solution of clinical problems. Interested residents should be given the opportunity to spend additional time on the service to study particular problems that have challenged them. Dissection in the anatomy laboratory is essential. It is suggested that each resident be assigned a specific area for dissection and be required to present his specimens in detail at a monthly meeting. If available, an animal laboratory affords an opportunity for basic research in many areas. For example, response of the animal foot pad to trauma, infection, foreign materials, surgery, and denervation will provide answers to similar problems in the human.

Part VIII
APPENDICES AND INDEX

APPENDIX 1

SUGGESTED COURSE OUTLINE FOR RESIDENT STUDY OF THE ADULT FOOT AND ANKLE

F. William Wagner, Jr., M.D.

I. *The Normal Foot*
(Children and Adults)
   1. Embryology
   2. Gross anatomy
   3. Growth
   4. Histology
   5. Variations in normal measurement

II. *Biomechanics of the Foot and Ankle* (Children and Adults)
   1. Energy and work loads
   2. Imbalance and stress and strain
   3. Kinematics
   4. Kinetics
   5. Lubrication

III. *Neuromuscular and Neurologic Diseases Affecting the Foot* (Children and Adults)
   1. Amyotrophic lateral sclerosis
   2. Cerebral palsy
   3. Cerebrovascular accidents
   4. Charcot-Marie-Tooth disease
   5. Diabetes mellitus
   6. Friedreich's ataxia
   7. Hypertensive neuropathy
   8. Interdigital neuroma
   9. Leprosy (Hansen's disease)
   10. Multiple sclerosis
   11. Muscular dystrophy
   12. Myelodysplasia
   13. Neurotrophic arthropathy
   14. Poliomyelitis
   15. Tarsal tunnel syndrome
   16. Tuberous sclerosis

IV. *Circulatory Disturbances*
   1. Arterial aneurysms
   2. Diffuse angiodysplastic syndromes
   3. Distal arterial occlusive disease
   4. Hypercoagulable conditions
   5. Hyperviscosity conditions
   6. Infections
   7. Lymphedema
   8. Proximal arterial occlusive disease
   9. Reflex dystrophy; reflex causalgia; sympathetic dystrophy
   10. Thrombosis
   11. Trauma
   12. Vascular tumors
   13. Venous and lymphatic insufficiency

V. *Dermatologic Disorders, Including Nails*
   1. Affections Peculiar to Nails and Soft Tissue Adjacent to the Nail
      a. Onychia

1831

b. Onychogryphosis
   i. Ingrown toenail
c. Onychomycosis
d. Onychoptosis
   i. Calloused nail groove
e. Paronychia
f. Trauma
g. Tumors
     i. Chondroma
    ii. Epithelioma
   iii. Glomus tumor
   iv. Melanoma
    v. Pyogenic granuloma
   vi. Sarcoma
  vii. Synovial cysts
 viii. Verruca

2. Ainhum disease
3. Congenital diseases
  a. Anonychia
  b. Congenital ectodermal defect
  c. Pachyonychia congenita
  d. Polydactyly, syndactyly
4. Dermatophytosis (dermatomycosis)
5. Eccrine poroma
6. Epidermal cyst
7. Glomus
8. Hypersensitivity reactions
9. Keloids
10. Manifestations of systemic diseases
  a. Eczema
  b. Epidermolysis bullosa
  c. Ichthyosis
  d. Lues, tuberculosis, leprosy
  e. Mee's lines (arsenic poisoning)
  f. Pityriasis rubra pilaris
  g. Psoriasis
  h. Pyogenic infectious disease
  i. Scleroderma
11. Nevus
12. Onychodystrophies
  a. Beau's lines
  b. Dystrophia unguis mediana canaliformis
  c. Koilonychia
  d. Leukonychia
  e. Onychauxis, onychogryphosis
  f. Onycholysis
13. Parasitic infections
14. Pyogenic infections
15. Verruca plantaris (vulgaris)
16. Viral infections (molluscum contagiosum)

VI. *Tumors*
1. Angiosarcoma
2. Benign/malignant giant cell tumors
3. Chondrosarcoma
4. Ewing's sarcoma
5. Fibroma
6. Fibromatosis
7. Fibrosarcoma
8. Ganglion
9. Hemangioma
10. Intramedullary fibrosarcoma
11. Lipoma
12. Liposarcoma
13. Lymphangioma
14. Multiple myeloma
15. Neurofibroma
16. Neurogenic sarcoma
17. Osteogenic sarcoma
18. Osteoid osteoma
19. Paget's disease
20. Paget's osteogenic sarcoma
21. Plantar fascial fibromatosis
22. Pseudo tumors
23. Reticulum cell sarcoma
24. Rhabdomyosarcoma
25. Secondary/metastatic bone tumors
26. Synovial sarcoma
27. Unicameral bone cyst
28. Xanthoma

VII. *Infectious and Noninfectious Inflammatory Disorders*
1. Bursitis
  a. Acute simple
  b. Chronic serous
  c. Pyogenic
2. Coccidioidal infections
3. Foreign body
4. Gas gangrene (*Clostridium welchii*)
5. Leprosy
6. Lues
7. Mycetoma
8. Plantar fasciitis
9. Tetanus (*Clostridium tetani*)
10. Tuberculosis

VIII. *Rheumatoid Foot*
1. Acute disease; systemic treatment
2. Chronic disease; deformity progression

3. Claw toes
4. Hammer toes
5. Joint resections, fusions, replacements
   a. Timing and technique
6. Rheumatoid nodules
7. Tendon rupture
8. Tenosynovitis

IX. *Hallux Valgus, Hallux Rigidus, Hallux Varus, Metatarsus Primus Varus*
1. Bunions
2. Examination, diagnosis, evaluation
3. Pathologic anatomy and first metatarsophalangeal joint
4. Sesamoids—osteochondrosis, fracture, traumatic sesamoiditis
5. Surrounding soft-tissue structures
6. Treatment
   a. Nonoperative
   b. Operative

X. *Forefoot and Toe Deformities*
1. Calluses, clavi, keratoses
2. Claw toes
3. Corns
   a. Hard
   b. Soft
4. Gigantism, with or without macrodactyly
5. Hammer toes
6. Interdigital neuroma
7. Intractable plantar keratosis
8. Joplin's neuroma
9. Metatarsalgia
10. Splayfoot deformity
11. Supernumerary toes
12. Syndactylism
    a. Congenital
    b. Acquired
13. Tailor's bunion (bunionette)
14. Varus deformity of the fifth toe

XI. *Gout and Periarticular Alterations*
1. Burns
2. Calcific deposits
3. Calcinosis circumscripta
4. Gout
   a. Acute
   b. Subclinical

5. Hemophilia
6. Pseudogout
7. Pulmonary hypertrophic osteoarthropathy

XII. *Amputations, Fusions, and Arthroplasties*
1. Ankle joint arthrodeses and ankle joint replacements
2. Arthroplasty/implant replacement of metatarsophalangeal joints
3. Creation of toe syndactyly
4. Disarticulations of interphalangeal and metatarsophalangeal joints
5. Grice procedure—extraarticular subtalar arthrodesis
6. Interphalangeal and metatarsophalangeal joint fusions
7. Metatarsal head resections
8. Phalangectomy (partial and total)
9. Removal of talus, removal of os calcis (partial and complete)
10. Subtalar and triple arthrodeses
11. Syme, Pirogoff, Boyd, and Vasconcellos amputations
12. Tarsal and metatarsal fusions
13. Toe and ray resections
    a. Central
    b. Lateral
    c. Medial
14. Transmetatarsal amputations
15. Lisfranc and Chopart amputations

XIII. *Fractures and Dislocations*
1. Fractures and fracture-dislocations of the ankle
2. Fractures and fracture-dislocations of the talus
3. Fractures of the os calcis
   a. Classifications, types, treatment methods, selection of treatment
4. March fracture
5. Metatarsal fractures
6. Metatarsophalangeal fractures and dislocations
7. Phalangeal fractures and dislocations

8. Sesamoid fractures and bipartite sesamoids
9. Tarsal fractures and dislocations

XIV. *Hindfoot Problems*
 1. Calcaneal spur, fasciitis, bursitis
 2. "Pump-bump"
 3. Rupture of tendo Achillis

XV. *Sports Injuries*
 1. Fractures of the accessory bones
  a. Accessory navicular
  b. Os trigonum
  c. Sesamoids
 2. March fracture
 3. Nerve entrapment syndromes
 4. Sprains and strains
 5. Stress fractures
  a. Tibia
  b. Fibula

XVI. *Clubfoot—Treatment of Late Residuals in the Adult*
 1. Flat-topped talus
 2. Loss of subtalar motion
 3. Metatarsal head pressure
  a. Base of fifth metatarsal pressure
 4. Residual equino varus

XVII. *Cavus Feet*
 1. Etiology
  a. Cerebral palsy
  b. Friedreich's ataxia
  c. Idiopathic types
  d. Mental retardation
  e. Multiple sclerosis
  f. Myelodysplasia
  g. Neuromuscular dystrophies
  h. Poliomyelitis
  i. Progressive muscular atrophy
  j. Tumors of the spinal canal
  k. Charcot-Marie-Tooth disease

 2. Treatment
  a. Operative
  b. Nonoperative

XVIII. *Flatfoot or Pes Planus*
 1. Biomechanical studies
 2. Classification
  a. Etiologic types
   i. Acquired: (1) Articular; (2) external tibial tarsi; (3) ligamentous; (4) muscle imbalance; (5) osseous—fractures or disease of the talus and os calcis; (6) postural or static
   ii. Congenital: (1) Hypermobile; (2) rigid (congenital vertical talus, tarsal coalitions)
  b. Clinical types
   i. Flexible—normal peroneals
   ii. Painful, nonpainful
   iii. Rigid—normal peroneals
   iv. Rigid—spastic peroneals
 3. Roentgenographic criteria
 4. Treatment
  a. Nonoperative
   i. Active passive stretching
   ii. Casting
   iii. Corrective orthoses
   iv. Corrective footwear
   v. Exercise
  b. Operative
   i. Arthrodesis
   ii. Combination—arthrodesis and osteotomy
   iii. Osteotomy
   iv. Tendon transfer

SUGGESTED COURSE OUTLINE FOR RESIDENT STUDY OF CHILD'S FOOT AND ANKLE

F. William Wagner, Jr., M.D.

I. *The Normal Foot.* See preceding section on Adult Foot and Ankle.

II. *Biomechanics of the Foot and Ankle.* See preceding section on Adult Foot and Ankle.

III. *Neuromuscular and Neurologic Diseases Affecting the Foot.* See preceding section on Adult Foot and Ankle.

IV. *Genetic Disturbances Affecting the Foot*
  1. Mendelian disorders
    a. Autosomal dominant
      i. Apert's syndrome
      ii. Brachydactyly
      iii. Calcaneonavicular bar
      iv. Marfan's syndrome
      v. Multiple epiphyseal dysplasia
      vi. Nail-patella syndrome
      vii. Polydactyly
      viii. Syndactyly
      ix. Talocalcaneal coalition
    b. Autosomal recessive
      i. Carpenter's syndrome
      ii. Congenital insensitivity to pain
      iii. Diastrophic dwarfism
      iv. Friedreich's ataxia
      v. Smith-Lemli-Opitz syndrome
  2. Chromosomal disorders
    a. Review of chromosome study techniques and nomenclature
      i. Trisomy D
      ii. Trisomy E
      iii. Trisomy G
      iv. Mongolism: (1) Non-dysjunction; (2) translocation
  3. Multifactorial conditions
    a. Clubfoot
    b. Meningomyelocele

V. *Congenital Deformities of the Foot*
  1. Ball-and-socket ankle joint
  2. Convex pes valgus (vertical talus, rocker bottom, flatfoot)
  3. Dysmelia
  4. Hallux valgus and bunion
  5. Hallux varus
  6. Metatarsus primus varus
  7. Metatarsus varus
  8. Split foot
    a. Lobster claw
  9. Talipes calcaneovalgus
  10. Talipes equinovalgus
  11. Talipes equinovarus
    a. Pathologic anatomy

            i. Skeletal
            ii. Soft-tissue
        b. Roentgenographic findings
        c. Treatment
            i. Nonoperative
            ii. Operative
    12. Talipes varus
    13. Tarsal coalitions
        a. Calcaneocuboid
        b. Calcaneonavicular
        c. Cubonavicular
        d. Talocalcaneal
        e. Talonavicular
        f. Variations and combinations

VI. *Pes Cavus*
    1. Clinical and roentgenographic
       features
    2. Etiology and pathogenesis
    3. Treatment
        a. Soft-tissue procedures
        b. Osseous procedures

VII. *Pronated Feet (Valgus, Flatfeet)*
    1. Treatment
        a. Shoe corrections and inserts
        b. Surgical management

VIII. *Hallux Rigidus*
    1. Etiology
    2. Roentgenographic features
    3. Treatment
        a. Nonoperative
        b. Operative

IX. *Hammer Toes and Claw Toes*
    1. Pathologic anatomy
    2. Treatment
        a. Nonoperative
        b. Operative

X. *Miscellaneous Toe Problems*
    1. Congenital curly (varus) toe
    2. Congenital overriding fifth toe
        a. Treatment
            i. Nonoperative
            ii. Operative
    3. Macrodactyly
        a. Etiology
        b. Treatment
            i. Nonoperative
            ii. Operative

    4. Mallet toe
    5. Microdactyly
    6. Polydactyly
    7. Syndactyly

XI. *Tumors of the Foot*
    1. Soft-tissue
        a. Fibroma, fibromatosis
        b. Ganglion
        c. Hemangioma
        d. Lipoma
        e. Lymphangiectasis
    2. Osseous (occasional occurrence)
        a. Aneurysmal bone cyst
        b. Chondroma,
           Chondroblastoma
        c. Exostosis, osteoma
        d. Metastatic (rare to foot)
        e. Multiple hereditary
           exostosis
        f. Unicameral bone cyst

XII. *Skin and Nail Lesions*
    1. Corn
        a. Hard
        b. Soft
    2. Ingrowing nail
    3. Plantar wart

XIII. *Fractures.* See also preceding
      section on Adult Foot and Ankle
      for specific bones
    1. Fractures involving the distal
       epiphysis of the tibia and fibula
        a. Salter and Harris
           Classification
            i. Type I
            ii. Type II
            iii. Type III
            iv. Type IV
            v. Type V
    2. Mechanism of injury
        a. Abduction
        b. Adduction
        c. Axial compression
        d. Direct violence
        e. External rotation
        f. Plantar flexion

GUIDE TO BASIC LITERATURE ON THE FOOT

F. William Wagner, Jr., M.D.

The following list represents a guide to the basic literature on the foot. It was begun by members of the Educational Committee of the American Orthopedic Foot Society (Alice Garrett, M.D., Chairman; Michael M. Donovan, M.D.; Robert B. Elliott, M.D.; and Robert M. Walters, M.D.). There are obviously many more articles in both the English and foreign language literature, and there may be many omissions in this list. However, it is expected that the interested reader will continue his or her search from the bibliography of the articles that he or she reads.

BASIC BOOKS AND ARTICLES

Banks, S. W., and Laufman, H.: An Atlas of Surgical Exposure of the Extremities. Philadelphia, W. B. Saunders Company, 1953.

Bateman, J. E. (ed.): Proceedings of the American Orthopaedic Foot Society. Orthop. Clin. North Am., 4(1):1, 1973.

Bateman, J. E. (ed.): Proceedings of the American Orthopaedic Foot Society. Orthop. Clin. North Am., 5(1):1, 1974.

Bateman, J. E. (ed.): Symposium on pitfalls in foot surgery. Orthop. Clin. North Am., 7(4):1, 1976.

Bateman, J. E. (ed.): Foot Science. Philadelphia, W. B. Saunders Company, 1976.

Burgess, E. M., Romano, R. L., and Zettl, J. H.: The Management of Lower Extremity Amputations. Washington, D. C., Superintendent of Documents: U. S. Government Printing Office, August 1969.

Committee on Prosthetic-Orthotic Education, Division of Medical Science, National Research Council, National Academy of Sciences: The Geriatric Amputee: Principles of Management. Washington, D.C., 1971.

Crenshaw, A. H. (ed.): Campbell's Operative Orthopaedics, 5th ed. St. Louis, C. V. Mosby Co., 1971.

DePalma, A. F. (ed.): Clin. Orthop. 16:1, 1960.

Dickson, F. D., and Diveley, R. L.: Functional Disorders of the Foot, 3rd ed. Philadelphia, J. B. Lippincott Co., 1953.

Erlacher, P. J.: Die Technik des Orthopadischen Eingriffs. Wien, J. Springer, 1928, p. 482.

Ferguson, A. B., Jr.: Orthopedic Surgery in Infancy and Childhood. Baltimore, Williams and Wilkins, 1968.

Frankel, V. H., and Burstein, A. H.: Orthopaedic Biomechanics. Philadelphia, Lea and Febiger, 1970.

Giannestras, N. J. (ed.): Static Deformities of the Foot. Clin. Orthop., 70:1, 1970.

Giannestras, N. J.: Foot Disorders: Medical and Surgical Management, 2nd ed. Philadelphia, Lea and Febiger, 1973.

Gocht, H., Debrunner, H., and Vogel, F. C.: Orthopädische Therapie. 1925, p. 340.

Hauser, E. D. W.: Diseases of the Foot. Philadelphia, W. B. Saunders Co., 1960.

Hohmann, G.: Fuss und Bein, 5th ed. Munich, J. F. Bergmann, 1951, p. 541 (and later editions).

Hohmann, G., Hackenbroch, M., Lundemann,

K.: Handbuch der Orthopadie, Vol. IV, Part 2. Stuttgart, Thieme, 1961, pp. 741–1390. (Desirable bibliography.)

Jaffe, H. L.: Metabolic Degenerative and Inflammatory Diseases of Bone and Joints. Philadelphia, Lea and Febiger, 1972.

Keith, A.: The history of the human foot and its bearing on orthopedic practice. J. Bone Joint Surg., 11:10, 1929.

Kelikian, H.: Hallux Valgus, Allied Deformities of the Forefoot and Metatarsalgia. Philadelphia, W. B. Saunders Company, 1965.

Klenerman, L.: The Foot and Its Disorders. Oxford, Blackwell Scientific Publications, 1976.

Köhler, A.: Borderlands of the Normal and Early Pathologic in Skeletal Roentgenology, 10th ed. (translated and edited by J. T. Case). New York, Grune and Stratton, 1956.

Lake, N. C.: The Foot, 4th ed. London, Ballière, Tindall and Cox, 1952.

Lange, F.: Lehrbuch de Orthopadie und Traumatologie, 3 Vol. Stuttgart, Enke, 1960–68.

Lelièvre, J.: Pathologie du Pied. Paris, Masson et Cie, 1967.

Levin, M. E., and O'Neal, L. W.: The Diabetic Foot, 2nd ed. St. Louis, C. V. Mosby Co., 1973.

Lewin, P.: The Foot and Ankle: Their Injuries, Diseases, Deformities and Disabilities, 4th ed. Philadelphia, Lea and Febiger, 1959.

Mann, R. E. (ed.): DuVries' Surgery of the Foot, 4th ed. St. Louis, C. V. Mosby Co., 1978.

Manual of Orthopaedic Surgery. Chicago, American Orthopaedic Association, 1966.

Method of Measuring and Recording. Chicago, American Academy of Orthopaedic Surgeons, 1965.

Mital, M. A., and Pierce, D. S.: Amputees and Their Prostheses. Boston, Little, Brown and Co., 1971.

Morton, D. J.: The Human Foot. New York, Columbia University Press, 1936.

Morton, D. J.: Human Locomotion and Body Form. Baltimore, Williams and Wilkins, 1952.

Radin, E. L., Simon, S. R., Rose, R. M., and Igor, L. P.: Practical Biomechanics for the Orthopedic Surgeon. New York, John Wiley and Sons, 1979.

Rockwood, C. A., Jr., and Green, D. P.: Fractures. Philadelphia, J. B. Lippincott Co., 1975.

Schuster, O. N.: Foot Orthopaedics, 2nd ed. Albany, J. B. Lyon Co., 1939.

Tachdjian, M. O.: Pediatric Orthopedics, Vols. I and II. Philadelphia, W. B. Saunders Company, 1972.

Urist, M. R. (ed.): AOFS surgery of the foot. Clin. Orthop., 85:1, 1972.

Walsham, W. J., and Hughes, W. K.: Deformities of the Human Foot. New York, William Wood and Co., 1895.

Watson-Jones, R.: Fractures and Joint Injuries, 5th ed. (J. N. Wilson [ed.]) London, Churchill Livingstone, 1976.

THE NORMAL FOOT—CHILD AND ADULT

Acton, R. K.: Surgical anatomy of the foot. J. Bone Joint Surg., 49A:555, 1967.

Anderson, M., Blais, M., and Green, W. T.: Growth of the normal foot during childhood and adolescence. J. Phys. Anthrop., 1950.

Bardeen, C. R.: Development and variations of the nerves and the musculature of the inferior extremity and of the neighboring regions of the trunk in man. Am. J. Anat., 6:259, 1906–07.

Bardeen, C. R., and Lewis, W. H.: Development of limbs, body-wall, and back in man. Am. J. Anat., 1:1, 1901.

Barnett, C. H.: Valgus deviation of the distal phalanx of the great toe. J. Anat., 4:265, 1905.

Barnett, C. H., Davies, D. V., and MacConaill, M. A.: Synovial Joints. Springfield, Charles C Thomas, 1961.

Barnett, G. H., and Napier, J. R.: The axis of rotation of ankle joint in man. Its importance upon the form of the talus and the mobility of the fibula. J. Anat., 86:1, 1952.

Bautrier: Cited in Meyer, M., Cuny, J., and Trensz, F.: L'os tibial externe et ses divers aspects radiologiques. Strasbourg Méd., 85:24, 1927.

Bjornson, R. G. B.: Developmental anomaly of the lateral malleolus simulating fracture. J. Bone Joint Surg., 38A:128, 1956.

Blais, M. M., Green, W. T., and Anderson, M.: Lengths of the growing foot. J. Bone Joint Surg., 38A:998, 1956.

Blechschmied, W.: Die Architektur des Fersenpolsters. Jahrbuch Morphol. Mikroshop Anat. 73:20, 1934. (Embryology and anatomy of the fat pads of the foot.)

Braus, H.: Anatomie des Menschen ein Lehrbuch für Studierende und Arzte, Fortgeführt von Cust Elze. 3 Aufl. Berlin, Springer, 1954.

Browne, D.: A mechanical interpretation of certain malformations. Adv. Teratol., 2:11, 1967.

Burman, M. S., and Lapidus, P. W.: The functional disturbances caused by the inconstant bones and sesamoids of the foot. Arch. Surg., 22:936, 1931.

Caffey, J.: Pediatric X-ray Diagnosis, 5th ed. Chicago, Year Book Medical Publishers, 1967, p. 744.

Cihak, R.: Ontogenesis of the Skeleton and Intrinsic Muscles of the Human Hand and

Foot. Berlin and New York, Springer-Verlag, 1972.

Corning, H. K.: Lehrbuch der Topographiscen Anatomie für Studierende und Arzte. 24 Aufl., 14–15 ed. Munchen, Bergmann, 1949.

Dubois, J. P., and Levanne, J. A.: Anatomie Descriptive du Pied Humain. Paris, Libraire Maloine, 1966, p. 429.

Duchenne, G. B.: Physiology of Motion (translated and edited by E. B. Kaplan). Philadelphia, J. B. Lippincott Co., 1949.

Dwight, T.: A Clinical Atlas, Variations of the Bones of the Hands and Feet. Philadelphia, J. B. Lippincott Co., 1907.

Dyment, P. G., and Bogan, O. M.: Pediatricians' attitudes concerning infants' shoes. Pediatrics, 50:655, 1972.

Elftman, H.: A cinematic study of the distribution of pressure in the human foot. Anat. Rec., 59:481, 1934.

Elftman, H.: The transverse tarsal joint and its control. Clin. Orthop., 16:41, 1960.

Elftman, H., and Manter, J. T.: The axes of the human foot. Science, 80:484, 1934.

Elftman, H., and Manter, J. T.: The evolution of the human foot, with especial reference to the joints. J. Anat., 70:56, 1935.

Faber, A.: Os tibiale externum bie erbgleichen Zwillingen. Erbatz, 4:83, 1934.

Feist, J. H., and Mankin, H. J.: The tarsus. Radiology, 79:250, 1962.

Féré, C. H., and Deniker, M.: Note sur des exostosis symétriques des scaphoides tarsiens. Rev. Chir., 29:544, 1904.

Fick, Rudolf, Gustav: Handbuch der Anatomie und Mechanik der Gelenke unter Gruchsichligung der Bewegenden Muskeln. 1904, Vol. 1, p. 512; 1910, Vol. 2, p. 376; Vol. 3, p. 688 Jena, Fisher. (Rare book.)

Francillon, M. R.: Untersuchungen zur anatomischen und klinischen Bedeutung des Os tibiale externum. Z. Orthop. Chir., 56:61, 1932.

Fraser, F. C.: Taking the family history. Am. J. Med., 34:585, 1963.

Frohse, F., Fisher, M. F.: Die Muskeln des Menschlichen Armes. Jena, Fisher, 1908 and 1913, p. 693.

Gardner, E., Gray, D. J., and O'Rahilly, R.: Anatomy, 4th ed. Philadelphia, W. B. Saunders Company, 1975.

Gardner, E., Gray, D. J., and O'Rahilly, R.: The prenatal development of the skeleton and joints of the human foot. J. Bone Joint Surg., 41A:847, 1959.

Geist, E. S.: The accessory scaphoid bone. J. Bone Joint Surg., 7:570, 1925.

Goergen, T. G., Danzig, L. A., Resnick, D., and Owen, C. A.: Roentgenographic evaluation of the tibiotalar joint. J. Bone Joint Surg., 59A:874, 1977.

Gottlieb, C., and Berenbaum, S. L.: Pirie's bone, accessory ossicle on the dorsum of the astragalus — often bilateral. Radiology, 55:423, 1950.

Grant, J. C. B.: Atlas of Anatomy, 6th ed. Baltimore, Williams and Wilkins, 1969.

Gray, H.: Gray's Anatomy of the Human Body, 28th ed. (edited by C. M. Goss). Philadelphia, Lea and Febiger, 1966.

Grodinsky, M.: A study of the fascial spaces of the foot and their bearing on infections. Surg. Gynecol. Obstet., 49:737, 1929.

Haliburton, R. A., Sullivan, C. R., Kelly, P., and Peterson, L. F. A.: Extra-osseous and intra-osseous blood supply of the talus. J. Bone Joint Surg., 40A:1115, 1958.

Hall, M. C.: The normal movement at the sub-talar joint. Can. J. Surg., 2:287, 1959.

Henke, F., Lubarsch, D., and Rössle, R. (founding eds.): Handbuch der Speciellen Pathologischen, Anatomie und Histologie, Vol. 19. Berlin, Springer, Part I — Bone, Muscle, Tendons, Sheaths, Bursa, 1929, p. 678; Part II — Joints and Bones, 1934, p. 680; Part III — Bones and Joints, 1937, p. 824; Part IV — Bones, 1939; Part V — Special Pathology of Parts of the Skeleton, 1939.

Harding, V. V.: Time schedule for the appearance and fusion of a secondary center of ossification of the calcaneus. Child Dev., 23:181, 1952.

Hartmann: Die Schnenscheiden und Synovialsacke des Fusses (Mit Tafel XII–XV). Morphol. Arbeit. 5:241, 1896. (The bursae and synovial sheaths of the foot.)

Harty, M.: The position of the foot in walking. Lancet, 2:275, 1953.

Hicks, H. J.: Mechanics of the foot. J. Anat., 87:345, 1953.

Hoerr, N. D., Pyle, S. L., and Francis, C. C.: Radiographic Atlas of Skeletal Development of the Foot and Ankle. Springfield, Illinois, Charles C Thomas, 1962.

Hohmann, G.: Fuss und Bein, 5th ed. Munisch, J. F. Bergmann, 1951.

Holland, C. T.: On rarer ossifications seen during x-ray examinations. J. Anat., 55:235, 1921.

Hollinshead, W. H.: Anatomy for Surgeons, Vol. 3. New York, Harper and Row, 1969.

Hoppenfeld, S.: Physical Examination of the Spine and Extremities. New York, Appleton-Century-Crofts, 1976, pp. 197–235.

Hubay, C. A.: Sesamoid bones of the hands and feet. Am. J. Roentgenol., 61:493, 1949.

Inge, G. A. L., and Ferguson, A. B.: Surgery of the sesamoid bones of the great toe. Arch. Surg., 27:466, 1933.

Inkster, R. G., et al.: The Anatomy of the Locomotor System. London, Oxford University Press, 1956.

Jahss, M. H.: Geriatric aspects of the foot and ankle. In Rossman, I., et al. (eds.): Clinical Geriatrics. Philadelphia, J. B. Lippincott Co., 1971, pp. 327–339.

Jahss, M. H.: Unusual diagnostic problems of the foot. Clin. Orthop. 85:42, 1972.

Kelikian, H.: The dynamic and circulatory relations of the ankle. A. A. O. S. Instructional Course Lectures, Vol. 9. Ann Arbor, J. W. Edwards, 1952, p. 347.

Kelly, R. O., et al.: Ultrastructure and growth of human limb mesenchyme (HLM 15) in vitro. Anat. Rec., 175:657, 1973.

Kewenter, Y.: Die Sesambeine des I. Metatarsophalangealgelends des Menschen. Acta Orthop. Scand., Suppl. 2:1, 1936.

Kidner, F. C.: The prehallux (accessory scaphoid) in its relation to flatfoot. J. Bone Joint Surg., 11:831, 1929.

Kidner, F. C.: The prehallux in relation to flatfoot. J. A. M. A., 101:1539, 1933.

Kienböck, R., and Müller, W.: Os tibiale externum and Verletzung des Fusses. Z. Orthop. Chir., 66:257, 1937.

Köhler, A.: Borderlands of the Normal and Early Pathologic in Skeletal Roentgenology, 10th ed. (translated and edited by J. T. Case). New York, Grune and Stratton, 1956, pp. 571–707.

Lapidus, P. W.: Subtalar joint. Its anatomy and mechanics. Bull. Hosp. Joint Dis., 16;179, 1955.

Le Double, A. F.: Traité Des Variations du Systeme Musculaire de l'Homme. Paris, Schleicher Frères, 1897, 2me tome.

MacAlister, A.: Muscular anomalies in human anatomy. Trans. R. Irish Acad., 25:118, 1872.

Manter, J. T.: Movements of the subtalar and transverse tarsal joints. Anat. Rec., 80:397, 1941.

Marti, T.: Kasuistischer Beitrag zum Studium des Os tibiale externum. Praxis, 51:828, 1962.

McDougall, A.: The os trigonum. J. Bone Joint Surg., 37B:257, 1955.

Meyer, M., Cuny, J., and Trensz, F.: L'os tibial externe et ses divers aspects radiologiques. Strasbourg Méd., 85:24, 1927.

Milaire, J.: Histochemical observations on the developing foot of normal oligosyndactylous (OS/+) and syndactylous (sm/sm) mouse embryos. Arch. Biol. (Liege), 78:223, 1967.

Monahan, J. J.: The human pre-hallux. Am. J. Med. Sci., 160:708, 1920.

Morrison, A. G.: The os paracuneiform. Some observations of an example removed at operation. J. Bone Joint Surg., 35B:254, 1953.

Niederecker, K.: Der Plattfuss. Stuttgart, Ferdinand Enke, 1959.

Olivier, G.: Formation du Squelette des Membres. Paris, Vigot, 1962.

O'Rahilly, R.: A survey of carpal and tarsal anomalies. J. Bone Joint Surg., 35A:626, 1953.

O'Rahilly, R., Gardner, E., and Gray, D. J.: The skeletal development of the foot. Clin. Orthop., 16:7, 1960.

O'Rahilly, R., Gray, D. J., and Gardner, E.: Chondrification in the hands and feet of staged human embryos. Contrib. Embryol. Carneg. Inst., 36:183, 1957.

Pfizner, W.: Beiträge zur Kenntnis des menschilichen Extremitätenskeletts, VII. Die Variationen in Aufbau des Fuffskeletts. Schwalbe's Morph. Arb., 6:245, 1896.

Powell, H. P. W.: Extra center of ossification for the medial malleolus in children. Incidence and significance. J. Bone Joint Surg., 42B:107, 1961.

Roche, A. F., and Sunderland, S.: Multiple ossification centers in the epiphyses of the long bones of the human hand and foot. J. Bone Joint Surg., 41B:375, 1959.

Ross, S. E., and Caffey, J.: Ossification of the calcaneal apophysis in healthy children: Some normal radiologic features. Stanford Med. Bull., 15:224, 1957.

Schultz, A. H.: The skeleton of the trunk and limbs of higher primates. Hum. Biol., 2:303, 1930.

Schurman, D. J.: Ankle-block anesthesia for foot surgery. Anesthesiology, 44:348, 1976.

Selby, S.: Separate centers of ossification of the tip of the internal malleolus. Am. J. Roentgenol., 86:496, 1961.

Shands, A. R., Jr.: The accessory bones of the foot. South. Med. Surg., 93:326, 1931.

Shands, A. R., Jr., and Wentz, I. J.: Congenital anomalies, accessory bones, and osteochondritis in the feet of 850 children. Surg. Clin. North Am., 33:1643, 1953.

Sirry, A.: The pseudocystic triangle in the normal os calcis. Acta Radiol., 36:516, 1951.

Steindler, A.: Lectures on the Interpretation of Pain in Orthopaedic Practice. Springfield, Illinois, Charles C Thomas, 1960, pp. 606–658.

Strasser, H.: Lehrbuch der Muskel und Gelenkmechanik, Vols. I–IV. 1908–1917, Vol. I — Allgermeiner; Vol. II — Der Stamm; Vol. III—Die unter extremitat. Berlin, Springer.

Straus, W. L., Jr.: Growth of the human foot and its evolutionary significance. Contrib. Embryol., 19:93, 1927.

Trolle, D.: Accessory Bones of the Human Foot. Copenhagen, Munksgaard, 1948.

Vinning, P.: Variations of the digital skeleton of the foot. Clin. Orthop., 16:26, 1960.

von Lanz, T., and Wachsmuth, W.: Praktische Anatomie. Bein und Statik, Vol. I. Berlin, Springer, 1938, p. 485.

Weseley, M. A., and Barenfeld, P. A.: Thoughts on in-toeing and out-toeing, pathogenesis and treatment. Bull. Hosp. Joint Dis., 32:182, 1971.

Wright, D. G., Desai, S. M., and Henderson, W. H.: Action of the subtalar and ankle-joint complex during the stance phase of walking. J. Bone Joint Surg., 46A:361, 1964.

Zadek, I.: The significance of the accessory tarsal scaphoid. J. Bone Joint Surg., 8:618, 1926.

Zadek, I., and Gold, A. M.: The accessory tarsal scaphoid. J. Bone Joint Surg., 30A:957, 1948.

BIOMECHANICS OF THE FOOT AND ANKLE — CHILD AND ADULT

Basmajian, J. R., and Stecko, G.: The role of muscles in arch support of the foot. J. Bone Joint Surg., 45A:1184, 1963.

Basmajian, J. R., and Bentzon, J. W.: An electromyographic study of certain muscles of the leg and foot in the standing position. Surg. Gynecol. Obstet., 98:662, 1954.

Berry, F. R., Jr.: Angle variation patterns of normal hip, knee and ankle in different operations. Berkeley, California, Prosthetic Devices Research Project, Institute of Engineering Research, University of California, Berkeley, Series 11, Issue 15, The Project, May 1951.

Close, J. R., and Inman, V. T.: The action of the ankle joint. Berkeley, California, Prosthetic Devices Research Project, Institute of Engineering Research, University of California, Berkeley, Series 11, Issue 22, The Project, April 1952.

Close, J. R., and Inman, V. T.: The action of the subtalar joint. Berkeley, California, Prosthetic Devices Research Project, Institute of Engineering Research, University of California, Berkeley, Series 11, Issue 24, The Project, May 1953.

Cunningham, D. N.: Components of floor reactions during walking. Berkeley, California, Prosthetic Devices Research Project, Institute of Engineering Research, University of California, Berkeley, Series 11, Issue 14, The Project, November 1950.

Frankel, V. H., and Burstein, A. H.: Orthopedic Biomechanics. Philadelphia, Lea and Febiger, 1970.

Griffin, P. P., Wheelhouse, W. W., Shiavi, R., and Boss, W.: Habitual toe-walkers. A clinical and electromyographic gait analysis. J. Bone Joint Surg., 59A:97, 1977.

Grundy, M., Tosh, P. A., McLeish, R. D., and Smidt, L.: An investigation of the centres of pressure under the foot while walking. J. Bone Joint Surg., 57B:98, 1975.

Haworth, B.: Dynamic posture in relation to the foot. Clin. Orthop., 16:74, 1960.

Hicks, J. H.: The function of the plantar aponeurosis. J. Anat., 85:414, 1951.

Hicks, J. H.: The mechanics of the foot. I. The joints. J. Anat., 87:345, 1953.

Hicks, J. H.: The mechanics of the foot. II. The plantar aponeurosis and the arch. J. Anat., 88:25, 1954.

Inman, V. T.: Human locomotion. Can. Med. Assoc. J., 94:1047, 1966.

Inman, V. T.: Influence on the ankle of the proximal limb. Artif. Limbs, 13:59, 1969.

Inman, R. E., and Inman, V. T.: Anthropometric studies of the human foot and ankle. Bull. Prosthet. Res., 10–11:97, 1969.

Laurin, C., and Mathieu, J.: Sagittal mobility of the normal ankle. Orthop. Clin. North Am., 108:99, 1975.

Mann, R. A.: Biomechanics of the foot. In Atlas of Orthotics: Biomechanical Principles and Application. St. Louis, C. V. Mosby Co., 1975.

Mann, R. A., and Inman, V. T.: Phasic activity of intrinsic muscles of the foot. J. Bone Joint Surg., 46A:469, 1964.

Manter, J. T.: Movements of the subtalar and transverse tarsal joints. Anat. Rec., 8:397, 1941.

McBeath, A. A., Bahrke, M., and Balke, B.: Efficiency of assisted ambulation determined by oxygen consumption measurement. J. Bone Joint Surg., 56A:994, 1974.

Morris, J. M.: Biomechanics of the foot and ankle. Clin. Orthop., 122:10, 1977.

Murray, M. P., et al.: Weight distribution and weight shifting activity during normal standing posture. Phys. Ther., 53:741, 1973.

Murray, M. P., and Clarkson, B. H.: The vertical pathways of the foot during level walking: Range of variability in normal men. J. Am. Phys. Ther. Assoc., 46:585, 1966.

Murray, M. P., Drongert, A. B., and Kory, R. C.: Walking patterns of normal men. J. Bone Joint Surg., 46A:335, 1964.

Perry, J.: The mechanics of walking: A clinical interpretation. Phys. Ther., 47:778, 1967.

Perry, J.: Kinesiology of lower extremity bracing. Clin. Orthop., 102:18, 1974.

Ralston, H. J.: Energy-speed relation and optimal speed during level walking. Int. Z. Angew. Physiol., 17:277, 1958.

Ryker, N. J., Jr.: Glass walkway studies of normal subjects during normal level walking. Berkeley, California, Prosthetic Devices Research Project, Institute of Engineering Research, University of California, Berkeley, Series 11, Issue 20, The Project, January 1952.

Sammarco, G. J., Burstein, A. H., and Frankel, V. H.: Biomechanics of the ankle: a kinematic study. Orthop. Clin. North Am., 4:75, 1973.

Saunders, J. B., de C. M., Inman, V. T., and Eberhart, H. D.: The major determinants in normal and pathological gait. J. Bone Joint Surg., 35A:543, 1953.

Schwartz, R. P., Heath, A. L., Morgan, D. W., and Towns, R. C.: A quantitative analysis of recorded variables in the walking pattern of "normal" adults. J. Bone Joint Surg., 46A:324, 1964.

Scott, J. R., Hulton, W. C., and Stohes, I. A. F.: Forces under the foot. J. Bone Joint Surg., 55B:335, 1973.

Steindler, A.: Mechanics of Normal and Pathological Locomotion. Springfield, Illinois, Charles C Thomas, 1935.

Steindler, A.: The pathomechanics of the static disabilities of the foot and ankle. A. A. O. S. Instructional Course Lectures, Vol. 9. Ann Arbor, J. W. Edwards, 1952.

Steindler, A.: Kinesiology of the Human Body. Springfield, Illinois, Charles C Thomas, 1955.

Sutherland, D. H.: An electromyographic study of the plantar flexors of the ankle in normal walking on the level. J. Bone Joint Surg., 48A:66, 1966.

Sutherland, D. H., and Hagy, J. C.: Measurements of gait movements from motion picture film. J. Bone Joint Surg., 54A:787, 1972.

Viladot, A.: Metatarsalgia due to biomechanical alterations of the forefoot. Orthop. Clin. North Am., 4:165, 1973.

Water, R. L., Perry, J., Antonelli, D., and Hislop, H.: Energy cost of walking of amputees: The influence of level of amputation. J. Bone Joint Surg., 58A:42, 1976.

Wright, D. G., Desai, S. M., and Henderson, W. H.: Action of the subtalar and ankle-joint complex during the stance phase of walking. J. Bone Joint Surg., 46A:361, 1964.

NEUROMUSCULAR AND NEUROLOGIC DISEASES AFFECTING THE FOOT—CHILD AND ADULT

Alban, S. L., Alban, H., and Fixler, R. H.: Subtalar arthrodesis utilizing autogenous calcaneal grafts. J. Bone Joint Surg., 57A:133, 1975.

Alter, M.: Anencephalus, hydrocephalus, and spina bifida. Arch. Neurol., 7:411, 1962.

Anderson, M., and Messner, M. B.: Growth and prediction of growth in the lower extremities. J. Bone Joint Surg., 45A:1, 1963.

Baker, L. D., and Hill, L. N.: Foot alignment in the cerebral palsy patient. J. Bone Joint Surg., 46A:1, 1964.

Banks, H. H., and Green, W. T.: The correction of equinus deformity in cerebral palsy. J. Bone Joint Surg., 40A:1359, 1958.

Bleck, E. E.: Spastic abductor hallucis. Dev. Med. Child Neurol., 9:602, 1967.

Bradley, N., Miller, W. A., and Evans, J. P.: Plantar neuroma: analysis of results following surgical exision — 145 patients. South. Med. J., 69:853, 1976.

Carayon, A., Bourrel, P., Bourges, M., and Touze, M.: Dual transfer of the posterior tibial and flexor digitorum longus tendons for drop foot: report of thirty-one cases. J. Bone Joint Surg., 46A:144, 1967.

Carr, T. L.: The orthopaedic aspects of one hundred cases of spina bifida. Postgrad. Med. J., 32:201, 1956.

Classen, J. N.: Neurotrophic arthropathy with ulceration. Ann. Surg., 159:891, 1964.

Dawson, C. W., and Roberts, J.: Charcot-Marie-Tooth disease. J. A. M. A., 188:659, 1964.

Degenhardt, D. P., and Goodwin, M. A.: Neuropathic joints in diabetes. J. Bone Joint Surg., 42B:769, 1960.

Dennyson, W. G., and Fielford, G. E.: Subtalar arthrodesis, leg cancellous grafts and metallic internal fixation. J. Bone Joint Surg., 58B:507, 1976.

Drennan, J. C., and Sharrard, W. J. W.: The pathological anatomy of convex pes valgus. J. Bone Joint Surg., 53B:455, 1971.

Eichenholtz, S. N.: Charcot joints. J. Bone Joint Surg., 44A:1485, 1962.

Elsaby, N. I.: New method for correcting of traumatic foot-drop: case report. Plast. Reconstr. Surg., 50:614, 1972.

Gross, R. H.: A clinical study of the Batchelor subtalar arthrodesis. J. Bone Joint Surg., 58A:343, 1976.

Hayes, J. T., Gross, H. P., and Dow, S.: Surgery for paralytic defects secondary to myelomeningocele and myelodysplasia. J. Bone Joint Surg., 46A:1577, 1964.

Henry, A. K.: Extensile Exposure. Baltimore, Williams and Wilkins, 1963.

Hoadley, A. E.: Six cases of metatarsalgia. Chicago Med. Rec., 5:32, 1893.

Hsu, L. C. S., O'Brien, J. P., Yau, A. C. M. C., and Hodgson, A. R.: Batchelor's extra-articular subtalar arthrodesis. J. Bone Joint Surg., 58A:243, 1976.

James, C. C. M., and Lassman, L. P.: Spinal dysraphism. The diagnosis and treatment of progressive lesions in spina bifida occulta. J. Bone Joint Surg., 44B:828, 1962.

Japas, L. N.: Surgical treatment of pes cavus by tarsal V-osteotomy. J. Bone Joint Surg., 50A:927, 1968.

Kalanchi, A., and Evans, J. G.: Posterior subtalar fusion: a preliminary report on a modified Gallie's procedure. J. Bone Joint Surg., 59B:287, 1977.

Keck, C.: The tarsal tunnel syndrome. J. Bone Joint Surg., 44A:180, 1962.

Kopell, H. P., and Thompson, W. A. L.: Peripheral Entrapment Neuropathies. Baltimore, Williams and Wilkins, 1963.

Leonard, M. A.: The inheritance of tarsal coalition and its relationship to spastic flat foot. J. Bone Joint Surg., 56B:520, 1974.

Levin, M. E., and O'Neal, L. W.: The Diabetic Foot. St. Louis, C. V. Mosby Co., 1973.

Levitt, R. D., Canale, S. T., and Gartland, J. J.: Surgical correction of foot deformity in the older patient with myelomeningocele. Orthop. Clin. North Am., 5:19, 1974.

Lorber, J.: Incidence and epidemiology of myelomeningocele. Clin. Orthop., 45:81, 1966.

Mann, R. A.: Tarsal tunnel syndrome. Orthop. Clin. North Am., 5:109, 1974.

Menelaus, M. B.: Talectomy for equinovarus deformity in arthrogryposis and spina bifida. J. Bone Joint Surg., 53B:468, 1971.

Mooney, V., Perry, J., and Nickel, V. L.: Surgical and nonsurgical orthopaedic care of stroke. J. Bone Joint Surg., 49A:989, 1967.

Naide, M., and Schnall, C.: Bone changes in necrosis in diabetes mellitus. Differentiation of neuropathic from ischemic necrosis. Arch. Intern. Med., 107:124, 1961.

Perry, J., and Hoffer, M. M.: Preoperative and postoperative dynamic electromyography as an aid in planning tendon transfer in children with cerebral palsy. J. Bone Joint Surg., 59A:531, 1977.

Piper, C. A., and Murphy, T. O.: Care of the diabetic foot. Rev. Surg., 21:91, 1964.

Sharrard, W. J. W.: Paralytic deformity in the lower limb. J. Bone Joint Surg., 49B:731, 1967.

Sharrard, W. J. W., and Grosfield, I.: The management of deformity and paralysis of the foot in myelomeningocele. J. Bone Joint Surg., 50B:456, 1968.

Smith, T. K., Gregerson, G. G., and Samilson, R. L.: Orthopaedic problems associated with tuberous sclerosis. J. Bone Joint Surg., 51A:97, 1969.

Spencer, G. E., and Vignos, P. J., Jr.: Bracing for ambulation in childhood progressive muscular dystrophy. J. Bone Joint Surg., 44A:234, 1962.

Tinel, J.: Nerve Wounds (translated by F. Rothwell). New York, William Wood and Co., 1918, p. 317.

Tracy, W. H.: Operative treatment of the plantar-flexed inverted foot in adult hemiplegia. J. Bone Joint Surg., 58A:1142, 1976.

Treaner, W.: The hemiplegic posture and its correction. Clin. Orthop., 63:113, 1969.

Walker, G.: The early management of varus feet in myelomeningocele. J. Bone Joint Surg., 53B:462, 1971.

Williams, P. F.: Restoration of muscle balance of the foot by transfer of the tibialis posterior. J. Bone Joint Surg., 58B:217, 1976.

CIRCULATORY DISTURBANCES

Baffes, T. G., and Augustsson, M. H.: Changing concepts in hyperbaric oxygen therapy. Dis. Chest, 49:83, 1966.

Barrett, J. P., and Mooney, V.: Neuropathy and diabetic pressure lesions. Orthop. Clin. North Am., 4:43, 1973.

Bella, G. A., Finney, J. W., Aronoff, B. L., et al.: Use of intra-arterial hydrogen peroxide to promote wound healing. Part I. Regional intra-arterial therapy — technical surgical aspects. Am. J. Surg., 108:621, 1964.

Bessman, A. N., and Wagner, F. W., Jr.: Nonclostridial gas gangrene. J. A. M. A., 233:958, 1975.

Calloway, J. L.: Chronic leg ulcers. J. A. M. A., 186:1080, 1963.

Carter, S. A.: The relationship of distal systolic pressure to healing of skin lesions in limbs with arterial occlusive disease with special reference to diabetes mellitus. Scand. J. Clin. Lab. Invest., 31(Suppl. 128):239, 1973.

Degni, M., Toth, V., Lanfranchi, W., and Maia, A. C.: Chronic mural phlebitis. J. Cardiovasc. Surg., 6:496, 1965.

Deterling, R. A.: Is there a place for peripheral nerve crush? J. Cardiovasc. Surg., 3:329, 1962.

Dotter, C. T., Krippaehne, W. W., and Judkins, M. P.: Transluminal recanalization and dilatation in atherosclerotic obstruction of the femoral popliteal system. Am. Surg., 31:453, 1965.

Douglas, D. M., et al.: Late results of autogenous-vein grafting and lumbar sympathectomy in ischemic limbs. Lancet, 1:459, 1973.

Ellenberg, M., and Rifkin, H.: Diabetes Mellitus. New York, McGraw-Hill, 1970, p. 1031.

Fisher, D. A., and Morris, M. D.: Idiopathic edema and hyperaldosteronuria: postural venous plasma pooling. Pediatrics, 35:413, 1965.

Giannestras, N. J., Cranley, H., and Lentz, M.: Occlusion of the tibial artery after a foot operation under tourniquet. J. Bone Joint Surg., 59A:682, 1977.

Gillies, H., and Fraser, F. R.: The treatment of lymphedema by plastic operation. Bull. Med. J., 1:96, 1935.

Goldman, R. F., et al.: Effects of alcohol, hot drinks and smoking on hand and foot heat loss. Acta Physiol. Scand., 87:498, 1973.

Gundersen, J.: Segmental measurements of the systolic blood pressure in the extremities including the thumb and the great toe. Acta Chir. Scand. (Suppl.), *426*:1, 1972.

Hansteen, V., et al.: Induced hypertension in the treatment of severe ischemia of the foot. Circulation, *46*:976, 1972.

Hecker, S. P., Dramer, R. A., and Meigen, J. R.: Clinical value of venography of the lower extremity. Ann. Intern. Med., *59*:798, 1963.

Kane, W. J.: Diabetic foot problems — pathogenesis. Minn. Med., *56*:396, 1973.

Klenerman, L.: The tourniquet in surgery. J. Bone Joint Surg., *44B*:937, 1962.

Kostuik, J. P., Wood, D., Hornby, R., Feingold, S., and Mathews, V.: The measurement of skin blood flow in peripheral vascular disease by epicutaneous application of Xenon[133]. J. Bone Joint Surg., *58A*:833, 1976.

Kritter, A. E.: A technique for salvage of the infected diabetic gangrenous foot. Orthop. Clin. North Am., *4*:21, 1973.

Malan, E.: History and different clinical aspects of arteriovenous communications. J. Cardiovasc. Surg., *13*:491, 1972.

Malan, E., and Pugionisi, A.: Congenital angiodysplasias of the extremities. J. Cardiovasc. Surg., *5*:87, 1964.

Mali, J. W., Kuiper, J. P., and Hamers, A. A.: Macro-angiodermatitis of the foot. Arch. Dermatol., *92*:515, 1965.

Mannick, J. A., and Coffman, J. D.: Ischemic Limbs: Surgical Approach and Physiological Principles. New York, Grune and Stratton, 1973.

Mooney, V., and Wagner, F. W., Jr.: Neurocirculatory disorders of the foot and ankle. Clin. Orthop., *122*:53, 1977.

Presley, S. J., Paul, J., and Ranke, E. J.: Procaine in diabetic neuropathy. Am. J. Med. Sci., *243*:603, 1962.

Roberts, V. C., et al.: Blood flow in ischemic feet. Br. Med. J., *4*:114, 1971.

Schatz, I. J., Allen, E. V., Allen, C. V., and Litin, E. M.: Disability after real or alleged venous thrombosis. Postgrad. Med., *31*:358, 1962.

Schwindt, C. D., Lulloff, R. S., and Rogers, S. C.: Transmetatarsal amputations. Orthop. Clin. North Am., *4*:31, 1973.

Stephens, G. L.: Palpable dorsalis pedis and posterior tibial pulses. Arch. Surg., *84*:82, 1962.

Tanyol, H.: The concept of chemohemodynamics in the pathogenesis of primary varicose veins. Angiopatias (Brazilian Journal of Angiology), *3*:16, 1963.

Thornhill, H. I., Richter, R. W., Shelton, M. L., and Johnson, C.: Neuropathic arthropathy (Charcot forefeet) in alcoholics. Orthop. Clin. North Am., *4*:7, 1973.

Wagner, F. W., Jr.: Orthopedic rehabilitation of dysvascular lower limbs. Orthop. Clin. North Am., *9*:2, 325, 1978.

Wagner, F. W., Jr.: The diabetic foot and amputation of the foot. *In* Mann, R. A. (ed.): DuVries' Surgery of the Foot, 4th ed. St. Louis, C. V. Mosby Co., 1978.

Wagner, F. W., Jr.: Use of transcutaneous Doppler ultrasound in prediction of healing potential and selection of surgical level in dysvascular lower limbs. West. J. Med., *130*:59, 1979.

Wells, R.: The Microcirculation in Clinical Medicine. New York and London, Academic Press, 1973.

Wilgis, E. F., Jezic, D., Stonesifer, G. L., Jr., et al.: The evaluation of small-vessel flow. J. Bone Joint Surg., *56A*:1199, 1974.

Winsor, T.: Influence of arterial disease on the systolic blood pressure gradients of the extremity. Am. J. Med. Sci., *220*:117, 1950.

Yao, S. T.: New techniques in objective arterial evaluation. Arch. Surg., *106*:600, 1973.

Yao, S. T., and Bertran, J. J.: Application of ultrasound to arterial and venous diagnosis. Surg. Clin. North Am., *54*:23, 1974.

DERMATOLOGIC DISORDERS, INCLUDING NAILS

Allyn, B., and Waldorf, D. S.: Treatment of verruca with vaccinia. J. A. M. A., *203*:806, 1968.

Bean, W. B.: Nail growth: a twenty-year study. Arch. Intern. Med., *111*:476, 1963.

Bose, B.: A technique for excision of nail fold for ingrowing toenail. Surg. Gynecol. Obstet., *132*:511, 1971.

Dingman, R. O., and Graff, W. C.: The intractable plantar wart. Mich. State Med. Soc. J., *61*:297, 1952.

DuVries, H. L.: A new approach to the treatment of verruca plantaris (plantar wart). J. A. M. A., *152*:1202, 1953.

DuVries, H. L.: Verruca plantaris. J. A. M. A., *154*:1320, 1954.

Gibbs, R.: Skin Diseases of the Feet. St. Louis, Warren H. Green, 1974.

Jarrett, A., and Spearman, R. I. C.: The histochemistry of the human nail. Arch. Dermatol., *94*:652, 1966.

Lewis, B. L.: Microscopic studies of fetal and mature nail and surrounding soft tissue. Arch. Dermatol. Syph., *70*:732, 1954.

Lloyd-Davies, R. W., and Brill, G. C.: The aetiology and outpatient management of ingrowing toe-nails. Br. J. Surg., *50*:592, 1963.

Lusskin, R.: Serpentine sinus — a tract leading nowhere. J. Bone Joint Surg., *43A*:118, 1961.

Montgomery, R. M.: Dermatologic care of the painful foot. J. Bone Joint Surg., *46A*:1129, 1964.

Morris, J., Wood, M. G., and Samitz, M. H.: Eccrine poroma. Arch. Dermatol., 98:162, 1968.

Pardo-Costello, V.: Diseases of the Nails, 3rd ed. Springfield, Illinois, Charles C Thomas, 1960.

Reeves, R. J., and Jackson, M. T.: Roentgen therapy of plantar warts. Am. J. Roentgenol. Radium Ther. Nucl. Med., 76:977, 1956.

Rutledge, B. A., and Green, A. L.: Surgical treatment of plantar corns. U.S. Armed Services Med. J., 8:219, 1957.

Samman, P. D.: The Nails in Disease. London, William Heinemann Medical Books Ltd., 1965.

Van den Brenk, H. A. A., and Minty, C. C. J.: Radiation in the management of keloids and hypertrophic scars. Br. J. Surg., 47:595, 1960.

Zaias, N.: Embryology of the human nail. Arch. Dermatol. Syph., 87:37, 1963.

Zaias, N.: Onychomycosis. Arch. Dermatol., 105:263, 1972.

TUMORS

Ackerman, L. V., and Spjut, H. J.: Tumors of Bone and Cartilage. Washington, D.C., Armed Forces Institute of Pathology, 1962.

Appenzeller, J., and Weitzner, S.: Intraosseous lipoma of the os calcis — review of literature of intraosseous lipoma of extremities. Clin. Orthop., 101:171, 1974.

Barnett, L. S., and Morris, J. M.: Metastases of renal-cell carcinoma simultaneously to a finger and a toe. J. Bone Joint Surg., 51A:773, 1965.

Booher, R. J.: Lipoblastic tumors of the hands and feet. J. Bone Joint Surg., 47A:727, 1965.

Booher, R. J., and Pack, G. T.: Malignant melanoma of the feet and hands. Surgery, 42:1084, 1957.

Cameron, H. U., and Kostiuk, J. P.: A long-term follow-up of synovial sarcoma. J. Bone Joint Surg., 56B:613, 1974.

Coley, B. L.: Neoplasms of Bone, 2nd ed. New York, Hoeher, 1960.

Coley, B. L., and Higginbotham, N. L.: Secondary chondrosarcoma. Ann. Surg., 139:547, 1954.

Coventry, M. B., and Dahlin, D. C.: Osteogenic sarcoma: critical analysis of 430 cases. J. Bone Joint Surg., 39A:741, 1957.

Dahlin, D. C.: Bone Tumors, 2nd ed. Springfield, Illinois, Charles C Thomas, 1967.

Eisenstein, R.: Giant-cell tumor of tendon sheath. J. Bone Joint Surg., 50A:476, 1968.

Fahey, J. J., Stark, H. H., Donovan, W. F., and Drennan, D. B.: Xanthoma of the Achilles tendon: seven cases with familial hyperbetalipoproteinemia. J. Bone Joint Surg., 55A:1197, 1973.

Fielding, M. D. (ed.): Skin Tumors of the Foot: Diagnosis and Treatment. New York, Futura, 1974.

Giannestras, N. J., and Bronson, J. L.: Malignant schwannoma of the medial plantar branch of the posterior tibial nerve (unassociated with von Recklinghausen's disease): a case report. J. Bone Joint Surg., 57A:701, 1975.

Giannestras, N. J., and Diamond, J. R.: Benign osteoblastoma of the talus: a review of the literature and report of a case. J. Bone Joint Surg., 40A:469, 1958.

Goldenberg, R. R., Campbell, C. J., and Bonfiglio, M.: Giant cell tumor of bone. J. Bone Joint Surg., 52A:619, 1970.

Greenfield, G. B.: Radiology of Bone Diseases. Philadelphia, J. B. Lippincott Co., 1969.

Henderson, E. D., and Dahlin, D. C.: Chondrosarcoma of bone: a study of two hundred eighty-eight cases. J. Bone Joint Surg., 45A:1450, 1963.

Hutter, R. V. P., Worcester, J. N., Francis, K. C., et al.: Giant cell tumors of bone, benign and malignant clinicopathological analysis of the natural history of the disease. Cancer, 5:653, 1962.

Jaffe, H. L.: Tumors and Tumorous Conditions of the Bones and Joints. Philadelphia, Lea and Febiger, 1958.

Jahss, M. H.: Pseudotumors of the foot. Orthop. Clin. North Am., 5:67, 1974.

Jones, F. R., Soule, E. H., and Coventry, M. G.: Fibrous xanthoma of synovium (giant-cell tumor of tendon sheath, pigmented nodular synovitis). J. Bone Joint Surg., 51A:76, 1969.

Kaplan, R.: Neurilemoma in the foot. J. Bone Joint Surg., 48A:949, 1966.

Keller, R. B., and Baez-Giangreco, A.: Juvenile aponeurotic fibroma. Clin. Orthop., 106:198, 1975.

Larsson, S. E., and Lorentzon, R.: The incidence of malignant primary bone tumors in relation to age, sex, and site. J. Bone Joint Surg., 56B:534, 1974.

Larsson, S. E., Lorentzon, R., and Boquist, L.: Giant-cell tumor of bone. A demographic, clinical, and histopathological study of all cases recorded in the Swedish Cancer Registry for the years 1958 through 1968. J. Bone Joint Surg., 57A:167, 1975.

Larsson, S. E., Lorentzon, R., and Boquist, L.: Malignant hemangioendothelioma of bone. J. Bone Joint Surg., 57A:84, 1975.

Ledderhose: Zur Pathologie der Aponeurose des Fusses und der Hand. Arch. Klin. Chir., 55:694, 1897.

Lewis, G. M., and Wheeler, C. E., Jr.: Practical

Dermatology, 3rd ed. Philadelphia, W. B. Saunders Company, 1967.

Lichtenstein, L.: Bone Tumors, 4th ed. St. Louis, C. V. Mosby, 1972.

Macintosh, D. J., Price, C. H. G., and Jeffree, G. M.: Ewing's tumor. J. Bone Joint Surg., 57B:331, 1975.

Marsh, B. W., Bonfiglio, M., Brady, L. P., and Enneking, W. F.: Benign osteoblastoma: range of manifestations. J. Bone Joint Surg., 57A:1, 1975.

McKenna, R. J., Schwinn, C. P., Soong, K. Y., and Higginbotham, N. L.: Sarcomata of the osteogenic series (osteosarcoma, fibrosarcoma, chondrosarcoma, parosteal osteogenic sarcoma, and sarcomata arising in abnormal bone). An analysis of 552 cases. J. Bone Joint Surg., 48A:1, 1966.

McNeill, T. W., and Ray, R. D.: Hemangioma of the extremities. Review of 35 cases. Clin. Orthop., 101:154, 1974.

Mirra, J. M., and Marcove, R. C.: Fibrosarcomatous dedifferentiation of primary and secondary chondrosarcoma. A review of five cases. J. Bone Joint Surg., 56A:285, 1974.

Neer, C. S., Francis, K. C., Marcove, R. C., Terz, J., and Carbonava, P. N.: Treatment of unicameral bone cyst: a follow-up study of 175 cases. J. Bone Joint Surg., 48A:731, 1966.

Pandey, S.: Ewing's tumor of the talus. J. Bone Joint Surg., 52A:1672, 1970.

Poulsen, J. O.: Osteoid osteoma. Acta Orthop. Scand., 40:198, 1969.

Pritchard, D. J., Dahlin, D. C., Dauphine, R. T., Taylor, W. T., and Beabout, J. W.: Ewing's sarcoma: a clinicopathological and statistical analysis of patients surviving five years or longer. J. Bone Joint Surg., 57A:10, 1975.

Reddy, C. R. R. M., Roa, P. S., and Rajakumari, K.: Giant cell tumors of bone in South India. J. Bone Joint Surg., 56A:617, 1974.

Ross, J. A., and Dawson, E. K.: Benign chondroblastoma of bone. J. Bone Joint Surg., 57B:78, 1975.

Schajowicz, F., and Gallardo, H.: Chondromyxoid fibroma (fibromyxoid chondroma) of bone: a clinicopathological study of 32 cases. J. Bone Joint Surg., 53B:198, 1971.

Seda, T., Fukuda, H., Ishii, Y., Hanaoka, H., Yatabe, S., Takano, M., and Koibe, O.: Malignant transformation of benign osteoblastoma. A case report. J. Bone Joint Surg., 57A:424, 1975.

Sim, F. H., Dahlin, D. C., and Beabout, J. W.: Osteoid osteoma: diagnostic problems. J. Bone Joint Surg., 57A:154, 1975.

Simon, W. H., and Beller, M. L.: Intracapsular epiphyseal osteoid osteoma of the ankle joint: a case report. Clin. Orthop., 108:200, 1974.

Singh, R., Grewal, D. A., Bannerjee, A. K., and Bansal, V. P.: Haemangiomatosis of the skeleton, J. Bone Joint Surg., 56B:136, 1974.

Smith, R. W., and Smith, C. F.: Solitary unicameral bone cyst of the calcaneus. Review of twenty cases. J. Bone Joint Surg., 56A:49, 1974.

Smyth, M.: Glomus-cell tumors in the lower extremity: report of two cases. J. Bone Joint Surg., 53A:157, 1971.

Sterning, W. S.: Primary malignant tumors of the calcaneal tendon. J. Bone Joint Surg., 50B:676, 1968.

White, N. B.: Neurilemomas of the extremities. J. Bone Joint Surg., 49A:1605, 1967.

INFECTIOUS AND NONINFECTIOUS INFLAMMATORY DISORDERS

Altemeir, W. A., and Fullen, W. D.: Prevention and treatment of gas gangrene. J. A. M. A., 217:806, 1971.

Bingham, R., Fleenor, W. H., and Church, S.: The local use of antibiotics to prevent wound infection. Clin. Orthop., 99:194, 1974.

Campbell, C. H., Papademetriou, T., and Bonfiglio, M.: Melorheostosis. J. Bone Joint Surg., 50A:1281, 1968.

Carayon, A., Bourrel, P., Bourges, M., and Touze, M.: Dual transfer of the posterior tibial and flexor digitorum longus tendons for drop foot: report of 31 cases. J. Bone Joint Surg., 49A:144, 1967.

Charosky, C. B., and Marcove, R. C.: Salmonella paratyphi osteomyelitis. Report of a case simulating a giant cell tumor. Clin. Orthop., 99:190, 1974.

Christie, B. G. B.: The diagnosis and treatment of tenosynovitis. Br. J. Clin. Pract., 10:677, 1956.

DeHaven, K. E., and Evarts, C. M.: The continuing problem of gas gangrene: a review and report of illustrative cases. J. Trauma, 11:983, 1971.

Feigin, R. D., McAlister, W. H., San Joaquin, V. H., and Middlekamn, J. N.: Osteomyelitis of the calcaneus: report of eight cases. Am. J. Dis. Child., 119:61, 1970.

Gordon, S. L., Evans, C., and Greer, R. B., III: *Pseudomonas* osteomyelitis of the metatarsal sesamoid of the great toe. Clin. Orthop., 99:188, 1974.

Gristina, A. G., Rovere, G. D., and Shoju, H.: Spontaneous septic arthritis complicating rheumatoid arthritis. J. Bone Joint Surg., 56A:1180, 1974.

Hagler, D. J.: *Pseudomonas* osteomyelitis: puncture wounds of the feet. Pediatrics, 48:672, 1971 (letter to the editor).

Harris, J. R., and Brand, P. W.: Patterns of disintegration of the tarsus in the anaesthetic foot. J. Bone Joint Surg., 48B:4, 1966.

Hierholzer, G., Rehn, J., Knothe, H., and Masterson, J.: Antibiotic therapy of chronic posttraumatic osteomyelitis. J. Bone Joint Surg., 56B:721, 1974.

Houston, A. N., Roy, W. A., Faust, R. A., and Ewin, D. M.: Tetanus prophylaxis in the treatment of puncture wounds of patients in the Deep South. J. Trauma, 2:439, 1962.

Johanson, P. H.: *Pseudomonas* infections of the foot following puncture. J. A. M. A., 204:262, 1968.

Majid, M. A., Mathias, P. F., Seth, H. N., and Thirumalachar, M. J.: Primary mycetoma of the patella. J. Bone Joint Surg., 46A:1283, 1964.

Mansoor, I. A.: Typhoid osteomyelitis of the calcaneus due to direct inoculation: a case report. J. Bone Joint Surg., 49A:732, 1967.

Martini, M., Martin-Benkeddache, Y., Bekkechi, T., and Daoud, A.: Treatment of chronic osteomyelitis of the calcaneus by resection of the calcaneus. A report of 20 cases. J. Bone Joint Surg., 56A:532, 1974.

Miller, E. H., and Semian, D. W.: Gram-negative osteomyelitis following puncture wounds of the foot. J. Bone Joint Surg., 57A:535, 1975.

Minnefor, A. B., Oson, M. I., and Carver, D. H.: *Pseudomonas* osteomyelitis following puncture wounds of the foot. Pediatrics, 47:598, 1971.

Mukopadhaya, B., and Mishra, N. K.: Treatment of tuberculosis sinuses and abscesses of osteoarticular origin. J. Bone Joint Surg., 39B:326, 1957.

Nicholson, R. A.: Twenty years of bone and joint tuberculosis in Bradford. J. Bone Joint Surg., 56B:760, 1974.

Oyston, J. K.: Madura foot: a study of twenty cases. J. Bone Joint Surg., 43B:259, 1961.

Patzakis, M. J., Harvey, J. P., Jr., and Ivler, D.: The role of antibiotics in the management of open fractures. J. Bone Joint Surg., 56A:532, 1974.

Peterson, H. A., Tressler, H. A., Lang, A. G., and Johnson, E. W., Jr.: Osteomyelitis after puncture wounds of the foot. Minn. Med., 56:787, 1973.

Raff, M., and Dannaher, C. L.: Septic arthritis in adults. Report of a case and review of the literature. J. Bone Joint Surg., 56A:403, 1974.

Seal, P. V., and Morris, C. A.: Brucellosis of the carpus. J. Bone Joint Surg., 56B:327, 1974.

Warren, G.: Tarsal bone disintegration in leprosy. J. Bone Joint Surg., 53B:688, 1971.

Winn, W. A.: Coccidioidomycosis and amphotericin B. Med. Clin. North Am., 47:1131, 1963.

RHEUMATOID FOOT

Amuso, S. J., et al.: Metatarsal head resection in the treatment of rheumatoid arthritis. Clin. Orthop., 74:94, 1971.

Anderson, R. J.: The diagnosis and management of rheumatoid synovitis. Orthop. Clin. North Am., 6:629, 1975.

Aufranc, O.: Reconstructive surgery of the lower extremity in rheumatoid arthritis. A. A. O. S. Instructional Course Lectures. Miami, January 1961.

Barrett, J. P., Jr.: Plantar pressure measurements: rational shoe wear in patients with rheumatoid arthritis. J. A. M. A., 235:1138, 1976.

Barton, N. J.: Arthroplasty of the forefoot in rheumatoid arthritis. J. Bone Joint Surg., 55:126, 1973.

Bedi, S. S., and Ellis, W.: Spontaneous rupture of calcaneal tendon in rheumatoid arthritis after local steroid injection. Ann. Rheum. Dis., 29:494, 1970.

Benson, G. N., and Johnson, E. W.: Management of the foot in rheumatoid arthritis. Orthop. Clin. North Am., 2:733, 1971.

Bland, J. H., and Phillips, C. A.: Etiology and pathogenesis of rheumatoid arthritis and related multisystem diseases. Semin. Arthritis Rheum., 1:339, 1972.

Brattstrom, H., and Brattstrom, M.: Metatarso-phalangeal joints in rheumatoid arthritis. J. Bone Joint Surg., 50B:221, 1968.

Brattstrom, H., and Brattstrom, M.: Resection of the metatarso-phalangeal joint in rheumatoid arthritis. Acta Orthop. Scand., 41:213, 1970.

Campbell, C. J., Rinehart, W. T., and Kalenak, A.: Arthrodesis of the ankle. Deep autogenous inlay grafts with maximum cancellous bone apposition. J. Bone Joint Surg., 56A:63, 1974.

Chand, K.: Rheumatoid arthritis of the foot. Int. Surg., 58:12, 1973.

Clayton, M. L.: Surgery of the forefoot in rheumatoid arthritis. Clin. Orthop., 16:136, 1960.

Clayton, M. L.: Surgery of the lower extremity in rheumatoid arthritis. J. Bone Joint Surg., 45A:1517, 1963.

Clayton, M. L.: Surgical treatment of the rheumatoid foot. *In* Giannestras, N. J. (ed.): Foot Disorders: Medical and Surgical Management. Philadelphia, Lea and Febiger, 1967, pp. 319–340

Dixon, A. S.: The rheumatoid foot. Med. Trends Rheumatol., 2:158, 1971.

Ellison, M. R., Kelly, K. J., and Flatt, A. E.: The results of surgical synovectomy of the digital joints in rheumatoid arthritis. J. Bone Joint Surg., 53A:1041, 1971.

Fink, F. J., Jr.: Surgery of the foot in rheumatoid arthritis. Semin. Arthritis Rheum., 1:25, 1971.

Furey, J. G.: Plantar fasciitis. The painful heel syndrome. J. Bone Joint Surg., 57A:672, 1975.

Garner, R. W., Mowat, A. G., and Hazleman, B. L.: Wound healing after operation on patients with rheumatoid arthritis. J. Bone Joint Surg., 51B:134, 1973.

Hall, A. P.: The decision to operate in rheumatoid arthritis. Orthop. Clin. North Am., 6:675, 1975.

Hoffman, P.: An operation for severe grades of contracted or clawed toes. Am. J. Orthop. Surg., 9:441, 1911.

Hollander, J. L.: Arthritis and Allied Conditions, 8th ed. Philadelphia, Lea and Febiger, 1972.

Kelikian, H.: Hallux Valgus, Allied Deformities of the Forefoot and Metatarsalgia. Philadelphia: W. B. Saunders Company, 1965.

King, B. J., Jr., Novy, G. A., and Evans, E. B.: Palindromic rheumatism: an unusual cause of the inflammatory joint. Two case reports and a review. J. Bone Joint Surg., 56A:142, 1975.

Magyar, E., Talerman, A., Feher, M., and Wouters, H. W.: Giant bone cysts in rheumatoid arthritis. J. Bone Joint Surg., 56B:121, 1974.

Marmor, L.: Resection of the forefoot in rheumatoid arthritis. Orthop. Clin. North Am., 108:223, 1975.

Palmer, D. G.: Tendon sheaths and bursae involved by rheumatoid disease at foot and ankle. Australas. Radiol., 14:419, 1970.

Potter, T. A.: Talonavicular fusion with bone graft for spastic arthritic flat foot. Surg. Clin. North Am., 49:883, 1969.

Regnauld, B.: Surgery of the rheumatic forefoot. Acta Orthop. Belg., 35:557, 1971.

Ruddy, S.: Complement and properdin: biologic and clinical importance. Orthop. Clin. North Am., 6:609, 1975.

Sakallarides, H. T.: Ruptures of the tendons in rheumatoid arthritis and the surgical reconstruction. Int. Surg., 57:554, 1972.

Sledge, C. B.: Structure, development, and function of joints. Orthop. Clin. North Am., 6:619, 1975.

Thomas, W.: Surgery of the foot in rheumatoid arthritis. Orthop. Clin. North Am., 6:831, 1975.

Vainio, K.: The rheumatoid foot. A clinical study with pathological and roentgenological comments. Am. Chir. Gynaecol. Fenniae, 25(Suppl. 1), 1955.

Weissman, B., and Sosman, J. L.: The radiology of rheumatoid arthritis. Orthop. Clin. North Am., 6:653, 1975.

HALLUX VALGUS, HALLUX RIGIDUS, HALLUX VARUS, AND METATARSUS PRIMUS VARUS

A. A. O. S. Instructional Course Lectures. St. Louis, C. V. Mosby Co., 1972, Vol. 21, pp. 227–309.

Akin, O. F.: The treatment of hallux valgus — a new operative procedure and its results. Med. Sentinel, 33:678, 1925.

Bonney, G. L. N., and MacNab, I.: Hallux valgus and hallux rigidus: critical survey of operative results. J. Bone Joint Surg., 34B:366, 1952.

Butterworth, R. D., and Clay, B. R.: A bunion operation. Virginia Med. Monthly, 90:10, 1963.

Carr, C. R., and Boyd, B. N.: Correctional osteotomy for metatarsus primus varus and hallux valgus. J. Bone Joint Surg., 50A:1353, 1968.

Clayton, M. L.: Surgery of the forefoot in rheumatoid arthritis. J. Bone Joint Surg., 42A:523, 1960.

Colloff, B., and Weitz, E. M.: Proximal phalangeal osteotomy in hallux valgus. Clin. Orthop., 54:105, 1967.

Fitzgerald, J. A. W.: Review of long term results of arthrodesis of the metatarsophalangeal joint of the great toe. J. Bone Joint Surg., 50B:883, 1968.

Ford, L. T., and Gilula, L. A.: Stem fractures of the middle metatarsals following the Keller operation. J. Bone Joint Surg., 59A:117, 1977.

Gibson, M. C., and Piggott, H.: Osteotomy of the neck of the first metatarsal in the treatment of hallux valgus. J. Bone Joint Surg., 44:349, 1962.

Haines, R. W., and McDougall, A.: The anatomy of hallux valgus. J. Bone Joint Surg., 36B:272, 1954.

Hawkins, F. B.: Acquired hallux varus: cause, prevention and correction. Clin. Orthop. North Am., 76:169, 1971.

Hawkins, F. B., Mitchell, C. L., and Hendrick, D. W.: Correction of hallux valgus by metatarsal osteotomy. J. Bone Joint Surg., 27:387, 1945.

Henry, A. J., and Waugh, W.: The use of footprints in assessing the results of operations for hallux valgus accompanying Keller's operation and arthrodesis. J. Bone Joint Surg., 57B:478, 1978.

Hohmann, G.: Über Hallux Valgus und Spreiz-fuss, ihre Entstehungung Physiologische Behandlung. Arch. Orthop. Unfall. Chir., *21*:525, 1923. (Pathomechanics of splayfoot.)

Jahss, M.: Lelièvre bunion operation. A. A. O. S. Instructional Course Lectures, *21*:295, 1972.

Jamieson, E. S.: Hallux valgus. J. Bone Joint Surg., *34B*:328, 1952.

Jones, A. R.: Hallux valgus in the adolescent. Proc. R. Soc. Med., *41*:382, 1948.

Joplin, R. J.: Sling procedure for the correction of splay foot, metatarsus primus varus, and hallux valgus. J. Bone Joint Surg., *32A*:779, 1950.

Kelikian, H.: Hallux Valgus, Allied Deformities of the Forefoot and Metatarsalgia. Philadelphia, W. B. Saunders Company, 1965.

Keller, W. L.: Surgical treatment of bunions and hallux valgus. N.Y. Med. J., *80*:741, 1904.

Keller, W. L.: Further observations on the surgical treatment of hallux valgus and bunions. N.Y. Med. J., *95*:696, 1912.

Lapidus, P. W.: The author's bunion operation from 1931 to 1959. Clin. Orthop., *16*:119, 1960.

Mayo, C. M.: The surgical treatment of bunions. Ann. Surg., *48*:300, 1908.

McBride, E. D.: The surgical treatment of hallux valgus bunions. Am. J. Orthop., *5*:44, 1963.

McKeever, D. C.: Arthrodesis of the first metatarsophalangeal joint for hallux valgus and hallux rigidus and metatarsus primus varus. J. Bone Joint Surg., *34A*:129, 1952.

Miller, J. W.: Distal first metatarsal displacement osteotomy. Its place in the schema of bunion surgery. J. Bone Joint Surg., *56A*:923, 1974.

Miller, J. W.: Acquired hallux varus: a preventable and correctable disorder. J. Bone Joint Surg., *57A*:183, 1975.

Mitchell, C. L., et al.: Osteotomy, bunionectomy for hallux valgus. J. Bone Joint Surg., *40A*:41, 1958.

Piggott, H. H.: The natural history of hallux valgus in adolescents and early adult life. J. Bone Joint Surg., *42A*:749, 1960.

Raymakers, R., and Waugh, W.: Treatment of metatarsalgia with hallux valgus. J. Bone Joint Surg., *53B*:684, 1971.

Rix, R.: Modified Mayo operation for hallux valgus and bunion — a comparison with the Keller procedure. J. Bone Joint Surg., *50A*:1368, 1968.

Scheck, M.: Degenerative changes in the metatarsophalangeal joints after surgical correction of severe hammer toe deformities. J. Bone Joint Surg., *50A*:727, 1968.

Silver, D.: The operative treatment of hallux valgus. J. Bone Joint Surg., *5*:225, 1923.

Steindler, A.: Orthopaedic Operations. Springfield, Illinois, Charles C Thomas, 1940, p. 766.

Swanson, A. B.: Implant arthroplasty in disabilities of the great toe. Clin. Orthop., *85*:75, 1972.

Swanson, A. B.: Implant arthroplasty in disabilities of the great toe. A. A. O. S. Instructional Course Lectures, Vol. 21. St. Louis, C. V. Mosby Co., 1972.

Tangen, O.: Hallux valgus. Treatment by distal wedge osteotomy of first metatarsal (Hohmann-Thomasen). Acta Chir. Scand., *137*:151, 1971.

FOREFOOT AND TOE DEFORMITIES

Beals, R. K., and Bird, C. B.: Carpal and tarsal osteolysis. A case report and review of the literature. J. Bone Joint Surg., *57A*:681, 1975.

Chuinard, E. G., et al.: Claw foot deformity. J. Bone Joint Surg., *55*:351, 1973.

Cockin, J.: Butler's operation for an over-riding fifth toe. J. Bone Joint Surg., *50B*:78, 1968.

DuVries, H. L.: A new approach to the treatment of the verruca plantaris (plantar wart). J.A.M.A., *152*:1202, 1953.

Gillett, H. G. duP.: Incidence of interdigital clavus. A note on its location. J. Bone Joint Surg., *56B*:753, 1974.

Harris, R. I., and Beath, T.: Army Foot Survey, Vol. I. Ottawa, National Research Council of Canada, 1947.

Harty, M.: Metatarsalgia. Surg. Gynecol. Obstet., *136*:105, 1973.

Helal, B.: Metatarsal osteotomy of metatarsalgia. J. Bone Joint Surg., *57B*:187, 1975.

Jahss, M. H.: Diaphysectomy for severe acquired overlapping fifth toe and advanced fixed hammering of the small toes. *In* Bateman, J. E. (ed.): Foot Science. Philadelphia, W. B. Saunders Company, 1976, pp. 211–221.

Japas, L. M.: Surgical treatment of pes cavus by tarsal V-osteotomy. J. Bone Joint Surg., *50A*:927, 1968.

Joplin, R. J.: Surgery of the forefoot in the rheumatoid arthritic patient. Surg. Clin. North Am., *29*:847, 1969.

Joplin, R. J.: The proper digital nerve, vitallium stem arthroplasty, and some thoughts about foot surgery in general. Clin. Orthop., *76*:199, 1971.

Kelikian, H.: Hallux Valgus, Allied Deformities of the Forefoot and Metatarsalgia. Philadelphia, W. B. Saunders Company, 1965.

Kelikian, H., Clayton, L., and Loseff, H.: Surgical syndactylia of the toes. Clin. Orthop., *19*:208, 1961.

Kiehn, C. L., et al.: Treatment of the chronic painful metatarsal callus by a tendon transfer. Plast. Reconstr. Surg., 51:154, 1973.

Lapidus, P. W.: Spastic flat foot. J. Bone Joint Surg., 28:126, 1946.

Litchman, H. M., et al.: Morton's metatarsalgia. J. Int. Coll. Surg., 41:647, 1964.

Mann, R. A., et al.: Intractable plantar keratosis. Orthop. Clin. North Am., 4:67, 1973.

McDowell, F.: Plantar warts, plantar calluses, and such. Plast. Reconstr. Surg., 51:196, 1973.

Milgram, J. E.: Office measures for relief of the painful foot. J. Bone Joint Surg., 46A:1095, 1964.

Parrish, T. F.: Dynamic correction of claw toes. Orthop. Clin. North Am., 4:97, 1973.

Selakovich, W. G.: Medial arch support by operation: sustentaculum tali procedure. Orthop. Clin. North Am., 4:117, 1973.

Steindler, A.: Orthopaedic Operations. Springfield, Illinois, Charles C Thomas, 1940, p. 766.

Thomas, F. B.: Levelling the tread. J. Bone Joint Surg., 56B:314, 1974.

GOUT AND PERIARTICULAR ALTERATIONS

Bailey, R. W.: Calcinosis circumscripta — a local and metabolic study. J. Bone Joint Surg., 39B:584, 1957.

Bartels, E. C.: Unrecognized cases of gout. Lahey Clin. Found. Bull., 11:226, 1960.

Bauer, W., and Krane, S. M.: Diseases of Metabolism, 5th ed. Philadelphia, W. B. Saunders Company, 1964.

Bluhm, G. B., Riddle, N. J., Barkart, M. J., Duncan, H., and Sigler, J. W.: Crystal dynamics in gout and pseudogout. Med. Times, 97:135, 1969.

Crock, H. V., and Boni, V.: The management of orthopaedic problems in hemophiliacs. A review of 21 cases. Br. J. Surg., 48:8, 1960.

Evans, E. V., and Smith, J. R.: Bone and joint changes following burns. J. Bone Joint Surg., 41A:785, 1959.

Gatter, R. A., and McCarty, D. J.: Pseudogout syndrome. Clinical analysis of 30 cases. Arthritis Rheum., 6:271, 1963.

Gibbs, D. D., Schiller, K. F. R., and Stovin, P. G. I.: Lung metastases heralded by hypertrophic pulmonary osteoarthropathy. Lancet, 1:623, 1960.

Graham, W.: Gout and gouty arthritis. Postgrad. Med., 30:555, 1961.

Hamblen, D. L., Currey, H. L. F., and Key, J. J.: Pseudogout simulating acute suppurative arthritis. J. Bone Joint Surg., 48B:51, 1966.

Hollander, J. L.: Arthritis and Allied Conditions, 8th ed. Philadelphia, Lea and Febiger, 1972.

Kilburn, P.: Calcinosis: a review with report of four cases. Postgrad. Med., 33:555, 1957.

Krakoff, I. H., and Meyer, R. L.: Prevention of hyperuricemia in leukemia and lymphoma. J.A.M.A., 193:89, 1965.

Lapidus, P. W., and Guidotti, F. P.: Gout in orthopaedic practice. Clin. Orthop., 28:97, 1963.

Martel, W., Champion, C. K., Thompson, G. R., and Carter, T. L.: A roentgenologically distinctive arthropathy in some patients with the pseudogout syndrome. Am. J. Roentgenol., 109:587, 1970.

McCarty, D. J., Jr., and Silcox, D. C.: Gout and pseudogout. Geriatrics, 28:110, 1973.

Selye, H., Goldie, I., and Strebel, R.: Calciphylaxis in relation to calcification in periarticular tissue. Clin. Orthop., 28:181, 1963.

Ts'ai-Fan Yu, and Sutman, A. A. B.: Effect of allopurinol on serum and urinary uric acid in primary and secondary gout. Am. J. Med., 37:833, 1964.

Tulius, J. L., Melin, M., and Jurigian, P.: Clinical use of human prothrombin complexes. N. Engl. J. Med., 273:667, 1965.

Webb, J., Champion, D. G., Frecker, A. S., and Robinson, R. G.: Calcium pyrophosphate crystal synovitis with articular chondrocalcinosis. Med. J. Aust., 1:466, 1970.

Zitnan, D., and Sit'ai, S.: Chondrocalcinosis articularis (familiaris). Ann. Rheum. Dis., 22:142, 1963.

AMPUTATIONS, FUSIONS, AND ARTHROPLASTIES

Appoldt, F. A., and Bennett, L.: A preliminary report on dynamic socket pressures. Bull. Prosthet. Res., 10:68, 1967.

Baker, G. C. W., and Stableforth, P. G.: Syme's amputation. A review of 67 cases. J. Bone Joint Surg., 51B:482, 1969.

Bernau, A.: Long-term results following Lambrinudi arthrodeses. J. Bone Joint Surg., 59A:473, 1977.

Bonney, G. L. N., and MacNab, I.: Hallux valgus and hallux rigidus. A critical survey of operative results. J. Bone Joint Surg., 34B:366, 1952.

Brand, P. W.: Results of work at Public Health Service Hospital, Carville, Louisiana. In The Effect of Pressure on Soft Tissues. Washington, D.C., National Academy of Sciences, 1972.

Campbell, C. J., Rinehardt, W. T., and Kalevak, A.: Arthrodesis of the ankle. Deep autogenous inlay grafts with maximum cancellous bone apposition. J. Bone Joint Surg., 56A:63, 1974.

Clayton, M. L.: Surgery of the forefoot in rheumatoid arthritis. J. Bone Joint Surg., 42A:523, 1960.

Flint, M., and Sweetnam, R.: Amputations of all toes: a review of forty-seven amputations. J. Bone Joint Surg., *42B*:90, 1960.

Fowler, A. W.: A method of forefoot reconstruction. J. Bone Joint Surg., *41B*:507, 1959.

Harris, R. I.: Syme's amputation: the technical details essential for success. J. Bone Joint Surg., *38B*:614, 1956.

Harris, R. I.: The history and development of Syme's amputation. Artif. Limbs, *6*:4, 1961.

Hornby, R., and Harris, W. R.: Syme's amputation. Follow-up study of weight bearing in sixty-eight patients. J. Bone Joint Surg., *57A*:346, 1975.

Keller, W. L.: Surgical treatment of bunions and hallux valgus. N.Y. Med. J., *80*:741, 1904.

London, P. S.: Amputations of the fingers and toes. *In* Rob, C., and Smith, R. (eds.): Operative Surgery, 2nd ed. London, Butterworth and Co., 1969.

Magee, H. R., and Parker, W. R.: Replantation of the foot. Results after two years. Med. J. Aust., *1*:751, 1972.

Mayo, C. M.: The surgical treatment of bunions. Ann. Surg., *48*:300, 1908.

McKeever, D. C.: Arthrodesis of the first metatarsophalangeal joint for hallux valgus and hallux rigidus and metatarsus primus varus. J. Bone Joint Surg., *34A*:129, 1952.

McKittrick, L. S., McKittrick, M. B., and Risley, T. S.: Transmetatarsal amputation for infection of gangrene in patients with diabetes mellitus. Ann. Surg., *130*:826, 1949.

Monster, A. W.: Sensory augmentation in weight-bearing training. *In* The Effect of Pressure on Soft Tissues. Washington, D.C., National Academy of Sciences, 1972.

Morris, H. D.: Arthrodesis of the foot. Clin. Orthop., *16*:164, 1960.

Omer, G. E., Jr., et al.: Initial management of severe open injuries and traumatic amputations of the foot. Arch. Surg., *105*:696, 1972.

Schwindt, C. D., et al.: Transmetatarsal amputations. Orthop. Clin. North Am., *4*:31, 1973.

Selected articles from Artificial Limbs. Huntington, New York, R. E. Krieger Publishing Co., 1970.

Silver, D.: The operative treatment of hallux valgus. J. Bone Joint Surg., *5*:225, 1923.

Sizer, J. W., and Wheelock, F. C.: Digital amputations in diabetic patients. Surgery, *72*:980, 1972.

Srinivasan, H.: Syme's amputation in insensitive feet. J. Bone Joint Surg., *55*:558, 1973.

Stack, J. K.: Technical essentials in amputation. Surg. Clin. North Am., *38*:301, 1958.

Swanson, A. B.: Implant arthroplasty for the great toe. Clin. Orthop., *35*:75, 1972.

Swanson, A. B.: Implant arthroplasty in disabilities of the great toe. A. A. O. S. Instructional Course Lectures, Vol. 21. St. Louis, C. V. Mosby Co., 1972.

Taft, C. B.: Radiographic evaluation of stump-socket fit. Artif. Limbs, *13*:36, 1969.

Thompson, R. G.: Amputation in the lower extremity. J. Bone Joint Surg., *45A*:1723, 1963.

Tooms, R. E.: Amputations. *In* Crenshaw, A. H. (ed.): Campbell's Operative Orthopedics, 5th ed., Vol. 1. St. Louis, C. V. Mosby Co., 1971.

Wagner, F. W., Jr.: Amputations of the foot and ankle. Current status. Clin. Orthop., *122*:626, 1977.

Wheelock, F. C., Jr.: Transmetatarsal amputations and arterial surgery in diabetic patients. N. Engl. J. Med., *264*:316, 1961.

Wheelock, F. C., Jr., McKittrick, J. B., and Root, H. F.: Evaluation of the transmetatarsal amputation in patients with diabetes mellitus. Surgery, *41*:184, 1957.

Wilson, A. B., Jr.: Prostheses for Syme's amputation. Artif. Limbs, *6*:52, 1961.

FRACTURES AND DISLOCATIONS

Aitken, A.: Fractures of the os calcis treated with closed reduction. Clin. Orthop., *30*:67, 1963.

Boehler, L.: Technik der Knockenbruch Behandlung, 2nd ed. Wien, W. Manbrich, 1930. (More recent new editions.)

Bohler, L.: Treatment of Fractures, 5th ed. New York, Grune and Stratton, 1956.

Canale, S. T., and Kelly, F. B., Jr.: Fractures of the neck of the talus. Long-term evaluation of 71 cases. J. Bone Joint Surg., *60A*:143, 1977.

Cassebaum, W.: Fracture of Lisfranc's joint. Clin. Orthop., *30*:116, 1963.

Cassebaum, W.: Fracture of Lisfranc's joint. J. Trauma, *5*:718, 1965.

Cave, E. F.: Fractures of the os calcis: the problems in general. Clin. Orthop., *30*:64, 1963.

Dameron, T. B., Jr.: Fractures and anatomical variations of the proximal portion of the fifth metatarsal. J. Bone Joint Surg., *57A*:788, 1975.

Dart, D. E., and Graham, W. D.: The treatment of fractured calcaneum. J. Trauma, *6*:362, 1966.

DePalma, A.: The Management of Fractures and Dislocations, Vol. II. Philadelphia, W. B. Saunders Company, 1959.

Detenbeck, L. C., and Kelly, P. T.: Total dislocation of the talus. J. Bone Joint Surg., *51A*:283, 1969.

Essex-Lopresti, P.: The mechanism, reduction technique, and results in fractures of the os calcis. Br. J. Surg. *39*:395, 1951.

Gallie, W. E.: Subastragalar arthrodesis in fractures of the os calcis. J. Bone Joint Surg., *25*:731, 1943.

Hall, M. C., and Pennal, G. F.: Primary subtalar arthrodesis in treatment of severe fractures of the calcaneum. J. Bone Joint Surg., *43B*:336, 1960.

Harris, R. I.: Fractures of the os calcis. Treatment by early subtalar arthrodesis. Clin. Orthop., *30*:100, 1963.

Harty, M.: Anatomic considerations in injuries of the calcaneus. Orthop. Clin. North Am., *4*:179, 1973.

Hazelett, J. W.: Open reduction of fractures of the calcaneum. Can. J. Surg., *12*:310, 1969.

Horn, C. E.: Fractures of the calcaneum. Calif. Med., *108A*:209, 1968.

Jeffreys, T. E.: Lisfranc's fracture dislocation. J. Bone Joint Surg., *45B*:546, 1963.

Joy, G., Patzakis, M. J., and Harvey, J. P., Jr.: Precise evaluation of the reduction of severe ankle fractures. Technique and correlation with end results. J. Bone Joint Surg., *56A*:979, 1974.

Karlstrom, G., Lonnerholm, T., and Olerud, S.: Cavus deformity of the foot after fracture of the tibial shaft. J. Bone Joint Surg., *57A*:893, 1975.

Lapidus, P.: Mechanical anatomy of the tarsal joints. Clin. Orthop., *30*:20, 1963.

Lauge-Hansen, N.: Fractures of the ankle. II. Combined experimental surgical and experimental roentgenologic investigation. Arch. Surg., *60*:1957, 1950.

Lowry, M.: Avulsion fracture of the calcaneus. J. Bone Joint Surg., *51B*:494, 1969.

Maxfield, J. E.: Treatment of the calcaneal fractures by open reduction. J. Bone Joint Surg., *45A*:868, 1963.

McMaster, M.: Disability of the hindfoot after fracture of the tibial shaft. J. Bone Joint Surg., *58B*:90, 1976.

Mindell, E. R., Cisek, E. E., Kartalian, G., and Dziob, N. J.: Late results of injuries to the talus. J. Bone Joint Surg., *45A*:221, 1963.

Oh, W. H.: Progress in the treatment of fractures and dislocation of the talus, calcaneus and foot. Orthop. Rev., *16*:23, 1977.

Pennal, G. F., and Yadau, M. P.: Operative treatment of comminuted fractures of the os calcis. Orthop. Clin. North Am., *41*:197, 1973.

Pollack, W. J., and Parkes, J., III: Open skin grafting of war wounds. J. Bone Joint Surg., *51A*:926, 1969.

Sneppen, O.: Treatment of pseudoarthrosis involving the malleolus. A postoperative follow-up of 34 cases. Acta Orthop. Scand., *42*:201, 1971.

Sneppen, O.: Pseudoarthrosis of the lateral malleolus. Acta Orthop. Scand., *42*:187, 1971.

Spiegel, P. K., and Staples, O. S.: Arthrography of the ankle joint: problems in diagnosis of acute lateral ligament instability. Radiology, *114*:587, 1975.

Stewart, I. M.: Jone's fractures: fracture of the base of the fifth metatarsal. Clin. Orthop., *16*:190, 1960.

Turco, V. J.: Diastasis of the first and second tarsometatarsal rays: cause of pain in the foot. Bull. N.Y. Acad. Med., *40*:222, 1973.

Watson-Jones, R.: Fractures and Joint Injuries, 4th ed. Baltimore, Williams and Wilkins, 1955.

Yablon, I. G., Heller, F. G., and Shouse, L.: The key role of the lateral malleolus in displaced fractures of the ankle. J. Bone Joint Surg., *59A*:169, 1977.

Zayer, M.: Fractures of the calcaneus. A review of 110 fractures. Acta Orthop. Scand., *40*:530, 1969.

HINDFOOT PROBLEMS

Dickenson, P., Woodward, P. E., and Handler, D.: Tendo Achillis bursitis. J. Bone Joint Surg., *48A*:77, 1966.

Eggers, G. W. N.: Shoe pad treatment for calcaneal spur. J. Bone Joint Surg., *39A*:219, 1957.

Inglis, A. E., Scott, W. N., Sculco, T. P., and Patterson, A. H.: Ruptures of the tendo Achillis. An objective assessment of surgical and nonsurgical treatment. J. Bone Joint Surg., *56A*:990, 1976.

Mitchell, G. P.: Posterior displacement osteotomy of the calcaneus. J. Bone Joint Surg., *59B*:233, 1977.

Nellius, S. A., Nelsson, B. E., and Wistlin, N. E.: Incidence of Achilles tendon rupture. Acta Orthop. Scand., *47*:118, 1976.

SPORTS INJURIES

Brantigan, J. W., Pedegana, L. R., and Lippert, F. G.: Instability of the subtalar joint. Diagnosis by stress tomography in three cases. J. Bone Joint Surg., *59A*:321, 1977.

Chrisman, O. D., and Snook, G. A.: Reconstruction of lateral ligament tears of the ankle. An experimental study and clinical evaluation of seven patients treated by a new modification of the Elmslie procedure. J. Bone Joint Surg., *51A*:904, 1969.

Eckert, W. R., and Davis, E. A.: Acute rupture of the peroneal retinaculum. J. Bone Joint Surg., *58A*:670, 1976.

Jessing, P., and Hensen, E.: Surgical treatment of 102 tendo Achillis ruptures. Suture or tenotoplasty? Acta Chir. Scand., *144*:370, 1975.

Main, B. J., and Lovett, R. L.: Injuries of the mid-tarsal joints. J. Bone Joint Surg., *57B*:891, 1975.

Outland, T.: Sprains and separations of the inferior tibiofibular joint without important fracture. Am. J. Surg., 59:320, 1943.

Staples, O. S.: Ruptures of the fibular collateral ligaments of the ankle. Result study of immediate surgical treatment. J. Bone Joint Surg., 57A:101, 1975.

Vincelette, P., Laurin, C. A., and Lévesque, H. P.: Footballer's ankle and foot. Can. Med. Assoc. J., 107:872, 1972.

FLATFOOT OR PES PLANUS

Becker-Andersen, H., and Reimann, I.: Congenital vertical talus, re-evaluating early manipulative treatment. Acta Orthop. Scand., 45:130, 1974.

Cotton, C. L.: Surgical management of congenital vertical talus. J. Bone Joint Surg., 55B:566, 1973.

Jones, B. S.: Flat foot: preliminary report of operation for severe cases. J. Bone Joint Surg., 57B:279, 1975.

Sharrard, W. J. W.: Intoeing and flat feet. Br. Med. J., 1:88, 1971.

GENETIC DISTURBANCES AFFECTING THE FOOT

Berman, J. L., Rankin, J. K., Harrison, P. A., Donovan, D. J., Hogan, W. J., and Bearn, A. O.: Autosomal trisomy of a group 16-18 chromosome. J. Pediatr., 60:503, 1962.

James, J. I. P.: The orthopedic surgeon and research. J. Bone Joint Surg., 52B:14, 1970.

McKusick, V. A.: Human Genetics. Englewood Cliffs, New Jersey, Prentice-Hall, 1964.

McKusick, V. A.: Mendelian Inheritance in Man. Catalogs of Autosomal Dominant, Autosomal Recessive, and X-Linked Pheno Types, 3rd ed. Baltimore, The Johns Hopkins University Press, 1971.

McKusick, V. A.: Heritable Disorders of Connective Tissue. St. Louis, C. V. Mosby Co., 1972.

Nance, W. E.: Recent developments in genetics: controlled genes and the genetic code. J. Bone Joint Surg., 49A:183, 1971.

Nance, W. E., Elmore, S. M., and Hillman, J. W.: Genetics and orthopedics. J. Bone Joint Surg., 47A:1260, 1965.

Nance, W. E., and Engel, E.: Human cytogenetics: a brief review and presentation of new findings. J. Bone Joint Surg., 39A:1436, 1967.

Valentine, G. H.: The Chromosome Disorders — An Introduction for Clinicians. Philadelphia, J. B. Lippincott Co., 1969.

Yunis, J. J.: Human Chromosome Methodology. New York, Academic Press, 1965.

CONGENITAL DEFORMITIES OF THE FOOT

Talipes Equinovarus

Abrams, R. C.: Relapsed club foot. The early results of an evaluation of Dillwyn Evans' operation. J. Bone Joint Surg., 51A:270, 1969.

Adams, F. H.: Hereditary deformities in man. J. Hered., 36:2, 1945.

Adams, W.: A series of four specimens illustrating the morbid anatomy of congenital club-foot (talipes varus). Trans. Path. Soc. London, 6:348, 1854–1855.

Adams, W.: Club Foot, Its Causes, Pathology and Treatment. London, J. and A. Churchill, 1866.

Alberman, E. D.: The causes of congenital club foot. Arch. Dis. Child., 40:458, 1965.

Attenborough, C. G.: Severe congenital talipes equinovarus. J. Bone Joint Surg., 48B:31, 1966.

Beatson, R. R., and Pearson, J. R.: A method of assessing correction in club feet. J. Bone Joint Surg., 48B:40, 1966.

Bechtol, C. O., and Mossman, H. W.: Clubfoot. Embryological study of associated muscle abnormalities. J. Bone Joint Surg., 32A:827, 1950.

Bell, J. F., and Grice, D. S.: Treatment of congenital talipes equinovarus with the modified Denis Browne splint. J. Bone Joint Surg., 27:799, 1944.

Bentzon, P. G. K., and Thomasen, E.: On treatment of congenital clubfoot. Acta Orthop. Scand., 11:129, 1940.

Berman, A., and Gartland, J. J.: Metatarsal osteotomy for the correction of adduction of the forepart of the foot in children. J. Bone Joint Surg., 53A:498, 1971.

Bertelson, A.: Treatment of congenital club foot. J. Bone Joint Surg., 39A:599, 1957.

Bessel-Hagen, F. C.: Die Pathologie und Therapie des Klumfusses. Heidelberg, O. Peters, 1889.

Bissell, J. B.: The morbid anatomy of congenital talipes equinovarus. Arch. Pediatr., 5:406, 1888.

Blockey, N. J., and Smith, M. G. H.: The treatment of congenital club foot. J. Bone Joint Surg., 48B:660, 1966.

Blumenfeld, I., Kaplan, N., and Hicks, E. O.: The conservative treatment of congenital talipes equinovarus. J. Bone Joint Surg., 28:765, 1946.

Böhm, M.: Zur Pathologie und Röntgenologie des angeborenen Klumfusses. Munch. Med. Wochenschr., 55:1492, 1928.

Böhm, M.: The embryologic origin of clubfoot. J. Bone Joint Surg., 11:229, 1929.

Börnbeck, R.: Zur Pathologie des angeborenen Klumfusses. Orthop., 79:521, 1950.

Bost, F. C., Schottstaedt, E. R., and Larsen, I. J.: Plantar dissection. An operation to release the soft tissues in recurrent or recalcitrant talipes equinovarus. J. Bone Joint Surg., 42A:151, 1960.

Brockman, E. P.: Congenital Clubfoot (Talipes Equinovarus). New York, William Wood and Co., 1930.

Brockman, E. P.: Modern methods of treatment of clubfoot. Br. Med. J., 2:512, 1937.

Browne, D.: Talipes equinovarus. Lancet, 2:969, 1934.

Browne, D.: Congenital deformities of mechanical origin. Proc. R. Soc. Med., 29:1409, 1936.

Browne, D.: Congenital deformities of mechanical origin. Arch. Dis. Child., 30:37, 1955.

Browne, D.: Splinting for controlled movement. Clin. Orthop., 8:91, 1956.

Burrell, H. L.: A contribution to the anatomy of congenital equinovarus. Ann. Surg., 17:293, 1893.

Carpenter, E. B., and Huff, S. H.: Selective tendon transfers for recurrent club foot. South. Med. J., 46:220, 1953.

Cavanaugh, C. J.: Clubfoot and congenital hand anomalies. J. Hered., 44:53, 1953.

Clark, J. M. P.: Treatment of clubfoot. Early detection and management of the unreduced club foot. Proc. R. Soc. Med., 61:779, 1968.

Clark, M. W., D'Ambrosia, R. D., and Ferguson, A. B., Jr.: Congenital vertical talus. Treatment by open reduction and navicular excision. J. Bone Joint Surg., 59A:816, 1977.

Codivilla, A.: New procedure for surgical treatment of congenital pes equinus varus. Arch. Soc. Ital. Chir., 18:1906.

Codivilla, A.: Sulla cura del piedo equino varo congenito. Nuovo metodo de cura cruenta. Arch. Ortop., 23:245, 1906.

Compere, E. L.: Congenital talipes equinovarus. Surg. Clin. North Am., 15:767, 1935.

Crabbe, W. A.: Aetiology of congenital talipes. Br. Med. J., 2:1060, 1960.

Critchley, J. E., and Taylor, R. G.: Transfer of the tibialis anterior tendon for relapsed clubfoot. J. Bone Joint Surg., 34B:49, 1952.

Curtis, B. H., and Butterfield, W. L.: Surgical treatment of congenital clubfoot. In Delchey, J. (ed.): Dixième Congrès International de Chirurgie Orthopédique et de Traumatologie. Paris, 4–9 Septembre, 1966.

Bruxelles, Les Publications "Acta Medica Belgica," 1967, p. 1150.

Curtis, F. E., and Muro, F.: Decancellation of the os calcis, astragalus, and cuboid in correction of congenital talipes equinovarus. J. Bone Joint Surg., 16:110, 1934.

Dangelmajer, R. C.: A review of 200 clubfeet. Bull. Hosp. Special Surg., 4:73, 1961.

Denham, R. A.: Congenital talipes equinovarus. J. Bone Joint Surg., 49B:583, 1967.

Dittrich, R. J.: Pathogenesis of congenital club-foot. J. Bone Joint Surg., 12:373, 1930.

Dunn, H. K., and Samuelson, K. M.: Flat-top talus — a long term report of twenty club feet. J. Bone Joint Surg., 56A:57, 1974.

Dunn, N.: The treatment of congenital talipes equinovarus. Br. Med. J., 2:1, 216, 1923.

Dwyer, F. C.: The treatment of relapsed clubfoot by the insertion of a wedge into the calcaneus. J. Bone Joint Surg., 45B:67, 1963.

Elmslie, R. C.: The principles of treatment of congenital talipes equino-varus. J. Orthop. Surg., 2:669, 1920.

Evans, D.: Relapsed club foot. J. Bone Joint Surg., 43B:722, 1961.

Farill, J.: Tibioperoneal tenoplasty for congenital club-foot with peroneal insufficiency. J. Bone Joint Surg., 38A:329, 1956.

Flinchum, D.: Pathologic anatomy in talipes equinovarus. J. Bone Joint Surg., 35A:111, 1953.

Forrester-Brown, M.: The treatment of congenital equinovarus (club-foot). J. Bone Joint Surg., 17:661, 1935.

Forrester-Brown, M.: A clamp for stretching congenital club-feet. Lancet, 1:897, 1936.

Fredenhagen, H.: Der Klumpfuss, Vorkommen, Anatomie, Behandlung and Spätresultate. Z. Orthop., 85:305, 1954.

Fried, A.: Recurrent congenital club-foot. The role of the m. tibialis posterior in etiology and treatment. J. Bone Joint Surg., 41A:243, 1959.

Fripp, A. T.: The relapsed clubfoot. Proc. R. Soc. Med., 44:873, 1951.

Fripp, A. T.: The problem of the relapsed clubfoot (editorial). J. Bone Joint Surg., 43B:626, 1961.

Fripp, A. T., and Shaw, N. E.: Club-foot. Edinburgh and London, E. and S. Livingstone, Ltd., 1967.

Garceau, G. J.: Anterior tibial transposition in recurrent congenital club-foot. J. Bone Joint Surg., 22:932, 1940.

Garceau, G. J.: Recurrent clubfoot. Bull. Hosp. Joint Dis., 15:143, 1954.

Garceau, G. J., and Manning, K. R.: Transposition of the anterior tibial tendon in the treatment of recurrent congenital club-foot. J. Bone Joint Surg., 29:1044, 1947.

Garceau, G. J., and Palmer, R. M.: Transfer of the anterior tibial tendon for recurrent club-foot. A long-term follow-up. J. Bone Joint Surg., *49A*:207, 1967.

Gartland, J. J.: Posterior tibial transplant in the surgical treatment of recurrent club foot. A preliminary report. J. Bone Joint Surg., *46A*:1217, 1964.

Gelman, W. B.: Soft-tissue releasing procedure for persisting heel varus in the uncorrected clubfoot. Clin. Orthop., *16*:177, 1960.

Gunn, D. R., and Molesworth, B. D.: The use of the tibialis posterior as a dorsiflexor. J. Bone Joint Surg., *39B*:674, 1957.

Hamsa, W. R., and Burney, D. W., Jr.: Open correction of recurrent talipes equinovarus. A study of end-results. Clin. Orthop., 26:104, 1963.

Handelsman, J. E., Youngleson, J., and Malkin, C.: A modified approach to the Dwyer os calcis osteotomy in club foot. S. Afr. Med. J., 39:989, 1965.

Harry, N. M.: Denis Browne splints in the treatment of talipes equinovarus. Aust. N. Z. J. Surg., *10*:117, 1940.

Hauser, E. D. W.: Cohesive bandage for clubfoot in newborn infants. J.A.M.A., *138*:19, 1948.

Hauser, E. D. W.: Origin and etiology of clubfoot. Q. Bull. Northwest. Med. Sch., 28:274, 1954.

Hegdekatti, R. M.: Congenital malformation of hands and feet in man. J. Hered., *30*:191, 1939.

Helal, B., Gupta, S. K., and Gojansein, P.: Surgery for adolescent hallux valgus. Acta Orthop. Scand., 45:271, 1974.

Henke, W., and Reyher, C.: Studien über die Entwickelung der Extremitäten des Menschen inbesondere der Gelenkflachen. Sitzungsberichte d. k. Akademie d. Wissenschaflen Wiener Math. Naturwissenschaftliche Klasse, Ed. 3. 50:217, 1874.

Hersch, A.: The role of surgery in the treatment of club feet. J. Bone Joint Surg., *49A*:1684, 1967.

Heyman, C. H.: Ober operation for congenital club-foot. End-results in fifteen cases. Surg. Gynecol. Obstet., 49:706, 1929.

Heyman, C. H., Herndon, C. H., and Strong, J. M.: Mobilization of the tarsometatarsal and intermetatarsal joints for the correction of resistant adduction of the forepart of the foot in congenital clubfoot or congenital metatarsus varus. J. Bone Joint Surg., *40A*:299, 1958.

Heywood, A. W. B.: The mechanics of the hindfoot in clubfoot as demonstrated radiographically. J. Bone Joint Surg., *46B*:102, 1964.

Hirsch, C.: Observations on early operative treatment of congenital club-foot. Bull. Hosp. Joint Dis., *21*:173, 1960.

Hjelmstedt, A., and Sahlstedt, B.: Talar deformity in congenital clubfeet: anatomic and functional study with special reference to ankle joint mobility. Acta Orthop. Scand., *45*:628, 1974.

Hoffa, A.: Lehrbuch der Orthopädischen Chirurgie, 5th ed. Stuttgart, Ferdinand Enke, 1905, pp. 734–782.

Hüter, C.: Zu der Frage über das Wesen des angeborenen Klumpfüsses. Dtsch. Klin., *15*:487, 1863.

Idelberger, K.: Die Ergebnisse der Zwillingsforschung beim angeborenen Klumpfuss. Verh Dtsch. Orthop. Ges., 33:272, 1939.

Inclán, A.: Las anomalias de las inserciones tendinosas en la pathogenia del pié bot varo equino congénito. Rev. Orthop. Traumatol., 5:173, 1960.

Irani, R. N., and Sherman, M. S.: The pathologic anatomy of club feet. J. Bone Joint Surg., *45A*:45, 1963.

Jansen, K.: Treatment of congenital club foot. J. Bone Joint Surg., *39B*:599, 1957.

Jergesen, F. H.: The treatment of unilateral congenital talipes equinovarus with the Denis Browne splint. J. Bone Joint Surg., 25:185, 1943.

Johanning, K.: Excochleatio ossis cuboidei in the treatment of pes equinovarus. Acta Orthop. Scand., 27:310, 1958.

Kandel, B.: Suroplantar projection in the congenital clubfoot of the infant. Acta Orthop. Scand., 22:161, 1952.

Kaye, J. J., Ghelman, B., and Schuch, R.: Talonavicular joint arthrography for sustentaculum-tali tarsal coalitions. Radiology, *115*:730, 1975.

Kendrick, R. E., Sharma, N. K., Hassler, W. L., and Herndon, C. H.: Tarso-metatarsal mobilization for resistant adduction of the forepart of the foot. A follow-up study. J. Bone Joint Surg., *52A*:61, 1970.

Kite, J. H.: Non-operative treatment of congenital clubfeet. South. Med. J., *23*:337, 1930.

Kite, J. H.: The surgical treatment of congenital club-feet. Surg. Gynecol. Obstet., *61*:190, 1935.

Kite, J. H.: Principles involved in the treatment of club-foot. J. Bone Joint Surg., *21*:595, 1939.

Kite, J. H.: The Clubfoot. New York, Grune and Stratton, 1964.

Kite, J. H.: Errors and complications in treating foot conditions in children. Clin. Orthop., 53:31, 1967.

Kleiger, B.: Significance of the tibiotalar navicular complex in congenital clubfoot. J. Hosp. Joint Dis., 23:158, 1962.

Kocher: Zur Aetiologie und Therapie des pes

varus congenitus. Dtsch. Z. Chir., 9:329, 1879.

Kuhlman, R. F., and Bell, J. F.: A clinical evaluation of operative procedures for congenital talipes equinovarus. J. Bone Joint Surg., 39A:265, 1957.

Lange, M.: Orthopadische-Chirurgische Operationslehre. Munich, J. Bergman, 1951.

Larsen, B., Reimann, I., and Becker-Andersen, H.: Congenital calcaneovalgus: with special reference to treatment and its relation to other congenital foot deformities. Acta Orthop. Scand., 65:145, 1974.

LeNoir, J. L.: Congenital Idiopathic Talipes. Springfield, Illinois, Charles C Thomas, 1966.

Little, W. J.: A Treatise on the Nature of Club-foot and Analogous Distortions: Including Their Treatment Both With or Without Surgical Operation. London, W. Jeffs, 1839.

Lloyd-Roberts, G. C., and Clark, R. C.: Ball and socket ankle joint in metatarsus adductus varus (S-shaped or serpentine foot). J. Bone Joint Surg., 55B:193, 1973.

Lowe, L. W., and Hannon, M. A.: Residual adduction of forefoot in treated congenital club foot. J. Bone Joint Surg., 55B:809, 1973.

Lucas, I. S.: Surgical procedures in treatment of chronic clubfoot. West. J. Surg., 56:542, 1948.

Lusskin, H.: Nonrigid method of treatment for early clubfoot. J. Int. Coll. Surg., 14:444, 1950.

MacEwen, G. D., Scott, D. J., Jr., and Shands, A. R., Jr.: Follow-up survey of clubfoot treated at Alfred I. DuPont Institute. With special reference to the value of plaster therapy, instituted during earliest signs of recurrence, and the use of night splints to prevent or minimize the manifestations. J.A.M.A., 175:427, 1961.

Martin, J., and Pilcher, M. F.: Tendon transplantation in the prevention of foot deformities after poliomyelitis in children. J. Bone Joint Surg., 38A:633, 1956.

Mau, C.: Muskelbefunde und ihre Bedentung Beim angeborenen Klumfussleiden. Arch. Orthop. Unfallchir., 28:292, 1930.

McCauley, J. C., Jr.: Operative treatment of clubfeet. N.Y. J. Med., 47:255, 1947.

McCauley, J. C., Jr.: Surgical treatment of clubfoot. Surg. Clin. North Am., 31:561, 1951.

McCauley, J. C., Jr.: A release operation for problem clubfoot. N.Y. J. Med., 52:2997, 1952.

McCauley, J. C., Jr.: Treatment of clubfoot. A.A.O.S. Instructional Course Lectures, Vol. 16. St. Louis, C. V. Mosby Co., 1959.

McCauley, J. C., Jr.: Triple arthrodesis for congenital talipes equinovarus deformities. Clin. Orthop., 34:25, 1964.

McCauley, J. C., Jr.: Clubfoot. History of the development and the concepts of pathogenesis and treatment. Clin. Orthop., 44:51, 1966.

McCauley, J. C., Jr., and Krida, A.: Early treatment of equinus and congenital club foot. Am. J. Surg., 22:491, 1933.

Menelaus, M. B.: Talectomy in equinovarus deformity in arthrogryposis and spina bifida. J. Bone Joint Surg., 53B:468, 1971.

Middleton, D. S.: Studies on prenatal lesions of striated muscle as a cause of congenital deformity. Edinburgh Med. J. (N.S.), 41:401, 1934.

Miller, O. L.: Surgical management of pes calcaneus. J. Bone Joint Surg., 18:169, 1936.

Morita, S.: A method for the treatment of resistant congenital clubfoot in infants by gradual correction with leverage-wire correction and wire-traction cast. J. Bone Joint Surg., 44A:149, 1962.

Morris, R. H.: Skeletal traction as a method of treatment for certain foot deformities. Arch. Surg., 46:737, 1943.

Nagura, S.: Zur Ätiologie des angeborenen Klumpfusses. Z. Chir., 8:187, 1956.

Nagura, S.: Zur Frage der Vererbung des angeborenen Klumpfusses. Arch. Orthop. Unfallchir., 52:48, 1960.

Neel, J. V., Falls, H. T., and Test, A. R.: Pedigree of clubfoot. Am. J. Dis. Child., 79:442, 1950.

Nicholas, E. H.: Anatomy of congenital equinovarus. Boston Med. Surg. J., 36:150, 1897.

Ober, F. R.: An operation for the relief of congenital equinovarus deformity. Preliminary report. J.A.M.A., 65:621, 1915.

Ogston, A.: A new principle of curing clubfoot in severe cases in children a few years old. Br. Med. J., 1:1524, 1902.

Palmer, R. M.: The genetics of talipes equinovarus. J. Bone Joint Surg., 46A:542, 1964.

Pansini, A.: Indications and results of Codivilla operation in treatment of congenital club feet. Minerva Ortop., 16:158, 1965.

Parker, R. W.: Congenital Club-foot: Its Nature and Treatment. London, Lewis, 1887.

Parker, R. W., and Shattock, S. G.: The pathology and etiology of congenital club-foot. Trans. Path. Soc. London, 35:423, 1884.

Patterson, R. C., Parrish, H. J., and Hathaway, E. O.: Stabilizing operation on the foot. A study of the indications, techniques used and end results. J. Bone Joint Surg., 32A:1, 1950.

Penners, R.: Muskelanomalien bei angeborenen Klumpfüssen. Z. Orthop., 85:103, 1954.

Ponseti, I. V., and Smoley, E. M.: Congenital

club foot: the results of treatment. J. Bone Joint Surg., *45A*:261, 1963.

Primrose, D. A.: Talipes equinovarus in mental defectives. J. Bone Joint Surg., *51B*:60, 1969.

Reidy, J. A., Broderick, T. F., Jr., and Barr, J. S.: Tendon transplantations in the lower extremity. A review of end results in poliomyelitis. I. Tendon transplants about the foot and ankle. J. Bone Joint Surg., *34A*:900, 1952.

Salter, R. B.: Present trends in treatment of club feet. A.A.O.S. sound-slide program, 1965, No. 7.

Scarpa, A.: A memoir on the congenital club foot in children (translated from Italian by J. W. Wishart). Edinburgh, Constable and Co., 1818.

Scherb, R.: Zur Ätiologie Kongenitaler und Kongenital bedingter Fussdeformitäten mit besonderer Berücksichtingung des Pes equino-varus congenitus. Acta Chir. Scand., 67:717, 1930.

Schomburg, H.: Untersuchung der Entwicklung der Muskeln und Knochen des Menschlichen Fusses an Serienschnitten und Rekonstruktionen und unter Zuhülfenahme Makrosko-pischer Präparation. Gottinger, Kaestner, 1900.

Sell, L. S.: Tibial torsion accompanying congenital clubfoot. J. Bone Joint Surg., *23*:561, 1941.

Settle, G. W.: The anatomy of congenital talipes equinovarus: sixteen dissected specimens. J. Bone Joint Surg., *45A*:1341, 1963.

Singer, M.: Tibialis posterior transfer in congenital club foot. J. Bone Joint Surg., *43B*:717, 1961.

Singer, M., and Fripp, A. T.: Tibialis anterior transfer in congenital club foot. J. Bone Joint Surg., *40B*:252, 1958.

Somph, E., and Sulamad, M.: Early operative treatment of congenital club foot. Acta Orthop. Scand., *42*:513, 1971.

Steindler, A.: Stripping of the os calcis. J. Orthop. Surg., 2:8, 1920.

Stewart, S. F.: Club-foot: its incidence, cause and treatment. Anatomical-physiological study. J. Bone Joint Surg., *33A*:577, 1951.

Steytler, J. C. S., and Van der Walt, I. D.: Correction of resistant adduction of the forefoot in congenital clubfoot and congenital metatarsus varus by metatarsal osteotomy. Br. J. Surg., 53:558, 1966.

Swann, M., Lloyd-Roberts, G. C., and Catterall, A.: The anatomy of uncorrected clubfeet. J. Bone Joint Surg., *51B*:263, 1969.

Templeton, A. W., McAlister, W. H., and Zim, I. D.: Standardization of terminology and evaluation of osseous relationships in congenitally abnormal feet. Am. J. Roentgenol., 93:374, 1965.

Terry, R. J.: Sprengel's deformity and club-foot: an anthropological interpretation. Am. J. Phys. Anthropol., *17*:251, 1959.

Thomson, S. A.: Treatment of congenital talipes equinovarus with a modification of the Denis Browne method and splint. J. Bone Joint Surg., *24*:291, 1942.

Thomson, S. A.: The treatment of congenital club-foot. Nine years' experience with a modification of the Denis Browne method and splint. J. Bone Joint Surg., *31A*:431, 1949.

Thomson, S. A.: Modified Denis Browne splint for unilateral club-foot to protect the normal foot. J. Bone Joint Surg., *37A*:1286, 1955.

Turco, V. J.: Surgical correction of the resistant congenital club-foot—one-stage posteromedial release with internal fixation. A.A.O.S. Film No. 1293.

Turco, V. J.: Surgical correction of the resistant club foot. One-stage posteromedial release with internal fixation: a preliminary report. J. Bone Joint Surg., *53A*:477, 1971.

Wagner, L. C., and Butterfield, W. I.: Surgical release of contracted tissues for resistant congenital clubfoot. Am. J. Surg., *84*:82, 1952.

White, J. W., and Gulledge, W. H.: Skin-tight casts for treatment of club-foot. J. Bone Joint Surg., *33A*:475, 1951.

Widolfe, G. A.: Congenital club foot: better splint for conservative treatment. Med. J. Aust., *1*:846, 1973.

Wiley, A. M.: Club foot. An anatomical and experimental study of muscle growth. J. Bone Joint Surg., *41B*:821, 1959.

Wisbrun, W.: Neue Gesichtspunkte zum Redressement des angeborenen Klumpfusses und daraus sich ergebende Schlussfolgerungen bezüglich der Ätiologie. Arch. Orthop. Unfallchir., *31*:451, 1932.

Wynne-Davies, R.: Family studies and the cause of congenital clubfoot. J. Bone Joint Surg., *46B*:445, 1964.

Wynne-Davies, R.: Talipes equinovarus. A review of eighty-four cases after completion of treatment. J. Bone Joint Surg., *46B*:464, 1964.

Young, A. B.: Club foot treated by astragalectomy. Fifty year follow-up of a case. Lancet, *1*:670, 1962.

Zadek, I., and Barnett, E. L.: The importance of the ligaments of the ankle in correction of congenital clubfoot. J.A.M.A., 69:1057, 1917.

Metatarsus Varus

Berman, A., and Gartland, J. J.: Metatarsal osteotomy for the correction of adduction of the forepart of the foot in children. J. Bone Joint Surg., 53A:498, 1971.

Herndon, C. H.: Discussion of paper by Berman, A., and Gartland, J. J. J. Bone Joint Surg., 53A:505, 1971.

Heyman, C. H., Herndon, C. H., and Strong, J. M.: Mobilization of the tarsometatarsal and intermetatarsal joints for the correction of resistant adduction of the forepart of the foot in congenital clubfoot or congenital metatarsus varus. J. Bone Joint Surg., 40A:299, 1958.

Jacobs, J. E.: Metatarsus varus and hip dysplasia. Clin. Orthop., 16:203, 1960.

Kendrick, R. E., Sharma, N. K., Hassler, W. I., and Herndon, C. H.: Tarsometatarsal mobilization for resistant adduction of the forepart of the foot. J. Bone Joint Surg., 52A:61, 1970.

Kite, J. H.: Congenital metatarsus varus. Report of 300 cases. J. Bone Joint Surg., 32A:500, 1950.

Kite, J. H.: Congenital metatarsus varus. A.A.O.S. Instructional Course Lectures, 7:126. Ann Arbor, Michigan, J. W. Edwards, 1950.

Kite, J. H.: Congenital metatarsus varus. J. Bone Joint Surg., 49A:388, 1967.

Lusskin, R., and Lusskin, H.: A metatarsus varus splint for the pre-walker. J. Bone Joint Surg., 41A:363, 1959.

McCauley, J., Jr., Lusskin, R., and Bromley, J.: Recurrence in congenital metatarsus varus. J. Bone Joint Surg., 46A:525, 1964.

McCormick, D. W., and Blount, W. P.: Metatarsus adductovarus. "Skewfoot." J.A.M.A., 141:449, 1949.

Peabody, C. W., and Muro, F.: Congenital metatarsus varus. J. Bone Joint Surg., 15:171, 1933.

Ponseti, I. V., and Becker, J. R.: Congenital metatarsus adductus: the results of treatment. J. Bone Joint Surg., 48A:702, 1966.

Thomson, S. A.: Hallux varus and metatarsus varus. Clin. Orthop., 16:109, 1960.

Metatarsus Primus Varus and Hallux Valgus

Bonney, G., and MacNab, I.: Hallux valgus and hallux rigidus. A critical survey of operative results. J. Bone Joint Surg., 34B:366, 1952.

Carr, C. R., and Boyd, B. M.: Correctional osteotomy for metatarsus primus varus and hallux valgus. J. Bone Joint Surg., 50A:1353, 1968.

Cholmeley, J. A.: Hallux valgus in adolescents. Proc. R. Soc. Med. (Section of Orthopaedics), 51:903, 1958.

Ellis, V. H.: A method of correcting metatarsus primus varus. Preliminary report. J. Bone Joint Surg., 33B:415, 1951.

Haines, R. W., and McDougall, A.: The anatomy of hallux valgus. J. Bone Joint Surg., 36B:272, 1954.

Hardy, R. H., and Clapham, J. C. R.: Observations on hallux valgus. Based on controlled series. J. Bone Joint Surg., 33B:376, 1951.

Hardy, R. H., and Clapham, J. C. R.: Hallux valgus. Predisposing anatomic causes. Lancet, 1:1180, 1952.

Jones, A. R.: Hallux valgus in the adolescent. Proc. R. Soc. Med. (Section of Orthopaedics), 41:392, 1948.

Kelikian, H.: Hallux Valgus. Allied Deformities of the Forefoot and Metatarsalgia. Philadelphia, W. B. Saunders Company, 1965.

Keller, W. L.: Surgical treatment of bunion and hallux valgus. N. Y. Med. J., 80:741, 1904.

Keller, W. L.: Further observations on the surgical treatment of hallux valgus and bunions. N. Y. Med. J., 95:696, 1912.

Lapidus, P. W.: Operative correction of the metatarsus primus varus in hallux valgus. Surg. Gynecol., Obstet., 58:183, 1934.

McBride, E. D.: A conservative operation for bunions. J. Bone Joint Surg., 10:735, 1928.

McBride, E. D.: Hallux valgus, bunion deformity; its treatment in mild, moderate and severe stages. J. Int. Coll. Surg., 21:99, 1954.

McBride, E. D.: The McBride bunion hallux valgus operation. Refinements in the successive surgical steps of the operation. J. Bone Joint Surg., 42A:965, 1960.

Mitchell, C. I., Fleming, J. I., Allen, R., Glenney, C., and Sanford, G. A.: Osteotomy-bunionectomy for hallux valgus. J. Bone Joint Surg., 40A:41, 1958.

Piggott, H.: The natural history of hallux valgus in adolescence and early adult life. J. Bone Joint Surg., 42B:749, 1960.

Silver, D.: The operative treatment of hallux valgus. J. Bone Joint Surg., 5:225, 1923.

Simmonds, F. A., and Menelaus, M. B.: Hallux valgus in adolescents. J. Bone Joint Surg., 42B:761, 1960.

Tarsal Coalitions

Anderson, R. J.: The presence of an astragalo-scaphoid bone in man. J. Anat. Physiol., 14:452, 1880.

Anthonsen, W.: An oblique projection for roentgen examination of the talo-calcanean joint, particularly regarding intra-articular fracture of the calcaneus. Acta Radiol., 24:306, 1943.

Austin, F. H.: Symphalangism and related fusions of tarsal bones. Radiology, 56:882, 1951.

Badgley, C. E.: Coalition of the calcaneus and the navicular. Arch. Surg., 15:75, 1927.

Bargellini, D.: Fusione calcaneo-cuboidea e piede piatoo. Arch. Ital. Chir., 21:386, 1928.

Basu, S. S.: Naviculo-cuneo-metatarsophalangeal synostoses. Indian J. Surg., 25:750, 1963.

Bentzon, P. G. K.: Bilateral congenital deformity of the astragalocalcanean joint. Coalition calcaneonavicularis, mit besonderer Bezungnahme auf die operative Behandlung des durch diese Anomalie bedingten Plattfusses. Verh. Dtsch. Orthop. Ges., 23:269, 1929.

Bersani, F. A., and Samilson, R. L.: Massive familial tarsal synostosis. J. Bone Joint Surg., 39A:1187, 1957.

Blockey, N. J.: Peroneal spastic flat foot. J. Bone Joint Surg., 37B:191, 1955.

Boyd, H. B.: Congenital talonavicular synostosis. J. Bone Joint Surg., 26:682, 1944.

Braddock, G. T. F.: A prolonged follow-up of peroneal spastic flat foot. J. Bone Joint Surg., 43B:734, 1961.

Brobeck, O.: Congenital bilateral synostosis of the calcaneus and cuboid and of the triquetral and hamate bones. Report of a case. Acta Orthop. Scand., 26:217, 1957.

Bullitt, J. B.: Variations of the bones of the foot. Fusion of the talus and navicular, bilateral and congenital. Am. J. Roentgenol., 20:548, 1928.

Chambers, C. H.: Congenital anomalies of the tarsal navicular with particular reference to calcaneonavicular coalition. Br. J. Radiol., 23:580, 1950.

Conway, J. J., and Cowell, H. R.: Tarsal coalition: clinical significance and roentgenographic demonstration. Radiology, 92:799, 1969.

Cowell, H. R.: Extensor brevis arthroplasty. J. Bone Joint Surg., 52A:820, 1970.

Cruveilhier, J.: Anatomie Pathologique du Corps Humain, Tome I. Paris, 1829.

Del Sel, J. M., and Grand, N. E.: Cubonavicular synostosis: a rare tarsal synostosis. J. Bone Joint Surg., 41B:149, 1959.

Demarchi, E., Gambier, R., and Vespignani, L.: Les synostoses tarsiennes dans le pied plat valgus douloureux. J. Radiol., 36:665, 1955.

Devoldere, J.: A case of familial congenital synostosis in the carpal and tarsal bones. Arch. Chir. Neerl., 12:185, 1960.

Dwight, T.: A Clinical Atlas. Variations of the Bones of the Hands and Feet. Philadelphia, J. B. Lippincott Co., 1907.

Feist, J. H., and Mankin, H. J.: The tarsus. Radiology, 79:250, 1962.

Gaynor, S. S.: Congenital astragalocalcaneal fusion. J. Bone Joint Surg., 18:479, 1936.

Glessner, J. R., Jr., and Davis, G. L.: Bilateral calcaneonavicular coalition occurring in twin boys. A case report. Clin. Orthop., 47:173, 1966.

Grashey, R.: Articulatio talo-calcanea (Os sustentaculi). Roentgenpraxis, 14:139, 1942.

Hall, M. C.: The normal movement at the sub-talar joint. Can. J. Surg., 2:287, 1959.

Hark, F. W.: Congenital anomalies of the tarsal bones. Clin. Orthop., 16:21, 1960.

Harle, T. S., and Stevenson, J. R.: Hereditary symphalangism associated with carpal and tarsal fusion. Radiology, 89:91, 1967.

Harris, B. A.: Anomalous structures in the developing human foot (abstr.). Anat. Rec., 121:399, 1955.

Harris, R. I.: Rigid valgus foot due to talocalcaneal bridge. J. Bone Joint Surg., 37A:169, 1955.

Harris, R. I.: Peroneal spastic flat foot. A.A.O.S. Instructional Course Lectures, Vol. 15. Ann Arbor, J. W. Edwards, 1958.

Harris, R. I.: Retrospect: peroneal spastic flat foot (rigid valgus foot). J. Bone Joint Surg., 47A:1657, 1965.

Harris, R. I., and Beath, T.: Army Foot Survey. Ottawa, National Research Council of Canada 44, 1947.

Harris, R. I., and Beath, T.: Etiology of peroneal spastic flat foot. J. Bone Joint Surg., 30B:624, 1948.

Harris, R. I., and Beath, T.: John Hunter's specimen of talocalcaneal bridge. J. Bone Joint Surg., 32B:203, 1950.

Hayek, W.: Synostosis talonavicularis. Z. Orthop. Chir., 69:231, 1934.

Heikel, H. V. A.: Coalition calcaneonavicularis and calcaneus secundarius. A clinical and radiographic study of twenty-three patients. Acta Orthop. Scand., 32:72, 1962.

Hodgson, F. G.: Talonavicular synostosis. South. Med. J., 39:940, 1946.

Holl, M.: Beiträge zur chirurgischen Osteologie des Füsses. Arch. Klin. Chir., 25:211, 1880.

Isherwood, I.: A radiologic approach to the subtalar joint. J. Bone Joint Surg., 43B:566, 1961.

Jack, E. A.: Bone anomalies of the tarsus in relation to "peroneal spastic flat foot." J. Bone Joint Surg., 36B:530, 1954.

Jaubert de Beaujeu, A., Benmussa: Synostose, astragalo-scaphoïdienne congénitale, bilatérale et isolée. J. Radiol. Electrol., 23:348, 1939.

Johansoon, S.: A case of congenital ankylosis of the ankle joints and other malformations. Acta Orthop. Scand., 5:231, 1934.

Kadelbach, G.: Ein Beiträg zu den Fusswurzelsynostosen. Arch. Orthop. Unfallchir., 40:363, 1940.

Kendrick, J. I.: Treatment of calcaneonavicular bar. J.A.M.A., 172:1242, 1960.

Kirmisson, E.: Double pied bot varus par malformation osseuse primitive associé a des ankyloses congénitales des doigts et des orteils chez quatre membres d'une même famille. Rev. Orthop., 9:392, 1898.

Korvin, H.: Coalition Talocalcanea. Z. Orthop. Chir., 60:105, 1934.

Kozlowski, K.: Hypoplasie bilatérale congénitale du cubitus et synostose bilatérale calcanéocuboide chez une fillette. Ann. Radiol., 8:389, 1965.

LaGrange, M.: Anomalie du pied. Soudure des os du tarse et du métatarse. Progr. Med., 10:367, 1882.

Lapidus, P. W.: Bilateral congenital talonavicular fusion. Report of a case. J. Bone Joint Surg., 20:775, 1938.

Lapidus, P. W.: Spastic flat foot. J. Bone Joint Surg, 28:126, 1946.

Lisoos, I., and Soussi, J.: Tarsal synostosis with partial adactylia. Med. Proc., 11:224, 1965.

Lusby, H. I. J.: Naviculo-cuneiform synostosis. J. Bone Joint Surg., 41B:140, 1959.

Mahaffey, H. W.: Bilateral congenital calcaneocuboid synostosis. Case report. J. Bone Joint Surg., 27:164, 1945.

Maudsley, R. S.: Spastic pes varus. Proc. R. Soc. Med., 49:181, 1956.

Miller, E. M.: Congenital ankylosis of joints of hands and feet. J. Bone Joint Surg., 4:560, 1922.

Mitchell, G. P., and Gibson, J. M. C.: Excision of calcaneonavicular bar for painful spasmodic flat foot. J. Bone Joint Surg., 49B:281, 1967.

Nievergelt, K.: Positiver Vaterschaftsnachweis auf Grund Erbicher mit Bildungen der Extremitaten. Arch. Julius Klaus Stift., 19:157, 1944.

O'Donoghue, D. H., and Sell, L. S.: Congenital talonavicular synostosis. J. Bone Joint Surg., 25:925, 1943.

O'Rahilly, R.: A survey of carpal and tarsal anomalies. J. Bone Joint Surg., 35A:626, 1953.

O'Rahilly, R., Gardner, E., and Gray, D. J.: The skeletal development of the foot. Clin. Orthop., 16:7, 1960.

Outland, T., and Murphy, I. D.: Relation of tarsal anomalies to spastic and rigid flat feet. Clin. Orthop., 1:217, 1953.

Outland, T., and Murphy, I. D.: The pathomechanics of peroneal spastic flat foot. Clin. Orthop., 16:64, 1960.

Pearlman, H. S., Edkin, R. E., and Warren, R. F.: Familial tarsal and carpal synostosis with radial head subluxation. J. Bone Joint Surg., 46A:585, 1964.

Pfitzner, W.: Die Variationen im Aufbar des Fussekelts. Bertrage zur Kenntniss des menschlichen Extremitatenskelets. VII. Morphol. Arbeit., 6:245, 1896.

Rompe, G.: Ankylosen des Unteren Sprunggelenkes nach Offenem Unterschenkelbruch. Arch. Orthop. Unfallchir., 54:339, 1962.

Rothberg, A. S., Feldman, J. W., and Schuster, O. F.: Congenital fusion of astragalus and scaphoid: bilateral, inherited. N. Y. J. Med., 35:29, 1935.

Rutt, A.: Zur Genese der Coalitio calcaneo naviculare. Z. Orthop., 96:96, 1962.

Sanghi, J. K., and Roby, H. R.: Bilateral peroneal spastic flat feet associated with congenital fusion of the navicular and talus. A case report. J. Bone Joint Surg., 43A:1237, 1961.

Schreiber, R. R.: Talonavicular synostosis. J. Bone Joint Surg., 45A:170, 1963.

Seddon, H. J.: Calcaneo-scaphoid coalition. Proc. R. Soc. Med. (Section of Orthopaedics), 26:419, 1932.

Shands, J. R., and Wentz, I. J.: Congenital anomalies, accessory bones, and osteochondritis in the feet of 850 children. Surg. Clin. North Am., 33:1643, 1953.

Simmons, E. H.: Spastic tibialis varus with tarsal coalition. J. Bone Joint Surg., 47B:533, 1965.

Sloane, M. W. M.: A case of anomalous skeletal development in the foot. Anat. Rec., 96:23, 1946.

Slomann, H. C.: On coalition calcaneonavicularis. J. Orthop. Surg., 3:586, 1921.

Slomann, H. C.: On the demonstration and analysis of calcaneo-navicular coalition by roentgen examination. Acta Radiol., 5:304, 1926.

Solger, B.: Ueber abnorme Verschmelzung Knorpeliger Skelettheile Beim Fotus. Zentralbl. Allg. Pathol., 1:124, 1890.

Sutro, C.: Anomalous talocalcaneal articulation. Cause for limited subtalar movements. Am. J. Surg., 74:64, 1947.

Trolle, D.: Accessory Bones of the Human Foot (translated by E. Aagesen). Copenhagen, Munksgaard, 1948.

Vaughan, W. H., and Segal, G.: Tarsal coalition with special reference to roentgenographic interpretation. Radiology, 60:855, 1953.

Veneruso, L. C.: Unilateral congenital calcaneocuboid synostosis with complete absence of a metatarsal and toe. Case report. J. Bone Joint Surg., 27:718, 1945.

Wagoner, G. W.: A case of bilateral congenital fusion of the calcanei and cuboids. J. Bone Joint Surg., 10:220, 1928.

Waugh, W.: Partial cubo-navicular coalition as a cause of peroneal spastic flat foot. J. Bone Joint Surg., 39B:520, 1957.

Webster, F. S., and Roberts, W. M.: Tarsal anomalies and peroneal spastic flat foot. J.A.M.A., 146:1099, 1951.

Wray, J. B., and Herndon, C. N.: Hereditary transmission of congenital coalition of the calcaneus to the navicular. J. Bone Joint Surg., 45A:365, 1963.

Zock, E.: Ein Beiträg zu den Synostosen der Fusswurzel. Zentralbl. Chir., 78:845, 1953.

Zuckerkandl, E.: Ueber einen Fall von Synostose zwischen Talus und Calcaneus. Allg. Wein. Med. Zeitung., 22:293, 1877.

Convex Pes Valgus

Armknecht, P.: Orthopädische Lieden bei Zwillingen, Vergh. Dsch. Orthop. Ges., 26:62, 1931.

Aschner, B., and Engelmann, G.: Constitutronspathologie in der Orthopädie. Erbbiologie des peripheren Bewegungsapparates. Vienna, Julius Springer, 1928.

Bender, G., and Horvath, F.: Über eine seltene Entwicklungsanomalie des Talus und des Os Naviculare pedis. Fortschr. Roentgenstr., 94:281, 1961.

Berman, J. L., Rankin, J. K., Harrison, P. A., Donovan, D. J., Hogan, W. J., and Bearn, A. O.: Autosomal trisomy of a group 16-18 chromosome. J. Pediatr., 60:503, 1962.

Böhm, M.: Der Kongenitale Plattfuss. Zentralbl. Chir., 1932.

Camera, V.: A proposito del piedo piatoo valgo congenito. Arch. Ortop., 42:432, 1926.

Coleman, S. S., Martin, A. F., and Jarrett, J.: Congenital vertical talus: pathogenesis and treatment. J. Bone Joint Surg., 48A:1442, 1966.

Coleman, S. S., Stelling, F. H., and Jarrett, J.: Pathomechanics and treatment of congenital vertical talus. Clin. Orthop., 70:62, 1970.

Drennan, J. C., and Sharrard, W. J. W.: The pathologic anatomy of convex pes valgus. J. Bone Joint Surg., 53B:455, 1971.

Eyre-Brook, A.: Congenital vertical talus. J. Bone Joint Surg., 49B:618, 1967.

Grice, D. S.: The role of subtalar fusion in the treatment of valgus deformities of the feet. A.A.O.S. Instructional Course Lectures, Vol. 16. St. Louis, C. V. Mosby Co., 1959.

Gunz, E.: Die pathologische Anatomie der angeborenen Platfusses. Z. Orthop., 69:219, 1939.

Haliburton, R. A., Sullivan, C. R., Kelly, P., and Peterson, L. F. A.: The extra-osseous and intra-osseous blood supply of the talus. J. Bone Joint Surg., 40A:1115, 1958.

Hark, F. W.: Rocker-foot due to congenital subluxation of the talus. J. Bone Joint Surg., 32A:344, 1950.

Harrold, A. J.: Congenital vertical talus in infancy. J. Bone Joint Surg., 49B:634, 1967.

Haveson, S. B.: Congenital flatfoot due to talonavicular dislocation (vertical talus). Radiology, 72:19, 1959.

Henken, R.: Contribution à l'étude des formes osseuses du pied plat valgus congénital. Thèse de Lyon, 1914.

Herndon, C. H., and Heyman, C. H.: Problems in the recognition and treatment of congenital convex pes valgus. J. Bone Joint Surg., 45A:413, 1963.

Heyman, C. H.: The diagnosis and treatment of congenital convex pes valgus or vertical talus. A.A.O.S. Instructional Course Lectures, Vol. 16. St. Louis, C. V. Mosby Co., 1959.

Hohmann, G.: Fuss und Bein. Munich, J. F. Bergmann, 1934, pp. 26–33.

Hughes, J. R.: Congenital vertical talus. J. Bone Joint Surg., 39B:580, 1957.

Hughes, J. R.: Pathologic anatomy and pathogenesis of congenital vertical talus and its practical significance. J. Bone Joint Surg., 39B:580, 1957.

Joachimsthal: Euber pes valgus congenitus. Dtsch. Med. Wochenschr., 29:123, 1903.

Lamy, L., and Weissman, L.: Congenital convex pes valgus. J. Bone Joint Surg., 21:79, 1939.

Lange, F.: Plattfussbeschwerben und Plattfussbehandlung. Munch. Med. Wochenschr., 59:300, 1912.

Lloyd-Roberts, G. C., and Spence, A. J.: Congenital vertical talus. J. Bone Joint Surg., 40B:33, 1958.

Mau, C.: Muskelbefunde und ihre Bedeutung beim angeborenen Klumpfussleiden. Arch. Orthop. Unfallchir., 28:292, 1930.

Mead, N. C., and Anast, G.: Vertical talus. Clin. Orthop., 21:198, 1961.

Nové-Josserand: Formes anatomiques du pied plat. Rev. Orthop., 10:117, 1923.

Osmond-Clarke, H.: Congenital vertical talus. J. Bone Joint Surg., 38B:334, 1956.

Outland, T., and Hserk, H. H.: Congenital vertical talus. A.A.O.S. Instructional Course Lectures, Vol. 16. St. Louis, C. V. Mosby Co., 1959.

Parrish, T. F.: Congenital convex pes valgus accompanied by previously undescribed anatomic derangements. South. Med. J. 60:983, 1967.

Patterson, W. R., Fitz, D. A., and Smith, W. S.: The pathologic anatomy of congenital convex pes valgus. J. Bone Surg., 50A:458, 1968.

Rocher, H. L., and Pouyanne, L.: Pied plat congénital para subluxation sous-astragalienne congénitale et orientation verticale de l'astragale. Bordeaux Chir., 5:249, 1934.

Sharrard, W. J. W., and Grossfield, I.: The management of deformity and paralysis of the foot in myelomeningocele. J. Bone Joint Surg., 50B:456, 1968.

Sonnenburg: Klumpfuss. In Eulenburg: Real-Encyclopadie der gesamten Heilkunde, Aufl. 3, Bd. 12, s. 368. Wein, Urban und Schwarzenberg, 1897.

Stone, K. H., and Lloyd-Roberts, G. C.: Congenital vertical talus: a new operation. Proc. R. Soc. Med., 56:12, 1963.

Storen, H.: On the closed and open correction of congenital convex pes valgus with a vertical astragalus. Acta Orthop. Scand., 36:352, 1965.

Storen, H.: Congenital convex pes valgus with vertical talus. Acta Orthop. Scand., 94(Suppl.):1, 1967.

Wainwright, D.: The recognition and cure of congenital flat foot. Proc. R. Soc. Med., 57:357, 1964.

Ball-and-Socket Joint

Brahme, F.: Upper talar enarthrosis. Acta Radiol., 55:221, 1961.

Jacobs, P.: Some uncommon deformities of the ankle and foot. Br. J. Radiol., 35:776, 1962.

Lamb, D.: The ball-and-socket ankle joint. J. Bone Joint Surg., 40B:240, 1958.

Robins, R. H. G.: The ankle joint in relation to arthrodesis of the foot in poliomyelitis. J. Bone Joint Surg., 41B:337, 1959.

Schreiber, R. R.: Congenital and acquired ball-and-socket ankle joint. Radiology, 84:940, 1963.

Weston, W. J.: Congenital ball and socket ankle joint. Br. J. Radiol., 35:871, 1962.

Hallux Varus

Farmer, A. W.: Congenital hallus varus. Am. J. Surg., 95:274, 1958.

Kelikian, H., Clayton, L., and Loseff, H.: Surgical syndactylism of the toes. Clin. Orthop., 19:208, 1961.

McElvenny, R. T.: Hallux varus. Q. Bull. Northwest. Med. Sch., 15:277, 1941.

Thomson, S. A.: Hallux varus and metatarsus varus. Clin. Orthop., 16:109, 1960.

Split Foot (Lobster Claw)

Cowan, R. J.: Surgical problems associated with congenital malformations of the forefoot. Can. J. Surg., 8:29, 1965.

Meyerding, H. W., and Upshaw, J. E.: Heredofamilial cleft foot deformity (lobster-claw or split foot). Am. J. Surg., 74:889, 1947.

Phillips, R. S.: Congenital split foot (lobster claw) and triphalangeal thumb. J. Bone Joint Surg., 53B:247, 1971.

Potter, E. L., and Nadelhoffer, L.: A familial lobster claw. J. Hered., 38:331, 1947.

Stiles, K. A., and Pickard, I. S.: Hereditary malformations of the hands and feet. J. Hered., 34:341, 1943.

Vogel, F.: Verzogerte Mutation biem Mescchen, einige kritische Bemerkungen zu Ch.

Auberbachs Arbeit. Ann. Hum. Genet., 22:132, 1958.

Walker, J. C., and Clodius, L.: The syndromes of cleft lip, cleft palate and lobster-claw deformities of hands and feet. Plast. Reconstr. Surg., 32:627, 1963.

PES CAVUS

Alvik, I.: Operative treatment of pes cavus. Acta Orthop. Scand., 23:137, 1953.

Barenfeld, P. A., Weseley, M. S., and Shea, J. M.: The congenital cavus foot. Clin. Orthop., 79:119, 1971.

Barwell, R.: Pes planus and pes cavus: an anatomical and clinical study. Edinburgh Med. J., 3:113, 1898.

Bentzon, P. G. K.: Pes cavus and the m. peroneus longus. Acta Orthop. Scand., 4:50, 1933.

Bertrand, P.: Le pied creux essentiel. Discussion-symposium. Rev. Chir. Orthop., 53:423, 1967.

Beykirch, A.: Ein Beltrag zur Atiologie und Therapie des Klauenhohlfusses. Z. Orthop. Chir., 52:41, 1929.

Brewerton, D. A., Sandifer, P. H., and Sweetman, D. R.: "Idiopathic" pes cavus, an investigation of its etiology. Br. Med. J., 5358:659, 1963.

Brockway, A.: Surgical correction of talipes cavus deformities. J. Bone Joint Surg., 22:895, 1940.

Cole, W. H.: The treatment of claw-foot. J. Bone Joint Surg., 22:895, 1940.

Coonrad, R. W., Irwin, C. E., Gucker, T. III, and Wray, J. B.: The importance of plantar muscles in paralytic varus feet; results of treatment by neurectomy and myoneurectomy. J. Bone Joint Surg., 38A:563, 1956.

Duchenne, G. B.: Physiology of Motion (translated and edited by E. B. Kaplan). Philadelphia, W. B. Saunders Company, 1959, p. 384.

Dwyer, F. C.: Osteotomy of the calcaneum for pes cavus. J. Bone Joint Surg., 41B:80, 1959.

Fowler, B., Brooks, A. L., and Parrish, T. F.: The cavovarus foot. J. Bone Joint Surg., 41A:757, 1959.

Frank, G. R., and Johnson, W. M.: The extensor shift procedure in the correction of clawtoe deformities in children. South. Med. J., 59:889, 1966.

Garceau, G. J., and Brahms, M. A.: A preliminary study of selective plantar-muscle denervation for pes cavus. J. Bone Joint Surg., 38A:553, 1956.

Hackenbroch, M.: Der Hohlfuss. Berlin, J. Springer, 1928, p. 83.

Hallgrimsson, S.: Pes cavus, seine Behandlung

und Einige Bennerkungen uber seine Aetiologie. Acta Orthop. Scand., *10*:73, 1939.

Hammond, G.: Elevation of the first metatarsal bone with hallux equinus. Surgery, *13*:240, 1943.

Heyman, C. H.: The operative treatment for clawfoot. J. Bone Joint Surg., *14*:334, 1932.

Hibbs, R. A.: An operation for "claw-foot." J.A.M.A., 73:1583, 1919.

Hughes, W. K.: Talipes cavus. Br. Med. J., 2:902, 1940.

Ingelrans, P.: Le pied creux essentiel. Discussion-symposium. Rev. Chir. Orthop., 53:422, 1967.

Japas, I. M.: Surgical treatment of pes cavus by tarsal V-osteotomy. Preliminary report. J. Bone Joint Surg., *50A*:927, 1968.

Jones, R.: The soldier's foot and the treatment of common deformities of the foot. Part II: Claw-foot. Br. Med. J., *1*:749, 1916.

Kelikian, H.: Hallux Valgus, Allied Deformities of the Forefoot and Metatarsalgia. Philadelphia, W. B. Saunders Company, 1965.

Kleinberg, S., Horwitz, T., and Sobel, R.: Pes cavus. Bull. Hosp. Joint Dis., *10*:252, 1949.

Lambrinudi, C.: An operation for claw-toes. Proc. R. Soc. Med., *21*:239, 1927.

McElvenny, R. T., and Caldwell, G. D.: A new operation for correction of cavus foot. Fusion of first metatarsocuneiform-navicular joints. Clin. Orthop., *11*:85, 1958.

Meary, R.: Le pied creux essentiel. Symposium. Rev. Chir. Orthop., *53*:389, 1967.

Mills, G. P.: The etiology and treatment of claw foot. J. Bone Joint Surg., *6*:142, 1924.

Parkin, A.: Causation and mode of production of pes cavus. Br. Med. J., *1*:1285, 1891.

Rütt, A.: Der Hohlfuss. *In* Handbuch der Orthopadie, Bd. IV/2. Stuttgart, Thieme, 1961, pp. 1068–1095.

Saunders, J. T.: Etiology and treatment of clawfoot. Arch. Surg., *30*:179, 1935.

Scheer, G. E., and Crego, C. H., Jr.: A two-stage stabilization procedure for correction of calcaneocavus. J. Bone Joint Surg., *38A*:1247, 1956.

Schnepp, K. H.: Hammer-toe and claw-foot. Am. J. Surg., *36*:351, 1937

Siffert, R. S., Forster, R. I., and Nachamie, B.: "Beak" triple arthrodesis for correction of severe cavus deformity. Clin. Orthop., *45*:101, 1966.

Stauffer, R. N., Nelson, G. E., and Bianco, A. J., Jr.: Calcaneal osteotomy in treatment of cavo varus foot. Mayo Clin. Proc., *45*:624, 1970.

Steindler, A.: Stripping of the os calcis. J. Orthop. Surg., *2*:8, 1920.

Steindler, A.: The treatment of pes cavus. Arch. Surg., *2*:325, 1921.

Taylor, R. G.: The treatment of claw toes by multiple transfer of flexors into extensor tendons. J. Bone Joint Surg., *33B*:539, 1951.

PRONATED FEET

Basmajian, J. R., and Stecko, G.: The role of muscles in arch support of the foot. An electromyographic study. J. Bone Joint Surg., *45A*:1184, 1963.

Bettmann, F.: The treatment of flat-foot by means of exercise. J. Bone Joint Surg., *19*:821, 1937.

Butte, F. L.: Navicular-cuneiform arthrodesis for flat-foot. J. Bone Joint Surg., *19*:496, 1937.

Chambers, E. F. S.: An operation for correction of flexible flat feet of adolescents. West. J. Surg., *54*:77, 1946.

Chandler, F. A.: Children's feet, normal and presenting common abnormalities. Am. J. Dis. Child., 63:1136, 1942.

Clark, W. A.: A rebalancing operation for pronated feet. J. Bone Joint Surg., *13*:867, 1931.

Crego, C. H., Jr., and Ford, I. T.: An end-result study of various operative procedures for correcting flat feet in children. J. Bone Joint Surg., *34A*:183, 1952.

Grice, D. S.: An extra-articular arthrodesis of the subastragalar joint for correction of paralytic flat-feet in children. J. Bone Joint Surg., *34A*:927, 1952.

Haraldson, S.: Pes plano-valgus staticus juvenilis and its operative treatment. Acta Orthop. Scand., *35*:234, 1965.

Harris, R. I., and Beath, T.: Hypermobile flatfoot with short tendo Achillis. J. Bone Joint Surg., *30A*:116, 1948.

Harris, R. I., and Beath, T.: Spastic flatfoot. J. Bone Joint Surg., *30B*:624, 1948.

Helfet, A. J.: A new way of treating flat feet in children. Lancet, *1*:262, 1956.

Hicks, J. H.: The function of the plantar aponeurosis. J. Anat., 85:414, 1951.

Hicks, J. H.: The mechanics of the foot. I. The joints. J. Anat., 85:343, 1953.

Hicks, J. H.: The mechanics of the foot. II. The plantar aponeurosis and the arch. J. Anat., 88:25, 1954.

Hoke, M.: An operation for the correction of extremely relaxed flat feet. J. Bone Joint Surg., *13*:773, 1931.

Jack, E. A.: Naviculocuneiform fusion in the treatment of flat-foot. J. Bone Joint Surg., *35B*:75, 1953.

Jones, B. S.: Flat foot, a preliminary report of an operation for severe cases. J. Bone Joint Surg., *57A*:297, 1975.

Kidner, F. C.: The prehallux in relation to flat foot. J. Bone Joint Surg., *11*:831, 1929.

Koutsogiannis, E.: Treatment of mobile flat foot by displacement osteotomy of calcaneus. J. Bone Joint Surg., 53B:96, 1971.

Leavitt, D. G.: Subastragaloid arthrodesis for the os calcis type of flat-foot. Am. J. Surg., 59:501, 1943.

Leonard, M. H., Gonzalez, S., Breck, L. W., Basom, C., Palafox, M., and Kosick, Z. W.: Lateral transfer of the posterior tibial tendon in certain selected cases of pes planovalgus. Clin. Orthop., 40:139, 1965.

Miller, O. L.: A plastic flat foot operation. J. Bone Joint Surg., 9:84, 1927.

Purvis, G. D.: Surgery of the relaxed flat foot. Clin. Orthop., 57:221, 1968.

Rose, G. K.: Correction of the pronated foot. J. Bone Joint Surg., 40B:674, 1958.

Rose, G. K.: Correction of the pronated foot. J. Bone Joint Surg., 44B:642, 1962.

Rugtbeit, A.: Extra-articular subtalar arthrodesis according to Green-Grice in flat feet. Acta Orthop. Scand., 34:367, 1964.

Seymour, N.: The late results of naviculo-cuneiform fusion. J. Bone Joint Surg., 49B:558, 1967.

Seymour, N., and Evans, D. K.: A modification of the Grice subtalar arthrodesis. J. Bone Joint Surg., 50B:372, 1968.

Williams, P. F., and Menelaus, M. B.: Triple arthrodesis by inlay grafting — a method suitable for the undeformed or valgus foot. J. Bone Joint Surg., 59B:333, 1977.

Young, C. S.: Operative treatment of pes planus. Surg. Gynecol. Obstet., 68:1099, 1939.

Zadek, I.: Transverse wedge arthrodesis for the relief of pain in rigid flat-foot. J. Bone Joint Surg., 17:453, 1935.

HALLUX RIGIDUS

Bingold, A. C., and Collins, D. H.: Hallux rigidus. J. Bone Joint Surg., 32B:214, 1950.

Bonney, G., and MacNab, I.: Hallux valgus and hallux rigidus. A critical survey of operative results. J. Bone Joint Surg., 34B:366, 1952.

Breitenfelder, G.: Hallux rigidus Jugendlicher, Verh. Dtsch. Orthop. Ges., 80:313, 1951.

Cochrane, W. A.: An operation for hallux rigidus. Br. Med. J., 1:1095, 1927.

Glissan, D. J.: Hallux valgus and hallux rigidus. Med. J. Aust., 2:585, 1946.

Harrison, M. H. M., and Harvey, F. J.: Arthrodesis of the first metatarso-phalangeal joint for hallux valgus and rigidus. J. Bone Joint Surg., 45A:471, 1963.

Jack, E. A.: The aetiology of hallux rigidus. Br. J. Surg., 27:492, 1940.

Jansen, M.: Hallux valgus, rigidus and malleus. J. Orthop. Surg., 3:27, 1921.

Kelikian, H.: Hallux Valgus, Allied Deformities

of the Forefoot and Metatarsalgia. Philadelphia, W. B. Saunders Company, 1965.

Kessel, L., and Bonney, G.: Hallux rigidus in the adolescent. J. Bone Joint Surg., 40B:668, 1958.

Kingreen, O.: Zur Aetiologie des Hallux flexus. Zentralbl. Chir., 60:2116, 1933.

Lambrinudi, C.: Metatarsus primus elevatus. Proc. R. Soc. Med. (Section of Orthopaedics), 31:1273, 1938.

McMurray, T. P.: The treatment of hallux valgus and rigidus. Br. Med. J., 2:218, 1936.

Moynihan, F. J.: Arthrodesis of the metatarsophalangeal joint of the great toe. J. Bone Joint Surg., 49B:544, 1967.

Nilsonne, H.: Hallux rigidus and its treatment. Acta Orthop. Scand., 1:295, 1930.

Severin, E.: Removal of the base of the proximal phalanx in hallux rigidus. Acta Orthop. Scand., 17:77, 1947.

Steinhauser, W.: Osteochondrose der basalen epiphyse der Grundphalanx, Grosszehe und Hallux rigidus. Beitr. Ges. Orthop., 6:177, 1959.

Walsham, W. J., and Hughes, W. K.: The deformities of the human foot. London, Baillière, Tindall and Cox, 1895, pp. 512–514.

Waterman, H.: Die Arthritis deformans Grosszehengrundgelenkes. Z. Orthop. Chir., 48:346, 1927.

Watson-Jones, R.: Treatment of hallux rigidus. Br. Med. J., 1:1165, 1927.

HAMMER TOES AND CLAW TOES

Dickson, F. D., and Dively, R. L.: Operation for correction of mild claw foot, the result of infantile paralysis. J.A.M.A., 87:1275, 1926.

Ely, L. W.: Hammertoe. Surg. Clin. North Am., 6:433, 1926.

Forrester-Brown, M. F.: Tendon transplantation for clawing of the great toe. J. Bone Joint Surg., 20:57, 1938.

Girdlestone, G. R.: Physiotherapy for hand and foot. Journal of the Chartered Society of Physiotherapy, 32:176, 1947.

Glassman, F., Wallin, L., and Sideman, S.: Phalangectomy for toe deformities. Surg. Clin. North Am., 29:275, 1949.

Jones, R.: Notes on Military Orthopaedics. New York, P. B. Hoeber, 1917.

Krenz, L.: Die Hammerzehen und ihre Operation nacht Bocht. Arch. Orthop. Unfallchir., 21:459, 1923.

Lambrinudi, C.: An operation for claw-toes. Proc. R. Soc. Med., 21:239, 1927.

Lapidus, P. W.: Operation for correction of hammertoe. J. Bone Joint Surg., 21:977, 1939.

Merrill, W. J.: Conservative operative treatment of hammertoe. Am. J. Orthop. Surg., *10*:262, 1912.

Michele, A. A., and Krueger, F. J.: Operative correction for hammertoe. Mil. Surg., *103*:52, 1948.

Milgram, J. E.: Office measures for relief of the painful foot. J. Bone Joint Surg., *46*:1095, 1964.

O'Neil, J.: An arthroplastic operation for hammertoe. J.A.M.A., *57*:1207, 1911.

Pyper, J. B.: The flexor-extensor transplant operation for claw toes. J. Bone Joint Surg., *40B*:428, 1958.

Schig, S.: Hammertoe: a new procedure for its correction. Surg. Gynecol. Obstet., *72*:101, 1941.

Sharrard, W. J. W., and Smith, T. W. D.: Tenodesis of flexor hallucis longus for paralytic clawing of the hallux in childhood. J. Bone Joint Surg., *58B*:224, 1976.

Soule, R. E.: Operation for the cure of hammertoe. N.Y. Med. J., *91*:649, 1910.

Taylor, R. G.: An operative procedure for the treatment of hammer toe and claw toe. J. Bone Joint Surg., *22*:608, 1940.

Taylor, R. G.: The treatment of claw toes by multiple transfers of flexor into extensor tendons. J. Bone Joint Surg., *33B*:539, 1951.

Trethowan, W. H.: The treatment of hammertoe. Lancet, *1*:1257, 1925.

Young, C. S.: An operation for correction of hammertoe and claw toe. J. Bone Joint Surg., *20*:715, 1938.

MISCELLANEOUS TOE PROBLEMS

Castle, W. E.: Further data on webbed toes. Science, *55*:703, 1922.

Cockin, J.: Butler's operation for an overriding fifth toe. J. Bone Joint Surg., *50B*:78, 1968.

Goodwin, F. C., and Swisher, F. M.: The treatment of congenital hyperextension of the great toe. J. Bone Joint Surg., *25*:193, 1943.

Kelikian, H., Clayton, L., and Loseff, H.: Surgical syndactylia of the toes. Clin. Orthop., *19*:208, 1961.

Lantzounis, L. A.: Congenital subluxation of the fifth toe and its correction by a periosteocapsuloplasty and tendon transplantation. J. Bone Joint Surg., *22*:147, 1940.

Lapidus, P. W.: Transplantation of the extensor tendon for correction of the overlapping fifth toe. J. Bone Joint Surg., *24*:555, 1942.

McFarland, B.: Congenital deformities of the spine and limbs. *In* Platt, H. (ed.): Modern Trends in Orthopedics. New York, P. B. Hoeber, 1950.

Ogden, J. A.: An unusual case of polydactylism. Clin. Orthop., *84*:104, 1972.

Scrase, W. H.: The treatment of dorsal adduction deformities of the fifth toe. J. Bone Joint Surg., *36B*:146, 1954.

Sharrard, W. J. W.: The surgery of deformed toes in children. Br. J. Clin. Pract., *17*:263, 1963.

Stamm, T. T.: Surgery of the foot. *In* British Surgical Practice, Vol. 4. St. Louis, C. V. Mosby Co., 1948.

Sweetnam, R.: Congenital curly toes. An investigation into the value of treatment. Lancet, *2*:398, 1958.

Taylor, R. G.: The treatment of claw toes by multiple transfers of flexor with extensor tendons. J. Bone Joint Surg., *33B*:539, 1951.

Thompson, C. T.: Surgical treatment of disorders of the fore part of the foot. J. Bone Joint Surg., *46A*:1117, 1964.

Trethowan, W. H.: The treatment of hammertoe. Lancet, *1*:1257, 1312, 1925.

Wilson, J. N.: V-Y correction for varus deformity of the fifth toe. Br. J. Surg., *41*:133, 1953.

SKIN AND NAIL LESIONS

Branson, E. C., and Rhea, R. L., Jr.: Plantar warts. Cure by injection. N. Engl. J. Med., *248*:631, 1953.

Dickson, J. A.: Surgical treatment of intractable plantar warts. J. Bone Joint Surg., *30A*:757, 1948.

DuVries, H. L.: New approach to the treatment of intractable verruca plantaris (plantar wart). J.A.M.A., *152*:1202, 1953.

Heifetz, C. J.: Ingrown toe-nail. Am. J. Surg., *38*:298, 1937.

Heifetz, C. J.: Operative management of ingrown toe-nail. J. Missouri Med. Assoc., *42*:213, 1945.

Kopell, H. P., Winokur, J., and Thompson, W. A. L.: Ingrown toe-nail. New concept. N.Y. J. Med., *66*:1215, 1966.

Lapidus, P. W.: Orthopedic skin lesions of the soles and the toes. Clin. Orthop., *45*:87, 1966.

May, H.: The surgical treatment of intractable plantar warts. Surg. Clin. North Am., *31*:607, 1951.

McElvenny, R. T.: Corns — their etiology and treatment. Am. J. Surg., *50*:761, 1940.

Robinson, D. W.: Treatment of complications of plantar warts. Arch. Surg., *66*:434, 1953.

CONGENITAL HEMIHYPERTROPHY

Bryan, R. S., Lipscomb, P. R., and Chatterton, C. C.: Orthopedic aspects of congenital hypertrophy. Am. J. Surg., *96*:654, 1958.

Campbell, W. C.: Congenital hypertrophy: report of a case with diffuse neurofibromatosis. Surg. Gynecol. Obstet., *36*:699, 1923.

Carron, R.: L'hémihypertrophie congénitale. Pédiatrie, 6:969, 1951.

Carter, F. S., and Dockeray, M. C.: A case of congenital hemihypertrophy showing variations in bone age and development. Arch. Dis. Child., 28:321, 1953.

Crosby, E. H.: Hemihypertrophy totalis: case report. J. Bone Joint Surg., 17:1025, 1935.

Fordyce, A. D.: Hemi-hypertrophic alterne. Arch. Dis. Child., 3:300, 1928.

Friedberg, H.: Riesenwuchs des rechten Beines. Arch. Pathol. Anat., 40:353, 1867.

Gesell, A.: Hemihypertrophy and mental defect. Arch. Neurol. Psychiat., 6:400, 1921.

Gesell, A.: Hemihypertrophy and twinning. A further study of the nature of hemihypertrophy with report of a new case. Am. J. Med. Sci., 173:542, 1927.

Harwood, J., O'Flynn, E.: Right sided hemihypertrophy associated with pubertas praecox. Proc. R. Soc. Med., 28:857, 1935.

Kazanjian, V. H., and Sturgis, S. H.: Surgical treatment of hemiatrophy of the face. J.A.M.A., 115:348, 1940.

MacEwen, D. B., and Case, J. L.: Congenital hemihypertrophy. Clin. Orthop., 50:147, 1967.

Mayers, L. H.: Hemihypertrophy. Surg. Gynecol. Obstet., 43:746, 1926.

McFarland, B. L.: Hemihypertrophy. Br. Med. J., 1:345, 1928.

Morris, J. M., and MacGillivray, R. C.: Mental defect and hemihypertrophy. Am. J. Ment. Defic., 59:645, 1955.

Peabody, C. W.: Hemihypertrophy and hemiatrophy: congenital total unilateral somatic asymmetry. J. Bone Joint Surg., 18:466, 1936.

Penfield, W., and Robertson, J. S. M.: Growth asymmetry due to lesions of the postcentral cerebral cortex. Arch. Neurol. Psychiat., 50:405, 1943.

Peremans, G.: An unusual case of congenital asymmetry of the pelvis and lower extremities. J. Bone Joint Surg., 5:331, 1923.

Roget, J., Beaudoing, A., and Guilhot, J.: Un cas d'hémihypertrophie congénitale avec aspect anormal des cisternes de la base du crane. Pédiatrie, 10:195, 1955.

Rugel, S. J.: Congenital hemihypertrophy. Report of a case with postmortem observations. Am. J. Dis. Child., 71:530, 1946.

Sabanas, A. O., and Chatterton, C. C.: Crossed congenital hemihypertrophy. J. Bone Joint Surg., 37A:871, 1955.

Schwartzman, J., Grossman, L., and Dragutsky, D.: True total hemihypertrophy. Case report. Arch. Pediatr., 59:637, 1942.

Scott, A. J.: Hemihypertrophy: report of four cases. J. Pediatr., 6:650, 1935.

Silver, H. K., Kiyasu, W., George, J., and Deamer, W. C.: Syndrome of congenital hemihypertrophy, shortness of stature and elevated urinary gonadotropins. Pediatrics, 12:368, 1953.

Stoesser, A. U.: Hypertrophics of infancy and childhood. Am. J. Dis. Child., 35:885, 1928.

Wagner, H.: Hypertrophie der rechten Brust und der rechten oberen Extremität besonders der Hand und der Finger. Med. Jahrb. K.K. Osterreichischen Staates, 19:378, 1839.

Wakefield, E. G., and Hines, E. A.: Congenital hemihypertrophy. Am. J. Med. Sci., 185:493, 1940.

Ward, C. E., and Horton, B. T.: Congenital arteriovenous fistulas in children. J. Pediatr., 16:763, 1933.

Ward, J., and Lerner, H.: A review of the subject of congenital hemihypertrophy and a complete case report. J. Pediatr., 31:403, 1947.

Williams, J. A.: Congenital hemihypertrophy with lymphangioma. Arch. Dis. Child., 26:158, 1951.

Wisenberg, M.: Unusual case of hemigigantism. Can. Med. Assoc. J., 25:591, 1931.

AMPUTATIONS

Davidson, W. H., and Boline, W. H. O.: The Syme amputation in children. J. Bone Joint Surg., 57A:905, 1975.

Eilert, R. E., and Jayakumar, S. S.: Boyd and Syme ankle amputations in children. J. Bone Joint Surg., 58A:1138, 1976.

FRACTURES

Boehler, L.: Technik der Knochenbruch Behandlung, 2nd ed. Wien, Wilhelm Manbrich 1930. (And recent new editions.)

Mukherjee, S. K., Pringle, R. M., and Baxter, A. O.: Fracture of the lateral process of the talus. J. Bone Joint Surg., 56B:263, 1974.

Thomas, H. M.: Calcaneal fracture in childhood. Br. J. Surg., 56:664, 1969.

TERMINOLOGY UTILIZED IN THE FIELD OF PRESCRIPTION FOOTWEAR*

alignment. Adjusted in proper line.

anterior heel. Term for a specific type of metatarsal bar (similar to a metatarsal pad).

apex. Highest point or edge of a supporting element.

backpart. That portion of the last extending from the ball to the back.

back seam. Posterior seam joining the quarters of the uppers.

bal. Standard shoe with lace stays and tongue sewn at the throat.

balance. To support or arrange to equalize opposing forces.

ball. Widest part of the sole (at the metatarsal heads).

ball girth. The greatest dimension around the last passing through the ball break.

balloon. Expand or stretch out.

bar. A piece of material of indefinite size and shape that is long in proportion to its width.

bar, comma. A comma-shaped bar wedged laterally and posteriorly (e.g., Hauser type). Lateral wedge pronates forefoot.

bar, Denver. (Often referred to as a Denver heel). A wide metatarsal bar; the apex of this bar coincides with the posterior edge under the posterior half of the metatarsal shafts. Anterior edge is just proximal to the ball (metatarsal heads).

bar, Jones. A metatarsal bar placed between the innersole and outersole of a shoe.

bar, Mayo. A metatarsal bar with the anterior edge curved to approximate the position to the metatarsal heads.

bar, metatarsal. Any bar of rubber, leather, or synthetic material applied transversely across the bottom of the shoe sole, with the apex immediately posterior to the metatarsal heads.

bar, Thomas. A narrow metatarsal bar with abrupt anterior and posterior drop-off.

bar, transverse. A metatarsal bar.

blucher. A front-lace shoe pattern in which the tongue is part of the forepart and the quarters lap over the vamp or forepart. Lace stays are sewn at the sides rather than at the throat. Good for high-arched foot.

boot. High-quarter shoe in which the quarters cover the malleoli to any point up to the hip.

bottom. Plantar surface of the shoe, excluding the heel.

breast. Anterior surface of the heel.

breastline. An arbitrary line defining the forward boundary of the heel.

break. The wrinkle or crease formed in the vamp of a shoe when the shoe is flexed at the ball.

*Adapted by the editor from Weitsen, L. H., and Ullman, B. A.: Educational Committee of the Prescription Footwear Association, 1972.

brogue. Shoe of rugged construction and usually perforated and pinked with tips, foxing, and medallions on the toe-caps.

calfskin. Tanned calf skins, preferably of mellow, heavier weights; it is of finer texture and very durable.

Celastic. A pyroxylin material that can be molded and fixed into a rigid form.

chrome. A leather tannage using chromium salts, which impart greater strength, elasticity, and perspiration resistance.

chukka. A ¾ blucher boot pattern with two or three eyelets or a strap with a buckle.

closure. Method of inclosing, binding, or confining.

collar. A band of leather stitched to and encircling the top of a quarter of a shoe.

cone. The curved upper surface of the backpart of the last, which is divided by a V cut into a front and back cone.

cookie. A wafer-shaped piece of leather used in a shoe as a longitudinal arch support.

contralateral. Acting in conjunction with similar parts on an opposite side.

cordovan. A leather produced from the butt of a horsehide (a "fascia" between the hair and flesh sides).

corset. A reinforcement of firm leather or stays incorporated in the upper to support or restrict ankle motion.

counter. Reinforcement to preserve the shape of the backpart of the shoe (e.g., heel counter).

counter, long medial. Extended anteriorly beyond the breastline on the medial side (longitudinal arch).

counter, long lateral. Extended anteriorly beyond the breastline on the lateral side.

counter, upstanding. Extending up vertically above the malleoli.

crest. Ridge or prominence (as cushion or filling under the cavity under the phalanges).

cross. Opposite.

cross wedging. Combination wedging (as in medial heel and lateral sole).

crown. lateral curvature of the bottom of the last.

cuff. A band of leather stitched to the top of the quarter of a shoe to increase its height.

custom shoe. Custom-made shoe from plaster cast for severe deformities; can accommodate 1-inch-thick adjustable Levy mold (arch support).

doubler. An interlining placed between the vamp and vamp lining for additional body and shape reinforcement.

drop-off. The anterior vertical edge of a metatarsal or rocker bar.

Dutchman. Traditional term applied to wedges.

dynamic. Performing a regular function; forceful; energetic.

elevation. Raise of sole or heel.

elk. Chrome-tanned cattle-hide leather distinctive for softness and strength.

equalize. To balance opposing forces.

excavation. Hollowed-out cavity.

external. Outward part.

extra-depth shoe. One with extra depth to accommodate an arch support.

eyelet. A hole or metal ring used for lacing.

fiber. Any tough, strong, solid material composed of an animal, vegetable, or mineral threadlike substance.

filler. Any material—cork composition, felt, or rubber—placed between the innersole and outersole to provide leveling and cushioning.

flanged. A projected edge of sole or heel (medial and/or lateral) for stability.

flared. Spread out.

flexible. Pliable; yielding to pressure.

foot mold. An appliance that is full length and shaped to the plantar aspect of the foot.

forepart. That portion of the last extending from the ball break to the toe.

foxing. A piece of leather applied to the quarter or a perforated design in the quarter for decoration.

full grain. Leather in which the top grain has been left intact without correcting.

functional. Works properly.

girth. Dimension measured around the last.

Goodyear welt. A shoemaking process in which the joining of the upper, innersole, and outersole is accomplished with a leather welt strip to form a very firm attachment and a perfectly smooth innersole with no seams in contact with the foot and which is durable and easily repaired or modified.

goring. A woven elastic fabric inserted in the front or sides of a shoe upper, the expansion of which allows a larger opening to insert the foot.

grade. The change between sizes and/or widths of any portion of a last or pattern.

heel. (a) Back part of any covering of the foot. (b) Any solid part projecting downward from the back part of the shoe.

heel elevation. (orthopedic modification). Measured in a vertical line at the posterior of the heel from the treading or plantar surface to the heel point at the heel seat.

heel height. (commercial manufacturer's). Measured vertically from the treading or plantar surface to the heel seat at the breast or anterior surface of the heel—usually denoted in increments of eighths of an inch.

heel pad. Material placed in the shoe over the rough areas of the heel seat.

heel pitch. Inclination of the heel from the vertical at the posterior surface.

heel point. The rearmost point of a last at the heel seat.

heel seat. (a) Place to which the heel is attached. (b) Area on which the anatomic heel rests within the shoe.

heel-strike. Posterior heel contact against the treading surface.

heel types. (a) Spring heel ³/₈ to ⁶/₈ inch. Heel base lies under the outsole, eliminating a definite heel breast. (b) Flat heel ⁶/₈ to ¹⁰/₈ inch broad base. (c) Military heel ¹⁰/₈ to ¹³/₈ inch medium base. (d) Cuban heel ¹³/₈ to ¹⁴/₈ inch—narrower base than military heel. (e) Wedge heel ⁴/₈ to ¹⁴/₈ inch—extends from ball break backward to posterior heel surface as a solid wedge.

heel, special types. (a) Ashley heel—heel with breast set anteriorly with medial and lateral flares and pitched well forward to obtain additional longitudinal support, as well as medial and lateral stabilization (flanges). (b) Thomas heel—heel with medial side projected anteriorly for additional support; may be prescribed with medial flare and/or

wedge, as specified. (c) Calcaneal heel—long medial extension of the heel for heel spurs.

horseshoe correction. Outersole or arch support correction. Arms of the horseshoe extend beyond the first and fifth metatarsal heads. Central portion is proximal to the second, third, and fourth metatarsal heads.

inflare. To spread out or turn medially.

inlay. Any type of arch support or foot mold inserted in a shoe.

innersole. Sole conforming to the exact size and shape of the last bottom on which the foot rests.

insole. A supplementary sole made of any material and shaped as the original innersole that may be inserted within a shoe.

instep. (a) The arched, dorsal, middle portion of the human foot. (b) That part of the shoe over the anatomic instep.

internal. Interior or enclosed part.

iron. A measure of sole thickness (¹/₄₈ inch = 1 iron, e.g., 12 irons = ¹/₄ of an inch.

jimmy. A piece of material of felt, cork composition, or leather shaped as the forepart of an insole and inserted in a shoe to tighten it.

kidskin. A soft, strong leather of tanned baby goatskin.

lace stay. Portion of the upper containing eyelets for lacing.

lace-to-toe. Low or high quarter pattern with eyelets to the toe, usually a blucher, for easiest access.

lamelift. Sheet of natural cork used to laminate and shape into shortage elevations.

last. Model approximating the weight-bearing foot, made of wood or plastic, over which a shoe is formed or lasted. (a) Bunion last—rounded toe and wide at the ball to accommodate bunion. (b) Straight last—shoe with straight inner border. (c) Combination last—forefoot is relatively wide compared with the heel (e.g., for splayfoot).

last systems. Methods of proportional grading of last dimensions, (e.g., arithmetic, geometric, dynametric, DFC, Europoint).

leather. Animal skin tanned or otherwise dressed for use.

length. Dimension along the center line of

the last bottom from the toe point to the heel point.

linings. Material, usually of canvas, leather, or plastic, covering the inner portions of the shoe in contact with the foot to provide a smooth surface.

medallion. Perforated design used to decorate the toe of a shoe.

midsole. A sole placed between the innersole and the outersole.

moccasin. (a) Shoe of one-piece vamp quarter and sole and with stitched back seam and tongue. (b) A stitched and/or perforated circular design on the vamp of a shoe for decoration.

modification. An alteration or change.

mold, mould. That on which anything is shaped, modeled, or formed.

monk pattern. Low-quarter blucher with strap and buckle.

Morton's extension. Arch support extension beyond the head of the first metatarsal.

Napoleon tap. A sole placed under the original sole but undercut smaller than the original.

oak. Sole leather produce from hides and vegetable tanned with a combination of tanning materials.

orthopaedic shoe. One that is prescribed for functional accommodation or control or used in the therapeutic management of a particular abnormality. This would apply to any abnormal muscular, skeletal, vascular, or neurologic condition of the lower extremities.

outersole. Bottom sole of the shoe exposed to wear.

outflare. To spread out or turn laterally. An outflare shoe curves outward at forefoot and is used for flexible metatarsus adductus in infancy.

oxford. Low-quarter shoe; quarters extend to just below the malleoli.

pad. A cushion of any material used to prevent pressure or friction. (a) Metatarsal pad—usually a firm rubber pad put under sock lining posterior to the metatarsal heads. (b) Scaphoid pad—similar type of pad put in the arch of the shoe. (c) Sesamoid pad—similar to the metatarsal pad but with an extension behind the first metatarsal head.

patch. A piece of leather stitched or cemented to a shoe to cover a hole.

patterns. Templates of cardboard or fiberboard, brass bound, approximating the last as guide; these are used for cutting components of the uppers and linings to be incorporated in a shoe.

perforations. A series of punched holes for decoration or ventilation.

permanent. Fixed in place.

pinch. The wrinkle in the vamp and/or lining that may irritate or abrade the dorsum.

pinking. Edge of material serrated into angles or scallops for decoration.

plate. A flat piece of material (steel, aluminum, leather, or plastic) molded to form an arch support.

platform. Raised sole.

pocket. To form a pouch.

quarter. Posterior part or backpart of the uppers.

removable. Transferable from one place to another.

rigid. Firm; stiff; inflexible.

rocker. Curved base causing rocking instead of flexing action. (a) Metatarsal rocker bar — apex $1/4$ inch thick at the ball of the outersole; immobilizes for hallux rigidus. (b) Long sole rocker—stiff leather outersole rocker; often used with posterior heel elevation (SACH heel).

shank. Area of the shoe between the heel, breast, and ball. (a) Steel shank may be added between the innersole and the outersole for rigidity (e.g., hallux rigidus).

shank piece. Reinforcement of the shank (made of spring steel, wood, or plastic).

shell. Unfinished framework or base of an arch or full-length foot mold.

shoe horn. Instrument used to facilitate donning of a shoe.

side. Leather made of larger cattle hides.

size (shoe). Each half size (length) is $1/6$ inch different in length *and* $1/8$ inch different in circumference.

skive. To cut off in thin layers or to a fine edge.

sock lining. Lining covering the dorsal surface of the innersole.

splint. Any device designed to immobilize or limit motion.

splint, counter. A strip of flexible material attached to the counters of a shoe; used to limit internal rotation.

splint, Dennis-Browne. Any bar of rigid

material used to maintain the position of shoes and/or feet for correction of abnormal conditions of the feet, legs, or hips.

split. Leather obtained from the underside or flesh portion upon splitting of the original skin to get the desired weight or thickness.

split size. Different size shoes for foot inequality.

stabilize. To make steady.

stress. Pressure or strain caused by tension, compression, or shear or a combination of these forces.

suede. Flesh side of skin buffed to a velvety nap.

support. A reinforcement or arch used to control the stress of weight bearing areas.

tanning. Process of curing animal or reptile skins into leather.

tap. A sole placed under the original sole.

throat. The shallow part or entrance of the shoe, normally located at the waist or where the vamp and quarters meet at the base of the tongue.

toe-box. Reinforcement used to retain the original contour of the toe and guard against trauma or abrasion. A high toe-box is used for hammer toes.

toecap. An extra piece sewed to the vamp, covering the toe area.

toe crest. Transverse elevation in an arch support at the plantar base of the toes.

toe-off. To push off with the toes.

toe point. The foremost point of a last at the toe.

toe recede. Slope of the top surface of the last or shoe from toe point to the point of full toe thickness.

toe spring. Space between the outersole and base plane or horizontal treading surface measured vertically at the toe (allows rocker effect for toe-off). Same principle is used for sole elevations.

tongue. Strip of leather attached to the vamp, lying under the lacing or straps of a shoe.

toplift. Layer of material forming the plantar wearing surface of the heel.

torque. Twist or rotary force.

treadpoint. The point of the bottom forepart of the last or shoe in contact with the base plane or treading surface.

upper. Combined upper portions of the shoe, above the sole construction, including the outer surface materials, linings, and closures.

vamp. Anterior or forepart of the upper.

Velcro. Nylon hook and loop tape fasteners, that cling together on contact and are easily separated.

waist. The smallest dimension in girth between the ball and the instep.

wall. Medial and lateral perimeter of the forepart of the last or shoe; the relatively straight sides around the periphery of the last or shoe.

wedge. A piece of leather tapered to a thin edge; used to elevate one side of the sole or heel.

wedgie. Shoe with a rubber sole continuous with the heel; resilient and distributes weight bearing; good for anterior metatarsalgia. (a) Ripple sole —resilient rubber sole used for wedgies.

well. A hollowed area or hole; used in arch supports under calluses.

welt. A narrow strip of leather used to unite the upper, innersole, and outersole of a shoe by means of stitching.

width. Dimension across the ball area of the last or shoe at its widest point.

width (shoe). Each width is 1/4 inch different in circumference *and* 1/12 inch different in length.

wing tip. A perforated and pinked design, wing-shaped, decorating the vamp.

REFERENCES

1. Anderson, A. D.: The Shoe and Leather Lexicon, 15th ed. New York, 1952.
2. Carleton, F. J.: Shoes and Feet. West Chester, Pennsylvania, Charles H. Andress, 1940.
3. Diveley, R. L.: Foot appliances and shoe alterations. *In* American Academy of Orthopaedic Surgeons: Orthopaedic Appliances Atlas, Vol. 1. Ann Arbor, Michigan, J. W. Edwards, 1952, pp. 439–478.
4. Gibbard, L. C. (ed.): Charlesworth's Chiropodical Orthopaedics, 2nd ed. London, Baillière, Tindall and Cassell, 1968.
5. Jahss, M. H.: Shoes and shoe modifications. *In* American Academy of Orthopaedic Surgeons: Atlas of Orthotics. Biomechanical Principles and Application. St. Louis, C. V. Mosby Co., 1975, pp. 267–279.
6. Jahss, M. H.: Geriatric aspects of the foot and ankle. *In* Rossman, I. (ed.): Clinical Geriatrics, 2nd ed. Philadelphia, J. B. Lippincott Co., 1979, pp. 638–650.
7. Milgram, J. E.: Office measures for relief of the painful foot. Instructional Course Lectures. J. Bone Joint Surg., 46A:1095, 1964.
8. Sonderling, H.: Mechanics in modern foot therapy. *In* Gross, R. H.: Modern Foot Therapy, New York, Modern Foot Therapy Publishing Co., 1948, pp. 518–636.
9. Wickstrom, J., and Williams, R. A.: Shoe corrections and orthopaedic shoe supports. Clin. Orthop., 70:30, 1970.

INDEX

Page numbers in italics refer to illustrations.

Abduction, definition of, 125
Abductor digiti minimi, flaps of, for skin grafts, 955
Abductor hallucis, flaps of, for skin grafts, 955
  testing of, 292
Abnormal motion, definition of, 89
Abrasions, as acute foot infections, treatment of, 1401
Abscesses, of deep plantar space, treatment of, 1406
Accessory bones, anatomy of, 13, *14, 23, 25, 26*
  enumeration of, 123–125
  location of, 123–125, *123, 124*
  roentgenographic examination of, 98, 123–125, *123, 124*
Achilles tendinitis. See *Tendinitis, of Achilles tendon.*
Achilles tendon. See also *Heel cord.*
  anatomy of, *11, 19–21, 20–22, 23, 25, 27*
  bursitis of, in sports injuries, treatment of, 1595, *1596*
  fat pads of, 840
  granulomatous, in yaws, *1423*
  incisions in, *942, 943, 943*
  lengthening of, in Duchenne's muscular dystrophy,
      338–342, *340–342,* 345
    equinovarus deformity, 1116
    in equinus deformity, 1113
    in toe deformities, *1121*
    syndesmotomy and, 418, 420
  peroneal transfer to, for triceps surae paralysis, in
      poliomyelitis, 1151, *1151, 1152*
  problems of, in dancers, 1642, *1642.*
  rupture of, 1538–1541, *1539, 1540*
    diagnosis of, 1538
    in dancers, 1643.
    in geriatrics, 976
    physical examination for, 104
    spontaneous vs. traumatic, 1538
    treatment of, nonsurgical, 1538, 1540
      surgical, 805, *806*
        Bosworth method, 1539, *1539*
        Ma and Griffith percutaneous repair,
            1539–1541, *1540*
        vs. nonsurgical, 1538
  skin grafts for, 958
  tenosynovitis of, 856
  tightness of, in Sever's disease, 204
  tumors of, 866
  xanthomas in, *995, 996*
Achillobursitis, in geriatrics, 975
Achondrogenesis II, short life expectancy with, 234

Achondroplasia, 355, *356*
  clinical features of, 355
  pathogenesis of, 355
  radiographic features of, 356, *356*
Acrocephalopolysyndactyly, I and II, 237, *237*
Acromegaly, affecting foot, *1071,* 1072, *1072*
ACTH, in treatment of acute gouty arthritis, 1020
Active movement, assessment of, 540, *541*
Adduction, definition of, 125
Adductor hallucis, testing of, 292
Adductor tendon, ossification of, 835, *835*
Adductovarus deformity, of forefoot, hallux valgus and,
      599, *599*
  hallux varus and, *616,* 617
Adhesive neuritis, following surgery for hallux valgus,
      601, 602
Adhesive tendinitis, following surgery for hallux valgus,
      602
Adolescents, foot disorders in, evaluation of, 198
  Freiberg's infraction in, 208
Adult foot, 539–978
  dorsal view of, *18*
  lateral view of, *20*
  medial view of, *19*
  midsagittal section of, *11*
  plantar aspect, superficial muscles of, *23*
  posterior view of, *21*
Adult foot and ankle, suggested course outline for
  resident study of, 1831–1834
Adults, surgical considerations in, 151
Adventitious bursae, treatment of, 1406
Age factors, in choice of surgery, 151, 167
Ainhum, in small toes, at proximal interphalangeal joint,
      657, *657*
    clinical appearance, 656, *657*
    differential diagnosis, 657
    in Vohwinkel's disease, 657
    predominance in blacks, 656
    radiographic view, *657*
    treatment of, 657
"Air contrast" tomography, for talar fractures, 1465
Akin operation, in hallux valgus, 569, *569, 586, 601*
Albers-Schönberg disease, 365–367, *366.* See also
  Osteopetrosis.
Albright's syndrome, fibrous dysplasia in, 361, *1011*
Alcoholic neuropathy, peripheral, 1219–1223,
      1219–1222. See also *Neuropathy(ies).*

Alcoholic neuropathy (*Continued*)
  vs. diabetic neuropathy, 1219
Alcoholism, associated foot problems in, 1223
Allergic neuropathies, 1242
Allergies, history-taking for, 83
Allopurinol, for chronic gouty arthritis and tophaceous
    gout, 1020
  for secondary gout, 1022
Amelanotic melanoma, of hallux nail bed, 831, *831*
Amniocentesis, in experimental animals, clubfoot and,
    230
Amputation(s), 1364–1373, *1364–1372*. See also
    Prosthetics, Replantation, and under specific
    member.
  alternatives to, 1364, *1364, 1365*
  basic literature on, guide to, 1850, 1866
  Chopart, *1368, 1369, 1369, 1371,* 1392–1394, *1393*
    prostheses for, 1815, *1817*
  in children, 1684
  in clubfoot, 425
  in diabetic foot, 1392–1394, *1393–1395*
  in hammer toe, disadvantages of, 645
  Lisfranc, 1366, *1366,* 1369, *1370,* 1392–1394, *1394,*
    1395
  near-total, salvage of, 1364
  necessity for, 1364, *1364, 1365*
  of calcaneus, partial, results of, 1345, *1345*
  postoperative complications, 1369, *1369–1371*
  premature, of gangrenous tissue, 1328, *1329*
  Syme, 1366, *1367,* 1369, 1392. See also *Syme
    amputations.*
  tissue conservation in, 1365–1373, *1366–1372*
    flap formation, 1365, *1366, 1367*
    split-thickness skin grafts, *1368,* 1369, *1370*
    Steristrip closure, *1372,* 1373
    toes, *1371, 1373*
  vs. replantation, 1364, *1364, 1365*
Amyloidosis, EMG findings in, 73
Amyotrophic lateral sclerosis, electrodiagnosis in, 77
Amyotrophy, diabetic, 1217
Anatomy, 8–36
  early historical interest in, 1
  of Achilles tendon *11, 19–21, 20–22, 23, 25, 27*
  of ankle and foot joints, functional, 13, *14,* 38–43,
    39–42
  of calcaneocuboid joint, *12, 14, 15*
  of calcaneus, 10, *11, 12, 14, 23, 25, 27*
  of Chopart's joint, *12,* 15
  of cuboid, 10, *11, 12, 14, 27*
  of cuboideonavicular joint, 15
  of cuneiforms, 10–12, *11, 14*
  of cuneonavicular joint, 15
  of extrinsic muscles, 17–22, *18–21, 25–27*
  of human foot, ligaments, *11,* 13–17, *14*
    nerves, 24–31, *29*
    skin, 32
    vascular system, 31
    vs. hand, 1
  of humans vs. other primates, 6, *7*
  of interphalangeal joints, 17
    functional, 43
  of intrinsic muscles, 19, 22–24, *23, 25–27*
  of Lisfranc's joint, 15, *16*
  of metatarsophalangeal joints, *14, 16,* 17
    functional, 43
  of metatarsus, 12, *14, 16*
  of midtarsal joints, *12,* 15

Anatomy (*Continued*)
  of navicular, 10, *11, 12, 14*
    functional, 42
  of phalanges, 12, *14*
  of plantar aponeurosis, 17, *19, 26*
  of retinacula, at ankle, 17, *18–20*
  of sesamoid and accessory bones, 13, *14, 23, 25, 26,*
    662, 1459
  of subtalar joint, *11,* 13–15, *14*
    functional, 40–42, *41*
  of talocalcaneonavicular joint, *11, 12, 14,* 15
  of talus, 10, *11, 12, 14*
  of tarsometatarsal joints, 15, *16*
  of tarsus, 10–12, *11, 12, 14*
  of transverse tarsal joint, functional, 42, *42*
  surgical, 33
    dorsum, *18,* 33
    lateral aspect, *20,* 34
    medial aspect, *19,* 33
    plantar aspect, *11, 23,* 34
    posterior aspect, *21,* 34
    vs. standard, 33
Anemia, pernicious, clinical features and treatment of,
    1240
Anesthesia, hysterical, 1443. See also *Psychiatric
    aspects.*
  local block, 930
Anesthetic foot, footwear for, 1781
Aneurysm(s), of dorsalis pedis artery, in dancers, 1654,
    1655
  popliteal, resulting in acute arterial thrombosis, *1316,*
    1317, *1317*
  shower of microemboli from, *1314,* 1315
Angiosarcoma(s), 991
Ankle, 776–827
  abnormal, surgical correction of, 192
  anatomy of, 1544–1546, *1545, 1546*
    lateral, *1545*
    medial, *1545*
    posterior, *1546*
  and foot, in classical ballet and modern dance,
    1626–1660. See also *Dancing.*
    industrial injuries to, 1607–1625. See also
      Industrial injuries.
    sports injuries to, 1573–1606. See also *Sports
      injuries.*
  anterior, skin grafts for, 958
  arthritis of, leprosy and, 1419
  arthrodesis of. See *Arthrodesis(es)* and *Ankle
    fusion.*
  arthrography of. See *Arthrography.*
  arthroplasty of. See *Arthroplasty.*
  arthroscopy of. See *Arthroscopy.*
  axis of, anatomic position of, *429*
    axis of, relationship of, with knee axis, *39*
      with long axis of foot, *39*
  biomechanics of, 812
  bones of, surgical reconstruction, 802–804
  Charcot. See *Charcot foot* and *Charcot joint.*
  deformities of, in cerebral palsy, 282–334. See also
    Palsy, cerebral.
  development of, roentgenographic examination of,
    116–121, *119, 120*
  dislocations of, total, 1472–1474, *1473.* See also
    Ankle, injuries of and *Fractures, of ankle.*
  dorsiflexion of, excessive, in head trauma patient,
    treatment of, surgical, *1121, 1122*

Ankle (*Continued*)
  entrapment syndromes involving, treatment of,
    surgical, 804
  equinus contracture at, in Duchenne's muscular
    dystrophy, 336, *337*
  erythema multiforme of, *880*
  examination of, clinical, 89
  flail, fusion of, with subsequent knee instability, 82,
    82
  foot deformities and, 793
    acquired, 793
    at birth, 793
    normal foot contours vs. abnormal, 793
    poliomyelitis, 793
    tarsal coalition, 794
  fractures of, classification, 1546–1550, *1547–1550*. See
    also *Ankle, injuries of* and *Fractures, of ankle.*
  fracture-dislocations of, Weber classification, *1550,*
    1555–1559, *1555–1560*
  geriatric, and foot, traumatic injuries of, 976. See also
    Geriatric foot.
  hemophilia in, 1088–1093, *1088–1092*. See also
    Hemophilia.
  in dancers. See *Dancing.*
  incisions in, 159–161, *159–161*
  injuries of, 776–783, *777, 778, 780–782*. See also
    Ankle, trauma to; Dislocations; Fractures; and
    Sprains.
    classification, 1546–1550, *1547–1550*
      Ashhurst and Bromer, 1547
      Lauge-Hansen, 1547–1549, *1547–1549*, 1553
      mechanism of injury as basis of, 1547
      pronation-adduction, 1548, *1548*
      pronation-dorsiflexion, 1549
      pronation-eversion fracture, 1548, *1549*
      supination-adduction fracture, 1547, *1548*
      supination-eversion fracture, 1547, *1547*
      Weber, 1549, *1550*, 1555–1559, *1555–1560*
    complications of, residuals, 787–789
      adults vs. children, 789
      aseptic osteonecrosis, 788
      entrapment syndromes, 788
      infection, 787
      osteoporosis, 787
      peroneal nerve injury, 788
      Sudeck's post-traumatic osteoporosis, 787
      tarsal tunnel syndrome, 788
    in children, 1671–1673, *1672*. See also *Children*
      and *Growing foot.*
    industrial, 1610, *1611*. See also *Industrial injuries.*
    inversion, causing transchondral talus fractures,
      1464
    ligaments, 777–783, *777, 778, 780–782*
      chronic instability, 777, 779, *780–782*
        anterior talar, 780
        anteroposterior view, 780, *781*
        coexisting deformities and, 780
        inversion stress view, 779, *780–782*
        lateral view, 779, *780, 782*
        talar tilt, 779, *780*
      chronic sprain, 777, 778, *778*
      classification, 777
      dislocation, 780
      resulting complications from, 777, *777*
        abnormal healing, 777
        calcification or ossification, *777, 778*
        slipping peroneal tendon, 781

Ankle (*Continued*)
  injuries of, ligaments, resulting complications from,
      tibiofibular bars, *777, 778*
    mechanisms of, 776
    roentgenographic evaluation, 1550, *1557*
    traction, treatment of, surgical, 804
  instability of, anterior draw sign test for, 107, *108*
    chronic lateral, in sports injuries, 1589–1591, *1590.*
      See also *Sports injuries.*
  lateral aspect of, landmarks, *159*
  lichenification in, in atopic dermatitis, 871, *871*
  ligaments of, surgical reconstruction of, 799–802,
    800
  longitudinal deficiency of fibula and, 222
  normal, examination of, roentgenographic, technique,
    125–136, *126–135*
  motion of, 125
  osteoarthritis of, *149,* 150, 789–793, *790–792*. See also
    Osteoarthritis.
  prostheses for. See under *Prosthesis(es)* and
    Prosthetics.
  residuals of disease of, treatment of, 794–804,
      795–797, 800
    nonsurgical, medication, 795
      supports, 794
    surgical, 795–804, *795–797, 800*
      anterolateral incision, 797
      anteromedial incision, 797
      bone reconstruction, 802–804
      chronic sprains, 798
      lateral utility incision, 797, *796*
      ligament reconstruction, 799–802, *800*
      medial utility incision, 795, *795*
      posterior incision, 797, *797*
      talar trochlear osteochondral defects, 786, 799
  rheumatoid arthritis of, 1046–1055, *1047, 1048, 1050,*
    1053, 1054. See also *Rheumatoid arthritis.*
  sprains of. See *Sprains.*
  strapping of, 1726, *1726*. See also *Foot, pain in,*
    padding and devices.
  surgical approaches to, 159–161, *159–161*
  tendons of, lacerations in, 865, *865*
    surgical reconstruction, 805–807, *806*
      Achilles rupture, 805, *806*
      slipping peroneal tendon, 806
    in dancers, 1642–1648, *1642, 1644–1647.* See also
      Dancing.
  total replacement of, 1052–1055, *1053, 1054*. See also
    Rheumatoid arthritis, of ankle, treatment of,
    surgical.
  trauma to, 1543–1572. See also *Ankle, injuries of;*
    Dislocations; Fractures; and *Sprains.*
    historical background, 1543
  treatment of, surgical vs. nonsurgical, 1551
  tuberculosis of, 1408, *1408, 1409*. See also
    Tuberculosis.
  venomous snake bite of, 1460–1462. See also *Snake*
    bite.
Ankle fusion, optimum positions of, principles, 174, *175*
  surgical. See *Arthrodesis.*
Ankle joint,
  anatomy of, 13, *14,* 38–43, *39–42*
  arthrology of, 13, *14*
  arthroscopic division of, 141, *141*
  axes of, *402, 403, 429*
  breaks in, 388, *388, 390*
  dorsiflexion in, 40, *40,* 43, *44, 45*

Ankle joint (*Continued*)
  frontal, variations in, *39*
  in dancers. See *Dancing.*
  plantar flexion in, 40, *40*, 43, *44*, *45*
  primary destruction of, in tertiary syphilis, *1250*, 1251
  range of motion in, 40, *40*, 43, *44*, *45*
  rotational deformities of, 432
  severe comminuted fracture above, arterial occlusion
    and, 1322, *1322*
  subtalar joint and, axial relationship of, 40, 43, *44*
  synovectomy of, 1049–1051
  synovitis of, in dancers, 1648
Ankle pressures, and clinical states, correlation
  between, 1310
Ankylosing spondylitis, affecting foot, *1058*, 1059
  idiopathic, involving heel, 774
Ankylosis, bony, in rheumatoid arthritis, *1027*, 1031
  fibrous, as cause of peroneal spastic flatfoot, 743
  of joints, congenital vertical talus and, 444
Annular fibrosis, 832, *832*
Anterior draw sign, testing for, 107, *108*
Anterior horn cell disease, electrodiagnosis in, 77
  EMG findings in, 73
  motor units in, 70
Anterior tibial muscle. See *Tibialis anterior.*
Antibiotics, in burn injuries, 1692
    classification and action of, 1693
Aortoiliac reconstruction, techniques of, 1332–1335,
  1333–1335
Apodia, radiographic view, *238*
  Syme prosthesis for, 245
  treatment of, 245
Aponeurosis, plantar. See *Fascia, plantar.*
Appliances, for spina bifida foot, 278, *279*
Arch(es). See also specific structure.
  as stabilizing mechanisms, 52–55, *53–55*
  development of, in ballet and dance, 1628, *1628*, *1629*
  maintenance of, 22
Arch supports. See also *Foot, pain in, padding and*
    devices; Footwear; Orthosis(es); Orthotics; and
    Shoes, and shoe modifications.
  advantages of and mechanisms of relief, 1734
  correction and, specific, *1736*, *1738*, *1740*, *1740*, *1741*
  for corns and calluses, 1743
  importance of follow-up for, 1743, *1743*
  in dancers, 1655
  interrelationships of shoes and, 1733
  miscellaneous devices and, 1733–1744
  types of, 1734–1741, *1735–1738*, *1740*, *1741*
    miscellaneous, 1739
    rigid, 1734–1736, *1735*
    semi-rigid and soft, 1736–1739, *1736–1738*
Arterial bypasses, infrainguinal, 1336–1343, *1337–1343*
Arterial disobliteration, 1318–1320, *1318*, *1319*. See also
  Vascular diseases.
Arterial embolism, 1311–1315, *1312–315*. See also
  Vascular diseases, arterial occlusive.
Arterial occlusive disease, 1310–1318, *1310–1317*, 1322,
  1322, 1323. See also *Vascular diseases.*
Arterial reconstruction, edema of foot following, 1347
  results of, 1344–1347, *1345*, *1346*. See also *Vascular*
    reconstruction.
    after hallux amputation, 1345, *1345*
    after partial calcaneal amputation, 1345, *1345*
    and prognosis, 1344
    in femoropopliteal bypass, 1345, *1345*, *1346*
    with ischemic ulcer, 1345, *1346*

Arterial thrombosis, acute, 1315–1318, *1316*, *1317*. See
  also *Vascular diseases, arterial occlusive.*
Arteriosclerosis, vs. thromboangiitis obliterans,
  1347–1349
Arteriosclerosis obliterans, 82, 1324–1332, *1325–1331*
  arteries affected in, conduit vs. supply, 1324
  causing acute arterial thrombosis, 1315
  clinical signs of, *1315*, 1328–1330, *1329*, *1330*
    calcification, 1330, *1330*
    long-standing, 1328, *1329*
  clinical symptoms of, 1325–1328, *1325–1329*
    claudication, PVR examination of, 1325, *1325*
    gangrene, 1326–1328, *1327–1329*
    muscular involvement, 1326
    profound ischemia, 1326
    sensory changes, 1326
    ulceration, 1326, *1326*, *1327*
  diffuse nature of, 1324
  incidence of, 1324
  pathogenesis of, tobacco smoking, 1325
  peripheral, affecting foot, 84
  prognosis for, 1324
  sites affected in, in diabetics, 1324
    order of frequency of, 1324
  treatment of, nonsurgical, 1330–1332, *1331*
    control of diabetes, 1331
    daily hygiene and inspection, 1331, *1331*
    tobacco abstinence, 1331
Arteritis, in rheumatoid arthritis, vs. polyarteritis
  nodosa, 1224
Artery(ies), *18*, *19*, 31. See also under individual
  arteries.
  lesions of, 847
  of conduit and supply, characteristics of, 1324
Arthritis, gouty, acute, 1018–1020, 1019. See also *Gout.*
  in sickle cell disease, 1097, *1097*
  in children, variations of, 196
  in late childhood and adolescence, 199
  involving heel, 774
  of ankle, leprosy and, 1419
  of subtalar joint, as cause of heel pain, 976
  psoriatic, 1059–1061, *1059–1061*
    clinical features of, 1059, *1059*, *1060*
    involving heel, 774
    onset of, 1059
    radiographic features of, *1059*, 1060, *1060*, *1061*
    treatment of, 1061, *1061*
  rheumatoid, 1024–1057, *1025–1032*, *1036*, *1039–1048*,
    1050, *1053*, *1054*, *1056*. See also *Rheumatoid*
    arthritis.
  role of, in peroneal spastic flatfoot, 742, *743*
Arthritis mutilans, in psoriatic arthritis, 1060, *1060*
Arthorodesis(es), basic literature on, guide to, 1850
  for hyperlax foot, 241
  for peripheral nerve injuries, 1192
  Grice, 241, 1162, *1163*
  in cavus deformity, 482, *483*
  in drop foot, 190, *191*
  in hammer toe, technique of, 644
  in pes planus, indications and contraindications, 511
  in spina bifida, 261
  of ankle, 807–811, *808*, *1050*, 1051. See also *Ankle*
    fusion.
    complications of, 816
    contraindications for, 816
    different methods of, varying success rates, 813
    failed, pseudarthrosis following, 172, 823, *823*

Arthrodesis(es) (*Continued*)
  of ankle, in equinus deformity, severe, 190, *190*
    in surgical management of non-plantigrade foot,
      190–192, *190–192*
    in tuberculosis, 1408, *1409*
    nonunion following, 173, *174*
    pantalar, 810, 1051
      technique of, 761, 810
    period of immobilization required, 813
    postoperative care, 170
    supramalleolar osteotomy, 811
    talectomy, 810
      partial and fusion, 810
    talocrural, 807–811, *808*
      anterior approach, *808*, 809
      lateral approach, 807–809, *808*
      medial approach, *808*, 809
      posterior approach, *808*, 809
      transfibular approach, 807–809, *808*
    tibiocalcaneal, 810
    vs. total replacement, 811–816, 1055
      biomechanics, 812. See also *Ankle, biomechanics
        of.*
      surgical procedures, availability of, 813–815
        choice of, 815
          in rheumatoid patients, 815
          roentgenographic evaluation, 816
          tests for, 815
          young vs. old patients, 815
        gait analysis following, 814
  of first metatarsal-medial cuneiform joint, 714, *714*
  of first metatarsophalangeal joint, in hallux valgus,
    573, *574*
    postoperative care, 170
  of Lisfranc's joint, in metatarsalgia with cavus
    deformity, 677, *677*
  of midtarsal joint, in metatarsalgia with cavus
    deformity, 678, *678*
  of subtalar complex, indications and contraindications,
    754, *755–758*
  subtalar, extra-articular, in spinal muscular atrophy,
    349
    Grice technique, 1162, *1163*
    in calcaneal fractures, 1531
  tarsometatarsal truncated wedge, 716–718, *716*, *717*
  tibiocalcaneal, technique of, 810
  triple, 424
    in calcaneal fractures, 1531
    in cerebral palsy, technique of, 305–310, *306*, *307*
    in clubfoot, 244
    in non-plantigrade foot, 189, *189*
    in poliomyelitis, 188, *188*
    in spinal muscular atrophy, 349
    in subtalar complex, technique, 758–761, *759–761*
    in tarsal coalition, 533–535
    incisional landmarks, 159, *159*
    nonunion of talonavicular joint following, 723, *724*
    postoperative care, 170
Arthrography, of ankle joint, 136–138, *137*
  normal findings, 137, *137*
  technique of, 136
Arthrogryposis, congenital vertical talus and, 444
  neuropathic vs. myopathic, 454
  radiographic view, *440*
  tibialis anterior hypertrophy in, 440, *440*
Arthrogryposis multiplex congenita, 454–461, *455–460*
  clinical features of, 455–457, *455–458*

Arthrogryposis multiplex congenita (*Continued*)
  clinical features of, birth deformities, 455
    feet and ankles, 456, *456*, *458*
    hips, 456, *457*
    knees, 456
    mental retardation, 456
    muscles, *455*, 456
    skin, 456
    trunk and limbs, 455
    upper vs. lower limbs, 455
  congenital vertical talus and, *440–442*, 456, *458*
  electrodiagnosis in, 78
  etiology of, 454, *455*
    neuropathic vs. myopathic, 454, 456
  history of, 454
  incidence of, 455
  neurologic basis of, 254, *254*
  radiologic features of, *440*, 457, *459*
  talipes equinovarus in, 456, *458*
  treatment of, 452, 457–461, *460*
    childhood changes, 458
    closed reduction, 457–459
      maintenance following, 459
      technique, 458
    lateral column longer than medial, 458, 460
    manipulative, 457–459
    open reduction, 452, 459–461, *460*
      alternative procedures, 460
      technique, *452*, 459, *460*
  untreated, *456*
Arthrology, 11, *12*, 13–17, *14*, *16*
  of ankle joint, 13, *14*
  of calcaneocuboid joint, *12*, 14, *15*
  of cuboideonavicular joint, 15
  of cuneonavicular joint, 15
  of interphalangeal joints, 17
  of Lisfranc's joint, 15, *16*
  of metatarsophalangeal joints, *14*, *16*, 17
  of subtalar (talocalcaneal) joint, *11*, 13–15, *14*
  of talocalcaneonavicular joint, *11*, *12*, *14*, 15
  of talocrural joint, 13, *14*
  of tarsometatarsal joints, 15, *16*
Arthropathy, hemophilic, 1086, 1088, *1088*, *1089*
  clinical and degenerative changes in, 1088, *1088*,
    1089
  in ankle vs. other joints, 1088
  treatment of, surgical vs. nonsurgical, 1089
  neuropathic, 1248. See also *Charcot foot* and *Charcot
    joint.*
  pyrophosphate, 1022, *1022*. See also *Pseudogout.*
Arthroplasty(ies), basic literature on, guide to, 1850
  in ankle, total, 816–825, *817–825*, 1052–1055, *1053*,
    1054. See also *Rheumatoid arthritis, of ankle,
    treatment of, surgical.*
    complications following, 820–825, *821–825*
      in avascular necrosis of talus, 823, *823*, *824*
      in osteoarthritis, 820–822, *821*, *822*
      in pseudarthrosis of ankle fusion, 823, *823*
      in rheumatoid arthritis, 823–825, *824*, *825*
    contraindications for, 820–825, *821–825*
      in avascular necrosis of talus, 823, *823*, *824*
      in osteoarthritis, *821*, *822*, 822
      in pseudarthrosis of ankle fusion, 823, *823*
      in rheumatoid arthritis, *824*, 825, *825*
      prednisone, 824, *825*, 825
    postoperative care, 820
    prosthesis design, 816, *817*

Arthroplasty(ies) (*Continued*)
  in ankle, total, surgical technique, 817–820, *818–820*
  in forefoot, 1037–1043, *1039–1044, 1050*. See also
    Rheumatoid arthritis, of foot, treatment of,
    surgical.
  resection, 1043–1045
Arthroscopy, in post-traumatic arthritis, 142, *142*
  of ankle, complications of, 142
    history of, 139
    indications for, 142, *142*
    instrumentation, 139–142, *140*
    technique of, 139–142, *140, 141*
Arthrosis, of first metatarsophalangeal joint, following
  surgery for hallux valgus, 604, *604*
Articulation, intermetatarsal, 662, *663*
Aseptic necrosis. See also *Avascular necrosis.*
  of talus, 748, *748, 749*
Ashurst and Bromer classification, of ankle injuries, 1547
Astragalectomy, 1480
  for poliomyelitis, 757, *757*
Astragalus. See *Talus.*
Ataxias, cerebellar, 1236
  definition of, 283
  in cerebral palsy, 283
Athetosis, definition of, 283
  in cerebral palsy, 283
Athletic injuries, involving heel, 773
Atopic dermatitis, 871–873, *871–873*. See also
  Dermatitis.
Autoimmune diseases, dermatomyositis, 874, *874*
  lupus erythematosus, discoid, 873, *873*
    systemic, 874, *874*
    morphea, 874, *875*
    scleroderma, localized, 874, *875*
    systemic, 875, *876*
Autonomic nervous system, testing of, in neurologic
  examination of foot, 1110
Avascular necrosis, of foot, diagnosis of, 200
  of talar neck, following fracture, 1480, *1481*
  of tarsal navicular, 200–203, *202, 203*. See also
    Köhler's disease.
  steroid-induced, in renal osteodystrophy, 1076–1078,
    1077
Avulsion, of toenail, treatment of, 1450
Avulsion fractures, diagnosis of, differential, *1488*
  of cuboid, treatment of, *1491*
  roentgenographic view of, 97
Axes, of ankle and foot, anatomic position of, *429*
  of lower extremity, *402*, 403
  in normal stance phase, *430*
Axonal lesions, complete, electrodiagnosis in, 75
  mixed, electrodiagnosis in, 75
Axonotmesis, definition of, 75
  EMG findings in, 73
  nerve conduction studies in, 74

Babinski reflex, testing of, in neurologic examination of
  foot, 1109
Back, disorders of and pain in, in relation to neurologic
  examination of foot, 1108
Bacterial infections, that may affect feet, 887–890,
  888–890
  elephantiasis, 888, *888, 889*
  erysipelas, 888, *889*
  gram-negative, 888, *889*

Bacterial infections (*Continued*)
  that may affect feet, impetigo contagiosa, 887, *888*
    pitted keratolysis, 889, *890*
    streptococcal, 887, *888, 889*
Balance points, of foot, in ballet and dance, 1627, *1627,*
  1628
Ball-and-socket joint, basic literature on, guide to, 1862
Ballet, classical, and modern dance, foot and ankle in,
  1626–1660. See also *Dancing* and *Sports injuries.*
  injuries from, classification, 1573. See also *Dancing*
    and *Sports injuries.*
Balloon catheter, mechanisms of, for embolectomy,
  1318, *1319*
Basal cell nevus syndrome, affecting foot, 876, *876*
Baseball, footwear for, 1775
  injuries from, classification, 1573
Basic science, 1–194
Basketball, injuries from, classification, 1573
Batchelor-Brown arthrodesis, for hyperlax foot, 241
Becker's muscular dystrophy, 345. See also *Muscular*
  dystrophy.
Beriberi, as nutritional neuropathy, 1240
Bicycle spokes, injuries from, in children, 1683
Bicycling, injuries from, classification, 1573
Bifurcate ligament, *14*, 15
Big toe. See *Hallux.*
Biliary atresia, rickets and osteomalacia in, 1066, *1066*
Biomechanics, 37–67. See also *Pes planus.*
  forces during gait and, 46–50, *46–49*
  functional anatomy and, of ankle and foot injuries,
    38–43, *39–42*
  gait analysis, 57–67, *58–66*
  lower extremity and, transverse rotation of, 50–52,
    51, 52, 61–63
  muscle function and, 43–46, *44–46*
  of ankle, 812
  of anterior tarsus and Lisfranc's joint, 712
  of foot and ankle, basic literature on, guide to, 1841
  of metatarsals, 666–673, *666, 668–672*. See also
    Metatarsals and *Metatarsalgia.*
  of sesamoids, 671, *671*
  of step, 55–57, *56*
  stabilizing mechanisms and, 52–55, *53–55*
  walking cycle and, 37, *37, 38*
  whole body locomotion and, 37
Bipedalism, evolution of, speculation regarding, 4
Birth defects, minor foot disorders and, 197
Bismuth poisoning, 1070, *1070*
Black heel, etiology and clinical features of, 890, *890*
Blast injuries, treatment of, 1459
Blastomycosis, etiology of, 1417
  radiographic view of, *1417*
  sites of, 1418
  treatment of, 1418
Blisters, as acute foot infection, 1401
  infected, treatment of, 1405
  surgical principles and, 157
  treatment of, 1401, 1405
Blood flow, determination of, in vascular diseases, 1302,
  1304
Blood pressure, measurement of, in vascular diseases,
  1304, *1305*
Blood supply, decreased, physical examination for, 106
  in spina bifida, 260
  relation of to foot surgery, 146, *147*
"Blue toe" syndrome, 1315, *1315*
Body image, psychiatric aspects, 1433, *1434*

Boeck's sarcoid, acute synovitis of foot and, 844, *845*

Bone(s), calcification of, in osteomalacia, 1068, *1068*

  damage to, in leprosy, 1267, *1267*

  disease of, marble, vs. heavy-metal poisoning, 1070

    nutritional, 1064–1071, *1065–1071*. See also *Metabolic disorders, of bone.*

    Paget's, 1078–1083, *1078–1082*. See also *Paget's disease.*

  disorders of, metabolic, 1064–1078, *1065–1077*. See also *Metabolic disorders.*

  growth of, in fetus and postnatally, 1661, *1662*

    rate of, males vs. females, 116

  infarction of, in sickle cell disease, 1098–1101, *1098–1101*

  lesions of, in yaws, *1426*, 1427, *1427*

  normal anatomic variations of, 98

  of ankle, surgical reconstruction of, 802–804

  of small toes, in gout, 655, *655*

  resection of, in forefoot, classification of procedures, 1038

  transection of, principles of, 166

  tumors of, 996–1012, *997–1011*. See also *Tumors, of foot.*

    percentage of, 744

Bone dysplasias, 353–373.

  achondroplasia, 355, *356*

  classification of, endochondral bone formation, 353

    intramembranous bone formation, 353

  Ekman-Lobstein disease, 362, *364*

  enchondromatosis, 358–360, *359*

  epiphysealis hemimelica, 354, *355*

  fibrous, 360–362, *362*

  fragilitas ossium, 362, *364*

  hereditary multiple exostoses, 356–358, *357*

  Maffucci's syndrome, *359*, 360

  multiple osteocartilaginous exostoses, 356–358, *357*

  multiple osteochondromatosis, 356–358, *357*

  Ollier's disease, 358–360, *359*

  osteogenesis imperfecta, 362, *364*

  resorption, 364–372, *365–368, 370, 371*. See also *Bone dysplasias, sclerosing.*

  sclerosing, 364–372, *365–368, 370, 371*

    at sites of endochondral bone formation, Albers-Schönberg disease, 365–367, *366*

      osteopathia striata, 368, *368*

      osteopetrosis, 365–367, *366*

      osteopoikilosis, 367, *367*

      Voorhoeve's disease, 368, *368*

    at sites of intramembranous bone formation, Engelmann's disease, 368

      melorheostosis, 369–372, *371*

      progressive diaphyseal, 368

      Ribbing's disease, 369

    classification of, 365

    etiology of, 364

Bone grafts, open reduction and, in calcaneal fractures, 1528

Bone marrow, hyperplasia of, in sickle cell disease, 1097, *1098*

  tumors of, 1008, *1008*. See also *Tumors, of foot, bone.*

Bone procedures. See also *Osteotomy.*

  in cavus deformity, 480–483, *481–483*

  in clubfoot, 243

  in pes planus, *510*, 511–515, *512, 513*

Bone prominences, lateral, following calcaneal fractures, 1536

Bosworth operation, for repair of ruptured tendo Achillis, 1539, *1539*

Bowling, footwear for, 1775

Boyd procedure, in paraxial fibular hemimelia, 246

Brandes-Keller operation, as cause of first ray insufficiency syndrome, 687, *687*

Briquet's syndrome, 1439. See also *Psychiatric aspects.*

Brodén roentgenographic projection techniques, *1510, 1511, 1512*

Bromhidrosis, hyperhidrosis and, 896

  treatment of, 896

Bronx-Riverdale disease, Charcot neuropathy in, *1214*

Bullous dermatosis, dermatolytic, 878

  junctional, 878

Bunion(s), footwear for, *1760*, 1776, 1780

  in dancers, 1630–1633, *1632, 1633*. See also *Dancing.*

  in late childhood, 199

  of hallux, examination of, clinical, 93

    physical, 111, *112*

  orthoses for, 1741, *1742*

  shoe lasts for, 1723, *1723*

  shoe modifications for, 1759, *1760*

  tailor's, 95

    physical examination for, 111

  treatment of, in diabetics, 1383–1385, *1384*

    surgical, "blind," avoidance of, 154, *155*

      instruments for, 154–156, *155, 156*

      Mitchell procedure, contraindications for, 173, *173*

      sesamoid excision in, 162, *163*

  vs. hallux valgus, 545

"Bunion pain," in elderly patients, treatment of, 585, *585*

Burns, 1689–1702

  chemical, 1698–1701

    acid, pathophysiology and treatment of, 1699

    action of agent involved, 1698

    alkali, pathophysiology and treatment of, 1700

    treatment of, emergency, use of water, 1698

  deformities from, 1694–1696, *1695, 1697*

    dorsal, 1695, *1695*

    plantar, 1695

    prevention of, 1695

    treatment of, surgical, 1696, *1697*

  electrical, 1451, 1696–1698

    amperage and types of current involved, 1697

    arc-type, 1698

    entry wound, 1697

    exit wound, 1698

    levels of body resistance to, 1698

    treatment of, surgical, 1698

  from industrial injuries, 1613, *1613, 1614*. See also *Industrial injuries.*

  in children, 1684

  principles of care of, 1689

  radiation, 1701, *1701*

    chronic ulceration following, 1701, *1701*

    late effects of, 1701

    skin grafts for, 1701, *1701*

    types of, 1701

  thermal, 1689–1694, *1690, 1691, 1694*

    acute, management of, 1691–1694, *1694*

      antibiotic therapy, 1692

      assessment, 1691

      circulatory status, 1692

      wound care, 1692–1694, *1694*

        debridement and grafting, 1693

Burns (*Continued*)
  thermal, acute, management of, wound care,
      debridement and grafting, technique, 1694
    infection prevention, 1693
    progression prevention, 1693
  causes of, 1689
  pathophysiology of, 1689–1691, *1690, 1691*
    depth measurement, 1690, *1690*
    dermal ischemia, 1691
    partial- vs. full-thickness, 1689
    possible role of prostaglandins, 1691
    progressive nature, 1690
    zones of injury, 1690, *1691*
Bursa(e), 833, 848–854, *849–853.* See also *Bursitis.*
  adventitious, treatment of, 1406
  anatomic classification of, 848, *849, 850*
  caused by shoe vamp, 851, *851*
  pathologic, 848–854, *851–853*
    calcified and ossified, *833,* 853
    classification of, 851
    definition of, 848
    inflammatory, in gout, 853
      in rheumatoid arthritis, 853, *853*
    noninflammatory, pressure-induced, 851, *851, 852*
      spontaneous, *851,* 853, *853*
      traumatic, 852, *852*
    suppurative, 853
    under metatarsal heads, 852, *852*
  retrocalcaneal, physical examination of, 104, *105*
Bursata exostotica, *357, 358*
Bursitis. See also *Bursa(e).*
  calcaneal, 772
    physical examination for, 104, *105*
    treatment of, in geriatrics, 974
  in rheumatoid arthritis, 1031
  interdigital, in geriatrics, 973
  of Achilles tendon, in geriatrics, 975
    in sports injuries, treatment of, 1595, *1596*
  of peroneal tendon, physical examination for, 105, *106*
  padding and devices for pain in, 1731

Cachexia, diabetic neuropathic, 1217
Calcaneal petechiae. See *Black heel.*
Calcaneocuboid joint. See also *Subtalar complex.*
  anatomy of, 12, *14, 15*
  arthrology of, *12, 14, 15*
  roentgenographic view, anteroposterior and medial
    oblique, *1501,* 1511
  talonavicular joint and, as midtarsal joint, 1490. See
    also *Midtarsal joint, injuries of.*
  wedge resection of, in treatment of clubfoot, 243
Calcaneocuboid ligament, *14, 15*
Calcaneofibular ligament, 13, *14*
  rupture of, physical examination for, 108
Calcaneonavicular ligament, *14, 15*
Calcaneovalgus deformity, 252, *252*
  in spinal muscular atrophy, 349, *350*
  in utero, 1759
Calcaneovarus deformity, in spinal muscular atrophy, 349
Calcaneus. See also *Heel* and *Hindfoot.*
  amputation of, partial, results of, 1345, *1345*
  anatomy of, 10, *11, 12, 14, 23, 25, 27*
  apophysis of, in Sever's disease, 204, *204*
  bursitis of, 772
    physical examination for, 104, *105*
    treatment of, in geriatrics, 974

Calcaneus (*Continued*)
  deformity of, in Charcot foot, 1255, *1256, 1257*
    in Charcot-Marie-Tooth disease, *1234,* 1235
    in congenital vertical talus, 440, *440*
    in poliomyelitis, 1137, 1142
    in Riley-Day syndrome, *1258*
    in spina bifida, 252, 276, *276*
    in spinal dysraphism, *252,* 263
    in spinal muscular atrophy, 349
    in tuberculosis, *1410*
    pressure sore in, 276, *276*
    treatment of, surgical, *189,* 190, 252, 276, *276*
      in poliomyelitis, 1137, 1142
  eversion of, treatment of, surgical, in poliomyelitis,
    1142
  exostoses of, 772
  fractures of, 1497–1538. See also *Fractures.*
  fusion of, optimum position, 175
  incisions in, *160*
  inversion of, treatment of, surgical, in poliomyelitis,
    1142
  medial tubercle of, physical examination of, 103, *104*
  osteoma of, 745, *745*
    osteoid, 85, *86, 1000, 1001*
  osteomyelitis of, chronic, 862
  osteosarcoma of, *1003*
    following Paget's disease, *1082,* 1083
  osteotomy of, in pes cavus, 482, *482*
    rotation-displacement, 511–514, *512, 513*
  periostitis of, in geriatrics, 975
  roentgenographic examination of, 96
  rotation of, 50
  solitary bone cyst in, 997, *997, 998*
  spurs of, treatment of, nonsurgical, 767
    surgical, 767, *768*
  surgical approaches to, *160*
  talar facets of, *12, 15*
Calcaneus secundarium, location of, *123,* 124
Calcific tendinitis, of short flexor of hallux, 1460
Calcification, in arteriosclerosis obliterans, 1330, *1330*
  in subcutaneous lesions, 833, *833, 834*
    tuberculosis and, *834,* 835
    usual location of, *834, 834*
  of bursae, *833,* 853
  soft-tissue, vs. soft-tissue chondroma, 834, *834*
    vs. synovial sarcoma, 834, *834*
Calcinosis, tumoral, 1068
Calcinosis circumscripta, 1068
Calcinosis universalis, 1068
Calcitonin, for reflex sympathetic dystrophy syndrome,
  1290
Calf muscles, function of, 43–45, *44, 45*
  rupture of, incomplete, strapping for, 1728, *1728,*
    1729
Callosities, plantar, in geriatrics, 971
Callus(es), definition of, 1402
  etiology of, 1402
  in dancers, 1657, *1658*
  lateral, in fifth toe, 87, *94, 95*
  supports and devices for, and pretreatment, 1743
  treatment of, 1402
Camera's operation, in metatarsalgia with cavus
  deformity, 676
Cancer, neuropathy in, 1242
Candida albicans, in diabetes mellitus, affecting skin of
  foot, 876, *877*
Capsule, laxity of, 843

Capsule (*Continued*)
  synovium and, lesions of, 843–845, *843–845*
    acute transient synovitis of foot and ankle, 844,
      844, 845
    capsular exostoses, 845
    chronic subluxation of metatarsophalangeal and
      interphalangeal joints, 843, *843*
    in second metatarsophalangeal joint, 843
    spontaneous peritalar dislocation, 843, *844*
    synovial sinus, 845
Capsulitis, of metatarsophalangeal joints, 843
Capsulotomy, complete, in clubfoot, 243
  for peripheral nerve injuries, 1192, *1194*
Carcinoma, metastatic, and myeloma, in foot bone,
    1009, *1009*
  neuropathy in, 1242
Cartilage, tumors of, 1003–1008, *1004–1007*. See also
  Tumors, of foot.
Carville microcapsule slipper sock, 1285, *1285*
Cast application, for insensitive foot, 1279, *1279*
  principles of, 169, *169*
Causalgic syndrome (causalgia), 1292
  clinical aspects of, 1292
  definition of, 1292
  major and minor, 1445. See also *Psychiatric aspects.*
  pathogenesis of, 1293
  treatment of, 1293, 1298
Cavovarus deformity, hallux valgus and, case report,
    history, and analysis, *324–328*, 330
  treatment of, 331, 599, *600*
Cavus deformity, 252, 253, 463–485
  as cause of metatarsalgia, 674–678, *675, 677, 678.* See
    also *Metatarsalgia, causes of.*
  basic literature on, guide to, 1862
  biomechanics of, 733
  claw toes and, 465–467
    treatment of, 253, 277
  clinical evaluation of, 471
    auditory testing, 471
    cerebellar symptoms, 471
    gait, 472
    mental status, 471
    motor examination, 471
    sensory examination, 471
    tendon reflexes, 471
    vision testing, 471
  clinical view, *464*
  compensation for, 145, *145*
  correction with standing, *464*
  definition of, 463, *463, 464*
  electrodiagnosis in, 78, 472
  etiology of, 467–471
    cerebral palsy, 470
    Charcot-Marie-Tooth disease, 467, 1235, *1236*
    congenital spinal cord lesions, 470
    diseases underlying, 467
    hemispherical disorders, 470
    myelomeningocele, 470
    neuropathies, hereditary motor sensory, 468
      other, 468
    poliomyelitis, 468
    spina bifida, 470
    spinocerebellar degenerations, 469
      Friedreich's ataxia, 469
  fat pad atrophy in, 838
  gait in, vs. normal foot, *675*
  hammer toe and, 639

Cavus deformity (*Continued*)
  hammer toe and, footwear for, *1776, 1781*
  in children, 198
    surgery for, 186
  in hemophilia, *1091*
  in neurologic foot, 1211
  in poliomyelitis, 84, *84*, 468, 639, 1137, 1163–1167,
    1163–1167
  in spina bifida, *253*, 277
  in spinal dysraphism, *253*, 263
  laboratory studies in, 472
  ligaments of plantar surface and, 464, *465*
  mechanisms of, 465–467, *466, 467*
  metatarsalgia and, 674–678, *675, 677, 678*
    treatment of, 676–678, *677, 678.* See also
      Metatarsalgia.
  metatarsals in, 713
    increased weight bearing of, 179
  muscle biopsy in, 473, *473*
  muscular atrophy in, 466, *466, 467*
  osteotomies for, techniques, 480–482, *481, 482*,
    1163–1167, *1163–1167*
  peripheral nerve biopsy in, 474
  physical examination for, 110, *110*
  plantar standing view, *463*
  radiographic features of, *464*, 472, *483*
  spinal fluid tests for, 472
  symptoms of, 467
  surgical considerations in, 150
  treatment of, 474–483, *474, 476–483*
    goals, 474, *474*
    nonsurgical, 474
      physical therapy, 474
      shoe modifications, 474
    surgical, 475–483, *476–483*
      bone procedures, 480–483, *481–483*
        arthrodesis, 482, *483*
        osteotomy, calcaneal, 482, *482*
          dorsal, 480–482, *481*
          techniques, 1163–1167, *1163–1167*
      historical procedures, 476
      in poliomyelitis, 1137
      postoperative maintenance, 475, *476, 477*
      soft-tissue procedures, 477, *478*
        plantar fascia stripping, 477
        plantar fasciotomy, 478, *478*
      tendon transfers, 478–480, *479, 480*
        forefoot, 478
        hindfoot, 478–480, *479, 480*
    varying nomenclature for, 464
Center of gravity, displacement of, 46, *46*
  line of progression of, 48, *49*
  vertical force curve and, 47, *48, 66*
Central ray insufficiency syndrome, characteristics of,
    682
  congenital, 682
    treatment of, 682
  iatrogenic, treatment of, *683, 684*
  neurologic, 683
    treatment of, 683
Central ray overload syndrome, characteristics and
    treatment, 684
Cerebellar ataxias, 1236
Cerebral palsy. See *Palsy, cerebral.*
Cervical ligament, 13, *14*
Charcot foot, 183, *184*, 1177, 1248–1265. See also
    Charcot joint and *Neuropathic foot.*

Charcot foot (*Continued*)
  clinical features of, 1249–1252, *1249–1253*
    acute, 1249, *1249*
      vs. chronic, 1249–1251, *1249, 1250*
    by anatomic location, *1250,* 1251, *1251–1253*
    chronic, *1250,* 1251
    hypertrophic vs. atrophic, 1251
  complications of, 1252–1259, *1254–1258*
    deformity, 1255, *1256–1258*
      calcaneal, 1255, *1256, 1257*
      secondary to joint changes, 1255, *1257, 1258*
    presence of pain, 1255
    soft-tissue injury, *1250,* 1255–1259, *1257, 1258*
      Chopart's joint changes, 1255, *1257, 1258,* 1259
      ulceration, *1250,* 1259
    spontaneous fractures, 1253–1255, *1254, 1255*
  definition of, 1248
  diabetic, in rheumatoid arthritis, *1215*
  diagnosis of, differential, 1249
  in Lisfranc's joint, 184, *184, 1214*
  in motor neuritis, 1243, *1244*
  loss of motor vs. sensory function in, 1248
  metatarsal displacement in, 179, *184*
  microscopic findings in, 1252
  pseudo-, 1237, *1237*
  treatment of, 1259–1265, *1260–1263*
    control of neuropathy, 1259
    immobilization, 1259–1261, *1260, 1261*
    local debridement, 1259
    role of surgery, 1261–1265, *1262, 1263*
      contraindications, 1261, *1262, 1263*
      indications, 1264
      literature review, 1264
      postoperative management, 1265
Charcot joint. See also *Charcot foot.*
  diagnosis of, 1211
  in Bronx-Riverdale disease, *1214*
  in children vs. adults, 1213
  in diabetic foot, 82, 1379, *1379, 1380*
  in neurologic foot, 1211–1213, *1212–1215*
  pseudo-, *1212,* 1213
  treatment of, 1211
Charcot-Marie-Tooth disease, affecting foot, 84
  calcaneal deformity in, *1234,* 1235
  cavus deformity and, 198, 467, 1235, *1236*
  clinical features of, 1231–1235, *1234–1236*
  Dejerine-Sottas disease and, 1238
  electrodiagnostic studies in, 73, 78, 1236
  formes frustes, 1235
  hereditary sensory neuropathies and, 1227
  high longitudinal arch in, 91
  motor involvement in, wide variations of, 1235
  neurologic foot and, 1211
  pathologic changes in, 1236
  peripheral polyneuritis in, 1215
  severe, 1235, *1235*
  treatment of, surgical, 1235, *1235*
  ulceration in, 1236, *1236*
  with associated neuropathy, 1231–1236, *1234–1236*
Check-rein deformity, with tendon tethering, 861, *861*
Child(ren), foot and ankle of, suggested course outline
    for resident study of, 1835
  foot disorders in. See also *Children, trauma in* and
    Growing foot.
    classification of, 196
    early detection of, 195
    evaluation of, 198

Child(ren) (*Continued*)
  foot disorders in, identification of, 195–199, *197*
    racial variations, 196
  gait analysis in, 57, 63, 78
  surgical considerations in, 151
  trauma in, 1660–1688. See also *Children, foot
    disorders in* and *Growing foot.*
    and growth, 1661–1664, *1662–1664*
      bone replacement mechanism, 1661, *1662*
      epiphyseal and metaphyseal, 1662, *1662*
      of foot and lower extremities, 1661
      ossification, endochondral, *1662,* 1663, *1663,*
        1664
        epiphyseal blood vessels, 1663, *1663*
        growth plate divisions, zone of cartilage
          transformation, 1663, *1664*
        zone of growth, 1663, *1664*
        zone of ossification, 1664, *1664*
        osteogenesis vs. chondrogenesis, 1663, *1663*
        vs. periosteal, 1662, *1662*
      time of onset of congenital foot deformities in
        utero, 1661
    ankle injuries, fractures about, 1671–1673, *1672*
      classification of injury, 1671
      epiphyseal, complications of, 1673, *1674*
      miscellaneous, 1673
      severe, 1682
      sprains, 1681
        lateral ligament, 1681
        medial ligament, 1682
        tibiofibular ligament, 1682
      triplane, 1673
      types of, 1671–1673, *1672*
        fibular, 1671
        tibial, 1671–1673, *1672*
    environmental effects on growth plate and
      epiphysis, 1664–1666, *1665, 1666*
    epiphyseal injuries, 1668, *1668*
      bony, classification, 1669, *1669*
      effects of, 1668
      prognosis for, *1668,* 1669
    foot injuries, 1674–1685, *1676–1679, 1685*
      accessory bones, 1680
      Achilles tendinitis, 1681
      amputations, 1684
      athletic, 1681
      burns, 1684
      calcaneal fractures, 1675
      from bicycle spokes, 1683
      from freezing, 1684
      from power motors, 1683
      iatrogenic, 1685, *1685*
      in osteochondritis dissecans, *1666,* 1675
      limb replants, 1685
      Lisfranc joint dislocation, 1680
      metatarsal fractures, 1676–1680, *1678, 1679*
        Jones fracture, 1679
        transverse, 1679, *1679*
        trauma to heads, 1679
      metatarsophalangeal dislocation, 1680
      midfoot fractures and dislocations, 1680
      midtarsal, 1676, *1676, 1677*
      phalangeal fractures, 1680
      puncture wounds, 1682
      sagittal diastasis, 1682
      separation of first and second metatarsals, 1682
      skin loss, 1684

Child(ren) (*Continued*)
   trauma in, foot injuries, stress fractures, 1681
      talar fractures, 1674
      talar fracture-dislocation, 1675
     growth plate injuries, classification, 1669–1671,
      1669, 1670
     incidence of, 1660
      classification, 1660
      location of injury, 1661
     mechanisms of, 1666, *1667*
Chondroblastoma(s), 1005–1007, *1006*
Chondroma, soft-tissue, vs. soft-tissue calcification, 834,
   834
Chondromalacia, of sesamoids, 553, *554*
Chondromyxoid fibroma, *1006*, 1007
Chondrosarcoma(s), 1007, *1007*
   of small toes, 652, *653*
Chopart amputations, *1368, 1369, 1369, 1371,*
   1392–1394, *1393*
   prostheses for, 1815, *1817*
Chopart joint, anatomy of, *12, 15.* See also *Midtarsal*
   joint.
Christmas disease. See *Hemophilia(s).*
Chromosome 18q syndrome, short life expectancy with,
   234
Cigarette smoking, role of, as cause of arteriosclerosis
   obliterans, 1325
   as cause of thromboangiitis obliterans, 1347
   withdrawal of, in diabetics, 1383
Circulation, impaired, in diabetic foot, 1378, *1378*
Circulatory disturbances, basic literature on, guide to,
   1843
Circulatory status, assessment of, 539, *540*
Claudication, PVR examination of, in arteriosclerosis
   obliterans, 1325, *1325*
Clawfoot, in compartment syndrome, 1202
Claw toe(s). See also *Hammer toe(s).*
   basic literature on, guide to, 1864
   cavus deformity and, 465–467
     treatment of, 253, 277
   fixed, with metatarsophalangeal contracture,
     treatment of, surgical, classification of procedures,
     1035
   flexible, treatment of, surgical, classification of
     procedures, 1035
   hallux valgus and, treatment of, surgical, 1036
   hard corns and, physical examination for, 113, *113*
   in dancers, *1641*, 1642
   in rheumatoid arthritis, *1025, 1026, 1028, 1029*
   treatment of, in diabetics, 1383–1385, *1384*
     surgical, 644, 1281
      in poliomeylitis, 1137
   vs. hammer toe, 212, *212*, 639, *639*
Cleft foot, basic literature on, guide to, 1862
   congenital, clinical features of, 245
     treatment of, 245
Cleft hand and foot syndrome, radiographic view, *239*
Clubfoot. See also *Talipes equinovarus* and *Talipes,*
   inverted.
   amniocentesis in experimental animals and, 230
   complete, 384, *384,* 389
   constriction band syndrome and, 230
   heel cord function and, 728
   idiopathic, electrodiagnosis in, 78
   in diastrophic dwarfism, *236*
   in Pierre Robin syndrome, *239*
   overcorrected, surgery following, *180*

Clubfoot (*Continued*)
   pathogenesis of, prenatal positioning and, 8
   tibialis anterior tendon transfer for, 715, *715*
   treatment of, iatrogenic complications following, in
     children, 1685, *1685*
     results, 427
     surgical, aseptic necrosis of talus following, 748, *748*
      bone procedures, 243
      infection following, 153, *153*
      procedures for, 411
      talar avascular necrosis following, 173, *174*
      timing for, *149,* 150
   types of, classification, *376–379*
     composite plane grouping, *378, 379*
     coronal plane, *377*
     everted, *379*
     horizontal plane, *376*
     inverted, *379*
     sagittal plane, *377*
   variations of, 83
   vertical talus and, congenital, 444
Coccidioides immitis, 1416
Coccidioidomycosis, clinical features and treatment of,
   1416, *1417*
Cockayne's disease, characteristics of, 878
Colchicine, in treatment of acute gouty arthritis, 1020
Cold, injuries from, in children, 1684
   in forefoot and toes, 1450. See also *Injury(ies).*
Cold sensitivity, following cold injury, 1351
   in Raynaud's phenomenon, 1349–1351. See also
     Raynaud's phenomenon.
Cole's osteotomy, 1164, *1164, 1165*
Collagen disease(s), affecting foot, 84
   associated CNS diseases and, classification, 1224
   hand and foot vasculitis and, 83, *83*
   inflammatory tenosynovitis and, 855
   peripheral neuropathy in, 1223–1226, *1225*
     classification, 1224
Compartment syndrome(s), 1201–1203
   anterior, 1202
   etiology of, 1201
   fasciotomy in, indications for, 1201
   four-compartment involvement, 1202
   in adults vs. children, 1203
   in sports injuries, 1599
   isolated, of hand and foot, 1201
     peroneal, 1202
   leg and foot anatomy, 1201
   lower vs. upper extremities, 1201
   posterior, 1202
   tolerance levels of ischemia and, 1201
Compression by shoe, avoidance of, 1755, *1756*
Compression fracture(s), of navicular, treatment of, *1491*
   of talar body, 1483, *1484*
Compression injuries, neuropathies and, 1181, *1182*
   classification of, 1181
     Hoffmann-Tinel sign, 1182
Computerized axial tomography, uses of, 138
Condylectomy, partial, for soft corns, 630, *632*
Condyles, anatomy of, 659–666. See also *Metatarsals,*
   anatomy of.
Configuration, general examination of, 87, *87*
Congenital deformity(ies), 212–232
   basic literature on, guide to, 1853–1862
   constriction band syndrome, 228–230, *229.* See also
     Constriction band syndrome.
   convergent toes, 218

Congenital deformity(ies) (*Continued*)
curly toes, 214, *215*. See also *Curly toes.*
divergent toes, 218
hallux varus, 215, *216*, 616, *616*, *617*. See also *Hallux varus.*
hammer toe, 212–214, *212*, *213*. See also *Hammer toe(s).*
hemangioma, 219
longitudinal deficiency of fibula, 220–226, *221*, *224*. See also *Fibula, longitudinal deficiency of.*
longitudinal deficiency of tibia with intact fibula, 226–228. See also *Tibia, longitudinal deficiency of.*
lymphangioma, 220
macrodactyly, 218, *219*. See also *Macrodactyly.*
mallet toe, *212*, 214. See also *Mallet toe.*
microdactyly, 218
paraxial fibular hemimelia, 220–226, *221*, *224*. See also *Fibula, longitudinal deficiency of.*
polydactyly, 216–218, *217*. See also *Polydactyly.*
syndactyly, 218, *218*. See also *Syndactyly.*
varus toe, 214, *215*
tibial hemimelia, 226–228. See also *Tibia, longitudinal deficiency of.*
vertical talus, joint ankylosis and, 444
Congenital myopathies, 346
Constriction band syndrome, congenital, 228–230, *229*
abnormal pregnancy and, 228
associated anomalies and, 228
clinical features of, 229, 230
clubfoot and, 230
distal syndactyly and, 228, 230
etiology of, 228
historical background, 228
pathogenesis of, 228
treatment of, 230
Contact dermatitis, 891–894, *891–893*, 895. See also *Dermatitis, contact.*
Contracture(s), Dupuytren's, bilateral concurrent, weight-bearing and, 147, *148*
of plantar fascia, physical examination for, *109*, 110
equinus, at ankle, in Duchenne's muscular dystrophy, 336, *337*
of tendons, 866
Contusion(s), of forefoot and toes, definition of, 1449
diagnosis of, differential, 1449
treatment of, 1449
of toes, resulting in subungual hematoma, 1449
Convergent toes, congenital, treatment of, 218
Conversion hysteria, 1438–1444, *1442–1444*. See also *Psychiatric aspects, hysterical neurosis.*
Cord, spinal. See *Spinal cord.*
Corn(s), cause of, 1403
causing ulcers in diabetic foot, 1385, *1386*
definition of, 624, *624*, 1403
end, 624, 625, 634–636, *634–636*
causes of, 634, *634*
mallet toe and, 634, *634*
paraungual, 935
treatment of, nonsurgical, 936
surgical, 936
treatment of, palliative, 635, *635*
surgical, 164, 635, *636*
technique, 636, *636*
hard, 624–628, *624–628*
causes of, 624
claw toes and, physical examination for, 113, *113*
clinical features of, 624, *625*

Corn(s) (*Continued*)
hard, common location for, 624, *625*
hammer toe and, 113, *113*
miscellaneous considerations, 632–634
soft corns and, distal hemiphalangectomy for, 628
treatment of, 625–628, *626–628*
nonsurgical, 625, *626*
palliative, 625, *626*
surgical, 625–628, *627*, *628*
contraindicated in children, 628
principles of therapy, 628
technique, 626–628, *627*
flail toe following severance of extensor tendon, 628, *628*
in dancers, 1657, *1658*
paraungual, 935
treatment of, *636*, 651, *651*, *652*
periungual, 936
secondary to claw or hammer toes, physical examination for, 113, *113*
soft, 628–634, *629–632*
cause of, 628, *629*
common location of, 628, *629*, 631, *631*
definition of, 628, *629*
diabetes and, 95, *95*
diagnosis of, differential, 631–633
in fifth toe, 94, *95*
miscellaneous considerations, 632–634
physical examination for, 114, *114*
treatment of, nonsurgical, 629, 631
palliative, 629, 631
surgical, 629–632, *630–632*
common sites for, *632*
instruments, 632
local excision contraindicated, consequent secondary sinus tract formation, 631, *631*
partial condylectomy, *630*, 632
sites of incision, 629, *630*
when proximal toe dislocated, 629, *630*, 633
vs. fungal infections, 631, 633
supports and devices for, pretreatment and, 1743
treatment of, 1403
drug contraindications, 633
nonsurgical, in geriatrics, 968, *968*
orthoses, 633
postoperative care, 634
syndactylization, 631, 634
Corrective appliances, for spina bifida, 266
Cortical hyperostosis, caused by hypervitaminosis A, 1069
clinical features of, 1069
infantile, clinical features of, 1069
"Crab" yaws, *1423*
Cramps, leg, in neuropathic foot, 1210
Cranial nerves, in relation to neurologic examination of foot, 1108
Cretinism, 1073
Crush fractures, of hallux, 1458, *1458*
of talar body, treatment of, 1485
Crush injury(ies), metatarsal discombobulation in, 187, *187*
of forefoot and toes, definition of, 1450
treatment of, 1450
of midfoot, in childhood, 1676, *1676*
of midtarsal joint, treatment and prognosis, 1495
of navicular, vs. Köhler's disease, 1676, *1677*
treatment of, 1402

Crush injury(ies) (*Continued*)
  treatment of, surgical, 1298
Cryptococcosis, sites and clinical features of, 1415
Cryptococcus neoformans, 1415
Cuboid, anatomy of, 10, *11, 12, 14, 27*
  avulsion fracture of, treatment of, *1491*
  dislocation of, treatment of, *1493, 1493*
Cuboideonavicular joint, anatomy of, 15
  arthrology of, 15
Cuboideonavicular ligament, 15
Cuboides secundarium, location of, *123, 124*
Cuneiforms, anatomy of, 10–12, *11, 14*
  resections of, in poliomyelitis, 1140
Cuneonavicular joint, anatomy of, 15
  arthrology of, 15
Curled-under toes, 648, *648*
Curly toe(s), congenital, 214, *215*
  definition of, 214, *215*
  familial incidence of, 214
  treatment of, nonsurgical, 214
    surgical, 215
  vs. hammer toe, 214
Cushing-Lembert suture, *1144*
Cutaneous horn, clinical features of, 829, *830*
  definition of, 829
  treatment of, 829, *830*
Cutaneous nerves, dorsal, entrapment neuropathies in,
    1197
Cuticle, 914, *915, 916, 918*
  in human embryonic nails, 914
Cyanosis, of toe, caused by microemboli, 1315, *1315*
Cyst(s), and tumor-like lesions, 997–999, *997–999*. See
    also *Tumors, of foot, bone.*
  epithelial inclusion, vs. soft-tissue tumors, 981, *982*
  inclusion, of small toes, following Syme procedure,
    653, *655*
  mucous, of small toes, *655, 656*
Cystic lesions, in children, 196
  in late childhood and adolescence, 199

Dactylitis, in hemoglobin SC disease, 1102
  in sickle cell disease, 1099, *1099, 1100*
  syphilitic, treatment of, 1418
  tuberculous, clinical features of, 1410
Dancing, modern, and classical ballet, 1626–1659
    abnormal foot positions, 1639–1642, *1639–1641*
      rolling in, 1639–1641, *1640*
      rolling out, 1641, *1641*
      sickling, 1639, *1639, 1640*
      toe clawing, *1641, 1642*
    ankle joint in, anterior tibiofibular ligament
        strain, 1646
      osteophyte formation, treatment of, *1635,
        1636,* 1648
      synovitis, treatment of, 1648
    ankle tendon problems, 1642–1648, *1642,
        1644–1647*
      Achilles tendon, 1642, *1642*
        at gastrocnemius junction, 1643
        treatment of, 1642
      anterior tendons, tendinitis of tibialis anterior
        and extensor digitorum longus, 1648
      lateral compartment, tendinitis of peroneus
        brevis and peroneus longus, 1645–1648,
        1646, 1647

Dancing (*Continued*)
    modern, and classical ballet, ankle tendon problems,
        posteromedial compartment, 1643–1645,
        1644, 1645
      rupture of flexor hallucis longus, complete,
        1645
      partial, 1644, *1644, 1645*
      tendinitis of tibialis posterior, flexor
        digitorum longus, and flexor hallucis
        longus, 1643
      trigger toe, 1644, *1644, 1645*
    dancer's normal foot, 1630–1635, *1631–1633*
      bunions, 1630–1633, *1632, 1633*
        etiology of, *1632,* 1633
      hallux rigidus, clinical features and treatment
        of, 1634
      hallux valgus, 1629, *1629, 1632, 1633, 1633,*
        1641
      hammer toe, 1633, *1633*
      minor pain, treatment of, 1633
      splayfoot, clinical features and treatment of,
        1634
      "sur les pointes" position, 1630, *1631*
      surgical indications, 1634
    fatigue fractures in, 1637–1639, *1638*
      development of, 1637
      location of, 1637, *1638*
      through second metatarsal, 1637, *1638*
      treatment of, 1638
    foot trauma in, 1653–1655, *1653, 1655*
      aneurysm of dorsalis pedis artery, 1654, *1655*
      arch supports for, 1655
      dorsal cutaneous neuritis, 1654
      ligament and muscle sprains, 1654
      plantar fasciitis, 1654
      to fifth metatarsal, 1653, *1653*
        fracture of neck and shaft, 1653
        Jones fracture, 1653, *1653*
    forefoot injuries, 1655–1659, *1656–1658*
      calluses and soft corns, 1657, *1658*
      hallux, 1655–1657, *1656*
        flexion injury, 1656
        fractures of, 1655
        interphalangeal joint injury, 1657
        sesamoid injuries, 1655, *1656*
      nail problems, 1658, *1658*
      toe dislocations, 1657, *1657*
    fractures in, 1650–1654, *1650–1653*
      eversion, *1650, 1651, 1651*
      inversion, 1651, *1651, 1652*
      of talar dome, 1652, *1652*
    ligament injuries in, 1649
      eversion, 1650
      inversion, 1649
      strains, 1649
    os trigonum syndrome, 1648, *1649*
      diagnosis and treatment of, 1649, *1649*
    osteoarthritis in, 789
    roentgenographic characteristics, 1635–1637,
        1635–1637
      ankle, 1635, *1635*
      foot, 1636, *1636, 1637*
      ligament calcification, 1636, *1636*
      metatarsal thickening, 1636, *1636*
      osteochondritis dissecans, 1635, *1635*
      osteophyte formation, 1635, *1635, 1636,* 1648
      talar neck inclination, 1637, *1637*

Dancing (*Continued*)
   modern, and classical ballet, training for, 1626–1630,
      1626–1630
      arch development, 1628, *1628, 1629*
      balance points, 1627, *1627, 1628*
      basic foot positions, 1626, *1626*
      childhood developments, 1626
      congenital abnormalities, 1629, *1630*
Darier's disease, keratoses of sole in, *903, 904*
Debrisan, for wound debridement, 941, 947
   in diabetic foot, 1391
Deformity(ies), congenital, 212–232. See also *Congenital
   deformity(ies).*
   of foot. For other deformities, see under specific
      areas.
      classification of, in poliomyelitis, 1132. See also
        Poliomyelitis.
      combination possibility occurrences, *380*
      electrodiagnosis in, 78
      factors affecting, intrauterine molding, 254, *255*
        neurologic loss or absence, 253–258, *254*
        prolonged early development stages, 254
      gross, visible, in poliomyelitis, 1126. See also
        Poliomyelitis.
      in Becker's muscular dystrophy, 346. See also
        Muscular dystrophy.
      in cerebral palsy, 198, 282–334. See also *Palsy,
        cerebral.*
      in Duchenne's muscular dystrophy, 336–345,
        337–345. See also *Muscular dystrophy.*
      in Guillain-Barré syndrome, 351
      in fascio-scapulo-humeral muscular dystrophy, 346.
        See also *Muscular dystrophy.*
      in myotonic dystrophy, 347
      in scapulo-peroneal atrophy, 347
      in spinal muscular atrophy, 348, *348, 350.* See also
        Muscular atrophy.
      involving ankle, 793
      management of, 267
      pathogenesis of, 249–258, *250, 252–255, 257*
        motor activity at birth, 250
        neurologic loss and other factors, 253–258, *254,
          255, 257*
        neurologic patterns of paralysis, 251–253, *252,
          253*
      pathomechanics of, 381–392, *384, 385, 387–392.*
        See also *Talipes.*
      rotational, 432, 436. See also *Rotational
        deformities.*
      patterns of, factors affecting, external pressure, 257,
        257
        soft-tissue tension, 257
        neurologic loss and other factors affecting,
          253–258, *254, 255, 257*
        continuation after birth, 256
      postnatal changes in, 256
      varying terminology for, 375
   rotational, of lower extremity. See *Rotational
      deformities.*
Degloving injuries, treatment of, 1402
Dejerine-Sottas disease, Charcot-Marie-Tooth disease
   and, 1238
   EMG findings in, 73
de Lange's syndrome, clinical features of, *240*
   postoperative, *241*
   radiographic view, *240*
Deltoid ligament, *11, 13, 14*

Denervation, partial, with view to muscle rebalancing,
   268
   sympathetic, in diabetic polyneuropathy, 1218
Dermatitis, atopic, 871–873, *871–873*
   ankle lichenification in, 871, *871*
   associated conditions and, 871
   dryness and scaling in, 871, *872*
   eczema in, *872, 873*
   foot manifestations of, 871, *871–873*
   soap and detergent avoidance in, 872
   thickening caused by chronic scratching in, 872,
      872
   treatment of, 872
   vs. shoe dermatitis, 872
   vs. tinea pedis, 872
  contact, allergic, 891, *891*
   diagnosis of, 891–894
   from shoes, 894, *895.* See also *Dermatitis, shoe.*
   irritant, 891, *892, 893*
      from chemicals, 891, *892*
      from creams, 891, *892*
      from orthoses, 891, *893*
      from scalding, 891, *893*
   treatment of, 894
  factitial, self-inflicted injuries in, 1444. See also
      Psychiatric aspects.
  shoe, allergic nature of, 894, *895*
   clinical features of, 894, *895*
   diagnosis of, 894
   treatment of, 894
   vs. atopic dermatitis, 872
Dermatitis artefacta, self-inflicted injuries in, 1444. See
   also *Psychiatric aspects.*
Dermatofibrosarcoma protuberans, 986, *987*
Dermatoglyphic analyses, *197*
Dermatologic disorders, basic literature on, guide to,
   1844
Dermatomes, history and use, 944, 946, *946*
Dermatomyositis, affecting foot, 874, *874*
   peripheral neuropathies and, 1226
Dermatophytidic tinea pedis, 898, *900, 901*
Dermatosis, bullous, dermatolytic, 878
   junctional, 878
Dermis, of sole skin, anatomy of, 1400, *1400*
Dermopathy, diabetic, affecting foot, 877
Deutschländer's disease. See also *Fractures, march.*
   caused by first ray insufficiency syndrome, 688, *688*
   characteristics of, 688
   etiology of, 689
   evolutionary phases of, 689
   radiologic view of, 688, *688*
Development, of foot and ankle, roentgenographic
   examination of, 116–121, *117–120*
Developmental disorders, 200–211
   Freiberg's infraction, 207–210, *208, 209*
   Köhler's disease of tarsal scaphoid, 200–203, *202, 203*
   osteochondritis dissecans of talus, 204–207, *205–207*
   sesamoid osteochondritis, 210, *210*
   Sever's disease, 203, *204*
Diabetes. See also *Diabetic foot* and *Neuropathy,
   diabetic.*
   affecting foot, 84
   arteriosclerosis obliterans and, arterial sites affected
      in, 1324
   Charcot destruction in, in anterior tarsus and
      Lisfranc's joint, 718, *719*
   Charcot joint in, 1379, *1379, 1380*

Diabetes (*Continued*)
claw toes in, treatment of, 1383–1385, *1384*
control of, in arteriosclerosis obliterans, 1331, *1331*
electrodiagnosis in, 73
footwear for, 1781
history-taking for, 82
Lisfranc's joint destruction in, 1251, *1252*
Lisfranc's joint neuropathy in, 1255, *1257*
metatarsophalangeal destruction in, 1251, *1253*
midtarsal destruction in, 1251, *1251*
nerve conduction studies in, 73
small toe conditions and, 95, *95*
soft corns and, 95, *95*
subtalar neuroarthropathy in, *1258*
vs. syphilis, spontaneous fractures in, *1254*, 1255, *1255*
Diabetes mellitus, as cause of Charcot foot, 1248
skin of foot and, 876–878, *877, 878*
Candida albicans infections in, 876, *877*
diabetic dermopathy in, 877
digital bullous lesions in, 877
malum perforans in, 878, *878*
monilial paronychia in, 876, *877*
necrobiosis lipoidica diabeticorum in, 877, *877*
pruritus in, 878
Diabetic amyotrophy, 1217
Diabetic dermopathy, affecting foot, 877
Diabetic foot, 1377–1397. See also *Diabetes* and *Neuropathy, diabetic.*
EMG findings in, 73
historical perspective, 1377
pathophysiology of, 1377–1381, *1378–1381*
Charcot joints, 1379, *1379, 1380*
circulatory problems, 1378, *1378*
leukocyte changes, 1381
peripheral and CNS neuropathy, 1377
sensory involvement, 1378
skin changes, 1380, *1381*
source of infections, 1380
structural changes, 1380
wound healing, 1381
physical examination of, 1381–1383, *1382*
amputations, 1392–1394, *1393–1395*
treatment of, 1383–1394, *1384, 1386–1390, 1392–1395*
amputations, healing prognosis, 1396
prostheses for, 1394, *1395*
bunions and claw toes and, 1383–1385, *1384*
Debrisan, 1391
mal perforans ulcers and, 1385–1394, *1386–1390*
caused by corns and callosities, 1385, *1386*
causing secondary forefoot infection, 1387–1390, *1390*
in presence of gangrene, 1391, *1392, 1393*
large, 1387, *1387*
metatarsophalangeal involvement, 1387, *1389*
pinch grafts, 1387, *1389*
small, 1385
split-thickness grafts, 1387, *1387, 1388, 1390, 1391, 1392*
total debridement, 1391
patient education, 1383
tobacco withdrawal, 1383
whirlpool bath, 1391
Diabetic neuropathic cachexia, 1217
Diabetic neuropathy, 1210, 1217–1219, 1377–1397. See also *Diabetic foot* and *Neuropathy, diabetic.*

Diabetic polyneuropathy, sympathic denervation in, 1218
Diaphyseal dysplasia, progressive, clinical features of, 369
pathologic findings in, 369
radiographic features of, 369, *370*
Diaphyseal osteotomy, in first ray insufficiency syndrome, 698–700, *699*
Diaphysectomy, in hammer toe, 642, *642*
Jahss, 643
Diastasis, sagittal, in children, 1682
Diastematomyelia, spastic paraparesis in, 256
Diastrophic dwarfism, clubfoot and, *236*
hallux varus and, 216, *216*
Digital abnormality, in children, variations of, 196
Diphtheria, electrodiagnosis in, 73
Diplegia, spastic, case reports, 295–301, *295–297, 299, 300, 318–322, 319–321.* See also *Spastic diplegia.*
Dislocation(s), basic literature on, guide to, 1851
in sports injuries, 1588, *1588.* See also *Sports injuries.*
of ankle, total, 1472–1474, *1473.* See also *Ankle, injuries of* and *Fractures, of ankle.*
of forefoot and toes, general considerations, 1451, *1451*
of cuboid, treatment of, 1493, *1493*
of forefoot joints, 1452–1457, *1452–1456*
Lisfranc's joint, 1452, *1452–1455*
fracture-dislocations, diagrammatic views, 1452, *1453*
roentgenographic view, 1454, *1455*
treatment of, 1452, *1454, 1455*
inadequate, 1453, *1455*
types of, 1452, *1453*
in children, 1680
metatarsals, 179, *184, 187,* 1452, *1452–1455*
fractures and, 1453–1457
"march," 1457
"shatter," 1457
treatment of, 1456
metatarsal splitting, 1453, *1456*
navicular, 1453, *1456*
of metatarsophalangeal joint, in children, 1680
in dancers, 1657, *1657*
of midtarsal joint, plantar, *1494*
of sesamoids, in first ray insufficiency syndrome, 686
subtalar complex, peritalar and Chopart, 747
rheumatoid, *731,* 747
subtalar, 747
of subtalar joint, 1467–1472, *1468–1471*
anterior, 1471
treatment of, 1471
complications of, 1471
etiology and incidence of, 1467
lateral, 1479–1471, *1470*
roentgenographic view, *1470*
treatment of, 1470, *1470*
medial, 1468, *1468, 1469*
roentgenographic views, *1468, 1469*
treatment of, 1468, *1469*
posterior, 1471, *1471*
roentgenographic view, *1471*
treatment of, 1471
prognosis for, 1471
spontaneous, 843, *844*
total, 1472–1474, *1473*
of talocalcaneonavicular joint, 440, *440, 442*

Dislocation(s) (*Continued*)
  of talonavicular joint, in talar neck fractures, 1475, *1477*
    treatment of, 1479
  of talus, total, 1472–1474, *1473*
    complications of, 1472, 1474
    incidence of, 1472
    mechanism of injury, 1472, *1473*
    prognosis for, 1474
    treatment of, 1472–1474
      closed reduction, 1473
      open reduction, 1474
      postoperative, 1474
  of tendons, 865
    in sports injuries, 1591–1593, *1592, 1593*. See also *Sports injuries.*
  of toes, 1451–1459, *1451–1456, 1458*
    as cause of soft corns, 629, *630*, 633
    complex vs. simple, *1458*, 1459
    in dancers, 1657, *1657*
    traumatic, 1458, *1458*
    treatment of, 1459
  peritalar, 1467–1472, *1468–1471*. See also *Dislocations, of subtalar joint.*
Disobliteration, arterial, 1318–1320, *1318, 1319*. See also *Vascular diseases.*
Distal myopathies, 347
Distance runners, sports injuries in, 1601–1605, *1603*. See also *Sports injuries.*
Divergent toes, 647, *648*
  congenital, treatment of, 218
Doppler flowmeter, examination with, 947
Doppler ultrasound instruments, 1302, *1303*. See also *Vascular diseases, physiologic examination of.*
Dorsal cutaneous nerves, entrapment neuropathies in, 1197
Dorsal spurs, footwear for, 1780
Dorsalis pedis, anatomy of, 950
  aneurysm of, in dancers, 1654, *1655*
  flaps of, for skin grafts, 950–953, *951, 958*, 961. See also *Skin grafts.*
  palpation of, 106
  surgical bypass of, 1341, *1341*
Dorsiflexion, gait analysis and, *61*
  in ankle joint, 40, *40*, 43, *44, 45*
    excessive, in head trauma patient, *1121, 1122*
    inadequate, in poliomyelitis, 1137
    in stroke patient, 1114
  range of, tests for, 1716, *1717*
Dorsum pedis, anatomy of, surgical, *18*, 33
  incisions in, plastic surgery and, 943, *943*
  infections of, treatment of, 1406
Double-limb support, in walking cycle, 37
Down's syndrome, congenital vertical talus and, 444
  hallucal patterns in, 197
Dracunculus medinensis infestation, 1420, *1420*
Drop foot, ankle fusion in, 190, *191*
  avoidance of surgery in, 150
  physical examination for, 114, *115*
Dry skin, in geriatrics, 965
Duchenne's muscular dystrophy, 335–345, *337–345*. See also *Muscular dystrophy.*
Dupuytren's contracture, bilateral concurrent, weight-bearing and, 147, *148*
  of plantar fascia, physical examination for, *109*, 110
DuVries and Mann operation, in hammer toe, *643, 644*
Dwarfism, diastrophic, clubfoot and, *236*

Dwarfism (*Continued*)
  diastrophic, hallux varus and, 216, *216*
  hypothyroid, in children vs. adults, 1073
  metatrophic, short life expectancy in, 234
  thanatophoric, lethal nature of, 234, *234*
Dwyer's osteotomy, 1167, *1167*
Dysautonomia, clinical features of, 234
  familial, hereditary sensory neuropathies and, 1227
    self-inflicted injuries in, 1444
  limited life span with, 234
Dysesthesia, hysterical, 1443. See also *Psychiatric aspects.*
Dyshidrosis, affecting feet, 894
  clinical features of, 894
  differential diagnosis, 894
  treatment of, 894
Dysplasia(s), bone, 353–373. See also *Bone dysplasias.*
  definition of, 353
  fibrous, 360–362, *362*. See also *Fibrous dysplasia.*
  diaphyseal, progressive, 369, *370*
  resorption. See *Bone dysplasias.*
  sclerosing. See *Bone dysplasias.*
Dysplasia epiphysealis hemimelica, 354, 355, 1003, *1004*
  clinical features of, 354
  pathologic findings in, 354
  prognosis for, 354
  radiographic features of, 354, *355*
  treatment of, 354
Dysraphism, spinal, foot management in, 248–281. See also *Spinal dysraphism.*
Dystrophy, muscular. See *Muscular dystrophy.*
  myotonic. See *Myotonic dystrophy.*
  reflex sympathetic, 1287–1290, *1288*, 1445. See also *Psychiatric aspects* and *Reflex sympathetic dystrophy syndrome.*

Ectodermal ridge, studies on, 7
Eczema, in atopic dermatitis, 872, *873*
  vs. epidermophytosis, 94, *94*
Edema, brawny, following chronic venous insufficiency, 1356, *1357*
  doughy pitting, in transverse metatarsal arch, 93, *93*
  idiopathic, subcutaneous, 836, *836*
  of foot, following proximal arterial reconstruction, 1347
Egyptian foot, digital and metatarsal formulas for, *660*, 665
Ekman-Lobstein disease, 362, *364*. See also *Osteogenesis imperfecta.*
Elective surgery, standards for, 146
Electrical burns, 1451, 1696–1698. See also *Burns, electrical* and *Industrial injuries.*
Electrical hazards, protective footwear for, 1767, *1768*
Electrodiagnosis, 68–80
  as extension of clinical examination, 79
  clinical applications of, 73–79
    in amyotrophic lateral sclerosis, 77
    in anterior horn cell disease, 77
    in axonotmesis, 75
    in cerebral palsy, 78
    in entrapment syndromes, 76
    in foot deformities, 78
      arthrogryposis multiplex congenita, 78
      cavus deformity, 78, 472
      idiopathic clubfoot, 78

Electrodiagnosis (*Continued*)
  clinical applications of, in myelomeningocele,
      78
    in neurapraxia, 75
    in neuropathies, 73–75
    in neurotmesis, 75
    in peripheral nerve injuries, 75
      site localization, 76
    in radiculopathy, 77
    in upper motor neuron disease, 78
  electromyographic, 68–71, *69*
  electroneurographic, 71–73, *72*
  nerve conduction studies, 71–73, *72*
Electromyography, 68–71, *69*. See also *Electrodiagnosis*.
  in arthrogryposis multiplex congenita, 78
  in cerebral palsy, 63, 78
  in gait analysis, 60–66, *64, 65*
  in poliomyelitis, 64
  in stroke, 66
  indications for, 99
  technique of, 68, *69*
    during muscle contraction, maximal voluntary, 70
      minimal voluntary, 70
    during muscle rest, 68–70
    fasciculations, 69
    fibrillation potentials, 69
    muscle response to electrode insertion, 68
    positive short waves, 69
  vs. clinical assessment, 284
Electroneurography, 71–73, *72*. See also
    Electrodiagnosis.
Elephantiasis, affecting feet, clinical features and
    treatment, 888, *888, 889*
Embolectomy, early, 1318–1320, *1318, 1319*. See also
    Vascular diseases.
Embolism, arterial, 1311–1315, *1312–1315*. See also
    Vascular diseases, arterial occlusive.
Embryology, human, 7, *9*
    anlage positioning and development, 8, *9*
    duration, 8
    ectodermal ridge, 7
    limb buds, 7
    of toenails, 914, 921–925, *923–925*
Encephalopathy, static. See *Palsy, cerebral*.
Enchondroma(s), 1005, *1005, 1007*
  multiple, with hemiangiomas, in Maffucci's syndrome,
      1005
  of small toes, 652, *652*
Enchondromatosis, 358–360, *359*.
  clinical features of, 358
  pathogenesis of, 360
  pathologic findings in, 360
  radiographic features of, 358–360, *359*
End corn, 624, *625*, 634–636, *634–636*. See also *Corn,
    end*.
Endocrine disorders, classification of, 1209
Endocrine neuropathies, 1239
Engelmann's disease, 369, *370*.
Enlargement roentgenography, uses of, 138
Entrapment neuropathies, 1193–1200. See also
    Neuropathies, entrapment.
Entrapment syndromes. See *Neuropathies, entrapment*.
Eosinophilic granuloma, 1011, *1011*
Epidermis, of sole skin, anatomy of 1399, *1400*
Epidermolysis bullosa, clinical features of, 878, *879*
  diagnosis of, 879
  simplex, 878, *879*

Epidermolysis bullosa (*Continued*)
  terminologic classification of, 878
  treatment of, 879
Epidermophytosis, in small toes, 94, *94*
  vs. eczema, 94, *94*
Epiloia, periungual fibromas in, 912, *912*
Epiphysis, injuries of, in children, 1668, *1668*. See also
    Children, trauma in.
  trauma to, in children, 1664–1666, *1665*
Eponychium, 914, *915, 916, 918*
  in human embryonic nails, 914
Equinocavovarus deformity, spastic hemiparesis and,
    case report, history and surgical treatment, 312
Equinovalgus deformity, cerebral palsy and, 198
  hallux valgus and, case report, history and surgical
      treatment, 323–328, *324–328*
  in longitudinal deficiency of fibula, 222
  spastic hemiplegia and, case report,
      316, *316*
  spina bifida and, *252*, 273–276, *273, 275*
  spinal dysraphism and, *252*, 263
  treatment of, *252*, 273–276, *273, 275*
Equinovarus deformity. See *Clubfoot; Talipes, inverted;*
    and *Talipes equinovarus*.
Equinus contracture, at ankle, in Duchenne's muscular
    dystrophy, 336, *337*
Equinus deformity, ankle fusion in, surgery in, 190, *190*
  as cause of genu recurvatum, 794
  as cause of metatarsalgia, 674
  effect of on metatarsals, 179, 713
  extensor rigidity and, in head trauma patient, 1118,
      1119, 1120
    treatment of, nonsurgical, 1118, *1119*
      surgical, 1118, *1120*
  external pressure as factor in, 257, *257*
  hammer toes and, surgical considerations, 150, *150*
  hammer toes as sequelae to, 82
  in stroke patient, 1112–1114
    plantar flexion, 1112
    spasticity, 1112
    treatment of, surgical, 1113
  metatarsalgia and, 674
  of forefoot, 715–718, *716, 717*. See also *Tarsus,
      anterior, Lisfranc's joint and*.
  spastic diplegia and, case report, 332–334, *333*
    history and analysis, 332–334, *333*
    treatment, 334
  spina bifida and, *263*, 278
  spinal dysraphism and, *263*, *263*
    treatment of, *263*, 278
    surgical, in hemophilia, 1090, *1090*
      in poliomyelitis, 1135
      with subsequent knee instability, 82, *82*
  various levels of, 715
Erysipelas, affecting feet, clinical features and
    treatment, 888, 889
Erythema multiforme, clinical features of, 879, *880*
  differential diagnosis, 880
  treatment of, 880
Eversion, definition of, 125
  paralytic pes planus and, treatment of, surgical, in
      poliomyelitis, 1136
Eversion fractures, in dancers, *1650*, 1651, *1651*
Evolution, of human foot, 2–7, *3, 5, 7*
Ewing's sarcoma, bone marrow tumors in, 1008, *1008*
  treatment of, 1008
  vs. reticulosarcoma of bone, 1009

Examination, 81–102
    clinical, 86–96, 87, 91–95
        general, 87, 87
            configuration, 87, 87
            muscle power, 88
            neurologic, 88
            orthopaedic, 86
            peripheral neuropathies, 88
            sinus tracts, 88
            skin, 88
            vascular supply, 88
            walking, 87
        specific, ankle, 89
            Chopart's joint, 90, 91
            forefoot, 92, 92, 93
            hallux, 93
            heel and heel cord, 90
            longitudinal arch, 91
                flatfoot, 91
            midtarsus, 92
            small toes, 94, 94, 95
            sole, 95
            subtalar (talocalcaneal) joint, 90, 91
            transverse metatarsal arch, 92, 92, 93
            with differential diagnosis, 88–96, 91–95
    history-taking, 81–86, 82–84, 86
    photographic, 99–102. See also Photography.
    physical, by complaint, 103–115
        forefoot, 110–115, 111–115
        hindfoot, 103–107, 104–106
        midfoot, 107–110, 107–110
    radiographic. See Radiography.
    roentgenographic, 96–99, 116–138. See also
        Roentgenography.
    supplementary diagnostic aids in, 99
Excoriation, neurotic, self-inflicted injuries in, 1444,
    1445
Exercise(s), following sports injuries, 1576–1578, 1576
    noninvasive, and hyperemic tests, in vascular
        diseases, 1306, 1306, 1308, 1309
    stretching, for short heel cord, 1716, 1719
Exercise board, for dancers, 1646, 1646
Exostosis(es), capsular, 845
    hereditary, multiple, 356–358, 357. See also
        Osteochondromatosis, multiple.
    impingement, as stage in development of
        osteoarthritis, 789–792, 790, 791
    location of, in development of osteoarthritis, 789–792,
        790, 791
    marginal, in osteoarthritis of ankle, 789, 790, 791
    of calcaneus, 772
    of small toes, 652, 653
    osteocartilaginous, 1003, 1004
        multiple, 356–358, 357. See also Osteochondro-
            matosis, multiple.
    subungual, 1004, 1004, 1005
    tarsal, dorsal, 722
Extension, definition of, 125
Extensor digitorum brevis, flaps of, for skin grafts, 955
    tendinitis of, in dancers, 1648
    tendon transfer in, 288
    testing of, 288
        in poliomyelitis, 1131, 1132
Extensor hallucis brevis, ossification of, 835, 835
Extensor hallucis longus, laceration of, 864
    tendon transfer in, 287
    testing of, 287

Extensor hallucis longus (Continued)
    testing of, in poliomyelitis, 1130, 1131, 1131
Extensor tendon, severance of, flail toe following, 628,
    628
Extremities, disorders of, in relation to neurologic
        examination of foot, 1108
    lower, disorders of, in stroke and head trauma
        patient, 1112–1122, 1115–1117, 1119–1121. See
        also Head, trauma to and Stroke.
Eye(s), disorders of, in relation to neurologic
        examination of foot, 1108

Face, abnormalities of, in relation to neurologic
        examination of foot, 1108
Factors VIII and IX deficiency. See Hemophilia(s).
"Failed" foot, intractably painful, neurosurgical salvage
        of, 1295–1300, 1296, 1297, 1300
    case histories and discussion, 1298–1300
    clinical studies, 1298–1300
    differential spinal nerve blocks, 1296–1298, 1296,
        1297
    dorsal root rhizotomy as last resort, 1295
    pain from, differential diagnosis of, 1295
Falls, causing calcaneal fractures, 1499
Fascia, lesions in, 841, 841
    plantar fasciitis, 841
    plantar fibromatosis, 841, 841
    plantar, anatomy of, 17, 19, 26
    as stabilizing mechanism, 52–55, 54, 55
    contracture of, 842
        Dupuytren's physical examination for, 109, 110
        in poliomyelitis, 1162
    ossification of, 842
    palpation of, 108–110, 109
    rupture of, in distance runners and joggers, 1604
    stripping of, in cavus deformity, 477
Fasciculations, significance of, 69
Fasciitis, plantar, 841
    examination for, physical, 108–110,
        109
    in dancers, 1654
    in distance runners and joggers, 1604
    treatment of, in geriatrics, 975
Fascio-scapulo-humeral muscular dystrophy, foot
        deformities in, and treatment, 346. See also Muscular
        dystrophy.
Fasciotomy, indications for, in compartment syndromes,
        1201
    in venomous snake bite, 1461
    plantar, in cavus deformity, 478, 478
    technique of, in reperfusion syndrome, 1324
Fat necrosis, subcutaneous, 832, 833
Fat pads, Achilles, 840
    anatomy of, 837
    atrophy of, 840
    embryology of, 838, 838
    fibular, hypertrophy of, 839, 840
    hypertrophy of, 840, 841
    metatarsal, atrophy of, 838, 839
        surgical trauma to, 838, 838
    of heel, damage or atrophy in, 839, 839
    of longitudinal arch, 840
    physiology of, 838
    plantar, atrophy of, 176
        functions of, 176

Fatigue fractures, in dancers, 1637–1639, *1638.* See also *Dancing* and *Fractures, stress.*

Felty's syndrome, with rheumatoid arthritis and vasculitis, treatment of, *1225*

Femoral artery, common, surgical reconstruction of, *1335, 1335, 1336.* See also *Vascular reconstruction.*

Femoral rotation, gait analysis and, *62*

Femoropopliteal vein, surgical bypass of, *1338, 1338*

Femur, rotational deformities of, 429, 433–435, *434, 435*

    shortening of, longitudinal deficiency of fibula and, 222

Fetishism, regarding feet or shoes, 1447

Fibrillation potentials, significance of, 69

Fibrogenesis imperfecta, 1074, *1075*

Fibroma(s), chondromyxoid, *1006, 1007*

    of small toes, 653, *653*

    periungual, 912, *912*

        in epiloia, 912, *912*

        in tuberous sclerosis, 912, *912*

        vs. warts, 912

Fibromatosis(es), 984–986, *984–987.* See also *Tumors, of foot, soft-tissue.*

    of tarsus and metatarsus, 722, *722*

    plantar, 841, *841*

        associated lesions and, 841

        clinical features of, 841

        incidence of, 841

        location of, 841

        treatment of, 842

Fibrosarcoma, 986–988, *988*

Fibrosis, annular, 832, *832*

Fibrous ankylosis, as cause of peroneal spastic flatfoot, 743

Fibrous dysplasia(s), 360–362, *362*

    affecting foot bone, 1011, *1011*

    clinical course of, 361

    clinical features of, 361

    etiology of, 360

    in Albright's syndrome, 361, *1011*

    prognosis for, 362

    radiographic features of, 361, *362*

    sarcomas in, 362

Fibula, absence of, partial or complete, 220, *221.* See also *Fibula, longitudinal deficiency of.*

    fat pads of, hypertrophy of, 839, *840*

    fractures of, 780, 783, *783, 784*

        in children, 1671

        in dancers, 1637, *1638,* 1651, *1651*

    intact, with longitudinal deficiency of tibia, 226–228

    longitudinal deficiency of, congenital, 220–226, *221, 224*

        associated anomalies and, 220

        classification of, 220–222, *221*

        clinical features of, 222

        diagnosis of, differential, 222

        pathogenesis of, 220

        treatment of, 223–226, *224*

            nonsurgical, 223

            surgical, best age for, 225

                Syme amputation, 223–225, *224*

                Wagner operation, 223–225

Fibular. See also entries under *Peroneal.*

Fibular collateral ligament, role of in ankle stability, 1555

Fibular hemimelia, paraxial, 220–226, *221, 224.* See also *Fibula, longitudinal deficiency of.*

Fibular hemimelia (*Continued*)

    paraxial, clinical features of, 245

        treatment of, 245

First ray insufficiency syndrome, 684–702, *685, 687, 688, 691, 692, 694–696, 699, 701, 702*

    acute form, treatment of, 690

    alternative nomenclature for, 694

    causes of, 685–688, *685, 687*

        congenital alterations, 685, *685*

        flatfoot, 686

        iatrogenic, 686–688, *687*

            Brandes-Keller operation, 687, *687*

            hallux strength-diminishing operations, 687, *687*

            Hueter-Mayo operation, 686, *687*

            metatarsal osteotomy, 686

        relaxation of soft parts, 686

        sesamoid dislocation, 686

    characteristics of, 684

    chronic form, 689

        dorsal dislocation, 689

        hygroma pouch, 689

        hyperkeratosis, 689

        periostitis, *687,* 690

        treatment of, nonsurgical, 690–693, *691, 692*

            orthoses, 690, *691*

            pain-killing, 690

            physiotherapy, 691–693, *692*

            surgical, amputation of second ray, 697

                correction of shortening of first metatarsal, 697–702, *699, 701, 702*

                lengthening of first metatarsal, 697

                Lisfranc's joint arthroplasty, 697

                metatarsal alignment, 701, *701, 702*

                metatarsus primus varus, 693–697, *694–696.* See also *Metatarsus primus varus.*

                shortening of metatarsals other than first, 698–701, *699*

                    amputation of heads, 700

                    diaphyseal osteotomy, 698–700, *699*

    consequences of, 688–702, *688, 691, 692, 694–696, 699, 701, 702*

        decompensation of sudden onset, 688, *688*

        Deutschländer's disease, 688, *688.* See also *Deutschländer's disease.*

        march fracture, 688, *688*

    diagnosis of, differential, 690

    excess weight bearing in, 182

First ray overload syndrome, circumstances of appearance of, 679

    examination for, clinical, 679

        radiologic, 679, *680*

    treatment of, 680–682, *681, 682*

        nonsurgical, 680

        surgical, 680–682, *681, 682*

            extirpation of sesamoid, 682

            Jones operation, 680, *681, 682*

            osteotomy of metatarsal base, 681, *682*

Fissures, definition and location of, 1403, *1403*

    infected, of hallux, *1403*

    of sole, etiology and treatment of, 896

    treatment of, 1403

Fixation, internal, principles of, 166

Flail ankle, fusion of, with subsequent knee instability, 82, *82*

Flail foot, treatment of, 758

Flail toe, following severance of extensor tendon, 628, *628*

Flaps. See *Skin grafts.*
Flatfoot, 486–520. See also *Pes planus* and *Valgus deformity.*
    anterior. See *First ray insufficiency syndrome.*
    basic literature on, guide to, 1853
    cerebral palsy and, 198
    decompensated, tibialis anterior sling procedure for, 771, *771*
    heel cord function and, 728
    hypermobile, subtalar instability and, 736, *737*
    in first ray insufficiency syndrome, 686
    painful, treatment of, strapping, 1730, *1730*
    peroneal spastic, *740*, 741–744, *741–744*. See also *Spastic flatfoot, peroneal* and *Tarsal coalition.*
    predominance of in blacks, 91
    rigid or supple, physical examination for, 108, *109*
    spastic, 85, *86*, 91, 96, *97*. See also *Spastic flatfoot, peroneal.*
    transverse. See *First ray insufficiency syndrome.*
    variations of, in children, 196
    vs. normal foot, muscle function in, 45
        subtalar joint and, 40, *41*
Flexion, definition of, 125
    plantar, gait analysis and, *61*
        in ankle joint, 40, *40*, 43, *44*, *45*
        weakness of, in stroke patient, 1114
Flexor digitorum brevis, flaps of, for skin grafts, 956
Flexor digitorum longus, tendinitis of, in dancers, 1643
    tendon management in, 291
    testing of, 291
        in poliomyelitis, 1131, *1132*
Flexor hallucis longus, flaps of, for skin grafts, 954
    tendinitis of, in dancers, 1643
        physical examination for, 110, *110*
    tendon of, compression of, in osteoarthritis, *791*, *792*
        osteoarthritis, *791*, *792*
        management of, 291
    rupture of, in dancers, 1644, *1644*, *1645*
    tenosynovitis of, *855*, *856*, *857*, *859*
        in geriatrics, 973
    testing of, 291
        testing of, in poliomyelitis, 1131, *1132*
Fluorescein, dosage and side effects, 948
    examination with, 948
        to determine flap viability for skin grafts, 948
    safety of, 948
Foot, absence of. See *Apodia.*
    adult, 539–978. See also *Adult foot* and under specific disorders.
    anatomic segments of, 375, *375*
    axes of, *402*, *403*, *429*
    basic contours of, normal vs. abnormal, 793
    binding of, 1446
    deformities of. See *Deformities* and under specific conditions.
    development of, roentgenographic examination of, 116–121, *117*, *118*. See also *Children* and *Growing Foot.*
    dislocations of. See *Dislocations.*
    disorders of, evaluation of, in adolescence, 198
        in children, 198
        in newborns and infants, 196–198, *197*
            associated anomalies, 197
            dermatoglyphic analyses, 197, *197*
        minor, associated with birth defects, 197
            associated with pediatric malformation syndromes, 197

Foot (*Continued*)
    disorders of, orthotic and prosthetic management of, 1783–1826. See also *Orthosis(es)*, *Orthotics*, and *Prosthetics.*
    duplication of, amputation and dissection, 254, *254*
    dynamics of, 1761
    fractures of. See *Fractures.*
    functions of, biomechanics, 494–496, *494*, *495*. See also *Biomechanics* and *Pes planus.*
    geriatric, 964–978. See also *Geriatric foot.*
    growing, 98, 195–538. See also *Children.*
    in systemic disease, 1014–1448
    lateral, incisions in, *159*, *160*, 161
        landmarks, *159*
        surgical approaches to, *159*, *160*, 161
    management of, best use of existing muscles, 268
        joint instability, 269
        muscle rebalancing, 268
        pressure sores, 269
        principles, 267–270
            deformity, 267
        ulceration, 269
    medial, incisions in, 161, *161*
        surgical approaches to, 161, *161*
    pain in, padding and devices for relief of, 1703–1732. See also *Arch supports; Footwear; Orthosis(es); Orthotics;* and *Shoes, and shoe modifications.*
        bursitis, 1731
        deformities from sandals, 1720
        hallux rigidus gait, 1711–1715, *1712–1715*
        hammer toes, 1715, *1715*
        heel, 1731, *1732*
        history-taking and diagnosis as necessary preliminaries, 1703
        insoles and molds, *1719*, 1720–1722, *1721*, *1722*
        Morton's neuroma, 1709–1711, *1710*
        pads, 1704–1709, *1706–1708*
            construction of, 1704
            metatarsal, 1705–1708, *1706*, *1707*
            purposes of, 1704
            skin preparation and care for, 1704
            toe crest, 1708, *1708*
        shoes, 1722–1724, *1723*
            fitting of, 1724
        short heel cord, 1715–1720, *1716–1719*
            metatarsal deformity and, 1716, *1718*
            range of dorsiflexion tests, 1716, *1717*
            stretching exercises, 1716, *1719*
            toe crests and shoes for, *1718*, *1720*
            toe dorsiflexion gait, 1716, *1716*
        sole alterations, 1724–1726, *1725*
            rocker sole, 1724, *1725*
        strapping, 1726–1730, *1726*, *1728–1730*
            for hammer toe, 1729, *1729*, *1730*
            for incomplete rupture of calf muscles or heel cord, 1728, *1728*, *1729*
            for painful flatfoot, 1730, *1730*
            of ankle, 1726, *1726*
                inversional sprained, 1726
                suggestions for, 1727
        tendinitis, 1731
        tenosynovitis, 1731
    plantar, incisions in, *163–165*, 164
        surgical approaches to, *163–165*, 164
    plantigrade. See *Plantigrade foot.*
    position of, over- or undercorrection of, 293
    rotation of, gait analysis and, *63*

Foot (*Continued*)
  shortness of, treatment of, surgical, in poliomyelitis,
    1138
  tumors of, 979–1013. See also *Tumors.*
Foot service, organization of, 1827–1829
    inpatient division, 1829
    outpatient division, 1827–1829
    research and training, 1829
Football, injuries from, classification, 1573. See also
    Sports injuries.
  osteoarthritis in, 789
Footdrop, correction of, surgical technique, 1281
Footprint, changes in, in pes planus, 509, *509*
Footprint mat, Harris, 1284, *1284*, 1382, *1382*
Footwear. See also *Shoes, and shoe modifications.*
  faulty, 1761–1764.
  for adults, 1758–1760, *1759*, *1760*
  for children, 1756–1758
  for geriatrics, 966–968, *966*, *967*
  for hammer toe, 640, *640*
  for insensitive foot, 1781
  in sports. See *Shoes, and shoe modifications* and
    Sports injuries.
  postoperative, *619*, 620
  prescription, terminology of, 1867–1871
  protective. See *Industrial injuries, protection from*
    and *prevention of.*
Forceplate, in gait analysis, 66, *66*
Forefoot. See also under specific areas.
  abnormal, surgical correction of, 192
  adduction of without inversion, treatment of, surgical,
    in poliomyelitis, 1137
  adductovarus deformity of, hallux valgus and,
    treatment of, 599, *599*
    hallux varus and, *616*, 617
  arthroplasty in, 1037–1043, *1039–1044*, *1050*. See also
    Rheumatoid arthritis, of foot, treatment of,
    surgical.
  biomechanics of, in tiptoe position, 670, *670–672*
    toe function, 664
  bone resection in, classification of procedures, 1038
  classification of, 665
  complete absorption of, in hereditary sensory
    neuropathies, 1230, *1230*, *1231*
  contusions of, definition, diagnosis, and treatment of,
    1449
  crush injuries of, treatment of, 1450
  deformities of, basic literature on, guide to, 1849
    Hoffman-Clayton surgery in, 186, *186*
    in hemophilia, 1090, *1091*
  dislocations of, 1451–1459, *1451–1456*, *1458*. See also
    Dislocations.
  disorders of, in geriatrics, 968–973, *968–970*, *972*. See
    also *Geriatric foot.*
  equinus deformity of, 715–718, *716*, *717*. See also
    Tarsus, anterior, Lisfranc's joint and.
    treatment of, surgical, *145*, *188*, 188
  examination of, clinical, 92, *92*, 93
    physical, 110–115, *111–115*
    radiographic, 667, *668*
    roentgenographic, 97
  fractures of, 1451–1459, *1451–1456*, *1458*. See also
    Fractures.
  fusion of, optimum position, 175
  in spinal dysraphism, 262
  incisions in, *161*, *163*
  injuries of, 1449–1462. See also *Injuries.*

Forefoot (*Continued*)
  injuries of, in dancers, 1655–1659, *1656–1658*. See
    also *Dancing.*
  pliability of, assessment of, 540–543, *543*
  splaying of, biplanar, resilient, hallux valgus and,
    treatment of, 597, *597*
    rigid, hallux valgus and, treatment of, 598, *598*
    horizontal, hallux valgus in, treatment of, 587, *588*,
     589
    in dancers, 1634. See also *Dancing.*
    in rheumatoid arthritis, *1026*, 1028
    treatment of, surgical, 1034
    varying metatarsal stress in, *548–551*
  support of, biomechanics, 666–669, *668*, *669*. See also
    Metatarsals, biomechanics of.
  surgical approaches to, *161*, *163*
  tendon transfers in, in cavus deformity, 478
  tuberculosis in, 721, *721*
  ulcers of, treatment of, 1283
  upward displacement of, effect on weight bearing,
    179
  varus deformity of, effect on weight bearing, 183, *188*
    fixed, treatment of surgical, *188*, *188*, *191*
  wide, footwear for, 1781
  shoe modifications for, 1760
Foreign bodies, granulomas, 85, 95
  hairs, 897
  laceration by, surgical conversion of, 147, *147*
  pebbles and pellets, 897, *898*, *898*
  splinters, 897, *897*
  subcutaneous, 836, *836*, *837*
Fracture(s), avulsion, diagnosis of, differential, *1488*
  of cuboid, treatment of, *1491*
  roentgenographic view of, 97
  basic literature on, guide to, 1851, 1866
  care of, in hemophilia, 1088
  compression. See also *Compression injuries.*
    of navicular, treatment of, *1491*
    of talar body, 1483, *1484*
  crush. See also *Crush injuries.*
    of hallux, 1458, *1458*
    of talar body, treatment of, 1485
  in children. See *Children* and *Growing foot.*
  in dancers, 1650–1654, *1650–1653*. See also *Dancing.*
    eversion, *1650*, 1651, *1651*
    inversion, 1651, *1651*, *1652*
    fatigue, 1637–1639, *1638*
    stress, 1637–1639, *1638*
  in geriatrics, 976. See also *Geriatric foot.*
  in osteoporosis, 1065
  in spina bifida, 257, 260
  in sports injuries, 1578–1587, *1581–1587*. See also
    Sports injuries.
  "march," caused by first ray insufficiency syndrome,
    688, *688*. See also *Deutschländer's disease.*
    in transverse metatarsal arch, 93, *93*
    of metatarsals, 1457
  of ankle, classification, 1546–1550, *1547–1550*. See
    also *Ankle, injuries of.*
    in children, 1671–1674, *1672*, *1674*. See also
    Children and *Growing foot.*
    in geriatrics, 976
    pronation-adduction, 1548, *1548*
    pronation-dorsiflexion, 1549
    pronation-eversion, 1548, *1549*
    supination-adduction, 1547, *1548*
    supination-eversion, 1547, *1547*

Fracture(s) (*Continued*)
  of ankle, residuals of, fibula, *780, 783, 783, 784*
    inversion instability, *780, 783, 783*
    lateral rotation, *783, 784*
    talus, *786, 786*
      osteoarthritis, *786*
      osteochondritis dissecans, *786, 786*
      osteonecrosis, *786*
    tibia, *783, 784–786, 784, 785*
      anterior margin, *785*
      at medial malleolus, *784*
      fracture patterns, *784*
      inversion, *783, 784*
      lateral margin, *784, 785, 785*
      posterior margin, *785*
      resultant infection and deformity, *786*
      vertical axis compression, *785*
    treatment of, *1550–1570, 1551, 1552, 1555–1562,*
        1564, 1566–1570
      emergency, *1550, 1551*
      nonsurgical, modified Quigley traction, *1552,*
          1552
      open fractures, antibiotics, *1565*
      surgical, closed reduction, *1552–1555*
        mechanism of injury, abduction vs.
            adduction, *1553*
        postreduction care, *1554*
        roentgenographic criteria for, *1554*
        technique, *1553*
        vs. open, *1552*
      contraindications, *1552*
      open fractures, *1563–1565, 1564*
        debridement, *1563*
        internal fixation, *1564, 1564*
        postclosure complications, *1564*
        preoperative examination, *1563*
        wound classification, *1563*
      open reduction, *1555–1563, 1555–1562*
        fracture of distal end of tibia involving ankle
            joint, *1559–1562, 1561*
          anterior and posterior margins, *1561*
          cancellous bone grafts, *1562*
          internal fixation of tibia, *1562*
          Pilon fractures, *1561, 1561*
          reconstruction of lower articular surface of
              tibia, *1562*
          restoration of fibular length, *1562*
        postoperative care, *1562, 1562*
        role of fibular collateral ligament, *1555*
        technique, *1565–1570, 1566–1570*
          preoperative, *1566*
          type A fracture, *1566, 1566*
          type B fracture, *1566–1569, 1567–1568*
          type C fracture, *1569, 1569, 1570*
        Weber classification, type A fracture-
            dislocations, *1550, 1555, 1555, 1556*
          type B fracture-dislocations, *1550,*
              1556–1559, 1556–1558
          type C fracture-dislocations, *1550, 1559,*
              1559, 1560
  of calcaneus, *1497–1538*
    as cause of peroneal spastic flatfoot, *740, 741*
    classifications, *1511–1515*
      joint depression, *1503, 1514, 1515, 1516, 1526,*
          1527
      superomedial fragment and primary fracture,
          1513, 1516

Fracture(s) (*Continued*)
  of calcaneus, classification, tongue-type, *1504–1510,*
      1514, 1516
    clinical evaluation of, 1499
    crush, and arterial occlusion, treatment of, surgical,
        1323, 1323
    from falls, 1499
    in children, 1675
    in industrial injuries, 1612. See also *Industrial
        injuries.*
    in sports injuries, *1587, 1587*. See also *Sports
        injuries.*
    roentgenographic evaluation, *1500–1511, 1501,*
        1503–1510, 1512
      anteroposterior and medial oblique views, *1501,*
          1511
      anteroposterior oblique view, *1501, 1505,* 1511
      anteroposterior view, *1505,* 1511
      axial view, *1500–1502, 1501*
      lateral views, *1501, 1502–1511, 1503–1510*
        lateromedial, *1502–1511*
        mediolateral, *1501, 1502, 1503–1510*
      routine and special views, discussion, 1500
      special views, Brodén projections, *1510,* 1511,
          1512
    sequelae of, *1536–1538*
      lateral bony prominences, *1536*
      subtalar joint abnormalities, *1537*
    treatment of, *1515–1535, 1516–1518, 1520–1523,*
        1526, 1527, 1533, 1534
      anterior end, *1532–1535, 1534*
      body fractures with talar joint involvement, *1516,*
          1519–1532, 1520–1523, 1526, 1527
        discussion and evaluation, 1530
        open reduction and internal fixation with
            staples using medial approach, *1516,*
            1519–1528, 1520–1523, 1526, 1527
        postoperative results, *1525–1527*
        open reduction using lateral approach, *1516,*
            1528
        open reduction with bone grafts, *1516,* 1528
        open reduction without grafts, *1516,* 1529
        other methods, 1532
        reduction with sagittal pin, 1530
        subtalar arthrodesis, 1531
        triple arthrodesis, 1531
      body fractures without talar joint involvement,
          1516, 1519
      causes of, 1499
      classification, *1515, 1516*
        controversy regarding, *1497–1499*
      immediate active exercises without reduction or
          immobilization, 1535
      impacted fractures of lateral portion of posterior
          facet, *1523, 1532, 1533, 1534*
      nonsurgical, classification, 1497
      poor results following, 1497
      surgical, classification, 1497
      tuberosity fractures, *1516–1519, 1516–1518*
        avulsion, *1516, 1518, 1518*
        beak, *1516,* 1518
        posteroinferior, *1516–1518, 1516, 1517*
        posterosuperior, *1516, 1518, 1518*
      wide variations in, *1497–1499*
    with peroneal constriction, 861
  of fibula, *780, 783, 783, 784*
    in children, 1671

Fracture(s) (*Continued*)
  of fibula, in dancers, 1637, *1638*, 1651, *1651*. See also
    Dancing.
  of forefoot and toes, general considerations, 1451,
    1451
  of hallux, in sports injuries, 1578–1585, *1581–1585*.
    See also *Sports injuries.*
  of metatarsals, 179, *180*
    in children, 1676–1680, *1678, 1679*. See also
      Children, trauma in and *Growing foot.*
    in sports injuries, 1586, *1586*. See also *Sports
      injuries.*
    multiple, *187*
  of midfoot, in sports injuries, 1586. See also *Sports
    injuries.*
  of navicular, 1453, *1456*, 1491
  of sesamoids, in dancers, 1655, *1656*
    in sports injuries, *1581*, 1585. See also *Sports
      injuries.*
  of talus, 789, *786*. See also *Fractures, of ankle,
    residuals of.*
    as cause of peroneal spastic flatfoot, 742, *743*
    dome of, 1463–1467, *1465–1467*. See also
      Fractures, of talus, transchondral.
      in dancers, 1652, *1652*
      in children, 1674
      osteochondral, *1668*
    subtalar neck, complications of, 1480, *1481, 1482*
      prognosis for, 1480
      treatment of, excision of talus, 1480
        primary and secondary reconstruction
          procedures, 1481–1483, *1482*
    talar body, 1483–1489, *1484–1489*
      classification of, 1483, *1484*
      compression fractures, clinical features of, 1483
      compression fractures, treatment of, 1484
      crush fractures, treatment of, 1485
      incidence of, 1483
      lateral tubercle, 1486–1489, *1486–1489*
        clinical features and anatomy of, 1486, *1486,
          1487*
        diagnosis of, differential, 1487, *1488*
        incidence of, 1486
        mechanism of injury, 1487, *1487, 1488*
        prognosis for, 1489, *1489*
        treatment of, 1487–1489, *1489*
        types of, 1487, *1488*
      posterior tubercle, *1484*, 1485
        clinical features of, 1486
        incidence of, 1485
        treatment of, 1486
        vs. os trigonum, 1486
      shearing fractures, clinical features of, 1484, *1485*
        treatment of, 1484
    talar neck, 1475–1483, *1475–1477, 1479–1482*
      as threat to vascular supply, 1475, *1477*
      classification, Hawkins', 1475, *1475–1477*
        Group I, 1475, *1475*
        Group II, 1475, *1476*
        Group III, 1475, *1476*
        Group IV, 1475, *1476*
          injuries, 1479
      mechanism of injury, 1475
      plus talonavicular dislocation, 1475, *1477*
      treatment of, 1476–1480, *1479, 1480*
        and talonavicular reduction, 1479
        Group I injuries, 1476, *1477*

Fracture(s) (*Continued*)
  of talus, talar neck, treatment of, Group II injuries,
    1477, *1479*
      Group III injuries, 1478, *1479, 1480*
    transchondral (dome), 1463–1467, *1465–1467*
      caused by inversion ankle injury, 1464
      classification of, 1464, *1465*
      clinical features of, 1464
      etiology and sites of, 1463
      prognosis for, 1466
      radiographic assessment of, 1464
      treatment of, 1465
        nonsurgical, 1465
        postoperative, 1466
        surgical, 1465, *1466*
        technique, 1466, *1467*
  of tibia, 783, 784–786, *784, 785*. See also *Fractures,
    of ankle, residuals of.*
    distal end, involving ankle joint, treatment of,
      1559–1562, *1561*.
    in childhood, 1671–1673, *1672*
    Pilon, 1561, *1561*.
    Salter-Harris classification, *1670*
  of toes, 1451–1459, *1451–1456, 1458*
    fifth, proximal phalanx of, 1457
      treatment of, 1457
    hallux, crush fracture, 1458, *1458*
    multiple comminution, 1458
    second to fourth, 1457
      treatment of, 1458
  osteochondral, as cause of hallux rigidus, 608, *610*
  phalangeal, as cause of hallux rigidus, 608, *609, 610*
    in children, 1680
  "shatter," of metatarsals, 1457
  shearing, of talar body, 1484, *1484, 1485*
  spontaneous, in Charcot foot, 1253–1255, *1254, 1255*
    in diabetes vs. syphilis, *1254, 1255*, 1255
  stress, in children, 1681. See also *Children* and
    Growing foot.
    in dancers, 1637–1639, *1638*. See also *Dancing.*
    in distance runners and joggers, 1604. See also
      Sports injuries.
    in Paget's disease, 1082.
    in renal osteodystrophy, 1075, *1075*
    in sports injuries, 1598, *1599*. See also *Sports
      injuries.*
    of lesser metatarsals, following surgery for hallux
      valgus, 607
  subungual, 937
Fracture-dislocations. See also *Dislocations* and
    Fractures.
  of ankle, Weber classification, *1550*, 1555–1559,
    1555–1560
  of Lisfranc's joint, 1452, *1452–1455*.
  of metatarsals, 1453–1457
  of navicular, 1453, *1456*
  of talus, in children, 1675
Fragilitas ossium, 362, *364*. See also *Osteogenesis
    imperfecta.*
Freezing, injuries from, in children, 1684
Freiberg's infraction, 207–210, *208, 209*
  clinical findings in, 208
  etiology of, 208
  in late childhood, 199
  metatarsal heads in, 207, *208, 209*
  osteochondritis in, 210
  predominance of, in adolescents, 208

Freiberg's infraction (*Continued*)
  predominance of, in females, 207
  radiologic view, *208, 209, 209*
  treatment of, 209, *209*
Friedreich's ataxia, affecting foot, 84
  associated disorders and, 1236
  cavus deformity and, 198, 469
  clinical features of, 234, 1236
  electrodiagnosis in, 74, 78
  prognosis for, 234, 1236
  signs and symptoms of, 469
  treatment of, 234
Frostbite, clinical features and treatment of, 1450
  in children, 1684
Functional disorders, of foot, psychiatric aspects, 1429
Fungal infections, affecting feet, 898–901, *898–900*. See
    also *Tinea pedis*.
  vs. soft corns, 631, 633
Fusion(s), optimum positions of, principles, 174, *175*
  surgical, basic literature on, guide to, 1850. See also
    Arthrodesis(es).

Gaenslen split heel incision, 164, *165*
Gait, analysis of, 57–67, *58–66*
    dorsiflexion, *61*
    electromyographic, 60–66, *64, 65*
    femoral rotation, *62*
    foot rotation, *63*
    forceplate, 66, *66*
    frontal plane motion, *60*
    hip flexion-extension, *60*
    hip joint rotation, *62*
    in cerebral palsy, 57, 63, 78
    in children, 57, 63, 78
    in poliomyelitis, 64
    in stroke, 66, 1112
    in total joint replacement, 57
    knee flexion-extension, *61*
    knee joint rotation, *62*
    pelvic obliquity, *60*
    pelvic rotation, *62*
    pelvic tilt, *60*
    photometric, 58–60, *59*
    plantar flexion, *61*
    sagittal plane motion, *60, 61*
    tibial rotation, *63*
    transverse plane motion, *62, 63*
    visualization of subject in, 58–60, *58–63*
      camera layout, 58, *58*
      lateral view, *59*
  center of gravity displacement and, 46, *46*
  changes in, in geriatrics, 965
  examination of, in poliomyelitis, 1126
  forces during, 46–50, *46–49*
    forward-aft shear, 47, *49*, 66
    medial-lateral shear, 48, *49*, 66
    torque, 48, *49*
    vertical, 47, *47, 48*, 66
  in cavus deformity vs. normal foot, *675*
  metatarsal biomechanics and, 671–673, *672*
  normal, muscle function in, 43, *44*
    vs. pathologic, 38
  speed of, effect of, 46–48
Ganglia, tarsal, dorsal, 723
Gangosa, in yaws, 1424

Gangrene, in arteriosclerosis obliterans, 1326–1328,
    1327–1329
  in diabetic foot, 1391, *1392, 1393*
  treatment of, danger of premature amputation, 1328,
    1329
  venous, in phlegmasia cerulea dolens, *1358*
Gastrocnemius, medial, flap elevation technique for skin
    grafts, 956, *957*
  transfer of, in poliomyelitis, *1166*, 1167
Gastrocnemius-soleus, as most common site of muscle
    hemorrhage in hemophilia, 1087, *1089*
Genetic deformities, shoe modifications for, 1760
Genetic disturbances, affecting foot, basic literature on,
    guide to, 1853
  generalized, 233–246
    achondrogenesis II, 234
    acrocephalopolysyndactyly, 237, *237*
    chromosome 18q syndrome, 234
    cleft foot, 245
    cleft hand and foot syndrome, 237, *239*
    clubfoot, 242
    de Lange's syndrome, 237, *240, 241*
    Duchenne pseudohypertrophic muscular dystrophy,
      234
    dwarfism, diastrophic, *236, 237*
      metatrophic, 234
      thanatophoric, 234, *234*
    dysautonomia, 234
    Friedreich's ataxia, 234
    hyperlax foot, 241
    lethal, severe foot deformities and, 233, *234*
    longitudinal deficiencies, 245
    Marfan's syndrome, 235
    Menkes' syndrome, 234
    Moebius syndrome, 237, *238*
    neurofibromatosis, 234
    Pierre Robin syndrome, 237, *239*
    polydactyly, *235*, 237, *237*, 244
    polysyndactyly, *236*, 237
    syndactyly, 245
    talipes equinovarus, 242
    transverse deficiencies, 245
  nonfatal, listing, 237
Genu recurvatum, caused by equinus deformity, 794
  treatment of, surgical, in poliomyelitis, 1153, *1154*
Genu valgum, shoe modifications for, 1759
  splints for, 435, *435*
  treatment of, surgical, in poliomyelitis, 1161
Genu varum, shoe modifications for, 1759
  treatment of, surgical, in poliomyelitis, 1161
Geriatric foot, 964–978
  ankle and, fractures of, 976
    traumatic injuries of, 976
  compensatory walking habits and, 965
  degenerative changes in, 965
  disorders of, forefoot, 968–973, *968–970, 972*
    corns, treatment of, nonsurgical, 968, *968*
    hammer toes, treatment of, nonsurgical, 968–970,
      969
    interdigital bursitis, 973
    metatarsophalangeal joint, treatment of, 971
    overlapping toes, treatment of, nonsurgical, 969,
      970
    plantar callosities, 971
    relief of painful pressure, 971, *972*
    toenails, *969, 970*
      causes of, 970

Geriatric foot (*Continued*)
  disorders of, forefoot, treatment of, nonsurgical, 970
    heel pain, 974–976
      Achilles tendon rupture and, 976
      achillobursitis, 975
      associated disorders and, 975
      calcaneal bursitis, 974
      calcaneal periostitis, 975
      causes and location of, 974
      from subtalar joint arthritis, 976
      lipoatrophy, 974
      marginal callus, 976
      plantar fasciitis, 975
      sinus tarsi syndrome and, 976
    incidence of, 964
    midfoot, 973
      dorsal ganglion, 973
      osteoarthritis of first metatarsocuneiform joint, 973
      rupture of tibialis anterior tendon, 973
      tenosynovitis, of flexor hallucis longus tendon, 973
      of peroneus longus tendon, 973
    osteoarthritis, infrequency of, 965
    warts, reduced incidence of, 965
  dry skin in, 965
  in institutionalized vs. active individuals, 964
  shoes for, 966–968, *966, 967*
Giant cell tumor(s), in foot bone, treatment of, 1009, *1010*
Gigantism, of hallux, in alcoholic peripheral neuropathy, 1219, *1221*
Girdlestone operation, inadvisability of, in hammer toe, 214
Girdlestone-Taylor operation, in curly toe, 215
Glomangioma(s), 991, *991, 992*
Glomerulonephritis, chronic, renal osteodystrophy and, 1075, *1076*
Golf, footwear for, 1775
Gonococcal infections, clinical features and progress of, 1419
  treatment of, 1420
Gonorrhea, acute synovitis of foot in, 844, *844*
Goundou, in yaws, 1424, *1425*
Gout, 84, 1014–1023. See also *Pseudogout.*
  arthritis and, acute, 1018–1020, *1019*
    clinical findings, 1018, *1019*
    diagnosis of, 1019
    prevention of recurrence of, 1020
    treatment of, 1019
    chronic, tophaceous gout and, 1020–1022
      clinical findings, 1020
      treatment of, pharmacologic, 1020
        surgical, 1021
          indications for, 1021
          techniques, 1021
  basic literature on, guide to, 1850
  characteristics of, 1014
  chondrocalcinosis and, 1022, *1022.* See also *Pseudogout.*
  diagnosis of, 99
  hereditary nature of, 1014
  historical background of, 1014
  in sickle cell disease, 1097, *1097*
  inflammatory bursae in, 853
  onset of, 84
  pathogenesis of, 1014

Gout (*Continued*)
  pathogenesis of, excretion of uric acid vs. urea, 1015
    hyperuricemia, 1014
    uric acid, as end product of purine metabolism, 1015
      excretion of, normal vs. abnormal, 1015
      relationship with, 1014
      storage of in tophi, 1015
  pyrophosphate arthropathy and, 1022, *1022.* See also *Pseudogout.*
  secondary, 122
  small toe involvement in, 655, *655,* 656
  synovitis induced by urate crystal deposits and, pathologic findings and pathogenesis, 1015–1018, *1016–1018*
  tenosynovitis and, inflammatory, 855
  tophaceous, chronic, clinical appearance of, *1017*
    histologic view, *1017, 1018*
    radiographic appearance, *1016*
    chronic gouty arthritis and, 1020–1022. See also *Gout, arthritis and.*
    presenting as symmetric polyarthritis, 1020
  tophi in, tendon tumors and, 866, *866*
  urate deposition in, 115–1018, *1016–1018*
  vs. pseudogout, 1022
Grafts, bone, open reduction and, in calcaneal fractures, 1528
  skin. See *Skin grafts.*
Gram-negative bacteria, affecting feet, clinical features and treatment of, 888, *889*
  foreign-body, 85, 95
Granuloma(s), eosinophilic, 1011, *1011*
Granuloma annulare, *830, 831*
  clinical features of, 880, *881, 882*
  differential diagnosis, 880
  treatment of, 880
Granuloma pyogenicum, of hallux, 831, *831*
  periungual and subungual, 932, *934*
Granulomatosis, in yaws, 1421, *1421–1423*
Granulomatous infections, 1399, 1407–1419, *1407–1417.* See also *Infections, of foot.*
Gravity, role of, in changes in deformity, 256
Great toe. See *Hallux.*
Greek foot, digital and metatarsal formulas for, *660,* 665
Grice arthrodesis, 1162, *1163*
  for hyperlax foot, 241
Griseofulvin, side effects of, in toenail treatment, 911
Groin, flaps of, for skin grafts, 961
Growing foot, 195–538. See also *Children.*
Growth hormone, disorders of, 1071, *1071, 1072.* See also *Metabolic disorders, of bone.*
Guanethidine, for reflex sympathetic dystrophy syndrome, 1290
Guillain-Barré syndrome, clinical features of, 349–351
  electrodiagnosis in, 73
  foot deformities in, 351
    early and late, 351
    treatment of, 351
Guinea worm infestation, 1420, *1420*
Gummatous osteomyelitis, 1418
Gummatous periostitis, 1418
Gymnastics, injuries from, classification of, 1573. See also *Sports injuries.*

Hair growth, on dorsum, 33

Hallux, 539–621
  amputation of, arterial reconstruction following, 1345,
    1345
  bunion of, examination for, physical, 111, 112
  check-rein deformity of, 861, 861
  cutaneous horn on, 830
  examination of, clinical, 93
    bunions, 93
    hallux rigidus, 93
    hallux valgus, 93
    ingrown toenails, 93
  extension test, 502, 502
  fissures of, infected, 1403
  flexion-extension in, 672
  floppy, following surgery for hallux valgus, 607
  fractures of, crush, 1458, 1458
    in sports injuries, 1578–1585, 1581–1585. See also
      Sports injuries.
  fusion of, optimum position, 175
  gigantism of, in alcoholic peripheral neuropathy,
    1219, 1221
  granuloma pyogenicum in, 831, 831
  hemorrhage in, treatment of, 1091
  injuries of, in dancers, 1655–1657, 1656. See also
    Dancing.
  knuckling of, following surgery for hallux valgus, 605
  nail bed of, amelanotic melanoma of, 831, 831
  nail deformities of, tubular or circular, 651, 651
  overriding, 551, 552
  paronychia of, treatment of, 1405
  patterns of, dermatoglyphic analysis, 197
  sesamoid derangement and, 613–616, 614. See also
    Sesamoids.
  sesamoids of, anatomy of, 1459
  short flexor of, calcific tendinitis of, 1460
  sloughing of, following surgery, 172
  tendons of, spontaneous rupture of, 864, 864
  treatment of, surgical, approaches to, 160, 161, 162,
    163
    as cause of first ray insufficiency syndrome, 687,
      687
    incisions, 160, 161, 162, 163
      interphalangeal joint, 162
      metatarsophalangeal joint, 162
      nail, 162
      proximal phalanx and, 162
      sesamoids, 162, 163
    postoperative, dressing, 618, 620
      footwear, 619, 620
    preoperative assessment, 539–545, 540–544
      active and passive movements, 540, 541, 542
      circulatory status, 539, 540
      contraindications, 539
      pliability of forefoot, 540–543, 543
    preoperative preparation, 545
      roentgenographic, 543–545, 544
    strength-diminishing, as cause of first ray
      insufficiency syndrome, 687, 687
  ulcers of, chronic plantar, 1404
    subungual, 1210, 1210
    treatment of, 1281
  underslung, 551, 552
Hallux elevatus, treatment of, 618–620
Hallux extension test, for pes planus, 502, 502
Hallux extensus, treatment of, 618–620
Hallux flexus, vs. hallux rigidus, 618
Hallux rigidus, 608–613, 609–612

Hallux rigidus (Continued)
  basic literature on, guide to, 1848, 1864
  classification of, 608
  clinical features of, 608, 611
  etiology of, 608, 609, 610
  examination for, physical, 111, 112
  footwear for, 1779, 1780
  gait in, foot pads and devices for, 1711–1715,
    1712–1715
  in dancers, 1634. See also Dancing.
  primary vs. secondary, 608
  radiographic features of, 608, 609, 610
  treatment of, surgical, 608–613, 612, 1036
    postoperative care, 613
  varying nomenclature for, 608
  vs. hallux flexus, 618
Hallux valgus, 545–608
  adductovarus deformity of forefoot and, treatment of,
    599, 599
  arthritis of first metatarsophalangeal joint and, with
    metatarsalgia of first metatarsal head, treatment
    of, 595
    with metatarsus primus varus, treatment of, 594,
      595
    with axial rotation of hallux and taut long extensor,
      treatment of, 595–597, 596
    treatment of, 594, 595
  basic literature on, guide to, 1848, 1858
  bilateral, with metatarsal adductovarus deformity, 551
  biplanar forefoot splaying and, resilient, treatment of,
    597, 597
    rigid, treatment of, 598, 598
  "bunion pain" in, treatment of, in elderly patients,
    585, 585
  caused by medial sesamoid excision, 852, 852
  cavovarus deformity and, 324–328, 330, 599, 600
  cerebral palsy and, 322–332, 324–328, 331
    incidence of, 322
    treatment of, 323
  claw toes and, treatment of, surgical, 1036
  clinical features of, 322
  conditions associated with, case reports, 323–332,
    324–328, 331
    cavovarus deformity, 324–328, 330
      analysis, 330
      history, 330
      treatment, 324–328, 330
    equinovalgus deformity, 323–328, 324–328
      history, 323, 324
      surgical treatment, 323–328, 326
    spastic diplegia, 324–328, 328–330
      etiology, 329
      foot analysis, 329
      history, 328
      recognition of, 329
      treatment, 329
    spasticity and athetosis in cerebral palsy,
      330–332, 331
      history, 330, 331
      treatment, 331
  definition of, 545
  development of, 322
  evolution of, 551–558, 552–557
    arthritis in first metatarsophalangeal joint, 553–557,
      556, 557
    axial rotation, 551, 553
    fibular toe drift, 551, 552

Hallux valgus (*Continued*)
  evolution of, in rheumatoid arthritis, 551, 552
    metatarsal hyalin divestment, 553, *556*
    metatarsal sagittal groove, 553, *556*
    metatarsalgia, 557
    osteophytic growth, 555–557, *557*
    sesamoid shift, 551–553, *554*
    subluxation at first metatarsophalangeal joint,
      congruous or incongruous, 553, *555*
  examination for, physical, 111, *112*
  fixed, claw toes and, treatment of, surgical, 1036
  footwear for, *1776, 1780*
  hammer toe and, 212
  in ballet and dance, 1629, *1629, 1632, 1633, 1633,*
    1641. See also *Dancing.*
  in horizontally splayed forefoot, treatment of, 587,
    588, 589
    with moderate metatarsalgia under second
      metatarsal head, treatment of, 587–589, *588*
  in rheumatoid arthritis, 551, 552, *1026*, 1029, *1029*
  incongruity of first metatarsophalangeal joint and,
    treatment of, 595, *595*
  interphalangeal, acquired, 584
    congenital, 583
    treatment of, 583, *583*
  isolated, treatment of, surgical, 1036
      classification of procedures, 1035
  juvenile, treatment of, 584, *584*
  metatarsalgia and, 557, 607
  metatarsus primus valgus and, with osteophyte
    emanation from first metatarsal head, treatment of,
    593, *594*
  metatarsus primus varus and, basic literature on,
    guide to, 1858
    treatment of, 586, *587*. See also *Hallux valgus,
    without metatarsus primus varus.*
    with axial rotation of hallux, treatment of, 591, *592*
    with bowstrung extensor hallucis longus tendon,
      treatment of, 589, *591*
    with metatarsalgia and plantar bulging of central
      metatarsal heads, treatment of, 589, *590*
    with overriding or underslung great toe, treatment
      of, 591–593, *593*
  pes planus and, 518, *518*
  role of metatarsals in, 545–551, *548–551*
  treatment of, surgical, 558–608
    Akin operation, 569, *569*, 586, 601
    arthrodesis of first metatarsophalangeal joint, 573,
      574
    conditioning factors and tenets, 558
    extracapsular osteotomies of first metatarsal,
      566–569, *567, 568*
    Hoffman operation, 577, *578*, 598, 599
    Hueter-Mayo-Stone resection, 577, *578*, 605
    Keller operation, 569, *570*, 593
      Lelièvre modification, 571–573, *572*
      modified, 570, *571*, 594, 595, 596, 604, *604*,
        607, 615
    Lapidus operation, 563, *564*, 604
    McBride operation, 561–563, *562*, 602–604, *602*,
      607, 615, 618
    Mitchell operation, 563–566, *565*, 604, *605*
    partial and total replacement of first
      metatarsophalangeal joint, 573–577, *575, 576*
    postoperative complications, 601–608, *601–606*.
      See also *Hallux valgus, treatment of,
      surgical, sequelae and salvage.*

Hallux valgus (*Continued*)
  treatment of, surgical, postoperative complications,
      adhesive neuritis, *601*, 602
    adhesive tendinitis, 602
    arthrosis of first metatarsophalangeal joint, 604,
      604
    floppy hallux, 607
    hallux varus, 602, *602*
    hallux varus extensus, 603, *603*
    incisional hazards, 601
    infections, 601
    knuckling of hallux, 605
    metatarsalgia, 607
    osteotomized first metatarsal, malunion of, *606*,
      607
      nonunion of, 605, *605*
    recurrence, 602
    snapping medial sesamoid, *603*, 604
    stress fracture of lesser metatarsals, 607
  postoperative dressing, *618. 620*
  procedure appraisal, 558
  recommended procedures for individual
    deformities, 583–599, *583–600*
  sequelae and salvage, 599–608, *601–606*. See also
      *Hallux valgus, treatment of, surgical,
      postoperative complications.*
    errors of surgeon, 599–601
    prolonged recovery period, 601
  Silver operation, 559, *560*
    modified, 559–561, *561*, 586, 602–605, 607,
      618
  supplementary procedures, 577–583, *579–582*
  varieties of, 545, *546, 547*
  vs. bunion, 545
  without metatarsus primus varus, treatment of, 585,
    586. See also *Hallux valgus, metatarsus primus
    varus and.*
Hallux varus, 616–618, *616, 617*
  acquired, treatment of, 618
  adductovarus deformity of forefoot and, *616*, 617
  basic literature on, guide to, 1848, 1862
  congenital, 215, *216*, 616, *616, 617*
    adductovarus deformity of forefoot and, *616*, 617
    associated deformities, 215
    basic literature on, guide to, 1862
    diastrophic dwarfism and, 216, *216*
    preaxial polydactyly, 617, *617*
    primary, 215, *216*
    skeletal affections and, 216, *216*
    treatment of, 216, 617
    types of, 215, *216*
  definition of, 215
  diastrophic dwarfism and, 216, *216*
  following surgery for hallux valgus, 602, *602*
  secondary, as postoperative complication, *173*
Hallux varus extensus, following surgery for hallux
  valgus, 603, *603*
Hammer toe(s). See also *Claw toe(s).*
  acquired, 212
    vs. congenital, 84
  associated with recurrent trauma, treatment of, 1459
  basic literature on, guide to, 1864
  causes of, 639, *640*
  cavus deformity and, 639
    footwear for, *1776, 1781*
  congenital, 212–214, *212, 213*
    vs. acquired, 84

Hammer toe(s) (*Continued*)
  definition of, 212, *212*, 638, *639*
  equinus forefoot and, as sequelae of, 82
    surgical considerations, 150, *150*
  examination of, radiographic, 96, *96*
  hallux valgus and, 212
  hard corns and, physical examination for, 113, *113*
  in dancers, 1633, *1633*. See also *Dancing.*
  in late childhood, 199
  in poliomyelitis, 639
  metatarsal displacement and, 178
  metatarsophalangeal joint in, 94
  orthoses for, 1741, *1742*
  pads and devices for relief of pain in, 1715, *1715*
  rheumatoid arthritis and, 94, *1025*, *1026*, 1028,
    1029
  treatment of, in adolescents, 213, *213*
    in children, 213
    in infants, 213
    indications for, 640
    nonsurgical, in geriatrics, 968–970, *969*
      strapping, 1729, *1729*, *1730*
    other deformities and, 640, *640*
    palliative, *626*, 640, *640*
    surgical, 94, 213, *213*, 640–646, *641–645*
      amputation, disadvantages of, 645
      arthrodesis technique, 644
      contraindicated procedures, 650
      diaphysectomy, Jahss procedure, 643
        of proximal phalanx, 642, *642*
      DuVries and Mann procedure, *643*, 644
      failure of, salvage procedures, 645, *645*, 650
      interphalangeal fusion, 644, *644*
      metatarsal head resection, 642, *642*
      metatarsophalangeal joint, 214
        risks of, 643
      postoperative care, 170
      proximal hemiphalangectomy, 640, *641*
      ray excision, disadvantages of, 645
      syndactylization, 641, *641*
      waist resection of proximal phalanx, 642, *642*
  types of, 94
  valgus deformity and, 640, *640*
  vs. claw toe, 212, *212*, 639, *639*
  vs. curly toe, 214
  vs. mallet toe, 212, *212*
  with pressure over tip, treatment of, surgical,
    classification of procedures, 1035
Hamstrings, testing of, in poliomyelitis, *1128*, 1129
  transfer of, in poliomyelitis, 1155–1161, *1156–1158*,
    1160, *1161*
    general rules, 1155–1157
    technique, *1156–1158*, 1157–1161, *1160*, *1161*
Hand, evolutionary modifications of, 6
Hand-foot syndrome, in hemoglobin SC disease, 1102
  in sickle cell disease, 1099, *1099*, *1100*
Hand-foot-and-mouth disease, affecting feet, 886, *887*
Hansen's disease, affecting foot, 1418
Hard corns, in small toes, 624–628, *624–628*, 632–634.
  See also *Corns, hard.*
Harris footprint mat, 1284, *1284*, 1382, *1382*
Head, abnormalities of, in relation to neurologic
  examination of foot, 1107
  trauma to, lower extremity disorders and, *1116*,
    1117–1122, *1119–1121*
    equinovarus deformity, treatment of, surgical,
      1122

Head (*Continued*)
  trauma to, lower extremity disorders and, equinus
    deformity and extensor rigidity, 1118,
    1119, *1120*. See also *Equinus deformity.*
    excessive ankle dorsiflexion, treatment of,
      surgical, *1121*, 1122
    toe deformities, 1118–1121, *1121*. See also *Toes,*
      deformities of.
  neurologic recovery from, 1117
  vs. stroke, surgical considerations, 1118
Heavy-metal poisoning, 1069–1071, *1070*, *1071*. See also
  Poisoning.
Heel. See also *Calcaneus* and *Hindfoot.*
  adult, 764–775
  black, etiology and clinical features of, 890, *890*
  corrective footwear for, 1777, *1778*
  disorders of, arthritic, 774
    idiopathic ankylosing spondylitis, 774
    metabolic disturbances, 774
    psoriatic, 774
    Reiter's syndrome, 774
    rheumatoid (sero-positive), 774
    classification, 766
  examination of, clinical, 90
  fat pads of, damage or atrophy in, 839, *839*
  fissures of, etiology and treatment of, 896
  in rheumatoid arthritis, valgus deformity, 1029, *1030*
    varus deformity, *1030*, 1031
  injuries of, industrial, 1611. See also *Industrial*
    injuries.
  jogger's, 773, 1605
  Kaposi's sarcoma under, 831, *832*
  lateral, incisions in, *160*, 165
    surgical approaches to, *160*, 165
  lipoatrophy of, treatment of, in geriatrics, 974
  medial, incisions in, *161*, 165
    surgical approaches to, *161*, 165
  narrow, footwear and shoe modifications for, 1760,
    1781
  painful, associated disorders and, 975
    etiology of, 766–774
      arthritic disorders, 774
      athletic injuries, 773, 1605
      lateral, 772
      medial, 767–772
      plantar, 766
      posterior, 772
    from athletic injuries, treatment, nonsurgical, 773
      surgical, 773
    in distance runners and joggers, 1605
    in geriatrics, 974–976. See also *Geriatric foot.*
    lateral, 772
    mechanisms of, 764–766, *765*, *766*
      lateral, 764, *765*
      medial, 764, *765*
      plantar, 764, *765*
      posterior, 766, *766*
    medial, 767–772, *769–771*
      calcaneal branch neurodynia, 770, *770*
        treatment of, nonsurgical, 770
          surgical, 770, *770*
      tarsal tunnel syndrome, 767–770, *769*
        treatment of, nonsurgical, 769
          surgical, 769, *769*
      tibialis posterior tendon disorders, 770–772, *771*
        treatment of, surgical, 771, *771*
    padding and devices for relief of, 1731, *1732*

Heel (*Continued*)
  painful, plantar, 766, 767, 768
    calcaneal spurs, 767
      treatment of, nonsurgical, 767
        surgical, 767, 768
    fasciitis, 766
      treatment of, 766, 767
    posterior, 772
      Achilles tendinitis, 772
        treatment of, nonsurgical, 773
          surgical, 773
      calcaneal bursitis, 772
      calcaneal exostoses, 772
    syndrome, 1200
      treatment of, nonsurgical, 1405
  posterior, incisions in, 166
    surgical approaches to, 166
  skin grafts for, 958
  ulcers of, in arteriosclerosis obliterans, 1326, *1326*,
    1327
    treatment of, nonsurgical, 1283, *1283*
      surgical, 1283
Heel cord. See also *Achilles tendon*.
  calcaneus and, trauma to, 1497–1538. See also
    Calcaneus.
  deformity of, treatment of, surgical, 190
  examination of, clinical, 90
  function of, relation to clubfoot, 728
    relation to flatfoot, 728
  gouty tophi about, 866, *866*
  ossification of, 857, *860*, 866
  pain in, mechanisms of, 766, *766*
  rupture of, incomplete, strapping for, 1728, *1728*
    spontaneous, 864
  shortening of, pads and devices for, 1715–1720,
    1715–1719. See also *Foot, pain in, padding and
    devices*.
  tendinitis in, 857, *859*, 860
  tight, shoe modifications for, 1759
Heel space, infections of, treatment of, 1406
Heel spur syndrome, examination for, physical, 85, 103,
  104
  soft-tissue ossification and, 835, *835*, 836
Helomata dura, in small toes, 624–628, *624–628*,
  632–634. See also *Corns, hard*.
Helomata mollia, in small toes, 628–634, *629–632*. See
  also *Corns, soft*.
Hemangioendothelioma(s), 991
  malignant, affecting foot bone, *1010*, 1011
Hemangioma(s), 989–991, *990*, *991*
  congenital, capillary vs. cavernous, 219
    cavernous, treatment of, surgical, 220
  in Maffucci's syndrome, *990*, 991
  of foot bone, 1009–1011, *1010*
Hemangiopericytoma(s), 991
Hemarthrosis, acute, treatment of, 1087
Hematologic disorders, affecting foot, summary of, 1084
Hematoma(s), ossifying, post-traumatic, in sports
  injuries, 1600
  subungual, resulting from contusions, 1449
  surgical principles and, 157
Hemianesthesia, hysterical, 1444. See also *Psychiatric
  aspects*.
Hemihypertrophy, congenital, basic literature on, guide
  to, 1865
Hemimelia, paraxial fibular, congenital, 220–226, *221*,
  224. See also *Fibula, longitudinal deficiency of*.

Hemimelia (*Continued*)
  tibial, congenital, 226–228. See also *Tibia,
    longitudinal deficiency of*.
Hemiparesis, spastic. See *Spastic hemiparesis*.
Hemiphalangectomy, distal, for combined hard and soft
  corns, 628
  in hammer toe, 640, *641*
Hemiplegia, as hysterical motor disorder, 1441. See also
  Psychiatric aspects.
  in stroke patient, 1112
  spastic. See *Spastic hemiplegia*.
Hemodynamic physiology, invasive measurements of,
  1303, 1307–1310, *1310*
Hemoglobin SC disease, dactylitis in, 1102
  incidence and diagnosis of, 1102
  vs. sickle trait, 1102
Hemoglobinopathy(ies), 1095–1106
  definition of, 1095
  hemoglobin SC disease, 1102
  leg ulcers, 1104, *1105*
  osteomyelitis and, 1102–1104, *1104*
  sickle cell disease, 1096–1102, *1097–1101*. See also
    Sickle cell disease.
  sickle trait, 1102
  summary of, 1095
  thalassemia syndromes, 1102, *1103*
Hemoglobins, normal vs. variant, 1095, *1095*
Hemophilia(s), 1084–1094, *1088–1093*
  A vs. B, 1085
  antibody formation in, 1086
  as congenital coagulative disorders, 1084
  cavus deformity in, *1091*
  clinical features of, 1084
  equinus deformity in, 1090, *1090*
  etiology of, Factor VIII vs. Factor IX deficiency, 1085
  in foot and ankle, 1088–1093, *1088–1092*
    forefoot problems, 1090, *1091*
    hemophilic arthropathy, 1086, 1088, *1088*, *1089*.
      See also *Hemophilic arthropathy*.
    muscle hemorrhage, 1089, *1090*
      treatment of, nonsurgical, 1089
        surgical, 1090
  incidence of, 1085
  orthopaedic considerations in, 1086–1088
    acute hemarthrosis, treatment of, 1087
    conservative rehabilitation, 1087
    fracture care, 1088
    hemophilic arthropathy, 1086, 1088, *1088*, *1089*
    pseudotumor formation, 1088, 1090–1093,
      1091–1093
    soft-tissue hemorrhage, 1087
  procoagulant activity levels in, 1085
  severe vs. moderate, 1085
  therapy for. See also *Hemophilia, treatment of*.
    analgesic, 1086
    replacement materials, cryoprecipitate, 1085
      fresh frozen plasma, 1085
      lyophilized concentrates, 1085
      whole blood, 1085
    treatment of. See also *Hemophilia, therapy for*.
      anti-inflammatory agents, 1086
      methods, 1086
      surgical, 1086
Hemophilic arthropathy, 1086, 1088, *1088*, *1089*.
  clinical and degenerative changes in, 1088, *1088*, *1089*
  in ankle vs. other joints. 1088
  treatment of, surgical vs. nonsurgical, 1089

Hemorrhage, intraosseous, as cause of pseudotumors, *1092*, 1093
  muscle, in hemophilia, 1089, *1090*
  soft-tissue, in hemophilia, 1087
Heparin, in acute venous thrombosis, 1354
Hereditary sensory neuropathy, 1226–1231, *1228–1234*.
  See also *Neuropathy(ies)*.
Hernias, muscle, in sports injuries, diagnosis and
  treatment of, 1600
Herpes zoster, affecting feet, 886, *886*
Hersage, for nerve trauma, 1183
Heyman-Herndon-Strong procedure, in clubfoot, 243
Higgs operation, in hammer toe, *644*
Hindfoot. See also *Calcaneus, Heel,* and *Talus*.
  abnormal, surgical correction of, 192
  basic literature on, guide to, 1852
  deformities of, in rheumatoid arthritis, 1045, *1046*
  examination of, physical, 103–107, *104–106*
  fractures of, in sports injuries, 1587, *1587*. See also
    Fractures and *Sports injuries*.
  in spinal dysraphism, 262
  incisions in, *161*
  longitudinal deficiency of fibula and, 222
  surgical approaches to, *161*
  tendon transfers in, in cavus deformity, 478–480, *479,
    480*
Hip(s), deformities of, effect on metatarsal weight
  bearing, 183, *183*
  dislocation of, congenital, congenital vertical talus
    and, 444
  flexion contracture of, treatment of, surgical, in
    poliomyelitis, 1162
  flexion-extension of, gait analysis and, *60*
  "windblown," in utero, 1758, *1759*
Hip joint, rotation of, deformities of, 433
  gait analysis and, *62*
History-taking, 81–86, *82–84, 86*
  anatomic and pathologic relationships, 81
  differential diagnosis, 81
  etiology, 81
  foot/ankle–hip/knee relationships, 81, *82*
  general conditions affecting foot, 84
  hypertensive patients, 85
  local foot complaints, 84–86, *86*
    foreign-body granulomas, 85
    gout, 84
    osteoid osteoma, 84, *86*
    plantar heel spur syndrome, 85
    spastic flatfoot, 85, *86*
    subtalar, 86, *86*
    Sudeck's atrophy, 85
  pathologic sequelae, 82
  prior infections, 85
  prior surgery, 85
  prior trauma, 85
  systemic review, 82–84, *83, 84*
    allergies, general, 83
      drug, 83
    arteriosclerosis obliterans, 82
    cardiac decompensation, 82
    Charcot's diabetic arthropathy, 82
    clubfoot varieties, 83
    collagen disease, 83, *83*
    congenital or hereditary multiple-system conditions,
      83
    contraindications for surgery, 82
    diabetes, 82

History-taking (*Continued*)
  systemic review, lymphatic stasis, 82
    neurologic conditions, 84
    occupational, 83
    poliomyelitis, 84, *84*
    sesamoiditis vs. osteochondritis, 83, *83*
    vasculitis of hands and feet, 83, *83*
Hockey, ice, footwear for, 1774
"Hockey-stick" incisions, contraindications for, 147, *147*
Hoffmann operation, in hallux valgus, 577, *578*, 598, 599
Hoffmann-Clayton procedure, modified, in rheumatoid
  arthritis, 186, *186*
  postoperative care, 170
Hoffmann-Tinel sign, nerve regeneration and, 1182
Hoover test, for hysterical motor disorders, 1441, *1442*.
  See also *Psychiatric aspects*.
Hormonal disorders, 1071–1073, *1071–1073*. See also
  Metabolic disorders, of bone.
Horn, cutaneous, clinical features of, 829, *830*
  definition of, 829
  treatment of, 829, *830*
Hueter-Mayo operation, as cause of first ray
  insufficiency syndrome, 686, *687*
Hueter-Mayo-Stone resection, in hallux valgus, 577,
  578, 605
Human foot, anatomy of, 8–36. See also *Anatomy*.
  arthrology of, *11, 12*, 13–17, *14, 16*. See also
    Arthrology.
  development of. See *Embryology*.
  embryology of, 7, *9*. See also *Embryology*.
  evolution of, 2–7, *3, 5, 7*
  innervation of, *18, 19*, 24–31, *29*. See also under
    individual nerves.
  myology of, 17–24, *18–21, 23, 25–27*. See also
    Myology.
  osteology of, 8–13, *11, 12, 14, 23, 25, 26*. See also
    Osteology.
  prenatal, rotation of, 8, *9*
Hypalgesia, testing for, in neurologic examination of
  foot, 1110
Hyperemic testing, and noninvasive exercises, in
  vascular diseases, 1306, *1306, 1308, 1309*
Hyperesthesia, hysterical, 1443, *1444*. See also
  Psychiatric aspects.
Hyperhidrosis, affecting feet, 895
  associated conditions and, 896
  bromhidrosis and, 896
  etiology of, 896
  treatment of, 896
Hyperkeratosis(es), in first ray insufficiency syndrome,
  689
  plantar, in yaws, *1423*
  vs. warts, 905
Hyperkeratotic psoriasis, on soles, 883, *885*
Hyperlax foot, associated anomalies and, 241
  treatment of, 241
Hypermobile foot, treatment of, 505–515, *506–510, 512,
  513*. See also *Pes planus*.
Hypermobility, of joints, congenital, 497, *497, 499, 500*
Hyperostosis, cortical, caused by hypervitaminosis A,
  1069
  clinical features of, 1069
  infantile, clinical features of, 1069
Hyperplasia, bone marrow, 1097, *1098*
Hyperpronated foot, treatment of, 505–515, *506–510,
  512, 513*. See also *Pes planus*.
Hyperthyroidism, 1072, *1072*

Hyperuricemia, in gout, 1014
  tophaceous, 1020
  in sickle cell disease, *1097*, 1101
  theoretical bases for, 1015
Hypervitaminosis A, as cause of cortical hyperostosis, 1069
Hypervitaminosis D, as cause of bone calcification, 1068, *1068*
  vs. heavy-metal poisoning, 1070
Hypesthesia, hysterical, 1443. See also *Psychiatric aspects.*
  testing for, in neurologic examination of foot, 1109
Hypochondriasis, 1437. See also *Psychiatric aspects.*
Hyponychium, *915–918*, 919
Hypophosphatasia, 1073
Hyposensitive foot, footwear for, 1781
Hypospadias, congenital vertical talus and, 444
Hypothyroid dwarfism, in children vs. adults, 1073
Hypothyroidism, 1073
Hypovitaminosis C, 1068, *1069*. See also *Scurvy.*
Hypovitaminosis D, 1065–1068, *1066–1068*. See also *Rickets.*
  rickets and, 1065–1067, *1066, 1067*
    clinical features of, 1066
    radiographic features of, 1066, *1066, 1067*
    treatment of, 1066, *1067*
Hysteria, conversion, 1438–1444, *1442–1444*. See also *Psychiatric aspects, hysterical neurosis.*
Hysterical dysesthesia, 1443. See also *Psychiatric aspects.*
Hysterical hemianesthesia, 1444. See also *Psychiatric aspects.*
Hysterical hyperesthesia, 1443, *1444*. See also *Psychiatric aspects.*
Hysterical hypesthesia, 1443. See also *Psychiatric aspects.*
Hysterical motor disorders, 1441–1443, *1442, 1443*. See also *Psychiatric aspects.*
Hysterical neurosis, 1438–1444, *1442–1444*. See also *Psychiatric aspects.*
Hysterical paresthesias, 1443. See also *Psychiatric aspects.*
Hysterical sensory disorders, 1443, *1444*. See also *Psychiatric aspects.*

Ice hockey, footwear for, 1774
Ice skating, footwear for, 1774
Idiopathic edema, subcutaneous, 836, *836*
Immersion foot, clinical features and treatment of, 1450
Impetigo contagiosa, clinical features and treatment of, 887, *888*
Impingement syndrome, in sports injuries, 1593–1595, *1594, 1595*. See also *Sports injuries.*
  marginal exostoses in, 789–792, *790, 791*
Incisional neuroma, treatment of, surgical, 1298
Indomethacin, in treatment of acute gouty arthritis, 1020
Industrial injuries, incidence of, 1607–1609, *1608*
  prevention of, 1621–1625, *1621, 1623, 1624*
    home injuries and, 1623–1625, *1624*
    safety programs, 1622, *1623*
    safety shoes, 1621, *1621*
  protection from, 1614–1621, *1615, 1616, 1618–1620*
    occupational comparisons, *1615, 1616*
    shoe toecaps, 1618, *1618–1620*

Industrial injuries (*Continued*)
    protection from, statistics and legislation, 1614–1617, *1615, 1616*
  specifically job-related, 1612–1614, *1613, 1614*
    "aviator's astragalus," 1612
    burns and thermal injuries, 1613, *1613, 1614*
      chemical, 1613, *1614*
      electrical, 1613, *1614*
      scalding water, 1613, *1613*
    calcaneal fractures, 1612
  statistics and discussion, 1607–1609, *1608*
  to ankle, 1610, *1611*
    causes and clinical features of, 1611, *1611*
    protection from, 1621
    treatment of, 1611
  to heel, causes of, 1611
    treatment and prognosis, 1611
  to metatarsal region, 1609, *1610*
    causes and clinical features of, 1609, *1610*
    protection from, 1619–1621, *1620*
    treatment of, 1610
  to sole, 1611, *1612*
    clinical features and treatment of, 1612
    protection from, 1617, *1618*
    puncture wounds, incidence of, 1612, *1612*
  to toes, incidence and treatment of, 1609
Industry, safety shoes for, 1764–1769, *1765, 1766, 1768–1770*. See also *Shoes, and shoe modifications.*
Infants, foot disorders in, evaluation of, 196–198, *197*
Infarction, skeletal, in sickle cell disease, 1098–1101, *1098–1101*. See also *Sickle cell disease.*
Infection(s), classification of, 1209
  of foot, 1398–1420
    acute, 1401–1407, *1403–1405*
      abrasions, 1401
      blisters, 1401
      calluses, 1402
      corns, 1403
      fissures, 1403, *1403*
      painful heel, 1405
      purulent, 1405–1407. See also *Infections, of foot, purulent.*
      tenosynovitis, 1405
      ulcers, 1401
        chronic, over bony prominences, 1404, *1405*
          plantar, 1403, *1404*
      wounds, 1402
        crush injuries, 1402
        degloving injuries, 1402
        puncture, 1402
    chronic, 1407–1420, *1407–1417, 1419, 1420*
      granulomatous, 1407–1419, *1407–1417*
        leprosy, 1418. See also *Leprosy.*
        mycosis, 1411–1418, *1411–1417*. See also *Mycosis.*
        sarcoidosis, 1418. See also *Sarcoidosis.*
        syphilis, 1418. See also *Syphilis.*
        tuberculosis, 1407–1411, *1407–1410*. See also *Tuberculosis.*
      nongranulomatous, 1419, *1419, 1420*
        parasitic infestations, 1420, *1420*
        pyogenic, 1419, *1419*. See also *Infections, of foot, pyogenic.*
    gonococcal, clinical features and progress of, 1419
      treatment of, 1420
    granulomatous, 1407–1419, *1407–1417*. See also *Infections, of foot, chronic.*

Infection(s) (*Continued*)
  of foot, granulomatous, causes of, 1399
    insensitive 1278–1280, *1279*
    pain as factor in, absence vs. presence of, 1398
    purulent. See also *Infections, of foot, pyogenic.*
      adventitious bursae, 1406
      deep plantar space abscesses, 1406
      dorsum, 1406
      heel space, 1406,
      infected blister, 1405
      paronychia, 1405
      plantar interdigital subcutaneous space, 1406
      pulp space, 1406
      web space, 1406
    pyogenic. See also *Infections, of foot, purulent.*
      causative bacteria, 1419
      causes of, 1399
      causing squamous cell epithelioma, 1419, *1419*
      etiology of, 1419
      treatment of, surgical and nonsurgical, 1419
    routes of, 1399–1401, *1399–1401*
      hematogenous, 1399, *1399*
      skin anatomy, 1399–1401, *1400*
        dermis, 1400, *1400*
        epidermis, 1399, *1400*
        vs. other body skin, 1399
      space anatomy, 1401, *1401*
    socioeconomic and climatic origins of, 1398
Infectious and noninfectious inflammatory disorders,
  basic literature on, guide to, 1846
Infestations, parasitic, affecting foot, 1420, *1420*
Inflammatory disorders, infectious and noninfectious,
  basic literature on, guide to, 1846
Infrainguinal artery, surgical reconstruction of,
  1335–1343, *1335–1343*. See also *Vascular
  reconstruction.*
Ingrown toenail(s), 925–930, *926–930*. See also
  Toenail(s), ingrown.
Injury(ies). See also *Trauma.*
  crush, 1402, 1450. See also *Crush injury(ies).*
  degloving, treatment of, 1402
  electrical, industrial, 1613, 1614
  from blast, treatment of, 1459
  in the home, prevention of, 1623–1625, *1624*
  industrial, 1607–1625. See also *Industrial injuries.*
  of forefoot and toes, 1449–1462
    classification of, 1449
    contusions, 1449
    crush injuries, 1402, 1450
    electrical burns, 1451, 1613, *1614*
    fractures and dislocations, 1451–1459, *1451–1456,
      1458*. See also *Dislocations* and *Fractures.*
    from blast, 1459
    from cold, 1450
      frostbite, 1450
      immersion foot, 1450
      trench foot, 1450
    ligamentous sprains, 1449
    miscellaneous, 1459
    recurrent trauma associated with hammer toe,
      1459
    sesamoiditis, 1459. See also *Sesamoiditis.*
    tennis toe, 1459
    toenail avulsion, 1450
    venomous snake bite, 1460–1462. See also *Snake
      bite.*
  of midfoot, 1463–1496

Injury(ies) (*Continued*)
    of midtarsal joint, 1490–1495, *1490–1495*. See also
      Midtarsal joint.
    of talus, 1463–1496. See also *Talus.*
    self-inflicted, 1444, *1445*. See also *Psychiatric aspects.*
    sports, to foot and ankle, 1573–1606. See also *Sports
      injuries.*
    thermal, industrial, 1613, *1613, 1614*. See also
      Industrial injuries.
    traumatic, of vascular supply to foot, 1320–1324,
      1322, 1323. See also *Vascular diseases.*
Innervation, of human foot, *18, 19*, 24–31, *29*. See also
  under individual nerves.
Insensitive foot, causes of, 1266
    footwear for, 1781
    including leprosy, 1266–1286. See also *Leprosy.*
    ulcers of, 1268–1285, *1268–1274, 1276–1279,
      1282–1285*. See also *Ulcers.*
Interdigital bursitis, in geriatrics, 973
Intermetatarsal articulation, 662, *663*
Internal fixation, principles of, 166
Interosseous talocalcaneal ligament, *11*, 12
Interphalangeal fusion, Higgs procedure, *644*
    in hammer toe treatment, 644, *644*
    Tierny procedure, *644*
Interphalangeal joint(s), anatomy of, 17
    functional, 43
    arthrology of, 17
    in claw toe, 212, *212*
    in curly toe, 214
    in hammer toe, 94, 212, *212*
      treatment of, surgical, 213, *213*
    in mallet toe, 212, *212*
    in varus toe, 214
    surgery in, 162
In-toeing, in children, variations of, 196, 198
Intraspinal disease, progressive, indications for, 256
Intrauterine molding, as factor affecting foot deformities,
      254, 255
    muscle imbalance and, as factors in deformity, 256
Intrinsic muscles, as stabilizing mechanisms, 55, *55*
Inversion, caused by peroneal palsy, treatment of,
      surgical, in poliomyelitis, 1137
    definition of, 125
    of subtalar joint, 45, *46*
Inversion fractures, in dancers, 1651, *1651, 1652*
Inverted talipes, 374–428. See also *Talipes, inverted.*
Ischemia, acute, diagnosis of, following traumatic
      vascular injuries, 1312, 1322
    signs and symptoms of, 1312
    chronic, of foot, 1324–1332, *1325–1331*. See also
      Arteriosclerosis obliterans.
    dermal, in thermal burns, 1691
    diagnosis of, vs. venous thrombosis, 1312
    profound, in arteriosclerosis obliterans, 1326
    tolerance levels of, compartment syndromes and, 1201
Ischemic neuropathies, classification of, 1177
    nerve injuries and, 1180, *1180, 1181*

Jahss diaphysectomy, in hammer toe, 643
Japas' osteotomy, 1165
Jogger's heel, 773
Jogger's toe, 1605
Jogging, changes in walking cycle during, 38, *38*
    footwear for, 1774

Jogging (*Continued*)
　injuries from, classification, 1574.
　　sports, 1603–1605. See also *Sports injuries.*
Joint(s). See also under individual joints.
　ankylosis of, congenital vertical talus and, 444
　axes of, anatomic and biomechanical correlations,
　　727–729, *728, 729*
　　with tendon relationships, 728, *728*
　flexibility of, maintenance of, surgical considerations
　　and, 150, *150,* 179
　hypermobility of, congenital, 497, *497, 499, 500*
　instability of, management of, 269
　involvement of in rheumatoid arthritis, 1025–1027,
　　1027
　of forefoot, dislocations of, 1452–1457, *1452–1456.* See
　　also *Dislocations.*
　replacement of, total, gait analysis in, 57
　surgery in, in pes planus, 510, 511–515, *512, 513*
Jones, Ellis, technique, for slipping peroneal tendon,
　807
Jones fracture, of fifth metatarsal, in children, 1679
　in dancers, 1653, *1653*
Jones operation, in first ray overload syndrome, 680,
　681, 682
Jones sling operation, for tendon dislocations, 1592,
　1593
Jones suspension procedure, contraindications for, 150,
　179
Juvenile rheumatoid arthritis, 1054–1057, *1056.* See also
　Rheumatoid arthritis.

Kaposi's sarcoma, 992, *992*
　clinical features of, 880–883, *882*
　diagnosis of, 883
　granulomatous, 831, *832*
　treatment of, 883
Keller and Silver operation, postoperative care, 170
Keller operation, in hallux valgus, 569, *570,* 593
　　Lelièvre modification, 571–573, *572*
　modified, 570, *571,* 594, *595, 596,* 604, *604,* 607,
　　615
Keller-Brandes operation, as cause of first ray
　insufficiency syndrome, 687, *687*
Kelly operation, for tendon dislocations, 1592, *1592*
Keratin, excessive, 828
　formation of, 828, *829*
　　following skin grafts, 829
Keratoderma climactericum, 904, *904*
Keratodermia blennorrhagica, in Reiter's syndrome,
　1057
Keratolysis, pitted, affecting feet, clinical features and
　treatment of, 889, *890*
Keratolysis exfoliativa, clinical features and diagnosis of,
　901, *901*
　treatment of, 901
Keratoma(s), plantar, 930–932, *931*
　　etiology and clinical features of, 932, *933*
　　treatment of, 932
Keratosis(es), 828, *829*
　causes of, 829
　　weight-bearing, 147, *148*
　of soles, 901–904, *902–904*
　　affecting palms also, 902
　　arsenical, *903,* 904
　　diffuse, 902, *902, 903*

Keratosis (*Continued*)
　of soles, diffuse, dominant vs. recessive inheritance,
　　902, *902, 903*
　　in mal de Meleda, 903, *903*
　　in Unna-Thost disease, 902, *902*
　　noninherited, 903
　　guttate, 904
　　odd-shaped, 904, *904*
　　punctate, 903, *903*
　　　dominant vs. recessive inheritance, 903, *903*
　treatment of, 904
Keratosis palmaris et plantaris hereditarium, 902, *902*
Kidneys, failure of. See *Renal failure.*
　osteodystrophy of, 1075–1078, *1075–1077.* See also
　　Osteodystrophy, renal.
Kite slipper cast, in congenital clubfoot, 242
Knee, axis of, relationship with ankle axis, 39
　deformities of, affecting foot, surgical correction of, in
　　poliomyelitis, 1152–1162, *1154, 1156–1158, 1160,
　　1161.* See also *Poliomyelitis, of foot, treatment of,
　　surgical.*
　　rotational, 431, 435
　flexion-extension of, gait analysis and, *61*
　longitudinal deficiency of fibula and, 222
　pain in, in distance runners and joggers, 1603
Knee joint, rotation of, gait analysis and, *62*
Knuckling, of hallux, following surgery for hallux valgus,
　605
Koenen's periungual fibromas, 912, *912*
Köhler's disease, of tarsal navicular, 200–203, *202, 203*
　age of incidence of, 200
　clinical findings in, 201
　in late childhood, 199
　occurrence in both feet, 201
　predominance in boys, 200
　prognosis for, 203
　radiologic view, 201, *202, 203*
　trauma as etiologic factor in, 201
　treatment of, 201–203, *203*
　varying nomenclature for, 200
　vs. crush injuries of navicular, 1676, *1677*

Laceration, of tendons, 864, *865.* See also *Tendons,
　tears of.*
Lapidus operation, in hallux valgus, 563, *564,* 604
Larsen's syndrome, subtalar instability in, 735, *736*
Lasts, and shoe manufacture, 1750–1752, *1750, 1751*
Lateral ligament, 13, *14*
Lateral rotation, definition of, 125
Latissimus dorsi, flaps of, for skin grafts, 961
LaTorre prosthesis, 1394, *1395*
Lauge-Hansen classification, of ankle injuries,
　1547–1549, *1547–1549,* 1553
Lead poisoning, 1070, *1070*
　electrodiagnosis in, 73
Leg(s), cramps in, in neuropathic foot, 1210
　duplication of, amputation and dissection, 254, *254*
　muscles of, transfer of, in poliomyelitis, 1142–1152,
　　1143–1152. See also *Poliomyelitis, of foot,
　　treatment of, surgical.*
　ulcers of, in sickle cell disease, 1104, *1105.* See also
　　Ulcers.
Leg pain syndromes, in sports injuries, 1596–1601,
　1598, 1599. See also *Sports injuries.*

Lelièvre's operation, in metatarsalgia with cavus
    deformity, 677
  in metatarsus primus varus, technique, 694–697,
    694–696
  postoperative care, 170
Leprosy, 1266, 1267. See also Insensitive foot.
  affecting foot, clinical features of, 886, 1266, 1418
    in Hansen's disease, 1418
  as cause of foot insensitivity, 1266
  bone damage in, 1267, 1267
  clinical features of, 886, 1266, 1418
  effect of on lower extremities, 1267
  EMG findings in, 73
  in arthritis of ankle, 1419
  lepromatous, 1266
  loss of sensation in, 1267
  nerve damage in, 1267
  neuropathic foot and, radiographic features of, 1266,
    1267
  peripheral neuropathy in, 1240–1242
    anatomic distribution, 1241
    clinical features of, 1241
    diagnosis of, differential, 1241
    lepromatous vs. tuberculoid, 1241
    treatment of, 1241
  treatment of, 1267
  tuberculous, 1266
Lesch-Nyhan syndrome, self-inflicted injuries in, 1445
Lesions, extradural, 1237, 1237
  interruptive, nerve disorders and, 1178, 1178
  intradural, 1237, 1237
  irritative, nerve disorders and, 1179
  of muscles, 845, 846, 847. See also Muscles.
  of nerves, 834, 848, 848
  of skin, 828–832, 829–832. See also Skin, lesions of.
  of spinal cord, 84, 470
  of spine, classification of, 1209
  of tendons, 854–867, 855, 856, 858–866. See also
    Tendons.
  of toenails, basic literature on, 1865
  of veins, 846, 847
  paraungual, treatment of, 636, 651, 651, 652
  periungual, 911, 911, 912.
  soft-tissue, miscellaneous, 828–868
  subcutaneous, 832–837, 832–838. See also
    Subcutaneous lesions.
  subungual, 651, 911, 911, 912
  tumor-like, and tumors, classification of, 983
Lichenification, in ankle, in atopic dermatitis, 871, 871
Ligamentous sprains, 1449
  treatment of, 1450
Ligaments, anatomy of, 11, 13–17, 14. See also under
    individual ligaments.
  calcification of, in dancers, 1636, 1636
  injury of, in ankle, 777–783, 777, 778, 780–782. See
    also under Ankle, injuries of.
    in dancers, 1649.
  laxity of, 843
  lesions of, 836, 842
    multiple traction spurs, 836, 842
    traction periostitis, 842
  of ankle, surgical reconstruction of, 799–802, 800
  of plantar surface of foot, 464, 465
  sprains of, 1449
    in dancers, 1654
    treatment of, 1450
Limb(s), buds of, defects of, multiple causes of, 233

Limb(s) (Continued)
  congenital anomalies of, 233
  defects of, rehabilitative surgery for, indications and
    contraindications, 233
  embryology of, 7, 233
Limb-girdle syndrome, clinical features of, 346
Lipoatrophy, of heel, treatment of, in geriatrics, 974
Lipoma(s), 988, 989
  within tendon sheaths, 857, 858
Liposarcoma(s), 988, 989
Lisfranc amputations, 1366, 1366, 1369, 1370,
    1392–1394, 1394, 1395
Lisfranc's joint, anatomy of, 15, 16
  functional, 711, 712
  anterior tarsus and, disorders of, 711–726. See also
    Tarsus, anterior.
  arthrodesis of, in metatarsalgia with cavus deformity,
    677, 677
  arthrology of, 15, 16
  arthroplasty in, 697
  breaks in, 386, 387, 388, 389–391
  Charcot foot in, 184, 184, 1214
  fracture-dislocations of, 1452, 1452–1455. See also
    Dislocations and Fractures.
  in diabetes, destruction of, 1251, 1252
    neuropathic involvement of, 1255, 1257
  neuropathic changes in, 1379, 1380
  pyarthrosis of, 721, 721
  rocker-bottom deformity in, 713, 713
Literature on foot, guide to, 1837–1866
  amputations, 1850, 1866
  arthrodeses, 1850
  arthroplasties, 1850
  basic books and articles, 1837
  biomechanics of foot and ankle—child and adult,
    1841
  cavus deformity, 1862
  circulatory disturbances, 1843
  claw toes, 1864
  congenital deformities, 1853–1862
    ball-and-socket joint, 1862
    cleft foot, 1862
    hallux varus, 1862
    lobster claw, 1862
    metatarsus primus varus and hallux valgus, 1858
    metatarsus varus, 1857
    split foot, 1862
    talipes equinovarus, 1853–1857
    tarsal coalitions, 1858–1861
    valgus deformity, convex, 1861
  congenital hemihypertrophy, 1865
  dermatologic disorders, including nails, 1844
  dislocations, 1851
  flatfoot, 1853
  forefoot and toe deformities, 1849
  fractures, 1851, 1866
  fusions, 1850
  genetic disturbances, 1853
  gout and periarticular alterations, 1850
  hallux rigidus, 1848, 1864
  hallux valgus, 1848, 1858
  hallux varus, 1848, 1862
  hammer toes, 1864
  hindfoot, 1852
  infectious and noninfectious inflammatory disorders,
    1846
  metatarsus primus varus, 1848, 1858

Literature on foot (*Continued*)
  guide to, nail lesions, 1865
    neuromuscular and neurologic diseases—child and
      adult, 1842
    normal foot—child and adult, 1838–1841
    pes planus, 1853
    pronated feet, 1863
    rheumatoid foot, 1847
    skin lesions, 1865
    sports injuries, 1852
    toe problems, miscellaneous, 1865
    tumors, 1845
"Lobster claw," basic literature on, guide to, 1862
  congenital, clinical features of, 245
    treatment of, 245
Long muscles of foot, action of, modifying factors, 734
  control of on subtalar complex, 734
Longitudinal arch, elevation of, windlass mechanisms
    and, 52–54, *54*
  examination of, clinical, 91
  fat pad of, 840
  high, associated disorders and, 91
    effect on weight bearing, 179, *181*
    maintenance of, in treatment of Köhler's disease,
      202, *203*
  strain of, footwear for, 1780
  subtalar stability and, 735–738, *735–737.* See also
    Subtalar complex.
Longitudinal axis, metatarsal break and, *50, 52*
Longitudinal deficiencies, paraxial fibular hemimelia,
    245
  paraxial tibial hemimelia, 246
  treatment of, 245
Lower extremity, axes of, *402, 403*
  in normal stance phase, *430*
  disorders of, in stroke and head trauma patient,
    1112–1122, *1115–1117, 1119–1121.* See also
    Head, trauma to and *Stroke.*
    rotational. See *Rotational disorders.*
  muscles of, electromyographic study of, 63–66, *65*
  transverse rotation of, 50–52, *51, 52, 61–63*
Lues. See *Syphilis.*
Lumbosacral syringomyelia, hereditary sensory
    neuropathies and, 1227
Lunula, of nails, *915, 916,* 919
Lupus arthritis, as cause of peroneal spastic flatfoot, 743,
    743
Lupus erythematosus, discoid, affecting foot, 873, *873*
    vs. psoriasis, *873, 873*
  systemic, affecting foot, 874, *874*
Lymphangiomas, congenital, 220
Lymphatic drainage, 32

Ma and Griffith operation, for percutaneous repair of
    ruptured Achilles tendon, 1539–1541, *1540*
Macrodactyly, congenital, 218, *219*
  diagnosis of, differential, 218
  of foot vs. hand, 218
  of small toes, 649, *650*
    causes of, 649
    treatment of, surgical, 218, 650
Macroemboli, 1311, *1312, 1313.* See also *Vascular
    disease, arterial occlusive.*
Madura foot. See *Madura mycosis.*
Madura mycosis, 1411, *1411–1416*

Maduromycosis. See *Madura mycosis.*
Maffucci's syndrome, *359,* 360
  enchondromas and hemangiomas in, *990, 991,* 1005
Mal de Meleda, diffuse keratoses of soles in, 903, *903*
Mal perforans ulcers, in diabetes, 1255, *1257.* See also
    Diabetic foot.
Malformation syndromes, pediatric, minor foot disorders
    and, 197
Malingering, diagnosis of, differential, 1445
Malleolus(i), fractures of, in dancers, 1651, *1651, 1652*
  medial and lateral, skin grafts for, 958
Mallet toe, 624, *625,* 636–638, *636, 637*
  causes of, 636
  congenital, *212,* 214
  definition of, 212, *214,* 636
  end corn and, 634, *634*
  in children vs. adults, 214
  metatarsophalangeal joint in, 212, *212,* 214
  treatment of, nonsurgical, 214, 638
    surgical, technique, 214, *637, 638*
  vs. hammer toe, 212, *212*
Malum perforans, diabetes mellitus and, 878, *878*
Marble bone disease, vs. heavy-metal poisoning, 1070
"March" fracture(s), caused by first ray insufficiency
    syndrome, 688, *688.* See also *Deutschländer's
    disease.*
  in transverse metatarsal arch, 93, *93*
  of metatarsals, 1457
Marfan's syndrome, clinical features of, 235
  longitudinal arch sagging in, *735, 736*
  prognosis for, 235
  subtalar instability in, *735,* 736
Marie's disease, 1071, *1072, 1072*
Marrow hyperplasia, in sickle cell disease, *1097, 1098*
Massive osteolysis syndrome, 1293
Mayer-Bunnell suture, 1145
McBride operation, in hallux valgus, 561–563, *562,*
    602–604, *602,* 607, 615, 618
  postoperative complication of, *173*
McElvenny and Caldwell's osteotomy, 1165, *1166*
McFarland and Scrase operation, modified, for
    contracted overlapping fifth toe, 647, *647*
Medial ligament, 13, *14*
Medial rotation, definition of, 125
Medullostomy, tarsal, radiographic views, in
    Duchenne's muscular dystrophy, *344*
Melanoma, amelanotic, of hallux nail bed, 831, *831*
Melanosarcoma, periungual and subungual, *934,* 935,
    935
Melorheostosis, clinical features of, 369, *371*
  pathologic findings in, 369–372
  prognosis for, 372
  radiographic features of, 369, *371*
Meningomyelocele, neuropathic foot and, treatment of,
    1261, *1261*
Menkes' syndrome, short life expectancy in, 234
Mental retardation, in arthrogryposis multiplex
    congenita, 456
  in congenital vertical talus, 444
Metabolic disorders, classification of, 1209
  of bone, 1064–1078, *1065–1077*
    classification of, 1064
    hormonal disorders, 1071–1073, *1071–1073*
      cretinism, 1073
      growth hormone, 1071, *1071, 1072*
        acromegaly, *1071,* 1072, *1072*
        deficiency of, 1071

Metabolic disorders (*Continued*)
  of bone, hormonal disorders, growth hormone, excess of, 1071
    hyperthyroidism, 1073
    myxedema, 1073
    parathyroid hormone, 1072, *1072*
      hyperparathyroidism, 1072, *1072*
      hypothyroidism, 1073
      pseudohypoparathyroidism, *1072*, 1073
      thyroid hormone, 1073
        hypothyroid dwarfism, children vs. adults, 1073
    nutritional diseases, 1064–1071, *1065–1071*
      calcinosis curcumscripta, 1068
      calcinosis universalis, 1068
      heavy-metal poisoning, 1069–1071, *1070, 1071*
      hypervitaminosis A, 1069
      hypovitaminosis C, 1068, *1069*. See also *Scurvy.*
      hypovitaminosis D, 1065–1068, *1066–1068*
        osteomalacia, 1066–1068, *1066, 1067*
          genetic forms of, 1073–1075, *1073–1075*. See also *Osteomalacia.*
        rickets, 1065–1067, *1066, 1067*. See also *Rickets.*
      osteoporosis, 1064, *1065*
      tumoral calcinosis, 1068
      renal osteodystrophy, 1075–1078, *1075–1077*. See also *Osteodystrophy, renal.*
      vs. Paget's disease, 1078
Metabolic neuropathies, 1238
Metacarpals, osteitis of, in yaws, *1422*
  periostitis of, in yaws, *1422*
Metastable foot, treatment of, 505–515, *506–510, 512, 513*. See also *Pes planus.*
Metatarsal(s), 659–710
  alignment of, surgical, in first ray insufficiency syndrome, 701, *701, 702*
  anatomy of, 659–666, *660–665*
    common characteristics, 659–661, *660, 661*
      angles, 661, *661*
      arches, 661, *661*
      Fick angle, 659, *660*
      formulas, 659–661, *660*
      regional pathology, 659
    fifth, 663
    first, 663, *671*
    intermetatarsal articulation, 662, *663*
    mobility, 663, *664*
    particularities, 663, *664, 671*
    sesamoids, 662
    toes, 664–666, *665*
    topographic, 664, *664*
    trabecular systems, 661, *662*
  arch of, transverse, examination of, clinical, 92, *92, 93*
    in splay foot syndrome, 92
    "march" fracture in, 93, *93*
    plantar warts and, 93
    weight-bearing role of, 177, *177, 178*
  bases of, osteotomy of, first ray overload syndrome and, 681, *682, 686*
    relationship, 16
  biomechanics of, 666–673, *666, 668–672*
    during gait, 671–673, *672*
    forefoot in tiptoe position, 670, *670–672*
    forefoot support, 666–669, *668, 669*
      anatomy, 667
        comparative, 667

Metatarsal(s) (*Continued*)
  biomechanics of, forefoot support, embryology, 667
    examination, clinical, 667
      plantar print, 667, *669*
      radiographic, 667, *668*
    theories of, 666, *666*
  in anterior tarsus and Lisfranc's joint, 712
  break in, long axis of foot and, 50, *52*
  deformities of, in short heel cord, 1716, *1718*
  destruction of, in yaws, *1426, 1427*
  discombobulation of, in crush injuries, 187, *187*
  dislocations of, 179, *184, 187,* 1452, *1452–1455*. See also *Dislocations.*
  displacement of, 178, *179, 180*
    dorsal, as cause of rocker bottom in Lisfranc's joint, 713, *713*
    in Charcot foot, 179, *184*
    in Lisfranc's dislocation, 179, *184*
    in poliomyelitis, 178, *179, 180*
    plantar, in hammer toe, 178
  effect of Mitchell bunion procedure on, *181, 182*
  fat pads of, weight bearing and, 838, *838, 839*
  fifth, anatomy of, 663
    avulsion of styloid process of, physical examination for, 110, *111*
    trauma to, in children, 1679
    in dancers, 1653, *1653*
  first, anatomy of, 663, *671*
    correction of shortening of, amputation of last four metatarsal heads, 700
      amputation of second ray, 697
      lengthening, 697
      Lisfranc's joint arthroplasty, 697
      metatarsal alignment, 701, *701, 702*
      shortening of remaining metatarsals, 698–701, *699*
        diaphyseal osteotomy, 698–700, *699*
    extracapsular osteotomies of, in hallux valgus, 566–569, *567, 568*
    lengthening of, in first ray insufficiency syndrome, 697
    osteotomy of, malunion following surgery for hallux valgus, *606, 607*
    nonunion following surgery for hallux valgus, 605, *605*
    skin ulceration under, in alcoholic neuropathy, 1219, *1219, 1221*
  first and second, traumatic separation of, in children, 1682
  fractures of, 179, *180*
    in children, 1676–1680, *1678, 1679*. See also *Children, trauma in* and *Growing foot.*
    in sports injuries, 1586, *1586*. See also *Sports injuries.*
    multiple, *187*
  fracture-dislocations of, 1453–1457
  fusion of, optimum position, 175
  heads of, amputation of, 185, *185, 186*
    in first ray insufficiency syndrome, 700
    transmetatarsal, prostheses for, 1815, *1816*
    in Freiberg's infraction, 207, *208, 209*
    resection of, in hammer toe, 642, *642*
    risks of, 643
    skin grafts for, 962
  hyalin divestment of, in hallux valgus, 553, *556*
  in cavus deformity, 713
  in equinus deformity, 179, 713

Metatarsal(s) (*Continued*)
  in rheumatoid arthritis, 713
  in surgical management of non-plantigrade foot, *180,*
    185–188, *185–187*
  incisions in, *160, 162*
  injuries of, industrial, 1609, *1610.* See also *Industrial*
    injuries.
    protection from, 1619–1621, *1620.*
  lesser, stress fracture of, following surgery for hallux
    valgus, 607
  mobility of, 663, *664*
  osteocartilaginous exostosis in, *1004*
  osteomyelitis of, treatment of, *1666*
  osteotomy of, 424
    as cause of first ray insufficiency syndrome, 686
    nonunion following, 172, *173*
    postoperative care, 170
  pads for, 1705–1708, *1706, 1707.* See also *Foot, pain*
    in, padding and devices.
  pathologic bursae under, 852, *852*
  pathomechanics of, 673–702. See also *Metatarsalgia.*
  plantigrade foot and, 177–183, *177–185,* 188, *191*
  pliability of, assessment of, 540–543, *543*
  relative length of, in pes planus, 500, *500*
  role of, in hallux valgus, 545–551, *548–551*
    in stable posture, 500, *501*
  safety footwear for, *1766, 1767*
  sagittal groove in, in hallux valgus, 553, *556*
  second, fatigue fracture through, in dancers, 1637,
    1638. See also *Dancing.*
    interspace syndrome, clinical features of, 707
      etiopathology of, 707
      treatment of, 707
  shaft of, length of, effect on weight bearing, 182
  shortening of, surgical, in first ray insufficiency
    syndrome, 697–702, *699, 701, 702*
  splitting of, in forefoot dislocation, 1453, *1456*
  surgical approaches to, *160, 162*
  thickening of, in dancers, 1636, *1636*
  varying stress borne by, *548–551*
  weight-bearing role of, 177, *177, 178*
  weight sharing among, 500, *501*
Metatarsalgia, anterior, predominance in females, 92
    symptoms of, 88, 92, *92*
  causes of, 673–686, *673–675,*
    biomechanical alterations, 673, *673*
      irregular distribution of metatarsal load, 678–702
        central ray insufficiency syndrome, 682–684,
          683. See also *Central ray insufficiency*
          syndrome.
        central ray overload syndrome, characteristics
          and treatment, 684
        first ray insufficiency syndrome, 684–702, *685,*
          687, 688, 691, 692, 694–696, 699, 701, 702.
          See also *First ray insufficiency syndrome.*
        first ray overload syndrome, 679–682, *680–682.*
          See also *First ray overload syndrome.*
      overload of anterior support, 673–678, *673–675,*
        677, 678
        in cavus deformity, 674–678, *675, 677, 678*
          gait cadence, 675, *675*
          treatment, 676–678, *677, 678.* See also
            Metatarsalgia, cavus deformity and,
            treatment of.
        in equinus deformity, 674
        too high shoe heel, 674, *674*
    Morton's disease, 702

Metatarsalgia (*Continued*)
  cavus deformity and, treatment of, 676–678, *677, 678*
    nonsurgical, 676
    surgical, 676–678, *677, 678*
      skeletal, 677, *677, 678*
        Lelièvre's operation, 677
        Lisfranc's joint arthrodesis, 677, *677*
        midtarsal joint arthrodesis, 678, *678*
      soft tissues, 676
        Camera's operation, 676
        Steindler's operation, 676
  examination for, physical, 113
  flexible, treatment of, surgical, 1036
  footwear for, *1776, 1781*
  hallux valgus and, 557, 607
  Morton's, symptoms of, 1198
    treatment of, nonsurgical, 1199
    surgical, 1200
  pathomechanics of, 673–702
  treatment of, nonsurgical, orthoses, 690, *691*
Metatarsocuneiform joint, first, disorders of, in
    geriatrics, 973
Metatarsophalangeal joint(s), anatomy of, *14, 16,* 17
    functional, 43
  arthrology of, *14, 16,* 17
  Charcot, 1211, *1213*
  chronic diabetic Charcot changes in, *1222*
  destruction of, in diabetes, 1251, *1253*
  dislocation of, in children, 1680
    in dancers, 1657, *1657*
  disorders of, treatment of, in geriatrics, 971
  examination of, roentgenographic, 98
  fifth, chronic subluxation of, 843, *843*
  first, arthritis in, 553–557, *556, 557*
    arthrodesis of, in hallux valgus, 573, *574*
      postoperative care, 170
    arthrosis of, following surgery for hallux valgus,
      604, *604*
    gout in, *1016, 1019*
    subluxation of, congruous or incongruous, 553, *555*
    fusion of, optimum position, 175
  in claw toe, 212, *212*
  in hammer toe, 94
    treatment of, surgical, 214
  in mallet toe, 212, *212,* 214
  involvement of, in alcoholic peripheral neuropathy,
    1219, *1220–1222*
  mal perforans ulcers and, in diabetic foot, 1387, *1389*
  osteoarthritis of, occupational, 83
  replacement of, partial or total, in hallux valgus,
    573–577, *575, 576*
  second, capsulitis or synovitis of, 843
  synovitis of, in rheumatoid arthritis, *1025, 1027, 1028*
    treatment of, surgical, 1034
  treatment of, surgical, 162
Metatarsus, anatomy of, 12, *14, 16*
Metatarsus adductus, in utero, 1759
Metatarsus primus varsus, basic literature on, guide to,
    1848, 1858
  effect of on weight bearing, 182
  hallux valgus and, basic literature on, guide to, 1858
  static vs. dynamic, 549
  treatment of, surgical, "fibrous cerclage" and sesamoid
    anchoring, 694–697, *694–696*
    osteotomy, 693
    setting with soft material, 694
Metatarsus varus, basic literature on, guide to, 1857

Metatrophic dwarfism, short life expectancy in, 234
Microcephalia, congenital vertical talus and, 444
Microdactyly, congenital, 218
  of small toes, 648
Microemboli, 1312–1315, *1314, 1315.* See also *Vascular diseases, arterial occlusive.*
Midfoot. See also under specific areas.
  crush injuries of, in childhood, 1676, *1676*
  deformities of, in rheumatoid arthritis, 1045, *1046*
  disorders of, in geriatrics, 973. See also *Geriatric foot.*
  examination of, physical, 107–110, *107–110*
  fractures of, in sports injuries, 1586. See also *Sports injuries.*
  injuries of, 1463–1496
Midtarsal joint. See also *Subtalar complex.*
  anatomy of, *12,* 15
    functional, 42
  arthrodesis of, in metatarsalgia with cavus deformity, 678, *678*
  breaks in, 386–391, *388*
  changes of, in Charcot foot, 1255, *1257, 1258, 1259*
  destruction of, in Charcot foot, 1251, *1251*
  disarticulation of, *12*
  dislocation of, plantar, *1494*
  examination of, clinical, 90, *91*
  in subtalar complex, 732–734, *733*
  injuries of, 1490–1495, *1490–1495*
    classification of, 1490
    crush, 1494
      treatment and prognosis, 1495
    diagnosis of, 1490, *1490*
    lateral, 1493, *1493, 1494*
      fracture sprains, treatment of, 1493
      fracture subluxations, treatment of, 1493, *1493*
      swivel dislocation, 1494, *1494*
    longitudinal, clinical features of, 1492
      treatment of, 1492
    medial, 1490–1492, *1491, 1492*
      fracture sprains, treatment of, 1490
      fracture subluxation and dislocation, treatment of, 1490–1492, *1491*
      swivel dislocations, treatment of, 1492, *1492*
    plantar, 1494, *1494, 1495*
      fracture sprains, 1494
      fracture subuxation and dislocation, treatment of, 1494, *1494, 1495*
  laxity of, subtalar instability and, 736, *736*
  neuropathic changes in, *1379,* 1380
    in Charcot foot, 1255–1259, *1257, 1258*
    in diabetes, *1251*
  range of motion in, axes of, 733
    in pes planus, 733, *733*
Midtarsus, abnormal, surgical correction of, 192
  examination of, clinical, 92
  incisions in, *160,* 162
  osteoarthritis in, 92
  surgical approaches to, *160,* 162
Military footwear, 1769–1771, *1770–1773*
Mitchell bunion surgery, contraindications for, 173, *173*
  postoperative effect of on metatarsal weight bearing, *181,* 182
Mitchell operation, in hallux valgus, 563–566, *565,* 604, *605*
Mitral valvular disease, arteriographic view, *1318*
Moebius syndrome, associated anomalies and, 238

Moldable Podiatric Compound, for relief of painful pressure in geriatrics, 972, *972*
Molo, for relief of painful pressure in geriatrics, 972, *972*
Mononeuritis multiplex, polyarteritis nodosa and, 1225
  rheumatoid arthritis and, 1225
Mononeuropathy, diabetic, 1217
Mononeuropathy multiplex, 1217
Monoplegia, as hysterical motor disorder, 1441. See also *Psychiatric aspects.*
Morphea, affecting foot, 874, *875*
  vs. necrobiosis lipoidica diabeticorum, 874, *875*
Morton's disease, 702–707, *704, 705, 707.* See also *Morton's metatarsalgia, Morton's neuroma,* and *First ray insufficiency syndrome.*
  clinical features of, 703
  definition of, 703
  diagnosis of, differential, 703
  etiopathology of, 705, *705*
  microscopic view, 704, *704*
  pathologic anatomy of, 704, *704*
    treatment of, nonsurgical, 706
      surgical, 706, *707*
  varying nonmenclature for, 703
Morton's metatarsalgia, symptoms of, 1198
  treatment of, nonsurgical, 1199
    surgical, 1200
Morton's neuroma, examination for, physical, 113
  foot pads for, 1709–1711, *1710*
  treatment of, surgical, 1034
Morton's syndrome. See *First ray insufficiency syndrome.*
Motion, abnormal, definition of, 89
  of foot and ankle, definitions of, 125
  range of. See *Range.*
Motor activity, types of, at birth, 250
Motor disorders, hysterical, 1441–1443, *1442, 1443.* See also *Psychiatric aspects.*
Motor neuritis, 1242–1244, *1243, 1244.* See also *Neuritis, motor.*
Motor neuron disease, upper, electrodiagnosis in, 78
Motor power, assessment of, 264
Motor sensory neuropathies, hereditary, as cause of cavus deformity, 468
Motor system, disorders of, in relation to neurologic examination of foot, 1108
Motor unit disease, 335–352
  Becker's muscular dystrophy, 345
  classification of, 335
    clinical, 336
  congenital myopathies, 346
  definition of, 335
  distal myopathies, 347
  Duchenne's muscular dystrophy, 335–345, *337–345*
  fascio-scapulo-humeral muscular dystrophy, 346
  Guillain-Barré syndrome, 349–351
  limb-girdle syndrome, 346
  myotonic dystrophy, 347
  scapulo-peroneal atrophy, 347
  spinal muscular atrophy, 347–349, *348, 350*
Motor units, activation of, during voluntary muscle contraction, 70
  amplitude of, as affected by disease, 70
  duration of, as affected by disease, 70
  in anterior horn cell disease, 70
  in primary muscle disease, 70
  shape of, as affected by disease, 70

Motor units (*Continued*)
  varying muscle fibers in, 71
Multiple sclerosis, peripheral polyneuritis in, 1216
Muscle(s). See also under individual muscles.
  abnormalities of, congenital, 846
  atrophy of. See *Muscular atrophy*.
  biopsy of, in cavus deformity, 473, *473*
    in neurologic examination of foot, 1111
  contraction of, speed of, relationship to spasticity, 286
    voluntary, during electromyography, 70
  disorders of, in relation to neurologic examination of
    foot, 1108
  dissection of, plantar, 25–27
  dystrophy of. See *Muscular dystrophy*.
  extrinsic, anatomy of, 17–22, *18–21, 25–27*
  fibers of, varying, in motor units, 71
  function of, 43–46, *44–46*
    ankle and subtalar joint axial relationships and, 43,
      44
    dorsiflexion vs. plantar flexion, 43, *44*
    in normal foot vs. flatfoot, 45
  hernias of, in sports injuries, diagnosis and treatment
    of, 1600
  hypertrophy of, 846, *846*
  imbalance of, intrauterine molding and, as factors in
    deformity, 256
  intrinsic, anatomy of, *19*, 22–24, *23, 25–27*
  lesions of, 845, *846, 847*
    atrophy, 845. See also *Muscular atrophy*.
    congenital abnormalities, 846
    hypertrophy, 846, *846*
    myositis ossificans, 846, *847*
  rebalancing of, management of, partial denervation,
    268
      tendon elongation, 268
      tendon transfers, 268
  sprains of, in dancers, 1654
  tension in, relationship to spasticity, 286
  testing of, abductor hallucis, 292
    adductor hallucis, 292
    anterior tibial, 288
    extensor digitorum longus, 288, 1131, *1132*
    extensor hallucis longus, 287, *1130*, 1131, *1131*
    flexor digitorum longus, 291, 1131, *1132*
    flexor hallucis longus, 291, 1131, *1132*
    hamstrings, *1128*, 1129
    in cerebral palsy, 287–293
    in poliomyelitis, 1127–1132, *1128–1132*
    individual foot and leg muscles, 287
    peronei, 1130, *1131*
    peroneus longus and brevis, 289
    plantars, 292
    posterior tibial, 289
    quadriceps, 1128, *1128*
    tibialis anterior, 1130, *1130*
    tibialis posterior, 1129, *1129*
    triceps surae, 1129, *1129*
Muscle force, relationship to spasticity, 286
Muscular atrophy, 845
  in cavus deformity, 466, *466, 467*
  in neuropathic foot, 1210
  peroneal, 1231–1236, *1234–1236*. See also *Charcot-
    Marie-Tooth disease*.
  spinal, 347–349, *348, 350*
    bony procedures for, 349
    clinical features of, 348
    foot deformities in, 348, *348, 350*

Muscular atrophy (*Continued*)
  spinal, foot deformities in, calcaneal, 349
    calcaneovalgus, 349, *350*
    calcaneovarus, 349
    equinovarus, 349
    tiptoe standing, 348, *348*
    prognosis for, 348
    varying nomenclature for, 348
Muscular dystrophy, Becker's, 345
  clinical features of, 345
  foot deformities in, 346
  prognosis for, 346
  treatment of, 346
  Duchenne's, 335–345, *337–345*
    age of onset, 335
    clinical features of, 335
    foot deformities in, 336
      early ambulatory, 336, *337*
        treatment of, 336, *337, 338*
      late ambulatory, 337, *338, 339*
        treatment of, 338
    progression and prognosis, 336
    pseudohypertrophic, short life expectancy in, 234
    treatment of, 336–345, *337, 338, 340–343*
      surgical procedures, 338–343, *340–342*
        Achilles tendon lengthening, 338–342,
          340–342, 345
          with posterior tibial tendon transfer,
            339–342, *341, 342*
        percutaneous tarsal medullostomy and soft-
          tissue release, 343, *344*
        percutaneous tarsal osteoclasis, 342
        postoperative orthoses, 342, *343*
      wheelchair deformities, early, 343, *344, 345*
        late, 343–345
  fascio-scapulo-humeral, clinical features of, 346
    foot deformities in, 346
    treatment of, 346
Musculoskeletal system, heritable disorders of, causes
  of, 233
Mycetoma, 1411–1415, *1411–1416*. See also *Mycosis, of
  foot*.
Mycetoma pedis. See *Mycosis, of foot*.
Mycosis, of foot, 1411–1418, *1411–1417*
  blastomycosis, 1417, *1417*
    clinical features and treatment of, 1418
    etiology of, 1417
    radiographic view, *1417*
  coccidioidomycosis, clinical features and treatment
    of, 1416, *1417*
  cryptococcosis, sites and clinical features of, 1415
  etiology of, 1411
  Madura, 1411, *1411–1416*
  mycetoma, 1411–1415, *1411–1416*
    associated infections and, 1411, *1415*
    clinical features of, 1411–1415, *1412*
    etiology of, 1411
    micrographic view, *1416*
    radiographic view, *1413–1415*, 1415
    treatment of, 1415
Myelodysplasia, spinal dysraphism and, foot
  management in, 248–281. See also *Spinal
  dysraphism*.
  principles, 267–270
  in experimental animals, 254
Myeloma, and metastatic carcinoma, in foot bone, 1009,
  1009

Myelomeningocele, cavus deformity and, 470
  congenital vertical talus and, 444
  deformities in, 255, *255*
  EMG findings in, 78
  pes planus and, 515
  treatment of, surgical, 515
Myology, of human foot, 17–24, *18–21, 23, 25–27*
    extrinsic muscles, 17–22, *18–21, 25, 27*
    intrinsic muscles, *19,* 22–24, *23, 25–27*
Myopathy(ies), congenital, 346
  EMG findings in, 73
  distal, 347
  nerve conduction studies in, 74
Myositis ossificans progressiva, 846, *847*
  vs. parosteal osteogenic sarcoma, 846, *847*
Myotonia congenita, vs. myotonic dystrophy, 347
Myotonic dystrophy, clinical features of, 347
  foot deformities in, 347
  treatment of, 347
  vs. myotonia congenita, 347
Myxedema, 1073

Nail(s). See also *Toenails.*
  embryology of, 914, 921–925, *923–925*
    longitudinal thumb section, *923, 924*
  growth of, foot vs. hand, 33
  human, dorsal diagram, *916*
    longitudinal section, *916, 918*
    sagittal section, *915*
    structures of, *915*
  lunula of, *915, 916,* 919
  onychogenic areas for, *917*
Nail bed, anatomy of, 914–919, *915*
  of hallux, amelanotic melanoma of, 831, *831*
Nail plate, anatomy of, 914–919, *915*
Narcotics addicts, self-inflicted injuries in, 1445
Navicular. See also *Köhler's disease.*
  accessory, 725
  anatomy of, 10, *11, 12, 14*
  blood supply to, 201
  compression fracture of, treatment of, *1491*
  fracture-dislocation of, 1453, *1456*
  giant cell tumor of, 722, *722*
  hematogenous osteomyelitis of, 719–721, *721*
  in congenital vertical talus, 440, *440*
  tarsal, adult, aseptic necrosis of, 719, *720*
    Köhler's disease of, 200–203, *202, 203.* See also
      Köhler's disease.
  tuberculosis of, radiographic view, *1409*
Naviculectomy, in congenital vertical talus, 448,
  449–451, 453
Naviculomedial cuneiform joint, fusion of, congenital, *96*
Naviculomedial cuneiform synostosis, as cause of
  peroneal spastic flatfoot, 741, *742*
Necrobiosis lipoidica diabeticorum, affecting skin of foot,
  877, *877*
  vs. morphea, 874, *875*
Necrosis, aseptic, of talus, 748, *748, 749*
  avascular, of foot, diagnosis of, 200
    of talar neck, following talar fracture, 1480, *1481*
    of tarsal navicular, 200–203, *202, 203.* See also
      Köhler's disease.
    steroid-induced, in renal osteodystrophy,
      1076–1078, *1077*

Neoplasms, benign, in children, 196
  in late childhood and adolescence, 199
  malignant, in children, 196
  in late childhood and adolescence, 199
Nerve(s). See also *Neurologic disorders, Neurologic*
  foot, Neuropathic foot, and *Neuropathy(ies).*
  blood supply of, 1171
  cranial, in relation to neurologic examination of foot,
    1108
  damage to. See *Nerves, trauma to.*
  disorders of, 1177–1200, *1178, 1180–1182, 1184–1187,*
    1189–1191, 1193–1195
    classification of, 1177
    entrapment neuropathies, 1193–1200. See also
      Neuropathy(ies), entrapment.
    injuries and traumatic neuropathies, 1178–1182,
      1178, 1180–1182
      compression injuries, 1181, *1182*
      interruptive lesions, 1178, *1178*
        axon regeneration and reinnervation of motor
          end plates, 1179
        clinical significance of degree of injury, 1178
      irritative lesions, 1179
      ischemic, 1180, *1180, 1181*
    painful heel syndrome, 1200
    trauma and neuropathies due to trauma, treatment
      of, 1182–1193, *1184–1187, 1189–1191,*
      1193–1195. See also *Nerve(s), trauma to.*
  injuries of, associated with traumatic vascular injuries,
    1321
    classification of, 1177
    degrees of, 1178, *1178*
    peripheral, orthopaedic reconstruction and releases
      for, 1192, *1193–1195*
    traumatic neuropathies and, 1178–1182, *1178,*
      1180–1182. See also *Nerve(s), disorders of.*
  lesions of, *834,* 848, *848*
  medial and lateral plantar, entrapment neuropathies
    in, 1198
  of human foot, *18, 19,* 24–31, *29.* See also under
    individual nerves.
  peripheral, biopsy of, in cavus deformity, 474
    in neurologic examination of foot, 1111
    tumors of, 992, *993*
  plantar interdigital, entrapment neuropathies in,
    1198–1200
  roots of, spinal, supplying sensory function of foot,
    1295, *1296*
  structure of, anatomy of, 1170, *1170*
  trauma to, avoidance of, 153, *159*
    in leprosy, 1267
    neuropathies due to trauma and, treatment of,
      1182–1193, *1184–1187, 1189–1191,*
      1193–1195
      examination, 1182
      neurolysis, 1183–1188, *1186, 1189–1191,*
        1193–1195. See also *Neurolysis.*
      orthopaedic reconstruction and releases, 1192,
        1193–1195
        timing of procedures, 1192
      orthoses, 1189–1192
      peroneal, *1172,* 1183, *1185–1187, 1189–1191*
      physical modalities, 1188–1192
      posterior tibial, 1183
      prevention, 1183
      sciatic nerve, 1183, *1184, 1185*

Nerve blocks, spinal, differential, technique of, 1296–1298, *1296*, *1297*
Nerve conduction studies, 71–73, *72*. See also *Electrodiagnosis* and *Electromyography.*
Nervous system, autonomic, testing of, in neurologic examination of foot, 1110
Neurapraxia, definition of, 75
  EMG findings in, 73
  nerve conduction studies in, 74
Neuritis, adhesive, following surgery for hallux valgus, *601*, 602
  dorsal cutaneous, in dancers, 1654
  iatrogenic, 1244
  monosensory, peripheral, 1244
    definition and clinical features of, 1244
    iatrogenic, 1244
    treatment of, 1244
  motor, 1242–1244, *1243*, *1244*
    associated disorders and, 1243
    Charcot changes in, 1243, *1244*
    spinal pathology in, 1243, *1243*
    traumatic, 1243, *1243*
    treatment of, 1243
  peripheral, forms of, 1205
Neuroanatomy, of foot and leg, 1171–1174, *1172*, *1174*
  peroneal nerve, common, 1172, *1172*
    deep, 1173, *1174*
    superficial, 1173, *1174*
  posterior tibial nerve, 1173
  saphenous nerve, 1172
Neuroarthropathy, subtalar, in diabetes, *1258*
Neurofibroma(s), 992, *992*
Neurofibromatosis, affecting foot, 84
  clinical features of, 234
  congenital vertical talus and, 444
  fat pad and subcutaneous hypertrophy in, *840*, 841
  limited life span in, 234
Neurogenic sarcomas, 993
Neurilemoma(s), 993, *993*
Neurologic disorders. See also *Nerve(s)*, *Neurologic foot*, *Neuropathic foot*, and *Neuropathy(ies)*.
  affecting foot, basic literature on, guide to, 1842
  of foot, examination of, 1107–1111
    ancillary studies, 1110
      blood, 1110
      electrodiagnostic, 1110
      muscle biopsies, 1111
      peripheral nerve biopsies, 1111
      radiography, 1110
      urine, 1110
    in relation to generalized body disorder, 1107
    physical, 110, *110*
    primary aspects, 1107–1110
      autonomic nervous system, 1110
      back disorders, 1108
      cranial nerves, 1108
      extremities, 1108
      eye disorders, 1108
      head and face abnormalities, 1107
      motor system, 1108
      reflexes, 1109
      sensory perception, 1109
        hypalgesia, 1110
        hypesthesia, 1109
        joint position, 1110
        perianal, 1110

Neurologic disorders (*Continued*)
  of foot, examination of, primary aspects, sensory perception, touch, 1109
      vibratory, 1110
    skin, 1107
    tongue disorders, 1108
Neurologic foot. See also *Nerve(s)*, *Neurologic disorders*, *Neuropathic foot*, and *Neuropathy(ies)*.
  cavus deformity in, 1211
  diagnosis of, Charcot joints, 1211–1213, *1212–1215*
    familial and hereditary, 1213
    sensory and proprioceptive, 1211
  incidence of, ethnic, 1215
Neurologic function, fluctuations in after first year, significance of, 256
Neurologic loss, as factor in deformity, 253–258, *254*, *255*, *257*
Neurologic patterns of paralysis, 251–253, *252*, *253*
Neurolysis, for nerve trauma, 1183–1188, *1186*, *1189–1191*, *1193–1195*
  hersage, 1183
  indications, 1186
  surgical techniques, 1187, *1189–1191*
Neuroma(s), iatrogenic, 1244
  incisional, treatment of, surgical, 1298
  interdigital, plantar, 702–707, *704*, *705*, *707*. See also *Morton's disease.*
  symptoms of, 1198
  treatment of, nonsurgical, 1199
    surgical, 1200
  monosensory, peripheral, 1244
  Morton's. See *Morton's neuroma.*
Neuromuscular diseases, affecting foot, basic literature on, guide to, 1842
Neuropathic arthropathy, 1248. See also *Charcot foot* and *Charcot joint.*
Neuropathic degeneration, 724
Neuropathic foot. See also *Charcot foot*, *Nerve(s)*, *Neurologic disorders*, *Neurologic foot*, and *Neuropathy(ies)*.
  diagnosis of, cavus deformity and, 1211
    Charcot-Marie-Tooth disease and, 1211
    differential, 1208–1215, *1210*, *1212–1215*
    leg cramps, 1210
    muscular atrophy, 1210
    soft-tissue atrophy, 1210, *1210*
    ulcers, 1208–1210
  examination of, 1208–1215, *1210*, *1212–1215*
  in leprosy, radiographic features of, 1266, *1267*
  meningomyelocele and, treatment of, 1261, *1261*
  treatment of, immobilization, 1259–1261, *1260*, *1261*
Neuropathy(ies). See also *Nerve(s)*, *Neurologic disorders*, *Neurologic foot*, and *Neuropathic foot.*
  alcoholic, vs. diabetic, 1219
  allergic, 1242
  axonal, EMG findings in, 73
    nerve conduction studies in, 74
    vs. demyelinating, electrodiagnosis in, 73
  carcinoma and, 1242
    nerve conduction studies in, 74
  demyelinating, EMG findings in, 73
    vs. axonal, electrodiagnosis in, 73
  diabetic, 1210, 1217–1219, 1377–1397. See also *Diabetes* and *Diabetic foot.*
    amyotrophy, 1217
    classification of, 1217

Neuropathy(ies) (*Continued*)
  diabetic, diagnostic basis for, 1218
    mononeuropathy, 1217
    mononeuropathy multiplex, 1217
    neuropathic cachexia, 1217
    polyneuropathy, 1217
      sympathetic denervation in, 1218
    treatment of, surgical, 1298
    ulcers, 1218
    vs. alcoholic neuropathy, 1219
    weight-bearing factors and, 148
  differentiation among, 73–75
  direct infiltration, classification of, 1209
  electrodiagnosis in, clinical applications, 73–75
  endocrine, 1239
  entrapment, 1193–1200
    clinical features of, 1193–1195
    definition of, 76
    dorsal cutaneous nerves, 1197
    electrodiagnosis in, 76
    EMG findings in, 76
    etiology of, 1193
    following ankle injury, 788
    interdigital neuroma, 1198
    medial and lateral plantar nerves, 1198
    Morton's metatarsalgia, 1198
    nerve conduction studies in, 76
    peroneal nerve, 1195
      deep, 1197
      superficial, 1196
    plantar interdigital nerves, 1198–1200
    posterior tibial nerve, 1197
    sural nerve, 1200
    tarsal tunnel syndrome, 1197
    treatment of, 804, 1195
  footwear for, 1781
  hereditary motor sensory, cavus deformity and, 468
  hereditary sensory, 1226–1231, *1228–1234*
    Charcot changes in, 1230, *1232–1234*
    clinical features of, 1227
    complete forefoot absorption in, 1230, *1230*, *1231*
    congenital indifference to pain in, 1227
    congenital vs. familial, 1226
    familial dysautonomia and, 1227
    infection in, secondary virulent, of foot and ankle, *1229*, *1230*
    overlap syndromes and, Charcot-Marie-Tooth disease, 1227
      lumbosacral syringomyelia, 1227
      Refsum's disease, 1227
      with spinal cord involvement, 1227
    Riley-Day syndrome and, 1227
    treatment of, 1228–1231, *1228–1234*
      surgical, 1229
    ulceration in, *1228*, *1229*
  interstitial, 1237
    classification of, 1209
    hypertrophic polyneuritis, progressive, 1238
    multiple, 1237
  ischemic, classification of, 1177
    nerve injuries and, 1180, *1180*, *1181*
  leprous, 1240–1242
  metabolic, 1238
    primary vs. secondary, 1238
  nutritional, 1239
    associated disorders and, 1240
    beriberi, 1240

Neuropathy(ies) (*Continued*)
  nutritional, definition and classification of, 1240
    pellagra, 1240
    pernicious anemia, 1240
    vitamin deficiency, 1240
  peripheral, affecting foot, 1169–1204
    associated manifestations and, 1176
    blood supply of nerves, 1171
    Charcot deformity, 1177
    compartment syndromes, 1201–1203
    nerve disorders, 1177–1200, *1178*, *1180–1182*, *1184–1187*, *1189–1191*, *1193–1195*. See also *Nerve(s), disorders of.*
    nerve structure, 1170, *1170*
    neuroanatomy of foot and leg, 1171–1174, *1172*, *1174*. See also *Neuroanatomy.*
    neurologic examination, 1174–1176
    pain, 1176
    symptomatology, 1174
  alcoholic, 1219–1233, *1219–1222*
    clinical features of, 1219, *1219*
    hallucal gigantism in, 1219, *1221*
    metatarsophalangeal involvement, 1219, *1220–1222*
    rarity of Charcot changes in, 1219–1223
    skin ulcerations in, 1219, *1219–1221*
    soft-tissue atrophy in, 1210, *1210*
    treatment of, nonsurgical, 1219–1223
      surgical contraindications, 1219
    vs. vitamin deficiency neuropathy, 1223
    weight-bearing factors and, 148, *148*
  carcinoma and, 1242
  classification of, 1209
  CNS diseases and, classification, 1224
  collagen disorders and, classification, 1224
    dermatomyositis, 1226
    mononeuritis multiplex, 1225
    periarteritis nodosa, 1226
    polyarteritis, 1226
    polyarteritis nodosa, 1225
    polymyositis, 1226
    Raynaud's phenomenon, 1223
    scleroderma, 1226
    Sjögren's syndrome, 1226
    SLE, 1226
  definition of, 1205
  diabetic, weight-bearing factors and, 148
  diagnosis of, 1205
  electrodiagnostic studies in, 1216
  hereditary sensory, 1226–1231, *1228–1234*
  in leprosy, 1240–1242. See also *Leprosy.*
  in rheumatoid arthritis and other collagen disorders, 1223–1226, *1225*
  interstitial, 1237
  metabolic, 1238
    renal failure, 1238
      clinical types of, 1238
      diagnosis of, 1239
      treatment of, surgical vs. nonsurgical, 1239
  mild sensory vs. severe, 1224
  miscellaneous, and neuropathy-like syndromes, 1205–1247
  monosensory neuritis and neuromas, 1244
  motor neuritis, 1242–1244, *1243*, *1244*. See also *Neuritis, motor.*
  pathologic findings of, 1225
  polyneuritis, 1215–1217. See also *Polyneuritis.*

Neuropathy(ies) (*Continued*)
peripheral, rheumatoid arthritis and, clinical features
of, 1224, *1225*
treatment of, 1226
sensory and proprioceptive systems and, 1206–1208
pain, forms of, 1206
proprioceptive fibers, 1207
temperature discrimination, 1207
tendon reflexes, 1207
touch and pressure, 1207
vascular and hematologically related, 1240
with spinal cord disorders, 1231–1237, *1234–1237.*
See also *Spinal cord, disorders of.*
rheumatoid, classification of, 1032
sensory, hereditary and congenital, classification of,
1209
shoe modifications for, 1760
subdivision by class of nerve fiber, 74
toxic, 1242
classification of, 1209
traumatic, classification of, 1177
nerve injuries and, 1178–1182, *1178, 1180–1182.*
See also *Nerve(s), disorders of.*
treatment of, 1182–1193, *1184–1187, 1189–1191,*
1193–1195. See also *Nerve(s), trauma to.*
vascular and hematologically related, 1240
vitamin deficiency, vs. alcoholic, 1223
Neuropathy-like syndromes, and miscellaneous
peripheral neuropathies, 1205–1247. See also
Neuropathies, peripheral.
classification of, 1209
Neurosis, hysterical, 1438–1444, *1442–1444.* See also
Psychiatric aspects.
Neurosurgical salvage, of intractably painful "failed"
foot, 1295–1300, *1296, 1297, 1300.* See also *"Failed"*
foot.
Neurotic excoriation, self-inflicted injuries in, 1444,
1445
Neurotmesis, definition of, 75
EMG findings in, 73
nerve conduction studies in, 74
Neurovascular damage, avoidance of, 153, *153*
Newborns, foot disorders in, evaluation of, 196–198,
197
Nicotine, role of, in arteriosclerosis obliterans, 1325
in thromboangiitis obliterans, 1347
withdrawal of, in diabetics, 1383
Non-plantigrade foot, avoidance of, 183, *184*
after ankle fusions, 184
after massive trauma, 184
after triple arthrodesis, 184
in Charcot's disease, 183, *184*
management of, surgical, *180,* 185–193, *185–192*
ankle arthrodesis, 190–192, *190–192*
calcaneus, 189, *190*
equinus forefoot with metatarsal calluses, *145,*
188, *188*
fixed varus forefoot, 188, *188, 191*
heel cord, 190
metatarsals, *180,* 185–188, *185–187*
midtarsal cavus deformity with metatarsal
calluses, 189, *189*
supramalleolar osteotomy, 190–192, *191*
triple arthrodesis, 189, *189*
Nonunion, following ankle fusion, 173, *174*
following metatarsal osteotomy, 172, *173*
Normal foot, definition of, 116

Normal foot (*Continued*)
in children and adults, basic literature on, guide to,
1838–1841
motion of, 125
Normal foot and ankle, examination of,
roentgenographic, 116–138, *126–135.* See also
Roentgenography.
Nuclear scanning, uses of, 138
Nutritional diseases, of bone, 1064–1071, *1065–1071.*
See also *Metabolic disorders, of bone.*
Nutritional neuropathies, 1239. See also
Neuropathy(ies).

Occlusion, arterial, 1310–1318, *1310–1317,* 1322, *1322,*
1323. See also *Vascular diseases.*
Occupational factors, in choice of surgery, 149, 168
Ollier's disease. See *Enchondroma(s)* and
Enchondromatosis.
Onychauxis, in geriatrics, 970
Onychogryphosis, *931, 932, 933*
in geriatrics, 970
Onychoma, definition and treatment of, 830, *927, 927,*
928, 930
Onychocryptosis, in geriatrics, rarity of, 970
Onychomycosis, in geriatrics, 971
of toenails, dermatologic management of, 911. See
also *Toenails.*
Orthopaedic reconstruction, for peripheral nerve injury,
1192, *1193–1195*
"Orthopaedic syndrome," progressive foot deformity in,
257
Orthosis(es), 154, *154,* 155. See also *Arch supports;*
Foot, pain in, padding and devices; Footwear;
Orthotics; and *Shoes, and shoe modifications.*
as cause of irritant contact dermatitis, 891, *893*
definition of, 1733
for corns, 633
for distance runners, 1602, *1603*
for sports injuries, 1602, *1603*
for toes, 1741–1743, *1742*
for weight bearing, 506, *506, 507*
in Duchenne's muscular dystrophy, 342, *343*
in first ray insufficiency syndrome, 690, *691*
in hammer toe, 1741, *1742*
in Köhler's disease, 202, *203*
in metatarsalgia, 690, *691*
in nerve trauma, 1189–1192
in pes planus, 506, *506, 507*
in spina bifida, 278, *279*
in stroke patient, dispensation with, 1117
interrelationships of shoes and, 1733
Orthotic and prosthetic management, of foot disorders,
1783–1826. See also *Orthosis(es), Orthotics,* and
Prosthetics.
Orthotic foot management, 1703–1829
Orthotics, 1783–1812. See also *Arch supports; Foot,*
pain in, padding and devices; Footwear;
Orthosis(es); and *Shoes, and shoe modifications.*
care of children and, 1820, *1821–1823*
components and systems, 1798–1812, *1798–1804,*
1806–1812
ankle-foot orthoses, 1799–1812, *1800–1804,*
1806–1812, 1821–1823
metal double-bar, 1799–1801, *1800–1802, 1821*
indications for, 1801

Orthotics (*Continued*)
   components and systems, ankle-foot orthoses, molded
        spiral, 1804, *1804*, *1823*
      indications and criteria for, 1805
     patellar-tendon-bearing, 1806–1812, *1807–1812*,
        1815, *1817*
      indications and criteria for, 1812
     posterior leaf-spring, 1801–1804, *1803*
      indications and criteria for, 1804
     solid, 1805, *1806*, *1822*, *1823*
      indications and criteria for, 1806
    foot orthoses, 1798, *1798*, *1799*
     indications for molded shoe insert, 1799
   development of prescription, 1787–1793, *1789–1792*
    assessment systems, *1789–1792*, 1793
    evaluation, 1786–1793
    management process, 1786
    Orthotic Service, 1787
   foot disorders amenable to, classification of, 1787
   functional electrical stimulation and, 1819, *1820*
   functional terminology of, 1783
   lower-limb orthoses and, classification of, 1784
   plastics used in fabrication, 1784–1786
    advantages of, 1786
    indications for, 1786
    technique of, 1793–1796, *1794*, *1795*
   postfabrication delivery, check-out, and training,
    1796–1798
   recent developments in, 1783
Os calcis. See *Calcaneus.*
Os intermetatarseum, location of, *123*, 124, *124*
Os supranaviculare, location of, *123*, 124
Os sustenaculi, location of, *123*, 124
Os tibiale externum, location of, *123*, 124
Os trigonum, impingement of. See *Os trigonum
    syndrome.*
   location of, *123*, *123*
Os trigonum syndrome, in dancers, diagnosis and
    treatment of, 1648, *1649*
   vs. fracture of posterior talar tubercle, 1486
Os vesalianum, location of, *123*, 124
Ossification, endochondral, *1662*, 1663, *1663*, *1664*. See
    also *Children, trauma in.*
    vs. periosteal, in children, 1662, *1662*
   in heel cord, 857, *860*, 866
   in subcutaneous lesions, 835, *835*, *836*
   of bursae, 853
   of plantar fascia, 842
   soft-tissue, 835, *835*, *836*
    as traction spurs at tendon insertions, 835, *835*, *836*
Osteitis, of metacarpals, in yaws, *1422*
Osteitis deformans, 1078–1083, *1078–1082*. See also
    Paget's disease.
Osteoarthritis, caused by talar fractures, 786
   characteristics of, 789
   degenerative, as cause of peroneal spastic flatfoot, 741
   early difficulties of recognition of, 789
   in dancers, 789
   in football players, 789
   in geriatric foot, infrequency of, 965
   of ankle, *149*, *150*, 789–793, *790–792*
    advanced, 792, *792*
    characteristics of, 789
    impingement syndrome, 789–792, *790*, *791*
    marginal exostoses in, 789, *790*, *791*
    pathologic elements of, 792, *793*
    rarity in conjunction with poliomyelitis, 794

Osteoarthritis (*Continued*)
   of ankle, subchondral sclerosis as advanced sign of,
    792, *792*
    talar pseudocysts following injury, 792
   of first metatarsocuneiform joint, in geriatrics, 973
   of first metatarsomedial cuneiform joint, 714, *714*
   of first metatarsophalangeal joints, occupational, 83
   of midtarsus, 92
   of subtalar complex, 737, *737*, 740
   patterns of, in relation to mechanical stress, 794
   total ankle arthroplasty for, complications and
    contraindications, 820–822, *821*, *822*
Osteoblastoma(s), 1000, *1002*
   vs. osteosarcoma, *1002*
Osteocartilaginous exostosis, 1003, *1004*
Osteochondral fractures, as cause of hallux rigidus, 608,
    610
Osteochondritis, in children, variations of, 196
   in Freiberg's infraction, 210
   in late childhood, 198
   of sesamoids, 210, *210*
    etiology of, 210
    radiologic view, *210*
    treatment of, 210
   vs. sesamoiditis, 83, *83*
Osteochondritis dissecans, arthroscopy in, 142, *142*
   as cause of hallux rigidus, 608, *610*
   as indication for arthroscopy, 142, *142*
   aseptic necrosis of talus and, 748
   causes of, 1669
    talar trochlear fractures, controversy regarding, 786,
     786
   in children, *1666*, 1675
   in dancers, 1635, *1635*
   of talus, 204–207, *205–207*
    clinical findings in, 204
    diagnosis of, 204, *205*
    radiologic view, 204, *205–207*
    treatment of, in adolescent, 205, *207*
     in younger child, 204, *206*
     surgical, 205, *207*
Osteochondroma(s), 1003, *1004*
   of tibia, 357, *358*
Osteochondromatosis, multiple, 356–358, *357*
    clinical features of, 356–358, *357*
    radiographic features of, *357*, 358
Osteodystrophy, renal, 1075–1078, *1075–1077*
    avascular necrosis and, steroid-induced, 1076–1078,
     1077
    bone changes in, 1075
    chronic glomerulonephritis, 1075, *1076*
    severe, 1076, *1076*
    stress fractures in, 1075, *1075*
Osteogenesis imperfecta, clinical features of, 362
   pathologic findings in, 363
   prognosis for, 363
   radiographic features of, 363, *364*
   treatment of, 363
Osteoid osteoma. See *Osteoma, osteoid.*
Osteogenic sarcoma, parosteal, vs. myositis ossificans,
    846, *847*
Osteology, 8–13, *11*, *12*, *14*, *23*, *25*, *26*
   of human foot, metatarsus, 12, *14*, *16*
    phalanges, 12, *14*
    sesamoid and accessory bones, 13, *14*, *23*, *25*, *26*
    tarsus, 10–12, *11*, *12*, *14*
Osteolysis, in Paget's disease, 1081, *1081*

Osteolysis (*Continued*)
massive, 1293
Osteoma, of calcaneus, 745, *745*
osteoid, 84, 999, *1000, 1001*
of calcaneus, 85, *86*
subungual, 936
subungual, 937, *937*
Osteomalacia, 1066–1068, *1066, 1067*. See also
Hypervitaminosis D.
diagnosis of, 1067
drug-induced, treatment of, 1082
genetic forms of, 1073–1075, *1073–1075*
fibrogenesis imperfecta, 1074, *1075*
hypophosphatasia, 1073
renal resistance to parathyroid hormone, 1073, *1073*
vitamin D-resistant rickets, 1074, *1074*
gross deformities in, 1067, *1067*
in adults, 1068
in children, 1067, *1067*
osteosclerosis and, 1073, *1073*
renal osteodystrophy and, 1075, *1075*
rickets and, in biliary atresia, 1066, *1066*
treatment of, osteotomy, 1068
vs. rickets, 1067
Osteomyelitis, chronic, of calcaneus, *862*
gummatous, 1418
hematogenous, of navicular, 719–721, *721*
hemoglobinopathies and, 1102–1104, *1104*
in sickle cell disease, 1102, *1104*
Salmonella, 1103, *1104*
skeletal infarction and, *1100,* 1101
treatment of, 1103
of metatarsals, treatment of, *1666*
Osteonecrosis, aseptic, as residual of ankle injury, 788
caused by talar fractures, 786
Osteopathia striata, clinical features of, 368
radiographic features of, 368, *368*
Osteopetrosis, clinical features of, 366
definition of, 365
pathologic findings in, 367
prognosis for, 367
radiographic features of, 366, *366*
vs. heavy-metal poisoning, 1070
Osteophyte(s), formation of, in dancers, 1635, *1635,*
1636, 1648
growth of, in hallux valgus, 555–557, *557*
Osteopoikilosis, clinical features of, 367
pathologic findings in, 368
radiographic features of, 367, *367*
Osteoporosis, as residual of ankle injury, 787
bone marrow hyperplasia and, in sickle cell disease,
1098
definition of, 1064
diagnosis of, 1065
etiology of, 1064
fractures in, 1065
in rickets, 1066, *1066*
in scurvy, 1069, *1069*
of foot and ankle, frequent occurrence of, 1064
pathologic view of, 1065, *1065*
spotty, roentgenographic features of, *1291*
Sudeck's post-traumatic, 787
surgical problems in, 1065
transient painful, 1290–1292, *1291*
alternate terminology for, 1290
clinical aspects of, 1290–1292, *1291*
diagnosis of, differential, 1292

Osteoporosis (*Continued*)
transient painful, roentgenographic features of, 1291,
1291
treatment of, 1292
vs. reflex sympathetic dystrophy syndrome, 1291
treatment of, 1065
Osteosarcoma(s), 1000–1003, *1002, 1003*
extraskeletal, 1000, *1003*
in Paget's disease, 1000, *1003*
of calcaneus, following Paget's disease, *1082,* 1083
vs. osteoblastoma, *1002*
Osteosclerosis, osteomalacia and, 1073, *1073*
Osteotomy(ies), Cole's, 1164, *1164, 1165*
diaphyseal, in first ray insufficiency syndrome,
698–700, *699*
dorsal, in cavus deformity, 480–482, *481*
Dwyer's, 1167, *1167*
extracapsular, of first metatarsal, in hallux valgus,
566–569, *567, 568*
in cavus deformity, techniques, 1163–1167, *1163–1167*
in metatarsus primus varus, 693
in osteomalacia, 1068
in pes planus, *510,* 511–515, *512, 513*
in subtalar complex, 758
Japas', 1165
McElvenny and Caldwell's, 1165, *1166*
of calcaneus, in cavus deformity, 482, *482*
in clubfoot, 244
of metatarsal(s), 424
as cause of first ray insufficiency syndrome, 686
base of, in clubfoot, 243
in first ray overload syndrome, 681, *682*
central, 698–700, *699*
first, malunion following surgery for hallux valgus,
606, 607
nonunion following surgery for hallux valgus, 605,
605
nonunion following, 172, *173*
postoperative care, 170
of tibia, rotational, 425
opening wedge, contraindications for, 152
supramalleolar, in surgical management of non-
plantigrade foot, 190–192, *191*
technique of, 811
tarsal, 424
Japas technique, 480, *481*
Overlapping toes. See *Toes, overlapping.*

Pacini corpuscles, visualization of, 176, *176*
Padding and devices, for relief of foot pain, 1703–1732.
See also *Arch supports; Foot, pain in; Footwear;
Orthosis(es); Orthotics;* and *Shoes, and shoe
modifications.*
Paget's disease, of bone, 1078–1083, *1078–1082.*
active and inactive phases in, 1080
affecting tibia, *1078,* 1079–1081, *1079–1081*
vs. other bones, 1081
age of onset, 1078
diagnosis of, 1081, *1081*
osteolytic changes, 1081, *1081*
progressive nature of, 1081
etiology of, 1079
evaluation of, 1081
alkaline phosphatase tests, 1081
bone scans, 1081
pain as presenting symptom, 1081

Paget's disease (*Continued*)
　of bone, evaluation of, stress factors, 1082
　　　weight-bearing, 1082
　　malignancy following, *1082*, 1083
　　morphologic changes in, *1078, 1079, 1079*
　　osteosarcoma and, 1000, *1003, 1082*, 1083
　　temporal sequence of site involvement in, 1080,
　　　1080
　　treatment of, 1082
　　varying pathologic changes in, 1080, *1080*
　　varying sites for, 1078
　　vs. other metabolic disorders, 1078
Pain, absence of. See *Insensitive foot.*
　chronic, psychiatric aspects, 1430–1437, *1434, 1437.*
　　See also *Psychiatric aspects.*
　forms of, in peripheral neuropathies, 1206
　from "failed" foot, differential diagnosis of, 1295
　in foot infections, absence vs. presence of, 1398
　in heel, 1200
　　treatment of, 1405
　indifference to, congenital, in hereditary sensory
　　neuropathies, 1227
　intractable, from "failed" foot, neurosurgical salvage
　　of, 1295–1300, *1296, 1297, 1300.* See also *"Failed"*
　　foot.
　relief of, padding and devices for, 1703–1732. See also
　　Arch supports; Foot, pain in; Footwear;
　　Orthosis(es); Orthotics; and *Shoes, and shoe*
　　modifications.
Painful heel syndrome, 1200
Palsy, cerebral, cavus deformity and, 470
　clinical assessment of, 284
　definitions of, 282–284
　　ataxia, 283
　　athetosis, 283
　　deformity, mild, 283
　　　moderate, 283
　　　severe, 283
　　spasticity, 283
　EMG findings in, 78
　equinovalgus deformity and, 198
　equinovarus deformity and, treatment of, surgical,
　　189, *189*
　etiology of, 284
　flatfoot and, 198
　foot and ankle deformities in, 282–334
　foot position in, over- or undercorrection of,
　　293
　gait analysis in, 57, 63, 78
　hallux valgus and, 322–332, *324–328, 331.* See also
　　Hallux valgus.
　involving lower extremities, case reports, 293–322
　　specific problems in, 293–322
　　　spastic diplegia, 295–301, *295–297, 299, 300,*
　　　　318–322, 319–321
　　　spastic hemiparesis, 293–295, 310–313
　　　spastic hemiplegia, 313–315, 316–318, *316–318*
　　　tetraparesis, 301–310, *301–304, 306, 307,* 315
　pes planus and, treatment of, surgical, 514
　spastic, neurophysiologic aspects of, 285. See also
　　Spasticity.
　spasticity and athetosis in, hallux valgus and, case
　　report, 330–332, *331*
　treatment goals, 285
　muscle testing in, 287–293. See also *Muscles, testing*
　　of.
　peroneal, treatment of, *1189–1191,* 1192, *1195*

PAM (procaine penicillin in aluminum monostearate),
　for yaws, 1427
Papules, piezogenic, 833, *833,* 905, *905*
Parakeratin, 828
　neurologic patterns of, 251–253, *252, 253*
　　asymmetric, 251
　　normal, 251
　　paraparesis, spastic, 251
　　paraplegia, flaccid, complete, 251
　　　incomplete, 251, *252, 253*
　　　mixed, complete, 251
　　　spastic, complete, 251
Paraparesis, spastic, 251
　progressive, 256
Paraplegia, as hysterical motor disorder, 1441. See also
　　Psychiatric aspects.
　flaccid, complete, 251
　　incomplete, 251, *252, 253*
　mixed, complete, 251
　spastic, complete, 251
Parasitic infestations, affecting foot, 1420, *1420*
Paratendinitis, vs. peritendinitis, 854
Paratenosynovitis, 854
Parathyroid hormone, disorders of, 1072, *1072.* See also
　　Metabolic disorders, of bone.
　renal resistance to, in osteomalacia, 1073, *1073*
Paraungual lesions, treatment of, 636, 651, *651, 652.*
　See also *Toenails.*
Paraxial fibular hemimelia, 220–226, *221, 224.* See also
　　Fibula, longitudinal deficiency of.
　clinical features of, 245
　treatment of, 245
Paraxial tibial hemimelia, clinical features of, 246
　treatment of, 246
Paresthesias, hysterical, 1443. See also *Psychiatric*
　　aspects.
Paronychia, monilial, in diabetes mellitus, affecting skin
　　of foot, 876, 877
　of hallux, treatment of, 1405
Paronychium, anatomy of, 919
Parosteal osteogenic sarcoma, vs. myositis ossificans,
　　846, *847*
Pars peronaea metatarsalis primi, location of, *123,* 124
Passive movement, assessment of, 540, *542*
Patella, congenital absence of, congenital vertical talus
　　and, 444
　longitudinal deficiency of fibula and, 222
Pathomechanics, of foot deformities, 381–392, *384, 385,*
　　387–392. See also *Talipes, inverted.*
　of metatarsals, 673–702. See also *Metatarsalgia.*
Patient evaluation, preoperative importance of, 149
Pediatrician, role of, in identifying foot disorders,
　　195–199, *197.* See also *Children.*
Pellagra, as nutritional neuropathy, 1240
Pelvis, obliquity of, gait analysis and, *60*
　rotation of, deformities of, 429
　　gait analysis and, *62*
　tilt of, gait analysis and, *60*
Periarteritis nodosa, peripheral neuropathies and, 1226
Periarticular alterations, basic literature on, guide to,
　　1850
Perionychium, anatomy of, 919
Periostitis, calcaneal, in geriatrics, 975
　gummatous, 1418
　in first ray insufficiency syndrome, 687, 690
　of metacarpals, in yaws, *1422*
　psoriatic, of medial cuneiform, 718, *718*

Periostitis (*Continued*)
  traction, 842
Peripheral nerves, injury to, electrodiagnosis in, 75
  surgical decompression of, electromyography
    following, 76
Peripheral neuropathies, affecting foot, 1169–1204. See
    also *Nerves, disorders of* and *Neuropathies,
    peripheral.*
  miscellaneous, and neuropathy-like syndromes,
    1205–1247. See also *Nerves, disorders of* and
    Neuropathies, peripheral.
Peritalar dislocations, 1467–1472, *1468–1471.* See also
    Dislocations, of subtalar joint.
Peritalar joint. See *Talocalcaneonavicular joint.*
Peritendinitis, vs. paratendinitis, 854
Periungual corn, 936. See also *Toenails.*
Periungual lesions, 911, *911, 912.* See also *Toenails.*
Pernicious anemia, clinical features and treatment of,
    1240
Peroneal. See also entries under *Fibula* and *Fibular.*
Peroneal artery, surgical bypass of, *1338,* 1339, *1339,
    1340*
Peroneal constriction, with calcaneal fracture, 861
Peroneal muscular atrophy, 1231–1236, *1234–1236.* See
    also *Charcot-Marie-Tooth disease.*
Peroneal nerve, common, anatomy of, 1172, *1172*
  deep, anatomy of, 1173, *1174*
  entrapment neuropathies in, 1195–1197
  injury to, following ankle injury, 788
    physical examination for, 114
  superficial, anatomy of, 1173, *1174*
  trauma to, treatment of, surgical, 1183, *1185–1187,
    1189–1191*
Peroneal palsy, treatment of, *1189–1191,* 1192, *1195*
Peroneal spastic flatfoot, 740, 741–744, *741–744.* See
    also *Spastic flatfoot, peroneal* and *Tarsal coalition.*
Peroneal tendon(s), bursitis of, physical examination for,
    105, *106*
  slipping, treatment of, surgical, 806
  tendinitis of, physical examination for, 105, *106*
  transfer of, in poliomyelitis, 1143–1146, *1143–1147*
Peroneal tubercle, enlargement of, physical examination
    for, 105, *106*
Peronei, testing of, in poliomyelitis, 1130, *1131*
Peroneus brevis, deforming effects of, management of, 289
  flaps of, for skin grafts, 953
  pseudotumor of, 859
  tendinitis of, in dancers, 1645–1648, *1646, 1647*
  testing of, 289
Peroneus longus, deforming effects of, management of,
    289
  tendinitis of, in dancers, 1645–1648, *1646, 1647*
  tenosynovitis of, in geriatrics, 973
  testing of, 289
  transfer of, to Achilles tendon, for triceps surae
    paralysis, 1151, *1151, 1152*
Peroneus tertius, testing of, in poliomyelitis, 1131, *1131*
"Persian slipper" foot, in congenital vertical talus, 441,
    441
Pes cavus, 463–485. See also *Cavus deformity.*
Pes planus, 486–520. See also *Flatfoot* and *Valgus
    deformity.*
  basic literature on, guide to, 1853
  biomechanical considerations, 489–496, *489–495.* See
    also *Pes planus, pathology of, biomechanics.*
  axial relationships, 489, *490*
  extrinsic articulations, *492–494,* 493

Pes planus (*Continued*)
  biomechanical considerations, extrinsic articulations,
    calcaneo-contact, *492, 493*
  plantar aponeurosis, *493, 493, 494*
  foot functions, 494–496, *494, 495*
  intrinsic articulations, 489–493, *489–492*
    linkage, 489
    subtalar "stool" structure, 490, *492*
    types of stability, 490–492, *491*
  definition of, 486
  diagnostic difficulties in, 486–489, *487, 488*
  examination of, clinical, 501–504, *502, 504*
    abnormal joint laxity, 503
    Achilles tendon length, 503
    appearance, 502
    calcaneal angle, 503
    hallux extension test, 502, *502*
    history, 502
    intrinsic imbalance, 503
    line of great toenail, 503
    patellar line, 502
    range of motion, 503
    shoe wear, 503
    sole skin thickening, 503
    special tests, 503, *504*
  hallux valgus and, 518, *518*
  hypermobile, 497, *497,* 499, *500*
    radiographic view of, 733, *733*
    treatment of, nonsurgical, footwear, *750*
  joint axes in, 728
  metatarsals in, relative length of, 500, *500*
  midtarsal range of motion in, 733, *733*
  paralytic, treatment of, surgical, in poliomyelitis, 1136
  pathology of, 496–501, *496, 497, 499–501, 504, 513*
    biomechanics, 496, *496, 504, 513.* See also *Pes
      planus, biomechanical considerations.*
    unbalanced metastable foot, 496, *496*
    unbalanced stable foot, 496
    morbid anatomy and etiology, 497–501, *497,
      499–501*
    unbalanced metastable foot, 497–499, *497, 499,
      500*
    unbalanced stable foot, 499–501, *500, 501*
  radiologic examination of, 504, *504, 505*
  role of tibialis anterior in, 728, *729*
  terminology for, 486, 519
  treatment of, 505–518, *506–510, 512, 513, 515–518*
    unbalanced, metastable, hypermobile
        hyperpronated foot, 505–515, *506–510,
        512, 513*
      neonatal, 505
      surgical, 509–515, *510, 512, 513*
        additional steps in cerebral palsy, 514
        bones, *510,* 511–515, *512, 513*
        joints, *510,* 511–515, *512, 513*
        myelomeningocele, 515
        rarity of, 509
        tendons, *510,* 511–515, *512, 513*
        variety of, 510, *510*
      weight bearing, 505–509, *506–509*
        footprint changes, 509, *509*
        line of force application, 505, *506, 507*
        orthoses, 506, *506, 507*
        pronatometer, 506, *507*
        shoe inserts, 508, *508*
    unbalanced stable foot, 515–518, *515–517*
      monitored posture changes, 515, *515*

Pes planus (*Continued*)
  treatment of, unbalanced stable foot, results, *516, 517, 517*
    shoe inserts, 515–518, *515–517*
  variations of, in children, 196
Pes valgus. See *Flatfoot* and *Valgus deformity.*
Petechiae, calcaneal, 890, *890*
Phalanges, absence of, 245
  anatomy of, 12, *14*
  fractures of, as cause of hallux rigidus, 608, *609, 610*
    in children, 1680
Phenol, injection of, for equinus deformity, 1118, *1120*
Phlebitis, saphenous, progressive, venous thrombosis in, 1352
Phlegmasia cerulea dolens, treatment of, surgical, 1358, *1358*
  venous gangrene following, *1358*
Phosphorus poisoning, 1070, *1071*
Photography, of foot, 99–102, 264, *264.*
  clinical, 99
  for publication, 102
  general optical principles, 100
  in office, 101
  in operating room, 100
  x-ray and copy work, 101
Photomicroscopy, 102
Physician-patient relationships, psychiatric aspects, 1431–1433
Pierre Robin syndrome, clubfoot in, *239*
  radiographic view, *239*
Piezogenic papules, 833, *833,* 905, *905*
Pigeon toe, in children, variations of, 196, 198
Pillow splint, as emergency treatment for ankle fractures, 1550, *1551*
Pilon fractures, of distal tibia, 1561, *1561*
Pitted keratolysis, of soles, clinical features and treatment of, 889, *890*
Plantar aponeurosis. See *Fascia, plantar.*
Plantar fascia. See *Fascia, plantar.*
Plantar fasciitis. See *Fasciitis, plantar.*
Plantar flexion. See *Flexion, plantar.*
Plantar interdigital neuroma, 702–707, *704, 705, 707.*
  See also *Morton's disease.*
Plantar ligaments, *14, 15, 464, 465*
Plantar muscles, testing of, 292
Plantigrade foot, functions of, 175
  metatarsals and, 177–183, *177–185, 188, 191*
  mobilization vs. immobilization, 183
  proprioception in, 176, *176*
  surgical achievement of, 175–193, *176–192*
  surgical principles and, 144–194. See also *Surgical principles.*
  toes and, 177
Plastic surgery, 939–963
  contaminated or infected wounds and, diagnosis of, 940
    management, 940–942
      enzymatic agents, 941
      sugar derivatives, 941
      wet-to-dry dressings, 941
  incisions and, 942–944, *942, 943*
    danger areas, 942, *942*
    dorsum, 943, *943*
    posterior aspect, *942, 943, 943*
    sole, *942, 943*
  skin grafting and, 944–962, *946, 951, 957.* See also *Skin grafts.*

Plastic surgery (*Continued*)
  soft-tissue coverage and, general principles, 939
Podoscope, *1274*
Poisoning, arsenical, in keratoses of soles, *903, 904*
  heavy-metal, 1069–1071, *1070, 1071*
    affecting leg and foot bones, 1069
    bismuth, 1070, *1070*
    lead, 1070, *1070*
    phosphorus, 1070, *1071*
    vs. hypervitaminosis D, 1070
    vs. marble bone disease, 1070
    vs. osteopetrosis, 1070
  lead, 73, 1070, *1070*
Poliomyelitis, and foot, 84, *84,* 1123–1168
  examination of, 1125–1133, *1128–1132*
    clinical, 1125–1133, *1128–1132*
    deformities, classification of, 1132
    degree of manual correction of, 1133
    electromuscular, 1125
    gait, 1126
    general inspection, 1126
    gross visible deformities, 1126
      muscle testing, 1127–1132, *1128–1132*
        extensor digitorum longus, 1131, *1132*
        extensor hallucis longus, *1130,* 1131, *1131*
        flexor digitorum longus, 1131, *1132*
        flexor hallucis longus, 1131, *1132*
        hamstrings, *1128,* 1129
        peronei, 1130, *1131*
        peroneus tertius, 1131, *1131*
        power rating, 1127
        quadriceps, 1128, *1128*
        tibialis anterior, 1130, *1130*
        tibialis posterior, 1129, *1129*
        triceps surae, 1129, *1129*
      radiographic studies, 1133
      standing, 1126
      walking aids, 1126
    galvanofaradic, 1125
  metatarsal displacement in, 178, *179, 180*
  residual, general rules for surgery, 1138
  treatment of, 1133–1167
    hot packs, 1134
    initial stage, 1133
    leg muscles affecting foot, 1134
    nonsurgical, 1133–1135
    prevention of deformities, 1135
    recovery stage, 1135
    spasmodic stage, 1133
    surgical, 1135–1167
      adduction of forefoot without inversion, 1137
      calcaneus and cavus deformity, 1137
      calcaneus deformity, 1137
      cavus deformity with normal long muscles, 1137
      claw toes, 1137
      equinus, 1135
      equinus from lack of power in muscles, 1136
      eversion and paralytic pes planus, 1136
      general rules, 1138
      inversion caused by peroneal palsy, 1137
      lack of dorsiflexion power, 1137
      paralysis resulting in flatfoot only, 1136
      shortness of foot, 1138
      techniques, 1139–1167, *1141, 1143–1152, 1154, 1156–1158, 1160, 1161, 1163–1167*
        alternative, 1162–1167, *1163–1167*

Poliomyelitis (*Continued*)
  and foot, treatment of, surgical, techniques,
        contracture of plantar fascia, 1162
       correction of knee deformities, 1152–1162,
         1154, 1156–1158, 1160, 1161
         back knee, 1153, *1154*
         flexion contracture, 1153–1155
         genu recurvatum, 1153, *1154*
         genu valgum and varum, 1161
         hamstrings transfer, 1155–1161,
           1156–1158, 1160, 1161
         hyperextension, 1153, *1154*
       flexion contracture of hip, 1162
       foot stabilization, 1139–1142, *1141*
        bone blocks, 1142
        calcaneus deformity, 1142
        cuneiform resections, 1140
        eversion or inversion of calcaneus, 1142
        first metatarsal segment, 1141, *1141*
       osteotomies for cavus deformity, 1163–1167,
        1163–1167
       transfer of leg muscles, 1142–1152,
        1143–1152
        peroneal tendon, 1143–1146, *1143–1147*
        peroneus longus to Achilles for triceps
          surae paralysis, 1151, *1151, 1152*
        tibialis anterior, 1146–1149, *1148, 1149*
        tibialis posterior, 1149–1151, *1149, 1150*
  ankle and foot deformities in, 793
  astragalectomy for, 757, *757*
  bodily distribution of, 1123
  calcaneal deformity in, 1137, 1142
  cavus deformity in, 84, *84*, 468, 639, 1137,
    1163–1167, *1163–1167*
  claw toes in, treatment of, surgical, 1137
  definition of, 1123
  diagnosis of, 1124
    differential, 1124
  electromyography in, 64
  equinus deformity in, 1135
  gait analysis in, 64
  hammer toe in, 639
  high longitudinal arch in, 91
  in ankle, rarity of osteoarthritis in conjunction with,
    794
  in children vs. adults, 793
  incidence of, 1123
  metatarsal displacement in, 178, *179, 180*
  muscles affected by, 1125
  pathology of, 1124
  phases of, 1124
  pes planus in, paralytic, 1136
  residuals of, and resulting proneness to fracture, 794
    present-day, 793
  surgical considerations in, 151, *151*
  triple arthrodesis in, 188, *188*
  viral origin of, 1123
Polyarteritis, peripheral neuropathies and, 1226
Polyarteritis nodosa, mononeuritis multiplex and, 1225
  vs. rheumatoid arthritis, 1224
Polydactyly, associated deformities and, 216
  axial and post-axial, radiographic view, *235*
  clinical features of, 244
  congenital, 216–218, *217*
  definition of, 216. *217*
  hereditary nature of, 216
  preaxial, hallux varus and, 617, *617*

Polydactyly (*Continued*)
  treatment of, surgical, 217, 244
    optimal age for, 217
    techniques, 217
Polymyositis, peripheral neuropathies and, 1226
Polyneuritis, hypertrophic, progressive, 1238
  peripheral, 1215–1217
    as part of wider CNS involvement, 1216
    definition of, 1215
    distribution of, 1215
    examination for, 1215
    motor vs. sensory involvement, 1216
    varying characteristics of, 1216
Polyneuropathy, diabetic, 1217
  sympathetic denervation in, 1218
Polysyndactyly, radiographic view, *236*
Pompholyx, affecting feet, 894. See also *Dyshidrosis.*
Popliteal aneurysm(s), resulting in acute arterial
    thrombosis, *1316, 1317, 1317*
  shower of microemboli from, *1314,* 1315
Popliteal artery, surgical bypass of, 1337–1339, *1337,
    1339*
Popliteal thrombosis, acute, 1318
Porphyria, acute synovitis of ankle and, 844, 845
Posterior tibial muscle. See *Tibialis posterior.*
Posterior tibial nerve. See *Tibial nerve, posterior.*
Posterior tibial syndrome, in distance runners and
    joggers, 1603
Posteromedial release, Turco, in treatment of clubfoot,
    242
Postoperative care, principles of, 169
Postoperative complications, early, 171, *172*
  late, 172–174, *173, 174*
Postoperative dressings, 168
Post-traumatic arthritis, as indication for arthroscopy,
    142, *142*
Posture changes, monitoring of, 515, *515*
Power motor injuries, in children, 1683
Prednisone, in rheumatoid arthritis, as contraindication
    for total ankle arthroplasty, 824, 825, *825*
Pregnancy, abnormal, constriction band syndrome and,
    228
Prescription footwear, terminology of, 1867–1871
Pressure, center of, line of, 48, *49*
Pressure and shear stress, evaluation of, in insensitive
    foot, 1284, *1284, 1285*
Pressure necrosis, in insensitive foot, *1268, 1269, 1269*
Pressure prints, in equinovarus vs. normal foot, 265,
    266
Pressure sores, in calcaneus deformity, 276, *276*
  in equinovarus deformity, 271,. *271*
  management of, 269
Primary muscle disease, motor units in, 70
Primates, living, feet of, plantar view, *7*
  phylogenetic tree of, *3*
Probenecid, in treatment of chronic gouty arthritis and
    tophaceous gout, 1020
Procaine penicillin in aluminum monostearate (PAM),
    for yaws, 1427
Profunda femoris, surgical reconstruction of, 1332–1336,
    1333–1336. See also *Vascular reconstruction.*
Pronated foot, basic literature on, guide to, 1863
Pronation, definition of, 125
  footwear for, 1781
Pronatometer, principles of, in pes planus, 506, *507*
Propranolol, for reflex sympathetic dystrophy syndrome,
    1290

Proprioceptive system, peripheral neuropathies and, 1206–1208
Prostaglandins, possible role of in thermal burn injuries, 1691
Prosthesis(es). See also *Prosthetics*.
    for ankle, design of, 816, *817*
        varying success rates, 814
    LaTorre, 1394, *1395*
Prosthetic and orthotic management, of foot disorders, 1783–1826. See also *Orthosis(es)*, *Orthotics*, and *Prosthesis(es)*.
Prosthetics, 1812–1819. See also *Amputation(s)* and *Prosthesis(es)*.
    care of children and, 1821, *1823, 1824*
    components and systems, partial tarsal amputations, 1815, *1817*
        toe amputations, 1815
        total foot amputation, 1816–1819, *1818, 1819*
        transmetatarsal amputations, 1815, *1816*
    current ratio of lower-limb amputations, 1813
    development of ankle-foot prescriptions, 1814
    functional electrical stimulation, 1819, *1820*
    materials used in ankle-foot prostheses, 1814
    recent developments in, 1812
    terminology of, 1813
Pruritus, in atopic dermatitis, 872, *872*
    in diabetes mellitus, affecting foot, 878
Pseudarthrosis, following arthrodesis, 172
Pseudochromidrosis plantaris, 890, *890.*
Pseudogout. See also *Gout*.
    characteristics of, 1022, *1022*
    histologic view of, *1022*
    pathogenesis of, 1023
    treatment of, 1023
    vs. gout, 1022
    vs. uric acid gout, 1023
Pseudohypoparathyroidism, *1072*, 1073
Pseudolipoma, in tendons, 857
Pseudotumors, in hemophilia, 1088, 1090–1093, *1091–1093*
    intraosseous hemorrhage as cause of, *1092*, 1093
    of tendons, *859*, 866
    treatment of, *1092*, 1093
Psoriasis, affecting foot, 84
    as cause of peroneal spastic flatfoot, 743, *743*
    clinical features of, 883, *883–885*
    diagnosis of, 885
        differential, 883–885
    hyperkeratotic, on soles, 883, *885*
    of foot vs. other locations, 883
    osseous and articular forms of, *718*, 723
    pustular, 883
    small toe involvement in, 656, *656*
    tendon rupture in, 864, *864*
    treatment of, 885
    vs. discoid lupus erythematosus, 873, *873*
    vs. rheumatoid arthritis, 885
    "white," 883
Psoriatic arthritis, 1059–1061, *1059–1061*. See also *Arthritis, psoriatic*.
Psychiatric aspects, 1429–1448
    causalgia, definition and etiology of, 1445
        major, 1445
            clinical features of, 1445
            treatment of, 1446
        minor, 1446
            clinical features of, 1446

Psychiatric aspects (*Continued*)
    causalgia, minor, treatment of, 1446
    chronic pain patient, 1430–1437, *1434, 1437*
        body image, 1433, *1434*
        cognitive factors, 1430
        description of, 1430
        emotional factors, 1431
        interpersonal factors, 1431
        physician-patient relationship, 1431–1433
        psychiatric consultation, 1433
        psychiatric treatment, 1434–1437, *1437*
            behavioral analysis, 1435
            case report, 1436, *1437*
            range of, 1435
            role of family, 1435
            self-"diagnosis," 1430
    conversion reactions, 1438–1444, *1442–1444*. See also *Psychiatric aspects, hysterical neurosis*.
    foot and shoe psychology, 1446
        fetishism, 1447
        foot binding, 1446
        symbolism, 1446
    functional foot disorders, 1429
        diagnosis of, 1430
        hysterical symptoms of, 1430
    hypochondriacal patient, 1437
        definition of, 1437
        recognition of, 1438
        vs. hysterical patient, 1438
    hysterical neurosis, conversion type, 1438–1444, *1442–1444*
        current theories and findings, 1440
        definition of, 1439
            Briquet's hysteria, 1439
            conversion reaction or hysteria, 1439
            hysterical personality, 1440
        history, 1438
        motor disorders, 1441–1443, *1442, 1443*
            case report, 1442, *1443*
            clinical features of, 1441
            Hoover test, 1441, *1442*
            testing for, 1441, *1442*
        predominance in females, 1440
        sensory disorders, 1443, *1444*
            clinical features of, 1443, *1444*
            location of, 1443
    malingering, 1445
    reflex sympathetic dystrophies, 1445
    self-inflicted injuries, 1444, *1445*
        dermatitis artefacta, 1444
        factitial dermatitis, 1444
        in Lesch-Nyhan syndrome, 1445
        in narcotics addicts, 1445
        in Riley-Day syndrome, 1444
        malingering, 1445
        neurotic excoriation, 1444, *1445*
Psychology, of foot and shoe, 1446. See also *Psychiatric aspects*.
Pulp space, infection of, treatment of, 1406
Puncture wounds, of foot, in children, 1682
    of sole, 1612, *1612*. See also *Industrial injuries*.
    treatment of, 1402
Purulent infection, 1405. See also *Infections, of foot*.
Pus, subungual, 1210, *1210*
Pyarthrosis, of Lisfranc's joint, 721, *721*
Pyoderma gangrenosum, treatment of, alternatives to amputation, 1365, *1365*

Pyogenic infections, 1399, 1419, *1419*. See also *Infections, of foot.*
Pyrophosphate arthropathy, 1022, *1022*. See also *Pseudogout.*

Quadriceps, testing of, in poliomyelitis, 1128, *1128*
Quigley traction, modified, for ankle fractures, 1552, *1552*

Radiation burns, 1701, *1701*. See also *Burns.*
Radiculopathy, definition of, 77
  electrodiagnosis in, 77
Radiography, in detection of rotational deformities, *396*, 399, 401–403, *401, 402*
  intraoperative, 170
  postoperative, 170, *171*
  preoperative, 170, *170, 171*
Ram's horn deformity. See *Onychogryphosis.*
Range of motion, in ankle joint, 40, *40*, 43, *44, 45*
  in subtalar joint, 40, *41*, 43, *44*
  in transverse tarsal joint, 42, *42*
Ray(s). See *First ray insufficiency syndrome* and *First ray overload syndrome.*
  excision of, in hammer toe treatment, disadvantages of, 645
Raynaud's disease, vs. Raynaud's phenomenon, 1349
Raynaud's phenomenon, 1349–1351
  clinical features of, 1349
  definition of, 1349
  diagnosis of, differential, 1350
  in association with other collagen diseases, 1350
  predominance in females, 1350
  systemic scleroderma and, affecting foot, 875, 876
  treatment of, 1350
  vs. Raynaud's disease, 1349
Reflex sympathetic dystrophy syndrome, 1287–1290, *1288*, 1445. See also *Psychiatric aspects.*
  alternate terminology for, 1287
  clinical aspects of, 1287–1289, *1288*
  diagnosis of, differential, 1289
  following injuries, 1288, *1288*
  roentgenographic features of, *1288*, 1289
  treatment of, 1289
    nonsurgical, 1290
    surgical, 1290
  vs. transient painful osteoporosis, 1291
Reflexes, testing of, in neurologic examination of foot, 1109
Refsum's disease, hereditary sensory neuropathies and, 1227
Reiter's syndrome, 1057–1059, *1057, 1058*
  characteristics and etiology of, 1057
  clinical features of, 1057, *1057*
  involving heel, 774
  radiographic view of, 1057, *1057, 1058*
  treatment of, nonsurgical, 1057
Relapse, of corrected inverted talipes, pathomechanics of, 383
Renal failure, associated with peripheral neuropathy, 1238
  clinical types of, 1238
  diagnosis of, 1239
  treatment of, surgical vs. nonsurgical, 1239

Renal osteodystrophy, 1075–1078, *1075–1077*. See also *Osteodystrophy, renal.*
Reperfusion syndrome, clinical features of, 1323
  following traumatic vascular injuries, 1323
  treatment of, compartmental decompression, 1324
    fasciotomy, 1324
Replantation, of foot, 1358–1364, *1360, 1362, 1364, 1365*. See also *Amputation.*
  basic principles, 1363
  case reports, 1359–1363, *1360, 1362*
  history of, 1358
  near-total amputation, 1364
  surgical considerations, 1359–1363, *1360, 1362*
  theoretical considerations, 1359
  vs. amputation, 1364, *1364, 1365*
Resection arthroplasty, 1043–1045
Resorption dysplasias. See *Bone dysplasias.*
Retentive treatment, 426
Reticulosarcoma(s), of bone, 1008, *1008*
  vs. Ewing's sarcoma, 1009
Retinacula, anatomy of, flexor, 17, *19*
  inferior extensor, 17, *18–20*
  peroneal, 17
  superior extensor, 17, *18, 20*
Rhabdomyosarcoma(s), 988
Rheumatoid arthritis, 84, 1024–1057, *1025–1032, 1036, 1039–1048, 1050, 1053, 1054, 1056*
  as cause of peroneal spastic flatfoot, 742
  biplanar forefeet splaying in, *550*
  bony ankylosis in, *1027*, 1031
  claw toes in, *1025, 1026, 1028, 1029*
  diabetic Charcot ankle in, *1215*
  diagnosis of, 99
  footwear for, 1760, *1776, 1781*
  hammer toe in, 94, *1025, 1026, 1028, 1029*
  heel involvement in, sero-positive, 774
  inflammatory bursae in, 853, *853*
  joint involvement in, different clinical types of, bony ankylosis, 1027, *1027*
    loose *1026*, 1027
    stiff, *1025*, 1027
  juvenile, 1054–1057, *1056*
    clinical features of, 1055, *1056*
    treatment of, 1055, *1056*
  level excision of metatarsal heads and necks in, 185, *185, 186*
  metatarsals in, 713
  mononeuritis multiplex and, 1225
  of ankle, 1046–1055, *1047, 1048, 1050, 1053, 1054*
    incidence of, 1046
    radiologic changes vs. clinical function, *1047, 1048*, 1049
    treatment of, 1049–1055, *1050, 1053, 1054*
      nonsurgical, 1049
      surgical, 1049–1055, *1050, 1053, 1054*
        arthrodesis, *1050*, 1051
        pantalar arthrodesis, 1051
        synovectomy of ankle joint, 1049–1051
        talectomy, 1052
        total replacement arthroplasty, 1052–1055, *1053, 1054*
          contraindications for, 824, 825, *825*, 1052
          incidence of, 1052
          indications for 1052
          postoperative results, 1052
          vs. arthrodesis, 1055

Rheumatoid arthritis (*Continued*)
  of foot, 1024–1046, *1025–1032, 1036, 1039–1046*
    clinical features of, *1025–1031,* 1027–1031
      bursitis and nodules, 1031
      classification of areas involved, 1027
      claw toes, *1025, 1026,* 1028, *1029*
      forefoot splaying, *1026,* 1028
      hallux valgus, *1026,* 1029, *1029*
      hammer toes, *1025, 1026,* 1028, *1029*
      swan-neck toe deformity, 1028, *1029*
      synovitis of metatarsophalangeal joints, *1025,* 1027, *1028*
      tarsal joint involvement, *1027,* 1029–1031, *1030*
      tenosynovitis, 1031, *1031*
    incidence of, 1024
    treatment of, nonsurgical, 1032, *1032*
      surgical, 1033–1046, *1036, 1039–1046*
        anesthesia for, 1034
        antibiotics and, 1034
        indications, 1033
        preoperative radiography for, 1034
        priorities with other joints, 1033
        procedures, 1034–1046, *1036, 1039–1046*
          choice of, 815
          classification of, for forefoot bone resection, 1038
          comparison of, 1037
          flexible metatarsalgia, 1036
          forefoot arthroplasty, 1037–1043, *1039–1044, 1050*
            complications of, 1042, *1044, 1045*
            postoperative dressings, 1040, *1040*
            results of, 1040–1042, *1041–1043*
            technique, 1037–1040, *1039*
            with both feet involved, 1037
          forefoot splaying, 1034
          hallux rigidus, 1036
          hallux valgus, fixed, and claw toes, 1036
            isolated, 1036
          isolated toe deformity, 1034–1036, *1036*
            classification, 1035
          midfoot and hindfoot, 1045, *1046*
          Morton's neuroma, 1034
          painful nodule, 1034
          painful synovitis of metatarsophalangeal joints, 1034
          resection arthroplasty, 1043–1045
        purpose of, 1036
  peripheral neuropathy in, 1223–1225, *1225*
    clinical features of, 1224, *1225*
    treatment of, 1226
  shoe modifications for, 1760
  small toe involvement in, 656
  special problems in, neuropathies, 1032
    rheumatoid vasculitis, 1031. *1225*
  tendon rupture in, 864
  typical forefoot in, *178*
  valgus deformity in, *1026, 1029, 1030*
  varus deformity in, *1030,* 1031
  vs. collagen diseases, 1027
  vs. polyarteritis nodosa, 1224
  vs. psoriasis, 885
  with Felty's syndrome and vasculitis, treatment of, 1225
Rheumatoid foot, basic literature on, guide to, 1847
Rheumatoid neuropathies, classification of, 1032

Rheumatoid vasculitis, diagnosis and treatment of, 1031, *1225*
Rhizotomy, dorsal root, for causalgia, 1298
  for crush injuries, 1298
  for diabetic neuropathy, 1298
  for intractably painful "failed" foot, 1295
Ribbing's disease, 369
Rickets, 1065–1067, *1066, 1067.* See also *Hypovitaminosis D.*
  nutritional, epiphyseal changes in, 1066, *1066*
    osteoporosis in, 1066, *1066*
    treatment of, 1066, *1067*
  osteomalacia and, in biliary atresia, 1066, *1066*
  vitamin D-resistant, 1074, *1074*
  vs. osteomalacia, 1067
Rickettsial disease, affecting feet, 886
Riley-Day syndrome, heredity sensory neuropathies and, 1227
  self-inflicted injuries in, 1444
  talar and calcaneal deformity in, *1258*
Rocker-bottom foot, in Lisfranc's joint, 713, *713*
  pathomechanics of 386, *388, 390*
  types of, 406, *406*
Rocky Mountain spotted fever, affecting feet, 886, *887*
Roentgenography, 96–99, 116–138
  enlargement, uses of, 138
  general principles, 96, *96*
  in talipes, 375
  of accessory bones and normal variants, 98
  of ankle, technique of, routine views, 127, *127, 128*
    anteroposterior, 127, *127*
    lateral, 127, *127*
    oblique, 128, *128*
  of foot, technique of, routine views, 125–127, *126*
    dorsoplantar, 125, *126*
    lateral, 125, *126*
    oblique, *126,* 127
  of normal foot and ankle, 116–138
    accessory bones, 123–125, *123, 124*
    alternative techniques, 138
    anteroposterior view, 119–121, *119, 120*
    characteristics, 121, *121, 122*
      anteroposterior view, 121, *121*
      dorsoplantar view, 122, *122*
      lateral view, 121, *122*
    development of, 116–121, *117–120*
      dorsoplantar view, 116, *117*
      lateral views, 117–119, *118*
    motion of, 125
    sesamoid bones, 122, 123, *126, 129*
    technique of, 125–136, *126–135*
      motion views, extension, 132, *132*
        flexion, 132, *132*
        pointe position, 133
        tiptoe, 133, *133*
      special views, 128–130, *128–130*
        sesamoid, 129, *129*
        subtalar joint, *126,* 129, *129, 130*
        toes, 128, *128*
      standing full weight-bearing views, 130–132, *131*
        amputation view, 131
        anterior tangential, 130, *131*
        anteroposterior, *121,* 130
        dorsoplantar, *122,* 130
        lateral, *122,* 130
        posterior tangential 131, *131*

Roentgenography (*Continued*)
  of normal foot and ankle, technique of, stress views,
      133–136, *134, 135*
        anterior transpositional, *135,* 136
        eversion, 135
        extension, *132,* 136
        flexion, 136
        inversion, *134, 135, 135,* 136
        lateral rotation, 133–135, *134*
  special views, 96–98, *97*
Rotation, in prenatal period, 8, *9*
  lateral, definition of, 125
  medial, definition of, 125
Rotational deformities, of lower extremity, detection of,
      radiographic, *396, 399,* 401–403, *401, 402*
  in infants and children, 428–437, *428–430, 434, 435*
    axes of reference, 429, *429, 430*
    habitual problems, 436
    orientation planes, *428*
    treatment of, 433–436, *434, 435*
      femur, 433–435, *434, 435*
      foot, 436
      hip joint, 433
      knee joint, 435
      shoe corrections, 436
      tibia, 435
    types of, 429–433
      ankle joint, 432
      femur, 430
      foot, 432
      knee, 431
      pelvis, 429
      spine, 429
      tibia, 432
Rothmann-Makai syndrome, subcutaneous fat necrosis
      in, 832
Ruffini corpuscles, visualization of, 176, *176*
Ruiz-Mora operation, for contracted overlapping fifth
      toe, 646
Running, changes in walking cycle during, 38, *38*
  footwear for, 1774
  sports injuries in, 1601–1605, *1603.* See also *Sports
      injuries.*
Rupture, of Achilles tendon, 1538–1541, *1539, 1540.*
      See also *Achilles tendon.*
  of heel cord or calf muscles, incomplete, strapping
      for, 1728, *1728, 1729*
  of plantar fascia, in distance runners and joggers, 1604
  of tendons, acute, in sports injuries, 1591. See also
      Sports injuries.

Saber shin, in yaws, 1424, *1424*
Sagittal plane, motion of, in gait analysis, 60, *61*
Salter-Harris classification, of epiphyseal injuries,
      1669–1671, *1669, 1670*
Sandals, deformities from, 1720
Saphenous nerve, anatomy of, 1172
Saphenous vein, surgical complications involving, in
      infrainguinal arterial reconstruction, 1338, 1343
  thrombophlebitis of, 1352
Sarcoidosis, affecting foot, clinical features of, 1418
  radiographic and histological features of, 1418
Sarcoma(s), clear cell, 995
  Ewing's. See *Ewing's sarcoma.*
  in fibrous dysplasia, 362

Sarcoma(s) (*Continued*)
  Kaposi's. See *Kaposi's sarcoma.*
  neurogenic, 993
  parosteal osteogenic, vs. myositis ossificans, 846, *847*
  synovial, 994, *995*
  synovial, vs. soft-tissue calcification, 834, *834*
Scabies, affecting feet, 909, *910*
  contagious nature of, *909,* 910
  diagnosis of, 910
  etiology and usual locations of, 910
  treatment of, 910
Scalding, as cause of irritant contact dermatitis, 891, *893*
Scaphoid. See also *Navicular.*
  tarsal, Köhler's disease of, 200–203, *202, 203.* See also
      Köhler's disease.
Scapulo-peroneal atrophy, characteristics of, 347
  foot deformities in, 347
  treatment of, 347
Scarpa's foot, 384, *384,* 389
Schwannoma(s), 993, *993*
  malignant, 993
Sciatic nerve, trauma to, treatment of, surgical, 1183,
      1184, 1185
Scleroderma, localized, affecting foot, 874, *875*
  peripheral neuropathies and, 1226
  systemic, affecting foot, *875,* 876
Sclerosing dysplasias. See *Bone dysplasias.*
Sclerosis, multiple, peripheral polyneuritis in, 1216
  subchondral, as sign of advanced osteoarthritis, 792,
      792
  tuberous, periungual fibromas in, 912, *912*
Scurvy, 1068, *1069.*
  clinical features of, 1068
  diagnosis of, 1069
  epiphyseal separation in, 1069, *1069*
  osteoporosis in, 1069, *1069*
  treatment of, 1069
Sensation, loss of, testing for, 177
Sensibility, assessment of, 264, *265*
Sensory disorders, hysterical, 1443, *1444.* See also
      Psychiatric aspects.
Sensory function, of foot, spinal nerve roots supplying,
      1295, *1296*
Sensory neuropathy, hereditary, 1226–1231, *1228–1234.*
      See also *Neuropathy(ies)*
Sensory perception, testing of, in neurologic
      examination of foot, 1109
Sensory system, peripheral neuropathies and,
      1206–1208
"Serpentine" foot, 252
  treatment of, *252,* 273
Sesamoid(s), accessory bones and, anatomy of, 13, *14,
      23, 25, 26,* 662, 1459
  anatomic relations of, 613–615, *614*
  anchoring of, "fibrous cerclage" and, in metatarus
      primus varus, 694–697, *694–696*
  biomechanics of, 671, *671*
  chondromalacia of, 553, *554*
  derangement of, 613–616, *614*
    bipartition, 613
    numerical variations, 613
    sesamoidectomy, 615
      postoperative care, 616
      sequelae of and salvage following, 615
  dislocation of, in first ray insufficiency syndrome, 686
  examination of, roentgenographic, *122, 123, 126, 129,
      129*

Sesamoid(s) (*Continued*)
  excision of, rarity of, 162, *163*
  extirpation of, in first ray overload syndrome, 682
  fractures of, in dancers, 1655, *1656.*
    in sports injuries, *1581*, 1585. See also *Sports injuries.*
  growth pattern of, 613
  injuries of, 1459. See also *Sesamoiditis.*
    in dancers, 1655, *1656*
  medial, excision of, as cause of hallux valgus, 852, *852*
    snapping, following surgery for hallux valgus, *603*, 604
  of hallux, anatomy of, 1459
    surgery in, 162, *163*
  osteochondritis of, 210, *210*. See also *Osteochondritis.*
  radiologic view of, in first ray overload syndrome, 679, *680*
  shift of, in hallux valgus, 551–553, *554*
Sesamoidectomy, 615
Sesamoiditis, 1459
  etiology and clinical features of, 1460
  examination for, physical, 113
  in dancers, 83, 1655, *1656*
  occupational, 83, 1655, *1656*
  treatment of, nonsurgical, 1460
    surgical, 1460
  vs. osteochondritis, 83, *83*
Sever's disease, 203, *204*
  age of incidence of, 204
  clinical findings in, 203
  in late childhood, 198
  predominance in boys, 204
  radiologic view, 204, *204*
  treatment of, 204
Shatter fractures, of metatarsals, 1457
Shear, forward-aft, during gait, 47, *49*, 66
    measured by forceplate, 66, *66*
  medial-lateral, during gait, 48, *49*, 66
    measured by forceplate, 66, *66*
Shearing fractures, of talar body, 1484, *1484*, *1485*
Shin, saber, in yaws, 1424, *1424*
Shin splints, in sports injuries, definition of, 1596
  diagnosis and treatment of, 1597
Shingles, affecting feet, 886, *886*
Shoes, and shoe modifications, 1745–1782. See also
    *Arch supports; Foot, pain in, padding and
    devices; Footwear; Orthosis(es); and Orthotics.*
  basic requisites, 1754–1756, *1756*
    avoidance of compression, 1755, *1756*
    "complementing" the foot, 1755
    conformity and attachment, 1754
    fitting, 1754
  correction heels, 1777, *1778*
  correction shoes, 1775–1777, *1775*, *1776*
    for adults, 1775–1777, *1776*
    for children, 1775, *1775*
    for rotational deformities, 436
  faulty footwear, 1761–1764
    chisel last shoe, 1762
    foot dynamics, 1761
    heavy, 1763
    high-heeled shoes, 1762
    negative heel, 1763
    "nonbreathing" materials, 1763
    "nonbreathing" socks, 1764
    platform shoes, 1763
    pointed-toe shoes, 1762

Shoes (*Continued*)
  and shoe modifications, faulty footwear,
    slippery, 1764
    unyielding materials, 1763
  for adults, 1758–1760, *1759*, *1760*
    developmental deformities, bunions, 1759, *1760*
      contracted plantar structures, 1759
      genu valgum and varum, 1759
      leg length discrepancies, 1759
      narrow heel and wide forefoot, 1760
      short first metatarsal and long lesser toes, 1760
      tight heel cords, 1759
    genetic deformities, 1760
    neuropathies, 1760
    position-in-utero deformities, calcaneovalgus feet, 1759
      metatarsus adductus, 1759
      "windblown hips," 1758, *1759*
    rheumatoid arthritis, 1760
    trauma, 1760
  for children, 199, 1756–1758
  general aspects of therapy, 1780–1782
    anesthetic feet, 1781
    bunions, *1760*, *1776*, 1780
    cavus deformity with hammer toes, *1776*, 1781
    diabetes, 1781
    dorsal spurs, 1780
    hallux rigidus, *1779*, 1780
    hallux valgus, *1776*, 1780
    hyposensitive feet, 1781
    longitudinal arch strain, 1780
    metatarsalgia, *1776*, 1781
    narrow heel and wide forefoot, 1781
    neuropathies, 1781
    plantar heel spurs, *1778*, 1781
    pronation, 1781
    rheumatoid arthritis, *1776*, 1780
    smelly feet, 1781
  history, 1745, *1746*
  insole, *1761*, 1779. See also *Arch supports.*
  manufacture, 1746–1754, *1746*, *1747*, *1750*, *1751*, *1753*
    common shoe terminology, 1748
    lasts, 1750–1752, *1750*, *1751*, 1777
    principal parts, 1746–1748, *1746*, *1747*
    process of, 1753
    sizes, 1749
    upper patterns, 1752, *1753*
    welt shoes, Bal and blucher patterns, *1747*, 1748
  materials and linings, 1760, *1761*
  military footwear, 1769–1771, *1770–1773*
  outsole, 1777–1779, *1779*
  safety shoes for industry, 1764–1769, *1765*, *1766*, *1768–1770*. See also *Industrial injuries.*
    conductive shoes, 1767
    electrical hazards shoes, 1767, *1768*
    for women, 1769, *1769*, *1770*
    metatarsal safety, *1766*, 1767
    National Safety Council, 1764
    puncture-resistant soles, 1768, *1768*
    with steel toecaps, 1765–1767, *1765*, *1766*
      compression testing, 1765–1767, *1766*
      impact testing, 1765, *1765*
    Z41 Committee, 1764
  sizing, 1760
  sports footwear, 1771–1775. See also *Sports injuries.*

Shoes (*Continued*)
  and shoe modifications, upper, 1780
    variations of, 1780, *1780*
  dermatitis from, 894, 895. See also *Dermatitis, shoe.*
  design and texture of, for insensitive foot, 1275–1278, *1276–1278*
  inserts for, for unbalanced stable foot, 515–518, *515–517*
    in pes planus, 508, *508*, 515–518, *515–517*
  interrelationships of orthoses and, 1733
  protective. See *Industrial injuries, prevention of* and *protection from;* and *Shoes, and shoe modifications.*
Sickle cell disease, 1095, 1096–1102, *1097–1101*
  clinical presentation of, 1097, *1097*
    age of onset, 1097
    gout, 1097, *1097*
    marrow hyperplasia, 1097, *1098*
    other musculoskeletal manifestations and, *1097,* 1101
    skeletal infarction, 1098–1101, *1098–1101*
      bilateral involvement, 1099
      dactylitis, 1099, *1099, 1100*
      early changes, 1099, *1099*
      late changes, 1099, *1100*
      osteomyelitis and, *1100,* 1101
      sites of, 1098
      treatment of, 1101
  dactylitis in, 1099, *1099, 1100*
  diagnosis of, 1096
  incidence of, 1096
  inheritance of, 1096
  leg ulcers of, 1104, *1105*
  osteomyelitis in, *1100,* 1101–1103, *1104*
    treatment of, 1103
  pathophysiology of, *1095,* 1096
  treatment of, 1101
Sickle trait, incidence and diagnosis of, 1102
  vs. hemoglobin SC disease, 1102
Sickling, in dancers, 1639, *1639, 1640*
Silastic implants, contraindications for, 147, *147*
Silver operation, in hallux valgus, 559, *560*
  modified, 559–561, *561, 586,* 602–605, 607, 618
Sinus, synovial, 845
Sinus tarsi, palpation of, 107, *107*
Sinus tarsi syndrome, heel pain and, in geriatrics, 976
Sinus tracts, examination of, general clinical, 88
Sjögren's syndrome, peripheral neuropathies and, 1226
Skeletal infarction, in sickle cell disease, 1098–1101, *1098–1101.* See also *Sickle cell disease.*
Skew foot, pathomechanics of, 391, *392*
Skiing, footwear for, 1774
  injuries from, classification of, 1573. See also *Sports injuries.*
Skin, 869–913
  composition of, 32
  diseases of, classification according to primary and secondary lesions, 870
    nonsystemic, that may affect feet, 887–910, *888–893, 895, 897–909*
      bacterial infections, 887–890, *888–890*
      black heel, 890, *890*
      contact dermatitis, 891–894, *891–893, 895*
      dyshidrosis, 894
      fissures, 896
      foreign bodies, 897, *897, 898*
      fungal infections, 898–901, *898–900*
      hyperhidrosis, 895

Skin (*Continued*)
  diseases of, nonsystemic, that may affect feet,
      keratolysis exfoliativa, 901, *901*
      keratoses of soles, 901–904, *902–904*
      piezogenic papules, 905, *905*
      scabies, *909,* 910
      shoe dermatitis, 894, 895
      warts, plantar and ordinary, 905–910, *906–908*
    ointments vs. creams vs. lotions, 872
    systemic infectious, that may affect feet, 886, *886, 887*
      differential diagnosis, 886
      hand-foot-and-mouth disease, 886, *887*
      herpes zoster, 886, *886*
      leprosy, 886
      rickettsial disease, 886
      Rocky Mountain spotted fever, 886, *887*
      shingles, 886, *886*
      smallpox, 886
    systemic or generalized, commonly affecting feet, 871–887, *871–887*
      atopic dermatitis, 871–873, *871–873*
      autoimmune diseases, 873–876, *873–875*
      basal cell nevus syndrome, 876, *876*
      diabetes mellitus, 876–878, *877, 878*
      epidermolysis bullosa, 878, *879*
      erythema multiforme, 879, *880*
      granuloma annulare, 880, *881, 882*
      Kaposi's sarcoma, 880–883, *882*
      psoriasis, 883–886, *883–885*
  examination of, general clinical, 88
    neurologic, 1107
    Wood's light, 871
  incisions in, general principles of, 157, *163*
  lesions of, 828–832, *829–832*
    basic literature on, guide to, 1865
    differential diagnosis of, 829
    nontumorous masses, 828–831, *829, 830*
      cutaneous horn, 829, *830*
      foreign body inclusions, 830
      granuloma annulare, 830, *831*
      keratosis, 828, *829*
      onychoma, 829, *830*
    primary, classification according to disease, 870
      vs. secondary, 869
    secondary, classification according to disease, 870
    viral and tumor involvement, 831, *831, 832*
      benign and malignant, 831, *831, 832*
        amelanotic melanoma, 831, *831*
        granuloma pyogenicum, 831, *831*
        Kaposi's sarcoma, 831, *832*
        warts, 831
  loss of, in children, 1684
  of foot, anatomy of, 1399–1401, *1400.* See also *Infections.*
    biopsies from, 870
    dorsal vs. plantar, 869
Skin grafts, 944–962, *946, 951, 957.* See also *Plastic surgery.*
  flaps and, 949–958, *951, 957, 958–962*
    "axial" cutaneous, 949–953, *951*
      dorsalis pedis, 950–953, *951*
        advantages and disadvantages, 952
        design and anatomic pitfalls, 950
        technique of flap elevation, 951
    cross-leg, 956–958, *957, 960*

Skin grafts (*Continued*)
  flaps and, cross-leg, medial gastrocnemius elevation
        technique, 956, *957*
    stabilization and transection timing, 957
  local "random," 949, 960
  muscular, 953–956
    long leg muscles, 953–955
      flexor hallucis longus, 954
      peroneus brevis, 953
      soleus, *954*
    small foot muscles, 955
      abductor digiti minimi, 955
      abductor hallucis, 955
      extensor digitorum brevis, 955
      flexor digitorum brevis, 956
  for burns, deformities from, technique, 1696, *1697*
    electrical, 1698
    radiation, 1701, *1701*
    thermal, 1693
  history of, 944
  keratosis following, 829
  pinch, in diabetic foot, 1387, *1389*
  problem areas for, 958–962
    Achilles tendon, 958
    anterior ankle, 958
    heel, 958
    medial and lateral malleoli, 958
    metatarsal heads, 962
    sole, 959–962
      resurfacing techniques, 959–961
        cross-leg flaps, 960
        dermal overgrafting, 959
        free flap reconstruction, 960–962
          dorsalis pedis, 961
          groin, 961
          latissimus dorsi, 961
        full-thickness, 959
        local flaps, 960
        split-thickness, 959. See also *Skin grafts, split-
            thickness.*
  special methods of evaluation for, 947–949
    arteriogram, 947
    Doppler flowmeter, 947
    fluorescein examination, 948. See also *Fluorescein.*
    venogram, 947
  split-thickness, following amputation, *1368, 1369,
        1370*
    in diabetic foot, 1387, *1387, 1388, 1390, 1391, 1392*
  techniques and pitfalls, 944–947, *946*
    calibrated dermatomes, 944, *944, 946*
    donor site, 946
    immobilization, 945
    recipient bed, 944
    sheet graft vs. mesh graft, 945
Sloughing, as postoperative complication, 171, *172*
Small toes, 622–658
  ainhum in, 656, *656, 657*
  anatomy of, 622–624, *623, 624*
    dorsal aponeurosis, 622, *623*
    extensor sling mechanism, 622–624, *623, 624*
    insertion of intrinsic muscles, 622, *623*
    orientation of lumbrical and interosseous muscles,
        622, *623*
  bones of, in gout, 655, *655*
  contracted overlapping fifth, 646, *646, 647*
  corns in, end, 624, *625,* 634–636, *634–636*
    hard, 624–628, *624–628,* 632–634

Small toes (*Continued*)
  corns in, soft, 628–634, *629–632*
  cysts of, mucous, 655, *656*
  deformities of, hammer toe, 638–646, *639–645.* See
      also *Hammer toe.*
    mallet toe, 624, *625,* 636–638, *636, 637.* See also
        Mallet toe.
    uncommon, 647–650, *648, 650*
      curled-under toes, 648, *648*
      divergent toes, 647, *648*
      macrodactyly, 649, *650*
      microdactyly, 648
      overlapping and underlapping, 648, *648*
      trigger toe, 649
  diseases of, systemic, 656, *656*
  disorders of, ungual, 651, *651, 652*
  examination of, clinical, 94, *94, 95*
    chronic eczema, 94, *94*
    epidermophytosis, 94, *94*
    fifth toe, lateral calluses, *87,* 94, *95*
    hammer toe, 94
    soft corn, 94, *95*
    tailor's bunion, 95
  flexion-extension in, *672*
  fusion of, optimum position, 175, *175*
  helomata dura in, 624–628, *624–628,* 632–634. See
      also *Corns, hard.*
  helomata mollia in, 628–634, *629–632.* See also
      Corns, soft.
  incisions in, *160,* 163, *163*
    distal interphalangeal joint, 164
    end corn approach, 164
    metatarsophalangeal level, 163
    middle phalanx diaphysis, 164
    proximal interphalangeal level, 163
    proximal phalanx diaphysis and, 163
    tip of toe, 164
    web space, 164
  infections in, 656
  lacerations of, 864
  lesions in, paraungual, *636,* 651, *651, 652*
    subungual, 651
  surgical approaches to, *160,* 163, *163*
  tumors and tumor-like conditions of, 652–656,
        652–655
    chondrosarcoma, 652, *653*
    cysts, inclusion, following Syme procedure, 653,
        655
      mucous, 655, *656*
    enchondromas, 652, *652*
    exostoses, 652, *653*
    fibromas, 653, *653*
    gouty bone involvement, 655, *655*
    pigmented villonodular kenosynovitis, 653, *654*
  ulceration in, 656
Smallpox, affecting feet, 886
Smelly feet, footwear for, 1781
Snake bite, venomous, of foot and ankle, 1460–1462
      identification of rattlesnakes, 1460
      treatment of, hospital tests, 1461
        immediate, 1461
        incision and suction, 1461
        indications for fasciotomy, 1461
        various responses to, 1460
Soccer, footwear for, 1775
  injuries from, classification, 1574. See also *Sports
      injuries.*

Socks, "nonbreathing," 1764
Soft corns, in small toes, 628–634, 629–632. See also
  Corns, soft.
Soft-tissue atrophy, in alcoholic peripheral neuropathy,
  1210, 1210
Soft-tissue lesions, miscellaneous, 828–868
  arteries, 847
  bursae, 833, 848–854, 849–853. See also Bursae.
  capsule and synovium, 843–845, 843–845. See also
    Capsule.
  fascia, 841, 841. See also Fascia.
  fat pads, 837–841, 838–840. See also Fat pads.
  ligaments, 836, 842. See also Ligaments.
  muscles, 845, 846, 847. See also Muscles.
  nerves, 834, 848, 848
  of skin, 828–832, 829–832. See also Skin, lesions of.
  subcutaneous, 832–837, 832–838. See also
    Subcutaneous lesions.
  tendons, 854–867, 855, 856, 858–866. See also
    Tendons.
  veins, 846, 847. See also Veins.
Soft-tissue surgery, 412–424, 413–416, 418, 421
  general remarks, 419–424, 421
  in treatment of clubfoot, 242
  joint operations, 412–424, 413–416, 418, 421
    syndesmotomy, 412–419, 413–416, 418
  tendon operations, 424. See also Tendon(s).
Soft-tissue tension, as factor in deformity, 257
Sole, examination of, clinical, 95
    foreign-body granulomas, 95
  fissures of, etiology and treatment of, 896
  footwear and devices for, 1724–1726, 1725
  incisions in, plastic surgery and, 942, 943
  injuries of, industrial, 1611, 1612. See also Industrial
    injuries.
    protection from, 1617, 1618
  infections of, fungal, 898, 898, 899
  keratoses of, 901–904, 902–904. See also Keratosis(es).
  psoriasis of, hyperkeratotic, 883, 885
  sensation in, 176
  skin grafts for, 959–962. See also Skin grafts.
  skin of, anatomy of, 1399–1401, 1400
  tendon lacerations in, 864, 865
  Trichophyton infections of, 898, 898
  warts on, 905–910, 906–908. See also Warts.
Soleus, flaps of, for skin grafts, 954
Spastic diplegia, case reports, 295–301, 295–297, 299,
    300, 318–322, 319–321
  analysis, 296, 297, 319, 321
  history, 295–297, 295, 296, 318–321, 319
  postoperative views, 296, 297, 319–321
  preoperative assessment, 295–297, 295, 296
  treatment, surgical, 297–301, 296, 297, 299, 300,
    319–321, 321
    special aspects of technique, 298–301, 299, 300
  equinus deformity and, case report, history and
    analysis, 332–334, 333
    treatment, 334
  etiology of, 284
  hallux valgus and, case report, 324–328, 328–330
    foot analysis, 329
    history, 328
    recognition and etiology, 329
    treatment, 329
Spastic flatfoot, 85, 86, 91, 96, 97
  abnormal subtalar complex and, 740, 740
  causes of, 91

Spastic flatfoot (Continued)
  causes of, 740, 741–744, 741–744
    arthritis, 742, 743
    degenerative osteoarthritis, 741
    fibrous ankylosis, 743
    fractures and dislocations, 740, 741, 743
    Sudeck's atrophy, 744, 744
    tarsal coalition, 741, 741, 742
  incidence of, vs. tarsal coalition, 523
  roentgenographic view, 96, 97
Spastic hemiparesis, case report, 293–295
  history, 293
  treatment, 295
    analysis, 294
  equinocavovarus deformity and, case report, history
    and surgical treatment, 312
  with equinovarus deformity, case report, 310–312
    history, 310
    technical management, 311
    tendon transfer analysis, 311
    treatment analysis, 310
Spastic hemiplegia, case reports, 313–318, 316–318
  effects of tendon transfer, 314, 316, 318
  equinovalgus deformity, 316, 316
  foot deformity analysis, 313, 316, 316, 317, 317
  night splinting, importance of, 318, 318
  treatment, 313–318, 318
Spastic tetraparesis, case report, 315
  analysis and history, 315
  surgical treatment, 315
  tendon transfer, 315
Spasticity, characteristics of, 285
  definition of, 283
  in cerebral palsy, 283
    hallux valgus and, case report, 330–332, 331
  in stroke patient, 1112
  neurophysiologic aspects of, 285
    muscle contraction speed, 286
    muscle excursion, 286
    muscle force, 286
    muscle tension, 286
Spina bifida. See also Spinal dysraphism.
  affecting foot, 84
  arthrodesis in, 261
  associated anomalies and, common etiologic factors,
    249
  calcaneus deformity and, treatment of, 252, 276, 276
  cavus deformity and, treatment of, 253, 277, 470
  corrective appliances for, 266
  deformities in, factors affecting, fractures, 257
  early literature on, 249
  equinovalgus deformity and, treatment of, 252,
    273–276, 273, 275
  equinus deformity and, treatment of, 263, 278
  factors affecting, intrauterine molding, 254, 255
  high longitudinal arch in, 91
  in breech presentation infant, 255, 255
  in experimental animals, 259
  in foot, appliances for, 278, 279
    pathologic changes in, 258–261
      blood supply, 260
      fractures, 260
      motor function, 260
      muscle imbalance, 259
      nerve function, 260
      sensory function, 260
      similarities with normal spine, 258

Spina bifida (*Continued*)
  individual deformities in, treatment of, 270–279, *271,*
    273, 275, 276, 279
  normal feet in, 270
  reflex activity in paralyzed muscles in, 250
  treatment of, choice of, 248
    early vs. late, 248
  valgus deformity and, *252, 263,* 272
    convex, treatment of, *252,* 273–276, *273, 275*
  varus deformity and, treatment of, 250, *250, 252, 263,*
    270–272, *271*
  vertical talus and, treatment of, *252,* 273–276, *273,*
    275
Spina ventosa, clinical features of, 1410
Spinal cord, abnormalities in, correlation with limb
    changes, 259
  disease of, neurologic correlation, 250
  disorders of, with associated neuropathy, 1231–1237,
    1234–1237
    cerebellar ataxias, 1236
    degenerative cord lesions, 1231–1236, *1234–1236*
      Charcot-Marie-Tooth disease, 1231–1236,
      1234–1236
      Friedreich's ataxia, 1236
    intra- and extradural lesions, 1237, *1237*
  injury to, causing motor neuritis, 1243, *1243*
  involvement of, in hereditary sensory neuropathies,
    1227
  lesions of, affecting foot, 84
    congenital as cause of cavus deformity, 470
Spinal dysraphism. See also *Spina bifida.*
  associated anomalies and, 249
  deformities in, factors affecting, fractures, 257
  foot assessment in, 261–267, *262–266*
    at birth, 261
    corrective appliances, 266
    deformity classification, *252, 253,* 262–264, *263*
      calcaneus, *252, 263*
      cavus, *253, 263*
      equinovalgus, *252, 263*
      equinovarus, *263, 263*
      equinus, *263, 263*
      forefoot, 262
      hindfoot, 262
      toes, 262
      valgus, *263, 263*
      varus, *263*
      vertical talus, *252, 263*
    motor activity, 262, *262*
    photography, 264, *264*
    root innervation, 262, *262*
    sensibility, 264, *265*
    weight-bearing capabilities, 265, *266*
  foot management in, 248–281
    principles, 267–270
  neurologic loss and other factors affecting, 253–258,
    254, 255, 257
  neurologic patterns of paralysis and, 251–253, *252,*
    253
  treatment of, early vs. late, 248
  types of, similarity of deformities in, 261
Spinal muscular atrophy, 347–349, *348, 350.* See also
  Muscular atrophy.
Spinal nerve blocks, differential, technique of,
  1296–1298, *1296, 1297*
Spine, deformities of, rotational, 429
  early closure of, arguments for, 248

Spine (*Continued*)
  lesions of, classification of, 1209
  muscular atrophy in, 347–349, *348, 350.* See also
    Muscular atrophy.
Spinocerebellar degeneration, as cause of cavus
    deformity, 469
  lesions contributing to, 469
Spirochetal diseases. See *Yaws.*
SPLATT (split anterior tibial tendon trànsfer) procedure,
    for equinovarus deformity, 1113
  for equinus deformity, 1116
  for toe deformities, *1121*
  for varus deformity, 1115, *1115*
  postoperative results of, *1121*
Splayfoot, biplanar, resilient, hallux valgus and,
    treatment of, 597, *597*
  rigid, hallux valgus and, treatment of, 598, *598*
  horizontal, hallux valgus and, treatment of, 587, *588,*
    589
  in dancers, 1634. See also *Dancing.*
  in rheumatoid arthritis, *1026,* 1028
  tranverse metatarsal arch in, 92
  treatment of, surgical, 1034
  varying metatarsal stress in, *548–551*
Splint(s), at night, 318, *318, 337, 338*
  Denis Browne, 409
  femoral rotator, 434, *434*
  genu valgum corrective, 435, *435*
  pillow, as emergency treatment for ankle fractures,
    1550, *1551*
Splinters, treatment of, 897, *897*
Split foot, basic literature on, guide to, 1862
Spondylitis, ankylosing, affecting foot, *1058,* 1059
  idiopathic, involving heel, 774
Sports, footwear for, 1771–1775. See also *Shoes, and*
  shoe modifications.
Sports injuries, basic literature on, guide to, 1852
  to foot and ankle, 1573–1606
    bursitis of Achilles tendon, clinical features of, 1595
      treatment of, 1596, *1596*
    classification of, 1573
    dislocations, 1588, *1588*
    examination, physical, 1574
      auscultation, 1574
      inspection, 1574
      palpation, 1574
      percussion, 1574
     roentgenographic, 1574
    fractures, 1578–1587, *1581–1587*
     of hallux, 1578–1585, *1581–1585*
      etiology of, 1578
      mechanism of injury, 1581, 1582, *1582*
      treatment of, nonsurgical, 1582, *1583, 1584*
       surgical, *1581,* 1583, *1584, 1585*
      valgus deformity and, 1582, *1583*
     of hindfoot, 1587, *1587*
     of metatarsals, 1586, *1586*
     of midfoot, 1586
     of sesamoids, *1581,* 1585
     of small toes, 1586
    history-taking, 1574
    impingement syndrome, 1593–1595, *1594, 1595*
     clinical and roentgenographic features of, 1594,
      1594
     etiology of, 1593
     treatment of, surgical, 1594, *1595*
    in distance runners, 1601–1605, *1603*

Sports injuries (*Continued*)
  to foot and ankle, in distance runners, Achilles
        tendinitis, 1604
    anatomic factors, 1601
    heel pain, 1605
    knee pain, 1603
    orthoses, 1602, *1603*
    plantar fasciitis, clinical features and treatment of,
      1604
    posterior tibial syndrome, 1603
    running surfaces, 1602
    rupture of plantar fascia, clinical features and
      treatment of, 1604
    shoes, 1601
    stress fractures, 1604
    training errors, 1601
  in joggers, 1603–1605. See also *Sports injuries, to
    foot and ankle, in distance runners.*
  jogger's toe, 1605
  leg pain syndromes, 1596–1601, *1598, 1599*
    classification of, 1596
    compartment syndromes, 1599
      acute, signs and symptoms of, 1599
        treatment of, 1599
      chronic, signs and symptoms, 1600
        treatment of, 1600
    muscle hernias, diagnosis and treatment of, 1600
    post-traumatic ossifying hematoma, diagnosis of,
      1600
      treatment of, 1600
    shin splints, definition of, 1596
      diagnosis of, 1597
        differential, 1597
      treatment of, 1597
    stress fractures, 1598, *1599*
      clinical and roentgenographic features of, 1599,
        1599
      diagnosis of, differential, 1598
      treatment of, 1599
    tenosynovitis, 1601
    tibial stress syndrome, 1597, *1598*
      diagnosis of, differential, 1597
      roentgenographic features of, 1598, *1598*
      treatment of, 1598
  sprains, clinical features of, 1588
    treatment of, nonsurgical, 1589
      surgical, for chronic lateral ankle instability,
        1589–1591, *1590*
        postoperative care, 1590
        technique, 1589, *1590*
  static problems, 1595
  tendons, 1591–1593, *1592, 1593*
    acute rupture of, 1591
    dislocations of, 1591–1593, *1592, 1593*
      treatment of, surgical, 1592, *1592, 1593*
      vs. sprains, 1592
    stenosis of tendon sheath, 1591
    tenosynovitis, 1591
  treatment of, 1575–1578, *1576–1580*
    acute phase, 1575
      compression, 1575
      early gentle motion, 1575
      elevation, 1575
      ice therapy, 1575
      rest, 1575
      recovery phase, ultrasound, 1575
      whirlpool, 1576

Sports injuries (*Continued*)
  to foot and ankle, treatment of, rehabilitation phase,
      1576–1578, *1576–1580*
    initial stage, 1576
    proprioceptive exercises, 1576
    protection, 1578, *1578–1580*
    strengthening exercises, 1576–1578
    stretching exercises, *1576*, 1578
Sprain(s), in sports injuries, 1588–1591, *1590*. See also
    Sports injuries.
  of ankle, chronic, 777, 778, 788
    treatment of, surgical, 798
    diagnostic difficulties and treatment, 1726, 1726
    examination of, physical, 107, *107, 108*
    in children, 1681. See also *Children, trauma in.*
    in sports injuries, 1589–1591, *1590*. See also *Sports
      injuries.*
    strapping for, 1726, *1726*. See also *Foot, pain in,
      padding and devices.*
  of ligaments, 1449
    in dancers, 1654
    treatment of, 1450
  of muscles, in dancers, 1654
Spurs, dorsal, footwear for, 1780
  heel, *1778, 1781*
Squamous cell epithelioma, 1419, *1419*
Squared foot, digital and metatarsal formulas for, *660*,
  665
Stability, types of, 490–492, *491*
Stabilizing mechanisms, 52–55, *53–55*
  arches of foot, 52–55, *53–55*
  intrinsic muscles, 55, *55*
  plantar fascia, 52–55, *54, 55*
  talonavicular joint, 55, *55*
Stable foot, unbalanced, treatment of, 515–518, *515–517*
Stance phase, of walking cycle, 37, *37*, 43, *44*, 55–57, *56*
Static encephalopathy. See *Palsy, cerebral.*
Steindler's operation, in metatarsalgia with cavus
  deformity, 676
Step, biomechanics of, 55–57, *56*
Strapping, 1726–1730, *1726, 1728–1730*. See also *Foot,
  pain in, padding and devices.*
Streptococcal infections, clinical features and treatment
  of, 887, 888, 889
Stress fractures. See *Fractures, stress.*
Stroke, electromyography in, 66
  lower extremity disorders and, 1112–1117, *1115–1117*
    equinovarus deformity, 1116, *1116*. See also *Talipes
      equinovarus.*
    equinus deformity, 1112–1114. See also *Equinus
      deformity.*
    gait analysis, 66, 1112
    hemiplegia, 1112
    inadequate dorsiflexion, 1114
    orthosis-free walking, 1117
    plantar flexion weakness, 1114
    spasticity, 1112
    toe deformities, 1117, *1117*. See also *Toe(s),
      deformities of.*
    varus deformity, 1114–1116, *1115*. See also *Varus
      deformity.*
    vs. head trauma, surgical considerations, 1118
Subcutaneous lesions, 832–837, *832–838*
  annular fibrosis, 832, *832*
  calcification and, 833, *833, 834*
  fat necrosis, 832, *833*
  foreign bodies, 836, *836, 837*

Subcutaneous lesions (*Continued*)
  idiopathic edema, 836, *836*
  miscellaneous tumors, 837, *838*
  ossification and, 835, *835, 836*
  piezogenic papules, 833, *833*
Subluxation, of metatarsophalangeal joint, fifth, chronic, 843, *843*
  first, congruous or incongruous, 553, *555*
Subtalar coalition, as cause of peroneal spastic flatfoot, 741, *742*
Subtalar complex, 727–763. See also *Subtalar joint.*
  abnormal, examination of, clinical, 740, *740*
      peroneal spastic flatfoot, 740, *740.* See also
        Spastic flatfoot, peroneal.
    radiographic changes in, *740, 741*
  anatomic and biomechanical clinical correlations, joint axes, 727–729, *728, 729*
  angles of talar head and neck, 731, *732*
  arthrodesis in, pantalar, technique, 761
    triple, technique, 758–761, *759–761*
  aseptic necrosis of talus and, 748, *748, 749*
  Charcot involvement of, 748, *749*
  composition of, 729
  deformity of, secondary and late effects of, 737, *739*
      hallux valgus following hypermobile pes planus, 739
      hammer toe following cavus deformity, 739
      osteoarthritis, 737, *740*
  dislocations of, *731,* 746, *747.* See also *Dislocations.*
  examination of, clinical, 729
  functions of, 738
  infections of, 745, *745, 746*
    differential diagnosis, 745
    location, 746, *746*
    synovial cavities, anatomy, 745, *746*
  instability of, surgery for, 758
  irregularity of, *149*
  long muscle foot control on, 734
  midtarsal joint and, 732–734, *733*
    talocalcaneal (subtalar), 733, *733*
    talonavicular, 732
  osteoarthritis of, 737, *737, 740*
  pain in, treatment of, nonsurgical, 750–752, *750, 751*
      ankle orthoses, 751, *751*
      footwear, 750, *750, 751*
      steroids, 752
    surgical, 752–757, *753, 754, 756*
      arthrodesis, *754, 755–757*
        contraindications, 756
        indications, 756
      concomitant ankle pathology, *753, 754*
      contraindications, 755
      controversy regarding, 752
      neurectomy, 755, *756*
      sinus tarsi excision, 755
  peritalar rheumatoid dislocation of foot and, 731, *731*
  range of motion of, 729, 735
  solid fusion of, *753*
  stability of, longitudinal arch and, 735–738, *735–737*
      Chopart's joint laxity, 736, *736*
      hypermobile flatfoot, 736, *737*
      Larsen's syndrome, 735, *736*
      ligamentous laxity, *735,* 736
      Marfan's syndrome, *735,* 736
      peritalar laxity, 736, *736*
      range of motion variations, 735
      sustentacular anomalies, 736, *737, 737*

Subtalar complex (*Continued*)
    stability of, longitudinal arch and, talar neck elongation, 737, *737*
  subtalar and peritalar joints, 730–732, *731, 732*
    areas of controversy regarding surgery, 730
    axial route and variations, 730
    range of motion, 730, *731*
  surgery involving, 752–758, *753, 754, 756, 757*
    relief of deformity, 757, *757*
      arthrodesis, 757, *757*
      astragalectomy, 757, *757*
      naviculectomy, 757
    relief of pain, 752–757, *753, 754, 756.* See also
      Subtalar complex, pain in.
    stabilizing procedures, 758
      arthrodesis, 758
      for flail foot, 758
      osteotomy, 758
  systemic diseases involving, 748–750, *750*
  tuberculosis in, *746*
  tumors of, 744, *745*
    benign vs. malignant, 744
  weight-bearing forces on and distributed by, 738, *738*
Subtalar joint. See also *Subtalar complex.*
  abnormalities of, following calcaneal fractures, 1537
  anatomy of, *11, 13–15, 14*
    functional, 40–42, *41*
  ankle joint and, axial relationship of, 40, 43, *44*
  arthritis of, as cause of heel pain, 976
  arthrology of, *11, 13–15, 14*
  axial variations in, 40, *41*
  axis of, 489, *490*
  breaks in, 388, *389*
  Charcot involvement of, 748, *749*
  conditions of, 86, *86*
  dislocations of, 1467–1472, *1468–1471.* See also
    Dislocations.
  effect of triceps surae on, 45, *46*
  examination of, clinical, 90, *91*
    roentgenographic, 96, *97*
      technique, *126,* 129, *129, 130*
  in normal vs. flatfoot, 40, *41*
  in rheumatoid arthritis, 1029, *1030*
  in subtalar complex, 733, *733*
  in tarsal coalition vs. normal foot, 529–531
  in tuberculosis, *746*
  inversion of, 45, *46*
  primary destruction of, in syphilis, 1251, *1251*
  range of motion in, 40, *41,* 43, *44*
  torque conversion of, 489, *490*
Subungual exostosis, 1004, *1004, 1005*
Subungual lesions, 911, *911, 912.* See also *Toenails.*
  treatment of, 651
Sudeck's atrophy, 85, 1287–1290, *1288.* See also *Reflex sympathetic dystrophy syndrome.*
  as cause of peroneal spastic flatfoot, 744, *744*
  tuberculosis and, 744, *744*
Sudeck's post-traumatic osteoporosis, as residual of ankle injury, 787
Sulfinpyrazone, in treatment of chronic gouty arthritis and tophaceous gout, 1020
Supination, definition of, 125
Sural nerve, entrapment neuropathies in, 1200
Surgery, choice of, 167
    indications and contraindications, 146, 156
    occupational factors, 149, 168
    elective, in elderly patients, 156

Surgery (*Continued*)
  in children vs. adults, indications and
    contraindications, 151
  plastic, 939–963. See also *Plastic surgery*
  principles of, age of patient, 151
    armamentarium, 154–156, *154–156*
    bone transection, 166
    cast application, 169, *169*
    excess surgery, 166, *167*
    general considerations, 145, 148
    importance of follow-up, 145
    incisions and approaches, 159–166, *160, 161,*
      163–165
      ankle, 159–161, *159–161*
      foot, lateral, *159,* 160, 161
        medial, 161, *161*
      hallux, *160, 161, 162, 163*
      heel, lateral, *160,* 165
        medial, *161,* 165
        posterior, 166
      metatarsals, *160,* 162
      midtarsus, *160,* 162
      plantar aspect, *163–165, 164*
      small toes, *160, 163, 163*
    informed consent, 158
    instruments, 154–156, *155, 156*
    internal fixation, 166, *180, 185*
    joint flexibility, 150, *150, 179*
    landmarks, 158, *159*
    miscellaneous, 157
    nerve damage avoidance, 153, *159*
    neurovascular damage avoidance, 153, *153*
    opening wedge osteotomy, 152
    optimum fusion position, 174, *175*
    outmoded surgery, 168
    patient evaluation, 149
    plantigrade foot and, 144–194
    postoperative, care, 169
      complications, 171–174, *171–174*
      dressings, 168
    preoperative medication, 154
    procedure selection, 167
    radiography, 170, *170, 171*
    relation of blood supply to, 146, *147*
    role of surgeon and, 144
    techniques and, 156–158, *163*
      blisters, 157
      hematomas, 157
      skin incisions, 157, *163*
    tendon transfer, 152
    timing, 149, *149*
    truncated wedge, 151, *151, 190*
    weight-bearing factors, 147, *148*
    wound closure, 168
Surgical anatomy, 33. See also *Anatomy.*
Swing phase, of walking cycle, 37, *37,* 43, 44, 55–57, *56*
Syme amputation(s), *1366, 1367, 1369, 1392*
  for end corn, 636
  for paraungual lesions, *636,* 651, *651, 652*
  for subungual lesions, 651
  heel pad damage in, 839
  in longitudinal deficiency of fibula, 223–225, *224*
  in longitudinal deficiency of tibia with intact fibula,
    227
  in paraxial fibular hemimelia, 246
  inclusion cysts of small toes following, 653, *655*
  postoperative advantages of, 225

Syme amputation(s) (*Continued*)
  prostheses for, 1816–1819, *1818, 1819*
  technique of, 225
Sympathetic dystrophies, reflex, 1445. See also
  Psychiatric aspects.
Syndactylization, in hammer toe, 641, *641*
  in treatment of corns, 631, 634
Syndactyly, congenital, 218, *218*
  treatment of, 218
  constriction band syndrome and, 228, 230
  treatment of, 245
Syndesmotomy, 412–419, *413–416, 418.* See also
  Talipes, inverted, treatment of.
Synovectomy, of ankle joint, 1049–1051
  with tenosynovectomy of foot, 1049
Synovial cavities, in subtalar complex, anatomy of, 745,
  746
Synovial sarcoma(s), 994, *995*
  vs. soft-tissue calcification, 834, *834*
Synovial sinus, 845
Synovial tissue, tumors of, 993–995, *994, 995*
Synovioma(s), 994, *995*
Synovitis, acute transient, of foot and ankle, 844, *844,*
    845
    Boeck's sarcoid and, 844, *845*
    gonorrhea and, 844, *844*
    porphyria and, 844, *845*
  in dancers, treatment of, 1648
  induced by urate crystal deposits, pathologic findings
    and pathogenesis of, in gout, 1015–1018, *1016–1018*
  occupational, 83
  of ankle joint, in dancers, 83, 1648
  of metatarsophalangeal joints, 843
    in rheumatoid arthritis, 1025, 1027, *1028*
    treatment of, surgical, 1034
  of talonavicular joint, in Köhler's disease, 201
  pigmented villonodular, diffuse and localized, 993,
    994
Synovium, capsule and, lesions of, 843–845, *843–845.*
  See also *Capsule.*
Syphilis, affecting foot, congenital vs. acquired, 1418
    treatment of, 1418
  as cause of Charcot foot, 1248
  Charcot foot in, surgical contraindications, *1262, 1263*
  dactylitis in, treatment of, 1418
  destruction of subtalar joint in, *1251, 1251*
  tertiary, destruction of ankle joint in, *1250,* 1251
  vs. diabetes, spontaneous fractures in, *1254, 1255,*
    1255
Syringomyelia, as cause of Charcot foot, 1248
  lumbosacral, hereditary sensory neuropathies and,
    1227
Systemic disease, 1014–1448
Systemic lupus erythematosus, peripheral neuropathies
  and, 1226

Taches noires, 890, *890*
Tailor's bunion, 95
  examination for, physical, 111
TAL (tendo-Achillis lengthening) procedure, for equinus
    deformity, 1113
  for toe deformities, *1121*
  postoperative results of, *1121*

Talar trochlear osteochondral defects, treatment of, surgical, *786, 799*

Talectomy, partial, and fusion, technique of, 810
technique of, 810

Talipes. See also *Deformities, of foot.*
inverted, 374–428. See also *Clubfoot* and *Talipes equinovarus.*
classification of, 374–381, *375–380*
combination possibility occurrence of deformities, *380*
composite plane, *378, 379*
computer analysis, 381
coronal plane, *377*
horizontal plane, *376*
initial types of clubfoot and flatfoot, *379*
mathematical premise, 375–381, *376–380*
sagittal plane, *377*
segmental, *380,* 381
diagnosis of, radiologic, 392–407, *393, 394, 396–402, 404–407*
examination of, radiologic, 392–407, *393, 394, 396–402, 404–407*
abnormal views, 403–407, *404–407*
curved first metatarsal mechanism, 406, *407*
rocker-bottom feet, 406, *406*
short first metatarsal mechanism, 406, *407*
talar external rotation break, 406, *407*
type I, 403, *404*
type II, 404, *404*
type III, 404, *405*
type IV, 405, *405*
apparatus, 392, *393, 394*
normal views, 395–403, *396–402*
anteroposterior, 395–398, *396–398*
coronal, 400
cuboid sign, 400, *400, 421*
detection of rotational deformities, *396, 399, 401–403, 401, 402*
horizontal plane, 395–398, *396–398*
lateral, 398–400, *399, 400*
sagittal plane, 398–400, *399, 400*
value of, 393–395
roentgenographic, *375,* 419
incidence of, 381
pathomechanics of, 381–392, *384, 385, 387–392*
conversion feet, 383
degree of deformity, 382
degree of rigidity, 382
initial types, *378, 379,* 384–392, *384, 385, 387–392*
latent adaptive segmental deformities, 382
relapse, 383
segmental breaks, 382
types of, 383
segmental deviations, *380,* 382
skew foot, *391, 392*
terminology, 382
type I, 384–388, *384, 385, 387, 388*
complete clubfoot, 384, *384*
planar system, 384
rotatory motions, 384, *385*
Scarpa's foot, 384, *384*
segmental breaks in, 386–388, *387, 388*
ankle joint, 388, *388*
Chopart's joint, 386–388, *388*
rocker-bottom foot, 387, *388*
Lisfranc's joint, 386, *387, 388*

Talipes (*Continued*)
inverted, pathomechanics of, type I, segmental breaks in, Lisfranc's joint, curved first metatarsal mechanism, 386, *387, 388*
locked middle segment, 386, *387*
rocker-bottom foot, 386, *388*
short first metatarsal mechanism, 386, *387, 388*
subtalar joint, 388
vs. type II, 385, 389, *421*
type II, 389, *389*
complete clubfoot, 389
segmental breaks in, 389
ankle joint, 390
Chopart's joint, 389
Lisfranc's joint, 389
subtalar joint, 389
type III, 390, *390*
segmental breaks in, 390
type IV, 390, *391*
segmental breaks in, 391
treatment of, 407–427, *410, 413–416, 418, 421*
nonsurgical, 408–410, *410*
cast, 409, *410*
Denis Browne splint, 409
manipulation, 409
traction, 408
results of, 427
retentive, 426
surgical, 410–426, *413–416, 418, 421*
bone surgery, 424
amputation, 425
metatarsal osteotomy, 424
rotation osteotomy of tibia, 425
soft-tissue surgery and, 426
tarsal osteotomy, 424
triple arthrodesis, 424
medial release, 420–423
roentgenography during, 419
soft-tissue surgery, 412–424, *413–416, 418, 421*
bone surgery and, 426
general remarks, 419–424, *421*
joint operations, 412–424, *413–416, 418, 421*
syndesmotomy, 412–419, *413–416, 418*
anterior ankle joint, *413,* 418
instruments for, 412, *414*
lateral Chopart, *413,* 417
lateral Lisfranc, *413,* 417
lateral subtalar, *413,* 418, *418*
medial Chopart, 412–415, *413*
medial Lisfranc, *413,* 415–417
medial subtalar, 412, *413, 414–416*
with Achilles tendon lengthening, 418, 420
tendon operations, 424
use of tourniquets, 419
varying terminology for, 375

Talipes cavus, 463–485. See also *Cavus deformity.*

Talipes equinovarus, 252, *252.* See also *Clubfoot* and *Talipes, inverted.*
arthrogryposis multiplex congenita and, 456, *458*
basic literature on, guide to, 1853–1857
cerebral palsy and, treatment of, surgical, 189, *189*
congenital, 242–244
treatment of, nonsurgical, early, 242
surgical, bony procedures, 243
soft-tissue procedures, 242

Talipes equinovarus (*Continued*)
  congenital, treatment of, surgical, tendon transfers, 243
    varying types of, 242
  differing forms of, 253
  external pressure as factor in, 257, *257*
  hysterical, 1442, *1443*. See also *Psychiatric aspects.*
  in children, variations of, 196
  in head trauma patient, treatment of, surgical, 1122
  in normal and abnormal spine, similarities, 258
  in stroke patient, 1116, *1116*
    treatment of, surgical, SPLATT procedure, 1116
  pressure sores in, 271, *271*
  radiographic view, 264, *265*
  spastic hemiparesis and, case report, 310–312
    history, 310
    technical management, 311
    tendon transfer analysis, 311
    treatment analysis, 310
  spinal dysraphism and, 258, 263, *263*
  spinal muscular atrophy and, 349
  treatment of, special technical considerations, 311
  vs. normal foot, pressure prints of, 265, *266*
Talocalcaneal joint. See *Subtalar joint.*
Talocalcaneonavicular joint, anatomy of, *11, 12, 14, 15,*
  439, 440
  arthrology of, *11, 12, 14, 15*
  dislocation of, 440, *440, 442*
  open reduction of, 449–454, *451–453*. See also *Talus,*
    vertical, congenital.
Talocrural joint. See *Ankle joint.*
Talofibular ligament, 13, *14*
  anterior, rupture of, physical examination for, 107,
    107, 108
Talonavicular joint. See also *Subtalar complex.*
  as stabilizing mechanism, 55, *55*
  calcaneocuboid joint and, as midtarsal joint, 1490. See
    also *Midtarsal joint, injuries of.*
  dislocation of, in talar neck fractures, 1475, *1477*
    treatment of, 1479
  in subtalar complex, 732
  nonunion of, after triple arthrodesis, 723, *724*
  synovitis of, in Köhler's disease, 201
Talonavicular ligament, *14, 15*
Talonavicular synostosis, as cause of peroneal spastic
  flatfoot, 741, *741*
Talus. See also *Heel* and *Hindfoot.*
  anatomy of, 10, *11, 12, 14*
  aseptic necrosis of, 748, *748, 749*
    as osteochondritis dissecans, 748
    following fractures, 748, *749*
    following surgery, 748, *748, 749*
  avascular necrosis of, as contraindication for total
    arthroplasty, 823, *823, 824*
    following naviculectomy, 448, *451*
    following clubfoot surgery, 173, *174*
  chondroblastomas in, 1005–1007, *1006*
  deformity of, in Riley-Day syndrome, *1258*
    major, in talipes equinovarus, 258
  dislocations of, total, 1472–1474, *1473*. See also
    Dislocations.
  excision of, 1480
    in poliomyelitis, 1480
  fractures of, 786, *786*. See also *Fractures* and
    Fractures, of ankle, residuals of.
    dome of, 1463–1467, *1465–1467*. See also
      Fractures, of talus, transchondral.
    in dancers, 1652, *1652*

Talus (*Continued*)
  fractures of, talar body, 1483–1489, *1484–1489.* See
    also *Fractures, of talus.*
    talar neck, 1475–1483, *1475–1477, 1479–1482.* See
      also *Fractures, of talus.*
  fracture-dislocations of, in children, 1675
  head of, angles of, 731
  injuries of, 1463–1496.
    "aviator's astragalus," 1612
    classification of, 1463
    incidence of, 1463
    subtalar dislocations, 1467–1472, *1468–1471.* See
      also *Dislocations, of subtalar joint.*
  neck of, angles of, 731, *732*
    in dancers, 1637, *1637*
  osteochondritis dissecans of, 204–207, *205–207.* See
    also *Osteochondritis dissecans.*
  subluxation of, despite strapping, *1726, 1727*
  systemic diseases involving, 748–750, *750*
  tuberculosis and, radiographic view, *1409*
  vascular supply of, threatened by talar neck fractures,
    1475, *1477*
  vertical, clinical features and treatment of, 252,
    273–276, *273, 275*
    congenital, 439–454, *440–443, 445–447, 449–453*
      anatomy, 439, *440*
        talocalcaneonavicular joint dislocation, 440, *440*
      arthrogryposis multiplex congenita and, *440–442,*
        456, 458
      associated conditions and, 444
      bilateral, *458*
      clinical features of, 441, *441, 447*
      clubfoot and, 444
      etiology of, 442–444, *443*
      history of, 439
      incidence of, 440, 444, *445, 446*
      radiologic features of, *440, 441, 442, 443*
      treatment of, 440, 445–454, *445–447, 449–453*
        childhood changes, 445–447, *447*
        early, importance of, 445
        medial column longer than lateral, 447, *447*
        nonsurgical, closed reduction, technique, 448
          manipulative, 445, 448
            Becker-Anderson and Reimann, 445
        surgical, naviculectomy, 448, *449–451, 453*
          open reduction, postoperative, 448, *453, 454*
            technique, *440, 449–454, 451–453*
              anterolateral incision, 451–454, *452, 453*
              medial incision, *440, 450, 451, 452*
          vs. closed, 445
          varying procedures, 447
    pathogenesis of, prenatal poisitioning and, 8
    spina bifida and, 252, 273–276, *273, 275*
    spinal dysraphism and, 252, *263*
Tarsal bones, tuberculosis of, 1408–1410, *1409, 1410.*
  See also under *Tuberculosis.*
Tarsal coalition, 521–538. See also *Spastic flatfoot,*
  peroneal.
  anatomy and, 524–526
  as cause of peroneal spastic flatfoot, 741, *741, 742*
  associated conditions and, 536
  basic literature on, guide to, 1858–1861
  complications of, 794
  diagnosis of, differential, 536
    radiologic, 528–532, *528–532*
      calcaneonavicular, 531, *532*
      cartilaginous, 532, *532*

Tarsal coalition (*Continued*)
  diagnosis of, radiologic, Harris-Beath view, 528, *528*
    lateral oblique view, *531*
    lateral view, *529, 530*
    secondary signs, 531, *532*
    talar beaking, *529, 530*
    tomographic, 532
    vs. normal foot, *529–531*
  etiology of, 522, *522,* 525
    accessory ossicle theory, 522
    genetic basis, 522
  history of, 521
  incidence of, 523
    bilateral, 523
    subtalar vs. calcaneonavicular, 524
    talonavicular, 524
    vs. peroneal spastic flatfoot, 523
  longitudinal definition of fibula and, 222
  massive, 753
  signs and symptoms of, 526–528
    age and cause of presentation, 527
    appearance postfusion, 527
    restriction of motion, 526
    unreliability of flatfoot appearance as guide, 526
  treatment of, 532–536, *533*
    calcaneonavicular, 532–535, *533*
      manipulative, 532
      surgical, 533–535, *533*
        criteria for resection, 534
        postoperative results, 533–535
    subtalar, 535
      manipulative, 535
      surgical contraindications for resection, 535
Tarsal joint(s), axial relationships of, *42*
  involvement of, in rheumatoid arthritis, *1027,*
    1029–1031, *1030*
  transverse, functional anatomy of, 42, *42*
    range of motion of, everted vs. inverted foot, 42, *42*
Tarsal medullostomy, radiographic views, in Duchenne's
  muscular dystrophy, *344*
Tarsal tunnel, tendon tethering in, 857, *862, 862*
Tarsal tunnel syndrome, *834, 848, 848*
  clinical features of, 767–769
  following ankle injury, 788
  in leprosy, 1241
  symptoms of, 1197
  treatment of, nonsurgical, 769
    surgical, 769, *769*
Tarsometatarsal fusion, postoperative care, 170
Tarsometatarsal joint(s), anatomy of, 15, *16*
  arthrology of, 15, *16*
Tarsus, amputation of, partial, prostheses for, 1815,
  1817
  anatomy of, 10–12, *11, 12, 14*
    calcaneus, 10, *11, 12, 14,* 23, 25, 27
    cuboid, 10, *11, 12, 14,* 27
    cuneiforms, 10–12, *11, 14*
    navicular, 10, *11, 12, 14*
    talus, 10, *11, 12, 14*
  anterior, definition of, 711
    Lisfranc's joint and, anatomy of, functional, 711,
      712
      pathologic, 713, *713*
        in cavus deformity, 713
        in children, 713
        in equinus deformity, 713
        in rheumatoid arthritis, 713

Tarsus (*Continued*)
  anterior, Lisfranc's joint and, anatomy of, pathologic,
      rocker-bottom deformity, 713
      rotatory deformities, 713
  biomechanics of, 712
  disorders of, 711–726
    accessory navicular, 725
    aseptic necrosis of adult tarsal navicular, 719,
      720
    Charcot destruction in diabetes, 718, *719*
    congenital and hereditary, 718
    dorsal tarsal exostoses, 722
    dorsal tarsal ganglia, 723
    effects of footwear, 715
    first metatarsomedial cuneiform joint, 713, *714*
      osteoarthritis of, 714, *714*
      postoperative fusion of, 714, *714*
    forefoot equinus deformity, 715–718, *716, 717.*
      See also *Equinus deformity.*
      treatment of, tarsometatarsal truncated
        dorsal wedge arthrodesis, 716–718, *716,*
        717
    infections, 719–721, *721*
      hematogenous osteomyelitis of navicular,
        719–721, *721*
      pyarthrosis, 721, *721*
      tuberculosis, 721, *721*
    lever arms of foot, 714, *715*
    miscellaneous, 722–725, *724*
    neuropathic degeneration, 724
    neuropathic involvement, 718, *719*
    nonunion of talonavicular joint after triple
      arthrodesis, 723, *724*
    psoriasis, 718, 723
    systemic, 718, *718*
    tumors, 721, 722
  incisions in, *160*
  navicular of, adult, aseptic necrosis of, 719, *720*
    Köhler's disease of, 200–203, *202, 203.* See also
      Köhler's disease.
  osteotomy of, 424, 480, *481*
  scaphoid of, Köhler's disease of, 200–203, *202, 203.*
    See also *Köhler's disease.*
  surgical approaches to, *160*
Temperature contrasts, in damaged vs. undamaged foot,
  1273, *1273*
Tendinitis, Achilles, 857, *859, 860*
  examination for, physical, 104, *105*
  in children, 1681
  in dancers, 1642
  in distance runners and joggers, 1604
  treatment of, nonsurgical and surgical, 773
  adhesive, following surgery for hallux valgus, 602
  calcific, of short flexor of hallux, 1460
  definition of, 857
  in dancers, of extensor digitorum longus, 1648
    of flexor digitorum longus, 1643
    of flexor hallucis longus, 1643
    of peroneus brevis, 1645–1648, *1646, 1647*
    of peroneus longus, 1645–1648, *1646, 1647*
    of tibialis anterior, 1648
    of tibialis posterior, 1643
  in heel cord, 857, *859, 860.* See also *Tendinitis,*
    Achilles.
  padding and devices for relief of pain in, 1731
  peroneal, physical examination for, 105, *106*
Tendinitis crepitans, 857

Tendo Achillis. See *Achilles tendon.*

Tendo calcaneus. See *Achilles tendon.*

Tendon(s). See also under individual tendons.

abnormalities of, congenital, 866

in dancers, 1642–1648, *1642, 1644–1647.* See also *Dancing.*

contractures of, 866

dislocations of, 865

in sports injuries, 1591–1593, *1592, 1593.* See also *Sports injuries.*

elongation of, in muscle rebalancing, 268

injuries of, in sports, 1591–1593, *1592, 1593.* See also *Sports injuries.*

insertions of, traction spurs at, soft-tissue ossification and, 835, *835, 836*

lesions of, 854–867, *855, 856, 858–866*

etiologic and pathologic classification of, 854

paratenosynovitis, 854

tenosynovitis, 854–857, *855, 856, 858, 859*

tethering, 857–862, *861, 862.* See also *Tendons, tethering of.*

of ankle, surgical reconstruction of, 805–807, *806.* See also *Ankle, tendons of.*

pseudotumors of, *859,* 866

reflexes of, in peripheral neuropathies, 1207

ruptures of, 862–865, *862–865.* See also *Tendons, tears of.*

sheath of, stenosis of, in sports injuries, 1591. See also *Sports injuries.*

surgery in, in pes planus, *510,* 511–515, *512, 513*

lengthening, 424

release, 424

plantar, 424

shortening, 424

tenodesis, 424

transfer, indications and contraindications, 424

tears of, 862–865, *862–865*

laceration, 864, *865*

at ankle level, 865, *865*

at metatarsophalangeal level, 864, *865*

of extensor hallucis longus, 864

of small toes, 864

of sole, 864, *865*

treatment results, 865

rupture, spontaneous, 862–864, *862–864*

of heel cord, 864

of tibialis anterior, 862, *862*

of tibialis posterior, 863, *863*

secondary to rheumatoid arthritis and psoriasis, 864, *864*

treatment of, 863, *863*

traumatic, *835,* 865

tethering of, 857–862, *861, 862*

complete, 861, *861, 862*

in tarsal tunnel, 862, *862*

with check-rein deformity, 861, *861*

partial constriction, peroneal constriction with calcaneal fracture, 861

tarsal tunnel, 857

trigger toes, 857

thickening of, 857, *859, 860*

transfer of. See also under individual muscles or tendons.

about subtalar axes, complexities of, 734

extensor digitorum longus, 288

extensor hallucis longus, 287

for peripheral nerve injuries, 1192, *1193, 1194*

Tendon(s) *(Continued)*

transfer of, in cavus deformity, 478–480, *479, 480*

in clubfoot, 243

tibialis anterior, 715, *715*

in compartment syndromes, 1202

in footdrop, technique of, 1281

in muscle rebalancing, 268

in poliomyelitis, 1143–1146, *1143–1147.* See also *Poliomyelitis.*

in spastic hemiparesis, 311

in spastic hemiplegia, 314, 316, 318

in spastic tetraparesis, 315

in talipes equinovarus, congenital, 243, 311

indications and contraindications, 424

principles of, 152

SPLATT procedure, 1113, 1115, *1115, 1121*

tibialis anterior,•288, 715, *715*

tibialis posterior, with Achilles tendon lengthening, in Duchenne's muscular dystrophy, 339–342, *341, 342*

tumors of, 865, *866*

gouty tophi and, 866, *866*

surgical complications, 866

Tennis, footwear for, 1774

injuries from, classification of, 1574

Tennis toe, clinical features and treatment of, 1459

Tenodesis, 424

Tenosynovectomy, of foot, with synovectomy of ankle joint, 1049

Tenosynovitis, 854–857, *855, 856*

classification of, 854

in rheumatoid arthritis, 1031, *1031*

in sports injuries, 1591, 1601

inflammatory, 855, *855*

mechanical, bone and shoe friction, *851,* 856, *862*

chronic passive stretching, 856

overuse, 855, *856*

of flexor hallucis longus, 857, *859*

in geriatrics, 973

of peroneus longus, in geriatrics, 973

padding and devices for relief of pain in, 1731

pigmented vollinodular, of small toes, 653, *654*

tendinitis and, 857, *859, 860*

treatment of, 1405

tuberculous, 1411

varying terminology for, 854

with lesions between tendons and their sheaths, 857, *858, 859*

lipoma and pseudolipoma, 857, *858*

miscellaneous, 857, *859*

partial rupture, 857

reduplication and accessory tendons, 857

Tethering, of tendons, 857–862, *861, 862.* See also *Tendons.*

Tetraparesis, spastic. See *Spastic tetraparesis.*

static and dynamic, cerebral palsy and, case report, 301–310, *301–304, 306, 307*

history, 301–304, *301*

postoperative views, *303, 304*

preoperative assessment, *302,* 304

surgical procedures, *303, 304, 305*

treatment analysis, 305

triple arthrodesis technique, 305–310, *306, 307*

Thalassemia syndromes, 1102, *1103*

clinical features of, *1102,* 1103

diagnosis of, 1102

incidence of, geographical, 1102

Thalessemia syndrome (*Continued*)
  major vs. minor, 1102
  sickle cell, 1102
  treatment of, 1102
Thanatophoric dwarfism, lethal nature of, 234, *234*
Thermal burns, 1689–1694, *1690, 1691, 1694.* See also
  Burns.
Thermal injuries, industrial, 1613, *1613, 1614.* See also
  Industrial injuries.
Thromboangiitis obliterans, 1347–1349, *1348, 1349*
  angiographic appearance of, 1348, *1349*
  clinical features of, 1348, *1348*
  diagnosis of, differential, 1347–1349
  incidence of, 1347
  pathogenesis of, tobacco smoking, 1347
  pathologic findings in, 1347
  prognosis for, 1349
  treatment of, 1349
  vs. arteriosclerosis, 1347–1349
Thrombosis, arterial, acute, 1315–1318, *1316, 1317.* See
  also *Vascular diseases, arterial diseases.*
  venous, 1351–1356, *1353–1355.* See also *Venous
    thrombosis.*
Thyroid hormone, disorders of, 1073. See also *Metabolic
  disorders, of bone.*
Tibia, fractures of, 783, 784–786, *784, 785.* See also
  Fractures of tibia, and *Fractures, of ankle,
    residuals of.*
  longitudinal deficiency of, congenital, with intact
    fibula, 226–228
      associated anomalies and, 226
      classification of, 226
      familial occurrence of, 226
      treatment of, surgical, 227
        Syme amputation, 227
  longitudinal deficiency of fibula and, 222
  osteochondroma of, 357, 358
  osteotomy of, rotational, 425
  Paget's disease in, *1078,* 1079–1081, *1079–1081*
  posterior syndrome in, in distance runners and
    joggers, 1603
  rotation of, in gait analysis, *63*
  deformities of, 432, 435
Tibial artery, anterior, surgical bypass of, 1339–1341,
  1340
  posterior, palpation of, 106
  surgical bypass of, *1340,* 1341, *1342*
Tibial hemimelia, 226–228. See also *Tibia, longitudinal
  deficiency of.*
  in de Lange's syndrome, *240*
  paraxial, clinical features of, 246
    treatment of, 246
Tibial nerve, posterior, anatomy of, 1173
  entrapment neuropathies in, 1197
  trauma to, treatment of, 1183
Tibial stress syndrome, in sports injuries, 1597, *1598.*
Tibialis anterior, idiopathic thickening of, *860*
  insertion of, variations in site and extent of, role in
    pes planus, 728, *729*
  nerve conduction studies in, 74
  paralysis of, resulting in flatfoot, treatment of,
    surgical, in poliomyelitis, 1136
  sling procedure and, for decompensated flatfoot, 771,
    771
  spontaneous rupture of, 862, *862*
  tendinitis of, in dancers, 1648
  tendon transfer in, 288

Tibialis anterior (*Continued*)
  tendon transfer in, in clubfoot, 715, *715*
  testing of, 288
    in poliomyelitis, 1130, *1130*
  transfer of, in poliomyelitis, 1146–1149, *1148, 1149*
  weakness of, physical examination for, 114, *115*
Tibialis anterior tendon, rupture of, in geriatrics, 973
Tibialis posterior, disorders of, 770–772, *771*
  treatment of, surgical technique, 771, *771*
  spontaneous rupture of, 863, *863*
  tendinitis of, in dancers, 1643
  tendon laceration of, *865*
    tendon management in, 290
  tenosynovitis of, 855, *855*
  testing of, 289
    in poliomyelitis, 1129, *1129*
  transfer of, in poliomyelitis, 1149–1151, *1149, 1150*
    with tendo Achillis lengthening, technique of, in
      Duchenne's muscular dystrophy, 339–342, *341,
      342*
Tibiocalcaneal ligament, 13, *14*
Tibiofibular ligament, 13, *14*
  anterior, strain of, in dancers, 1646
Tibionavicular ligament, *11,* 13, *14*
Tibiotalar joint, arthroscopic view of, *141*
  longitudinal deficiency of fibula and, 222
Tibiotalar ligament, *11,* 13, *14*
Tierny operation, in hammer toe, *644*
Tinea pedis, 898–901, *898–900*
  skin examination for, 898–900
  varieties of, dermatophytidic, 898, *900*
    treatment of, 901
    dry, 898, *898, 899*
      differential diagnosis, 900
      treatment of, 900
    wet, of sole, 898, *899*
      of web spaces, 898, *899*
      treatment of, 900
  vs. atopic dermatitis, 872
  vs. soft corns, 631, 633
Tiptoe position, biomechanics of, 670, *670–672*
Tiptoe standing, in spinal muscular atrophy, 348, *348*
Tobacco, role in arteriosclerosis obliterans, 1325
    thromboangiitis obliterans, 1347
  withdrawal of, in diabetics, 1383
Toe(s). See also *Forefoot.*
  adult, longitudinal section of, *918*
  amputation of, prostheses for, 1815
    tissue conservation in, *1371,* 1373
  anatomy of, 664–666, *665*
  "blue," syndrome, 1315, *1315*
  clawing of. See *Claw toe(s).*
  contusions of, definition, diagnosis, and treatment of,
    1449
    resulting in subungual hematoma, 1449
  convergent, congenital, treatment of, 218
  crest pads for, *1708, 1708.* See also *Foot, pain in,
    padding and devices.*
  curly, congenital, 214, *215.* See also *Curly toe(s).*
  cyanosis of, caused by microemboli, 1315, *1315*
  deformities of, basic literature on, guide to, 1849
    in head trauma patients, 1118–1121, *1121*
      treatment of, surgical, 1120, *1121*
        contraindications, 1120
    in rheumatoid arthritis, 1034–1037, *1036*
    in stroke patients, 1117, *1117*
      curling, *1116,* 1117, *1117*

Toe(s) (*Continued*)
  deformities of, in stroke patients, treatment of,
      surgical, 1117, *1117*
    isolated, treatment of, surgical, 1034–1036, *1036*
      classification of procedures, 1035
    swan-neck, in rheumatoid arthritis, 1028, *1029*
  dislocations of, 1451–1459, *1451–1456, 1458*. See also
      Dislocations and *Fractures*.
  divergent, 647, *648*
    congenital, treatment of, 218
  examination of, roentgenographic, 98
    roentgenographic technique, 128, *128*
  fifth, contracted overlapping, 646, *646*, *647*
    treatment of, nonsurgical, 646
      surgical, 646, *647*
        McFarland and Scrase modification, 647, *647*
        Ruiz-Mora technique, 646
  examination of, clinical, lateral calluses, 87, 94, 95
  first, osteoporotic, 1065, *1065*
    valgus deformity of, causing hammer toe, 640, *640*
  flail, following severance of extensor tendon, 628, *628*
  forefoot and, injuries of, 1449–1462. See also
      Injury(ies).
  fractures of, 1451–1459, *1451–1456, 1458*. See also
      Dislocations and *Fractures*.
  function of, vital role in biomechanics, 664
  great. See *Hallux*.
  hammer, 638–646, *639–645*. See also *Hammer toe(s)*.
  in spinal dysraphism, 262
  injuries of, 1449–1462. See also *Injuries*.
    crush, treatment of, 1450
    industrial, 1609
      protection from, 1618, *1618–1620*
    sports, 1573–1606. See also *Sports injuries*.
  jogger's, 1605
  miscellaneous problems of, basic literature on, guide
      to, 1865
  orthoses for, 1741–1743, *1742*
  overlapping, 646–649, *646*, *647*
    treatment of, nonsurgical, in geriatrics, 969, *970*
    with metatarsophalangeal capsular contracture,
        treatment of, surgical, 649
  pigeon, in children, variations of, 196, 198
  plantigrade foot and, 177
  small, 622–658. See also *Small toes*.
  trigger, 649, 857
    in dancers, 1644, *1644, 1645*
  underlapping, 648, *648*
  webbing of, congenital, 218, *218*
Toecaps, protective, 1618, *1618–1620*. See also
    Industrial injuries.
Toenails, 914–938. See also *Nails*.
  anatomy of, 914–919, *915–918*
    comparative and evolutionary, 919, *919–922*
    distal groove, 914, *915, 918*
    distal ridge, 914–919
    eponychium, 914, *915, 916, 918*
    hyponychium, *916–918*, 919
    layers, 914
    lunula, *916*, 919
    nail bed, 914–919
    nail plate, 914–919
    paronychium, 919
    perionychium, 919
  attrition of, 914
  avulsion of, treatment of, 1450
  changes in, in psoriatic arthritis, 1059, *1059, 1060*

Toenails (*Continued*)
  composition of, 914
  deformities of, hypertrophic thickening, 932
    miscellaneous, 932, *933*
    onychogryphosis, *931*, 932, *933*
    periungual and subungual lesions, granuloma
        pyogenicum, 932, *934*
      melanosarcoma, *934*, 935, *935*
    tubular, 932, *933*
    tubular or circular, 651, *651*
  disorders of, dermatologic, basic literature on, guide
      to, 1844
    management of, 911
      griseofulvin, 911
        side effects, 911
    in geriatrics, 969, *970*. See also *Geriatric foot*.
    paraungual corns, 935
      end corn, 935. See also *Corn, end*.
    periungual and subungual lesions, 911, *911, 912*,
        932–935, *934, 935*
      fibromas, 912, *912*
        treatment of, 912
      in small toes, *636*, 651, *651, 652*
      miscellaneous, 936, *937*
      osteoma, 937, *937*
        osteoid, 936
      warts, 911, *911*
        treatment of, surgical, 912
    periungual corns, 936
    subungual fracture, 937
    tubular or circular, in small toes, 651, *651*
  embryology of, 914, 921–925, *923–925*
    vs. fingernails, 923
  evolution of, human vs. nonhuman, 919, *919–922*
  growth of, vs. fingernails, 925
  incurvation of, in geriatrics, *969*, 970
  infections of, subungual, 935
  ingrown, 925–930, *926–930*
    abscessed, treatment of, saucerization, 926, *926*
    clinical features of, 925
    examination of, clinical, 93
      physical, 114, *114*
    pathology of, 926, *926*
    treatment of, historical, 925
      nonsurgical, 926
      surgical, avoidance of nail bed tissue curettage,
          928
        avulsion, 927, *929, 933*
        complete and permanent removal, 928–930,
            929, 930
        regrowth following, 928
        sloughing following, *172*
        wedge resection, 926, *927*
  lesions of, basic literature on, 1865
  local block anesthesia for, 930
  plantar keratoma and, 930–932, *931*
  problems of, in dancers, 1658, *1658*
  subungual exostosis and, 1004, *1004, 1005*
Tomography, "air contrast," for talar fractures, 1465
  uses of, 138
Tongue, disorders of, in relation to neurologic
    examination of foot, 1108
Tophaceous gout, *1016–1018*, 1020–1022. See also *Gout*.
Torque, during gait, 48, *49*
  measured by forceplate, 66, *66*
Tourniquet, avoidance of, 147
Toxic neuropathies, 1209, 1242

Trabecular systems, of metatarsals, 661, *662*
Track sports, footwear for, 1775
  injuries from, classification of, 1574
Traction, Quigley, modified, for ankle fractures, 1552, *1552*
Traction periostitis, 842
Traction spurs, at tendon insertions, soft-tissue ossification and, 835, *835*, *836*
  multiple, 835, *836*, 842
Transient painful osteoporosis syndrome, 1290–1292, *1291*. See also *Osteoporosis*.
Transverse deficiencies, absent phalanges, 245
  apodia, 245
  through forefoot, 245
Transverse plane, motion of, in gait analysis, 62, *63*
Transverse rotation, of lower extremity, 50–52, *51*, *52*, *61–63*
Trauma. See also *Injury(ies)*.
  to calcaneus and heel cord, 1497–1542. See also *Achilles tendon*, *Calcaneus*, and *Heel cord*.
  to child's foot and ankle, 1660–1688. See also *Children* and *Growing foot*.
  to foot and ankle, 1449–1702
Traumatic neuropathies, classification of, 1177
  nerve injuries and, 1178–1182, *1178*, *1180–1182*. See also *Nerve(s)*, *disorders of*.
  treatment of, 1182–1193, *1184–1187*, *1189–1191*, *1193–1195*. See also *Nerve(s)*, *trauma to*.
Travase, in treatment of problem wounds, 941
Trench foot, clinical features of, 1450
Treponema pallidum, in syphilis, 1418
Treponema pertenue, causing yaws, 1420
Trevor-Fairbank disease, 354, *355*. See also *Dysplasia epiphysealis hemimelica*.
Triceps surae, effect of, on subtalar joint, 45, *46*
  paralysis of, peroneal transfer for, in poliomyelitis, 1151, *1151*, *1152*
  testing of, in poliomyelitis, 1129, *1129*
Trichophyton infections, 898, *898*, *899*
Trigger toe(s), 649, 857
  in dancers, 1644, *1644*, *1645*
Trochlea tali, fractures of, 1483–1489, *1484–1489*. See also *Fractures of talus*.
Truncated wedge principle, apex fallacy and, 151, *151*, *190*
Tuber calcanei, fractures of, 1516–1518, *1516*, *1517*. See also *Fractures of calcaneus*.
Tuberculosis, 1407–1411, *1407–1410*
  dactylitis in, clinical features of, 1410
  in subtalar complex, *746*
  leprosy and, 1241
  lesions of, untreated progress of, 1407
  lower extremity involvement in, 1407
  micrographic view, 1407, *1407*
  of ankle, 1408, *1408*, *1409*
    clinical features of, 1408
    radiographic view of, 1408, *1408*, *1409*
    Sudeck's atrophy and, 744, *744*
    synovial vs. osseous forms, 1408
    treatment of, surgical vs. nonsurgical, 1408, *1409*
  of calcaneus, radiographic view, *1410*
  of foot, routes taken, 1407
    spina ventosa, clinical features of, 1410
    tenosynovitis and, 1411
    treatment of, chemotherapy, 1407
  of forefoot, 721, *721*
  of navicular, radiographic view, *1409*

Tuberculosis (*Continued*)
  of talus, radiographic view, *1409*
  of tarsal bones, 1408–1410, *1409*, *1410*
    locational spread of, 1408
    treatment of, nonsurgical, 1408
    surgical, 1410
  soft-tissue calcification and, *834*, 835
Tuberous sclerosis, periungual fibromas in, 912, *912*
Tumor(s), basic literature on, guide to, 1845
  bone, percentage of, 744
  of anterior tarsus and Lisfranc's joint, 721, *722*
  of foot, 979–1013
    biopsy, 980
    bone, 996–1012, *997–1011*. See also *Tumors, of foot, cartilage*.
      benign and malignant, classification of, 996
      aneurysmal bone cyst, diagnosis and treatment, 997–999, *998*, *999*
      cysts and tumor-like lesions, 997–999, *997–999*
        solitary bone cyst, 997, *997*, *998*
        in calcaneus, 997, *997*, *998*
        treatment of, 997
      eosinophilic granuloma, 1011, *1011*
      fibrous dysplasias, 1011, *1011*
      giant cell, 1009, *1010*
      of navicular, 722, *722*
      hemangioendothelioma, *1010*, 1011
      marrow, 1008, *1008*
        Ewing's sarcoma, 1008, *1008*
        reticulosarcoma, 1008, *1008*
      metastatic carcinoma and myeloma, 1009, *1009*
      osteoblastic, 999–1003, *1000–1003*
        osteoblastoma, 1000, *1002*
        osteoid osteoma, diagnosis and treatment of, 999, *1000*, *1001*
        osteosarcoma, 1000–1003, *1002*, *1003*
      vascular, 1009–1011, *1010*
    cartilage, 1003–1008, *1004–1007*. See also *Tumors, of foot, bone*.
      chondroblastoma, 1005–1007, *1006*
      chondromyxoid fibroma, *1006*, 1007
      chondrosarcoma, 1007, *1007*
      dysplasia epiphysealis hemimelica, 1003, *1004*
      enchondroma, 1005, *1005*, *1007*
      osteocartilaginous exostosis, 1003, *1004*
      osteochondroma, 1003, *1004*
      subungual exostosis, 1004, *1004*, *1005*
    classification of, 983
    clinical and laboratory evaluation of, 980
      angiography, 980
      arteriography, 980
      CAT scan, 980
      radioisotope scan, 980
      tomography, 980
      xerography, 980
    definition of, 979
    soft-tissue, 981–996, *982–995*
      benign and malignant, incidence and rarity of, 982
      classification of, 983
      clear cell sarcoma, 995
      fibrous lesions and tumors, dermatofibrosarcoma protuberans, 986, *987*
        fibromatoses, 984–986, *984–987*
          aggressive, 985, *986*
          calcifying, 985, *985*
          cicatricial, 984

Tumor(s) (*Continued*)
 of foot, soft tissue, fibrous lesions and tumors,
   fibromatoses, extra-abdominal desmoid,
   985, *986*
  in melorheostosis, 985, *987*
  juvenile aponeurotic, 985, *985*
  nodular fasciitis, 985
  plantar, 984, *984*
  pseudosarcomatous, 985
 fibrosarcoma, 986–988, *988*
  vs. fibrous tissue in other lesions, 979, 983,
   983, *984*
   collagen in other tissues, 984
   degeneration with calcification, 984, *984*
   degenerative changes, 983, *983*
   fibroma, 979, 984
   reparative and granulomatous, 983
 lipoblastic, 988, *989*
  lipoma, 988, *989*
  liposarcoma, 988, *989*
 muscle tissue, angiomyoma, 988
  rhabdomyosarcoma, 988
 onset and etiology of, 981
 peripheral nerves, 992, *993*
  neurilemoma, 993, *993*
  neurofibroma, 992, *992*
  neurogenic sarcoma, 993
  schwannoma, 993, *993*
   malignant, 993
 synovial tissues, 993–995, *994*, *995*
  pigmented villonodular synovitis, 993, *994*
   diffuse, 993, *994*
   localized, 993, *994*
  synovial sarcoma, 994, *995*
  synovioma, 994, *995*
 vascular, 989–992, *990–992*
  angiosarcoma, 991
  glomangioma, 991, *991*, *992*
  glomus tumor, 991, *991*, *992*
  hemangioendothelioma, 991
  hemangioma, 989–991, *990*, *991*
  hemangiopericytoma, 991
  Kaposi's sarcoma, 992, *992*
 vs. epithelial inclusion cysts, 981, *982*
  xanthoma, 995, *996*
 vs. nontumorous lesions, 979, *979*
 of peripheral nerves, 992, *993*
 of skin, benign and malignant, 831, *831*, *832*
 of small toes, 652–656, *652–655*. See also *Small toes.*
 of subtalar complex, 744, *745*
 of tendons, 865, *866*
 subcutaneous, 837, *838*
 tumor-like lesions and, classification of, 983
Tumoral calcinosis, 1068
Turco procedure, in clubfoot, 242
"Turf-toe," as sports injury, *1581*, *1582*, *1582*

Ulcer(s), as acute foot infections, 1401
 as sign of peripheral neuropathy, 1210
 causes of, 1208
 chronic, as late effect of radiation burns, 1701, *1701*
  over bony prominences, 1404, *1405*
  plantar, 1403, *1404*
 diabetic, 1218
  caused by corns, 1385, *1386*

Ulcer(s) (*Continued*)
 extensive, in hallux valgus, 556
 in arteriosclerosis obliterans, 1326, *1326*, *1327*
 in Charcot foot, *1250*, 1259
 in Charcot-Marie-Tooth disease, 1236, *1236*
 in neuropathic foot, 1208–1210, 1218
 in yaws, 1421–1424, *1421*, *1423*
 ischemic, arterial reconstruction following, results of,
   1345, *1346*
  vs. stasis ulcers, 1326, 1357, *1357*
 mal perforans, in diabetes, 1255, *1257*. See also
   Diabetic foot.
 malleolar, 1404, *1405*
 of hallux, treatment of, 1281
 of heel, treatment of, nonsurgical, 1283, *1283*
  surgical, 1283
 of insensitive foot, 1268–1285, *1268–1274*, *1276–1279*,
   1282–1285
  damage from infection, 1278–1280, *1279*
   importance of bed rest, 1279
   plaster casts for, 1279, *1279*
  degree of insensibility, 1268
  evaluation of pressure and shear stress, 1284, *1284*,
   1285
  level and type of mechanical stress, 1268–1278,
   1268–1274, *1276–1278*
   damage from high stress, 1270, *1270*
    prevention of, 1271
   damage from low stress, 1268, 1269, *1269*, *1270*
    prevention of, 1270, *1270*
    site of, 1269, *1269*
   damage from moderate stress, 1270–1278,
    1271–1274, *1276–1278*
    daily number of steps, 1275
    length of stride, *1274*, 1275
    repetitive, 1271–1275, *1273*
    shoe design and texture, 1275–1278, *1276–1278*
  newly healed, 1280
  recurrence of, 1280
  specific situations and role of surgery, 1280–1284,
   1282, *1283*
   footdrop, correction of, technique, 1281
   in forefoot, 1283
   in heel, 1283, *1283*
   in lateral border of foot, 1282, *1282*
   in plantigrade foot, 1280
   problem of infections and, 1280
 of leg, etiology of, 1104
  in sickle cell disease, 1104, *1105*
   clinical features of, 1104, *1105*
   radiologic changes in, 1105
   treatment of, surgical vs. nonsurgical, 1105
 of plantigrade foot, treatment of, surgical, 1280
 painless, 1208
 sites of, 1210
 stasis, following chronic venous insufficiency, 1357,
   1357
  vs. ischemic, 1326, 1357, *1357*
 treatment of, 269, 1402
Ulnar hemimelia, in de Lange's syndrome, *240*
Ultrasound, Doppler, instruments, 1302, *1303*. See also
   Vascular diseases, examination of, physiologic.
 in deep venous thrombosis, 1353, *1353*
Unbalanced foot, treatment of, 505–515, *506–510*, *512*,
   513. See also *Pes planus.*
 stable, treatment of, 515–518, *515–517*
Underlapping toes, 648, *648*

Unna-Thost disease, diffuse keratoses of soles in, 902, *902*
Urate deposition, in gout, 1015–1018, *1016–1018*

Valgus deformity. See also *Flatfoot* and *Pes planus.*
  convex, 252, *252*
    basic literature on, guide to, 1861
    neurologic abnormalities in, 258
    spina bifida and, 252, 273–276, *273, 275*
    treatment of, 252, 273–276, *273, 275*
  from sports injury, 1582, *1583.* See also *Sports injuries.*
  of first toe, causing hammer toe, 640, *640*
  rheumatoid arthritis and, *1026, 1029, 1030*
  spina bifida and, 252, 263, 272. See also *Valgus deformity, convex.*
  spinal dysraphism and, 263, *263*
  treatment of, *252, 263, 272*
Valgus index, *487, 488, 489*
Valgus knee, effect of on metatarsal weight bearing, 183
Varus deformity, in diabetic foot, *1380*
  in stroke patient, 1114–1116, *1115*
    muscular involvement, 1114
    treatment of, nonsurgical, 1114, *1115*
      SPLATT procedure, 1115, *1115*
  rheumatoid arthritis and, *1030,* 1031
  spina bifida and, 250, *250, 252, 263,* 270–272, *271*
  spinal dysraphism and, 263
  treatment of, 250, *252,* 263, 270–272, *271*
Varus toe, congenital, 214, *215.* See also *Curly toe.*
Vascular diseases, 1301–1376
  amputations and, 1364–1373, *1364–1372.* See also *Amputation* and *Replantation.*
  and elective vascular reconstruction affecting foot, standard surgical approaches, 1332–1344, *1333–1343.* See also *Arterial reconstruction* and *Vascular reconstruction.*
  arterial disobliteration, 1318–1320, *1318, 1319*
    early embolectomy, balloon catheter for, 1318, *1319*
      choice of artery for, 1319
  arterial occlusive, 1310–1318, *1310–1317*
    acute arterial thrombosis, 1315–1318, *1316, 1317*
      arising from popliteal aneurysms, *1316, 1317, 1317*
      arteriographic view, *1316,* 1318
      caused by arteriosclerosis obliterans, 1315
      causes of, 1315–1317
      clinical features of, 1316, *1317*
      femoropopliteal involvement, 1317
      gradual onset of, 1317
      popliteal entrapment and, 1318
    acute vs. chronic, 1310
    embolism, 1311–1315, *1312–1315*
      macroemboli, 1311, *1312, 1313*
        common sites of, 1311
        diagnosis of, vs. venous thrombosis, 1312
        ischemic onset, 1311
          signs and symptoms of, 1312
        PVR tracings of, 1312, *1313*
      microemboli, 1312–1315, *1314, 1315*
        affecting digital circulation, 1315, *1315*
        "blue toe" syndrome and, 1315, *1315*
        causing toe cyanosis, 1315, *1315*
        common sites of, 1312, *1314*
        shower of from popliteal aneurysm, *1314,* 1315

Vascular diseases (*Continued*)
  arterial occlusive, location of, effect on foot, 1310, *1311*
  arteriosclerosis obliterans, 1324–1332, *1325–1331.* See also *Arteriosclerosis obliterans.*
  chronic ischemia of foot, 1324–1332, *1325–1331.* See also *Arteriosclerosis obliterans.*
  cold sensitivity, Raynaud's phenomenon and, 1349–1351. See also *Raynaud's phenomenon.*
  examination of, physiologic, 1301–1310, *1303–1306, 1308–1310*
    criteria for effectiveness of, 1302
    Doppler ultrasound, instruments, 1302, *1303*
      to determine blood flow, 1302, *1304*
      to measure arterial blood pressure, 1304, *1305*
    functions of laboratory tests, 1302
    invasive measurements of hemodynamic physiology, *1303,* 1307–1310, *1310*
    measurement of walking distance, 1301
    method of approach, 1301
    noninvasive exercise and hyperemic tests, 1306, *1306, 1308, 1309*
      correlation between ankle pressures and clinical states, 1310
      interpretation of data from, 1307, 1310
    physiologic vs. anatomic aspects, 1302
    pulse volume recorder, *1305,* 1306
    qualitative and quantitative, 1302
    wave-form analysis, 1304–1306, *1305*
  foot replantation and, 1358–1364, *1360, 1362, 1364, 1365.* See also *Amputation* and *Replantation.*
  Raynaud's phenomenon, cold sensitivity and, 1349–1351. See also *Raynaud's phenomenon.*
  thromboangiitis obliterans, 1347–1349, *1348, 1349.* See also *Thromboangiitis obliterans.*
  traumatic injuries of vascular supply to foot, 1320–1324, *1322, 1323*
    acute arterial occlusion, 1322, *1322, 1323*
    acute ischemia, diagnosis of, 1312, 1322
    arterial laceration, 1320
    associated with nerve injuries, 1321
    importance of history-taking, 1321
    increased incidence of, 1320
    pulsatile flow determination, 1321
    reperfusion syndrome, 1323. See also *Reperfusion syndrome.*
    severe bleeding following, 1320
    treatment of, digital pressure and compression, 1321
      presurgical, 1322
      surgical, 1323, *1323*
  venous foot disorders, 1351–1358, *1353–1355, 1357, 1358.* See also *Venous disorders.*
Vascular disorders, classification of, 1209
Vascular injuries, traumatic, nerve injuries and, 1321
Vascular neuropathies, 1240
Vascular reconstruction, affecting foot, standard surgical approaches, 1332–1344, *1333–1343.* See also *Arterial reconstruction.*
  aortoiliac reconstruction, 1332–1335, *1333–1335*
  infrainguinal arterial reconstruction, 1335–1344, *1335–1343*
    bypasses, 1336–1343, *1337–1343*
      common femoral and profunda femoris, 1336–1338, *1337*
      dorsalis pedis artery, 1341, *1341*
      femoropopliteal thromboendarterectomy, 1343, *1343*

Vascular reconstruction (*Continued*)
  affecting foot, standard surgical approaches,
        infrainguinal arterial reconstruction,
        bypasses, femoropopliteal vein, 1338, *1338*
        intraoperative angiography and, *1342*, *1343*
        peroneal artery, *1338*, 1339, *1339*, *1340*
        popliteal artery, 1337–1339, *1337*, *1339*
        saphenous vein complications, 1338, 1343
        tibial arteries, 1339–1341, *1340*, *1342*
     common femoral and profunda femoris, 1335,
       1335, *1336*
     nonautogenous materials, 1343
Vascular supply, examination of, general clinical, 88
  threat to, from talar fractures, 1475, *1477*
  to foot, traumatic injuries of, 1320–1324, *1322*, *1323*.
    See also *Vascular diseases*.
Vascular system, 31
  arteries, *18*, *19*, 31
  lymphatic drainage, 32
  veins, 32
Vasculitis, autoimmune, inflammatory, classification of,
  1209
  in rheumatoid arthritis and Felty's syndrome,
    treatment of, *1225*
  of hands and feet, 83, *83*
  rheumatoid, diagnosis and treatment of, 1031, *1225*
Veins, 32. See also under individual veins.
  lesions of, 846, *847*
Venography, techniques of, in deep venous thrombosis,
  1354, *1354*, *1355*
Venous disorders, 1351–1358, *1353–1355*, *1357*, *1358*
  chronic insufficiency, 1356–1358, *1357*
    pathogenesis of, 1356
    permanent brawny edema following, 1356, *1357*
    stasis ulcer following, 1357, *1357*
    treatment of, 1357
      alternatives to amputation, 1364
  phlegmasia cerulea dolens, 1358, *1358*
  venous thrombosis, 1351–1356, *1353–1355*
    acute, iliofemoral, 1352
      treatment of, 1354–1356, *1355*
        bed rest, 1354, *1355*
        elastic supports, 1356
        heparin, 1354
    associated diseases and, 1351
    common sites of, 1351
    deep, diagnosis of, 1352–1354
      laboratory tests for, 1352–1354, *1353–1355*
      symptoms and signs of, 1352–1354, *1353–1355*
    etiology of, 1351
    in progressive saphenous phlebitis, 1352
    vs. ischemia, 1312
Verrucae vulgares, 905, *906*
Vertebrae, fusion of, congenital vertical talus and, 444
Vertical force, measured by forceplate, 66, *66*
Vertical talus. See *Talus, vertical.*
Visualization of subject, in gait analysis, 58–60, *58–63*
Vitamin deficiency(ies), 1240
  classification of, 1209
Vohwinkel's disease, ainhum of small toes in, 657
Voorhoeve's disease, clinical features of, 368
  radiographic features of, 368, *368*

Wagner operation, in longitudinal deficiency of fibula,
  223–225

Waist resection, of proximal phalanx, in hammer toe,
  642, *642*
Walking cycle, 37, *37*, *38*
  changes in, during walking, jogging, and running, 38,
    38
  complete, schematic diagram of, *56*
  events of, 38, *38*, 55–57, *56*
  gait analysis and, *60–63*
  normal vs. pathologic gaits, 38
  phases of, 37, *37*, *38*, 43, *44*, 55–57, *56*
  vertical force curve and, 47, *47*, *48*, 66
Warts, causes of, 831
  flat, dorsal, 905, *908*
  mosaical appearance of, *907*
  multiple, 905, *907*
  neurovascular, 905
  paring of, pinpoint bleeding following, 905, *908*
  periungual and subungual, 911, *911*
    vs. fibromas, 912
  plantar, about metatarsal heads, 93
    and ordinary, 905–910, *906–908*
    clinical appearance of, 905, *906*, *907*
    etiology of, 905
  reduced incidence of in geriatrics, 965
  treatment of, 831
    surgical vs. nonsurgical, 908–910
  viral, 905, *906*
  vs. hyperkeratoses, 905
  vs. periungual fibromas, 912
Watson-Jones tenodesis, for ankle ligament
    reconstruction, 799–801, *800*
    modification of, author's, *800*, 801
      Lee, *800*, 801
    for slipping peroneal tendon, 807
Web spaces, anatomy of, 1401, *1401*
  infections of, fungal, 898, *899*
    treatment of, 1406
    Trichophyton, 898, *899*
Webbing, congenital, of toes, 218, *218*
Weber classification, of ankle injuries, 1549, *1550*,
  1555–1559, *1555–1560*
Weight bearing, anatomic factors determining, 182, *182*,
  185
  capabilities of, measurement of, 265, *266*
  decrease of, factors governing, 178–183
  dynamics of, 1761
  factors of, 147, *148*
  forces of, dispersion of in foot on talar loading, 738,
    738
    on and distributed by subtalar complex, 738, *738*
  in neuropathies, alcoholic, 148, *148*
    diabetic, 148
  increase of, factors governing, 178–183
  metatarsal fat pads and, 838, *838*, *839*
  on sole, 95
  pes planus and, 505–509, *506–509*
  plantigrade foot and, 175
Welt shoes, Bal and blucher patterns, *1747*, *1748*
Wheelchair deformities, early and late, in Duchenne's
  muscular dystrophy, 343–345, *344*, *345*
Whitman arch support, 1734, *1735*
"Windblown hips," in utero, 1758, *1759*
Windlass mechanism, plantar fascia and, 52–54, *54*
Wood's light examination, of skin, 871
Working cycle, electromyography and, 63
Wounds, causing foot infections, 1402
  closure of, principles of, 168

Wounds (*Continued*)
    management of, in plastic surgery, 940–942. See also
       Plastic surgery.
Wrestling, injuries from, classification of, 1574

Xanthoma(s), *995, 996*
   in Achilles tendon, *995, 996*
Xeroroentgenography, uses of, 138

Yaws, 1420–1428, *1421–1427*
   bone lesions in, *1426,* 1427, *1427*

Yaws (*Continued*)
   "crab," *1423*
   diagnosis of, 1421
   etiology of, controversy regarding, 1420
   gangosa in, 1424
   goundou in, 1424, *1425*
   phases of, primary, 1421, *1421*
   incidence of, geographical, 1421
   saber shin in, 1424, *1424*
   stages of, secondary, 1421, *1422*
     tertiary, 1421–1427, *1423–1427*
   treatment of, 1427

Z-plasty, contraindications for, 147, *147*